Equine Neurology

Equine Neurology

SECOND EDITION

Martin Furr

Marion duPont Scott Equine Medical Center
Virginia-Maryland Regional College of Veterinary Medicine
Leesburg, USA

Stephen Reed

Rood and Riddle Equine Hospital
Lexington, USA

WILEY Blackwell

This edition first published 2015 © 2015 by John Wiley & Sons, Inc.

First edition, 2008 © Blackwell Publishing Professional

Editorial Offices

1606 Golden Aspen Drive, Suites 103 and 104, Ames, Iowa 50014-8300, USA

The Atrium, Southern Gate, Chichester, West Sussex, PO19 8SQ, UK

9600 Garsington Road, Oxford, OX4 2DQ, UK

For details of our global editorial offices, for customer services and for information about how to apply for permission to reuse the copyright material in this book please see our website at www.wiley.com/wiley-blackwell.

Library of Congress Cataloging-in-Publication Data

Equine neurology / [edited by] Martin Furr, Stephen Reed. – Second edition.
     p. ; cm.
   Includes bibliographical references and index.
   ISBN 978-1-118-50147-4 (cloth)
1. Horses–Diseases.   2. Nervous system–Diseases.   3. Veterinary neurology.   I. Furr, Martin, editor.
II. Reed, Stephen M., editor.
   [DNLM: 1. Central Nervous System Diseases–veterinary.   2. Horse Diseases–diagnosis.
3. Nervous System Diseases–veterinary. SF 959.N47]
   SF959.N47E68 2015
   636.1′08968–dc23

                                    2015007228

A catalogue record for this book is available from the British Library.

Wiley also publishes its books in a variety of electronic formats. Some content that appears in print may not be available in electronic books.

Cover image: istockphoto-neuron-impulses 10-01-07 © ChristianAnthony

Set in 8.5/10.5pt Meridien by SPi Global, Pondicherry, India
Printed and bound in Singapore by Markono Print Media Pte Ltd

1 2015

Contents

Contributors List

Monica Aleman, MVZ Cert, PhD, Dip ACVIM
(Internal Medicine, Neurology)
College of Veterinary Medicine
University of California
Davis, USA

Frank Andrews, DVM, MS, Dip ACVIM
School of Veterinary Medicine
Louisiana State University
Baton Rouge, USA

Joseph J. Bertone, DVM, MS, Dip ACVIM
College of Veterinary Medicine
Western University
Pomona, USA

Fabio Del Piero, DVM, PhD, Dip ACVP
School of Veterinary Medicine
Louisiana State University
Baton Rouge, USA

Tom Divers, DVM, Dip ACVIM
College of Veterinary Medicine
Cornell University
Ithaca, USA

Martin Furr, DVM, Dip ACVIM, PhD
Marion duPont Scott Equine Medical Center
Virginia-Maryland Regional College of Veterinary
Medicine
Leesburg, USA

Katherine Garrett, DVM, Dip ACVS
Rood and Riddle Equine Hospital
Lexington, USA

Lutz S. Goehring, DVM, MS, PhD, Dip ACVIM
College of Veterinary Medicine
Ludwig Maximillians University
Munich, Germany

Caroline Hahn, DVM, MSc, PhD, Dip ECEIM,
Dip ECVN, MRCVS
Royal (Dick) School of Veterinary Studies
The University of Edinburgh
Midlothian, UK

Richard Hepburn, BVSc, MS, Cert EM(Int Med),
Dip ACVIM, MRCVS
B & W Equine Hospital
Gloucestershire, UK

Melissa Hines, DVM, Dip ACVIM
College of Veterinary Medicine
University of Tennessee
Knoxville, USA

Katherine A. Houpt, VMD, PhD, Dip ACVB
College of Veterinary Medicine
Cornell University
Ithaca, USA

Daniel K. Howe, PhD
Gluck Equine Center
University of Kentucky
Lexington, USA

Amy L. Johnson, DVM, Dip ACVIM
New Bolton Center
University of Pennsylvania School of Veterinary Medicine
Kennett Square, USA

Craig Johnson, BVSc, PhD, DVA, Dip ECVA
Institute of Veterinary, Animal and Biomedical Sciences
Massey University
Palmerstown North, New Zealand

Véronique A. Lacombe, DVM, PhD, Dip ACVIM,
Dip ECEIM
Center for Veterinary Health Sciences
Oklahoma State University
Stillwater, USA

Maureen T. Long, DVM, MS, PhD, Dip ACVIM
College of Veterinary Medicine
University of Florida
Gainesville, USA

Robert J. MacKay, BVSc, PhD, Dip ACVIM
College of Veterinary Medicine
University of Florida
Gainesville, USA

Jerry Masty, DVM, MS, PhD
College of Veterinary Medicine
The Ohio State University
Columbus, USA

Yvette S. Nout-Lomas, DVM, MS, PhD, Dip ACVIM, Dip ACVECC
College of Veterinary Medicine
Colorado State University
Fort Collins, USA

Kirstie Pickles, BCMS, MSc, Dip ECEIM, PhD
Scarsdale Equine Veterinary Practice
Derby, UK

Stephen Reed, DVM, MS, Dip ACVIM
Rood and Riddle Equine Hospital
Lexington, USA

John L. Robertson, VMD, PhD
Virginia Tech
Virginia-Maryland Regional College of Veterinary Medicine
Leesburg, USA

Adriana G. Silva, DVM, MS
Faculty of Veterinary Medicine
University of Montreal
Saint Hyacinthe, Canada

George M. Strain, PhD
School of Veterinary Medicine
Louisiana State University
Baton Rouge, USA

Ramiro E. Toribio, DVM, MS, PhD, Dip ACVIM
College of Veterinary Medicine
The Ohio State University
Columbus, USA

Tim Vojt, MA
College of Veterinary Medicine
The Ohio State University
Columbus, USA

Carissa L. Wickens, PhD
Department of Animal Sciences
University of Florida
Gainesville, USA

Preface

It has been 6 years since the publication of the first edition of *Equine Neurology*, and new information continues to accumulate about equine neurology; hence, it seems timely to offer the second edition of this work. Our goal in the first edition was to provide a comprehensive review of the field of equine neurology and to structure a textbook that provided not only the clinical descriptions of various equine neurologic disorders but also foundation material to assist in understanding neurologic dysfunction in general. With the second edition, we have attempted to continue in this same theme, with the basic organization remaining the same—however, all chapters have been reviewed, modified, and updated—some a little and others more substantially. In addition, we have added chapters on imaging of the nervous system, neuronal physiology, sleep disorders, head shaking, differential diagnosis of muscle trembling and weakness, and cervical articular process joint disease. The chapters on equine neuropathology and electrodiagnostic evaluation have been substantially expanded. The major change is the inclusion of videos illustrating many of the described conditions. These videos were selected to be representative and high-quality instructional videos to aid the reader in their understanding of the text and equine nervous system disease in general.

We wish to acknowledge the hard work and talent of the many individuals who contributed to this work. The time commitment necessary to produce high-quality chapters is substantial, and this edition would not have been produced without their hard work and input. We hope that you read and study this text, use it aid your clinical work, and most of all enjoy learning about equine neurology.

Martin Furr
Stephen Reed

Video Clips Demonstrating Clinical Signs

This book is accompanied by a companion website:

www.wiley.com/go/furr/neurology

The website includes:

• Web exclusive videos

Foundations of Clinical Neurology

SECTION 1

Foundations of Clinical
Nephrology

1 Overview of Neuroanatomy

Caroline Hahn[1] and Jerry Masty[2]

[1] Royal (Dick) School of Veterinary Studies, The University of Edinburgh, Midlothian, UK
[2] College of Veterinary Medicine, The Ohio State University, Columbus, USA

In order to evaluate a patient with a neurologic disorder, a basic understanding of the structure and function of the nervous system is necessary. The goal of this chapter is not to expose the reader to intricate and perhaps daunting detail but rather to present a basic overview of neuroanatomy, highlighting some of the peculiarities of equine neuroanatomy. A basic understanding of the nervous system from an anatomic and functional perspective is an absolute prerequisite to interpreting the neurological examination and to assess if there is indeed a lesion in the nervous system and, if so, where the lesion is located (the "anatomic diagnosis").

Organization of the nervous system

The nervous system is organized into central and peripheral divisions. The central nervous system (CNS) is composed of the brain and spinal cord and is located within the skull and vertebral column. The peripheral nervous system (PNS) is formed by neuronal cell processes that extend from the central axis to the periphery. There are also collections of neuronal cell bodies in the periphery ("ganglia") that contribute to the components of the peripheral system. Functionally, the nervous system is divided into the somatic nervous system, a system under voluntary control that innervates skeletal muscle and whose sensory branch reaches consciousness, and the autonomic nervous system, which is concerned with subconsciously regulating visceral smooth muscle structures. Both the somatic and nervous system and CNS have central and peripheral motor and sensory components.

Development

The nervous system begins as a thickening of the embryonic layer identified as ectoderm. The initial growth of the neural ectoderm forms a thickened layer of cells identified as the neural plate. The neural groove is evident as a depression in the neural plate. As continued growth of the developing system occurs, neural folds develop at the margins of the neural plate caused by migration of the cells in a dorsal direction. Eventually, the neural folds meet and fuse at the dorsal midline thereby forming a cylindrical structure identified as the neural tube. This simplified explanation of the formation of the neural tube is shown in Figure 1.1.

As the neural tube is forming, cells in the region of the neural folds pinch off and migrate throughout the developing body. These are the neural crest cells that differentiate to become various structures in the adult: spinal ganglia, sensory ganglia associated with some of the cranial nerves, autonomic ganglia associated with various body systems, cells of the adrenal medulla and, interestingly, melanocytes.

Closure of the neural tube begins in the midsection of the developing embryo and progresses in a cranial and caudal direction. The opening at each end of the tube is identified as the neural pore. If complete closure of either neural pore is arrested during development, congenital malformations may be evident after birth such as anencephaly, which results in decreased formation of the cerebral hemispheres. In extreme conditions, the hemispheres may be completely absent. Failure of closure of the caudal neuropore results in spina bifida. This condition presents as varying degrees of lack of closure and fusion of the neural tissue and the bony tissue of the vertebral canal that would normally enclose the caudal portion of the spinal cord.

To understand the basic generalized arrangement of the adult nervous system, certain facets of development should be kept in mind. As the neural tube completes its closure, it becomes a fluid-filled cylindrical structure that serves as the template for further development of the adult structures. Segments of the neural tube undergo differential growth to become the adult divisions and

Equine Neurology, Second Edition. Martin Furr and Stephen Reed.
© 2015 John Wiley & Sons, Inc. Published 2015 by John Wiley & Sons, Inc.
Companion website: www.wiley.com/go/furr/neurology

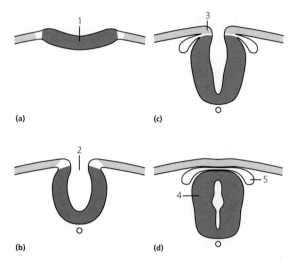

Figure 1.1 Stages of neural tube formation. (a) Thickening of cells to form neural plate (1) (b) Indentation formed by the neural groove (2) (c) Closure of the neural tube produced by neural folds (3) (d) Neural tube (4) closure completed with formation of neural crest cells (5) Circle in (b–d) represents the notochord.

structures of the nervous system. As the process of differential growth occurs, the fluid-filled center of the embryonic neural tube follows this pattern of differential growth to become the ventricular system of the nervous system.

Embryonic vesicles

The adult brain is divided into five regions that have their beginnings localized to specific areas of the developing neural tube. As the embryonic brain is developing, it is characterized by vesicle formation (swellings) that begins to divide the developing brain topographically into separate regions. There is a primary stage of development where three vesicles are observed. This is followed by a secondary stage where five vesicles subsequently form from the initial three. Upon further differentiation and growth, these five vesicles give rise to the five topographic regions of the adult brain.

From rostral to caudal, the vesicles of the primary stage are identified as the prosencephalon (forebrain), mesencephalon (midbrain), and rhombencephalon (hindbrain). With continued differential growth at the rostral end of the neural tube, the prosencephalon develops into the telencephalon (cerebrum) and diencephalon (thalamus). At the caudal end of the tube, the rhombencephalon gives rise to the metencephalon (pons and cerebellum) and the more caudally positioned myelencephalon (medulla oblongata) (Figure 1.2).

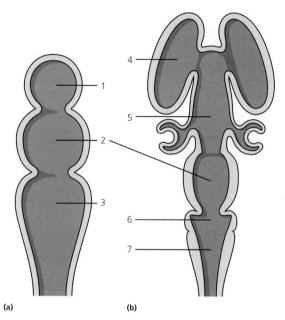

Figure 1.2 Embryonic brain vesicles. (a) Primary vesicle stage; (b) secondary vesicle stage. 1, Prosencephalon; 2, mesencephalon; 3, rhombencephalon; 4, telencephalon; 5, diencephalon; 6, metencephalon; 7, myelencephalon.

Ventricular system

The fluid-filled cavity of the developing neural tube follows the differential growth pattern of the neural tissue through the vesicle stages into the formation of the adult brain. Therefore, a portion of the ventricular system is found at all levels of the adult brain as shown in Figure 1.3.

The right and left lateral ventricles follow the growth of the cerebral hemispheres of the cerebrum as they expand dorsally and caudally over the developing brainstem. The interventricular foramen interconnects each lateral ventricle with the third ventricle. The third ventricle, located in the thalamus, is shaped somewhat like an upright tire, encircling the interthalamic adhesion (the connection of the left and right halves of the thalamus across the midline of the brainstem). In the midbrain, the ventricular system is present as the narrow, tubular mesencephalic aqueduct. Cerebrospinal fluid (CSF), principally produced by the choroid plexus in the lateral and third ventricles, flows through the mesencephalic aqueduct to enter the relatively large fourth ventricle. The fourth ventricle is a somewhat diamond-shaped depression of the dorsal medulla oblongata, mostly hidden by the overlying cerebellum. CSF leaves the fourth ventricle through lateral apertures at the junction between the midbrain and the medulla oblongata and enters the subarachnoid space that surrounds the brain and spinal cord. CSF can also

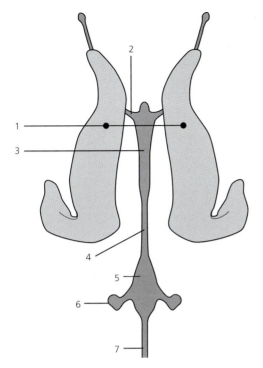

Figure 1.3 Dorsal view of ventricular system. 1, Lateral ventricles; 2, interventricular foramen; 3, third ventricle; 4, mesencephalic aqueduct; 5, fourth ventricle; 6, lateral aperture; 7, extension of ventricular system into central canal of spinal cord.

enter the central canal of the spinal cord through the median aperture of the caudal extent of the fourth ventricle; there is therefor bulk flow of CSF from a cranial to caudal direction with some modification of the fluid content during this passage. Hence, CSF collected at the lumbosacral junction has slightly different reference values compared with CSF collected at the atlantooccipital site (see Table 1.1).

Organization of gray and white matter in the CNS

The two main components of the CNS are the brain and the spinal cord. In turn, the brain and spinal cord are formed by numerous glial cells, a rather smaller number of neurons, and neuronal processes (axons, with or without surrounding myelin). Cell bodies of neurons and their unmyelinated processes have a somewhat gray appearance and not surprisingly form the gray matter of the nervous system. White matter of the nervous system is formed by myelinated axons of the neurons. The gray and white matter of the nervous system is organized differently in the brain and spinal cord: gray matter of the cerebrum is found either on its surface where it is identified as cortical gray matter or as collections of neuronal cell bodies located deep to the surface, the basal nuclei. Neurons within a particular cluster generally perform the same function and in the CNS are called nuclei.

Table 1.1 Functional classification of the cranial nerves.

Cranial nerve	Number	Function
Sensory		
Olfactory	CN I	Olfaction
Optic	CN II	Vision
Vestibulocochlear	CN VIII	Balance and hearing
Motor		
Oculomotor	CN III	Extraocular eye muscles
		Parasympathetic to eye
Trochlear	CN IV	Extraocular eye muscles
Abducens	CN VI	Extraocular eye muscles
Accessory	CN XI	Pharyngeal and laryngeal muscles; cervical muscles
Hypoglossal	CN XII	Lingual muscles
Mixed		
Trigeminal	CN V	General sensation to face; motor to muscles of mastication
Facial	CN VII	Taste sensation; motor to muscles of facial expression; parasympathetic for salivation and lacrimation
Glossopharyngeal	CN IX	Pharyngeal sensation; taste; swallowing muscles; parasympathetic for salivation
Vagus	CN X	Sensation pharynx and larynx; swallowing; parasympathetic for thoracic and abdominal organs

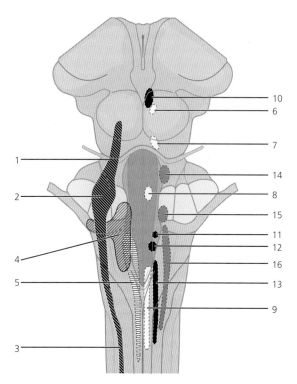

Figure 1.4 Schematic view of the dorsal brainstem. Sensory nuclei are indicated on the left, motor nuclei on the right. Motor nuclei with similar shading form functional groups for target structures as described in the text. 1, Mesencephalic nucleus of the trigeminal nerve; 2, pontine sensory nucleus of the trigeminal nerve; 3, spinal nucleus of the trigeminal nerve; 4, vestibular and cochlear nuclei; 5, solitary nucleus; 6, oculomotor nucleus; 7, trochlear nucleus; 8, abducens nucleus; 9, hypoglossal nucleus; 10, parasympathetic nucleus of the oculomotor nerve; 11, parasympathetic nucleus of the facial nerve; 12, parasympathetic nucleus of the glossopharyngeal nerve; 13, parasympathetic nucleus of the vagus nerve; 14, motor nucleus of the trigeminal nerve; 15, motor nucleus of the facial nerve; 16, nucleus ambiguus.

The white matter of the cerebrum is organized into bundles that form a system of conduction pathways to, from, and within the cerebrum. Three types of white matter fiber systems are recognized, consisting of projection fibers, commissural fibers, and association fibers. The critically important projection fibers carry information to and from the cerebrum to form connections with the brainstem and spinal cord, principally through the internal capsule. Commissural fibers carry information across the midline between the left and right cerebral hemispheres, mostly through the prominent corpus callosum. Association fibers form more subtle pathways that connect structures within one hemisphere, within and between lobes. A lobe of

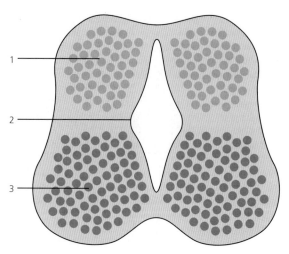

Figure 1.5 Neuron segregation in the developing spinal cord (schematic). 1, Alar plate containing sensory neurons; 2, sulcus limitans; 3, basal plate containing motor neurons.

the brain refers to a region of the cortex that tends to have some functional specificity and is named topographically for the overlying bone of the skull. Therefore, the frontal, parietal, occipital, and temporal lobes are identified deep to the skull bone of the same name.

Gray matter in the brainstem is arranged in columns of cells with broadly similar functions, often broken into nuclei of neurons with an even more specific function. Thus, the ventrally located somatic motor column of neurons is arranged into nuclei that innervated specific cranial nerves associated with specific functions, such as cranial nerve V for innervation of the muscles of mastication and cranial nerve VII for innervation of muscles of facial expression. A similar arrangement is evident for the medially located column consisting of parasympathetic autonomic neurons innervating, for example, the constrictor muscles of the pupil (cranial nerve III) or the lacrimal glands (cranial nerve VII) (see Figure 1.4). Furthermore, more dorsal structures tend to be sensory while those on the ventral aspect tend to have motor functions: this arrangement is followed through into the gray columns of the spinal cord, whereby the neurons of the dorsal horns are principally sensory, while the ventral horns comprise motor neurons. In the thoracic and lumbar segments of the spinal cord, an additional column is present in a lateral position approximately midway between the dorsal and ventral columns. This lateral horn of gray matter contains cell bodies that function as the presynaptic (preganglionic) lower motor neurons (LMNs) in the autonomic nervous system.

The anatomic segregation of sensory and motor cells can be appreciated in the embryonic spinal cord as shown in Figure 1.5. The dorsal half of the developing gray

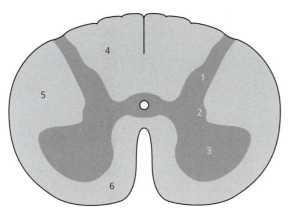

Figure 1.6 Arrangement of gray and white matter in the spinal cord. 1, Dorsal gray column; 2, lateral gray column; 3, ventral gray column; 4, dorsal funiculus; 5, lateral funiculus; 6, ventral funiculus.

matter is identified as the alar plate; neurons in this region will become the sensory neurons in the dorsal gray column in the adult spinal cord. The ventral half of the gray matter is referred to as the basal plate; neurons in this region will become the motor neurons in the ventral column of gray matter. The hollow portion of the embryonic tube will persist in the adult spinal cord as its central canal. There is a slight evagination within the central embryonic cavity identified as the sulcus limitans, and this serves as a dividing line between the sensory and motor neurons of the developing spinal cord.

Spinal cord white matter (Figure 1.6) meanwhile is located superficial to the gray columns and is arranged into large bundles called funiculi, which are organized by function. Dorsal funiculi for the most part carry sensory information to the forebrain, lateral funiculi connect the spinal cord and the cerebellum, and ventral funiculi principally consist of somatic motor axons on their way to synapse with LMNs in the ventral horn of the spinal cord.

Organization of gray and white matter in the PNS

The PNS is located peripheral to the skull and vertebral column. By convention, a cluster of neuronal cell bodies located outside the CNS is called a ganglion and consist of somatic sensory and autonomic motor neurons, that is, there are no somatic motor neurons outside of the CNS. Equine spinal ganglia are easily identified on dissection, while those associated with the sensory branches or cranial nerves tend to be much smaller. An exception is the trigeminal ganglion in the base of the skull, which is comparatively enormous.

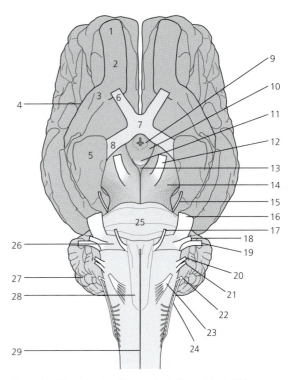

Figure 1.7 Ventral view of the brain (schematic). 1, Olfactory bulb; 2, olfactory peduncle; 3, lateral olfactory tract; 4, lateral rhinal sulcus; 5, piriform lobe; 6, optic nerve; 7, optic chiasm; 8, optic tract; 9, tuber cinereum; 10, hypothalamus; 11, mammillary body; 12, oculomotor nerve; 13, interpeduncular fossa; 14, crus cerebri; 15, trochlear nerve; 16, trigeminal nerve; 17, abducent nerve; 18, facial nerve; 19, vestibulocochlear nerve; 20, glossopharyngeal nerve; 21, vagus nerve; 22, accessory nerve; 23, hypoglossal nerve; 24, spinal root of accessory nerve; 25, transverse fibers of the pons; 26, trapezoid body; 27, cerebellum; 28, pyramid; 29, ventral median fissure.

The white matter of the peripheral system is composed of axons covered by Schwann cells and may be myelinated or unmyelinated, somatic or autonomic.

Gross anatomy of the CNS

An overview of the surface anatomy of the brain is described here. Readily observed structures of each of the five adult divisions of the brain will be highlighted. From rostral to caudal, the divisions of the brain are the medulla oblongata, pons and cerebellum, midbrain, thalamus, and cerebrum. As each division is described, the reader should refer to the diagrams of the ventral surface of the brain (Figure 1.7), the dorsal surface of the brainstem (Figure 1.8), and the median section of the brain (Figure 1.9) to see the location of the referenced structures.

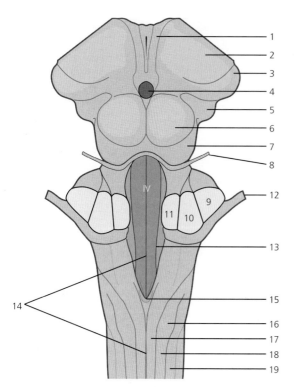

Figure 1.8 Dorsal view of the brainstem (schematic). 1, Stria habenularis thalami; 2, thalamus; 3, lateral geniculate body; 4, pineal body; 5, medial geniculate body; 6, rostral colliculus; 7, caudal colliculus; 8, trochlear nerve; 9, middle cerebellar peduncle; 10, caudal cerebellar peduncle; 11, rostral cerebellar peduncle; 12, vestibulocochlear nerve; 13, sulcus limitans; 14, median sulcus; 15, obex; 16, cuneate tubercle; 17, fasciculus gracilis; 18, fasciculus cuneatus; 19, spinal tract of the trigeminal nerve.

Cerebrum (telencephalon)

The telencephalic vesicle in the developing embryo gives rise to the cerebrum, formed by the left and right cerebral hemispheres. The cerebrum is the large superstructure that is connected to, and covers, the rostral brainstem. On the ventral surface, the olfactory bulbs are located at the rostral limit of each hemisphere. Olfactory receptors located in the nasal cavity transmit impulses along the olfactory nerve ((cranial nerve (CN) I) to synapse in the olfactory bulbs. The name olfactory "nerve" is actually a misnomer since it consists entirely of CNS tissue but in humans is so diminutive as to resemble a nerve. The olfactory tract is visible on the ventral surface in its position between the olfactory bulbs and the piriform lobe of the cerebrum. These olfactory structures contribute to the formation of that part of the cerebrum identified as the rhinencephalon for processing olfactory information; this is demarcated from the rest of the cerebral cortex by the lateral rhinal sulcus.

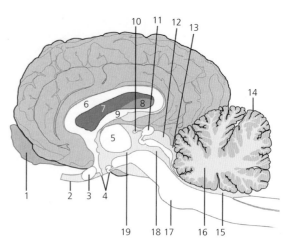

Figure 1.9 Median section of the brain (schematic). 1, Olfactory bulb; 2, optic nerve; 3, optic chiasm; 4, hypothalamus (pituitary gland removed); 5, interthalamic adhesion; 6, corpus callosum; 7, lateral ventricle; 8, hippocampus; 9, fornix; 10, habenula; 11, pineal body; 12, rostral colliculus; 13, caudal colliculus; 14, cerebellum; 15, fourth ventricle; 16, arbor vitae (cerebellar white matter); 17, pons; 18, mesencephalic aqueduct; 19, third ventricle.

The surface of the cerebrum is characterized by ridges identified as gyri and grooves identified as sulci. The left and right cerebral hemispheres are separated along the midline by the longitudinal cerebral fissure, while the caudal aspect of each hemisphere is separated from the cerebellum by the transverse cerebral fissure. The surface of the cerebrum is divided into lobes that are named topographically for the overlying bone of the skull: the cerebral lobes are thus identified as frontal, parietal, temporal, and occipital, each with broad functional specificities but no very detailed anatomical delineation. A greatly simplified listing of cerebral function suggests the following associations: the frontal lobe in horses is likely the motor cortex and association area involved in planning actions and movement. The parietal lobe is found just caudal to the motor cortex and consists of somesthetic regions and cognitive association areas involved in perceiving sensory input, while auditory information is processed in the temporal lobe ventrolateral to the parietal lobe. The occipital lobe processes visual information.

CSF within the respective cerebral hemispheres is contained in the left and right lateral ventricles, which intercommunicate at the midline with the third ventricle through the small interventricular foramen.

Thalamus (diencephalon)

The thalamus is located rostral to the midbrain and is part of the forebrain and not the brainstem. Strictly speaking, the anatomical structure is best termed the diencephalon, which is composed of five separate parts: thalamus, epithalamus, metathalamus, hypothalamus, and subthalamus. The largest portion of this however is the thalamus, and it is reasonable to refer to this structure by that name.

On the ventral surface of the thalamus is found the hypothalamus, bounded by the mammillary bodies caudally and the optic chiasm rostrally. The pituitary gland is attached to the hypothalamus by the tuber cinereum, a slightly elevated ridge of hypothalamic tissue between the two landmarks identified earlier, but because it is firmly adhered to the skull the pituitary is rarely removed along with the brain. The mammillary bodies appear as the two small prominences and are the most caudally located structures of the ventral surface of the thalamus. These act as relay stations interconnecting olfactory, behavioral, and autonomic areas of the brain. The optic nerve (CN II) fibers enter at the rostral edge of the diencephalon and form the optic chiasm. Calling this structure a "nerve" is, strictly speaking, incorrect as it is merely an extension of the brain with axons surrounded by oligodendrocytes not Schwann cells.

The dorsal surface of the thalamus is visible once the cerebrum has been removed. The left and right lateral geniculate nuclei are dorsocaudal projections at the most caudal margin of the thalamus and are vital relay stations that send information into the cerebrum. Slightly ventral to each lateral geniculate nucleus on either side are the medial geniculate nuclei, which send auditory information to the cerebrum. On the caudal dorsal surface of the thalamus is found a small unpaired prominence so important in regulating mare seasonal reproduction, the pineal gland.

At the level of the thalamus, the ventricular system resembles a tire, which encircles the median section of the thalamus. This is where the left and right divisions of the thalamus are joined across the midline by thalamic tissue identified as the interthalamic adhesion. A midsagittal view of the brainstem in Figure 1.9 reveals the third ventricle encircling the interthalamic adhesion.

Midbrain (mesencephalon)

A further prominent division of the brain is midbrain. Ventrally it is covered by conspicuous bundle fibers, known as the crus cerebri. These relatively large bundles are formed by fibers of the motor system as they pass through the midbrain to reach the pyramids in the caudal portions of the brainstem. The oculomotor nerve (CN III) emerges from the ventral surface of the mesencephalon. The mesencephalic aqueduct is that part of the ventricular system located in the mesencephalon and interconnects the third and fourth ventricles.

The dorsal surface of the mesencephalon is characterized by two pairs of rounded prominences, the rostral and caudal colliculi ("hillock"). Each rostral colliculus serves as a synaptic site in the pathway for visual

reflexes, while the caudal colliculus serves as a synaptic site in the pathway for auditory reflexes activity. The region of the midbrain dorsal to the mesencephalic aqueduct is known as the tectum, and tectospinal tracts running from the tectum to LMNs in the spinal tract regulate movement associated with auditory reflexes and visual reflexes.

The other cranial nerve associated with the midbrain is the trochlear nerve (CN IV), and unusually the fibers from that nucleus emerge from the *dorsal* surface of the mesencephalon and cross to reach the *opposite* ventral surface of the brainstem as it travels toward the orbit.

Pons (ventral metencephalon)

Moving caudally, the next division of the brain is the pons. The ventral surface is formed by the transverse fibers of the pons, a wide bundle of fibers that transmits information from the forebrain to the cerebellum. As the transverse fibers of the pons move laterally and dorsally, they form the middle cerebellar peduncle, which can be seen entering into the cerebellum. The only nucleus in the pons is the prominent motor nucleus of the trigeminal nerve. It innervates the muscles of mastication and is not infrequently affected by *Sarcocystis neurona* (the causative agent of equine protozoal myeloencephalitis). The large trigeminal nerve (CN V) leaves the ventral surface of the pons at the rostral edge of the transverse fibers of the pons.

Cerebellum (dorsal metencephalon)

The cerebellum ("little brain") is the superstructure seen on the dorsal surface of the pons. Embryologically this is part of the metencephalon; however, it is not considered part of the brainstem. The role of the cerebellum is to monitor sensorimotor information that travels through the nervous system, and it acts to integrate this information to produce smooth, coordinated movement. It is separated from the cerebrum by an intervening space in which lies the bony tentorium cerebelli, an immovable object under which the brain can herniate with devastating consequences should disease result in swelling of the neural structures rostral or caudal to it.

Anatomy of the cerebellum

The cerebellar surface is divided into a midline strip, the vermis, and the tissues lateral to the vermis are the left and right cerebellar hemispheres. The cerebellar surface is characterized by alternating grooves and ridges of tissue identified as the sulci and folia, respectively. As a general guideline, the primary fissure separates the rostral lobe of the cerebellum from the caudal lobe on the dorsal surface. On the ventral surface, the caudolateral fissure separates the caudal lobe of the cerebellum from the flocculonodular lobe (Figure 1.10).

Figure 1.11a, b shows that the anatomic arrangement of the gray and white matter in the cerebellum

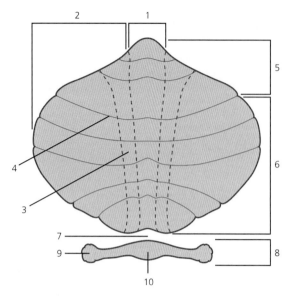

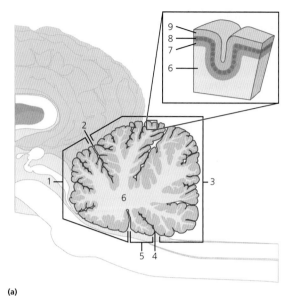

Figure 1.10 Schematic view of the cerebellum indicating anatomic regions. The cerebellum has been "unfolded" with the flocculonodular lobe positioned at the bottom of the diagram. 1, Vermis; 2, hemisphere; 3, intermediate hemisphere; 4, primary fissure; 5, rostral lobe; 6, caudal lobe; 7, caudolateral fissure; 8, flocculonodular lob; 9, flocculus; 10, nodulus.

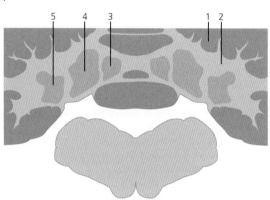

Figure 1.11 (a) Schematic view of the sagittally sectioned cerebellum. Inset shows cerebellar cortical layers. 1, Rostral lobe; 2, primary fissure; 3, caudal lobe; 4, caudolateral fissure; 5, flocculonodular lobe; 6, white matter (arbor vitae); 7, granular layer; 8, Purkinje cell layer; 9, molecular layer. (b) Schematic view of transversely sectioned cerebellum dorsal to the brainstem. 1, Cerebellar gray matter; 2, cerebellar white matter; 3, fastigial nucleus; 4, interpositus nucleus; 5, lateral nucleus.

is analogous to the arrangement that was seen in the cerebrum. Gray matter composed of a staggering number of small neurons covers the cerebellar cortical surface that surrounds the deeper white matter. The cortical gray matter is dived into three layers. From superficial to deep, these layers are identified as the molecular, Purkinje, and granular layer. Significantly, Purkinje fibers are the only neurons whose axons send efferent information from the cerebellar cortex. Subcortical gray matter is innervated by the Purkinje neurons and appears as three pairs of cerebellar nuclei embedded in the white matter. From medial to lateral, these deep cerebellar nuclei are identified as the fastigial, interpositus, and lateral nuclei, respectively.

Three pairs of cerebellar peduncles connect the cerebellum to the brainstem. From lateral to medial, these stalk-like connections are identified as the middle, caudal, and rostral cerebellar peduncles ("feet"), respectively (Figure 1.8). The peduncles are named based on their connections to the brainstem, not on their position relative to each other. Therefore, the middle cerebellar peduncle is the most lateral of the three and has been described previously as fibers that represent the continuation of the transverse fibers of the pons carrying information into the cerebellum. The caudal cerebellar

peduncle is so named because it is formed by various tracts that pass through the caudal portion of the brainstem to reach the cerebellum. The most medial of the cerebellar peduncles is the rostral cerebellar peduncle. It solely carries efferent fibers originating in the cerebellum that travel rostrally into the brainstem. As a general rule of thumb, the caudal cerebellar peduncle carries a majority of fibers that represent afferent tracts entering the cerebellum, and the rostral cerebellar peduncle primarily carries fibers that represent efferent tracts leaving the cerebellum.

Functional organization of the cerebellum

While the cerebellum is a complex structure in terms of its role in the nervous system, a simplified overview can be presented to gain a fundamental understanding of cerebellar function. The cerebellum receives general proprioceptive information from the periphery along with information from both the pyramidal and extra motor systems. Information about head position and movement also enters the cerebellum.

The Purkinje cells in the cortex monitor and process all the incoming information. When activated as a result of the net summation of all the afferent impulses, the Purkinje cells send normally inhibitory impulse to the appropriate cerebellar nuclei. The cerebellar nuclei in turn stimulate upper motor neurons (UMNs) in the brainstem, which in turn project to LMNs in the spinal cord as well as the cerebral cortex to produce coordinated movement.

While there is some degree of overlap, it is possible to correlate functional areas of the cerebellar lobes with the type of movement that is regulated and coordinated. The flocculonodular lobe (Figure 1.10) on the ventral surface of the cerebellum maintains balance and equilibrium and controls head and conjugate eye movements through the input of the vestibular system. This part of the cerebellum is identified as the vestibulocerebellum. The vermis and paravermal areas of the cerebellum coordinate activity for muscle tone and posture control and functionally are identified as the spinocerebellum. Finally, the cerebellar hemispheres lateral to the intermediate zone are known as the cerebrocerebellum as they coordinate voluntary and highly skilled movement.

Neurologic signs of cerebellar dysfunction

Although this is a greatly simplified explanation of cerebellar connections, it is through these complex interactions that the cerebellum monitors motor, proprioceptive, and vestibular (balance) information to maintain muscle tone and equilibrium and produce smooth, coordinated movement. The clinical signs of cerebellar disease can be related to the area of the cerebellum that has been affected and results in loss of its regulatory ability. The most common signs of cerebellar dysfunction relate to the function of the spinocerebellum and a loss of inhibition of UMNs due to a loss of inhibitory Purkinje cell output. This results in increased range of movement (hypermetria) and increased tone (spasticity). If the vestibulocerebellum is involved either directly or indirectly by altered input from the vestibular system, then vestibular signs such as a swaying posture, wide-based stance, nystagmus, and ventral strabismus may be noted. A loss of feedback pathways between the cerebrocerebellum and the forebrain results in asynchrony in movements and clinical signs of overshooting of body parts as well as tremor that is exacerbated as the animal attempts to make a voluntary movement (intention tremor).

Medulla oblongata (myelencephalon)

The medulla oblongata is the most caudal part of the brainstem located between the trapezoid body rostrally and the junction of the brainstem with the spinal cord at the level of the emergence of the first cervical spinal nerve. The ventral median fissure divides the ventral surface into right and left halves. Immediately adjacent to the fissure are the fiber bundles identified as the pyramids. The pyramids consist of descending motor fibers traveling through the brainstem. Given the lack of a corticospinal tract in equids (see "Descending tracts of the spinal cord"), it is likely that the pyramidal tracts consist of fibers destined for LMNs in cranial nerve nuclei, the so-called corticonuclear fibers. The rectangular-shaped trapezoid body at the rostral edge of the medulla oblongata is formed by fibers associated with the auditory system. The fibers of cranial nerves VI through XII exit the brainstem on the ventral surface of the medulla oblongata.

The caudal portion of the medulla oblongata is a tubular structure, but the rostral portion is open dorsally and forms the fourth ventricle. Three white matter fiber bundles occupy the dorsal surface beneath the ventricle: the bundle closest to the midline is the fasciculus gracilis, formed by fibers that carry conscious proprioceptive impulses from the pelvic limb to the forebrain via the thalamus. Just lateral to the fasciculus gracilis is the fasciculus cuneatus, which transmits similar fibers arising from the thoracic limbs. Moving laterally, the next bundle is the spinal tract of the trigeminal nerve; this tract is formed by fibers that carry nociceptive information from the head to conscious perception by the forebrain.

The rostral portion of the fourth ventricle lies in the dorsal pons, and the caudal half makes up the dorsal portion of the rostral medulla oblongata. The roof of the fourth ventricle is formed by the rostral and caudal medullary velum. These are a thin membranous covering made up of ependymal and pial cells of the meninges, respectively, located rostral and caudal to the cerebellum, respectively, and function to prevent the escape of CSF into the subarachnoid space. The caudal angle of the fourth ventricle forms a topographic landmark identified as the obex, and the groove along the midline in the floor of the ventricle that separates the two halves of the medulla oblongata is called the median sulcus.

Topographic features of the spinal cord

Since a large number of neurologic cases presenting to clinicians do so due to lesions to the spinal cord, it behooves clinicians to have a good understanding of the functional neuroanatomy relating to this structure. The white matter of the spinal cord is formed by ascending and descending pathways that transmit sensory and motor information through the nervous system. Ascending pathways originate in the spinal cord and travel to higher levels in the brain. Analogously, descending pathways that regulate motor activity originate in higher levels of the brain and descend through the CNS to reach spinal cord levels. Details of pathways are shown in Figure 1.12, but it is worth remembering that these represent extrapolations from other, better studied, species.

The spinal cord is divided into left and right halves by the dorsal median sulcus and the ventral longitudinal fissure as shown in Figure 1.13. The spinal cord is composed of gray and white matter with the white matter superficial to the deeper embedded gray matter. Large bundles of white matter in the spinal cord are identified as funiculi. Each funiculus in turn is formed by smaller bundles of white matter, identified as the various ascending or descending tracts of the spinal cord. Spinal nerve roots enter and leave the spinal cord dividing it in a segmental manner.

The left and right dorsal roots enter the spinal cord at the dorsolateral sulcus; the large bundle of white matter located between the dorsal roots is the left and right dorsal funiculus. Fibers located in the dorsal funiculus of the spinal cord are predominately fibers for conscious proprioception heading to the thalamus and subsequently the forebrain. The dorsal funiculus is further divided by the intermediate sulcus into the fasciculus gracilis medially and the fasciculus cuneatus laterally: the fasciculus gracilis carries information related to conscious proprioception from the pelvic limb, while the fasciculus cuneatus carries information related to conscious proprioception from the thoracic limbs. The function of the dorsal funiculus is described in the section on conscious proprioception.

The lateral funiculus is the large bundle of white matter located between dorsal and ventral roots on either half of the spinal cord. The principle components of the lateral funiculus are the spinocerebellar tracts, that is, fibers running from the spinal cord to the cerebellum for subconscious proprioception. These are important components of the subconscious proprioceptive system discussed later.

The ventral funiculus is located between the ventral roots. It is also formed by a mixture of ascending and descending tracts. This principally consists of descending tracts carrying UMN axons to the LMNs further caudal in the spinal cord.

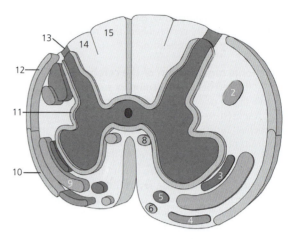

Figure 1.12 Position of ascending and descending tracts in the spinal cord (schematic). Descending tracts are numbered on the right; ascending tracts are numbered on the left. 2, Rubrospinal tract; 3, medullary reticulospinal tract; 4, lateral vestibulospinal tract; 5, pontine reticulospinal tract; 6, tectospinal tract; 8, medial longitudinal fasciculus; 9, spinothalamic tract; 10, ventral spinocerebellar tract; 11, fasciculus proprius (contains ascending and descending fibers); 12, dorsal spinocerebellar tract; 13, dorsolateral fasciculus (Lissauer's tract); 14, fasciculus cuneatus; 15, fasciculus gracilis.

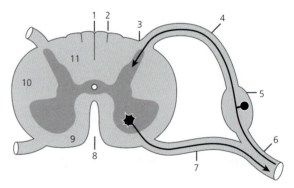

Figure 1.13 Spinal cord cross-section (schematic). The fiber of a sensory neuron is shown as it enters the spinal cord through the dorsal root. The fiber of a motor neuron is shown as it leaves the spinal cord through the ventral root. 1, Median sulcus; 2, dorsal intermediate sulcus; 3, dorsolateral sulcus; 4, dorsal root; 5, spinal ganglion; 6, spinal nerve proper; 7, ventral root; 8, ventral median fissure; 9, ventral funiculus; 10, lateral funiculus; 11, dorsal funiculus.

The peripheral nervous system

Peripheral nerves transmit a mix of sensory and motor information. Sensory impulses are detected by numerous and varied nerve receptors in the periphery

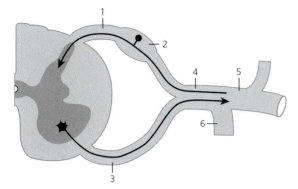

Figure 1.14 Spinal nerve anatomy. The dorsal root is formed by sensory neurons; the ventral root is formed by motor neurons. Arrowheads indicate sensory impulses travel toward the spinal cord and motor impulses travel toward the periphery. 1, Dorsal root; 2, spinal ganglion (dorsal root ganglion); 3, ventral root; 4, spinal nerve proper; 5, dorsal branch of the spinal nerve; 6, ventral branch of the spinal nerve.

and are transmitted toward the CNS, while motor impulses originate in LMNs of the CNS and travel through the peripheral nerves to provide motor innervation to somatic or visceral target structures of the body. The combined motor neuron soma, peripheral nerve, neuromuscular junction, and muscle are called a motor unit, and dysfunction of any portion of the motor unit will result in paresis with diminished reflexes and decreased muscle tone.

There are two broad categories of peripheral nerves: spinal nerves and cranial nerves. Both perform the same function of transmitting sensory and motor innervation between the CNS and peripheral structures, with the distinction between spinal and cranial nerves being simply their anatomic location. At the level of the spinal cord, each spinal nerve is attached to the cord by dorsal and ventral roots. The dorsal root of the spinal cord represents the equivalent of axonal processes that originated from sensory cell bodies located in the spinal ganglion, as shown in Figure 1.14. The ventral root is formed by axons that originated in large motor neuron soma located in the spinal cord ventral gray column and leave the spinal cord to innervate target structures in the periphery. The spinal nerve proper is a relatively short segment located at the level of the intervertebral foramen. At this level, the spinal nerve is composed of the intermingling of nerves of sensory nerve fibers from peripheral nerve receptors and the motor nerve fibers traveling to peripheral target structures. The spinal nerve divides into dorsal and ventral branches that carry sensory and motor impulses throughout the periphery.

Afferent function of peripheral nerves

Spinal and cranial peripheral nerves will transmit afferent (sensory) information from somatic and visceral structures. This includes impulses of nociception, temperature, touch, position, and movement, that is, nociception and proprioception, and autonomic impulses that originate within body viscera related to temperature; blood pressure; gas and chemical concentrations; and dilation, pressure, and movement of the body organs. For the spinal division of peripheral nerves, the sensory cell bodies are segmentally distributed and located in the spinal ganglia. Axons from these primary sensory cells generally synapse in the dorsal gray column and then ascend to higher centers in the nervous system.

Sensory information from the head is transmitted by specific cranial nerves (see Table 1.1). Proprioceptive and nociceptive information from the head travels through the trigeminal nerve (CN V). This information is processed through a column of cells in the brainstem identified as the trigeminal sensory nucleus. Sensory afferents for balance and equilibrium travel through the vestibular portion of the vestibulocochlear nerve and synapse in the brainstem in the vestibular nuclei. The cochlear division of the vestibulocochlear nerve carries auditory afferents that synapse in the brainstem cochlear nuclei. Autonomic afferent (via glossopharyngeal and vagus nerves) and taste fibers (via the facial nerve and glossopharyngeal nerve) synapse in another large sensory nucleus of the brainstem, the solitary nucleus. Afferent impulses for vision travel through the optic nerve (CN II) and synapse in the lateral geniculate nucleus of the thalamus. Sensory input for olfaction travels through the olfactory nerve (CN I) to synapse in the olfactory bulb of the rhinencephalon. These sensory cranial nerve nuclei are presented in Figure 1.4.

Efferent function of peripheral nerves

Motor neurons are distributed along the length of the spinal cord in the ventral gray column. Motor fibers leave the spinal cord to travel through the spinal nerve to provide innervation to the skeletal muscles in the body. Motor innervation to the muscles of the head travels through various cranial nerves. Motor nerve fibers travel through select cranial nerves to provide autonomic innervation. The cranial nerves with motor function originate from nuclei scattered throughout the brainstem. The cells of the motor nuclei are arranged in three fragmented columns that can be functionally organized based on their target structures, as described later and shown in Figure 1.4.

Autonomic system targets

The target structures for this group are glandular tissue and cardiac and smooth muscle cells that receive parasympathetic motor innervation via the cranial nerves. The efferent motor fibers originate in the parasympathetic motor nuclei of cranial nerves III, VII, IX, and X. A summary of cranial nerve function is found in Table 1.1.

Functional systems for clinicians

Neurological cases generally are presented to clinicians not with a complaint within a specific structure of the nervous system, instead clinical signs are primarily related to a functional system, be it paresis due to a lesion in the motor system, ataxia due to a deficit in general proprioception or the vestibular system, or a clinical sign related to the autonomic nervous system. Having an understanding of the organization of the nervous system provides the basis for understanding the disorders that affect the various components of the nervous system. The sensory and motor pathways (and associated clinical signs) that will be reviewed in the following sections include the somatic motor system (paresis), general proprioception (ataxia), nociception (pain perception), vestibular system (vestibular ataxia), and the autonomic system.

Somatic motor system

The control of voluntary movements is complex. Many different systems across numerous brain areas need to work together to ensure proper motor control. Neurons of the motor system send their axons from higher levels of the CNS to regulate and influence the activity of the motor neurons in the brainstem and spinal cord that leave the CNS to innervate target structures in the periphery. Motor neurons in the higher levels of the CNS are defined as upper motor neurons, and motor neurons that send their axons to provide motor innervation to peripheral targets are defined as lower motor neurons. The descending tracts of the spinal cord are formed by axons of UMNs that descend through the brain and spinal cord to provide a regulatory influence on the lower motor cells. The descending tracts of the spinal cord are shown opposite the ascending tracts in Figure 1.12. Unlike the autonomic system, there is only one LMN in this chain, that is, one UMN synapses (directly or indirectly) with one LMN, whose axon then influences a number of skeletal muscle fibers in the periphery. Damage to UMNs or LMNs result in the inability to initiate movement or bear weight (i.e., paresis), but the quality of the paresis is different for the two and will be described in the subsequent section.

In primates, the UMN system is organized into two components, the pyramidal motor system responsible for fine, isolated, precise and specific movements and the extrapyramidal system responsible for gross,

synergic movements, which require the activity of large groups of muscles. There is no evidence that horses have significant pyramidal tracts in the spinal cord, the only direct motor cortex to LMN pathways in equids likely terminates in the brainstem, and so this system will not be reviewed further.

Extrapyramidal motor organization

The extrapyramidal motor system is so named because the nuclei and tracts contained within this division do not contribute to formation of the pyramids seen on the ventral surface of the medulla oblongata. Anatomically, the extrapyramidal part of the motor system is composed of a myriad of nuclei and tracts located within all divisions of the brain. In general, the extrapyramidal system principally provides regulatory influence on the LMNs that are responsible for muscle tone and posture. The mechanism for the maintenance of muscle tone is further described in Chapter 36 and Figure 36.1.

UMN nuclei in the brain

Extrapyramidal structures are widespread throughout the CNS and provide multiple polysynaptic pathways to ultimately regulate the activity of LMNs. The cerebrum contains cortical and subcortical collections of extrapyramidal motor cells and further nuclei are found in the brainstem.

Motor neurons in the cerebral hemisphere are scattered in the cerebral cortex but also in the gray matter deep to the cortex in the basal nuclei. The nuclei of significance are the caudate nucleus, putamen, and globus pallidus. White matter between the caudate nucleus and the putamen appear grossly as stripes and the collective term for those two nuclei is the corpus striatum (Figure 1.15). Generally speaking, within the processing network of the corpus striatum, the caudate nucleus and the putamen act as afferent centers that receive and process information. The globus pallidus acts as an efferent center to send information to other extrapyramidal centers in the thalamus and brainstem.

Many motor nuclei are also found within the brainstem. In the midbrain, the major extrapyramidal nuclei are the red nucleus, the tegmental nucleus, and the substantia nigra. Of these three, the red nucleus is of particular importance. It gives rise to the rubrospinal tract that descends through the rest of the brainstem and the lateral funiculus in the spinal cord to reach the LMNs of the spinal cord. In the pons, a nuclear area deep in the reticular formation plays a role in extrapyramidal regulation and the medullary reticular nucleus is located in the reticular formation of the medulla oblongata.

Although the extrapyramidal motor system is characterized by numerous structures, descending regulation likely reaches the LMNs in the spinal cord mainly

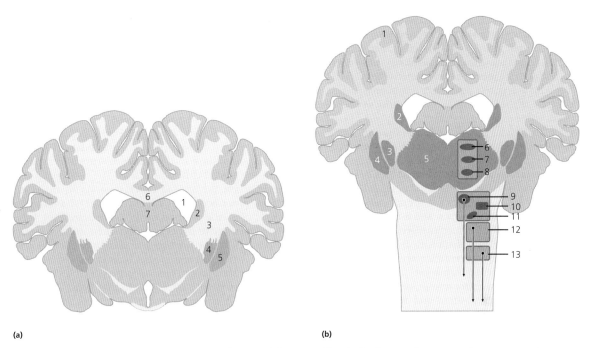

(a)

(b)

Figure 1.15 (a) Transverse section of the brain at the level of the mammillary body showing the corpus striatum. 1, Lateral ventricle; 2, caudate nucleus; 3, internal capsule; 4, globus pallidus (pallidum); 5, putamen; 6, corpus callosum; 7, hippocampus. (b) Schematic topographic organization of extrapyramidal motor centers. Nuclei 6, 7, and 8 are in the diencephalon; 9, 10, and 11 are in the midbrain; 12 is in the pons; and 13 is in the medulla oblongata. 1, Cerebral cortex; 2, caudate nucleus; 3, globus pallidus (pallidum); 4, putamen; 5, thalamus; 6, zona incerta; 7, endopeduncular nucleus; 8, subthalamic nucleus; 9, red nucleus (arrow represents rubrospinal tract that decussates and descends to spinal cord levels); 10, tegmental nucleus; 11, substantia nigra; 12, pontine reticular nucleus (arrow represents pontine reticulospinal tract that decussates and descends to spinal cord levels); 13, medullary reticular nucleus (arrow represents medullary reticulospinal tract that decussates and descends to spinal cord levels).

through three contralateral pathways, the rubrospinal tract of the midbrain, the pontine reticulospinal tract, and the medullary reticulospinal tract (See Figure 1.12).

Neurologic signs of UMN dysfunction

UMNs regulate LMNs, both initiating movement and, of principal importance in the extrapyramidal system, regulating tone. Indeed the vast majority of UMN axons function to inhibit extensor tone. A lesion that involves UMN structures or pathways essentially decreases or eliminates the regulatory control of the UMN on the LMN resulting in increased extensor tone and reflexes and diminished ability to initiate voluntary movements. The clinical signs that are considered to be hallmarks of UMN disease include hypertonus ("spasticity"), hyperreflexia (commonly examined in small animals but almost impossible to elicit in ambulatory adult horses), and UMN paresis. The most straightforward way to test for UMN paresis in horses is to firmly, and consistently, pull on the horse's tail as it is walking in a straight line; an animal with UMN paresis will not be able to initiate the ipsilateral limb extension required

to counteract this maneuver and particularly patients with acute spinal cord compression can be remarkably easy to pull over. UMN paresis differs from LMN paresis by the preservation, and often increase, of reflexes and muscle tone.

Somatic sensory systems

There are two principal sensory systems of the body, a system responsible for detecting body position and a system responsible for detecting the sensation of noxious stimuli. These two functional systems are defined as proprioception and nociception, respectively. The major pathways that monitor proprioception and nociception are described as follows.

General proprioception
Definition of general proprioception and ataxia

General proprioception is a sensory system that detects the state of the position and the movement in muscles and joints. The clinical sign resulting from a deficit in general proprioception is called "ataxia," an inconsistent gait with alterations in the rate, range, and force of movement. An ataxic gait is characterized by being inconsistent and having components of hypometria (too little joint movement, spasticity) and hypermetria (high striding) movement. Depending on the nature of the lesion, hypometria or hypermetria may predominate. Ataxia is purely due to a deficit in proprioception, not strength; however, since the majority of cases have spinal cord compression with lesions in the UMN system also, signs of both UMN paresis and ataxia are expressed together. Balance is a further proprioceptive system and a lesion in the vestibular system also results in ataxia, but an ataxia with somewhat different qualities (see Section on "Neurologic Signs of Vestibular System Dysfunction"). General proprioception consists of two separate components, one is the conscious proprioceptive pathway, which involves the transmission of proprioceptive information to the cerebral cortex; the other is for segmental reflex activity and transmitting proprioceptive information to the cerebellum. Broadly, conscious proprioception is the conscious awareness of body position and movement of body segments and monitoring of limb position while the animal is stationary. In horses, we assume that a deficit in replacing a limb in the correct position after, for example, spinning it in a circle is due to a deficit in conscious proprioception and is a component of an ataxic gait. The subconscious system monitors proprioception when the animal is in motion and a deficit is likely to result in the "swinging" movements particularly of the pelvic limbs when an ataxic horse is turned sharply.

General proprioception anatomy
General proprioceptive impulses from receptors in muscles and joints are relayed to higher centers where they can reach a state of conscious perception (forebrain) or remain at a subconscious level (cerebellum). The pathways for proprioception are formed by a chain of neurons with synapses at specific levels of the nervous system. For conscious proprioception there are three neurons in the chain, while for subconscious proprioception there are only two neurons in the pathway.

Conscious proprioception
Conscious proprioception is mediated by pathways in the dorsal column of the spinal cord through pathways that begin in joint receptors and end in the parietal lobe of the cerebral cortex; it enables the cortex to refine voluntary movements. The cell bodies of the neurons that are responsible for detecting proprioceptive changes are located in the dorsal root ganglia, and the dendrites of these neurons are modified to function as proprioceptors. The axons of the first-order cells project as part of the dorsal root of the spinal nerve and enter the white matter of the dorsal funiculus. As these axons turn and pass cranially through the spinal cord, they form the discrete fiber tract in the dorsal funiculus, identified as the fasciculus gracilis medially when information arises from the pelvic limbs, and in the more laterally placed fasciculus cuneatus for impulses from the thoracic limbs. These fibers ascend ipsilaterally until they reach their site of synapse in the caudal medulla oblongata at the level with the obex, at which point the axons in the fasciculus gracilis synapse with the bilateral gracilis nucleus and those in the fasciculus cuneatus synapse with the medial cuneate nucleus. The neurons in this nucleus are the second-order neurons in this conscious proprioceptive pathway. As the second-order axons cross the midline of the brainstem, they form the deep arcuate fibers and they then move rostrally and ascend in the brainstem as a component of a fiber bundle known as the medial lemniscus. The synapse with the third-order neuron occurs in the thalamus. These third-order neurons send their axons ipsilaterally through the internal capsule to their termination in the somesthetic cerebral cortex.

Subconscious proprioception
The cell body of the first-order neuron for subconscious proprioception is also in a spinal ganglion. The second neurons, however, with the exception of the small cuneocerebellar tract, are located not in the brainstem but in the dorsal horn of the spinal cord; these neurons send their axons to the cerebellum via the lateral funiculi of the spinal cord. The spinocerebellar tracts can be further subdivided into the dorsal and ventral spinocerebellar tracts carrying information from the pelvic limbs, and the more medially placed cuneocerebellar and rostral spinocerebellar tracts, which are related to information from the thoracic limbs. This arrangement may be one of the reasons why spinal cord compressions invariably have more severe clinical signs in the pelvic limbs compared with the thoracic limb: the pelvic limb tracts are more superficially placed and far more easily damaged. Subconscious proprioceptive information is ultimately relayed to the cerebellar cortex by axons that enter the caudal cerebellar peduncle to synapse in the cerebellar cortex.

Nociception
Fibers carrying impulses related to touch and noxious stimuli form the spinothalamic tract as they ascend through the spinal cord. "Tract" is actually a misnomer as, unlike in primates, this is a diffuse network of axons deep in the spinal cord with numerous ipsilateral and contralateral interconnections compared. Only a severe spinal cord lesion can damage this diffuse and multisynaptic pathway to the extent that limb nociception ("deep pain") is lost.

The first-order neuron is again located in the spinal ganglion. First-order axons ascend and descend in the cord traversing short intersegmental distance prior to synapsing with neurons in the substantia gelatinosa, a superficial gray matter layer of the spinal cord dorsal horn. Second-order axons immediately cross to the opposite side and form a diffuse spinothalamic tract in the contralateral funiculus. At the level of the thalamus, a synapse occurs on the third-order neuron in thalamus. Third-order axons enter into the formation of the internal capsule as they travel to their respective site of synapse in the somesthetic cortex.

Areas of innervation supplied by a single nerve are called an autonomous innervation zone, and knowledge of their distribution can be useful when testing for peripheral nerve damage (for reference, see Figure 33.4). Note that unlike humans and small animals equids do not have an autonomous zone for the radial nerve.

The vestibular system

Many equine neurological patients present with clinical signs related to vestibular dysfunction, most commonly a head tilt (see Figure 9.1), and clinicians need to be comfortable with this system. The vestibular system is a special sensory system of the body that monitors position, rotation, and movement of the head and subsequently adjusts body posture and eye position. Sensory receptors for balance and equilibrium are principally located in the semicircular canals of the inner ear and supported by proprioceptive information from the rest of the body and in horses particularly the dorsal roots of cranial cervical vertebrae. The visual system also has inputs into the vestibular nuclei. Impulses from the inner ear in response to head movement travel to the brainstem along the vestibular portion of the vestibulocochlear nerve (CN VIII), and the majority of the vestibular axons synapse in the brainstem on four pairs of vestibular nuclei in the very rostral medulla oblongata. In turn, axons from the vestibular nuclei project to the cerebellum, the brainstem nuclei that regulate the extraocular eye muscles, and the spinal cord. There is a very close connection between the vestibular nuclei and neurons in the cerebellum, particularly the flocculonodular lobe. This phylogenetically older part of the cerebellum is responsible for providing the sensorimotor coordination necessary to maintain balance and equilibrium.

Ascending projections from the vestibular nuclei pass rostrally through the brainstem to the motor nuclei of the extraocular eye muscles as the ascending limb of the medial longitudinal fasciculus. Appropriate stimulation of the eye muscles in response to these vestibular impulses initiated by head movement produces conjugate eye movement and dysfunction results in ventral strabismus (Figure 9.2) and spontaneous nystagmus.

The major fiber projection from the vestibular nuclei that enters the spinal cord forms the lateral vestibulospinal tract located in the ventrolateral funiculus of white matter as shown in Figure 1.12, while a smaller projection travels through the spinal cord in the ventral funiculus adjacent to the ventral median fissure. This smaller bundle forms the medial vestibulospinal tract, also identified as the descending limb of the medial longitudinal fasciculus, the tract that in the brainstem transmits vestibular control over cranial nerve nuclei. The two vestibulospinal tracts are responsible for regulating the extensor muscle tone necessary to maintain balance and posture. This is an important clinical concept: the vestibular system regulates ipsilateral antigravity tone. Vestibulospinal tract adjustments help to coordinate the activity of the limbs and trunks in response to head movements detected through the vestibular receptors in the inner ear.

Neurologic signs of vestibular system dysfunction

Classical vestibular signs include a head tilt, staggering ("vestibular ataxia"), circling, and nystagmus. The origin of the classical vestibular signs is anatomically interesting and can be explained by the unequal input into the vestibular nuclei and resulting loss of ipsilateral antigravity tone. For example, if a horse has a lesion on the right inner ear, then the vestibular nuclei would have unbalanced input, with left-side input being greater than the right. The brain would interpret the unbalanced input as indicating that the head is turning to the left resulting in decreased ipsilateral (i.e., right-sided) antigravity tone and increased antigravity extensor tone on the left. Thus the patient would tilt, stagger, and circle to the right. Even if the horse is at rest, the brain perceives the animal to be turning to the left due to the unbalanced input, and thus the eyes make rapid jerky movements to the left, before drifting back across the orbit again: so-called left-sided nystagmus, which, with rare exceptions, means that the lesion is on the opposite side of the vestibular system.

Lesions in the vestibular system may arise in the periphery (which practically means in the inner ear of the petrous temporal bone) or occasionally they may arise centrally in the brainstem, the vestibular portions of the cerebellum, or the relevant tracts in the cranial spinal cord. Thus, vestibular disease is called peripheral or central, respectively, and it is critical that clinicians differentiate the two by looking for other signs that may be evident in a central lesion. Broadly, this could include general proprioceptive ataxia, UMN paresis, or involvement of cranial nerves other than cranial nerve VII (which can be damaged by both central and peripheral lesions). Certain discrete central lesions disrupting cerebellar inhibition of vestibular nuclei can result in vestibular signs mimicking those from the opposite side; however, the other central deficits, for example, UMN paresis, will indicate the correct side of the lesion. Visual inputs also affect the vestibular nuclei, and (carefully) blindfolding in a horse with a marginal lesion and no otherwise-obvious vestibular signs can induce dramatic vestibular signs.

Autonomic nervous system: a two-LMN system

The autonomic nervous system differs from the somatic nervous system in that it is not under voluntary control and that the effectors are two LMNs, one in the CNS and one in ganglia in the periphery. Similar to the somatic system, it has UMNs situated in the brain and consists of motor and sensory systems. The autonomic sensory system is broadly similar to the somatic sensory system although it tends not to reach consciousness and it will not be discussed further here. The autonomic nervous system is responsible for the regulation of the visceral functions of the body. The classical representation of the autonomic system divides the system into two functional components, the sympathetic and parasympathetic divisions of the autonomic system. The key point to understanding the anatomic arrangement of autonomic innervation is the realization that the system is represented by a model composed of two neurons that synapse on each other prior to innervating a target structure. The site of synapse occurs in ganglia either close to the CNS, in the abdomen or pelvis, or indeed within a specific organ (such as the numerous submucosal and myenteric plexus neurons within the large and small intestines). The targets of autonomic innervation are cardiac muscle, smooth muscle, and glands. Sympathetic and parasympathetic innervation of the same structure is usually antagonistic. The sympathetic nervous system prepares the body for the classic "fight-or-flight" response. Parasympathetic innervation promotes "rest and recovery" functions of the body.

Sympathetic nervous system

Sympathetic innervation is provided through a chained network of two neurons that synapse on each other in a ganglion prior to reaching the target of innervation. The first neuron in this chain is identified as the presynaptic neuron of origin for the sympathetic system. The presynaptic soma is located in the lateral horn of the thoracic and lumbar segments of the spinal cord. For this reason, it is frequently called the thoracolumbar division of the autonomic nervous system. The presynaptic nerve fiber, that is, the axon of the

presynaptic soma, leaves the spinal cord to synapse on the second neuron in the chain identified as the postsynaptic soma.

The sympathetic postsynaptic soma is located in one of the ganglia of the sympathetic division of the system where it receives the synaptic contact of the presynaptic fiber. Sympathetic ganglia can be classified into two main groups, either paravertebral (parallel to the vertebral column) or prevertebral (some distance from the CNS) ganglia. A third group of sympathetic ganglia are found embedded in the organ to be innervated.

Prevertebral sympathetic ganglia are positioned approximately along the midline ventral to the vertebral column. They are wrapped around the origins of the major abdominal blood vessels that come from the aorta. The prevertebral ganglia are the celiacomesenteric ganglion and the caudal mesenteric ganglion. It is within these ganglia that the presynaptic axon synapses on the postsynaptic soma. In turn, the postsynaptic synaptic sends its axon into the periphery to reach the target of innervation.

The other main site of synapse for presynaptic sympathetic cells is in the paravertebral ganglia. These ganglia are located more laterally in relation to the position of the vertebral column. The paravertebral sympathetic ganglia are the cervical ganglia in the neck and the segmentally distributed ganglia along the sympathetic chain in the thoracic and abdominal cavities.

There are two pairs of cervical ganglia closely associated with the vagosympathetic trunk as it traverses the neck. The cranial cervical ganglia are located in the wall of the guttural pouch, and British pathologists have become adept at finding these as they are the principal biopsy site for the diagnosis of equine dysautonomia (grass sickness). The middle cervical ganglia are located near the thoracic inlet. In the species of major veterinary interest, the caudal cervical ganglion has fused with the most cranial ganglion of the sympathetic chain at the level of the first rib. This conjoined structure is identified as the cervicothoracic ganglion.

Due to the varying distribution of sympathetic ganglia, the presynaptic fibers can take several paths as they travel toward their ganglionic site of synapse with the second neuron in the chain (Figure 1.16). The third category of sympathetic ganglia is a miscellany of ganglia that are scattered along the aorta or are located near other organs. These ganglia can be identified individually as aortic ganglia, renal ganglia, and adrenal ganglia.

In the case of target structures in the head receiving sympathetic innervation, this becomes a relatively

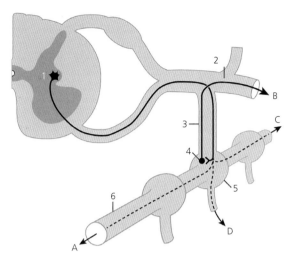

Figure 1.16 Model of sympathetic innervation. Presynaptic cells can synapse (A) on postsynaptic cells a few segments cranial in the sympathetic trunk; (B) on a postsynaptic cell at the segment where the postsynaptic fiber emerges; (C) on a postsynaptic cell caudal in the sympathetic trunk; (D) the presynaptic cell can bypass the sympathetic trunk ganglia and synapse in the prevertebral ganglia. 1, Presynaptic cell body; 2, spinal nerve; 3, ramus communicans; 4, postsynaptic cell body; 5, sympathetic trunk ganglion; 6, sympathetic trunk.

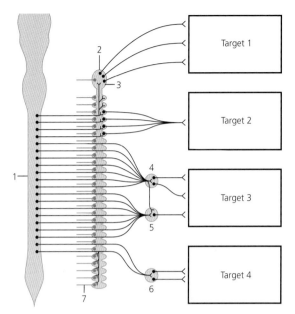

Figure 1.17 Sympathetic innervation targets. Structures receiving sympathetic innervation can be grouped as target areas in the body. Target 1 represents cranial structures such as ocular structures, the lacrimal gland, and the salivary glands. Target 2 represents the thoracic viscera. Target 3 represents abdominal viscera. Target 4 represents urinary and pelvic viscera. 1, Thoracolumbar origin of sympathetic innervation; 2, sympathetic trunk; 3, cervicothoracic ganglion; 4, celiac ganglion; 5, cranial mesenteric ganglion; 6, caudal mesenteric ganglion; 7, postganglionic sympathetic fibers to peripheral structures: vascular smooth muscle, arrector pili muscle, sweat glands.

long pathway. From the presynaptic cell body in the lateral horn of the spinal cord, the presynaptic fiber travels through the ventral root of the spinal nerve, enters the sympathetic chain, passes through the cervicothoracic ganglion and the ansa subclavia, through the middle cervical ganglion, through the vagosympathetic trunk in the cervical region, and finally reaches its site of synapse in the cranial cervical ganglion at the base of the skull. The postsynaptic cells in the cranial cervical ganglion then send their postsynaptic fibers to the target structures in the head such as the eye and salivary glands to provide sympathetic innervation. The sympathetic innervation scheme is shown in Figure 1.17.

Parasympathetic nervous system

The parasympathetic nervous system is also called the craniosacral division of the autonomic system. Anatomically, the parasympathetic system follows the two-neuron-chain model as described for the sympathetic system, but the presynaptic and postsynaptic cell bodies are located in different parts of the nervous system. The term "craniosacral" indicates the location of the presynaptic parasympathetic cell bodies

Table 1.2 Named ganglia associated with parasympathetic postganglionic nerve cell bodies.

Cranial nerve	Postganglionic cell body location
Oculomotor (CN III)	Ciliary ganglion
Facial (CN VII)	Mandibular or pterygopalatine ganglion
Glossopharyngeal (CN IX)	Otic ganglion
Vagus (CN X)	Terminal ganglion

within the nervous system. Presynaptic parasympathetic cell bodies are found in nuclei associated with specific cranial nerves and in the sacral portions of the spinal cord. The postsynaptic cell bodies are located in named ganglia associated with specific cranial nerves and in terminal ganglia throughout the body.

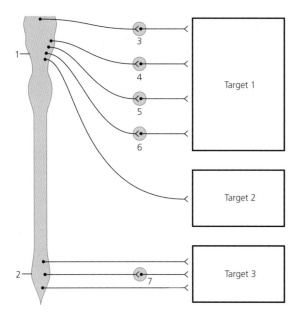

Figure 1.18 Parasympathetic innervation targets. Structures receiving parasympathetic innervation can be grouped as target areas in the body. Target 1 represents cranial structures such as ocular structures, the lacrimal gland, and the salivary glands that are innervated by cranial nerves. Target 2 represents the thoracic and abdominal viscera that are innervated by the vagus nerve. Target 3 represents urinary and pelvic viscera that are innervated by the pelvic nerve. 1, Parasympathetic cranial nerve nuclei of origin in the brainstem; 2, parasympathetic neurons in the sacral spinal cord; 3, ciliary ganglion; 4, pterygopalatine ganglion; 5, mandibular ganglion; 6, otic ganglion; 7, pelvic ganglion.

In the cranial portion of the parasympathetic division, presynaptic parasympathetic cell bodies are associated with four cranial nerves, the oculomotor nerve (CN III), the facial nerve (CN VII), the glossopharyngeal nerve (CN IX), and the vagus nerve (CN X). Collections of presynaptic parasympathetic cells form nuclei that are associated with each of the four cranial nerves identified earlier.

The postsynaptic cell bodies of three parasympathetic cranial nerves, the oculomotor nerve (CN III), the facial nerve (CN VII), and the glossopharyngeal nerve (CN IX), are located in named ganglia associated with those nerves. The postsynaptic cell bodies for the vagus nerve (CN X) and the sacral component of parasympathetic innervation will be located in terminal ganglia, as summarized in Table 1.2. Terminal ganglia are autonomic ganglia located in the wall of the target structure. For example, the submucosal and myenteric ganglia of the intestinal tract represent collections of postsynaptic parasympathetic cell bodies located in terminal ganglia (and coincidentally produce as much neurotransmitter as is produced in the brain!).

The sacral division of the parasympathetic nervous system follows the same organizational model of a two-neuron chain as seen with the parasympathetic cranial division of the system. Presynaptic parasympathetic cell bodies are located in the lateral horn of the sacral spinal cord. Presynaptic fibers exit the sacral spinal cord and synapse in the pelvic ganglion or in terminal ganglia of the pelvic viscera (Figure 1.18).

2 Cerebrospinal Fluid and the Blood–Brain Barrier

Martin Furr

Marion duPont Scott Equine Medical Center, Virginia-Maryland Regional College of Veterinary Medicine, Leesburg, USA

Cerebrospinal fluid (CSF) is a clear, colorless fluid that fills the brain's ventricular system, central canal of the spinal cord, and subarachnoid space. It penetrates and bathes all central nervous system (CNS) tissue and is contiguous with the CNS extracellular fluid [1]. The CSF functions to protect the brain from trauma and to maintain a consistent extracellular environment for the CNS. The CSF provides physical support (i.e., buoyancy) and cushioning of the CNS as a result of its specific gravity (1.004–1.006) and fluid pressure, which effectively reduces the weight of the brain 30-fold [2]. It also serves as a physiologic medium to transport a variety of compounds (neurotransmitters) and to regulate the chemical environment of the CNS ("sink-action"). Because the CSF bathes the entire CNS, diseases of the brain and spinal cord may result in changes in its composition, which can be used as a diagnostic aid. The production and composition of the CSF are highly dependent on the presence and normal functioning of the blood–brain barrier (BBB).

Blood–brain barrier

Structure

The concept of the BBB arose more than a century ago with the classic experiments of Ehrlich and Goldman, in which the dye trypan blue was injected intravenously and all organs subsequently demonstrated blue coloration when examined, with the exception of the brain [3]. Conversely, when the dye was administered intrathecally, the brain stained blue, but not other tissues [4]. Extensive studies have been performed subsequently to elucidate the anatomical basis for the BBB. It has been found that in addition to the BBB, the brain demonstrates a blood–CSF barrier as well. The BBB and blood–CSF barriers separate brain interstitial fluid and

CSF from the general circulation, respectively. These structures were once thought to be the same but extensive research has shown that the BBB and blood–CSF barriers are two independent membrane barriers with separate functions [5]. The BBB has a large surface area and separates the brain interstitial fluid from the general circulation. The blood–CSF barrier has approximately 5000-fold less surface area and is made up of the choroid plexus and other tiny regions of the ventricles [6]. The composition of brain interstitial fluid is determined by active transport of substances through the BBB, whereas the composition of the CSF is determined by secretory processes through choroid plexus epithelia. Because these two barriers are functionally separate, their anatomic compositions differ significantly. This may be the reason why extensive damage to brain parenchyma may result in minimal to no changes in CSF composition. The blood–CSF barrier separates the CSF from the general circulation and is the basis for the unique characteristics of this fluid. The BBB is found in almost all regions of the CNS and has unique anatomic characteristics. The BBB is composed of capillary endothelial cells, basal lamina, pericytes, astroglia, and perivascular macrophages. The blood–CSF barrier is composed of capillary endothelium, loose connective tissue, basal lamina, and ependymal cells. Certain (small) areas of the CNS do not have a BBB, including portions of the hypothalamus, area prostrema, and subfornical and subcommissural regions [7]. This observation has not been confirmed in horses; however, it is anticipated to be similar to other mammalian species. The endothelial tight junctions are of particular importance to the barrier function of the BBB. The electrical resistance of the BBB endothelial cells is approximately 2000 ohms/cm^2, as compared to 1–3 ohms/cm^2 in the mesenteric endothelium and 73 ohms/cm^2 for the choroid plexus endothelium [8]. Specific transendothelial

Equine Neurology, Second Edition. Martin Furr and Stephen Reed.
© 2015 John Wiley & Sons, Inc. Published 2015 by John Wiley & Sons, Inc.
Companion website: www.wiley.com/go/furr/neurology

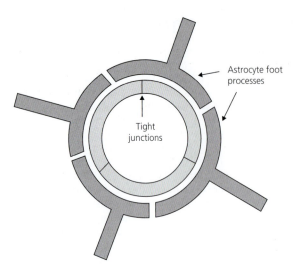

Figure 2.1 Schematic diagram showing the principal relationships that establish the blood–brain barrier. The inner ring is the endothelial cell layer with tight junctions and the outer ring demonstrates the close approximation of the astrocytes foot processes.

transport mechanisms are present in the endothelium for compounds which have particular importance for maintenance of brain function. For example, glucose is transported across the BBB by facilitated diffusion through a specific transport molecule, the glucose transporter-1 (GLUT-1). Deficiency of this transporter in people is associated with mental retardation and seizures, underscoring its importance to proper brain function [9]. Numerous other transport systems have been described.

The integrity of the BBB can be evaluated clinically by use of the albumin quotient (AQ) [10]. In normalcy, CSF albumin concentrations vary in direct proportion to the serum albumin concentration. This relationship is expressed mathematically as:

$$AQ = \left(\frac{albumin_{csf}}{albumin_{serum}}\right) \times 100 \qquad (2.1)$$

Iatrogenic blood contamination of the CSF samples, intrathecal hemorrhage, or inflammation/traumatic disruption of the BBB will result in an elevated AQ. A normal AQ value of less than 2.1 for mature horses and 1.8 ± 0.2 for foals is reported [10, 11].

Immunologic function

For many years, it was considered that the BBB was a passive physical barrier only; however, numerous investigations have demonstrated that the BBB is an active participant in determining the physicochemical properties of the CSF, by virtue of the presence of numerous specific transendothelial transport mechanisms, as described previously. In addition, the BBB has been demonstrated to have a major role in CNS inflammation; the endothelial cells, pericytes, and astroglial cells which compromise the BBB all have important immune functions. The BBB is perfectly positioned to act as an interface between the blood and CNS. Inflammatory cytokines and endotoxin have been demonstrated to influence BBB endothelial cells by upregulating their expression of adhesion and major histocompatibility complex (MHC) molecules. The functional outcome of endothelial cell activation is increased BBB permeability, formation of vasogenic edema, leukocyte extravasation, and vascular thrombosis. Pericytes contribute to microvascular reactivity, as well as being phagocytic, and express various adhesion molecules and MHC II receptors. Astrocytes interact with the endothelial cells and enhance their barrier function. Hence, the BBB is an active participant in the inflammatory process, rather than a passive physical barrier.

Cerebrospinal fluid

Formation

The CSF is produced as an ultrafiltrate of plasma and is actively secreted by ependymal cells and choroid plexus. While the majority of CSF is produced by the choroid plexus in the lateral ventricles, approximately 30–40% of CSF may be produced by the ependymal lining of the ventricles, the leptomeninges, and brain and spinal cord blood vessels [1]. Production is directly proportional to the transport of sodium via a Na-K ATPase in the brush border of the choroidal epithelium and is independent of vascular hydrostatic pressure. The CSF is formed at a constant rate, which in humans ranges from 0.32 to 0.37 ml/min [12, 13]. The rate varies with species and has been estimated to be 0.2–0.5 ml/min/g of choroid plexus tissue [2]. The rate of formation of CSF in the horse has not been determined.

The rate of CSF production can be altered by a variety of compounds. Carbonic anhydrase and Na-K ATPase inhibitors and hyperosmolality decrease production rate, while cholera toxin and adrenergic stimulation increase CSF production rate [2]. Osmotic agents and hypertonic solutions such as mannitol and dimethyl sulfoxide, when given intravenously, decrease CSF production in other species, but the effects of these compounds in the production of CSF in the horse have not been investigated.

Following formation, CSF flows into the third and fourth ventricles over the cerebral hemispheres and then exits caudally through foramina in the fourth ventricle to enter the subarachnoid space. Pulsation of blood in the choroid plexus forces the CSF in a cranial to caudal flow, and CSF is absorbed by collections of arachnoid villi in the dural sinuses or the cerebral veins. When CSF pressure exceeds venous pressure, these villi act as a one-way ball valve forcing CSF flow to the venous sinus.

Pressure

The production of CSF within the fixed volume compartment of the nervous system leads to a fluid pressure within the CNS. This intracranial pressure (ICP) can be determined by a variety of techniques. Monitoring of ICP has been found to have both prognostic and therapeutic benefits in human patients with a variety of disorders, including head trauma, subdural hematoma, and brain edema. Three physical components of the CNS interact to generate ICP: brain, blood vascular component, and CSF. The two major factors that determine ICP are the arterial pressure and the intracranial venous pressure. In accordance with the Monro–Kellie doctrine, given that the total cranial volume is fixed, an increase in the volume of one component must be compensated for by a decrease in the volume of at least one of the other components, or an increase in pressure must result (see Figure 2.2). Therefore, intracranial venous distention, associated with venous obstruction or increased central venous pressure, results in increased ICP. By this mechanism, occlusion of the external jugular veins will result in an increased ICP—this is the foundation of "Queckenstedt's test" for spinal occlusion. In this test, jugular occlusion should lead to an increase in the CSF pressure measured at the lumbar space. If this does not occur, then spinal subarachnoid blockage must exist. The Queckenstedt's maneuver can be used as an aid during spinal fluid collection.

The normal ICP for horses has been reported in only limited fashion. Using manometric techniques, the "opening pressure," that is, the pressure obtained before removal of any fluid, was reported to be 150–500 mm

H_2O (11.5–38.5 mm Hg) in the AO space, with a mean value of 308.8 mm H_2O (23.7 mm Hg) [14]. The AO CSF closing pressure, that is, the pressure after removal of a sample of CSF, was reported to be 75–400 mm H_2O (5.8–30.8 mm Hg) with a mean value of 223.5 mm H_2O (17.2 mm Hg) [14]. Lateral ventricle CSF pressure is similar to AO pressure and has been reported as 19.7 ± 2.4 mm Hg in anesthetized normal adult horses in lateral recumbency [15]. Head position has a profound effect upon CSF pressure, and in awake standing horses ICP was only 2 ± 4 mm Hg [16]. Lumbosacral CSF pressures are highly correlated to lateral ventricle CSF pressure ($r^2 = 0.94$), but specific values were not reported [15]. These authors did not detect a change in CSF pressure following the use of xylazine, but hypercapnia did increase CSF pressure markedly when the $PaCO_2$ increased to 80 mm Hg [15]. Using a subdural catheter and fluid-coupled transducer system, the ICP in a group of neonatal foals ranged from 5.8 to 9.5 mm Hg over the first 3 days of life [17].

Cerebral edema

Cerebral edema refers to an increase in the water content of the brain and is often, although not always, associated with increased ICP. Cerebral edema can be characterized as either cellular (cytotoxic), vasogenic, or interstitial in origin.

Cellular edema is characterized by swelling of all the cellular elements of the brain (neurons, glia, and endothelial cells) with an associated reduction on the volume of the brain extracellular fluid space. Cellular edema results from a failure of the energy-dependent

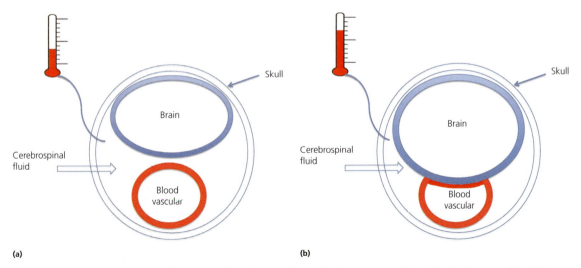

(a)   (b)

Figure 2.2 (a) and (b) The Monro–Kellie Doctrine describes the relationship between the solid and liquid elements of the CNS compartment and intracranial pressure. In (a), a normal balance of pressure is demonstrated, while in (b), the effects of increasing brain volume (i.e., from swelling) are schematized.

Table 2.1 Classification of mechanisms for development of cerebral edema.

	Vasogenic	Cellular	Hydrocephalic
Pathogenesis	Increased capillary permeability	Energy failure and cellular swelling	CSF outflow obstruction and increased total brain fluid
ECF composition	Plasma filtrate with protein	Water and sodium	Cerebrospinal fluid
Capillary permeability	Increased	Normal	Normal
Clinical conditions	Trauma, infarct, abscess, hemorrhage	Ischemia, hypoxia hypoosmolarity	

transmembrane sodium–potassium pumps, which allows the accumulation of sodium, chloride, and water in the cell. In addition, the energy failure that causes Na-K pump failure also promotes excessive neuronal depolarization, reduced neurotransmitter reuptake, and increased intracellular calcium concentrations. The end result of these events is neuronal cell death. Cellular edema is in general associated with the clinical conditions of hypoxia and ischemia, with probably the best equine example being hypoxic-ischemic encephalopathy of foals (reviewed in Chapter 34). In addition to hypoxia and ischemia, water intoxication can lead to cellular edema.

Vasogenic edema is characterized by increased permeability of brain capillary endothelial cells, with extravasation of macromolecules from the vasculature. Vasogenic edema is most commonly associated with tumor, trauma, abscess, infarction, lead intoxication, or severe ischemia. Often, the features of vasogenic and cellular edema coexist in a particular patient.

The final major pathophysiologic category of brain edema is interstitial edema, which is best observed in obstructive hydrocephalus. This obstruction results in transependymal movement of CSF, with a subsequent accumulation of brain interstitial fluid (Table 2.1) [18].

Composition

In normalcy, the CSF is clear and colorless with a viscosity similar to water. The CSF sample (minimum of 1 ml) should be examined for clarity and appearance in a clean, clear glass tube. A similar volume of clean water can be used for side-by-side comparison. Slight turbidity of the CSF will be noted at a cell count of above 400 cells/mm³ [18]. Tyndall's effect is described as a "snowy" or "sparkling" appearance when the fluid is observed and mildly agitated in direct sunlight. This appearance will be observed at cell counts below 400 cells/mm³. Turbidity is typically scored on a scale from 0 to 4+, with 0 being normal and 4+ being so turbid that newsprint cannot be read through the tube. Occasional small bits of epidural fat can be seen and are not considered significant (Table 2.2) [18].

Xanthochromia, a yellowish or occasionally yellow-orange discoloration of the fluid, arises due to the presence of bilirubin [18]. Most commonly this occurs following

Table 2.2 Turbidity scale for evaluation of cerebrospinal fluid.

Turbidity score	Description of appearance
0	Crystal clear
+1	Turbidity barely visible; faintly hazy or cloudy
+2	Turbidity clearly present; newsprint easily readable through sample
+3	Turbidity obvious; newsprint not easily readable through sample
+4	Almost opaque; newsprint not readable through sample

the rupture of red blood cells in the CSF but may occur due to hyperbilirubinemia. Xanthochromia takes 1–4 h to develop after a hemorrhagic event [19]. In humans, this discoloration may persist for up to 2–4 weeks after an extensive bleed. High total protein (over 150 mg/dl) may also cause a mild xanthochromia [19]. In neonatal foals, the CSF is slightly xanthochromic in foals up to 10 days of age [20]. Any xanthochromia greater than mild is considered abnormal, however.

The cellular composition of CSF in both adult horses and foals has been reported [14, 20, 23]. In normalcy, the CSF cell count is very low, with clinical reference values for white blood cells being 0–6 cells/μl for both adults and foals (Tables 2.3 and 2.4). Leukocytes are almost totally mononuclear cells, and neutrophils and eosinophils are almost never seen in normal horses, and should be regarded with suspicion, even if the total cell count is low. Due to the low concentration of protein, cells within the CSF deteriorate rapidly; hence, analysis should ideally occur within 1 h of collection. If the analysis of the CSF will be delayed, the sample should be split and one portion mixed with an equal volume of 40% ethanol until analysis.

Differential cell counts should be performed and require concentration methods due to the usually low number of cells in CSF. The sample can be filtered through a Millipore filter, or ideally prepared in a cytocentrifuge, then stained. Neutrophilic pleocytosis occurs in horses with infectious (bacterial or mycotic meningitis, Eastern equine

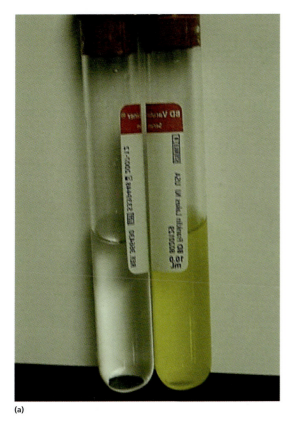

(a)

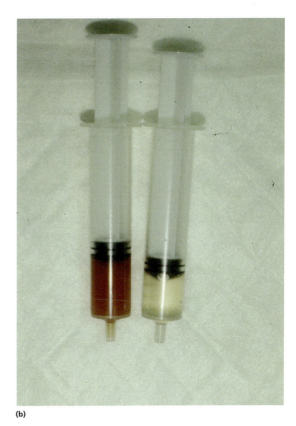

(b)

Figure 2.3 (a) and (b) The photograph (Figure 2.3a) demonstrates normal CSF on the left compared to xanthochromic CSF on the right. In Figure 2.3b, CSF contaminated with approximately 2500 RBC/μl is contrasted with blood-contaminated CSF (RBC count > 10,000 RBC/μl).

Table 2.3 Reference values for adult equine cerebrospinal fluid.

Parameter	Atlanto-occipital	Lumbosacral
Specific gravity [19]	1.004–1.008	1.004–1.008
Leukocytes (cells/μl) [14]	0–7	0–7
Erythrocytes (cells/μl)	<50	<50
Total protein (mg/dl) [21]	45–61	55–73
Immunoglobulin G (mg/dl) [10]	3.0–8.0	3.0–10.5
Albumin quotient [10]	1.0–2.1	0.9–2.4
Glucose (mg/dl) [14]	30–70% of plasma value	30–70% of plasma value
Lactic acid (mg/dl) [22]	1.92 ± 0.12	2.3 ± 0.21
Sodium (mEq/l) [14]	140–150	140–150
Potassium (mEq/l) [14]	2.5–3.5	2.5–3.5
Chloride (mEq/l) [14]	95–123	95–123
Calcium (mg/dl) [14]	2.5–6.0	2.5–6.0
Phosphorus (mg/dl) [14]	0.5–1.5	0.5–1.5
Urea nitrogen (mg/dl) [14]	5–20	5–20
Creatine kinase (IU) [14]	0–8	0–8
Lactate dehydrogenase (IU) [14]	0–8	0–8
Aspartate transferase (Sigma-Frankel units) [14]	15–50	15–50

Table 2.4 Reference ranges for equine neonatal cerebrospinal fluid.

Parameter	Atlanto-occipital	Lumbosacral
Leukocytes (cells/µl)	<5 [20]	
	1.3 ± 1.2 (AO site) [11]	0.9 ± 1.3 [11]
Erythrocytes (cells/µl)	46 ± 85 (range 0–317) [20]	
	208 ± 471 [11]	239 ± 349 [11]
Total protein (mg/dl)		
<48 h old	109 ± 9.7 [20]	
11–14 days old	81.0 ± 22.8 [20]	
21–22 days old	60.5 ± 22.4 [20]	
31–42 days old	58.5 ± 17.0 [20]	
7 days old	82.8 ± 19.2 [11]	83.6 ± 16.1 [11]
Immunoglobulin G (mg/dl) [11]	10.2 ± 5.5	9.9 ± 5.7
Albumin quotient [11]	1.86 ± 0.29	1.85 ± 0.51
IgG index5 [1]	0.52 ± 0.28	0.48 ± 0.27
Glucose (mg/dl) [20]		NR
<48 h old	98.8 ± 12.0	
11–14 days old	67.3 ± 12.0	
21–22 days old	65.3 ± 4.5	
31–42 days old	70.0 ± 5.4	
Sodium (mmol/l) [20]		NR
<48 h old	148.0 ± 7.2	
11–14 days old	152.2 ± 1.2	
21–22 days old	153.8 ± 2.5	
31–42 days old	151.7 ± 1.5	
Potassium (mmol/l) [20]		NR
<48 h old	3.01 ± 0.17	
11–14 days old	3.60 ± 1.12	
21–22 days old	3.06 ± 0.08	
31–42 days old	2.96 ± 0.07	
Magnesium (mg/dl) [20]		NR
<48 h old	2.43 ± 0.16	
11–14 days old	2.51 ± 0.08	
21–22 days old	2.65 ± 0.05	
31–42 days old	2.55 ± 0.05	

NR, not reported.

encephalitis, Western equine encephalitis, and Venezuelan equine encephalitis) or inflammatory conditions (trauma or chemical meningitis from hemorrhage or injection of ionic or nonionic contrast agents during a myelographic study) of the CNS. CSF lymphocytic pleocytosis is relatively uncommon in horses with nervous system disease [19]. Increased CSF lymphocyte counts may be seen in horses with CNS lymphoma and viral meningitis, specifically West Nile virus encephalitis. CSF eosinophilic pleocytosis is rare but has been reported in horses with verminous encephalitis due to *Halicephalobus* sp. [24].

In normalcy, the CSF does not contain circulating red blood cells, but they are commonly observed in CSF samples due to iatrogenic hemorrhage associated with CSF collection. Cerebrospinal fluid RBC concentrations up to 2000 cells/µl have been reported as normal by one author, although the mean number of CSF RBCs in that report was 195 cells/µl [14]. Higher numbers reported most likely reflect contamination from trauma during collection. The "acceptable" number of RBCs in CSF has decreased substantially in recent years and is considered to be a value of less than 50 RBC/µl by one author [25].

Interpretation of a CSF sample which contains blood is particularly challenging as it is difficult to determine if the elevated cell counts (both RBC and WBC) in the CSF are due to hemorrhage or simply from iatrogenic hemorrhage during collection. Horses with severe inflammatory disease and/or infections often have some component of blood in the CSF. Assuming that this is iatrogenic might lead to incorrect interpretation of the sample. To minimize the chances of this error, correction formulas have been proposed for both total protein and WBC count. These formulas have been evaluated and found to be not accurate or usable in a clinical setting [26–28] (Figure 2.4).

It has been demonstrated that blood contamination only minimally increases the CSF WBC count and total protein if the RBC count is less than 2000 RBC/µl; [28] hence this effect can almost be discounted unless the amount of blood is large. However, blood contamination has a profound effect upon CSF immunoassay (see Figure 2.5).

Plasma proteins gain access to the CSF primarily by diffusion across the blood–CSF barrier. This diffusion is

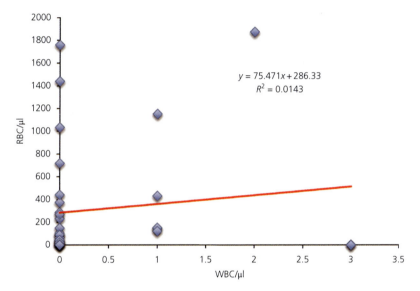

Figure 2.4 The relationship of RBC count and total WBC in normal CSF that was spiked with peripheral blood at various concentrations. Up to a value of 2000 RBC/µl, there was little effect upon total WBC count.

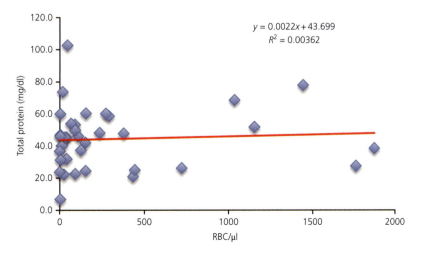

Figure 2.5 The relationship of RBC count and total protein in normal CSF that was spiked with peripheral blood at various concentrations. Up to a value of 2000 RBC/µl, there was little effect upon total protein concentration.

determined by the radius of the protein molecule which is directly related to the molecular weight [29]. Most of the blood proteins are represented in the CSF; however, the relative proportions of each are altered as a reflection of the filtering function of the BBB. Normal CSF total protein concentration is roughly 1/100th that of the blood plasma.

Several methods exist to assay total CSF protein. These include turbidometric, spectrophotometric, Lowry, biuret, dye binding, and immunologic methods [19]. Each of these methods has different characteristics of sensitivity and specificity and will generate slightly different assay results. Hence, it is important for the practitioner to utilize reference ranges reported by the particular laboratory that is performing the assay. The wide range of normal equine CSF total protein values that have been reported in the literature are largely a function of the various methods used, as well as inter-horse variability. Values from 10 to 120 mg/dl in healthy horses have been reported [14, 19], although the commonly reported reference range is 50–100 mg/dl for CSF taken from the lumbosacral (LS) space [19]. The total protein concentration differs depending upon the site of collection, with samples collected from the LS site having a slightly higher concentration than that from the atlanto-occipital (AO) site [14, 21]. In one study, the CSF total protein from the LS space was reported as 63.9 mg/dl (95% CI 54.7; 73.0 mg/dl), while the mean total protein from the same horses from the AO site was 53.2 mg/dl (95% CI 45.2; 61.3 mg/dl) [21]. In addition to the site of collection, it has been reported by one investigator that ponies have a higher CSF total protein than horse breeds (37.2 vs. 60.5 mg/dl) [14]. Breed-related differences have not been further examined and substantiated, however. The CSF total protein concentration of foals is higher than that of normal adult horses [20, 30]. Newborn foals (i.e., <2 days of age) had a mean CSF total protein of 109.0 mg/dl, with this value decreasing to adult values by the time the foals were 21 days of age [20].

An increase in CSF total protein is the single most useful change in the chemical composition of the CSF [18]. Protein concentrations are increased in diseases of the nervous system and occur due to increased permeability of the blood–CSF or BBB, increased protein synthesis within the CNS, obstruction of CSF flow, or tissue degeneration/necrosis. Obstructive diseases result in high protein concentrations due to enhanced resorption of water, as well as protein leakage. Complete spinal fluid block is associated with very high CSF protein concentrations and is referred to as "Froin's syndrome." Low CSF total protein is rarely found but can occur due to CSF leakage, removal of excessive quantities of CSF, increased ICP, or in cases of water intoxication.

The nature of specific proteins in equine CSF has been investigated by means of protein electrophoresis [21, 31, 32]. These studies found that the electrophoretogram varied based upon the supporting matrix used. When compared to protein electrophoresis of serum, CSF demonstrates a small prealbumin peak and the small α bands seen in serum are indistinct. The clinical significance of the prealbumin peak is not known. In one study comparing the CSF electrophoresis of normal horses and horses with cervical compressive myelopathy, differences were detected in affected horses. Post-β peaks were observed in 10 of 14 horses with cervical compression and in none of the normal horses [21]. In addition, the β-globulin fraction (composed of transferrin, plasminogen, complement, and hemopexin) was less in horses with cervical compression than normal horses. While these changes were suggested as a possible diagnostic method to screen for horses with cervical compressive disease, further work has not been pursued and this technique is not used clinically at this time (Figure 2.6 and Table 2.5).

Electrolyte composition of the CSF has been only sparsely reported, but in general the CSF sodium and chloride concentrations are similar to or slightly higher than serum values, while the potassium concentration is similar to or slightly lower than serum concentrations [14, 20, 30]. Magnesium concentration is slightly higher in CSF when compared to blood concentrations [20]. There does not appear to be any age-related effect upon electrolyte composition of the CSF in foals [20]. Measurement of electrolyte concentration has

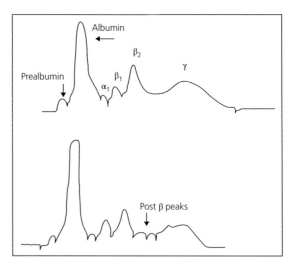

Figure 2.6 Electrophoretogram from a neurologically normal horse (top) and a horse with cervical compression (bottom). Note the two post-β-globulin peaks on the scan from the horse with cervical compression. (Used with permission from Ref. [21], © AVMA.)

Table 2.5 Protein fractions in equine cerebrospinal fluid.

Protein fraction	AO [21]	LS [21]	AO [32]	AO [31]
Total protein, mg/dl (95% CI)	53.2±3.8 (45.2; 61.3)	63.9±0.1 (54.7; 73.0)	9.2±3.7	40.1±0.1 (34.1; 46.2)
Prealbumin, mg/dl (95% CI)	1.3±0.2 (0.9; 1.6)	1.9±0.2 (1.4; 2.4)	0.19±0.2	NR
Albumin, mg/dl (95% CI)	20.3±1.6 (17.0; 23.5)	24.3±0.5 (21.0; 27.6)	3.99±1.68	15.3±1.2 (12.9; 17.6)
α1 globulin, mg/dl (95% CI)	1.8±0.3 (1.2; 2.4)	1.9±0.4 (0.9; 2.8)	0.48±0.24	5.2±0.9 (3.5; 6.9)
α2a globulin, mg/dl (95% CI)	NR	NR	0.31±0.15	6.7±0.4 (6.0; 7.4)
α2bc globulin, mg/dl (95% CI)	NR	NR	0.59±0.31	NR
β1 globulin, mg/dl (95% CI)	4.6±0.5 (3.5; 5.8)	6.0±0.7 (4.6; 7.5)	1.59±0.75	5.8±0.6 (4.7; 7.4)[a]
β2 globulin, mg/dl (95% CI)	10.9±0.9 (8.8; 12.8)	14.5±1.1 (12.0; 16.9)	0.7±0.32	NR
γ globulin, mg/dl (95% CI)	14.21±0.5 (11.1; 17.3)	15.3±1.5 (12.0; 18.6)	1.35±0.57	5.7±0.8 (4.6; 7.3)

NR, not reported.
[a] Values reported as B globulins only.

not been reported to be of utility in diagnosis of most neurologic diseases of horses.

CSF glucose concentration is closely correlated with blood glucose concentration; glucose enters the CSF by both active transport and passive diffusion [29]. A maximum CSF glucose concentration of about 200 mg/dl is proposed [29], but this has not been evaluated in the horse. Normal values for horse are 35–75% of plasma glucose and are usually found to be 30–70 mg/dl for the AO site and 40–75 mg/dl for the LS site. It is best to evaluate CSF glucose concentrations in concert with plasma or serum glucose concentration; however, there is a temporal delay of 1–3 h in changes of CSF glucose concentration following changes in plasma concentration [19].

Decreased concentration of CSF glucose (hypoglycorrhachia) is caused either by hypoglycemia, decreased active transport, and/or increased utilization. Bacterial meningitis is the most commonly recognized condition leading to increased utilization. This arises due to the combined effects of increased leukocyte metabolism, consumption of glucose by bacteria, and increased metabolic rate of CNS tissue. Erythrocytes also utilize glucose and subarachnoid hemorrhage may be associated with decreased CSF glucose concentration.

Lactic acid is produced by the anaerobic metabolism of glucose, and increased CSF lactate concentrations have been found to be associated with bacterial meningitis, Eastern equine encephalitis, head trauma, and brain abscesses [22]. Lactic acid is ionized and does not cross the BBB, while the lactate salt does diffuse across the blood–CSF barrier into the CSF. Reference ranges for CSF lactate have been described as well as values in various equine neurologic illnesses [19, 22]. A mild elevation (but not statistically significantly different from controls) in CSF lactate concentration was found in foals with bacterial

meningitis [22]. The use of CSF lactate and glucose concentrations to diagnose foals with bacterial meningitis is complicated by the fact that most of such foals are hypoglycemic and in circulatory shock and may have an elevated blood lactate in the absence of CNS disease.

Homeostatic mechanisms are present which contribute to the maintenance of a constant pH in the CSF and extracellular fluid of the nervous system. Cerebrospinal fluid pH remains stable over a fairly wide range of blood pH and is influenced by the function of the BBB. In addition, hydrogen ion-sensitive chemoreceptors present in the brainstem regulate respiration with direct effect upon arterial, and subsequently CSF, pH. The carbon dioxide/bicarbonate system is the major buffer in the CSF, due to the very low total protein present [18, 33]. In a group of healthy neonatal foals, the CSF was slightly more acidic (7.389) than corresponding arterial (7.452) or venous blood (7.422) [33]. The CSF pCO_2 (37.8 mm Hg) was slightly greater than the corresponding arterial blood (36.6 mm Hg) and slightly less than the corresponding venous blood (39.9 mm Hg) [33]. Acidity of CSF increased associated with an increased CSF pCO_2 after 75 min of hypercapnia. The authors concluded that the buffering capacity of the CSF is poor, related to the low protein concentration and the relatively poor permeability of the blood–CSF barrier [33].

The differing solubility of the BBB and blood–CSF barriers to CO_2 (high) and bicarbonate (low) can lead to unexpected changes in CSF pH in response to blood pH changes. Changes in the arterial CO_2 tension result in changes in CSF pH which parallel that of the blood [18, 33]. An abrupt increase in blood bicarbonate concentration, such as that associated with intravenous infusion of sodium bicarbonate to treat acidosis for example, can result in a paradoxical decrease in

CSF pH due to the rapid movement of CO_2 into the CSF, and the slower accumulation of bicarbonate. These paradoxical reactions are usually transient and last only a few minutes to hours [18]. Their significance in clinical practice is unknown and they may be only laboratory curiosities.

A number of enzymes have been reported to be present in the CSF and to have diagnostic utility. The most commonly discussed in the equine literature include creatine kinase (CK), lactate dehydrogenase (LDH), alkaline phosphatase (AP), and aspartate transaminase (AST). As most enzymes are relatively large molecules, there is very little diffusion across an intact and normal blood–CSF barrier, and increased concentrations of enzymes in the CSF are assumed to have arisen from the CNS. Potential sources of the increased enzyme activity in the CSF include diffusion across a damaged BBB or blood–CSF barrier, and release of enzymes from cells within the CNS such as inflammatory cells, microorganisms, and tumors, or directly from damaged nerve cells and myelin.

CK exists as three isoenzymes—CK-MM (CK1) for muscle, CK-MB (CK2) for cardiac muscle, and CK-BB (CK3) for nervous tissue. The CSF_{ck} has been reported to be a sensitive but nonspecific marker of nervous system disease [34, 35]. In humans, many conditions including trauma, inflammatory disease, global ischemia, microemboli, and tumors have been associated with increased concentration of CSF_{ck} [36–38]. Reference ranges for equine CSF_{ck} concentrations have been described; however, proper validation of the assay in CSF is lacking. CSF_{ck} activity is typically very low and increased values have been associated with neurologic disease in horses [39, 40]. In foals, increased CSF_{ck} was observed when compared to values in adults [30]. Increased CSF_{ck} activity was reported in horses with EPM, while CSF_{ck} activity in horses with cervical compressive myelopathy was within the reference range (i.e., below 6 IU/l) [39]. The authors suggested that CSF_{ck} values may therefore have value in the evaluation of horses with neurologic disease. Others have questioned this assessment and have found increased CSF_{ck} concentrations in horses following traumatic taps and in CSF samples contaminated with epidural fat [41]. Thus, contaminated CSF samples or those arising from difficult taps clearly have limitations, and increased enzyme activity in these cases should be interpreted with caution. However, CSF_{ck} may be a valid marker of CNS disease in CSF samples that are not blood contaminated or that did not result from a spinal tap that required multiple attempts.

Reference ranges for LDH and AP have been reported for the adult horse and are considered to be less than 8 IU, with a mean of 1.54 and 0.8 IU, respectively [14]. Aspartate transaminase has also been reported in equine CSF, with a mean activity of 30.7 Sigma-Frankel (SF) units. In foals, the concentration of these enzymes was higher than in a group of adults [30]. These enzymes have been very poorly studied in the horse, and little information is available regarding their evaluation in horses with neurologic disease. One report suggests that increased LDH activity may occur in horses with spinal lymphosarcoma [42].

The concentration of cholesterol and lipoproteins in equine CSF has been determined. Mean CSF cholesterol in mares was 13.56 mg/ml (9.8–17.5) [43]. Two major lipoproteins were detected in the CSF of horses: apolipoprotein A-1 (ApoA-1) and apolipoprotein E (apoE) [43]. The role of these compounds in the physiology of the nervous system is undetermined in the horse; however, these compounds are known to interact with a variety of receptors within the nervous system and presumably influence function and/or neuronal health. A number of fatty acids are also present in the CSF of normal horses. Isobutyric, isovaleric, phenylacetic, lauric, myristic, palmitic, oleic, and stearic acids were uniformly present in both normal horses and horses with neurologic disease [44]. Oleic, palmitic, and stearic acids predominated in equine CSF and no changes in the fatty acid profile could be detected in neurologically abnormal horses [44]. Hence, evaluation of CSF fatty acid profile appears to have little clinical value in equine neurologic disease.

Not surprisingly, a number of neurotransmitter compounds can be found within the CSF of horses, the primary compounds being homovanillic acid (HVA) and 5-hydroxyindolacetic acid (5-HIAA) [45]. Younger animals had greater CSF concentration of HVA than 5-HIAA, and mature horses had lower concentrations of CSF HVA than juvenile horses [46]. These compounds have not been investigated in horses with clinical disease at this time and their utility in clinical medicine is undetermined.

Indications for CF collection and assay interpretation

Analysis of CSF is a useful adjunct in the evaluation and diagnosis of neurologic disease in horses. Ideally, CSF collection and evaluation should be performed on any horse demonstrating undiagnosed neurologic abnormalities. In addition, CSF evaluation should be considered in horses with fever of unknown origin, as meningitis is an uncommon cause of fever in horses. It must be remembered, however, that it is not uncommon for the CSF composition to be normal even in horses with obvious neurologic disease. Several possible explanations for this exist including timing of the collection in relation to the clinical signs and pathologic changes, extradural or ventral root neuropathies, and sampling too far from the site of the lesion. Collection of CSF may occur early in disease before organic changes in the CSF occur, or late in the disease, after the organic changes have resolved.

Extradural lesions also do not result in changes in CSF parameters and include compressive lesions (cervical stenotic myelopathy, synovial cysts, and extradural tumors), peripheral neuropathies such as botulism and tetanus, and metabolic diseases. Furthermore, sampling too far from the site of the lesion may result in CSF results which differ from those that would be found if taken closer to the site of the lesion. Also, since CSF flows in a caudal direction, CSF collected rostral to a focal lesion may be normal.

On the other hand, inflammatory disease, or conditions that result in tissue necrosis, causes significant changes in the CSF. The observation that the CSF may be normal should not be considered as justification to forego spinal fluid collection, since normal CSF parameters have value in ruling out some diseases. Furthermore, it is not possible to predict in which clinical patient the CSF parameters will be of value or not, thus collection should be considered in all horses exhibiting neurologic disease.

Rarely are changes in CSF confirmatory of a specific diagnosis, rather they allow individual diseases to be grouped together into categories, such as acute and chronic inflammation, degeneration, and vasculitis. This allows the clinician to narrow the list of possible diagnoses to those that are known to produce changes that are consistent with the observed changes in the patient sample. The presence of bacteria, fungi, or neoplastic cells would be confirmatory evidence of a specific diagnosis.

Cerebrospinal fluid collection
Atlanto-occipital site
The technique for AO CSF collection has been previously described. The technique is simple, however and does require that the horse be anesthetized. This may or may not be advisable in all cases, and the benefits of collecting the fluid versus the risks of general anesthesia must be considered on a case-by-case basis. In most cases, an AO CSF sample can be collected quickly following short-acting injectable anesthesia.

After the horse is anesthetized, the poll is clipped and aseptically prepared, and the horse's head is flexed to expand the AO space. An 18-gauge, 3.5-inch spinal needle is inserted at the point at which a line is drawn between the cranial borders of the atlas intersect midline. The needle is directed toward the lower jaw and advanced until the dura is penetrated, usually at a depth of about 2–2.5 inches (5 cm) in the mature adult horse. It is important to ensure that the needle is advanced in the median plane, as it is possible to miss laterally if the needle is angled. Resistance to advancing the needle will increase as the needle penetrates the nuchal ligament, then will abruptly decrease, resulting in a characteristic "pop." The pop is more noticeable at the AO space than the LS, and needle advancement should cease immediately once it is felt. The stylet can then be withdrawn and fluid collected. The fluid should flow freely without the need for aspiration in most cases. If no fluid is present, the stylet should be replaced and the needle advanced in 1 mm steps, attempting collection between each step. Relatively large volumes of CSF (up to 90 ml) can be withdrawn from an adult horse, but usually 5 ml is adequate for analysis. In neonates, it is prudent to withdraw only 1–2 ml to minimize the risk of tentorial herniation.

The ultrasonic anatomy of the AO joint and space of the horse has been described, and a method for ultrasound-guided AO puncture described [47, 48]. While it is demonstrated that the AO puncture can be performed under ultrasound guidance, it is rarely if ever necessary, and this approach has not been shown to have any particular advantages.

Follow-up care after an AO CSF collection is minimal. Non-steroidal anti-inflammatory drugs can be given if there is neck soreness. It is advisable to keep the horse in a stall and feed them hay from a haynet or elevated rack for 1–2 days after the tap. This prevents the horse from putting its head down to graze, which appears to increase the degree of neck soreness following an AO puncture.

An alternative method for collection of CSF from the AO space in standing horses has been described [49]. In this method, the horse is restrained and heavily sedated, and the area on the lateral side of the AO space is clipped and prepared for sterile centesis. A 10–4 MHz microconvex curvilinear transducer, oriented dorsoventrally, is placed approximately 2 cm ventral to the mane at C1-2 and the subarachnoid space and the vertebral bodies of C1 and C2 are identified. An 18-gauge 3.5-inch spinal needle is inserted below the ultrasound probe and is directed dorsomedially under ultrasonic guidance into the subarachnoid space. Fluid does not normally spontaneously flow using this approach, and thus must be gently aspirated (Figure 2.7). In the case series (13 horses) in which this technique was described, no complications were noted, and RBC contamination was present in only the first two cases attempted. After this, RBC counts below 4 cells/μl were recovered in 8 of 11 horses. The technique is rapidly performed; however, experience is required and at present it does not appear to be a widely used technique.

Lumbosacral
The technique of CSF collection from the LS space is also well described in the literature. Horses can be restrained in a set of stocks (as is the authors preference), or restrained in the open. Stocks are advisable as they provide a degree of protection from reflexive kicks during the procedure. A nose twitch is applied and the horse sedated. Combinations of xylazine (250 mg IV)

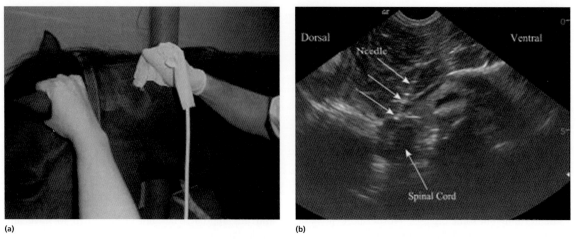

(a)   (b)

Figure 2.7 The photograph demonstrates the location and position of the ultrasound site (panel a) for standing C1-C2 CSF aspiration. Panel "b" shows the ultrasound image with proper needle placement. Reprinted from reference [49].

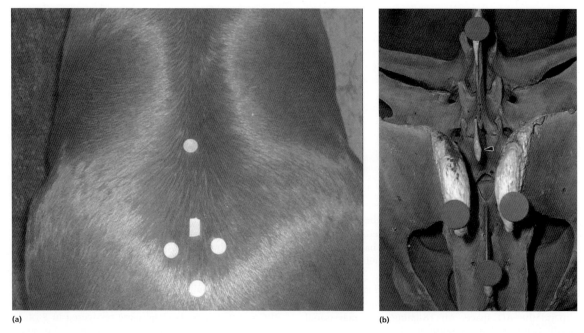

(a)   (b)

Figure 2.8 (a) and (b) The large dots demonstrate the palpable landmarks for the lumbosacral collection site and their corresponding anatomic sites. The dorsal spine at the arrow is not externally palpable in most horses, unless they are exceedingly thin. The insertion point for the needle is shown by the square marker.

and butorphanol (5 mg IV) for the 450 kg horse provide a good degree of sedation with a minimum degree of unsteadiness. Alternatively, detomidine (5–10 mg IV) can be used. The optimum site is the point on midline which is intersected by a line drawn between the cranial borders of the tuber sacrale. This is routinely determined by visual examination and palpation of the landmarks (Figure 2.8a, b). The ultrasonic anatomy of the site has been described, however, and ultrasound examination for landmarks may be beneficial for those horses which are obese and in which the landmarks are difficult to palpate. When using ultrasound guidance, the insertion site is on midline 0.5–1 cm cranial to the point at which the tuber sacrale are most superficial

[50]. The site should be clipped and scrubbed and the subcutaneous tissue infiltrated with local anesthetic. Following this, a small stab incision can be made with a #15 blade—this is advisable as it minimizes dulling of the spinal needle. A 6–8 inch, 18-gauge spinal needle is then inserted and stabilized at the skin surface using one hand, and the needle advanced with the opposite hand. The needle should be advanced steadily, not with jerking movements, and the operator must ensure that the needle is advanced straight down, without lateral or cranial–caudal deviations. It is sometimes useful to have an assistant stand well behind the horse and ensure that the needle is advancing perpendicularly to the horses back. If not, the needle should be withdrawn almost to the surface and redirected. If it is not withdrawn to the surface, the needle will follow the previous needle path. The LS space will be encountered at a depth of about 6 inches (13 cm) in most average-sized horses. As the needle approaches the space, increasing resistance will be felt, and then the resistance will abruptly decrease as the needle penetrates the ligamentum flavum. This is felt by the operator as a "pop" and is usually a good indication that the membranes have been penetrated and the needle is well positioned. Penetration of the membranes is often accompanied by a reaction from the horse, which may vary from no reaction at all, restlessness, a tail flick, stomping of the foot, or tightening of the caudal muscles. Occasionally, a very violent reaction can be seen; however, with proper sedation and a sharp spinal needle, these reactions are thankfully rare.

Persons restraining the horse should be made aware that these are possible, however.

Once the dura has been penetrated, the stylet can be removed and CSF may be collected by gentle aspiration using a 5 or 10 ml syringe. It is important to avoid placing strong negative pressure on the syringe, as this can lead to blood contamination of the subsequent sample or plugging of the needle with tissue. If negative pressure is present, the stylet should be replaced, the needle advanced, and collection attempted again.

If no fluid can be retrieved, and the operator has confidence that the needle is properly placed, then the needle can be advanced by 1 mm at a time, with fluid collection attempted again until fluid is recovered. Alternatively, the needle can be rotated 90°, with collection attempts repeated. Also, the horses head can be raised and held up for a few minutes, and both jugular veins occluded (Queckenstedt's maneuver) to increase ICP and promote caudal CSF movement.

If the needle contacts bone without feeling the characteristic "pop," or at a depth less than expected, the needle should be removed and redirected cranially or caudally until a proper needle depth is achieved or the space is penetrated (Figure 2.9).

When the sample is collected, the CSF should be withdrawn slowly with gentle aspiration. Iatrogenic blood contamination of the sample, rather than hemorrhage, is suggested if the blood is non-homogenously distributed in the sample. That is, typically a small "stream" of blood can be seen rising in the syringe, then swirling to

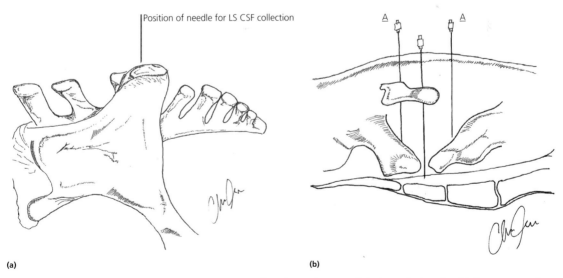

(a)   (b)

Figure 2.9 (a) and (b) The general position of the spinal needle is depicted in (a), while the sagittal section (b) demonstrates the position of the needle for a correct lumbosacral fluid collection. Needles labeled as "A" in (b) are placed too far cranially or caudally and demonstrate contact with bone at too shallow a depth, resulting in more needle exposed above the skin. When performing a lumbosacral fluid collection, this observation would suggest redirecting the needle until bone is contacted at progressively greater depths, indicating an approach to the LS space. (Drawings by Chris Furr.)

mix with the sample. In samples collected from horses with CNS hemorrhage, the blood is typically homogenously distributed and does not clear after multiple syringes have been removed (the "three tube test"). If the blood contamination remains uniform throughout the sample, it is most likely truly representative of the CSF. If gross blood is recovered, the needle should be discarded and a fresh needle used for a second attempt. Clear fluid can be recovered in these circumstances, although not in all cases. It should be recognized also that it may not be possible to enter the LS space in some animals due to calcification of the ligaments, for example.

Aftercare for horses following a LS spinal tap is minimal. The site should be kept clean and dry and observed for swelling or discharge. Phenylbutazone or similar analgesics are rarely necessary but may be useful if multiple attempts were needed to get the sample.

Other techniques

A technique has been described for accessing the cerebral ventricles of the horse via a trephination site through the frontal bone. The procedure was easily performed in anesthetized horses and has utility in physiological experimentation in the horse [51].

Complications

As in most procedures, complications may occur in a small percentage of individuals. Complications that may result from CSF collection include introduction of infectious agents into the CNS (septic meningitis), aseptic meningitis from hemorrhage, pain and swelling at the site of needle entry, or trauma associated with recovery from anesthesia. The author has occasionally seen horses flip over backward or fall during or following standing LS CSF tap. This usually occurs when the horse reacts badly or is severely ataxic during collection. Additional complications which may occur when collecting CSF from the AO space include spinal cord penetration ("pithing") if the needle is advance to deeply, herniation of the cerebellum, and fractures or worsening of neurologic signs after anesthetic recovery. Complication rates have not been reported following CSF collection in horses but are widely believed to be very low.

References

[1] Banks, W.J. (1981) Nervous system, in *Applied Veterinary Histology*, 1st edn (ed. W.J. Banks), Williams and Wilkins, Baltimore, pp. 277–303.

[2] Fishman, R.A. (1992) Physiology of the cerebrospinal fluid, in *Cerebrospinal Fluid in Diseases of the Nervous System*, 2nd edn (ed. R.A. Fishman), W.B. Saunders Co, Philadelphia, pp. 23–42.

[3] Ehrlich, P. (1906) *Uber die Beziehunger von chemische constitution. Vertheilung, und Pharmakologischer Wirkung. Reprinted and translated In: Collected Studies in Immunity*, John Wiley, New York, pp. 567–595.

[4] Goldman, E. (1913) Vital Faubung am Zentralnervensystem. *Abh Preuss Akad Wiss Phys-math K1*, 1, 1–60.

[5] Brigham, M.W. (1977) Morphology of the blood-brain interfaces. *Exp Eye Res*, 25, 1–25.

[6] Pardridge, W.M., Oldendorg, W.H., Cancilla, P. *et al.* (1986) Blood-brain barrier: interface between internal medicine and the brain. *Ann Intern Med*, 105, 82–95.

[7] Gross, P.M. and Weindl, S. (1987) Peering through the windows of the brain. *J Cereb Blood Flow Metab*, 7, 663–672.

[8] Butt, A., Jones, H.J. and Abbott, N. (1990) Electric resistance across the blood-brain barrier in anesthetized rats: a developmental study. *J Physiol*, 429, 47–62.

[9] DeVivo, D., Trifiletti, R., Jacobson, R. *et al.* (1990) Glucose transport deficiency causing persistent hypoglycorrhachia: a unique cause of infantile seizures and acquired microcephaly. *Ann Neurol*, 29, 414–415.

[10] Andrews, F., Maddux, J. and Faulk, B. (1990) Total protein, albumin quotient, IgG and IgG index determinations for horse cerebrospinal fluid. *Prog Vet Neurol*, 1, 197–204.

[11] Andrews, F.J., Geisesr, D.L., Sommardahl, C.S. *et al.* (1994) Albumin quotient, IgG concentration, and IgG index determination in cerebrospinal fluid of neonatal foals. *Am J Vet Res*, 55, 741–745.

[12] Masserman, J.H. (1934) Cerebrospinal fluid hemodynamics IV. Clinical experimental studies. *Arch Neurol Psychiatry*, 32, 523–553.

[13] Rubin, R.C. (1966) The production of cerebrospinal fluid in man and its modification by acetezolamide. *J Neurosurg*, 25, 430–436.

[14] Mayhew, I.G., Whitlock, R.H. and Tasker, J.B. (1977) Equine cerebrospinal fluid: reference values of normal horses. *Am J Vet Res*, 38, 1271–1274.

[15] Moore, R.M. and Trim, C.M. (1993) Effect of hypercapnia or xylazine on lateral ventricle and lumbosacral ccrebrospinal fluid pressures in pentobarbital-anesthetized horses. *Vet Surg*, 22, 151–158.

[16] Brosnan, R.J., LeCouteur, R.A., Steffey, E.U. *et al.* (2002) Direct measurement of intracranial pressure in adult horses. *Am J Vet Res*, 63, 1252–1256.

[17] Kortz, G.D., Madigan, J.E., Goetzman, B.W. *et al.* (1995) Intracranial pressure and cerebral perfusion pressure in clinically normal equine neonates. *Am J Vet Res*, 56, 1351–1355.

[18] Fishman, R.A. (1992) Composition of the cerebrospinal fluid, in *Cerebrospinal Fluid in Diseases of the Nervous System*, 2nd edn (ed. R.A. Fishman), W.B. Saunders, Philadelphia, pp. 183–252.

[19] Green, E., Constantinescu, G. and Kroll, R. (1993) Equine cerebrospinal fluid: analysis. *Compend Contin Educ Pract Vet*, 15, 288–301.

[20] Furr, M. and Bender, H. (1994) Cerebrospinal fluid variables in clinically normal foals from birth to 42 days of age. *Am J Vet Res*, 55, 781–784.

[21] Furr, M., Chickering, W.R. and Robertson, J. (1997) High resolution protein electrophoresis of equine cerebrospinal fluid. *Am J Vet Res*, 58, 939–941.

[22] Green, EM, Green SL. Cerebrospinal Fluid Lactic Acid Concentrations: Reference Values and Diagnostic Implications of Abnormal Concentrations in Adult Horses. Proceedings of the 18th Annual Meeting ACVIM, San Diego, CA, 1990;495–499.

[23] Beech, J. (1993) Cytology of equine cerebrospinal fluid. *Vet Pathol*, 20, 553–562.

[24] Darian, B.J., Belknap, J. and Nietfeld, J. (1998) Cerebrospinal fluid changes in two horses with central nervous system nematodiasis (Micronema deletrix). *J Vet Intern Med*, 2, 201–205.

[25] Furr, M., MacKay, R., Granstrom, D. *et al.* (2002) Clinical diagnosis of equine protozoal myeloencephalitis (EPM). *J Vet Intern Med*, 16, 618–621.

[26] Wilson, J.W. and Stevens, J.B. (1977) Effects of blood contamination on cerebrospinal fluid analysis. *J Am Vet Med Assoc*, 171, 256–260.

[27] Sweeney, C.R. and Russell, G.E. (2000) Differences in total protein concentration, nucleated cell count, and red blood cell count among sequential samples of cerebrospinal fluid from horses. *J Am Vet Med Assoc*, 217, 54–57.

[28] Furr, M. (2012) Effects of blood contamination on parameters of cerebrospinal fluid analysis. *J Vet Intern Med*, 26, 733.

[29] Kjeldsberg, C.R. and Krieg, A.F. (1984) Cerebrospinal fluid and other body fluids, in *Clinical Diagnosis and Management by Laboratory Methods*, 18th edn (ed. J.B. Henry), W.B. Saunders Co, Philadelphia, pp. 459–490.

[30] Rossdale, P.D., Cash, R.S.G. and Leadon, D.P. (1982) Biochemical constituents of cerebrospinal fluid in premature and full term foals. *Equine Vet J*, 14, 134–138.

[31] Kirk, G.R., Neate, S., McClure, R.C. *et al.* (1974) Electrophoretic pattern of equine cerebrospinal fluid. *Am J Vet Res*, 35, 1263–1264.

[32] Kristensen, F. and Firth, E.C. (1977) Analysis of serum proteins and cerebrospinal fluid in clinically normal horses, using agarose electrophoresis. *Am J Vet Res*, 38, 1089–1092.

[33] Geiser, D.R., Andrews, F., Rohrbach, B.W. *et al.* (1996) Cerebrospinal fluid acid-base status during normocapnia and acute hypercapnia in equine neonates. *Am J Vet Res*, 57, 1483–1487.

[34] Wilson, J.W. (1977) Clinical application of cerebrospinal fluid creatine phosphokinase determination. *J Am Vet Med Assoc*, 171, 200–202.

[35] Mass, A.I. (1977) Cerebrospinal fluid enzymes in acute brain injury. *J Neurol Neurosurg Psychiatry*, 40, 655–665.

[36] Nathan, M.J. (1967) Creatine phosphokinase in the cerebrospinal fluid. *J Neurol Neurosurg Psychiatry*, 30, 52–54.

[37] Vaagenes, P., Kjekshus, J., Siversten, E. *et al.* (1987) Temporal patterns of enzyme changes in cerebrospinal fluid in patients with neurologic complications after open heart surgery. *Crit Care Med*, 15, 726–731.

[38] Rabow, L., DeSalles, A.F., Becker, D.P. *et al.* (1986) CSF brain creatine kinase levels and lactic acidosis in severe head injury. *J Neurosurg*, 65, 625–629.

[39] Furr, M.O. and Tyler, R.D. (1990) Cerebrospinal fluid creatine kinase activity in horses with central nervous system disease: 69 cases (1984–1989). *J Am Vet Med Assoc*, 197, 245–248.

[40] Furr, M.O., Anver, M. and Wise, M. (1991) Intervertebral disk prolapse and diskospondylitis in a horse. *J Am Vet Med Assoc*, 198, 2095–2096.

[41] Jackson, C., DeLahunta, A., Divers, T.J. *et al.* (1996) The diagnostic utility of cerebrospinal fluid creatine kinase activity in the horse. *J Vet Intern Med*, 10, 246–251.

[42] Andrews, F.M. and Reed, S.M. (1990) The ancillary techniques and tests for diagnosing equine neurologic disease. *Vet Med*, December, 1325–1330.

[43] Puppione, D.L. and MacDonald, M.H. (2002) Characterization of lipoproteins in cerebrospinal fluid of mares during pregnancy and lactation. *Am J Vet Res*, 63, 886–889.

[44] Sweeney, R.W., Beech, J., Whitlock, R.H. *et al.* (1998) Analysis of fatty acids in equine cerebrospinal fluid using gas chromatography with electron capture detection. *J Chromatogr*, 494, 278–282.

[45] Vaughn, D.M. and Smyth, G.B. (1989) Different gradients for neurotransmitter metabolites and protein in horse cerebrospinal fluid. *Vet Res Commun*, 13, 413–419.

[46] Vaughn, D.M., Smyth, G.B., Whitmer, W.L. *et al.* (1989) Analysis of equine cisterna magna cerebrospinal fluid for the presence of some monamine neurotransmitters and transmitter metabolites. *Vet Res Commun*, 13, 237–249.

[47] Gollob, E., Edinger, H., Stanek, C. *et al.* (2002) Ultrasonographic investigation of the atlanto-occipital articulation in the horse. *Equine Vet J*, 34, 44–50.

[48] Audigie, F., Tapprest, J., Didierlaurent, D. *et al.* (2004) Ultrasound-guided atlanto-occipital puncture for myelography in the horse. *Vet Radiol Ultrasound*, 45, 340–344.

[49] Pease, A., Behan, A. and Bohart, G. (2011) Ultrasound-guided cervical centesis to obtain cerebrospinal fluid in the standing horse. *Vet Radiol Ultrasound*, 53, 92–95.

[50] Aleman, M., Borchers, A., Kass, P.H. *et al.* (2007) Ultrasound-assisted collection of cerebrospinal fluid from the lumbosacral space in equids. *J Am Vet Med Assoc*, 230, 378–384.

[51] Regodon, S., Franco, A., Lignereux, Y. *et al.* (1993) A new technique for accessing the cerebral ventricles of the horse. *Res Vet Sci*, 55, 389–391.

3 Immunology of the Central Nervous System

Martin Furr

Marion duPont Scott Equine Medical Center, Virginia-Maryland Regional College of Veterinary Medicine, Leesburg, USA

The immune system is key for the protection of the body from invasion by infectious organisms and other foreign substances in the environment. The nervous system is no different than other tissues in its requirement for immune protection, which is accomplished in much the same manner as other tissues. However, the unique nature of the nervous system requires that some of the normal immune mechanisms be altered within this tissue compartment. The study of immune reactions within the nervous system (neuroimmunology) has become a specialized field and is attended by a vast body of primary literature due to the complexity of the material and the importance of aberrant immune reactions in the pathophysiology of such important human diseases as multiple sclerosis, for example. The purpose of this chapter is to review the immunologic mechanisms in the nervous system and its application to equine disease.

Immune protection is accomplished via a number of defense mechanisms, which have broadly been described as physical (barrier) protection, innate immunity, and acquired immunity. Physical immunity is intended to exclude infectious or foreign material from the body and comprises of the skin, as well as "self-cleaning" mechanisms in the respiratory and gastrointestinal tract such as mucus flow and expectoration, coughing, sneezing, vomiting, and diarrhea—all processes intended to eliminate unwanted agents or material. These processes are important for protection of all body systems, including the nervous system. In addition, the central nervous system (CNS) is encased by tissue barriers such as the blood–brain barrier (BBB) (see Chapter 2 for extensive review) that minimizes the potential for foreign material to enter the CNS.

Innate immunity comprises a rapidly reacting, non-specific chemical and cellular response. The innate immune system lacks memory, and all responses are similar regardless of the stimulating agent. One primary action of the innate immune system is to initiate inflammation, which tends to focus the immune reactions to the area of infection or injury. Immunologic reactions result in increased blood flow, increased endothelial cell permeability, and extravasation of inflammatory cells (neutrophils and macrophages) which are key in clearing infection. In addition, complement and other immune defense proteins within the plasma are activated, resulting in death of the invading organisms. While beneficial in most circumstances, this inflammation is dangerous in the CNS, and control of inflammation is a unique adaptation of the CNS in mammals, which is discussed in detail in the following text.

Acquired (adaptive), or specific, immunity differs from innate immunity in that it results in memory of the invading antigen and responds specifically to that antigen more quickly and aggressively on subsequent encounters. Acquired immunity is first generated by an encounter with foreign antigen, which is trapped and processed by antigen presenting cells (mediated by the major histocompatibility cells (MHC) class II receptor) and then presented to other cells for recognition as foreign. Within the normal circulation, several cell types can perform this function, including dendritic cells and macrophages. B and T lymphocytes have receptors for foreign antigen and can bind the antigen and respond appropriately. This interaction most commonly occurs in lymph nodes. These responses include activation of cytotoxic T cells or production of specific antibody by B cells. This same process is required for immune protection and recognition in the CNS; however, an understanding of how this occurs has been slow to develop, as many of the necessary components for these interactions do not appear to be present in the CNS. For example, conventional lymphatics are not seen, and there are no "traditional" dendritic cells for antigen presentation. The mechanisms by which adaptive immunity is developed in the CNS continues to be an active area of investigation.

It has been known for many years that the immune response of the CNS differs from that in peripheral tissues. Foreign tissue transplanted into the brain survives for much longer than when the same tissue is transplanted into a peripheral tissue [1]. This led to the designation of the brain and CNS as an "immune privileged site", that is, a tissue in which the immune response to foreign antigen is inhibited [2]. Other immune privileged sites include the fetoplacental unit, the anterior chamber of the eye, and the testis. It is presumed that this mechanism of active immunosuppression has a survival role. Functional immunosuppression within the CNS is a means to limit the extent of inflammation and increase the likelihood of return to normal function of neurons and the CNS. As Leslie Brent states

> …It may be supposed that it is beneficial to the organism not to turn the anterior chamber of the eye, or the brain, into an inflammatory battlefield, for the immunological response is sometimes more damaging than the antigen insult that provoked it… [3]

This observation by Dr. Brent concisely and elegantly summarizes the importance of immunosuppression and control of inflammation in patients with inflammatory disease of the CNS.

The CNS is not, however, immunologically inept. This tissue can and does mount an effective immune response. This is supported by the observation that while tissue grafted into the CNS survives for prolonged periods, the tissue will be promptly rejected if the subject is immunized by prior exposure [1]. The specific characteristics of the immune response of immune privileged sites differ from that of other tissues. Specifically, antigen-specific inhibition of delayed-type hypersensitivity is induced, as well as an increased production of antigen-specific antibody [4, 5].

Initial interpretation of the diminished CNS immunoreactivity was attributed to the lack of conventional lymphatic vessels within the CNS. This was believed to isolate any antigen within the CNS from the peripheral immune system. It has been demonstrated, however, that there is significant contact of CNS antigen with the peripheral immune system. Up to 47% of antigen injected into the CNS appears in cervical and deep cervical lymph nodes [6]. Also, when antigen is directly placed within the CNS, antigen-specific antibodies appear in the serum, and antigen can be recovered in the deep cervical lymph nodes following injection [7, 8].

Another functional explanation for immune privilege within the CNS is the low concentration of MHC class II molecules expressed on cells of the CNS. As antigen presentation is required to initiate an adaptive immune response, the lack of antigen presenting cells within the CNS has been considered to be a key factor in the dampened immune response observed following CNS infection.

Although there is little constitutive secretion of MHC class II molecules, many cells of the CNS have been found to express MHC class II molecules when appropriately stimulated. Which cell type is the most important for antigen presentation *in vivo*, however, remains unconfirmed. In addition to escape from the CNS, soluble antigen can be presented to lymphocytes in the bloodstream by brain endothelial and choroid plexus cells [9], brain microvessel smooth muscle cells [10], as well as astrocytes and microglia [11, 12]. In addition, B cells are potent antigen presenting cells [13].

Another feature of the CNS and cerebrospinal fluid (CSF) that contributes to a diminished immune response is the observation that concentrations of complement are almost undetectable in normal healthy human subjects [14]. This has not been determined in the horse, but is likely to be similar to other species.

The nervous system parenchyma consists largely of two fixed cell populations: neurons and glial cells (Table 3.1). Neuron function is restricted to conduction of electrical information, although there is some evidence accumulating that neuronal activity can directly mediate inflammatory events. Glial cells have a supportive function. Glial cells differ from neurons in their lack of synaptic contacts, and they maintain the property of mitosis throughout life, and in particular as a response to injury [15]. Glial cells are subdivided into macro- and microglia.

Microglia are of mesodermal origin and invest the CNS at the time of embryonic vascularization of the CNS. Microglia maintain mobility, which is essential in responding to inflammation. Microglia are analogous to macrophages and migrate to areas of inflammation and are involved in phagocytosis, antigen presentation, and the production and release of inflammatory mediators. The mediators have an auto-, para- and possibly endocrine function, which signal to other cell populations (lymphocytes, polymorphonuclear cells, and astrocytes). Microglia are part of the reticuloendothelial system (RES) and are related in origin, function, and morphology to monocytes [12]. It is thought that they

Table 3.1 Functional classification of cells of the central nervous system.

Cell type	Function
Macroglia	
Oligodendrocyte	Produces myelin in CNS
Schwann cell	Produces myelin in PNS
Astrocyte	Antigen presentation, neurotransmitter recycling
Microglia	Antigen presentation, phagocytosis
Neuron	Conduction of electrical impulses

form a resident population of cells of the RES within the CNS. Whether there is a truly sequestered population of RES cells in the CNS, or whether they are continuously replaced by blood derived progenitors, is not clearly understood.

It appears from recent work that neurons can interact with microglia, and while the interactions are complex, it appears that neurons can stimulate the microglia to become activated or quiescent. Depending upon the cytokine milieu in the CNS at the time, this may result in a detrimental or beneficial phenotype [16, 17]. Such reactions have not been investigated in horses.

Macroglia consists of astrocytes and oligodendrocytes that are of ectodermal origin. Oligodendrocytes are responsible for the production of myelin within the CNS. The immunologic role of oligodendrocytes is less well defined. Oligodendrocytes appear to have limited ability to express MHC class II receptors, but they can produce interleukin-1 [18]. The immunologic function of astrocytes is also incompletely understood. The perivascular end-plates or "foot processes" of astrocytes ensheath the cerebral vasculature, restricting the passage of macrophages and other immune responsive cells, yet allowing the passage of activated T cells. As astrocytes are positioned at the interface between blood and the CNS, they can also influence the activity of invading cells [19]. Astrocytic responses can be detected within 24 h after a CNS infection or inflammatory event [20]. Astrocytes respond to the presence of IL-1 with the production of interferon (IFN)-γ and expression of MHC II molecules [21]. Tumor necrosis factor (TNF)-alpha induces astrocytes to express intracellular adhesion molecule 1, which is necessary for cellular migration through the BBB [22]. Hence, the astrocyte has a significant role in responding to and regulating immune responses within the CNS. Astrocytes are the most numerous cellular elements in the CNS, and they are among the first cells to respond to CNS injury by reactive gliosis and cellular swelling, which largely reflects hypertrophy and a minor component of astrocytic proliferation. This astrocytic cell swelling is associated with cytotoxic edema of the CNS, and these swollen astrocytes have been shown to release glutamate, which has been associated with excitotoxic neuronal cell injury. While this has not been demonstrated in horses, this is likely an important mediator of neuronal dysfunction in foals with hypoxic-ischemic encephalopathy and horses with head trauma.

In healthy mammals, the CNS contains T lymphocytes in such low concentrations that they are almost undetectable by immunohistochemical methods, yet are readily found in various inflammatory diseases [23]. B and T lymphocytes were noted in very low numbers in the spinal cord of normal horses (1 and 2% of nucleated cells, respectively) [24]. Lymphocyte numbers in CSF have also been examined and are also present in very low numbers. In human CSF, T cells predominate and are present in slightly higher proportions than in peripheral blood (72.9 vs. 63.8%, respectively) [25]. The proportion of B cells in human CSF varies among authors from <1 to 16% [25–27].

In the CSF of normal adult horses, T cells also predominate and are found in a higher proportion than in blood (67 vs. 79%) [28]. The CD4$^+$ lymphocyte phenotype predominates and is present in slightly lower numbers than in peripheral blood, while the CD8$^+$ subset proportion is slightly more than in blood (13.6 vs. 23.4%) [28].

The mechanisms by which lymphocytes are normally excluded from the CNS, yet are permitted to enter during disease, are poorly understood. The BBB is a functional and anatomical barrier between the CNS and the blood and acts as a significant barrier for cellular entry. Access to the CNS is strictly regulated, and the barrier guarantees a microenvironment that maintains CNS function. Increased permeability of the BBB is a pathologic event, which allows access of plasma proteins, complement factors, and inflammatory cells into the CNS. This is reflected as an increase in the albumin quotient (AQ), total protein, and cellularity of the CSF.

Even in the presence of a healthy BBB, there is a normal surveillance of the CNS by circulating lymphocytes, with fluorescein-labeled cells being found in CSF within 3 h of injection and peaking at 9–12 h after injection [23]. The time course for lymphocyte entry was similar for "activated" or unstimulated cells. In another study, it was found that lymphocytes enter the CSF in approximately the same time course as cells appear in the subcutaneous lymphatic fluid. Hence, it appears that cells do not need to be activated to allow entry into the CNS, and CNS lymphocytes appear to be a part of the normal recirculating pool [29]. In support of this concept, work in humans has found that CSF lymphocytes are primarily of memory phenotype (CD45RO$^+$) but show no evidence of recent activation [27]. Once primed cells recognize their cognate antigen within the CNS, however, they are retained and do not emigrate from the tissue, leading to a cellular pleocytosis within the CNS/CSF.

Of great clinical interest is the production of immunoglobulins in the CNS/CSF (intrathecal immunoglobulin synthesis), as this body fluid is often used in immunodiagnostic assays for conditions such as equine protozoal myeloencephalitis (EPM). In the stereotypical humoral immune response, B lymphocytes require physical contact with a helper T cell to initiate their response to an antigen. This occurs via the interaction of MHC class II molecules and antigen. Additional costimulation is required and is provided via the interaction of CD19/CD21 receptors and the CD40/CD40L receptors [30]. In peripheral tissues, this physical contact is accomplished by the interaction of B and T cells in lymph nodes. In neuroinflammatory disease or neuroinfections, the mechanism of antigen-specific activation of lymphocytes requires that processed antigen leave the CNS and consequently activate its antigen-specific lymphocytes outside the CNS, in lymph nodes draining the CNS intracellular fluid and CSF. Cells then traffic back into the CNS, under the influence of local adhesion factors, for local (intrathecal) immunoglobulin production. Once exposed to an antigen, memory B cells remain within the CNS and direct intrathecal activation of plasma cell with antibody production [13] (Figure 3.1).

Immunoglobulin concentrations in the CSF of normal horses was reported to be 10.2 ± 5.5 mg/dl (mean ± SD) from the AO space and 9.9 ± 5.7 mg/dl from the LS space in foals less than 10 days of age [31]. In normal adult horses, CSF IgG concentration was 18.5 ± 1.4 mg/dl (mean ± SD) in fluid collected from the AO space [8]. In another study, CSF IgG concentrations in normal adult horses was reported to be 0.056 ± 0.014 g/l (i.e., 5.6 ± 1.4 mg/dl) (mean ± SD) [32]. The concentration of other immunoglobulin subtypes has not been reported. Given that the normal serum concentration of IgG was 2740 ± 286 mg/dl (mean ± SEM) in one study, it is clear that there is a relative paucity of immunoglobulin in the

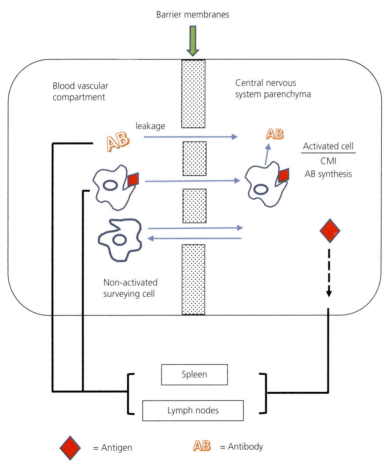

Figure 3.1 A schematic illustrating the basic interaction of antigen and immune response within the central nervous system (CNS). Antigen (represented by the red diamond) interacts with extracerebral lymphoid tissues and is processed, producing antigen-specific effector cells. The immune response loop is completed by the transbarrier movement of activated immune cells across intact brain-barrier membranes, which remain resident in the CNS and produce antigen-specific antibody within the CNS (intrathecal antibody production). Nonactivated cells will routinely survey the CNS but remain in the CNS only transiently if their cognate antigen is not encountered. The scheme recognizes the possibility that antigens in the brain are processed in some way yet to be established.

CNS and CSF in health [8]. Following neuroinfection, the concentration of immunoglobulin increases, with most immunoglobulin subtypes represented [33–35]. It has been suggested that isotype switching does not occur in the CNS [36], yet clear evidence of isotype switching of B cells within the CNS has been documented in a model of viral encephalitis in mice [37]. Presumably this also occurs in horses but has not been specifically investigated.

A number of methods have been proposed for the quantitative discrimination between a pathological CNS derived (i.e., intrathecal) immunoglobulin production and that which arises within the CSF from blood and protein leakage across a damaged BBB [38]. This distinction is of particular importance in the interpretation of diagnostic tests for neuroinfections, such as EPM. It has been demonstrated that antibodies are present in the CSF of normal horses in direct proportion (although lesser concentrations) to that in the serum (See Figure 3.2). Hence, discriminating between antibodies that are in the CSF from passive diffusion versus those that were actively produced within the CSF is of acute clinical importance.

In equine medicine, the IgG_{index} has been utilized as a method for estimating the excess amount of IgG within the CSF in disease of the nervous system [31, 32]. The IgG_{index} is a unitless number and is based upon the concept that the amount of IgG in the CSF is proportional to the amount of IgG in the serum and is hence dependant upon the barrier function of the BBB, as reflected by the AQ. This proportionality can be determined mathematically and related by the equation:

$$IgG_{index} = \left(\frac{IgG_{csf}}{IgG_{serum}} \right) \times \left(\frac{albumin_{serum}}{albumin_{csf}} \right) \qquad 3.1$$

From a study of normal adult horses, a value of 0.194 ± 0.046 (mean $\pm$ SD) was determined for CSF from the AO space and 0.194 ± 0.05 (mean $\pm$ SD) for the LS space [32]. From this study, an IgG_{index} value of greater than 0.27 was proposed to reflect intrathecal immunoglobulin synthesis [32]. For neonatal foals, an IgG_{index} of 0.519 ± 0.284 (mean $\pm$ SD) (AO site) and 0.482 ± 0.270 (mean $\pm$ SD) (LS site) was reported [31]. In another study, the IgG_{index} in normal adult horses was 0.45 ± 0.01 (mean $\pm$ SEM) [8]. The application of the IgG_{index} has not been rigorously applied to the evaluation of horses with CNS disease. In a model of neuroinflammation of the horse, the IgG_{index} did increase dramatically after antigen challenge of the CNS (Furr M, unpublished data). The IgG_{index} has been examined in horses with EPM, and conflicting results have been reported. In one large study of EPM (101 horses), it was found that the IgG_{index} was greater in horses with EPM than reported normal values and did decrease during treatment [39]. In addition, the magnitude of the IgG_{index} decreased during

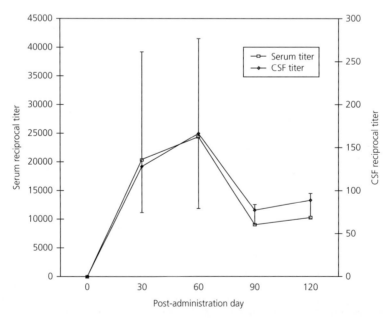

Figure 3.2 Serum and cerebrospinal fluid (CSF) anti-ovalbumin titers after IM administration of ovalbumin in six horses. Serum reciprocal titers are presented on the left axis and CSF reciprocal titers are presented on the right axis (mean $\pm$ SEM). (Reprinted with permission from Ref. [8].)

treatment and recovery. Due to its nonspecific nature, the IgG_{index} is currently considered to have no value in the diagnosis of EPM [40]. (Refer to Chapter 22 for a further discussion of the diagnosis of EPM.)

Other techniques that have been proposed to evaluate intrathecal antibody synthesis in the horse include the Goldmann-Witmer coefficient (C value) and the antibody index (AI). These methods have been proposed to be more sensitive and specific for diagnostic purposes than the IgG_{index} because they are calculated using antigen-specific immunoglobulin titers [41] (Figures 3.3 and 3.4). These are similar techniques that are based upon the premise that in the presence of a normal BBB and no intrathecal antibody production, the proportion of antigen-specific CSF IgG in relation to total IgG (or albumin concentration) in CSF will be equivalent to the corollary proportion in serum. Hence, any passive movement of immunoglobulin across the BBB would result in a ratio (CSF/serum) of less than or equal to 1. Intrathecal immunoglobulin production results in a disproportionately greater production of immunoglobulin in the CSF than serum, resulting in a calculated value greater than 1. The two methods differ only in the reference protein used; the AI uses albumin while the C value uses total IgG. Determination of these indices in six normal horses challenged with a novel antigen and sampled at five different times over 120 days found the AI to range from 0.51 to 0.75 and the C value to range from 1.0 to 1.7 [8]. The formulas for calculation of the AI and C value are (Figure 3.5):

$$AI = \frac{QAb}{QAlb},$$
3.2

where QAb (antibody quotient) is reciprocal CSF $titer_x \times 1000$/reciprocal serum $titer_x$ and QAlb (albumin quotient) is (CSF albumin concentration/serum albumin concentration) $\times 1000$.

C value = reciprocal CSF $titer_x \times$ total serum IgG/ total CSF IgG $\times$ reciprocal serum $titer_x$ 3.3

These techniques have been investigated in an equine model of neuroinflammation using intrathecal injection of ovalbumin. Ten days after injection, the AI for ovalbumin ($AI_{ovalbumin}$) had increased from 0.3 (preinjection) to 5.9. Similarly, the $C_{ovalbumin}$ increased from 0.6 (preinjection) to 7.5 10 days postchallenge. Titers for herpes virus were also determined and AI and C values calculated; the results demonstrated that the AI_{herpes} was 0.7 (i.e., normal) and the C_{herpes} increased to 1.7. These results suggest good specificity of these tests, with the ability to discriminate between active infection and passive antibody migration [41].

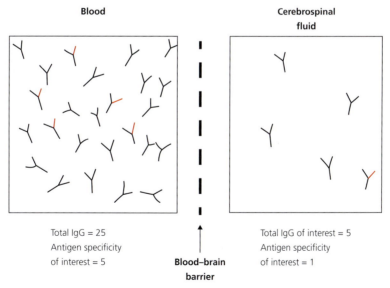

Figure 3.3 Schematic diagram demonstrating the principle of the antibody index and C value. In the normal condition, antibodies of various antigenic specificities are produced in the blood. For demonstration, the antigen-specific antibody of interest is indicated in red, while the other antibodies demonstrated are black. In the blood, there are 25 total IgG molecules, of which 5 are specific to the antigen of interest, resulting in a ratio of 5/25, or 0.2. A small number of these antibodies will cross into the CSF in a ratio equal to that in the blood, but in a much smaller concentration; hence five total IgG molecules with one of these having the specificity of interest (1/5, or 0.2). A ratio of the CSF/blood red antigen specificity then results in 1.

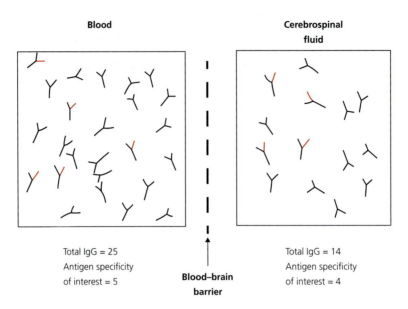

Figure 3.4 Schematic diagram demonstrating increased antibody index or *C* value in the CSF. In this example, the ratio of specific antibodies of interest, marked red, in the blood remains 0.2. However, with intrathecal antibody production, there are more antigen-specific antibodies present in the CSF than would be present by simple diffusion. Hence, in the CSF there are 14 total IgG molecules of which 4 are of the specificity of interest (4/14, or 0.28). The CSF/blood ratio is therefore 0.28/0.2, or 1.4. As this is greater than 1, intrathecal antibody production is confirmed.

It is obvious that the CNS has the functional capacity to respond to antigen, yet the response is altered, suggesting an active regulatory mechanism for immune privilege. The recognition that there were numerous immunoregulatory compounds (cytokines) responsible for the elegant coordination of the immune response has led to a search for such compounds within immune privileged tissues which might explain the observed phenomenon.

Within the CNS, and with an intact BBB, upregulation of the effector arm of the immune system differs from other sites of the body. One strategy employed in immune privileged sites is to create a local immunosuppressive microenvironment. This inhibitory milieu appears to be contributed to in part by immunosuppressive cytokines and substances present in biological fluids that bathe these sites. There are multiple mechanisms by which T-cell mediated processes can be suppressed. Responding lymphocytes can become functionally inactivated, or inactivated by initiating apoptotic cell death. A range of soluble substances have been identified, which have an *in vivo* and/or *in vitro* effect on the cells involved in defense mechanisms. Several substances with immunosuppressive properties were identified in brain tissue or CSF: alpha-melanocyte stimulating hormone, vasoactive intestinal peptide, calcitonin gene-related peptide,

somatostatin, and the cytokines transforming growth factor-β (TGF-β), IL-4, and IL-10 [42, 43]. Of these potential factors, only TGF-β has been investigated in the horse.

A pleiotropic hormone, members of the TGF-β family have the ability to influence many aspects of the immune response, including growth and differentiation of many hematopoietic lineages, proliferation and migration of mature immune cells, and regulation of immune responses [44]. For example, TGF-β inhibits interleukin 2 dependant proliferation, as well as secretion of IFN-γ, TNF-α and β, and interleukin 1, 2, and 3 [44, 45]. TGF-β suppresses MHC class II expression on cells induced by IFN-γ, thereby blocking one of the most important functions of IFN-γ [45]. While the predominant effect of TGF-β is immunosuppressive, it can lead to T-cell proliferation, block Fas-induced apoptosis, and expand the T_h2 CD4+T cell subset via inhibition of T_h1 products [45].

While not routinely found in the normal adult brain tissue, TGF-β is found in the CNS in a variety of disease states, including multiple sclerosis, Alzheimer's disease, and stroke. In the diseased brain, the source of TGF-β has been considered to arise from infiltrating T cells and macrophages, although it is now evident that microglia, astrocytes, and neurons can all produce at least some of the isoforms of TGF-β [46].

Patient values:

	Normal	Neuroinflammation
Serum IgG (mg/dl)	2420	3565
Serum albumin (mg/dl)	2350	3206
Serum titer$_x$	1:256	1:512
CSF IgG (mg/dl)	17.3	288.6
CSF albumin (mg/dl)	28.6	128.6
CSF titer$_x$	1:2	1:128

Normal horse:

$$AI = \frac{2 \times 1000/256}{(28.6 / 2350) \times 1000} = \frac{7.8}{12.1} = 0.64$$

$$C\ value = \frac{2 \times 2420}{7.3 \times 256} = \frac{4840}{4428} = 1.1$$

Horse with neuroinflammation:

$$AI = \frac{128 \times 1000/512}{(128.6 / 3206) \times 1000} = \frac{250}{40} = 6.25$$

$$C\ value = \frac{128 \times 3565}{288.6 \times 512} = \frac{456320}{147763} = 3.1$$

Values substantially greater than 1 in the horse with neuroinflammation confirms intrathecal production of antigen specific antibody for antigen X. C value and AI are usually similar, but are not expected to be exactly the same.

Figure 3.5 Example calculations for determining the antibody index and C value for equine cerebrospinal fluid.

It has been demonstrated that CSF will lead to suppressed lymphocyte blastogenesis and decreased IFN-γ production, and this effect was reversed by the application of anti-TGF antibodies [42, 43]. In horses, TGF-β2 has been documented to be present in the CSF and will stimulate IFN-γ production, rather than suppress it as was found in other species [47].

These findings confirm the immunomodulatory effects of CSF and suggest that immune privilege is maintained by the production of an immunosuppressive microenvironment. This environment is the product of the presence of immunosuppressive compounds within the CSF, combined with the presence of a BBB which mediates cellular infiltration into the CNS [48]. In general, the immune response within the CNS appears to be regulated in a manner that allows for control of infection, with a minimum of inflammation.

References

[1] Medewar, P. (1948) Immunity to homologous grafted skin III. The fate of skin homografts transplanted to the brain, to subcutaneous tissue, and to the anterior chamber of the eye. *Br J Exp Pathol*, 29, 58–69.

[2] Barker, C. and Billingham, R. (1977) Immunologically privileged sites. *Adv Immunol*, 25, 1–54.

[3] Cserr, H.F. and Knopf, P.M. (1992) Cervical lymphatics, the blood-brain barrier and the immunoreactivity of the brain: a new view. *Immunol Today*, 13, 507–512.

[4] Kaplan, H.J. and Streilein, J.W. (1977) Immune response to immunization via the anterior chamber of the eye. *J Immunol*, 118, 809–814.

[5] Panda, J. (1965) Immunologic response to subarachnoid and intracerebral injections of antigens. *J Immunol*, 94, 760–764.

[6] Cserr, H.F., Harling-Berg, C.J. and Knopf, P.M. (1992) Drainage of brain extracellular fluid into blood and deep cervical lymph and its immunological significance. *Brain Pathol*, 2, 269–276.

[7] Harling-Berg, C., Knopf, P.M., Merriam, J. *et al.* (1989) Role of cervical lymph nodes in the systemic humoral immune response to human serum albumin microinfused into rat cerebrospinal fluid. *J Neuroimmunol*, 25, 185–193.

[8] Furr, M. (2002) Antigen-specific antibodies in cerebrospinal fluid after intramuscular injection of ovalbumin in horses. *J Vet Intern Med*, 16, 588–592.

[9] Nathanson, J.A. and Chun, L.L. (1989) Immunological function of the blood-cerebrospinal fluid barrier. *Proc Natl Acad Sci U S A*, 86, 1684–1688.

[10] Fabry, Z., Waldschmidt, M.M., Moore, S.A. *et al.* (1990) Antigen presentation by brain microvessel smooth muscle and endothelium. *J Neuroimmunol*, 28, 63–71.

[11] Vidovic, M., Sparacio, S.M., Elovitz, M. *et al.* (1990) Induction and regulation of class II major histocompatability complex mRNA expression in astrocytes by interferon-gamma and tumor necrosis factor-alpha. *J Neuroimmunol*, 30, 189–200.

[12] Hickey, W.F. and Kimura, H. (1988) Perivascular microglia are bone marrow derived and present antigen *in vivo*. *Science*, 239, 290–292.

[13] Meinl, E., Krumbholz, M. and Hohlfeld, R. (2006) B lineage cells in the inflammatory central nervous system environment: migration, maintenance, local antibody production, and therapeutic modulation. *Ann Neurol*, 59, 880–892.

[14] Cserr, H.F., DePasquale, M., Harling-Berg, C.J. *et al.* (1992) Afferent and efferent arms of the humoral immune response to CSF-administered albumins in a rat model with normal blood-brain barrier permeability. *J Neuroimmunol*, 41, 195–202.

[15] Raine, C.S. (1994) Multiple sclerosis: immune system molecule expression in the central nervous system. *J Neuropathol Exp Neurol*, 53, 328–337.

[16] Noda, M. (2010) *Neuroimmune Biology: The Brain and Host Defense*, vol. 9, Elsevier BV, London, pp. 161–167.

[17] Biber, K., Neumann, H., Inoue, K. *et al.* (2007) Neuronal "On" and "Off" signals control microglia. *Trends Neurosci*, 30, 596–602.

[18] Benveniste, E.N. (1998) Cytokine actions in the central nervous system. *Cytokine Growth Factor Rev*, 9, 259–275.

[19] Aschner, M. (1998) Immune and inflammatory responses in the CNS: modulation by astrocytes. *Toxicol Lett*, 102, 283–287.

[20] Norenberg, M.D. (1996) *The Role of Glia in Neurotoxicity*, CRC Press, Boca Raton, pp. 93–107.

[21] Hellendall, R.P. and Ting, J.P. (1997) Differential regulation of cytokine-induced major histocompatability complex class II expression and nitric oxide release in rat microglia and astrocytes by effectors of tyrosine kinase, protein kinase C, and cAMP. *J Neuroimmunol*, 74, 19–29.

[22] Frohman, E.M., Frohman, T.C. and Dustin, M.L. (1989) The induction of intracellular adhesion molecule 1 (ICAM-1) expression on human fetal astrocytes by interferon-g, tumor necrosis factor-a, lymphotoxin, and interleukin-1: relevance to intracerebral antigen presentation. *J Neuroimmunol*, 23, 117–124.

[23] Hickey, W.F., Hsu, B. and Kimura, H. (1991) T-lymphocyte entry into the central nervous system. *J Neurosci Res*, 28, 254–260.

[24] Scott, P.R., Witonsky, S., Robertson, J. *et al.* (2005) Increased presence of T lymphocytes in central nervous system of EPM affected horses. *J Parasitol*, 91, 1499–1502.

[25] Moser, R., Robinson, J. and Prostko, E. (1976) Lymphocyte subpopulations in human cerebrospinal fluid. *Neurology*, 26, 726–728.

[26] Svenningsson, A. (1993) Adhesion molecule expression on cerebrospinal fluid T lymphocytes: evidence for common recruitment mechanisms in multiple sclerosis, aseptic meningitis, and normal controls. *Ann Neurol*, 34, 155–161.

[27] Svenningsson, A. (1995) Lymphocyte phenotype subset distribution in normal cerebrospinal fluid. *J Neuroimmunol*, 63, 39–46.

[28] Furr, M., Pontzer, C. and Gasper, P. (2001) Lymphocyte phenotype subsets in the cerebrospinal fluid of normal horses and horses with equine protozoal myeloencephalitis. *Vet Ther*, 2, 317–324.

[29] Seabrook, T., Johnston, M. and Hay, J. (1998) Cerebral spinal fluid lymphocytes are part of the normal recirculating pool. *J Neuroimmunol*, 91, 100–107.

[30] Tizard, I. (1996) *Veterinary Immunology*, W.B. Saunders, Co, Philadelphia, pp. 121–140.

[31] Andrews, F.M., Geiser, D.R., Sommardahl, C.S. *et al.* (1994) Albumin quotient, IgG concentration, and IgG index determinations in cerebrospinal fluid of neonatal foals. *Am J Vet Res*, 55, 741–745.

[32] Andrews, F., Maddux, J. and Faulk, B. (1990) Total protein, albumin quotient, IgG and IgG index determinations for horse cerebrospinal fluid. *Prog Vet Neurol*, 1, 197–204.

[33] Potasman, I., Resnick, L., Luft, B.J. *et al.* (1988) Intrathecal production of antibodies against *Toxoplasma gondii* in patients with toxoplasmic encephalitis and the acquired immunodeficiency syndrome. *Ann Intern Med*, 108, 49–51.

[34] Knopf, P.M., Harling-Berg, C.J., Cserr, H.F. *et al.* (1998) Antigen-dependent intrathecal antibody synthesis in the normal rat brain: tissue entry and local retention of antigen-specific B cells. *J Immunol*, 161, 692–701.

[35] Tyor, W.R. and Griffin, D.E. (1993) Virus specificity and isotype expression of intraparenchymal antibody-secreting cells during Sindbis virus encephalitis in mice. *J Neuroimmunol*, 48, 37–44.

[36] Tipold, A., Pfister, H., Zurbriggen, A. *et al.* (1994) Intrathecal synthesis of major immunoglobulin classes in inflammatory diseases of the canine CNS. *Vet Immunol Immunopathol*, 42, 149–159.

[37] Tyor, W.R., Moench, T.R. and Griffin, D.E. (1989) Characterization of the local and systemic B cell response

of normal and athymic nude mice with Sindbis virus encephalitis. *J Neuroimmunol*, 24, 207–215.

[38] Lefvert, A.K. and Link, H. (1985) IgG production within the central nervous system: a critical review of proposed formulae. *Ann Neurol*, 17, 13–20.

[39] Furr, M., Kennedy, T., MacKay, R. *et al.* (2001) Efficacy of ponazuril 15% oral paste as a treatment for equine protozoal myeloencephalitis. *Vet Ther*, 2, 215–222.

[40] Furr, M., MacKay, R., Granstrom, D. *et al.* (2002) Clinical diagnosis of equine protozoal myeloencephalitis (EPM). *J Vet Intern Med*, 16, 618–621.

[41] Furr, M. (2007) Humoral immune responses in the horse after intrathecal challenge with ovalbumin. *J Vet Intern Med*, 21, 806–811.

[42] Wilbanks, G. and Streilein, J. (1992) Fluids from immune privileged sites endow macrophages with the capacity to induce antigen-specific immune deviation via a mechanism involving transforming growth factor-beta. *Eur J Immunol*, 22, 1031–1036.

[43] Taylor, A. and Streilein, J. (1996) Inhibition of antigen stimulated effector T cells by human cerebrospinal fluid. *Neuroimmunomodulation*, 3, 112–118.

[44] Letterio, J. and Roberts, A. (1997) TGF-b: a critical modulator of immune cell function. *Clin Immunol Immunopathol*, 84, 244–250.

[45] Derynck, R. and Choy, L. (1998) *The Cytokine Handbook*, Academic Press, New York, pp. 593–636.

[46] Constam, D.B., Phillips, J., Malipiero, U.V. *et al.* (1992) Differential expression of transforming growth factor-beta 1 -beta 2 and beta 3 by glioblastoma cells, astrocytes, and microglia. *J Immunol*, 148, 1404–1410.

[47] Furr, M. and Pontzer, C. (2001) Transforming growth factor beta concentrations and interferon gamma responses in cerebrospinal fluid of horses with equine protozoal myeloencephalitis. *Equine Vet J*, 33, 721–725.

[48] Streilein, J.W. (1993) Immune privilege as the result of local tissue barriers and immunosuppressive microenvironments. *Curr Opin Immunol*, 5, 428–432.

4 Pharmaceutical Considerations for Treatment of Central Nervous System Disease

Véronique A. Lacombe[1] and Martin Furr[2]

[1] Center for Veterinary Health Sciences, Oklahoma State University, Stillwater, USA
[2] Marion duPont Scott Equine Medical Center, Virginia-Maryland Regional College of Veterinary Medicine, Leesburg, USA

Pharmaceutical treatment of diseases of the central nervous system (CNS) is occasionally necessary in equine practice. This includes treatment of bacterial, viral, fungal, or parasitic infections and the use of agents to minimize edema and drugs to control or limit inflammation, as well as to control seizures or to modify behavior.

Introduction to neuropharmacology

The presence of the blood–brain barrier (BBB) is of particular importance to CNS pharmacology as it directly influences the nature and extent of drug contact that can occur. It has been estimated that the BBB excludes >95% of all drugs from entering the brain from the blood [1]. The diffusion of compounds across the BBB is dependent on the physicochemical properties of the compounds, specifically lipid solubility, molecular weight, and electrical charge or ionization [2, 3]. In addition to the BBB, there are a number of other factors that influence the concentration of drugs within the CNS. Drugs that are highly protein bound will have diminished capacity to traverse the BBB [3, 4]. In contrast, drugs that are lipid-soluble, small in molecular size, and nonionized at the pH of the cerebrospinal fluid (CSF) will cross the BBB most readily [5]. It is also well recognized that meningeal inflammation will increase the penetration of many drugs into the CNS. It is important to recognize that brain tissue concentrations and CSF concentrations may not be the same, that is, there is compartmentalization. For example, brain tissue concentration of chloramphenicol following treatment is nine times the plasma concentration, yet CSF chloramphenicol concentration is only about 50% of simultaneous plasma concentration [4]. Brain tissue and CSF

concentrations of azithromycin differ markedly [6]. The elimination half-life for a drug in the CNS or CSF may differ markedly from that in serum and is frequently longer (allowing accumulation) [3]. Finally, the mechanism of bulk flow will remove chemicals from the CSF independent of their physicochemical properties.

In addition to the passive mechanisms described earlier, there are some active mechanisms of the BBB that influence CNS drug concentrations (Table 4.1). There is a low-capacity facilitated diffusion system in the BBB for some penicillin and cephalosporin antimicrobials that transports these drugs from the blood into the extracellular fluid of the CNS [7, 8]. In addition, there is also a mechanism for active efflux from the CSF for penicillins and other beta-lactam antimicrobials, macrolide antimicrobials, ivermectin, vinca alkaloids, digoxin, and dexamethasone among others, using the multidrug resistance transporter protein in the BBB [2, 7]. The activity or presence of this transporter in the horse has not been investigated.

Antibacterial drugs

There are few antibiotics used in the horse that readily achieve antibacterial concentrations in the CNS or CSF. Most information known about CSF antibiotic concentrations is extrapolated from humans and laboratory animals. As indicated earlier, a number of factors influence such concentrations, and direct extrapolation may not be accurate.

Penicillin achieves concentrations in the CSF that are roughly 10% of corresponding serum concentrations [9]. While meningeal inflammation does increase the proportion of penicillin that can cross the BBB, this is

Equine Neurology, Second Edition. Martin Furr and Stephen Reed.
© 2015 John Wiley & Sons, Inc. Published 2015 by John Wiley & Sons, Inc.
Companion website: www.wiley.com/go/furr/neurology

Table 4.1 Factors that influence CNS concentration of drugs.

Presence of BBB
Lipophilicity of compound
Protein binding
Physical size/radius
Molecular charge
Active transport
Active efflux
Bulk flow
Presence or absence of meningeal inflammation

variable and may not be adequate to result in therapeutic concentrations. Ampicillin achieves higher concentrations within the CSF than penicillin, however only in the presence of meningeal inflammation [10].

The third- and fourth-generation cephalosporins ceftazidime, cefotaxime, and cefepime achieve good CSF concentrations following peripheral administration and have a favorable spectrum of activity. Compounds in the cephalosporin class do not uniformly cross the BBB, however. Proper dosages and dose intervals for many of these drugs have not been established in the horse at this time. Ceftriaxone has been investigated in the horse, and a single IV dose of 50 mg/kg resulted in a CSF concentration of $0.6 \pm 0.14 \mu g/ml$ at 3 h after dosage and $0.4 \pm 0.31 \mu g/ml$ at 8 h after dosage [11]. The CSF concentration of ceftriaxone varied markedly between horses being studied, and the authors concluded that the variability was due to the presence of mild inflammation induced by an indwelling intrathecal catheter. The CSF concentrations achieved exceed the minimal inhibitory concentration (MIC) for many equine pathogens, making ceftriaxone an attractive choice for the treatment of bacterial meningitis in horses. It was suggested that a dose of 25 mg/kg IV BID would be adequate; however, this was not investigated specifically. Due to the cost, the use of ceftriaxone may be limited to use in foals and small ponies. Based upon pharmacokinetic studies in neonates, a dose of 25 mg/kg IV every 12 h was suggested for neonatal foals [12]. Cefotaxime has been used with success in foals with meningitis at a dose of 40 mg/kg QID [13, 14]. Specific CSF concentrations resulting from the dosage were not reported. Cephapirin could not consistently be found in the CSF of horses following intramuscular dosages of 20 mg/kg, and it is not likely to be useful in the treatment of CNS infections in horses [15]. Ceftiofur could not be detected in the CSF of mares following multiple doses (2 mg/kg body weight) [16]. Dosages for other cephalosporins must be extrapolated from those used in humans and may or may not be appropriate in horses. The expense of these antibiotics limits their use to the neonate in many cases.

Chloramphenicol has been extensively evaluated in the horse, and it has been used for the treatment of a number of equine infectious conditions [17]. Chloramphenicol has a favorable spectrum of activity for equine pathogens, and in humans the CSF concentration achieves almost 60% of serum concentrations when administered orally; [18] results in horses are similar [19]. The half-life of chloramphenicol in the horse is short following IV administration (0.43 h) [20] and somewhat longer after multiple oral doses (3.8 h) [19]. The metabolism and excretion of chloramphenicol in neonatal foals has been demonstrated to be similar to adult horses by 7 days of age [17, 21]. This short half-life makes frequent dosing necessary and limits its intravenous use. Dose recommendations vary widely but are commonly reported as 25–59 mg/kg orally every 6 h [22, 23]. The limitations on the use of chloramphenicol may make availability of this drug difficult in some circumstances.

Potentiated sulfonamide combinations such as trimethoprim/sulfamethoxazole (TMP/SMZ) or ormetoprim/sulfadimethoxine (OMP/SDM) are commonly used in the treatment of equine infections. At a dose of 2.5 mg/kg TMP and 12.5 mg/kg SMZ, CSF concentrations in one horse were $0.15 \mu g/ml$ TMP (28% of corresponding serum concentration) and $4.8 \mu g/ml$ SMZ (43% of corresponding serum concentration) [24]. These concentrations were not adequate to be effective against a number of equine pathogens reported by the authors. Although the authors suggested that there was evidence of accumulation of SMZ in the CSF, this was not confirmed. Meningeal inflammation does not appear to enhance the CSF concentration of TMP/SMZ [25, 26]; hence, use of this drug in CNS infections of the horse should be considered carefully and may not be optimum. The coadministration of intravenous dimethylsulfoxide (DMSO) had no effect upon CSF concentrations of TMP or SMZ [27]. Following dosing at 9.2 mg/kg ORM and 45.8 mg/kg SDM, OMP concentration in the CSF was $0.08 \pm 0.056 \mu g/ml$ and SDM concentration was $2.1 \pm 0.77 \mu g/ml$. This represents 47% (OMP) and 2.6% (SDM) of corresponding serum concentrations [27]. These concentrations are well below previously published minimum inhibitory concentrations for a number of equine pathogens [28, 29]. These values were derived from samples taken at only one time point and are not likely to constitute peak concentrations, however.

The use of sulfonamide drugs in the horse is known to be associated with a number of potential complications, including diarrhea and anemia. In addition, one report describes neurologic signs in four of six pony stallions following treatment with TMP/SMZ [30]. Clinical signs noted were clumsy thrusts and weakness and unsteadiness when mounting. Formal neurologic evaluations were not performed, unfortunately, but these signs are consistent with spinal ataxia [30]. This observation has not been further investigated, and its significance is unclear at this time.

Fluoroquinolones are highly lipid-soluble and have been reported to achieve high concentrations in the CNS following parenteral administration [31]. In dogs treated with enoxacin, good CSF concentrations were reported, and concentrations of pefloxacin in healthy dogs resulted in CSF concentrations that were 55% of those in serum [32]. The most commonly used fluoroquinolone in horses is enrofloxacin, and the CSF concentration was approximately 15 and 25% of corresponding serum concentrations at 74 and 84 h following treatment [33]. The concentration achieved at a dosage of 5 mg/kg BID PO exceeded the MIC for most equine pathogens (0.5 μg/ml) [33]. This drug would be a valuable compound in the treatment of bacterial meningitis; however, its use in foals is associated with a high risk of arthropathy, severely limiting its use in young foals. Very high doses of enrofloxacin (25 mg/kg IV) as a bolus dose have resulted in seizures in horses [34]. Giving the dose diluted or more slowly ameliorated the effect. This is assumed to result from transient high CSF concentrations and the binding of gamma amino butyric acid (GABA) receptors in the CNS.

Rifampin achieves high CSF concentrations, however must be administered concurrently with other antibiotics due to the rapid development of resistance [35]. Specific investigations in the horse are not reported. Metronidazole is highly lipophylic and it achieves high concentrations in the CSF of many species [36, 37]. Metronidazole is almost exclusively useful for anaerobic infections, which have not been reported in the CNS of the horse, hence its value is limited.

Parenteral administration of aminoglycoside antimicrobials does not result in measurable concentrations within the CNS [23, 38]. Administration of doxycycline at 10 mg/kg did not result in measurable concentrations of the drug within the CSF of horses [39]. Minocycline, however, at a dose of 2.2 mg/kg IV q12 h does result in

adequate CSF concentrations and may be useful for treatment of CNS infections [40]. Entry of erythromycin into the CNS and CSF is considered poor [3]. Treatment of humans with conventional doses of azithromycin has been found to result in high CNS tissue concentrations (up to 3.6 ± 3.81 μg/g tissue), which were 10 times the serum concentration [6]. Corresponding CSF azithromycin concentrations were minimal to undetectable [6]. Corresponding studies have not been performed in horses but would suggest that azithromycin may have value in the treatment of CNS abscesses caused by sensitive organisms (Table 4.2).

The optimal antimicrobial to use in equine CNS infections has not been established and must be determined based upon culture and sensitivity of the organism as well as knowledge of the pharmacology of the drug and its ability to enter the CNS and achieve an adequate concentration. It is unclear whether higher doses and longer intervals, or more frequent administration is most important in antimicrobial treatment of CNS infections [3]. In one study describing the treatment of human meningitis, antimicrobial combinations were most commonly used, including one or more third-generation cephalosporins, penicillin, ampicillin, and chloramphenicol [3]. It is reasonable to assume that due to the limited penetration of most antibiotics into the CSF of horse, combination therapy would be of value. This must be determined on a case-by-case basis accompanied by culture and sensitivity data.

One means to achieve high CSF concentrations of antibiotics is by direct injection into the CSF (intrathecal administration). Intrathecal treatment can be considered in cases in which the recovered organism is sensitive only to drugs that have poor penetration of the BBB. This method of treatment has been utilized in humans, particularly when treating resistant organisms, and high concentrations of antibiotics result [41, 42]. In humans, 5 mg of gentamicin intraventricularly, once per day, has been recommended [3]. No reports using intrathecal antibiotics in horses could be found, and the dose and frequency of treatment are totally unknown. Anecdotally, seizures have been reported in horses from this procedure, likely associated with the carrier and formulation of the compounds used.

Table 4.2 Relative drug concentrations in cerebrospinal fluid following parenteral dosing.

Good	Intermediate	Poor
Ceftriaxone	TMP/SMZ	Penicillin
Cefotaxime	OMP/S	Ampicillin
Chloramphenicol	Minocycline	Cephapirin
Rifampin		Ceftiofur
Metronidazole		Doxycycline
Enrofloxacin		

Categories reflect achievable concentrations relative to expected MICs of equine pathogens.

Antiviral drugs

Few antiviral drugs are available for use in the horse; however, acyclovir has been proposed for the treatment of equine herpesvirus-1 (EHV-1) myeloencephalopathy [43]. Acyclovir is an acyclic nucleoside analogue that has a good activity against herpes simplex virus type 1 and 2. Acyclovir has been shown to inhibit the replication of EHV-1 in Syrian hamsters at a dose of 100 mg/kg [44].

Oral availability of acyclovir is poor, and plasma concentrations after dosing with 20 mg/kg were below the limits of detection of the assay (<0.15 µg/ml) in one study [43] and below the effective concentration (EC_{50}) for EHV-1 in another study [45]. This is in contrast to another report in which multiple doses of the drug (10 mg/kg) resulted in plasma concentrations of 0.2–0.38 µg/ml [46]. These concentrations were effective for some but not all EHV-1 isolates *in vitro* [46]. Acyclovir has been used clinically at a dose of 20 mg/kg q8 h in one EHV-1 myeloencephalitis outbreak, but a clear benefit was not demonstrated [47]. Current evidence does not support the use of acyclovir in horses with EHV-1–associated disease.

Given the poor oral absorption of acyclovir, the use of the acyclovir prodrug valacyclovir is of interest as it appears to have much better bioavailability. Following oral administration, valacyclovir is converted to acyclovir and at a dose of 20 mg/kg body weight (BW) of valacyclovir, serum concentrations of acyclovir within the sensitive range for some strains of EHV-1 were obtained [45]. In another study, valacyclovir (40 mg/kg BW PO, q8 h) resulted in blood concentrations of acyclovir that exceeded the EC_{50} for one strain of EHV-1 for greater than 80% of the treatment time [48]. In this study, CSF concentrations of acyclovir were below the EC_{50} for EHV-1; however, the importance of this in treatment of affected horses is questionable as EHV-1 is not a neurotropic virus. Based upon these studies, an oral dose of 20–40 mg/kg, q8 h, is recommended for treatment of suspected susceptible infections [49]. However, in an infection study, valacyclovir had no effect upon clinical signs, viral shedding, or magnitude of viremia in EHV-1–infected ponies [50]. The utility of valacyclovir therefore remains undetermined in equine viral infections.

Anti-inflammatory drugs

The CNS is considered an "immune privileged site," in that response to infection of the CNS is less robust than that noted in other tissues. This restriction upon the degree of inflammation likely has survival benefit. In the treatment of CNS infections therefore, control of inflammation is of paramount importance. Control of inflammation is credited with improving outcomes in cases of human bacterial meningitis. Prostaglandins and thromboxanes are produced in the CNS in a number of clinical conditions, including seizures, inflammation, traumatic brain injury, and cerebral vascular disease [51]. The relative concentrations of and ability to generate eicosanoids appear to vary depending upon the region of the CNS affected, however [51]. While this topic has not been evaluated in the horse, it is presumed that a similar increase in prostanoid products would be found. From the preceding observations, a number of nonsteroidal anti-inflammatory drugs (NSAIDs) have been recommended in neuroinflammatory disease.

The NSAIDs ibuprofen, aspirin, and indomethacin increase survival in mice with Sandhoff's disease, an inflammatory neurodegenerative disorder [52]. These findings suggest that the NSAIDs should be useful in horses with neuroinflammation, as well as attenuating fever, myalgia, and perhaps improving appetite. No recommendations can be made at this time however, in regard to the specific NSAID to use or appropriate dosages. These should be determined on a case-by-case basis.

The use of corticosteroids in horses with neuroinflammation is controversial, as it is in people. It is well recognized that corticosteroids are effective in the treatment of cerebral edema and that they attenuate tissue injury by inhibiting host mediators at several steps in the inflammatory process [53]. Concern has been expressed regarding the potential for the immunosuppression associated with dexamethasone usage, allowing infection to progress. There is little to no empiric support of this concept, however. Extensive research has been conducted regarding the effects of steroids in CNS infections in humans and laboratory animals. In one study of bacterial meningitis in adults, treatment with dexamethasone was found to reduce the relative risk of death (0.48, 95% confidence interval (CI) 0.24–0.96, $P = 0.04$) when compared with no steroids [54], while another study found that the use of corticosteroids in human patients with bacterial meningitis reduced death, hearing loss, and neurologic sequelae [55]. A meta-analysis of randomized clinical trials also found that treatment with dexamethasone in people was beneficial and associated with low risk of side effects [56]. No comparable studies are reported in horses; however, it is assumed that the general beneficial effects upon cerebral inflammation would exist also. In horses, the risk of laminitis associated with corticosteroids use must be considered and assessed on an individual case basis; however, a short-term course of corticosteroids in horses with bacterial meningitis seems warranted.

The use of corticosteroids in viral disease is also controversial; however, corticosteroids have been used successfully in people with West Nile virus encephalitis [57] and have been proven beneficial in acute viral meningitis [58]. Furthermore, glucocorticoids have been found to be beneficial in people and experimental animals with herpes simplex encephalitis, and the use of glucocorticoids did not result in an increased viral load [59]. In fact, in another study, the use of corticosteroids alone was associated with a reduction in viral load by $63 \pm 13\%$ [60]. Similar studies have not been reported for horses with viral encephalitis; however, these studies provide compelling evidence for the value of corticosteroids in horses with viral-induced neuroinflammation. In horses with neurologic deficits due to viral encephalitis that are severe enough to require hospitalization, a short course of corticosteroids is strongly indicated.

Another commonly used anti-inflammatory drug in horses is DMSO. It is commonly recommended for treatment of horses with neuroinflammation; however, there is little evaluation of its use in the horse. Clinical experience suggests that it does have an anti-inflammatory effect, but this is difficult to establish conclusively. There is, however, a large body of work describing the effects of DMSO in neurologic disease in laboratory animal species, as well as its clinical use in humans. Calcium flux as a result of excitotoxic amine release is a well-recognized cause of neuronal cell death. It has been demonstrated that DMSO at concentrations that are associated with clinical treatment decrease excitotoxic cell death of neurons [61]. Further, DMSO has been shown to enhance the drug-induced blockade of calcium channels [62]. Intravenous DMSO at 1 mg/kg body weight, given as a 10% solution, has been shown to decrease intracranial pressure (ICP) by 45% in a model of brain edema in rabbits [63]. In addition, DMSO reduced neuronal cell death in an *in vivo* model of ischemia-reperfusion [64], rapidly decreased ICP in human patients suffering head trauma and improved cerebral perfusion pressure and neurologic outcomes [65]. It is expected that horses would have a similar response to DMSO, and a dose of 0.5–1 g/kg as a 10% solution (IV) 2 times per day is recommended in suspected cases of neuroinflammation. The drug should not be given at greater than a 20% solution as hemolysis can be seen at concentrations greater than 20%. Dosages of 4 g/kg IV were associated with toxic signs in 3 of 6 treated horses. Signs included muscle trembling, loose stool, and colic and abated quickly after cessation of the drug infusion [66].

Other compounds used to combat CNS edema include mannitol and hypertonic saline. Both compounds are considered to reduce cerebral edema primarily due to their hyperosmolar effects, but some evidence suggests slightly different mechanisms to the reduction of ICP [67]. Various concentrations of hypertonic saline have been investigated in cases of brain edema, with improvement noted in ICP following treatment with as low as 1.8% NaCl [68]. The beneficial effects of hypertonic saline persist even when followed by normal crystalloid solutions [69] and appear to be due to its ability to draw water from the cell, decreasing tissue pressure [69]. The recommended dose of hypertonic saline for horses with head trauma is 4–6 ml/kg of 5 or 7% NaCl as a bolus, which can then be followed by normal crystalloid solutions at a maintenance dose [70]. Isotonic fluids should not be given to horses with head trauma at high dose

rates, such as that used for circulatory shock, as this is likely to increase cerebral edema and ICP [71]. (Refer to Chapter 31 for further discussion of the treatment of CNS trauma.)

Mannitol is a hyperosmolar solution that has been used to reduce ICP. Mannitol is a 6-carbon nonmetabolizable polyalcohol with a molecular weight of 182 Da [72]. Several theories have been proposed to explain the effects of mannitol on ICP. The osmotic theory has the most support and states that the CNS shrinkage is a result of osmotically driven movement of fluid from the tissue into the vascular component. A variety of studies have confirmed that mannitol reduces water content of tissue (e.g., brain) [67]. Additional experimental work, however, has suggested that additional mechanisms may be involved in the reduction of ICP associated with mannitol. These theories include a reduction of CSF production, as well as direct vascular effects [73, 74]. It is likely that a combination of osmotic and other effects are present.

Dosages of mannitol of 1–2 g/kg body weight intravenously 2–4 times per day have been suggested for horses with suspected cerebral edema [75]. Rapid reduction of ICP is noted in experimental animals following bolus dosing of mannitol. A rebound effect may occur after treatment is stopped, and repeated dosing in experimental animals has lead to progressively reduced effects associated with accumulation of mannitol in tissues [67, 76]. Mannitol should not be used in horses in which subarachnoid or intraparenchymal hemorrhage is present, due to the potential to exacerbate bleeding or increase ICP.

Anticonvulsant drugs

Anticonvulsants are used to reduce the incidence, severity, or duration of seizures. Epileptical activity arises from an imbalance between excitatory and inhibitory neural transmitters, which induces an abnormal hypersynchronous electrical activity of neurons. The principle excitatory neurotransmitter in the brain is glutamate. A wave of depolarization reaching the presynaptic nerve terminal induces release of glutamate. Glutamate binds to *N*-methyl-D-aspartate (NMDA) receptors on the postsynaptic membrane, opening sodium and calcium channels and leading to entry of these ions into the postsynaptic neuron. This ionic movement leads to postsynaptic depolarization and generation of an excitatory postsynaptic potential [77]. In contrast, when GABA, the major inhibitory neurotransmitter, attaches to the postsynaptic $GABA_A$ receptor, chloride channels are opened. Chloride enters the postsynaptic neuron causing a state of hyperpolarization and an inhibitory postsynaptic potential. A failure of local surrounding inhibitory zones to prevent the spread of an initial focal epileptogenic activity allows the seizure focus to progress and spread diffusely throughout the cortex. By acting on pre- and postsynaptic ion channels, anticonvulsant drugs stabilize neuronal membranes and thereby limit the development and spread of the epileptical focus activity.

Only a few of the anticonvulsants available in humans have been proven to be clinically useful in horses. The most commonly used anticonvulsant drug in horses is phenobarbital, a barbiturate. Phenobarbital activates GABA-gated chloride channels, which increases intracellular chloride conductance and induces hyperpolarization of neuronal cells. Other mechanisms include inhibition of postsynaptic potentials produced by glutamate and inhibition of voltage-gated calcium channels at excitatory nerve terminals (Table 4.3). The overall result is an increase in the seizure threshold. Phenobarbital has very good bioavailability (i.e., ~100%) and is widely distributed into tissue [37, 79]. For acute management of seizures, phenobarbital is administered IV at an initial dose of 12–20 mg/kg, diluted in saline and given over 30 min, followed by 1–9 mg/kg q8–12 h. Maintenance therapy is usually administered by the oral route, with a proposed dose of 11 mg/kg once q24h in adults [79]. For further information on seizure management and therapeutic drug monitoring, please refer to Chapter 7. Primidone is a deoxybarbiturate, an analog of phenobarbital. There are only a few reports of its use in foals [80, 81].

Benzodiazepines (e.g., diazepam and midazolam) are the preferred drugs for the acute treatment of seizures, including status epileptics, because they rapidly cross the BBB due to their high lipid solubility. They specifically bind to GABA$_A$ receptors in the CNS and thereby activate GABA-gated chloride channels to increase

chloride conductance, making the cell more resistant to depolarization. Specific benzodiazepine binding sites have been identified in the brain, with the highest density being in the central cortex, the cerebellum, and the limbic system, as well as in peripheral tissues. Unlike barbiturates, benzodiazepines do not activate GABA receptors directly but require GABA to produce their effect [82]. Recommended dosage of diazepam is 0.05–0.2 mg/kg (~50 mg for an adult horse), given IV or IM, on an as-needed basis. Because of its short duration of action (10–15 min), repeated doses might be necessary. However, caution should be used as prolonged usage may cause respiratory depression or arrest in foals [83]. In horses that do not show response to initial bolus doses of diazepam, a constant-rate infusion of diazepam can be implemented at an initial rate of 0.1 mg/kg/h. Midazolam is a potent short-acting benzodiazepine that can be used on foals at 0.05–0.1 mg/kg IV or IM as well as a continuous-rate infusion [84].

Potassium bromide is one of the oldest used anticonvulsant drugs, although its mechanism is not well known. It is believed that potassium bromide hyperpolarizes neuronal membrane through its action on chloride channels and by its synergistic effect with barbiturates and benzodiazepines. It has been primarily used to treat seizures that are refractory to phenobarbital.

Phenytoin is a hydantoin derivative and is not commonly used in horses. Phenytoin appears to inactivate voltage-dependent neuronal sodium channels to prevent depolarization of the presynaptic neuronal membrane at the excitatory nerve terminal and thus to reduce release of glutamate, the excitatory neurotransmitter [77]. It also prevents the opening of the potassium channels, which leads to an increase in action potential

Table 4.3 Main mechanisms of action of anticonvulsant drugs used for horses and foals.

	Anticonvulsant drugs	Mechanisms of action			
		Decrease seizure onset		Decrease seizure spread	
		Enhanced Na$^+$ channel inactivation	Enhanced GABA-activated Cl$^-$ conductance	Reduced current through Ca^{2+} channels	Reduced glutamate-mediated excitation
Main	Benzodiazepines		++		
	Phenobarbital		++	+	+
	Bromide		++		
Alternative	Phenytoin	++			
	Primidone		++	+	+

Modified from Ref. [78], © Wiley.
++, postulated primary mechanism of action.

duration and in the refractory period. Because of its lidocaine-like effect in the heart, phenytoin has also been used to treat ventricular arrhythmias.

Carbamazepine is a sodium channel blocker that has been used to treat trigeminal neuralgia in humans. Carbamazepine (1.6–2.4 g, q6 h), in combination with cyproheptadine, has also been reported to be effective in treating horses with headshaking, without apparent side effects. There is no information on the pharmacokinetics of this drug [85].

Newer antiepileptic drugs have been introduced in veterinary medicine, with improved therapeutic indices (i.e., effective dose compared with toxic dose) with a reduction of the sedative and organ-toxic adverse reactions [78]. These drugs include felbamate, gabapentin, clorazepate, topiramate, and zonisamide and can be used as monotherapy or combined with bromide. However, the cost of these new antiepileptic drug therapies may prohibit their use in adult horse, and their clinical efficacy is currently unknown. For example, gabapentin is a synthetic GABA analog that crosses the BBB, although its main mechanism of action is due to the inhibition of the voltage-dependent calcium channels, thereby inhibiting excitatory neurotransmitter release (e.g., glutamate) [5]. A pharmacokinetic study in healthy horses showed that it is rapidly absorbed, with peak plasma levels occurring approximately 2 h following a single oral administration (5 mg/kg) in horses [86]. Although it is a useful adjunctive treatment for refractory and partial seizures in dogs, its clinical efficacy in epileptic horses is unknown.

Drugs affecting behavior

As with other domestic animals, horses exhibit many stereotypies (e.g., cribbing, weaving, and self-mutilation) and behavior disorders (e.g., aggressiveness). These adverse habits are most commonly managed by changes in husbandry; however, there is often a need for pharmacological alternatives. Please also refer to Chapter 36.

Antipsychotic drugs

Antipsychotic drugs, also referred as neuroleptics, refer to a number of structurally dissimilar drugs used in humans to treat most forms of psychosis. Although the exact mechanisms underlying stereotypies are not well known, it has been suggested that increased activity of dopamine, an important neurotransmitter in the basal ganglia and limbic portion of the brain, plays an important role [87, 88]. In addition, horses with stereotypies have higher dopamine D1 and D2 receptor densities in the nucleus accumbens than controls [89]. Because of their greater affinity for central dopamine receptor (primarily subtype D2) than dopamine itself, antipsychotic drugs decrease dopamine activity and synthesis. Dopamine depletion induces calming, depression, and extrapyramidal signs [90]. Antipsychotic drugs are not commonly used in veterinary behavioral medicine, with the exception of the phenothiazine tranquilizers (e.g., acepromazine), which are commonly used for sedation and restraint in equine practice. These drugs alter behavior pattern by reducing animal's general attendance to environment stimuli, inducing calming while maintaining arousability [82].

Acepromazine, a short-acting phenothiazine neuroleptic drug, is commonly used as a tranquilizer or preanesthetic agent in equine practice. It has also been suggested as a pharmacological aid for equine self-mutilation syndrome [91]. Although the exact mechanisms of action are not fully understood, phenothiazines block postsynaptic dopamine receptors in the CNS. They also have some antagonistic effects on alpha-adrenergic, histaminergic, serotonergic, and muscarinic receptors. At recommended doses (0.02–0.1 mg/kg IV), acepromazine produces calming, reluctance to move, and mild degree of ataxia [82]. The onset of action is fairly slow with peak effects reached within approximately 15 min and 1 h after IV and oral administration, respectively. As a CNS depressant, it blocks a range of central effects including respiratory response and locomotor activity. It also induces relaxation of the retractor penis muscle that causes penile prolapse lasting a few hours in males. Hypotension may also develop as a result of the alpha-1 adrenergic receptor blockage and a decrease in sympathetic tone. In addition, acepromazine may also lower the seizure threshold and potentiate seizures in predisposed animals.

Fluphenazine is a highly potent phenothiazine neuroleptic drug commonly used in humans with psychotic disorders. Because of its long-acting anxiolytic and sedative effects, fluphenazine decanoate has been used in an extra-label manner in young, nervous, or fractious performance horses making them more amiable during training and/or transport [92]. It has also been suggested as a pharmacological aid to reduce self-mutilation and other stereotypies [93]. However, this drug has a high potential for abuse when it is used to mask undesirable animal behavior/traits. In addition, severe adverse effects have been reported (see Chapter 34 for complete discussion of fluphenazine toxicity).

Serotonin reuptake inhibitors

Serotonin reuptake inhibitors are part of the general category of antidepressants. They include both the tricyclic antidepressants (e.g., imipramine and clomipramine) and the selective reuptake inhibitors (e.g., fluoxetine).

Abnormalities in central serotonin (5-hydroxytryptomine), a major neurotransmitter in the CNS, have been associated with mood disturbances, anxiety, aggression, and sexual drives [94, 95]. Therefore, tricyclic antidepressants, by blocking the uptake of serotonin and norepinephrine at presynaptic terminals, may enhance calm behavior. In contrast with humans and small animals, tricyclic antidepressants have limited use in horses and there is little information on the pharmacokinetics of these drugs. Amitriptyline (250 mg/day/horse orally), imipramine (500–1000 mg q12 h PO), and clomipramine (500–1000 mg q12 h PO) have been found clinically useful for self-mutilation stereotypies and to reduce anxiety in breeding males [90, 93]. Imipramine has also been recommended to control narcolepsy and cataplexy, although oral administration (250–750 mg orally) produces inconsistent results [96, 97]. Side effects of tricyclic antidepressants can include mild sedation and anticholinergic effects. At high doses (i.e., >2 mg/kg), imipramine can cause muscle fasciculations, tachycardia, hyperresponsiveness to sound, and hemolysis [98].

Selective serotonin reuptake inhibitors (SSRIs) bind to serotonin transporters and block the reuptake of serotonin by the presynaptic nerve terminal, therefore prolonging its exposure to receptors on the postsynaptic membrane [94]. In addition, they have little effect on the reuptake of norepinephrine and thereby are more specific than the tricyclic antidepressants [95]. In contrast with humans and small animals for whom SSRIs are widely used to treat a range of behavioral disorders, there is very limited study on their therapeutic effects and its use in horses is rather limited. Fluoxetine (Reconcile®, veterinary label; Prozac®, human label) is an SSRI with anxiolytic and anticompulsive effects that has been widely used to treat a range of human behavior, including depression, panic disorder, and obsessive–compulsive disorder. In horses, it has been used to manage aggression at a dose of 0.25–5 mg/kg orally q24 h [90]. However, it may require 4–6 weeks to become maximally effective. Please note that the administration of imipramine and fluoxetine in horses constitutes extralabel use and owners must be appropriately advised.

Anxiolytic drugs

The anxiolytic drugs include benzodiazepines, azapirones (e.g., buspirone), barbiturates, antidepressants, and antihistaminics [95].

In addition to their anticonvulsant effects (see previous section), benzodiazepines produce anxiolytic and muscle-relaxant effects. Diazepam (0.02–0.1 mg/kg IV) is commonly used in adult horses as a tranquilizer, a muscle relaxant, an anticonvulsant, and an adjunct to intravenous anesthesia [99]. Because it potentiates most common anesthetic agents, diazepam is usually coadministered with opioids and nonopioid analgesics to provide additive sedative effects [82, 99]. Peak drug effects are reached within 10 min after IV administration, 20–40 min after IM administration, and approximately 1 h after oral administration [82]. High doses (>0.2 mg/kg)

in adult horses may cause muscle weakness and ataxia, and recumbency may result [100]. Slow administration of a benzodiazepine antagonist (e.g., flumazenil and sarmazenil) could be used to treat overdoses of benzodiazepines or to reverse muscle weakness at the end of anesthesia [83, 99]. Diazepam (0.05–0.1 mg/kg, IV) has also been proven to be an effective and safe sedative drug in young foals [99].

Buspirone (Buspar®) is a partial agonist for serotonin receptor. Because this anxiolytic drug lacks sedative and muscle relaxant side effects, it might be a better drug for the treatment of anxiety disorders in horses, although there is very limited amount of information on its therapeutic effect [101]. It has been shown to improve behavior in horses demonstrating signs of self-mutilation syndrome the second hour following oral administration (0.5 mg/kg) [102].

Additional therapy for behavior modifications

Dopaminergic activity, which is increased during stereotypic behaviors, is modulated by many neurotransmitters including endogenous opioids and glutamate. Therefore, it has been shown that dextromethorphan, an NMDA receptor antagonist, at 1 mg/kg IV, reduced cribbing rate [88]. Similarly, opioid antagonists, such as naloxone, naltrexone, and nalmefene, have been successfully used to control self-mutilation and crib-biting in horses [102, 103].

Headshaking behavior in horses, which is characterized by an uncontrollable movement of the head and neck, has been associated with exposure to bright light and may resemble trigeminal neuralgia in humans. Cyproheptadine, an histamine (H-1)-blocking agent, is believed to be efficacious for the treatment of headshaking in some horses because of its serotonergic blocking antagonist properties [104, 105]. Serotonin plays a role in pain sensation, and cyproheptadine has been used to treat vascular/cluster headaches and hypersensitivity reactions in humans (e.g., rhinitis) [104, 105]. Cyproheptadine also has anticholinergic and sedative effects. There is no information on its pharmacokinetics in horses. Side effects of mild depression, anorexia, or lethargy have been reported [105]. Cyproheptadine is not an approved medication for use in performance horses (refer to Chapter 11 for further discussion of headshaking in horses).

Reserpine, an alkaloid extracted from *Rauwolfia serpentina* root, was one of the first modern tranquilizers; however, it was associated with severe side effects in humans. Reserpine is known as a noradrenergic depleting agent as it blocks a vesicular monoamine transporter, thereby inhibiting the uptake of norepinephrine and other monoamines into storage vesicles of sympathetic neurons. Although reserpine is not approved for use in horses, it is sometimes administered to horses as a sedative because of its efficacy at very low doses and long duration of action [37]. However, its use in horses is limited due to its side effects and toxicity, which include hypotension, bradycardia, and diarrhea [106–108].

References

[1] Pardrige, W.M. (1999) Non-invasive drug delivery to the human brain using endogenous blood-brain barrier transport systems. *Pharm Sci Technol Today*, 2, 49–59.

[2] de Vries, H.E., Kuiper, J., De Boer, A.G. *et al.* (1997) The blood-brain barrier in neuroinflammatory disease. *Pharmacol Rev*, 49, 143–155.

[3] Nau, R., Sorge, F. and Prange, H. (1998) Pharmacokinetic optimisation of the treatment of bacterial central nervous system infections. *Clin Pharmacokinet*, 35, 223–246.

[4] Brewer, B.D. (1984) Therapeutic strategies involving anti-microbial treatment of the central nervous system in large animals. *J Am Vet Med Assoc*, 185, 1217–1221.

[5] Hsu, W.H. and Riedesel, D.H. (2008) Drugs acting on the central nervous system, in *Handbook of Veterinary Pharmacology* (ed. W.H. Hsu), Wiley-Blackwell, Ames, pp. 81–103.

[6] Jaruratanasirikul, S., Hortiwakul, R., Tantisarasart, T. *et al.* (1996) Distribution of azithromycin into brain tissue, cerebrospinal fluid, and aqueous humor of the eye. *Antimicrob Agents Chemother*, 40, 825–826.

[7] Spector, R. (1986) Ceftriaxone pharmacokinetics in the central nervous system. *J Pharmacol Exp Ther*, 236, 380–383.

[8] Spector, R. (1986) Advances in understanding the pharmacology of agents used to treat bacterial meningitis. *Pharmacology*, 41, 113–118.

[9] Barling, R. (1978) The penetration of antibiotics into cerebrospinal fluid and brain tissue. *J Antimicrob Chemother*, 4, 203–227.

[10] Thea, D. (1989) Use of antibacterial agents in infections of the central nervous system. *Infect Dis Clin North Am*, 3, 553–570.

[11] Ringger, N.C., Pearson, E.G., Gronwall, R. *et al.* (1996) Pharmacokinetics of ceftriaxone in healthy horses. *Equine Vet J*, 28, 476–479.

[12] Ringger, N.C., Brown, M.P., Kohlep, S.J. *et al.* (1998) Pharmacokinetics of ceftriaxone in neonatal foals. *Equine Vet J*, 30, 163–165.

[13] Morris, D.D., Rutkowski, J. and Kent Lloyd, K.C. (1987) Therapy in two cases of neonatal foal septicemia and meningitis with cefotaxime. *Equine Vet J*, 19, 151–154.

[14] Gardner, S.Y., Sweeney, R.W. and Divers, T.J. (1993) Pharmacokinetics of cefotaxime in neonatal pony foals. *Am J Vet Res*, 54, 576–579.

[15] Brown, M.P., Gronwall, R.R. and Houston, A.E. (1986) Pharmacokinetic and body fluid and endometrial concentrations of cephapirin in mares. *Am J Vet Res*, 47, 784–788.

[16] Cervantes, C.C., Brown, M.P., Gronwall, R. *et al.* (1993) Pharmacokinetics and concentrations of ceftiofur sodium in body fluids and endometrium after repeated intramuscular injections in mares. *Am J Vet Res*, 54, 573–575.

[17] Page, S. (1991) Chloramphenicol 3: clinical pharmacology of systemic use in the horse. *Aust Vet J*, 68, 5–8.

[18] Friedman, C. (1979) Chloramphenicol disposition in infants and children. *J Pediatr*, 95, 1071–1077.

[19] Gronwall, R., Brown, M.P., Merritt, A.M. *et al.* (1986) Body fluid concentrations and pharmacokinetics of chloramphenicol given to mares intravenously or by repeated gavage. *Am J Vet Res*, 47, 2591–2595.

[20] Brown, M.P., Kelly, R.H., Gronwall, R.R. *et al.* (1984) Chloramphenicol sodium succinate in the horse: serum, synovial, peritoneal, and urine concentrations after single-dose intravenous administration. *Am J Vet Res*, 45, 578–580.

[21] Brumbaugh, G.W., Martens, R.J., Knight, H.D. *et al.* (1993) Pharmacokinetics of chloramphenicol in the neonatal horse. *J Vet Pharmacol Ther*, 6, 219–227.

[22] Knight, H.D. (1975) Antimicrobial agents used in the horse. *Proc Annu Meet Am Assoc Equine Pract*, 21, 131–145.

[23] Dowling, P.M. (2004) Antimicrobial therapy, in *Equine Clinical Pharmacology* (eds J.J. Bertone and L.J.I. Horspool), W.B. Saunders, Philadelphia, pp. 13–48.

[24] Brown, M.P., Gronwall, R. and Castro, L. (1988) Pharmacokinetics and body fluid and endometrial concentrations of trimethoprim-sulfamethoxazole in mares. *Am J Vet Res*, 49, 918–922.

[25] Levitz, R. and Quintaliani, R. (1984) Trimethoprim-sulfamethoxazole for bacterial meningitis. *Ann Intern Med*, 100, 881–890.

[26] Dudley, M., Levitz, R., Quintaliani, R. *et al.* (1984) Pharmacokinetics of trimethoprim-sulfamethoxazole in serum and cerebrospinal fluid of adult patients with normal meninges. *Antimicrob Agents Chemother*, 26, 811–814.

[27] Green, S.L., Mayhew, I.G., Brown, M.P. *et al.* (1990) Concentrations of trimethoprim and sulfamethoxazole in cerebrospinal fluid and serum in mares with and without a dimethyl sulfoxide pretreatment. *Can J Vet Res*, 54, 215–222.

[28] Brown, M.P., Gronwall, R.R. and Houston, A.E. (1989) Pharmacokinetics and body fluid and endometrial concentrations of ormetoprim-sulfadimethoxine in mares. *Can J Vet Res*, 53, 12–16.

[29] Adamson, P.J.W., Wilson, W.D., Hirsch, D.C. *et al.* (1985) Susceptability of equine bacterial isolates to antimicrobial agents. *Am J Vet Res*, 46, 447–450.

[30] Bedford, S.J. and McDonnell, S.M. (1999) Measurements of reproductive function in stallions treated with trimethoprim-sulfamethoxazole and pyrimethamine. *J Am Vet Med Assoc*, 215, 1317–1319.

[31] Cottagnoud, P. and Tauber, M. (2003) Fluoroquinolones in the treatment of meningitis. *Curr Infect Dis Rep*, 5, 329–336.

[32] Neer, T. (1988) Clinical pharmacologic features of fluoroquinolone antimicrobial drugs. *J Am Vet Med Assoc*, 193, 577–580.

[33] Giguere, S., Sweeney, R.W. and Belanger, M. (1996) Pharmacokinetics of enrofloxacin in adult horses and concentration of the drug in serum, body fluids, and endometrial tissues after repeated intragastrically administered doses. *Am J Vet Res*, 57, 1025–1030.

[34] Bertone, A.L., Tremaine, W.H., Macoris, D.G. *et al.* (2000) Effect of long-term administration of an injectable enrofloxacin solution on physical and musculoskeletal variables in adult horses. *J Am Vet Med Assoc*, 217, 1514–1521.

[35] Farr, M. (1982) Rifampin. *Med Clin N Am*, 66, 157–168.

[36] Anon (2004) Metronidazole, in *AHFS Drug Information* (ed. G. McEvoy), American Society of Health System Pharmacists, Bethesda, pp. 848–857.

[37] Dowling, P.M. (1999) Clinical pharmacology of nervous system disease. *Vet Clin North Am Equine Pract*, 15, 575–588.

[38] Neuwelt, E.A., Baker, D.E., Pagel, M.A. *et al.* (1984) Cerebrovascular permeability and delivery of gentamicin to normal brain and experimental brain abscess in rats. *J Neurosurg*, 61, 430–439.

[39] Bryant, J., Brown, M.P., Gronwall, R. *et al.* (2000) Study of intragastric administration of doxycycline: pharmacokinetics including body fluid, endometrial and minimum inhibitory concentrations. *Equine Vet J*, 32, 233–238.

[40] Nagata, S., Yamashita, S., Kurosawa, M. *et al.* (2010) Pharmacokinetics and tissue distribution of minocycline in horses. *Am J Vet Res*, 71, 1062–1066.

[41] Corpus, K., Weber, K. and Zimmerman, C. (2004) Intrathecal amikacin for the treatment of pseudomonal meningitis. *Ann Pharmacother*, 38, 992–995.

[42] Matasubara, H., Makimoto, A., Higa, T. *et al.* (2003) Successful treatment of meningoencephalitis caused by methicillin-resistant Staphylococcus aureus with intrathecal vancomycin in an allogenic peripheral blood stem cell transplant recipient. *Bone Marrow Transplant*, 31, 65–67.

[43] Wilkins, P., Papich, M. and Sweeney, R.W. (2005) Pharmacokinetics of acyclovir in adult horses. *J Vet Emerg Crit Care*, 15, 174–178.

[44] Rollinson, R. and White, G. (1983) Relative activities of acyclovir and BW 759 against Aujeskys disease and equine rhinopneumonitis viruses. *Antimicrob Agents Chemother*, 24, 221–226.

[45] Garre, B., Shebany, K., Gryspeerdt, A. *et al.* (2007) Pharmacokinetics of acyclovir after intravenous infusion of acyclovir and after oral administration of acyclovir and its prodrug valacyclovir in healthy adult horses. *Antimicrob Agents Chemother*, 51, 4308–4314.

[46] Wilkins, P. (2004) Acyclovir in the treatment of EHV-1 myeloencephalopathy. *Proc Annu Meet Am Coll Vet Intern Med*, 22, 170–172.

[47] Friday, P.A., Scarratt, W.K., Elvinger, F. *et al.* (2000) Ataxia and paresis with equine herpesvirus type 1 infection in a herd of riding school horses. *J Vet Intern Med*, 14, 197–201.

[48] Garre, B., Baert, K., Nauwynck, H. *et al.* (2009) Multiple oral dosing of valacyclovir in horses and ponies. *J Vet Pharmacol Ther*, 32, 207–212.

[49] Maxwell, L.K., Bentz, B.G., Bourne, D.W.A. *et al.* (2008) Pharmacokinetics of valacyclovir in the adult horse. *J Vet Pharmacol Ther*, 31, 312–320.

[50] Garre, B., Gryspeerdt, A., Croubels, S. *et al.* (2009) Evaluation of orally administered valacyclovir in experimentally EHV1-infected ponies. *Vet Microbiol*, 135, 214–221.

[51] Wolfe, L. and Horrocks, L. (1994) Eicosenoids, in *Basic Neurochemistry* (ed. C. Siegel), Raven Press, New York, pp. 475–490.

[52] Jeyakumar, M., Smith, D., Williams, I. *et al.* (2004) NSAIDs increase survival in the Sandhoff disease: synergy with N-butyldeoxynorimycin. *Ann Neurol*, 56, 642–649.

[53] Jafari, H. and McCracken, G. (1994) Dexamethasone therapy in bacterial meningitis. *Pediatr Ann*, 23, 82–88.

[54] de Gans, J. and van de Beek, D. (2002) Dexamethasone in adults with bacterial meningitis. *N Engl J Med*, 347, 1549–1556.

[55] Morris, A. (2004) Review: adjuvant corticosteroid therapy reduces death, hearing loss, and neurologic sequelae in bacterial meningitis. *Evid Based Med*, 9, 48.

[56] McIntyre, P., Berkey, C., King, S. *et al.* (1997) Dexamethasone as adjunctive treatment in bacterial meningitis. A meta-analysis of randomized clinical trials since 1988. *JAMA*, 278, 925–931.

[57] Pyrgos, V. and Younus, F. (2004) High dose steroids in the management of acute flaccid paralysis due to West Nile virus infection. *Scand J Infect Dis*, 36, 509–512.

[58] Nakano, A., Yamasaki, R., Miyazaki, S. *et al.* (2003) Beneficial effect of steroid pulse therapy on acute viral encephalitis. *Eur Neurol*, 50, 225–229.

[59] Meyding-Lamade, U., Oberlinner, C., Seyfer, S. *et al.* (2003) Experimental herpes simplex virus encephalitis: a combination therapy of acyclovir and glucocorticoids reduces long-term magnetic resonance imaging abnormalities. *J Neurovirol*, 6, 118–125.

[60] Thompson, K., Blessing, W. and Wesselingh, S. (2000) Herpes simplex replication and dissemination is not increased by corticosteroid treatment in a rat model of focal herpes encephalitis. *J Neurovirol*, 6, 25–32.

[61] Lu, C. and Mattson, M. (2001) Dimethyl sulfoxide suppresses NMDA and AMPA-induced ion currents and calcium influx and protects against excitotoxic death in hippocampal neurons. *Exp Neurol*, 170, 180–185.

[62] Wu, L., Karpinski, E., Wang, R. *et al.* (1992) Modification by solvents of the action of nifedipine on calcium channel currents in neuroblastoma cells. *Naunyn Schmiedebergs Arch Pharmacol*, 345, 478–484.

[63] James, H., Camp, P., Harbaugh, R. *et al.* (1982) Comparison of the effects of DMSO and pentobarbitone on experimental brain oedema. *Acta Neurochir (Wien)*, 60, 245–255.

[64] Phillis, J.N., Estevez, A.Z. and O'Regan, M.H. (1998) Protective effects of the free radical scavengers dimethyl sulfoxide and ethanol, in cerebral ischemia in gerbils. *Neurosci Lett*, 244, 109–111.

[65] Karaca, M., Bilgin, U., Akar, M. *et al.* (1991) Dimethyl sulfoxide lowers ICP after closed head trauma. *Eur J Pharmacol*, 40, 113–114.

[66] Appell, L., Blythe, L., Lassen, E. *et al.* (1992) Adverse effects of rapid intravenous DMSO administration in horses. *J Equine Vet Sci*, 12, 215–218.

[67] Berger, S., Schurer, L., Hartl, R. *et al.* (1995) Reduction of post-traumatic intracranial hypertension by hypertonic/hyperoncotic saline/dextran and hypertonic mannitol. *Neurosurgery*, 37, 98–108.

[68] Shackford, S., Zhuang, J. and Schmoker, J. (1992) Intravenous fluid tonicity: effect on intracranial pressure, cerebral blood flow, and cerebral oxygen delivery in focal brain injury. *J Neurosurg*, 76, 91–98.

[69] Gunner, W. and Jonasson, O. (1988) Head injury and hemorrhagic shock: studies of the blood brain barrier and intracranial pressure after resuscitation with normal saline solution, 3% saline solution and dextran-40. *Surgery*, 103, 398–402.

[70] Bertone, J.J. (1991) Hypertonic saline in the management of shock in horses. *Compend Contin Educ Pract Vet*, 13, 665–670.

[71] Crowe, D. (1992) Triage and trauma management, in *Veterinary Emergency and Critical Care Medicine* (eds R. Murtaugh and P. Kaplan), Mosby Year Book, St. Louis, p. 77.

[72] Kochevar, D.T. (2001) Diuretics, in *Veterinary Pharmacology and Therapeutics* (ed. H.R. Adams), Iowa State University Press, Ames, pp. 534–552.

[73] Hartwell, R.C. and Sutton, L.N. (1993) Mannitol, intracranial pressure, and vasogenic edema. *Neurosurgery*, 32, 444–450.

[74] Shapira, Y., Artru, A., Donato, T. *et al.* (1982) Effect of mannitol on cerebrospinal fluid dynamics and brain edema. *Anesthesiology*, 77, A782.

[75] Matthews, H. (1998) Spinal cord, vertebral, and intracranial trauma, in *Equine Internal Medicine* (eds S.M. Reed and W. Bayly), W.B. Saunders, Philadelphia, pp. 457–466.

[76] Kauffman, A.M. and Cardoso, E.R. (1992) Aggravation of vasogenic cerebral edema by multiple dose mannitol. *J Neurosurg*, 77, 584–589.

[77] Podell, M.L. (1998) Antiepileptic drug therapy. *Clin Tech Small Anim Pract*, 13, 185–192.

[78] Podell, M. (2001) Strategies of antiepileptic drug therapy. *Proc Annu Meet Am Coll Vet Intern Med*, 19, 430–431.

[79] Ravis, W.R., Duran, S.H., Pedersoli, W.M. *et al.* (1987) A pharmacokinetic study of phenobarbital in mature horses after oral dosing. *J Vet Pharmacol Ther*, 10, 283–289.

[80] Aleman, M., Gray, L.C., Williams, D.C. *et al.* (2006) Juvenile idiopathic epilepsy in Egyptian Arabian foals: 22 cases (1985–2005). *J Vet Intern Med*, 20, 1443–1449.

[81] May, C.J. and Greenwood, R.E. (1977) Recurrent convulsions in a thoroughbred foal: management and treatment. *Vet Rec*, 101, 76–77.

[82] Muir, W.W. (2008) Anxiolytics, nonopioid sedative-analgesics, and opioid analgesics, in *Equine Anesthesia* (eds W.W. Muir and J.A. Hubbell), W.B. Saunders, St. Louis, pp. 185–209.

[83] Norman, W.M., Court, M.H. and Greenblatt, D.J. (1997) Age-related changes in the pharmacokinetic disposition of diazepam in foals. *Am J Vet Res*, 58, 878–880.

[84] Magdesian, K.G. (2006) Intensive care medicine, in *The Equine Manual* (eds A.J. Higgins and J.R. Snyder), W.B. Saunders, Philadelphia, pp. 1255–1325.

[85] Newton, S.A., Knottenbelt, D.C. and Eldridge, P.R. (2000) Headshaking in horses: possible aetiopathogenesis suggested by the results of diagnostic tests and several treatment regimes used in 20 cases. *Equine Vet J*, 32, 208–216.

[86] Dirikolu, L., Dafalla, A., Ely, K.J. *et al.* (2008) Pharmacokinetics of gabapentin in horses. *J Vet Pharmacol Ther*, 31, 175–177.

[87] Dodman, N.H. (1998) Veterinary models of obsessive-compulsive disorder, in *Obsessive-Compulsive Disorders: Practical Management* (eds M.A. Jenicke, L. Baer and W.A. Minichiello), Mosby, St. Louis, pp. 318–334.

[88] Rendon, R.A., Shuster, L. and Dodman, N.H. (2001) The effect of the NMDA receptor blocker, dextromethorphan, on cribbing in horses. *Pharmacol Biochem Behav*, 68, 49–51.

[89] McBride, S.D. and Hemmings, A. (2005) Altered mesoaccumbens and nigro-striatal dopamine physiology is associated with stereotypy development in a non-rodent species. *Behav Brain Res*, 159, 113–118.

[90] Crowell-Davis, S.L. (2009) Aggression in horses, in *Current Therapy in Equine Medicine* (eds E. Robinson and K.A. Sprayberry), W.B. Saunders, St. Louis, pp. 112–115.

[91] Dodman, N.H., Shuster, L., Patronek, G.J. *et al.* (2004) Pharmacologic treatment of equine self-mutilation syndrome. *Int J Appl Res Vet Med*, 2, 90–98.

[92] Baird, J.D., Arroyo, L.G., Vengust, M. *et al.* (2006) Adverse extrapyramidal effects in four horse given fluphenazine decanoate. *J Am Vet Med Assoc*, 229, 104–110.

[93] Mc Donnell, S.M. (2008) Practical review of self-mutilation in horses. *Anim Reprod Sci*, 107, 219–228.

[94] Mohammad-Zadeh, L.F., Moses, L. and Gwaltney-Brant, S.M. (2008) Serotonin: a review. *J Vet Pharmacol Ther*, 31, 187–199.

[95] Sherman, B.L. and Papich, M.G. (2011) Drugs affecting animal behavior, in *Veterinary Pharmacology and Therapeutics* (eds J.E. Riviere and M.G. Papich), Blackwell, Ames, pp. 509–538.

[96] Hines, M.T., Schott, H.C. and Byrne, B.A. (1992) Adult-onset narcolepsy in the horse. *Proc Annu Meet Am Assoc Equine Pract*, 38, 289–296.

[97] Mayhew, I.G. (1983) Coma and altered states of consciousness, in *Large Animal Neurology* (ed. I.G. Mayhew), Lea and Febinger, Philadelphia, pp. 133–146.

[98] Peck, K.E., Hines, M.T., Mealey, K.L. *et al.* (2001) Pharmacokinetics of imipramine in narcoleptic horses. *Am J Vet Res*, 62, 783–786.

[99] Shini, S. (2000) A review of diazepam and its use in the horse. *J Equine Vet Sci*, 20, 443–449.

[100] Muir, W.W., Sams, R.A., Huffman, R. *et al.* (1982) Pharmacodynamic and pharmacokinetic properties of diazepam in horses. *Am J Vet Res*, 43, 1756–1762.

[101] Crowell-Davis, S. and Murray, T. (2006) Azapirones, in *Veterinary Psychopharmacology* (eds S. Crowell-Davis and T. Murray), Wiley-Blackwell, Ames, pp. 111–118.

[102] Dodman, N.H., Shuster, L., Court, M.H. *et al.* (1987) Investigation into the use of narcotic antagonists in the treatment of a stereotypic behavior pattern (crib-biting) in the horse. *Am J Vet Res*, 48, 311–319.

[103] Dodman, N.H., Shuster, L., Court, M.H. *et al.* (1988) Use of a narcotic antagonist (nalmefene) to suppress self-mutilative behavior in a stallion. *J Am Vet Med Assoc*, 192, 1585–1586.

[104] Bell, A.J. (2004) Headshaking in a 10-year-old thoroughbred mare. *Can Vet J*, 45, 153–155.

[105] Madigan, J.E., Kortz, G., Murphy, C. *et al.* (1995) Photic headshaking in the horse: 7 cases. *Equine Vet J*, 27, 306–311.

[106] Lloyd, K.C., Harrison, I. and Tulleners, E. (1985) Reserpine toxicosis in a horse. *J Am Vet Med Assoc*, 186, 980–981.

[107] Bidwell, L.A., Schott, H.C. and Derksen, F.J. (2007) Reserpine toxicosis in an aged gelding. *Equine Vet Educ*, 29, 341–343.

[108] Memon, M.A., Usenik, E.A., Varner, D.D. *et al.* (1988) Penile paralysis and paraphimosis associated with reserpine administration in a stallion. *Theriogenology*, 30, 411–419.

5 Fundamental Neurophysiology

Craig Johnson[1] and Caroline Hahn[2]

[1] Institute of Veterinary, Animal and Biomedical Sciences, Massey University, Palmerstown North, New Zealand
[2] Royal (Dick) School of Veterinary Studies, The University of Edinburgh, Midlothian, UK

Any understanding of the dysfunction of the nervous system is grounded in a thorough understanding of the physiological principles that underlie its normal function. This chapter will outline the important features of the structure and function of the neuron and its immediate environment. The focus throughout will be on aspects of cellular neurophysiology that are essential in understanding the pathophysiology of neurological diseases particular to the equine.

Ionic gradients and membrane potentials

The plasma membrane that surrounds all animal cells is responsible for the sequestration of some charged particles within the cytoplasm and the virtual elimination of others from the cytoplasm. These differential concentrations are maintained by active transport of ions across the membrane and the differing degrees to which the membrane is permeable to them. The resulting concentration gradients lead to the development of a potential difference across the membrane, known as the membrane potential.

The origin of the membrane potential

The lipid bilayer of the plasma membrane is very impermeable to charged particles, but it contains a number of transmembrane proteins that facilitate the movement of ions between the cytosol and the extracellular fluid. The ionic pump sodium–potassium–ATPase is the primary driver of this process exchanging sodium and potassium ions across the membrane. The resting membrane is very impermeable to sodium ions but less so to potassium ions, which diffuse back out of the cell through another transmembrane protein, the potassium channel. Potassium ions are driven out of the cell by their increased concentration on the inside, but this process is opposed by the electrical gradient that develops as they leave. The resting membrane potential is the electrical potential

across the plasma membrane when the opposing forces of diffusion and electrical attraction are balanced and the cell is at equilibrium. This exchange of sodium and potassium ions is the single most energy-demanding process in the body and accounts for between 10 and 40% of an animal's total ATP usage.

The magnitude of the membrane potential

The membrane potential reflects the balance of ions across the plasma membrane, and its magnitude depends on the relative permeability of the membrane to each of them. The more permeable the membrane is to a particular ion, the more closely the membrane potential will reflect the equilibrium potential of that ion. The resting membrane is approximately 20 times more permeable to potassium than to sodium and so the potential is much more influenced by the equilibrium potential of potassium (−90 mV) than that of sodium (+55 mV). Some cells are more permeable to sodium ions than others, and in these cells the membrane potential will be less negative because they are relatively more influenced by the equilibrium potential of sodium. The magnitude of the resting membrane potential has consequences on the way in which a particular cell functions because of the concept of the threshold potential that leads to the development of an action potential in excitable tissues (see later). Cells with membrane potentials close to threshold such as smooth muscle fibers and cardiac myocytes are able to generate action potentials more easily than cells such as lower motor neurons where the membrane potential is much more negative than the cell's threshold.

Action potentials

A number of cell types, collectively called the excitable tissues, express sodium channels in their plasma membranes. At rest, these channels are closed and impermeable to

Equine Neurology, Second Edition. Martin Furr and Stephen Reed.
© 2015 John Wiley & Sons, Inc. Published 2015 by John Wiley & Sons, Inc.
Companion website: www.wiley.com/go/furr/neurology

sodium, but under certain circumstances they can transiently undergo a conformational change and open. This dramatically increase the cell's permeability to sodium, and the sudden increase in sodium permeability alters the potential of the cell from its resting membrane potential to a potential much closer to the equilibrium potential of sodium, forming the basis of the action potential. Sodium channels are either voltage-gated and open when the membrane potential of the plasma membrane reaches a threshold or chemically gated containing receptor sites for a specific neurotransmitter that opens the channel.

Action potentials (Figure 5.1) are propagated when the membrane potential of a particular area of a neuron reaches threshold. The opening of voltage-gated sodium channels in this region causes a reversal of the membrane potential (depolarization), and this leads to adjacent areas of the membrane reaching threshold and so themselves depolarizing. In this way, the action potential moves along the neuron as a propagated wave. In the period immediately following the propagation of an action potential, sodium channels become refractory and so the membrane potential returns to normal values due to the diffusion of the exchanged ions from the immediate area of the plasma membrane and ultimately their return across the plasma membrane by the action of sodium–potassium–ATPase. This refractory period means that neurons have a maximum rate at which they can propagate action potentials.

The rate at which action potentials travel depends on a number of factors, the most relevant being whether a nerve fiber is myelinated (see later) and the diameter of the axon, the thicker the axon, the faster the action potential is propagated. Action potentials in unmyelinated neurons typically travel at a speed of up to $2\,ms^{-1}$. In myelinated neurons, action potential propagation speeds can be up to $120\,ms^{-1}$.

The neuron

The neuron is a very specialized cell. It usually has a very elongated form and the ability to convey information from one end to the other and to neighboring cells via synapses. The following discussion will be in two parts, the first will consider the neuron's ability to transmit information through the integration and conduction of action potentials and the second will consider various metabolic aspects of neuronal function. There are many variations on the form of the neuron and so the concept of the generalized neuron (Figure 5.2) is often used when outlining the way in which information is transferred.

Neurons are stimulated by specific excitants and inhibitors that alter the membrane potential in specific regions of the cell. These electrical changes are summated over regions of the cell body and dendritic arborization. A long extension of the neuron, the axon, extends from a region called the axon hillock and if the changes in membrane potential result in this region reaching threshold, then an action potential is propagated along the axon to the secretory unit or synapse at

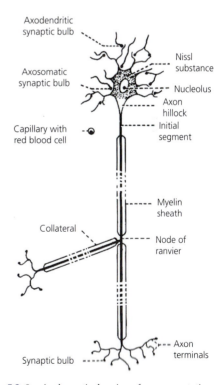

Figure 5.2 Semi-schematic drawing of a representative neuron. The capillary and red blood cell indicate relative size. Broken lines indicate shortening. (Reproduced from Ref. [2], © Wiley.)

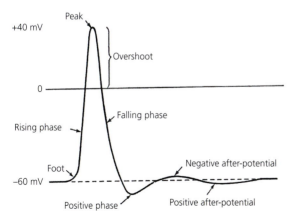

Figure 5.1 Diagram demonstrating the action potential. (Reproduced from Ref. [1], © Cambridge.)

the far end. This synapse in turn secretes a neurotransmitter that acts as an excitant or inhibitor for another neuron, muscle fiber, or gland.

Structure of the axon

The axon is an elongation of the neuron (the longest axons in the horse can be up to 3 m in length) and is a very specialized structure dedicated to the transfer of action potentials from one end to the other. Many axons are surrounded by multilayered fatty coatings of myelin that provide electrical insulation between the axon and the extracellular fluid surrounding it. These myelin sheaths are formed and maintained by Schwann cells in the peripheral nervous system and oligodendrocytes in the central nervous system (CNS). The axon is only in electrical contact with the extracellular fluid at the nodes between adjacent sheaths, and these can be spaced as far as 1.5 mm apart. This arrangement means that myelinated axons can only undergo action potentials at nodes. The action potential jumps along from node to node by saltatory conduction and can result in nerve conduction velocities as high as $120\,\text{ms}^{-1}$.

The synapse

Synapses are connections between neurons that allow information to be passed from one to the other. In general, neurons receive synaptic connections projected from many others. For example, a single lower motor neuron can receive synaptic connections from as many as 200,000 other neurons. Electrical synapses are direct electrical connections that contain channels passing between the neurons, but these are unusual in mammals and will not be considered further. The majority of mammalian synapses are chemical and employ neurotransmitters to transmit information. Figure 5.3 illustrates the neuromuscular junction, a specialised synapse connecting the lower motor neuron and its muscle fascicle. This is one of the most intensively studied synapses in the body and is the basis of much of our understanding of synaptic function.

Structure of chemical synapses

Chemical synapses consist of a presynaptic nerve terminal, a synaptic cleft between the neurons, and a protein-rich density adjacent to the postsynaptic membrane that often forms a protrusion of the postsynaptic membrane known as a dendritic spine. The presynaptic nerve terminal contains many vesicles of neurotransmitter that are bound to the cytoskeleton. The arrival of an action potential at the nerve terminal causes voltage-gated calcium channels present in that region of the plasma membrane to open leading to an increase in calcium permeability and an influx of calcium into the cytosol. This influx of calcium

triggers a series of events that ultimately lead to the fusion of some of the vesicles with the plasma membrane and the discharge of their neurotransmitters into the synaptic cleft. Once free in the cleft, the neurotransmitters diffuse toward the postsynaptic membrane and act as ligands for its receptors. A large number of neurotransmitters are used by different synapses including small molecules such as acetylcholine, biogenic amides such as serotonin or noradrenaline, amino acids such as glutamate, and neuropeptides such as the enkephalins.

Function of chemical synapses

The postsynaptic membrane contains receptors for the neurotransmitter, which can be of two kinds, ionotrophic or metabotrophic. Ionotrophic receptors consist of chemically gated ion channels that allow the influx of cations (usually sodium ions) in the case of excitatory synapses. In the case of inhibitory synapses, chemically gated ion channels allow the influx of anions (usually chloride ions) or the efflux of cations (usually potassium ions). Ionotrophic synapses contribute to alterations in the membrane potential of the local region of postsynaptic cell and so contribute to that cell's integration of information via excitatory or inhibitory postsynaptic potentials. Ionotrophic receptors typically take approximately 1 ms to activate and their effects last for approximately 50 ms. Metabotrophic receptors do not contain ion channels but affect the function of the postsynaptic neuron through second messenger systems often utilizing G-proteins. These systems do not contribute directly to the integration of information but can alter the responsiveness of the postsynaptic cell and are responsible for changes that take seconds to minutes to activate and can last for minutes or hours.

Fate of neurotransmitters

Following release into the synaptic cleft and stimulation of the postsynaptic receptor, neurotransmitters are removed from the cleft in readiness for the arrival of another action potential. Neurotransmitters are either lysed by enzymes present in the cleft or taken back up into the nerve terminal and stored in vesicles for reuse. In general, small molecules that do not require much energy to synthesize are destroyed, while more complex molecules are taken up by nerve terminals. For example, acetylcholine is cleaved by the enzyme acetylcholinesterase, but the amines are returned to vesicles for reuse. The neuroactive peptides are neither returned to the presynaptic nerve terminal nor broken down by specific enzymes. They diffuse away from their site of action and are lysed by tissue peptidases.

Synaptic blockade

Failure of synaptic transmission can have many causes including electrolyte imbalances, specific neurotoxins, and drugs. Synaptic blockade can occur due to interference

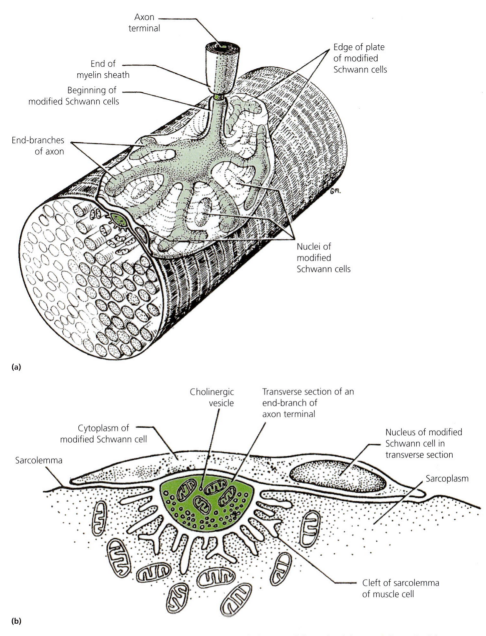

Figure 5.3 (a) Diagram of a skeletal muscle fiber and its motor end plate. Each branch of the axonal terminal forms a synaptic contact with the muscle fiber. (Reproduced from Ref. [2], © Wiley.) (b) Diagram of a synaptic contact with a motor end plate. This figure demonstrates an enlargement of a diagrammatic transverse section through the synaptic contact between an end branch of the axonal terminal and the underlying sarcolemma. (Reproduced from Ref. [2], © Wiley.)

with the process of synaptic transmission in a number of ways, four of which are clinically significant:

Presynaptic blockade: This kind of blockade occurs when the vesicles in the presynaptic nerve terminal are prevented from being released into the synaptic cleft.

This is characteristic of many neurotoxins such as botulinum and tetrodotoxin as well as electrolyte disturbances including hypocalcemia and hypermagnesemia. It can occur as a side effect of some drugs including the aminoglycoside antibiotics.

Competitive antagonism: This kind of blockade is seen with the use of nondepolarizing neuromuscular blocking agents that are sometimes used during clinical anesthesia. The neuromuscular blocker is a competitive antagonist at the postsynaptic acetylcholine receptor.

Direct depolarization: This kind of blockade is seen when drugs such as suxamethonium chloride are used clinically. These drugs stimulate the acetylcholine receptors of the postsynaptic membrane of the neuromuscular junction but are not rapidly metabolized and so remain active. Following initial stimulation, there is a prolonged refractory period of muscle paralysis. This drug is no longer widely used in equine anesthesia, and so its effects are of mostly historical interest.

Indirect depolarization: This is seen when the neurotransmitter is not removed from the synaptic cleft sufficiently rapidly to allow its effects to wane. Functionally it is similar to a direct depolarizing blockade. Examples of this include the action of antiacetylcholinesterases such as organophosphates, which allow acetylcholine to accumulate at the neuromuscular junction, and the monoamine oxidase inhibitors, which reduce the breakdown of the biogenic amines.

Metabolic aspects of neuronal function

Vesicles

The vesicles that manage the storage and release of neurotransmitters in the synaptic cleft are manufactured in the endoplasmic reticulum of the neuronal soma. They are transported to the presynaptic nerve terminal by means of the fast axonal transport system. This is an ATP-requiring process that transports the vesicles via a series of interaction between proteins in the surface membrane of the vesicle and proteins attached to the neuronal cytoskeleton. Once they arrive at the nerve terminal, the vesicles remain attached to the cytoskeleton until they are activated by calcium ions and fuse with the cell membrane discharging their neurotransmitter into the synaptic cleft. Following the release of neurotransmitter, vesicles containing small-molecule neurotransmitters are reformed by separation from the neuronal cell membrane, refilled with neurotransmitter, and attached to the cytoskeleton. This cycle of discharge and reformation occurs over a time frame of approximately 30s and continues throughout the life span of the vesicle. After several cycles of neurotransmitter release and reformation, degraded vesicles are returned to the neuronal soma to be broken down.

The various processes in the life cycle of the vesicle involve complex interactions that are managed by interactions between proteins on the outer surface of the vesicle, the inner surface of the cell membrane, and the cytoskeletal structure. Many of these interactions are energy-dependant and are driven by ATP. Many disease processes interfere with the vesicular lifecycle; for example, botulinum toxin induces the degradation of synaptosomal-associated protein-25 (SNAP-25) necessary for vesicular fusion to the cell membrane. This degradation prevents neurotransmitter release and leads to failure of synaptic conduction.

Molecular biology of neurotransmitters

Neurotransmitters are signaling molecules that are involved in the transmission of information across chemical synapses. The definition of a neurotransmitter is somewhat imprecise, but a molecule must usually fulfill four criteria to be considered a neurotransmitter (Table 5.1)

Three main classes of neurotransmitter are found in the mammalian nervous system: small molecules, neuroactive peptides, and unconventional transmitters. There are only a few small-molecule neurotransmitters including acetylcholine; biogenic amines such as adrenaline, dopamine, and serotonin; and some amino acids such as glutamate and adenosine. In contrast, more than 50 peptide molecules can act as neurotransmitters including somatostatin, vasopressin, β-endorphin, substance P, calcitonin, etc. The unconventional neurotransmitters include such molecules as nitric oxide, ATP, and hydrogen sulfide. These molecules have actions resembling those of the more conventional neurotransmitters, but often they do not fulfill all of the four criteria.

Small-molecule and peptide neurotransmitters differ in a number of ways including their site of synthesis, the type of vesicle in which they are stored, and the mechanism of their release. Neuroactive peptides require protein synthetic mechanisms for their manufacture and so are only formed in the neuronal soma. Conversely, the small-molecule neurotransmitters are mostly manufactured locally within nerve terminals. Following their

Table 5.1 Criteria for a chemical to be considered a neurotransmitter.

It is synthesized by the neuron
It is present in the synaptic cleft in sufficient quantities to have an effect on the postsynaptic neuron of effector organ
When administered exogenously in reasonable concentrations, it exactly mimics the effect of the endogenously released transmitter
A specific mechanism exists for its removal from the site of action

release into the synaptic cleft, small-molecule neurotransmitters or their components are rapidly taken back into the presynaptic neuron and concentrated back into vesicles. There are no reuptake mechanisms for neuroactive peptides, rather they diffuse away from the site of action and are degraded by extracellular peptidases. Neuroactive peptides are stored in dense-core vesicles that are manufactured and filled with neurotransmitter in the Golgi apparatus. They lack several proteins that are required for vesicle recycling and so are used only once in contrast to the recycling of vesicles containing small-molecule neurotransmitters outlined earlier. The process of neurotransmitter release and reformation for vesicles containing small molecules is specialized and unique to their situation. Vesicles containing neuroactive peptides release them using the same secretory mechanism that is utilized by other cellular secretory processes.

Composition of extracellular fluid

The extracellular fluid of the CNS is protected by the blood–brain barrier (BBB), and so its composition is more similar to cerebrospinal fluid (CSF) than it is to plasma. There are a variety of transport mechanisms that control the movement of molecules across this barrier and many of these are specific to this location. Consequently, the extracellular fluid of the CNS shows many differences to that of the rest of the body. In particular, it has very low protein content, approximately 2/3 of the glucose concentration, fewer ionic cations, and a more acidic pH. The production, composition, and analysis of CSF are discussed in detail in Chapter 2.

The differences between the extracellular environment of the CNS and that of the body can be problematical in certain disease conditions because different CSF components equilibrate across the BBB at different rates. For example, CO_2 equilibrates rapidly but bicarbonate ions much more slowly. This means that a developing acidosis can be transiently more severe within the CNS space as CO_2 can increase more rapidly than the compensating bicarbonate buffering system. In extreme cases, this can cause neuronal dysfunction and lead to the development of cerebral edema.

Glia

The glia comprise all the cells of the nervous system that are not neuronal. There are several major types of glia in the CNS each serving a number of specific purposes. The following section will primarily focus on the microglia that are responsible for immunological function within the CNS as an understanding of their role is important in the consideration of many clinical syndromes.

Astrocytes

These are the most abundant glial cells. They undertake a number of roles such as removal of neurotransmitters and regulation of extracellular ion concentrations that help to control the environment of the neurons. Although they do not form the BBB themselves, it is thought that they are responsible for initiating the change in the capillary endothelial cells within the CNS that leads to the formation of this structure.

Oligodendrocytes

The oligodendrocytes form myelin sheaths around CNS neurites. Their role is equivalent to that of the Schwann cells in the peripheral nervous system.

Ependymal cells

These cells line the cavities of the CNS. They secrete CSF and have ciliated membranes that aid with its circulation. It is also possible that they act as neural stem cells.

Radial glia

These are very important in the developing nervous system. Most glia of this type do not persist postnatally.

Microglia

Microglia are macrophages that have become resident in the CNS. The presence of the BBB means that large structures have difficult access into the CNS; this includes infective agents such as bacteria and viruses but also large protein molecules such as antibodies. For this reason, the CNS is considered to be an immunologically privileged area. The microglia are the first and main form of active immune response in the CNS. Microglia perform the functions of scavenging foreign material and damaged cells from the CNS and perform the roles of recognition and phagocytosis as well as acting as antigen-presenting cells. The absence of antibodies requires them to be extremely sensitive to even small changes in the CNS environment, and this is achieved by the expression of unique membrane proteins including potassium channels that respond to very small alterations in extracellular potassium concentration.

Microglia originate from the bone marrow and are part of the monocyte cell lineage. They travel to the CNS as monocytes and further differentiate into microglia *in situ*. The BBB is relatively difficult for cells to cross and so unlike monocytes, microglia have an extremely long life span in their downregulated form. Once activated, they proliferate extremely rapidly to deal with any infections or foreign material. In extreme cases of CNS infection, the BBB is damaged and the microglia are joined by other immune cells such as macrophages and myeloid progenitor cells. Once the infection has subsided, BBB integrity is restored and only microglia are present in the later stages of the response. The wide role of microglia requires them to be very flexible, and they can undergo a variety of structural changes depending upon their location and current role. They are divided into six subtypes, which are as follows:

Amoeboid: In this form, microglia are mobile and phagocytic. They are able to scavenge cellular debris but do not act as antigen-presenting cells. This form is particularly prevalent in the developing CNS and in areas of plasticity and remodeling.

Ramified: This is the resting form of microglia. It is found throughout the CNS and has the appearance of a small cellular body with long branching ramifications. The cell body is relatively motionless, while the ramifications move through the surrounding area of the cell surveying for foreign material. The ramified form is unable to express many of the proteins required for immunological function and maintains a constant presence of potential response to infection while preserving a very low-level immune environment.

Activated (nonphagocytic and phagocytic): The nonphagocytic activated form is seen as microglia move from the ramified to the fully active state. Following stimulation by cytokines, cell necrosis factors, lipopolysaccharides or a number of other microenvironmental stimuli, they undergo morphological and functional changes and begin to express cytotoxic factors. The phagocytic form is the fully activated form. It has an amoeboid appearance and performs all the immunogenic roles of the microglia. In the face of immunological challenge, activated phagocytic microglia are capable of rapid proliferation.

Gitter cells: These are the eventual result of the process of phagocytosis. The cell takes on a granular appearance and persists as a means of sequestrating the foreign material in an inactive state. Gitter cells are characteristic of healed areas of infection.

Perivascular: Perivascular microglia perform all the functions of normal microglia in the area around the basal lamina of the vascular tree. They are embedded into the walls of the blood vessels. Unlike other microglia, they are regularly replaced by precursor cells from the bone marrow.

Juxtavascular: Juxtavascular microglia make contact with the basal lamina of the blood vessels but are not embedded within them. Both perivascular and juxtavascular microglia express immunological proteins even at low levels of activation.

A further discussion of the immune response of the CNS is found in Chapter 3.

References

[1] Aidley, D. (1998) *The Physiology of Excitable Cells*, 4th edn, Cambridge University Press, New York.
[2] King, A.S. (1999) *Physiological and Clinical Anatomy of the Domestic Animals*, vol. 1, Blackwell Science, Oxford.

Further Reading

Kandel, E.R., Schwartz, J.H., Jessell, T.M., Siegelbaum, S.A. and Hudspeth, A.J. (eds) (2012) *Principles of Neural Science*, 5th edn, McGraw-Hill, New York.
Kaur, C. and Eng-Ang, L. (2012) *Microglia: Biology, Functions and Roles in Disease*, Nova Publishers, New York.
Kettenmann, H. and Ransom, B.R. (eds) (2012) *Neuroglia*, 3rd edn, Oxford University Press, Oxford.
Siksou, L., Triller, A. and Serge, M. (2011) Ultrastructural organization of presynaptic terminals. *Curr Opin Neurobiol*, 21, 261–268.

SECTION 2
Clinical Equine Neurology

6 Examination of the Nervous System

Martin Furr[1] and Stephen Reed[2]

[1] Marion duPont Scott Equine Medical Center, Virginia-Maryland Regional College of Veterinary Medicine, Leesburg, USA
[2] Rood and Riddle Equine Hospital, Lexington, USA

Many veterinarians feel that the evaluation of neurologic disease is a complicated and difficult procedure. In fact, neurologic examination is straightforward and relatively simple; interpretation requires knowledge of equine neurologic disorders, as well as a basic understanding of equine neuroanatomy. The key to a successful neurologic examination is to do the examination in a consistent and organized fashion. It is important to develop a routine and then do it the same way each time. This approach ensures that some parts of the examination are not forgotten, as well as increases the consistency of the examination as many horses performing the same maneuver are seen. A standardized examination form is a valuable aid in this, and it can be concise (Figure 6.1).

It is also important to recognize that the neurologic examination should not take place "in a vacuum"—it is only one part of a complete physical examination and will be used in concert with the other physical examination findings to reach a final conclusion about the horse. Musculoskeletal disease should always be considered. In horses demonstrating pelvic limb abnormalities, a rectal examination is often advisable to rule out the presence of pelvic injuries and to confirm the presence of aortic pulses. Signalment and history should not be overlooked. Determining vaccination history is important, as is housing and husbandry, the nature and quantity of feed, and if there has been any change in type of feed or hay and source, or new deliveries of foodstuffs. This information may help to elucidate the potential for feed-related toxicity. The owner or caretakers should be questioned about any other medical history or history of falls or injuries in the past. Often owners do not offer such information, as they are not aware of the potential connection between past (seemingly minor) events and current problems. The specific history of the illness should be determined regarding nature of onset and progression. This "severity vs. time" information finds acute onset in horses with trauma or infection, a slowly progressive course in horses with equine protozoal myeloencephalitis (EPM) or equine degenerative encephalomyelitis (EDEM), and a chronic fluctuating course in horses with cervical spinal cord compression.

The goals of the neurologic examination are (i) to determine if disease of the nervous system exists, (ii) to localize the lesion to a particular area of the nervous system, and (iii) to describe and record the responses as a baseline for future evaluations. In addition, repeated examinations over time may provide information that is useful in the diagnosis of various disorders. In general, one should attempt to explain all observed abnormalities with a single lesion; if this is not possible, then diffuse or multifocal disease is present. Finally, it is important to distinguish primary neurologic abnormalities from secondary changes (e.g., dehydration with associated mental dullness and muscular weakness) and their effects.

The specific order of examination is not of particular importance; however, a "nose-to-tail" approach is employed by most clinicians as being the most convenient. The evaluation is begun by a general observation of the horse, including its attitude and alertness, head and body position, position of the limbs, and symmetry of muscle development. The horse should be alert and should respond to the examiner and its environment. The horse should be observed from a short distance initially for any unusual behavior, presence of a head tilt, yawning, or muscle fasciculations. Subtle abnormalities are more easily seen when the horse is relaxed and may be hidden once the horse is handled. The horse's general posture and body position should be noted. The limbs should be evenly and squarely placed under the horse at each "corner of the horse's body"—abnormal limb position should alert the examiner to potential deficits of proprioception. If suspected, the presence of proprioceptive deficits should be further evaluated during the gait analysis.

Equine Neurology, Second Edition. Martin Furr and Stephen Reed.
© 2015 John Wiley & Sons, Inc. Published 2015 by John Wiley & Sons, Inc.
Companion website: www.wiley.com/go/furr/neurology

Neurologic Examination

Owner: _____   Horse: _____

Behavior/Mentation: _____

Head/Neck posture: _____

	Left	Right
Vision		
Menace		
Pupil/PCR		
Horners		
Strabismus		
Facial sens		
Facial symmetry		
Nystagmus: Resting Positional		
Head tilt		
Swallow/voice	Norm	Abnorm
Slap test	Norm	Abnorm
Tongue tone	Norm	Abnorm

Grade 0-No deficits

Grade 1-Just detected at a normal gait, but worsened by backing, turning, loin pressure or neck extension

Grade 2-Deficit easily detected at normal gait and exaggerated by backing, turning, swaying, loin pressure, and neck extension

Grade 3-Deficit very prominent on walking, with a tendency to buckle or fall with backing, turning, loin pressure, or neck extension

Grade 4-Stumbling, tripping, and falling spontaneously

Grade 5-Horse recumbent

Gait Assessment (0–5 as above)

	Thoracic Left	Thoracic Right	Pelvic Left	Pelvic Right
Paresis				
Ataxia				
Spasticity				
Dysmetria				

Neck and forelimbs	L	R	Hindlimbs	L	R	Tail and Anus	L	R
Muscle mass			Muscle mass			Muscle tone		
Sensation			Sensation			Sensation		
Hop			Placing			Reflexes		
Placing			Strength			Strength		

(Normal = 2, decreased=1, exaggerated = 3, absent = 0)

Comments:_____

Date:_____   Examiner:_____

Figure 6.1 An example of a neurologic examination form.

Behavior, mental status, and coordination of the head

The components of the neurologic examination include a general assessment of alertness and mentation; a cranial nerve examination; limb and placing responses; gait analysis; and tail, anal, and cutaneous trunci reflexes (Figure 6.2).

Changes in mentation or behavior can be difficult for the clinician to assess but are aided by careful observation and input from the owner or caretaker about the horses' normal behavior and any changes that may have occurred. Behavior is strongly influenced by variables such as age, breed, and gender, and these factors should be considered when making an assessment. Behavioral changes may be intermittent or continuous. Adopting abnormal postures or head pressing, however, are readily noted and are clear signs of cerebral disease. Head pressing or compulsive walking suggests diffuse

encephalopathy, while circling is associated with asymmetric forebrain lesions (Figure 6.3). Consciousness and mental alertness is mediated by the ascending reticular activating system of the central nervous system (CNS) and the cerebral hemispheres. Assessment of the state of consciousness is recorded in a decreasing continuum as alert, depression, stupor, semicomatose, or comatose. Horses that are mentally depressed react to their environment or stimulation in an inappropriate or diminished manner. Stupor describes a horse that appears asleep yet responds to sound, light, or noxious stimuli. Semicoma is the state of partial responsiveness to stimuli, and coma is the state of complete unresponsiveness to stimuli. The determination of state of consciousness is made by observation of the interaction with their external environment and their response to noxious stimuli such as a skin pinch.

The position and coordination of the head should be examined while the horse is at rest and relaxed. The head should be symmetrical and held straight upright when viewed from the front. Head posture and coordination

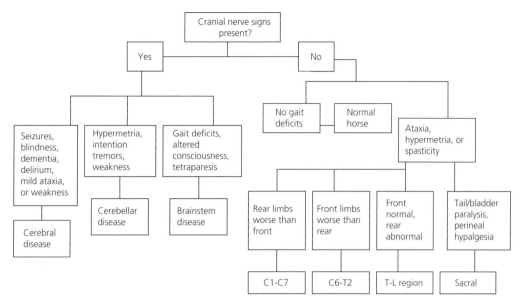

Figure 6.2 A flowchart demonstrating how the results of the neurologic examination can be used to aid the clinician in neuroanatomic localization. Ideally, the clinician should try to make one lesion explain all clinical signs. Combinations of clinical signs that cannot be explained by one site of disease imply diffuse or multifocal disease.

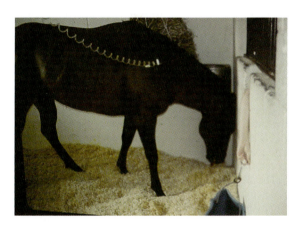

Figure 6.3 A horse with diffuse encephalitis demonstrating head pressing.

are controlled by the cerebellum and vestibular regions of the CNS in response to sensory input from the head, limbs, and trunk. Smooth coordination of head movements is controlled by the cerebellum, and cerebellar disease results in jerky, bobbing movements of the head, which are made worse when the horse attempts to prehend food. Lateral deviation of the head and neck should be differentiated from a head tilt. Lateral deviation of the head suggests asymmetrical forebrain disease, cervical soft tissue, or bone disease. When viewed from the side, the horse's head should be held higher than the withers; a lower resting position is seen in diseases

causing diffuse neuromuscular weakness (e.g., botulism) or cervical pain. The willingness of the horse to flex its neck should be determined by offering grain or grass and slowly withdrawing it to the point of the shoulder. Normal horses will follow the offered feed easily by lateral flexion of the neck. Horses with neck pain will either resist turning the neck and back up or turn the head on its side and flex at the poll to reach the feed. Passive flexion of the neck can be performed by pulling the horse head laterally; normal horses will have substantial freedom of movement and the head can be turned easily. Animals with neck pain will resist this or back up to (seemingly) relieve the pressure on their neck.

Cranial nerves

The tests listed in Figure 6.1 and Table 6.1 are sufficient to provide a complete evaluation of the cranial nerves and can be quickly performed during a routine physical examination.

Olfaction is not routinely tested, and vision is assessed by observation of the horse's movements in an unfamiliar environment or the presence/absence of a menace response. It should be noted, however, that cerebellar disease can result in a loss of the menace response in a visual horse. Other signs of cerebellar disease (such as intention tremors or hypermetric gait) should be present if this is the cause of the altered menace response. The menace response can be difficult

Table 6.1 Tests of cranial nerve function.

Test	Nerve tested	Abnormal response/interpretation
Menace	Optic, facial	No eye blink; blindness. Must differentiate blindness from facial nerve dysfunction
Pupillary light response	Optic, oculomotor	No response to bright light directed in eye
Horner's syndrome	Cervical sympathetic	Sweating around base of ear and eye, ptosis
Facial sensation	Trigeminal (sensory)	Failure to respond to stimulation of facial skin
Facial symmetry	Facial (motor)	Asymmetry of muzzle, with or without ear droop, food impacted in cheek
Palpebral reflex	Trigeminal, facial (motor)	Failure to blink
Nystagmus	Oculomotor, vestibular system	Central lesions associated with positional nystagmus; peripheral lesions are nonpositional
Swallow	Glossopharyngeal, vagus	Inability to swallow as determined by observation or passing of stomach tube
Tongue tone	Hypoglossal	Failure to withdraw tongue or tongue weak when pulled

to elicit in some circumstances, such as horses that are mentally depressed or are stoic. In addition to the menace test, one can test vision by walking the horse through a maze constructed of items that cannot injure the horse should it step in or on them. The fundus and optic disk should always be examined with an ophthalmoscope. Pupil size, position, and symmetry should be evaluated and the direct and consensual pupillary light response evaluated. In normalcy, a bright light directed into one eye should result in constriction of both the ipsilateral eye as well as the contralateral eye (consensual response). Observation of the consensual response is often difficult for one examiner to perform in large animals, hence the "swinging-light" test has been described [1]. From a distance of about 18 in, the light is shown alternately into each eye, and the more powerful, direct light response is seen as the beam reaches it. Due to the unequal crossing of optic nerve axons at the optic chiasm in horses, a lesion in the eye, optic nerve, or optic tract results in ipsilateral pupillary dilation. The swinging-light test takes advantage of the fact that the ipsilateral pupillary light response is more powerful than the contralateral (consensual) response. The pathway for this response involves the optic nerve and chiasma, then through the optic tracts in the midbrain to the oculomotor nuclei. The motor pathway arises from these nuclei, traveling via the oculomotor nerve to the ciliary ganglia, then to the pupillary constrictor muscles. The nerve tracts for the pupillary light response are within the brainstem and are not affected by lesions of the visual cortex. A widely dilated pupil in a visual eye suggests oculomotor nerve damage—there will be no direct or consensual light response (see video clips demonstrating clinical signs for videos).

The oculomotor nerve (cranial nerve (CN) 3) also innervates the extraocular muscles of the eye, and along with the trochlear (CN 4) and abducens nerves (CN 6) controls eye position. These nerves are tested by observation of eye position and motion and abnormalities of

the nerves results in an abnormal eye position (strabismus). When the nose is elevated, the eyes should move ventrally to maintain a horizontal gaze (the "Dolls eye" reflex). When the head is moved from side to side, the eyes should move slowly opposite the direction of the movement of the head, then move quickly in the direction of the head movement. This is referred to as a "normal vestibular" nystagmus, and its presence suggests an intact vestibular system, as well as normal function of CN 3 (Oculomotor N.), 4 (Trochlear N.), and 6 (Abducens N.). Spontaneous or positional nystagmus is always abnormal. Intact sympathetic innervation to the eye is evaluated by observation for Horner's syndrome. In this condition (see Chapter 9 for a more detailed discussion), disruption of sympathetic innervation results in pupillary constriction, ptosis of the upper eyelid, and protrusion of the nictitating membrane. Sweating of the cranial neck extending to the base of the ear is also associated. Mechanical deviations of the eye due to trauma, swelling, or periorbital disease may also occur and should be considered (Figures 6.4 and 6.5).

The head should be examined for facial symmetry, reflecting function of CN 7 (Facial N.), and facial sensation, which is solely mediated by CN 5 (Trigeminal N.). The motor branch of CN 5 is evaluated by observation of the ability to chew, as well as evaluation of the masseter and temporal muscles, which will atrophy if CN 5 is damaged. The head should also be examined for a head tilt, in which the poll is deviated toward the affected side. This reflects dysfunction of the vestibular system, which may be centrally or peripherally located. Central vestibular disease results in a nystagmus, which varies with different head positions ("positional nystagmus"), while peripheral vestibular disease is nonpositional. To further test the vestibular system, a blindfold can be applied and the horse observed for a head tilt. This may be valuable in subtle cases or those in which there has been some compensation. If a head tilt already exists, blindfolding is neither necessary nor advisable.

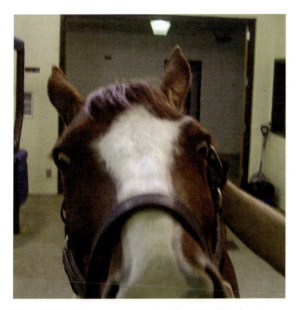

Figure 6.4 Strabismus can sometimes be elicited by elevating the patient's head and observing for a normal change in eye position. This horse demonstrates a mild ventral strabismus in the left eye.

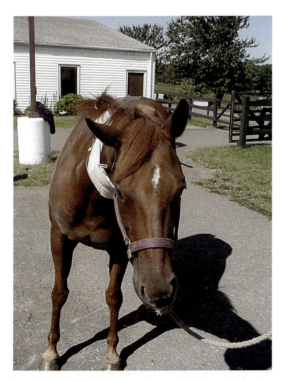

Figure 6.5 Right-sided facial paralysis and mild vestibular signs (body lean) associated with bacterial meningitis.

Swallowing is mediated by input from both the glossopharyngeal nerve (CN 9) and the vagus (CN 10). Swallowing can be evaluated by observation of normal mastication and swallowing, the "gag" reflex, or by passing a stomach tube. Pharyngeal function and the swallowing reflex can also be tested by observation with an endoscope. With the endoscope positioned in the pharynx, the wall of the pharynx and arytenoid cartilages can be touched with a probe and swallowing observed. The horse may be unable to swallow, or may swallow weakly, resulting in a dorsally displaced soft palate, which they are then unable to reduce. Stertorous breathing may be found in horses with bilateral pharyngeal or laryngeal paralysis.

Additional means to evaluate pharyngeal/laryngeal function include the "slap test" (laryngeal adductory test) [2]. In this test, the larynx is observed with an endoscope as the saddle area is slapped with moderate intensity. A normal response is an adductory flick of the contralateral arytenoid cartilage. Overstimulation (repeated slaps) results in a blunted laryngeal adductory response and should be avoided. Failure to demonstrate adductory laryngeal response after the slap test has been associated with cervical spinal cord lesions in a high percentage of cases [2]. In another report, however, the slap test was found to have a low sensitivity (50–58%) and specificity (69–75%) [3]. The test is difficult to interpret in young animals or horses with laryngeal hemiplegia. If an endoscope is not available, then the larynx can be palpated to detect contraction following the slap. This is less sensitive than the endoscopic method, however. Overall, the laryngeal adductory test appears to have very little utility in the evaluation of cervical spinal cord disease.

Tongue tone is dependent upon the function of the hypoglossal nerve (CN 12) and can be tested by grasping the tongue and applying gentle traction. Inability to resist or withdraw the tongue suggests hypoglossal nerve damage. Atrophy of the tongue has also been described secondary to hypoglossal nerve injury.

Skin, trunk, and cutaneous trunci reflexes

The cervical reflexes should be examined. The cervicoauricular reflex (also called cervicofacial) is elicited by lightly tapping the skin between the jugular groove and the crest at the level of C2. A positive response is for the horse to flick the ear forward. Other authors have also reported a pulling back of the lips ("smile" reflex) as well as the local muscle contraction and ear movement [1, 4]. An additional cervical reflex is the "local cervical" reflex noted between C3 and C6. Tapping the skin in the area between the crest and the jugular groove will result in local muscle contraction. This response is not as vigorous as the cutaneous trunci reflex over the trunk. Abnormalities of these reflexes have been noted in horses with cervical spinal cord disease [5]. Peripheral neuropathy due to arthritic compression of spinal nerves will also lead to an abnormal response.

The cutaneous trunci reflex is tested by stimulating the skin over the trunk, then observing for a "skin-flick" response. Perianal skin reactions should be evaluated, for loss of this response is characteristic of horses with herpes virus myeloencephalitis, for example. In addition, it may be altered in horses with cauda equina syndrome.

The tail carriage and anal tone and reflex should be examined. Normal tail carriage is straight down, with normal movement in all directions. Most normal horses will clamp the tail if it is grasped and raised. Stimulation of the anus should result in a strong tail clamp and sometimes a "squatting" position. Abnormalities of tail strength and anal reflex may be seen in horses with botulism or inflammation of the cauda equina. Elevated tail carriage is commonly seen in horses with equine lower motor neuron (LMN) disease. Hyperesthesia with skin damage and sensitivity can also be seen around the perianal region in horses with cauda equina; this may progress to hypalgesia.

Limb placement

These tests can be quickly performed and have value in detecting muscular weakness and conscious proprioceptive deficits. Abnormal limb positions, particularly a base-wide stance in the front limbs, may also be associated with vestibular disease. Limb placement tests are easier to perform and interpret on the front limbs. Typically, one front hoof is lifted then placed across the other front leg. Horses should quickly move the hoof back into a normal position or resist placement into an abnormal position. An abnormal response is to leave the hoof in this crossed position for a prolonged period (usually more than several seconds) or to attempt to move the foot back to a normal position but have difficulty in doing so. The demeanor and training of the horse must be carefully considered—a slow response in a 3-year-old Thoroughbred in race training is abnormal, but a similar response in an aged gelding may be normal. Placing the foot (either front or rear) in a base-wide position can also be performed, and the expected response is for the horse to return the foot into a normal position. Limb placement tests in horses appear to have a low sensitivity for the detection of abnormalities of the CNS, and these tests should be coupled with careful observation of foot placement during dynamic maneuvers (Figures 6.6 and 6.7).

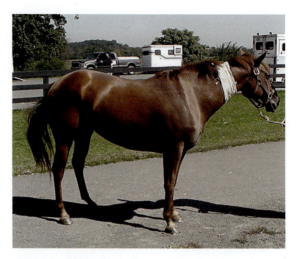

Figure 6.6 Adopting unusual postures at rest is a sign of conscious proprioceptive deficit, and the horse in this photo demonstrates a classic base-wide stance in the pelvic limbs.

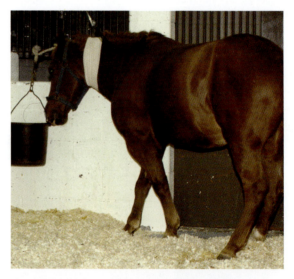

Figure 6.7 Conscious proprioceptive deficits expressed as crossed limbs in the thoracic limbs and a base-wide stance in the pelvic limbs. In addition, the pelvic limbs are placed too far cranially under the horse's body, which is typical of horses with conscious proprioceptive deficit.

Gait analysis

Gait is evaluated as an assessment of brainstem, spinal cord, and peripheral nerve function. Normal function of muscles, joints, and tendons is also necessary for a normal gait. The gait analysis is the process of evaluating the horse in motion at a walk and possibly trot and when the horse is asked to perform certain maneuvers that "challenge" specific functions of the nervous system. These include waking with the head elevated, downhill, backing, turning in tight circles, or moving over or around obstacles. Specific neurological abnormalities that are observed during this phase of the examination include ataxia, paresis and dysmetria or spasticity, and deficits of proprioception (see video clips demonstrating clinical signs for videos).

Ataxia

Ataxia refers to a lack of coordination of motor movements due to sensory dysfunction and may arise from disease of the vestibular system, cerebellum, or spinal cord [6]. Spinal ataxia seems to predominate in the horse, associated with interruption of proprioceptive (ascending) input to the cerebellum. Ataxia is a description of clinical signs, rather than a specific diagnosis, and it may occur alone or with spasticity or paresis. Ataxia arising from spinal cord disease is frequently associated with paresis [6], and it is often difficult to discriminate between the two deficits in clinical cases. Cerebellar ataxia is seen in foals with cerebellar abiotrophy, and rarely in inflammatory disease of the CNS, and is characterized by symmetric ataxia with intention tremors and retention of strength. Vestibular ataxia is usually associated with a head tilt and asymmetric ataxia (see Neuroanatomic discussion of ataxia in Chapter 1).

Ataxia is expressed in the horse as truncal sway, weaving during walking (i.e., placing feet out of line from one step to the next), crossing over when turning, or pivoting on the inside limb when spun. Additional signs include weaving of the affected limb during the swing phase of the stride resulting in abnormal foot placement. Many horses that are ataxic will also pace; this is significant only in breeds in which the pace is not a natural gait. Signs of ataxia are most noticeable at changes of speed and direction. Careful observation of the horse when turning in hand may reveal abducted or adducted foot placement, or pivoting. If abruptly pulled up from a trot in hand, ataxic horses will often crouch and go base-wide in the rear limbs. Signs of ataxia will be exacerbated when the horse is walked on a slope or with its head elevated.

Weakness

Weakness (paresis) is a deficiency of voluntary movement arising from a reduction in normal muscular power. Paresis can arise from damage to upper motor neurons (UMNs), LMNs, or muscle itself. UMN weakness results from disorders that affect the UMN or their axons in the cerebral cortex, subcortical white matter, brainstem, or spinal cord. UMN weakness is induced by decreased activation of LMNs and may be accompanied

Table 6.2 Clinical signs that help to differentiate upper motor neuron (UMN) and lower motor neuron (LMN) disease.

LMN weakness	UMN weakness
Flaccid	Spasticity
Decreased tone	Increased tone
Diminished reflex response	Exaggerated reflex response
Profound muscle atrophy	Minimal muscle atrophy
Fasciculations present	Fasciculations absent

by spasticity. LMNs are composed of the spinal cord grey matter, peripheral nerves, or neuromuscular junction. Differentiation between UMN and LMN disease may help with neuroanatomic localization and understanding the distribution of the lesion resulting in the observed clinical signs. For example, horses with both UMN and LMN abnormalities in different limbs must have multifocal disease. Table 6.2 describes clinical signs that can aid in the differentiation of UMN and LMN disease.

Weak horses have a low arc of foot flight, stumble, and have a poor response to the sway test. An additional sign of weakness in the horse is knuckling when going downhill or difficulty when hopping on one thoracic limb ("hop test"). The sway test demonstrates an animal's ability to resist being pushed off balance. When pushed at the withers, most adult horses should be able to resist or quickly step sideways if pushed off balance. Weak horses cannot resist and recover poorly (slowly) after being pushed sideways. A similar procedure is used in the rear limbs and is referred to as the "tail-pull." In this test, the horse is pulled sideways using the tail. Most adult horses can easily resist even a strong pull. This test should also be done when the horse is walking. As the horse is walking, the tail should be strongly pulled to the side then released; this should be repeated several times at different phases of the stride. Normal horses should quickly correct rear limb position with the next stride, while paretic horses are more easily pulled off balance, may take several strides to recover, or interfere while attempting to correct. Horses that demonstrate good rear limb strength standing still but are weak when walking usually have UMN weakness. This is in contrast to horses with LMN weakness, which are weak both when walking and standing still.

Horses with generalized weakness demonstrate a lowered head carriage, shuffling gait (i.e., dragging all four hooves), and reduced resistance to tail pulling and front limb hopping. Other signs of generalized weakness may include reduced tail clamp, slow eating, or dysphagia. In such horses, disease of the muscles or neuromuscular junction should be considered.

Dysmetria

Dysmetria refers to a gait in which the limb movements are either hypermetric or hypometric. A hypermetric/dysmetric gait is characterized with an exaggerated range of motion and excessive joint movement and is associated with cerebellar and spinal cord (spinocerebellar) disease. This can be expressed as limb stiffness and decreased joint flexion and gives the appearance of a "tin-soldier" walk. An exaggerated or prolonged flight phase can be observed in horses when going downhill or with the head elevated. Spasticity is an increase in muscle tone that primarily affects antigravity muscles. Spasticity is velocity-dependant and demonstrates a sudden release after reaching a maximum muscle tension (the "clasp-knife reflex"). Spasticity is generally associated with UMN disease and is due to the reduced inhibition of extensor motor neurons. Spasticity is most easily demonstrated in recumbent animals, but the "bouncing" gait seen in rear limbs of horses with cervical lesions may be an expression of spasticity and exaggerated extensor tone.

Proprioception

The characteristic of proprioception is the ability to recognize the position of the limbs, body, and head in space. Conscious proprioception is mediated by the cerebral cortex, while unconscious proprioception is integrated by the cerebellum. Tests of proprioception commonly used in small animals are difficult to evaluate or perform in the horse, and proprioception is best evaluated by dynamic observation. An exception to this generalization may be front limb hopping, which can be performed in the adult horse. In this test one front limb is held up, and the examiner pushes the horse sideways until the horse hops sideways to keep its balance. The authors have found this test difficult to interpret in clinical patients as muscle weakness can complicate the result. In addition, the examiner must choose the footing for performing this test with care to avoid injury to the horse or examiner should the horse fall. Another approach to testing proprioception is to place a limb in an unnatural position (i.e., very base-wide) and observe the horse for correction; failure to do so suggests a deficit of conscious proprioception. Clinical signs associated with proprioceptive loss include a base-wide stance, abnormal position of the limbs after coming to a stop, and truncal sway (if severe). When spun in a tight circle, the outside limb may be abducted, the horse may pivot on the affected limb, or cross the rear limb over the other. Extending (elevating) the head often increases the degree of incoordination and deficit. There is obvious overlap in the signs associated with proprioceptive deficit, dysmetria, and paresis, and discriminating the major component of the ataxia is often difficult (Figures 6.8 and 6.9).

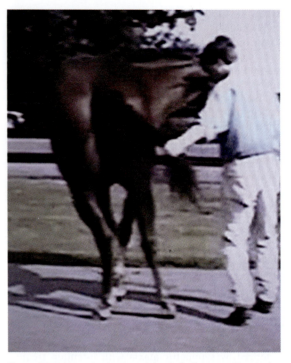

Figure 6.8 When spinning in a tight circle, horses with spinal ataxia will demonstrate various deficits. The horse in this photo demonstrates delayed movement of the rear limbs, resulting in the body "leaning." Normal horses will move the rear limbs sooner such that the leg remains under the horse's body as it turns.

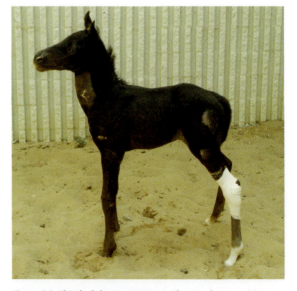

Figure 6.9 This foal demonstrates an abnormal "star-gazing" posture due to bilateral cortical blindness.

Examination procedure

Each examiner can establish their own approach to performing the gait analysis. The authors generally first observe the horse being led at a walk from the front, back, and side. It is helpful to walk alongside the horse, matching speed, and concentrate on detecting the various gait deficits. Each limb should be observed independently and is scored using a standardized scoring system. Use of this scoring system is important as it helps to localize neurologic deficits and serves as a "benchmark" in future examinations to monitor progress (Table 6.3).

The horse is then walked with the head elevated, and standing and walking tail-pulls are performed, followed by backing the horse. Backing will exacerbate proprioceptive deficits and ataxia, which are demonstrated by abnormal (usually base-wide) limb placement and dragging of the hooves. Limb placement, front limb hopping tests, tests of the cutaneous trunci reflex, and anal tone are evaluated next, and the horse is spun in a tight circle. It is important not to spin the horse for prolonged periods as this confuses the evaluation by making the horse dizzy. The spin should be limited to about three times around, after which the examiner should then stop and allow the horse several seconds to regain its balance. If necessary, the test can be repeated. The final test is to lead the horse down an incline with the head in a neutral position, then again with the head elevated. Walking the horse in a serpentine over a curb can also be done and is a good test of limb placement, strength, and coordination. Passive and active flexion of the neck should also be evaluated. If the neurologic signs are subtle, then jogging the horse on a straight line and in a circle are helpful to rule out musculoskeletal disease.

Table 6.3 Grading system for gait analysis.

Grade	Description
0	No neurologic deficits detected
1	Neurologic deficits just detected at a normal gait but worsened by backing, turning, loin pressure, or neck extension
2	Neurologic deficits easily detected at the walk and exaggerated by backing, turning, loin pressure, or neck extension
3	Neurologic deficits prominent at the walk, with a tendency to buckle or fall with backing, turning, loin pressure, or neck extension. Postural deficits noted at rest
4	Stumbling, tripping, and falling spontaneously at a normal gait
5	Horse recumbent

Modified from Ref. [7].

Recumbent patients

Neurologic evaluation of the recumbent patient presents unique challenges to the clinician. The effects of recumbency may alter responses and lead to complications such as peripheral neuropathies that are part of the primary diagnosis. In addition, fear and anxiety induced by recumbency, exhaustion from struggling, or dehydration may influence the results obtained. A general observation will reveal if the horse has normal mentation, suggesting a lesion caudal to C1. A general examination should be performed to determine if the horse has a musculoskeletal disorder such as a fractured limb or pelvis resulting in recumbency. Cardiovascular status should be evaluated as severe shock and dehydration can also result in diffuse weakness and recumbency. If the horse can attain a dog-sitting position, demonstrating good strength and coordination of the pectoral limbs, then the lesion is likely to be caudal to T2. Loss of pectoral limb strength while retaining the ability to lift the head and cranial neck suggests an extreme caudal cervical lesion, such as C6-T2. The Schiff–Sherrington phenomenon describes a condition of increased forelimb tone and flaccid paralysis of the hind limbs and has been seen in horses, associated with spinal cord lesions between T2 and L4 [8].

Specific spinal reflexes can be tested in recumbent horses. Spinal reflexes require only an intact sensory nerve, spinal cord segment(s), an intact peripheral motor nerve (LMN), and muscle. Perception of the stimulus requires intact ascending sensory pathways, and horses may have an intact reflex without perception of the stimulus. In the thoracic limbs, the flexor, triceps, and biceps reflexes can be evaluated.

The flexor (withdrawal) reflex is tested by clamping the skin over the distal limb and observing for withdrawal of the limb associated with flexion of the joints. In the thoracic limb, the reflex is mediated by sensory fibers in the median and ulnar nerves; spinal cord segments C6-T2; and motor fibers of the axillary, median, musculocutaneous, and ulnar nerves [9]. Peripheral nerve trauma from recumbency can lead to sensory nerve damage, and depression and/or exhaustion can lead to a diminished response, hence this reflex must be evaluated carefully.

The biceps reflex is tested by balloting the muscle belly of the biceps and brachialis muscles with a plexor and feeling for muscle contraction. This reflex is mediated by the musculocutaneous nerves and spinal cord segments C6 and C7. It is more readily detected in foals and may be difficult to detect in adult horses [9].

The triceps reflex is tested by slightly flexing the limb, putting the triceps muscle in slight tension, then balloting the distal portion of the triceps at its point of insertion. A positive reflex is the observation of triceps muscle contraction. The reflex pathway tested involves the radial nerve and spinal cord segments C7-T1.

The patellar reflex in the rear limbs can be tested in both foals and adults. In this test, the limb is moderately flexed, and the patellar tendon balloted with a heavy plexor or the examiner's hand in a "karate-chop" motion. A diminished response can be seen in horses with botulism or femoral nerve disease, among others. Exaggerated responses to any of these segmental reflexes are associated with UMN disease cranial to the site of the spinal cord segments tested by the reflex (Tables 6.4 and 6.5).

Table 6.4 Clinical abnormalities associated with different segments of the spinal cord.

Spinal segment	Clinical signs
C1–C5	Spastic gait, worse in rear limbs
	Proprioceptive deficits
	Weakness
	With or without Horner's syndrome
C6-T2	Proprioceptive deficits, worse in front than rear
	Weakness
	Muscle atrophy, thoracic limbs
	± Horner's syndrome
T3-L3	Proprioceptive deficits, rear
	Normal gait, front
	Rear limbs weakness
	Spasticity, pelvic limbs
S3–S5	Urinary incontinence
	Fecal retention
	Hypalgesia tail and perianal
	Normal thoracic and pelvic
Coccygeal	Decreased tail tone
	Hypalgesia caudal to lesion
	Normal front and rear limbs

Table 6.5 Clinical signs associated with disease of various anatomic regions of the nervous system.

Anatomic region	Predominant clinical signs
Cerebral cortex	Postural deficits, seizures, altered mentation, blindness
Brainstem	Ataxia, weakness, and dysmetria, mild to moderate. Dysphagia, anisocoria, or dilated pupils possible
Vestibular system	Ataxia, head tilt, postural deficits pronounced
Cerebellum	Ataxia and intention tremors
Spinal cord UMN	Paresis, ataxia, and dysmetria all present and mild to moderate. Spasticity is prominent
Peripheral nerve/LMN	Weakness predominates
	Postural deficits and ataxia mild

Examination of foals

The neurologic evaluation of foals presents some unique challenges to the equine practitioner [10]. Foal behavior, age-related changes in results, and the fact that foals are not in most cases trained to lead are complicating factors. The general examination procedure is similar for the foal; however, the gait evaluation must be accomplished with the foal at liberty following the mare. The normal newborn is usually standing by 2 h after birth. Although much time is spent down resting, the foal is readily arousable and is normally curious. Udder-seeking behavior is observed after arising. When restrained, the foal often struggles briefly then sinks limply into the examiner, which has been called "flopping." Restraint may stimulate biting or chewing movements. The normal foal holds its head in a slightly more upright and flexed position than adults, and head movements are somewhat jerky and exaggerated. Foals are somewhat hyperresponsive to tactile stimulation. Foals are visual from birth, but the menace response is not seen until about 2 weeks of age. A pupillary light response is present, and the pupil forms a slight ventro-medial angle to the palpebral fissure, which is not seen in adults, and which is lost by 1 month of age. The foal's gait shows exaggerated, short strides that are somewhat dysmetric, but that approach a normal adult gait by several weeks of age. This is highly variable among foals, however.

Foals can be placed in lateral recumbency to evaluate limb reflexes, which are in general exaggerated when compared with the normal adult. The triceps tendon and extensor carpi radialis tendon reflex are readily elicited in the newborn foal. A prominent crossed extensor reflex, as well as the extensor thrust reflex can be observed for the first day or two of life in normal foals.

Neurologic issues of the prepurchase examination

The neurologic examination should routinely be incorporated into the examination for purchase. The examination is performed in the same manner, and interpretation of any observed deficits is the same; however, an important feature is to be aware of the association between nervous system and musculoskeletal disease. This includes such problems as osteochondrosis of the stifle, hock, and shoulder joints, which often occur concurrently in horses with cervical stenotic myelopathy (CSM). Two common historical findings of particular interest are previous medial patellar desmotomy and/or bilateral bog spavin in early life. Bog spavin is highly associated with osteochondrosis of the distal tibia, while a prior patellar desmotomy may be performed due to quadriceps weakness secondary to neurologic disease [11]. The horse should be carefully examined for any breed-related neurologic illnesses, such as cerebellar abiotrophy in Arabians. Nutritional history and housing may be important in evaluating a horse's risk of developing equine LMN disease, which is associated with drylot housing and lack of fresh forage. Applying a blindfold to test for compensated head tilt is useful, particularly if there is any history of head injury or trauma. As in most other body systems, the horse may demonstrate some mild or inconclusive deficits during the neurologic examination. In many cases, these may be due to subtle musculoskeletal disease, rather than neurologic disease.

Differentiating neurogenic and musculoskeletal gait abnormalities

The differentiation of neurologic and musculoskeletal disease is often problematic. Normal response during the nervous system examination requires a sound musculoskeletal system; hence musculoskeletal disease will lead to abnormalities of the neurologic examination. In particular, multiple limb lameness or bilateral hind limb lameness will cause horses to stumble, interfere, or pivot when spinning. These cases are particularly challenging because the characteristic gait abnormalities associated with a particular lameness will be altered by the presence of lameness in other limbs. Careful observation of the horse's gait and application of a few basic principles can simplify the process, however.

In general, the horse with a musculoskeletal problem has a gait that is regularly irregular. That is, the horse may take an abnormal step or have abnormal placement; however, the abnormality is the same from step to step. In contrast, the gait in a horse with neurologic disease is irregularly irregular. The foot placement or step will vary from one step to the next. Furthermore, in horses with neurologic disease, the abnormality should be apparent in all phases of the gait examination, although particular maneuvers may make the signs more obvious. If a deficit is seen only during circling, for example, yet not detected during downhill, backing, or walking in a line, then hock soreness should be investigated.

Treatment of the horse with nonsteroidal anti-inflammatory drugs (NSAIDs) will minimize clinical signs of musculoskeletal disease yet will not commonly influence neurologic disorders. Hence, examination before and after treatment with NSAIDs can be a useful aid in some cases. Finally, the use of nerve blocks and joint anesthesia followed by a repeat nervous system examination can be done. If local anesthesia resolves the previously identified gait abnormality, then musculoskeletal disease must be the cause.

Examination of the peripheral nerves

Examination of the peripheral nerves is important in the neurologic examination. Of particular interest to veterinarians are those peripheral nerves that innervate the limbs. Typically, disease of the peripheral nervous system is usually unilateral and limited to a single limb or region. Evaluation is performed through direct observation of function or by reflex testing and is dependant upon knowledge of normal peripheral nerve anatomy and regions of innervation. Acute injury will result in functional loss (such as abduction of the shoulder joint or knuckling of a distal extremity), while chronic injury will result in atrophy of the affected muscle groups.

Sensation is tested by touching a region with a sharp instrument, and pain perception is tested by grasping the skin with forceps. Electrodiagnostic testing is more definitive and is described in detail in Chapter 14.

Neuroanatomic localization and case synthesis

Once the physical examination, history, and neurologic examination are complete, neuroanatomic localization of the nervous system abnormality is determined. Differential considerations can then be constructed and evaluated. The results of the neurologic examination should allow the examiner to determine which area or areas of the nervous system are affected. Basic neuroanatomic divisions are the cerebral cortex, brainstem, vestibular system, cerebellum, spinal cord, or peripheral nerve. In general, cranial nerve signs indicate a lesion rostral to the foramen magnum. A horse with a normal sensorium and no cranial nerve deficits has a lesion(s) caudal to the foramen magnum. Gait deficits are assigned a "score" based upon the criteria described in Table 6.3. Clinical signs associated with abnormalities of different segments of the spinal cord are presented in Table 6.4. In general, cervical lesions (C1–C6) result in proprioceptive deficits, paresis, and ataxia that involve all four limbs but are one grade worse in the pelvic limbs than the thoracic limbs. A gait deficit that is worse in the thoracic limbs than the pelvic limbs suggests a lesion within the region of the brachial intumescence (C7-T2). Neurologic gait deficits that involve the rear limbs with normal front limbs indicate a lesion in the thoracolumbar region. In general, the examiner should attempt to explain the neurologic deficits observed by a single lesion site; if this is not possible, multifocal disease must exist, which is important in differential diagnosis. In addition, the presence of symmetry or asymmetry must be evaluated. Some conditions, such as cervical compression, cauda equina syndrome, and EDEM are symmetrical, while others, especially equine protozoal myeloencephalitis (EPM), are characteristically asymmetric. The history of the neurologic disease should be considered, as some conditions have an acute onset (such as fracture) while others have a more chronic or insidious course (i.e., EPM). The presence of systemic disease, fever, and anorexia are important clues indicating the presence of an infectious disease, such as eastern equine encephalitis (EEE), western equine encephalitis (WEE), rabies, west nile virus (WNV), or meningitis. Once a neuroanatomic location is determined, then further specific diagnostic procedures can be selected as appropriate and performed.

References

[1] Mayhew, I.G. (2009) Neurologic Evaluation, in *Large Animal Neurology* (ed. I.G. Mayhew), Wiley-Blackwell Ltd, Ames, IA, pp. 11–46.

[2] Greet, T.R., Jeffcott, L.B., Whitwell, K.E. *et al.* (1980) The slap test for laryngeal adductory function in horses with suspected cervical spinal cord damage. *Equine Vet J*, 12, 127–131.

[3] Newton-Clarke, M.J., Divers, T.J., De lahunta, A. *et al.* (1994) Evaluation of the thoraco-laryngeal reflex ("slap test") as an aid to the diagnosis of cervical spinal cord and brainstem disease in horses. *Equine Vet J*, 26, 358–361.

[4] Reed, S.M. (1998) Neurologic examination, in *Equine Internal Medicine* (eds S.M. Reed and W.M. Bailey), W.B. Saunders Co, Philadelphia, PA, pp. 427–434.

[5] Rooney, J.R. (1973) Two cervical reflexes in the horse. *J Am Vet Med Assoc*, 162, 117–119.

[6] Oliver, J.E., Lorenz, M.D. and Kornegay, J.M. (1997) Ataxia of the Head and the Limbs, in *Handbook of Veterinary Neurology* (eds J.E. Oliver, M.D. Lorenz and J.M. Kornegay), W.B. Saunders Co, Philadelphia, PA, pp. 216–239.

[7] Mayhew, I., deLahunta, A., Whitlock, R. *et al.* (1978) Spinal cord disease in the horse. *Cornell Vet*, 68 (Suppl 6), 24–29.

[8] Chiapetta, J.R., Baker, J.C. and Feeney, D.A. (1985) Vertebral fracture, extensor hypertonia of thoracic limbs, and paralysis of pelvic limbs (Schiff-Sherrington syndrome) in an Arabian foal. *J Am Vet Med Assoc*, 186, 387–388.

[9] Hahn, C.N., Mayhew, I.G. and MacKay, R. (1999) Nervous System, in *Equine Medicine and Surgery* (eds P.T. Colahan, I.G. Mayhew, A.M. Merritt *et al.*), Mosby, Saint Louis, MO, pp. 863–996.

[10] Adams, R. and Mayhew, I.G. (1984) Neurological examination of newborn foals. *Equine Vet J*, 16, 306–312.

[11] Reed, S.M. (1992) The Neurologic Examination of the Horse for Purchase, in *Vet Clin of North America (Equine Practice)* (ed. G.M. Beeman), W.B. Saunders, Co, Philadelphia, PA, pp. 377–387.

7 Differential Diagnosis and Management of Horses with Seizures or Alterations in Consciousness

Véronique A. Lacombe[1] and Martin Furr[2]

[1] Center for Veterinary Health Sciences, Oklahoma State University, Stillwater, USA
[2] Marion duPont Scott Equine Medical Center, Virginia-Maryland Regional College of Veterinary Medicine, Leesburg, USA

The clinical problem of seizures in the horse is challenging for the veterinarian to diagnose and manage and is usually very distressing, if not downright dangerous to the owner or caretaker of adult horses. Like other problems of the central nervous system (CNS), the clinical expression of the disorder is often nonspecific, and the underlying cause may not be easily determined. This is particularly so in cases of recurrent seizures of adults, in which the horse may be clinically normal in the interictal period. Diagnosis and management is complicated by the fact that many horses (if not most) are unobserved for long periods of the day, hence inciting events may not be observed. The presence of seizures or other alterations in consciousness may be signaled by the observation of frequent superficial wounds or abrasions. Unexplained blindness or abrasions around the eyes and head are particularly evident in foals, as is impaction of soil or grass in the conjunctiva and lacerations or abrasions of the lips and mouth. This should alert the caretaker to the possibility of a seizure disorder and lead to increased observation. Caretakers must also be counseled about the potential for human injury from an adult horse suffering from a seizure. The strong inclination, among some horse-owners at least, to rush in and attempt to "control" the horse can lead to serious injury and must be avoided (see video clips demonstrating clinical signs for videos).

A seizure (from the Latin word *sacire*, "to take possession of") is a paroxysmal event that arises due to excessive discharges of the cerebrocortical neurons [1]. The abnormal electrical activity may arise in other portions of the brain or brainstem then spread to the cerebrum. The specific clinical presentation of the seizure depends upon the specific anatomic location and magnitude of the electrical discharge and is independent of the etiology [2]. Seizures, also known as fits or convulsions, are specific clinical events, and epilepsy is defined as reoccurring seizures from a chronic underlying process.

Clinical signs of seizures in horses can be variable, ranging from mild alterations in consciousness, or focal muscle fasciculations, to recumbency with tonic–clonic struggling. In this case, the movements are characterized by stiff, hypertonic limbs with repetitive, rhythmic struggling. The rhythmic patterned movements help to discriminate between a true seizure and merely aimless struggling from pain, anxiety, or severe orthopedic or muscle disease. In milder forms, horses do not always become recumbent and the presence of a seizure can be confirmed only by electroencephalography (EEG). There may be a prodromal phase (e.g., preictal or "aura") during which the horse is restless or distracted or demonstrates other changes in mentation. Following the seizure (e.g., postictal phase), there is usually a period of time during which the horse remains depressed and quiet and may be blind. The blindness is usually transient in adults but may persist for several days in foals [3] (see video clips demonstrating clinical signs for videos).

In the differential diagnosis of seizures in the horse, it is important to differentiate between true seizures (i.e., with a specific neural origin) and other disorders that may mimic seizures. Acute collapse without premonitory signs is most characteristic of a cardiovascular event, while muscle disease, circulatory shock, and botulism may lead to muscle tremors and flailing behavior that could be confused with a seizure. In addition, narcolepsy has been described in horses and may be confused with seizures. In animals with a true seizure, the muscle movements are repetitive and rhythmical, while movements that are misdirected and variable may be associated with a horse or foal struggling to right themselves. In addition, horses with seizures are nonarousable, while horses that are frightened and struggling are somewhat responsive to the examiner. Some factors that may aid in the differentiation of these two events in the horse are presented in Table 7.1. Nonneurologic disorders that can be confused with seizures are listed in Table 7.2.

Seizures in horses can be classified as being partial, generalized, or status epilepticus [4]. Partial seizures arise

from a discrete area of the cerebral cortex with resultant localized clinical signs that may include facial or limb twitching or self-mutilation. In addition, this category of seizure can progress and spread diffusely throughout the cortex—a phenomenon termed "partial seizure with secondary generalization." The progression of a very localized abnormal movement which then progresses to involve more of the extremity is termed "Jacksonian march" and represents a spread of the seizure focus over progressively larger areas of the cerebral cortex. [1] If consciousness is impaired, the seizure is termed a complex partial seizure. This type of seizure (complex partial) is commonly observed in neonatal foals and is commonly seen as "chewing-gum fits," jaw chomping, and lip smacking [5]. These are also referred to as "automatisms," which are involuntary automatic behaviors (see video clips demonstrating clinical signs for videos).

Generalized seizures arise from both cerebral hemispheres simultaneously and are further classified as primary generalized (i.e., generalized from the onset) or secondary generalized (i.e., secondary to a partial seizure). Although it is difficult in horses to determine if there was an initial focal seizure that progressed very rapidly to a generalized condition, careful observation of

Table 7.1 Clinical signs that can be used to differentiate between seizures and syncope.

Feature	Seizure	Syncope
Premonitory signs	Aura	Fatigue
Duration of unconsciousness	Minutes	Seconds
Duration of tonic or clonic movements	30 s or longer	None or a few seconds
Disorientation after event	Several minutes or longer	Recovery almost immediate

Table 7.2 Noncerebral clinical conditions that can be confused with seizure activity in adult horses and foals.

Disease	Comments
Cardiovascular disease	
Atrial fibrillation	Confirm by auscultation (irregularly irregular rhythm) and ECG
Ruptured chordae tendineae	Accompanied by the presence of pulmonary edema, abnormal auscultation
Myocardial infarction	Rarely observed; ECG abnormalities, irregular pulse
Aortic root rupture	Accompanied by pallor and very weak pulse quality
Pericarditis	Weak pulse, abnormal auscultation
Pericardial tamponade	Weak pulse, enlarged cardiac silhouette on radiography
Circulatory shock	
Hemorrhage	Cold extremities, weak pulse, elevated heart rate
Volume depletion	Pale mucus membranes, elevated heart rate
Electrolyte disorders	
Hypocalcemia	Muscle fasciculation, risus sardonicus
Hypomagnesemia	Muscle fasciculation, risus sardonicus, mania
Muscle disease	
Hyperkalemic period paralysis (HYPP)	Associated with hyperkalemia
Recumbency myopathy	History of recumbency, firm painful muscles
Other	
Botulism	Systemic flaccid paralysis and weakness of limbs and muscles of the head
Tetanus	Diffuse, symmetrical hypertonicity, limbs and muscles of head
Exertional rhabdomyolysis	Firm painful muscles, pigmenturia
Postanesthetic myelopathy	History of anesthesia with signs of spinal cord disease
Anaphylaxis	Cold extremities, weak pulse, elevated heart rate

the onset of seizures could allow the clinician to differentiate between primary and secondary generalized seizures and to better comprehend seizure development. Partial seizures appear to be the most common classification in horses [2]. Status epilepticus is characterized by a rapid succession of seizures and is considered uncommon in adult horses [3].

Seizures can be further classified by etiology as reactive (i.e., presence of a temporary systemic disease with a normal brain function), symptomatic (i.e., presence of identifiable structural brain lesion), or of unknown origin (i.e., cryptogenic) based on the results of the ancillary diagnostic tests as described later. Epilepsy of genetic origin appears to be very rare in the horse and has only been documented in Arabian foals with juvenile idiopathic epilepsy [6].

Seizures may arise from a wide range of causes, which are summarized in Table 7.3. Neonates appear to have a lower seizure threshold than adults, making them more susceptible to seizures. In neonatal foals, likely causes include hypoxic-ischemic encephalopathy, trauma, congenital disorders, and metabolic derangements. Persistent hyperammonemia should be considered in young Morgan horses, and severe pneumonia (with associated hypoxia) has been observed to result in seizures of weanling-age horses. The most common causes of seizures in adult horses are reported to be trauma, hepatoencephalopathy, and toxicity [3], although a large number of conditions have been reported to cause alterations in consciousness or seizures in adults as well.

Due to the numerous causes of seizures, a complete evaluation directed at eliciting both intracranial and extracranial causes should be pursued. In foals and young horses, it is important to note the breed, as Egyptian Arabs are reported to have benign seizure events while Morgan horses may have hyperammonemia. Travel and vaccination history should be obtained, as well as feed history and any recently administered pharmaceuticals. A physical examination should elucidate the presence of systemic, extracranial disease that may predispose to seizures. Cuts or scrapes on the head or evidence of bleeding from the nares or ears suggest trauma, while a concurrent or recent fever may signal an infectious disorder. A complete blood cell count and serum biochemistry analysis, which includes calcium and magnesium, are indicated. If evidence of systemic disorders or hepatic disease is found, further workup is indicated and may include liver function tests, liver biopsy, and determination of serum ammonia concentration. An arterial blood gas evaluation is indicated, particularly in foals, to rule out hypoxia or metabolic derangements. In the absence of systemic disease, intracranial disease must be assumed. Radiographs of the skull in both lateral and dorsoventral projection are indicated, followed by a cerebrospinal fluid (CSF) collection and evaluation. CSF collection from the atlanto-occipital space is ideal but may be contraindicated if the horse is showing signs of increased CSF pressure, such as mydriasis or papilledema. Bloody CSF is consistent with trauma, verminous migration, or tumors, while normal fluid can be seen in many conditions. CSF of normal neonates is slightly xanthochromic (up to 10 days of age) [7], but in older foals or adults it is consistent with prior hemorrhage and/or diffuse inflammatory conditions. Elevated total protein and cell counts are commonly seen in infectious conditions but are sometimes highly variable. Culture of the CSF is indicated if there is any suggestion of sepsis. Serologic testing of serum and CSF for the viral encephalitides is often warranted, as is testing for equine protozoal myeloencephalitis.

EEG is a useful ancillary test in many situations. It is a relatively simple and noninvasive neurophysiological technique, which is defined as the graphic recording of the rhythmic bioelectrical activity arising predominantly from the cerebral cortex. Although less work has been done in horses compared with humans and small animals, it has been found to have a good diagnostic potential [8]. EEG may be performed on awake or sedated animals or on animals under general anesthesia, and the

Table 7.3 Causes of seizure or altered states of consciousness in foals and adult horses.

Developmental/malformations	Infectious
Hydrocephalus	Bacterial meningitis/abscessation
Meningoencephalocele	Viral encephalitis
Dandy–Walker malformation	Verminous encephalitis
Undefined malformations	Mycotic encephalitis
Metabolic derangement	Amebic encephalitis
Hepatoencephalopathy	Equine protozoal myeloencephalitis
Hypocalcemia	**Toxic**
Hyponatremia	Metaldehyde
Hypoglycemia	Nardoo fern
Hypo-/hyperosmolality disorders	*Swainsonia*
Hyperammonemia	Locoweed
Neoplastic	*Datura* (jimsonweed)
Cholesterol granuloma	Buckeye (*Aesculus*)
Adenocarcinoma	*Solanum*
Lymphoma	*Fusarium*
Pituitary adenoma	Bromide
Iatrogenic	**Idiopathic**
Air embolism	Hypoxic-ischemic encephalopathy
Intracarotid injection	Benign epilepsy of Arabian foals
Postmyelography	Postanesthetic cerebral necrosis
Moxidectin overdose	Trauma
Fluphenazine	Hyperthermia
Enrofloxacin overdose	Hemorrhage

condition of recording greatly depends on the preference of the clinician. In humans and small animals, recordings on awake patients are optimal because the use of sedation and general anesthesia influences EEG patterns by altering cortical activity [9] but will significantly reduce artifacts caused by head, ear, and eye movements of the patient and caused by auditory and visual stimuli. To easily identify such bioelectrical artifacts on awake or lightly sedated horses, some clinicians simultaneously record electrooculographic, electromyographic, and electrocardiographic (ECG) activities as well as the horse's behavior [10]. However, since recording on alert animals is usually challenging, sedation or general anesthesia is usually preferred or required. Accurate interpretation of the EEG recording can provide information in regard to the presence (or absence) of cerebral disease and its nature. To this end, one should assess the background for abnormal frequency and amplitude, the presence of asymmetrical patterns between regions, and the presence of paroxysmal activity. The most common abnormalities associated with cerebral diseases are the change in either amplitude or frequency, or both [10]. For example, increases toward low-voltage fast activity or high-voltage slow activity have been observed and are suggestive of ongoing irritative processes or neuronal death in epileptic patients, respectively [11]. In addition, epileptiform paroxysmal activity, which is defined as abnormal paroxysmal transient events, such as spikes, sharp waves, and spike-and-wave discharges, supports the diagnosis of seizures. However, the lack of recording of epileptic activity does not automatically rule out seizures since the use of tranquilizers may increase the threshold for seizures and since the window of recording may not have been long enough to record interictal paroxysmal epileptiform discharges [12]. In addition, changes are not pathognomonic of a disease but rather reflect process occurring (e.g., acute vs. chronic, focal vs. diffuse, and inflammatory vs. degenerative). Therefore, the EEG is complementary, rather than an alternative, to other diagnostic tests and may allow the clinician to construct a list of differential diagnoses that helps identify the cause of the seizures in the light of the history, neurological examinations, and other diagnostic tests. The main limitations of this electrodiagnostic test are related to the facts that (i) only electrical activity arising from the superficial part of the cerebral cortex is recorded; (ii) the establishment of normal values remains difficult because frequency and amplitudes are state-dependent (i.e., the states of wakefulness, drowsiness, sleeping, and being sedated vs. anesthetized) and vary with age; (iii) it requires extensive expertise from the clinician to interpret the reading; and (iv) it is mostly limited to some large private practices and neurological referral institutions. Further discussion of EEG is found in Chapter 14.

Specialized imaging modalities (such as MRI or CT scan) may be useful, but availability is limited in adult horses and these procedures are expensive. In addition, although CT scan has superior capabilities for imaging bony structures and could reveal potential skull fractures that may remain undetected by conventional radiographs, it is less sensitive than MRI to image soft tissue structure, such as the brain [13, 14].

Management of horses with seizure disorders

The goals of treatment are to stop the seizure (if presently occurring), to correct the underlying disease (if determined), and to maintain a seizure-free status.

Anticonvulsant therapy

The immediate control of seizure-like activity is a priority as prolonged or recurring seizures may result in increased intracranial pressure and neuronal necrosis [15]. Prompt control of seizures is also important to minimize the possibility of further injury to the horse or any human caretakers. Seizures in neonates may also result in reduced arterial oxygenation, which may be important in some situations. The second goal is to eliminate or at least decrease the frequency of seizures by the use of long-acting anticonvulsant therapy, without unacceptable adverse effect associated with such therapy (Table 7.4).

Diazepam, a benzodiazepine anticonvulsant, has been routinely used for short-term (immediate) control of seizures. All benzodiazepines hyperpolarize neuronal cells by binding to the gamma-aminobutyric (GABA) receptor, thereby amplifying the action of GABA on chloride channels in the cell membrane. This increased chloride conductance hyperpolarizes the neuronal cell membrane, making the cell more resistant to depolarization. The overall result is an increase in the seizure threshold and a decrease in the electrical activity of the seizure focus [16]. Diazepam is distributed rapidly to the CNS after IV administration and has a short duration of action (10–15 min). Because of its short half-life, repeated doses must be used, as necessary. However, caution should be used as prolonged usage may cause respiratory depression or arrest in foals [17]. Furthermore, care should be taken when administering repeated doses to foals less than 21 days old because of the slower clearance of the drug reported in this age group compared with older foals and adults [17]. High doses (>0.2 mg/kg) in adult horses may cause muscle weakness and ataxia, and recumbency may result [18]. Furthermore, diazepam should be used with caution in horses or foals with hepatoencephalopathy as it may exacerbate clinical signs due to the upregulation of

Table 7.4 Guidelines for treating convulsing adult horses[a].

Regimen	Drug	Dosage	Route	Frequency
Control seizures: *Initial therapy*	Diazepam	0.05–0.2 mg/kg in 25–100 mg doses	IV or IM	As needed
	Phenobarbital	12–20 mg/kg initial dose (diluted in saline over 30 min), then 1–9 mg/kg	IV	q8–12 h after initial dose
	Phenytoin	1–5 mg/kg	IV or PO	q4 h for up to 24 h
	Pentobarbital	2–10 mg/kg	IV	To effect
	Chloral hydrate	33.3–133.3 mg/kg	IV	To effect
	Guaifenesin	88.9–133.3 mg/kg	IV	To effect
Prevent seizures: *Maintenance therapy*	Phenobarbital	5–11 mg/kg	PO	q12–24 h
	Potassium bromide	25–40 mg/kg	PO	q24 h
	Phenytoin	1–5 mg/kg	PO	q12 h
Control cerebrocortical edema	Dexamethasone	0.1–0.25 mg/kg	IV	q6–24 h
	Methylprednisolone	30 mg/kg followed by 15 mg/kg 2 and 6 h later, followed by a CRI (2.5 mg/kg/h) 100–1000 mg	IV IV	First dose within 4 h after trauma; CRI for 48 h
	DMSO	1.0 g/kg diluted as a 10% solution	IV	q12–24 h
	Mannitol	0.25–2 g/kg as a 20% solution	IV	q12–24 h
	Furosemide	1 mg/kg	IV, IM, SQ	q12 h
Antioxidant and NMDA receptor blockade therapy (*Efficacy not established*)	Alpha-tocopherol (vitamin E)	2,000 IU/adult 5,000–20,000 IU/adult	IM PO	Once, switch PO q24 h
	Ascorbic acid (vitamin C)	20 mg/kg	PO	q24 h
	Allopurinol	5 mg/kg	PO	q12 h
	Magnesium sulfate	50 mg/kg	IV slow	Once
Provide proper hydration and nutritional support	Cautious fluid therapy		IV	
	Oral feeding (if tolerated)			
Correct metabolic derangements (if needed)	Oxygen therapy		Nasal	
	Glucose supplementation		IV	
Minimize chances of trauma	Provide thick bedding, heavy padding, helmet, and leg wraps			

[a]Modified from Hines, Sihna and Cox, and MacKay [44, 53, 54].
CRI, constant rate infusion; IV, intravenously; IM, intramuscularly; PO, by mouth; SQ, subcutaneous.

benzodiazepine receptors [19]. In patients that do not respond to the initial course of bolus doses of diazepam, a constant-rate infusion of diazepam can be implemented at an initial rate of 0.1 mg/kg/h [15].

Midazolam is a potent short-acting benzodiazepine that has been utilized for anticonvulsant therapy in foals [20, 21] (Table 7.5). Midazolam has been recommended at the dose of 0.05–0.1 mg/kg IV or IM; the smallest effective dose should be used and can be repeated as needed. Midazolam can also be administered by continuous-rate infusion in foals with recurrent seizures (1–3 mg/h for a 50-kg foal) [20]. Midazolam has been proven to be highly effective for controlling status epilepticus and seizures that are refractory to phenobarbital

Table 7.5 Therapeutic guidelines for treating convulsing foals[a].

Regimen	Drug	Dosage	Route	Frequency
Control seizures: *Initial therapy*	Diazepam	0.1–0.4 mg/kg slow	IV	As needed
	Midazolam	0.05–0.1 mg/kg	IV or IM	As needed
	Phenobarbital	9–20 mg/kg loading dose (30 ml saline)	IV	
	Phenytoin	5–10 mg/kg	IV	
	Primidone	20–40 mg/kg	PO	To effect
	Pentobarbital	2–4 mg/kg	IV	To effect
	Chloral hydrate	66.6–222.2 mg/kg	IV	To effect
	Guaifenesin	To effect	IV	
Prevent seizures: *Maintenance therapy*	Phenobarbital	4–10 mg/kg	PO	q12h
		2–10 mg/kg	IV	q8–12h
	Phenytoin	1–5 mg/kg	PO, IM	q2–4h for 12h, then q6h or q12h
	Primidone	15 mg/kg	PO	q12h
Control cerebrocortical edema	Prednisolone	50–10 mg/kg	IV	
	DMSO	0.5–1.0 g/kg diluted in 10% solution	IV	q12h
Antioxidant and NMDA receptor blockade therapy (*Efficacy not established*)	Alpha-tocopherol (vitamin E)	500–4,000 units/foal	PO	q24h
	Ascorbic acid (vitamin C)	50–100 mg/kg	IV	q24h
	Allopurinol	40 mg/kg	PO	Within first 4h
	Magnesium sulfate (HIE)	50 mg/kg/h for the first hour diluted to 1% as a loading dose, then 25 mg/kg/h CRI	IV	CRI q24–48h
Provide respiratory support (if needed)	Oxygen supplementation	5–10 l/min	Nasal	
	Caffeine	*Loading dose*: 10 mg/kg *Maintenance dose*: 2.5–3.0 mg/kg	PO	
	Positive pressure ventilation		PO	q24h
Provide proper hydration and nutritional support	Cautious fluid therapy	Maintenance: 4–5 ml/kg/h	IV	
	Oral feeding (if tolerated)	Milk: 10–25% of foal's bw/day		
	Parenteral nutrition	—		
	Support body temperature	—		
Provide metabolic support	Glucose supplementation	—	IV	
	Electrolyte supplementation	—	IV or PO	
	Thiamine (HIE)	10 mg/kg	IV	q12h
Minimize chances of trauma	Provide thick bedding, heavy padding, head helmet, and leg wraps	—	—	—

[a] References [5, 44, 45, 60, 62].
HIE, hypoxic-ischemic encephalopathy; IM, intramuscularly; IV, intravenously; PO, by mouth.

and/or phenytoin in human infants. Limited pharmacological studies have been reported in horses; however, midazolam has a large volume of distribution and a fairly long T1/2 [22].

Some sedative drugs should be used with caution for emergency seizure management. For instance, xylazine reduces cerebral blood flow after transiently increasing

intracranial pressure, which may potentially exacerbate cerebral edema and worsen seizures [23]. Acepromazine is contraindicated since it may reduce the seizure threshold [3]. Historically, ketamine has also been contraindicated since it increases intracranial pressure and may exacerbate seizure-like activity [23]. However, ketamine also acts as an antagonist of *N*-methyl-D-aspartate (NMDA) receptors, which have been implicated in the pathogenesis of seizures in infants [24, 25]. In support of this, ketamine infusion has been proven to control seizure activity in a rodent model of status epilepticus refractory to phenobarbital [26], although the proof of a similar beneficial effect in a clinical setting is currently lacking [27]. Thus, the use of ketamine in the treatment of horses with seizures remains unclear.

Once the initial seizure has been controlled, it must be determined if prophylactic anticonvulsant therapy is warranted. This is a major commitment for the veterinarian and owners as the anticonvulsant may be administered for a minimum of several months before discontinuing. Furthermore, the owners must realize that seizure control does not necessarily imply complete elimination of the episodes but rather a decrease in the frequency and severity of the seizures. The decision to initiate anticonvulsant drug therapy depends on the underlying cause, seizure type, and frequency. Although rarely reported in horses, status epilepticus warrants the use of anticonvulsant therapy. With identified intracranial diseases, the therapy should be initiated at the onset of seizures. When no specific etiology has been determined, criteria for beginning maintenance anticonvulsant therapy include increased frequency, duration and/or severity (e.g., cluster of seizures, at least one seizure occurring at least every 2 months), or the presence of generalized repeated seizures resulting in recumbency or self-injury [28, 29]. A useful aid for determining the need for maintenance anticonvulsant therapy is to have the owners keep a log to document any observed seizures, with a recording of the date and time of day, duration, behavior of the horse in the interictal period, and any associated events that may be triggers. Video documentation of seizures is optimal if it can be performed under safe condition. In neonatal foals, if more than three doses of diazepam are needed over a few hours to control seizures, maintenance anticonvulsant therapy should be initiated (e.g., phenobarbital) due to their longer duration of action [19] (Table 7.5).

Options for anticonvulsant maintenance therapy include phenobarbital, bromide, phenytoin, and primidone. Phenobarbital is the drug of choice in horses. Although phenobarbital has been used to treat epilepsy for over 80 years, the mechanisms of action are not fully elucidated. The primary mechanism of action of phenobarbital is to facilitate neuronal stabilization via GABA receptors in postsynaptic neurons of inhibitory nerve terminals and increase intracellular chloride conductance (also refer to Chapter 4). Phenobarbital is well absorbed after oral administration, with a bioavailability close to 100% in horses [30]. The majority of the drug is metabolized in the liver with approximately 25% excreted as unchanged drug in horses [16]. Phenobarbital induces the hepatic cytochrome P450 enzyme complex,

resulting in a more rapid metabolism not only of phenobarbital but also of other concurrently administered drugs. For instance, the elimination half-life after a single oral dose of phenobarbital is reduced from 24 h (initial) to 11 h after 42 days of treatment in horses [31]. Therefore, dosage adjustment may be required after long-term therapy to maintain serum concentrations within the therapeutic window.

The half-life of phenobarbital in horses is shorter than in humans and small animals (~18 h with a range of 14–24 h for initial elimination half-life in adult, and approximately 12 h in foals after IV administration), in part because a smaller proportion of the drug is protein-bound [30–33].

The goal of any antiepileptic therapy is to achieve a therapeutic steady-state condition, which is usually reached within five to six elimination half-lives. Given the variability in half-life, clearance, and metabolism of phenobarbital, as noted earlier, therapeutic monitoring is necessary to ensure that adequate anticonvulsant concentrations are obtained and toxicity avoided. Thus, the peak concentration (which occurs 2 ± 1.5 h after oral dose administration in adults), and the lowest (trough) concentration (which occurs just before the next dose) should be determined 4–5 days after the initiation of treatment in adult horses and 3 days in foals [31]. The suggested therapeutic serum concentration in adult horses, as extrapolated from studies in humans and dogs, is 15–45 µg/ml (70–175 µmol/l) [16]. Monitoring of trough phenobarbital level should be done when seizure control is inadequate, when toxic side effects are seen, or after a dosage adjustment (Table 7.6). Furthermore, as mentioned earlier, dosage adjustment may be required after long-term therapy; we recommend, as a rule of thumb, serial monitoring of the trough phenobarbital concentration at 14, 45, and every 60 days after initiation of treatment, if the horse appears to be seizure-free. Although phenobarbital monitoring is important especially in cases with inadequate seizure control, the clinical response to therapy is as important in overall management. Thus, based on the initial clinical response (which varies between horses) and based on therapeutic serum concentrations (if needed), the dose of phenobarbital may be adjusted using the following formula:

$$\frac{[\text{Desired peak serum}]}{[\text{Measured peak serum}]} \times \text{old dose} = \text{New dose} [16]$$

The effects of hepatic induction and changes in body weight due to growth suggest that therapeutic monitoring is particularly important in foals. Furthermore, foals have altered distribution patterns and elimination characteristics of drugs due to greater extracellular fluid volume and lower concentrations of plasma-binding proteins compared with adults. Therefore, neonates may have

Table 7.6 Guide to maintenance anticonvulsant therapy to help control seizures in epileptic adult horses[a].

- Be certain that an epileptic seizure has occurred.
- The goal of this therapy is to eliminate or to reduce the frequency of seizures, without any adverse side effects.
- Set up realistic expectations with the owners. Warn owners that horse suffering from seizure disorders (even under anticonvulsant therapy) may not be safe to be around or to ride.
- Have the owners keep a diary of seizure activity and a medication record.
- Select a single anticonvulsant therapy (preferably start with phenobarbital).
- Begin at the recommended dose and adjust the dose until seizures are controlled without inducing toxicity (increasing the dose by 20% every 2 weeks has been proposed or adjust using formula described in text). The dosage must be titrated to the need of each individual horse.
- Monitor blood anticonvulsant concentrations, adjusting the dose to maintain the concentration within the therapeutic ranges (phenobarbital: 15–45 µg/ml; bromide: 1–3 mg/ml).
- If no toxic side effects are seen, do not begin decreasing the dose or altering the frequency of medication until after the horse has been seizure-free for at least 4 weeks.
- For economic and practical purposes, it is desirable to stop anticonvulsant maintenance therapy. Discontinue slowly; sudden withdrawal of drugs may precipitate seizures. If seizures reappear, continued and perhaps lifelong treatment must be considered. The horse should be reevaluated, perhaps including repeat electroencephalography.
- If the side effects are unacceptable (e.g., excessive sedation with phenobarbital or collapse with phenytoin) and seizures are not controlled with only one anticonvulsant therapy, reduce dose of the first drug by 20% or to nontoxic levels and begin a second drug at the recommended dose (e.g., potassium bromide).
- If the seizures are controlled with the administration of the two drugs for 6 months, slowly wean the patient off one drug at a time over 3 months. If seizures begin, raise the dose again.
- Beware of interactions when other drugs are used in patients on anticonvulsant therapy (e.g., tetracyclines, chloramphenicol, and ivermectin). Avoid use of drugs with known interactions.
- Treat the underlying disorders, if identified.

[a] Modified from Mayhew and Podell [15, 29, 38].

significant clinical effects at lower serum concentrations [34]. Indeed, an effective nontoxic therapeutic range of 5–30 µg/ml in foals has been reported [22].

In an emergency situation, intravenous phenobarbital should be used because it rapidly (within 20 min) provides a high serum concentration to stop seizures, as well as reduces cerebral metabolic rate [35]. An increase in cerebral oxygen consumption has been associated with seizure activity and will induce an increase in cerebral blood flow to match the enhanced oxygen demand, which may result in an increased intracranial pressure [36]. Thus reduction of metabolic rate is important particularly if cerebral edema is suspected. As a result of pharmacological studies in foals, it has been recommended to use a loading dose of 20 mg/kg (diluted in 30 ml of saline and infused IV over a 30-min period), followed by maintenance doses of 9 mg/kg IV q8h [33]. In adult horses, a parenteral loading dose of 12 mg/kg IV followed by 6.65 mg/kg IV (20 min infusion) q12h [32] is adequate to reach appropriate therapeutic concentrations. Maintenance therapy is usually administered by the oral route, with a proposed dose of 11 mg/kg once q24h in adults [30], although the half-life of phenobarbital is unknown after oral maintenance therapy in foals.

Overall, phenobarbital is well tolerated in horses. The major reported side effect is drowsiness. Sedation

may also occur in neonatal foals up to 8h after phenobarbital administration discouraging them from nursing [33]. Furthermore, phenobarbital may cause respiratory depression, bradycardia, hypotension, and hypothermia in neonatal foals, especially at larger doses. Therefore, the lowest effective concentration should be administered in conjunction with monitoring of serum drug concentration. Furthermore, foals receiving phenobarbital should have their body temperature, blood pressure, and respiratory rate monitored [37]. Veterinarians should also be aware of interactions if other drugs are prescribed in patients on anticonvulsant therapy. For instance, tetracyclines and chloramphenicol inhibit hepatic microsomal enzymes, thereby prolonging the effects of phenobarbital and phenytoin [38]. Furthermore, ivermectin, a GABA blocker, should not be given to horses and foals on anticonvulsant therapy because of the risk of breaks in seizure control that have occurred following its use [29, 38].

Bromide (sodium or potassium) is another anticonvulsant drug that can be used in the horse [22, 39]. Potassium bromide is the oldest anticonvulsant drug and was first used in 1857 to treat seizures in people. Potassium bromide has experienced a resurgence of use in the management of canine epilepsy, as well as in horses that were refractory to phenobarbital (e.g., inadequate control of seizures despite adequate to high serum phenobarbital levels). Although the mechanisms of action are not well known, bromide appears to compete with chloride ions to hyperpolarize (and thus stabilize) neuronal cell membranes [15]. It may also act synergistically with other drugs with GABAergic activity, such as barbiturates, to increase the seizure threshold. As the elimination half-life of bromide in horses is 3–5 days (shorter than in cows or dogs), it takes several weeks to achieve steady-state concentrations. Hence, potassium bromide should not initially be the sole agent used to treat ongoing seizures but rather administered in combination with phenobarbital, at an initial dose of 25–40 mg/kg/day PO [39, 40]. The suggested therapeutic concentration, based on a study in dogs, is 1–3 mg/ml when used as monotherapy and 1–2 mg/ml in combination with phenobarbital [41]. When used as monotherapy in horses, a loading dose of 120 mg/kg daily over 5 days followed by a maintenance dose of 40 mg/kg/day has been recommended [39]. Bromide toxicosis (bromism), which can occur in people with chronic oral administration, appears to be rare in horses. One study reported bromide toxicity in horses fed hay that contained bromide ion residue from accidental treatment with methyl bromide. Signs included lethargy, hind limb weakness, and ataxia or recumbency [42]. Overall, bromide administration appears to have few complications and is considered a safe therapeutic agent, although the clinical efficacy has not been evaluated for long-term management of horses with seizures [21]. Bromide will artificially increase the assayed concentration of serum chloride if not performed using an ion-specific electrode and should be suspected as the cause of apparent hyperchloridemia [40].

Although phenytoin is not routinely used as an anticonvulsant in horses, it may be considered as an alternative therapy if previous drugs are ineffective. Phenytoin appears to inactivate voltage-dependent neuronal sodium channels (refer to Chapter 4) [15]. The bioavailability of phenytoin in horses is quiet variable, hence serum phenytoin concentrations should be determined during treatment [43]. A serum steady-state concentration of 5–20 μg/ml is sufficient for effective seizure control based on human studies [43]. Side effects of phenytoin include prolonged depression in the foal, mild atrioventricular block, and decreased blood pressure [21, 44].

Sodium pentobarbital may be used to control seizures in horses or foals that are unresponsive to other drugs. Pentobarbital is not a true anticonvulsant; seizure control arises due to its anesthetic effects. This anesthetic agent has profound depressant effects on respiration with repeated doses. Doses of 2–10 mg/kg IV to effect are recommended and have been used [45]. Sodium

pentobarbital has little use in the management of seizures in adult horses but may be used in the short-term management (1–3 days) of seizures in neonatal foals.

Primidone is metabolized to phenobarbital, which is the main active metabolite, and to a smaller extent to phenylethylmalonamide, another active metabolite that may potentiate the anticonvulsant effects of phenobarbital. Although primidone has been reported anecdotally for treating foals with seizures [45, 46], its use is not advised to treat epileptic horses since pharmacokinetic properties and clinical effects are unknown.

Newer antiepileptic drugs have been introduced in veterinary medicine, with improved therapeutic indices (i.e., effective dose compared with toxic dose) with a reduction of the sedative and organ-toxic adverse reactions [47]. These drugs include felbamate, gabapentin, clorazepate, topiramate, and zonisamide and can be used as monotherapy or combined with bromide. For example, gabapentin, a structural analog of GABA, has been used as adjunctive therapy in humans and dogs for the treatment of partial seizures refractory to phenobarbital and bromide therapy [47]. However, the cost of these new antiepileptic drug therapies may prohibit their use in adult horse, and their clinical efficacy is currently unknown.

It is difficult to give a precise recommendation for when to terminate anticonvulsant therapy. The duration of the seizure-free period required before terminating anticonvulsant therapy is unknown and will depend upon the severity and frequency of the seizures prior to commencing therapy. As a general rule, the horse should be seizure-free for at least one month if the seizures were occurring every few days. If the seizures were less frequent and well-documented, then the seizure-free period should be a multiple of at least three times the duration of the seizure cycle. That is, if the horse was having a seizure roughly every 2 weeks, then the seizure-free period should be at least 6 weeks (2 weeks times 3). These are only guidelines, however, and each case must be determined individually. If therapy has reduced the severity or frequency of the seizures but not totally eliminated them, then termination of anticonvulsant therapy is not advised. Abrupt discontinuation of the anticonvulsant therapy may precipitate seizures, hence a protocol of tapering doses is recommended. In neonates, the dose can be decreased by one-fourth to one-half each day for a minimum of 3 days, then discontinued. In the adult that has been on anticonvulsant maintenance therapy long-term, a longer weaning period is suggested, decreasing the dose by 20% every other day for 1 week before stopping [28].

In humans and small animals, serial EEGs have been shown to be very useful in the management of epilepsy, in particular to monitor the need and response to treatment, to aid in establishing the probability of recurrence, and prognosis [48–51]. This practice has been limited in horses, however, based on our experiences as well as that of others; horses may be seizure-free on anticonvulsant therapy but still have an abnormal EEG [51]. Therefore, serial EEGs may provide valuable information on the progression or resolution of the disease and may help the clinician in determining if continued maintenance anticonvulsant therapy is necessary. For example, persistent paroxysmal activity on the EEG recording suggests the need for continued anticonvulsant medication.

Although rare, horses may suffer from status epilepticus, which may not be controlled effectively with regular anticonvulsant therapy. Although an anesthetic protocol for this patient population has not been investigated, general anesthesia may be induced by a combination of guaifenesin (50 mg/kg IV to effect as a 5% solution) and thiopental (5 mg/kg IV) as an initial bolus, followed by a continuous infusion of pentobarbital (0.005 mg/kg/min) for up to 24 h [52]. Supportive care under general anesthesia should include the use of a padded stall and broad-spectrum antibiotic treatment. Maintenance phenobarbital therapy should be administered throughout anesthesia. An endotracheal tube may be placed if ventilation is required. In cases where cerebral edema is suspected such as after head trauma, constant ventilatory control is crucial during the entire period of anesthesia to avoid an increase in cerebral blood flow and subsequent increase in intracranial pressure secondary to hypercapnia and/or hypoxia (e.g., $PaCO_2$ and PaO_2 should be maintained between 25–35 torr and 100–150 torr, respectively) [36]. Ventilation-induced hypocapnia has been proposed as a means to decrease intracranial pressure, but extreme hyperventilation (<25 torr) will result in poor cerebral perfusion [36, 53]. Furthermore, blood pressure should be maintained within the physiological range to sustain adequate cerebral perfusion. In cases of seizures refractory to all the aforementioned therapeutic interventions, gas anesthesia with isoflurane (which has the least effect on intracranial pressure) may be considered. This approach is only a reasonable option if there is compelling reason for the clinician to expect resolution of the inciting cause of the seizure or to provide time for conventional anticonvulsants to be administered and be fully effective. If severe generalized seizures have occurred with no response to anticonvulsant therapy, euthanasia should be recommended on humane grounds.

Finally, it should be recommended that horses not be ridden while on anticonvulsant therapy and the horses have remained free of seizures for at least several months after withdrawal of treatment. Breeding horses suffering from seizures may be considered as an alternative.

Ancillary therapy

The main principles of ancillary therapy in the treatment of equine seizures are as follows:
1 To control cerebral edema, CNS inflammation, and intracranial pressure
2 Decrease the production of oxygen-derived free radicals
3 Prevent posttraumatic autodestruction of nervous tissue
4 Provide appropriate supportive care

Control of inflammation can be achieved by the use of steroidal or nonsteroidal anti-inflammatory drugs. Glucocorticoids stabilize microvascular permeability and decrease seizure foci [16]. Dexamethasone is the most commonly used corticosteroid in horses, although it has been reported that high-dose prednisolone is more effective for recovery of small animals with neurological diseases [54]. In addition, short-acting glucocorticoids such as prednisolone sodium succinate are recommended in foals instead of long-acting corticosteroids [19]. Nonsteroidal anti-inflammatory drugs (e.g., flunixin meglumine, ketoprofen, vedaprofen, or phenylbutazone) have also been shown to be beneficial in the treatment of CNS inflammation in horses [16].

Dimethyl sulfoxide has anti-inflammatory properties, which may be beneficial in convulsing horses, because of its abilities to stabilize membranes and scavenge free radicals that are released during inflammatory and ischemic processes [55]. Dimethyl sulfoxide is indicated for the treatment of increased intracranial pressure and/or cerebral edema, for hypoxic-ischemic encephalopathy and for the acute treatment of equine protozoal myeloencephalitis (EPM) [56, 57]. Dimethyl sulfoxide at a dose of 1 g/kg is safe as a 10% diluted solution; however, concentrations greater than 20% may cause hemolysis, diarrhea, and muscle tremor.

Mannitol is also used to control cerebrocortical edema; however, it is contraindicated in cases of intracranial hemorrhage as it may exacerbate bleeding.

Other medications, which may be used for their antioxidant properties, include alpha-tocopherol (vitamin E) and ascorbic acid (vitamin C). Vitamin E has been recommended at a high dose (20,000 IU/adult) for horses suffering from brain trauma, although its clinical efficacy is not proven [53]. Similarly, the clinical efficiency of ascorbic acid, which has also NMDA receptor blockage properties, is unknown in horses. Finally, allopurinol, a xanthine oxidase inhibitor and thus an antioxidant, has been used in hypoxic-ischemic human neonates [58]. There are anecdotal reports of its use in equine neonates with hypoxic-ischemic encephalopathy and in adult horses suffering from brain injury after head trauma; however, its clinical efficiency is also unknown [53, 59, 60].

Supportive care

The primary principles of supportive care are to

1 Provide proper hydration and nutritional support (especially in horses and foals unable or unwilling to drink and/or eat), ensuring proper cerebral perfusion and adequate delivery of nutrients and oxygen to the brain

2 Provide metabolic support to minimize factors that trigger cell death

3 Treat skin trauma and limit injury associated with seizures or recumbency

Maintaining cerebral perfusion is achieved by careful administration of intravenous fluid, especially in horses with cerebral edema and in recumbent animals in which the metabolic rate is decreased. In foals, judicious administration of inotropes may be necessary to maintain adequate perfusion pressures.

In foals presenting in status epilepticus, maintaining a patent airway is the first priority. Foals with mild hypoxia should be maintained in sternal position as much as possible, and supported by intranasal administration of humidified oxygen. Other measures as necessary to ensure adequate oxygenation and perfusion should be employed and will be directed on an individual basis.

Any electrolyte and acid–base imbalance should be corrected, especially in case of renal or hepatic disease. Moderate to severe hypoglycemia secondary to impaired gluconeogenesis has been reported in horses suffering from hepatic encephalopathy, and glucose supplementation resulted in remission of neurological signs in some instances [61]. Although it rarely causes seizures in neonatal foals, hypoglycemia should be promptly corrected with a constant infusion of glucose.

It has been suggested that magnesium sulfate, an NMDA receptor antagonist, given as an infusion, may decrease the incidence of seizures in foals suffering from hypoxic-ischemic encephalopathy [37]. Given that magnesium sulfate improves neurologic outcome after brain impact injury in an animal model, it has also been proposed for the treatment of brain injury after head trauma in adults at a dose of 50 mg/kg (25 g/500-kg horse administered in the first 5–10 l of IV fluid) [53]. Thiamine administration may prevent glutamate-induced and NMDA receptor–mediated cell death in foals with hypoxic-ischemic encephalopathy [62]. Furthermore, thiamine is an essential coenzyme in glucose utilization by the brain, which will further provide metabolic support [15].

Finally, horses must be maintained and housed in a proper environment to enhance delivery of medication, ensure safety of attending personnel, and provide protection for the horse. The horse should be placed in a padded stall with heavy bedding and away from other horses. If tolerated by the horse, a protective helmet should be placed, especially on recumbent animals, which will prevent eye and head injuries. It is important to be sure that the helmet fits properly, as an ill-fitting helmet may lead to more problems than using no helmet. Maintaining horses with the potential for seizures in a sling is very dangerous and should be avoided. Security measures should be in place for all staff and owners to prevent injuries to persons treating horses with seizures. The immediate environment should be quiet and in some cases plugging the ears with cotton is helpful. The intensity of the lighting should not be suddenly increased, to minimize the potential effects of outside stimuli.

Treating the underlying cause

In horses with seizures, every effort should be made to identify the etiology and specific therapy directed toward that diagnosis employed. Specific treatment protocols for the numerous disorders that can lead to seizures in horses are detailed in other chapters within this text.

Narcolepsy

Narcolepsy is described as a syndrome of uncontrollable "sleep attacks" that are usually, but not always, accompanied by complete loss of muscle tone (cataplexy). Narcolepsy has been recognized in a variety of domestic animals, including horses. Originally described in the equine literature in 1924 in a group of Suffolk foals, it has been reported in a variety of other ages and breeds [63–68]. A familial association in Shetland ponies, American Miniature Horses, Lipizzans, and Suffolk horses has been proposed [63, 66–68].

The pathophysiology of narcolepsy is not well-described; however, abnormalities of various brain neurotransmitters have been proposed. These include dopamine, serotonin, and noradrenaline. More recent work has focused on the role of the histaminergic tuberomammillary nucleus network, which incorporates noradrenergic, serotonergic, cholinergic, histaminergic, hypocretin (orexin), and GABAergic signaling [69]. Alterations and manipulations of this system result in changes in the sleep/wakefulness cycle and are proposed to be key in the pathophysiology of narcolepsy [69]. These compounds have been poorly investigated in horses; however, in one foal with narcolepsy without cataplexy, hypocretin concentrations in the CSF were similar to a normal age-matched control; in addition, concentrations of homovanillic acid (a metabolic product of dopamine) and 5-hydroxy-indolacetic acid (5-HIAA, a metabolic product of serotonin) were also normal [70]. Hypocretin concentrations in the CSF were normal in three other foals with narcolepsy as well [67]. In another study of two foals with familial narcolepsy,

CSF concentrations of noradrenaline, 3-,4-dihydroxy-phenylacetic acid (a dopamine metabolite), and 5-HIAA were also considered normal [68]. In the familial form of the disease in dogs, hypocretin concentrations are normal, and abnormalities appear to arise due to a mutation in the hypocretin receptor [71]. Some investigators consider human narcolepsy to be an autoimmune disorder, with most cases linked to a specific human leukocyte antigen (HLA) haplotype [72, 73].

Clinical signs noted with the condition suggest two different forms of the disorder: a condition of foals and a condition that develops later in life [74]. The severity of clinical signs in newborn foals appears to be variable with some spontaneous recovery noted, with persistence in other cases, particularly Suffolk and Shetland foals. Clinical signs appear to vary between individuals and episode [74]. Most commonly, horses are noted to have a progressive lowering of the head, followed by a buckling of the forelimbs, from which horses recover or which may result in falling. In severe attacks, total recumbency with areflexia and rapid eye movement can be seen and provide the most compelling clinical evidence for a diagnosis. The ability to arouse the horse from this state varies. Once awake, the horses can regain their footing normally and appear to have normal neurologic examination. Horses remain neurologically normal between attacks. Clinical examination may find evidence of superficial trauma, particularly to the front of the fetlocks and carpi. The attacks can occur spontaneously but have also been reported to be incited by particular events such as saddling, grooming, or events that induce anxiety.

In its most severe form, the syndrome is characteristic; however, in less severe manifestations, diagnosis is challenging. It must be differentiated from syncope and seizures. Diagnosis is made based upon the observation of excessive drowsiness at inappropriate times, evidence of cataplexy, and/or the response to provocative testing with physostigmine (0.05–0.1 mg/kg slow IV) or reversal with atropine [64, 68, 70]. After administration of physostigmine, clinical signs should immediately worsen, while treatment with atropine (0.07 mg/kg IV) should lead to an improvement in clinical signs that may last for several hours. The diagnostic accuracy of these methods is questionable, at least anecdotally, however, as several horses with compelling clinical signs have failed to respond to provocative testing. Complete blood cell counts and serum biochemistry analysis, as well as CSF evaluation, are normal. Assay of CSF for hypocretin concentrations do not appear to have much value in diagnosis, as described earlier. EEG was unremarkable in the two foals in which it was performed [68].

Treatment with imipramine (250–750 mg orally for an adult or 0.5 mg/kg IM) has been suggested with variable success [64, 66, 68, 74]. In humans, imipramine simultaneously stimulates aminergic and inhibits cholinergic activity of the CNS, with good clinical effects for controlling cataplexy [75]. Limited studies of imipramine in horses are reported; however, a dose of 2 mg/kg IV resulted in neurologic abnormalities including muscle fasciculations and hyperexcitability, which lasted for several hours [75]. The prognosis is guarded, and some horses with adult-onset narcolepsy become unmanageable and dangerous, requiring euthanasia. The condition appears to be persistent in affected Suffolk and Shetland foals, but spontaneous recovery can be seen in other breeds.

References

[1] Lowenstein DH. Seizures and epilepsy. In: Hauser SL, Jameson JL, Kasper DL, et al. eds. *Harrisons Principles of Internal Medicine*, 16th ed. New York:McGraw-Hill;2005: 2357–2372.

[2] Lacombe VA, Mayes M, Mosseri S, et al. Distribution and predictive factors of seizure types in 104 cases. *Equine Vet J* 2014;46:441–445.

[3] Mayhew IG. Seizure disorders. In: Robinson NE, ed. *Current Therapy in Equine Medicine*. Philadelphia, PA:W.B. Saunders Co;1983:344–349.

[4] Andrews FA, Mathews H. Seizures, narcolepsy and cataplexy. In: Reed SM, Bayly W, eds. *Equine Internal Medicine*, 1st ed. Philadelphia, PA:W.B. Saunders Co;1998:451–457.

[5] Furr M. Perinatal asphyxia in foals. *Compend Contin Educ Pract Vet* 1996;18:1342–1351.

[6] Aleman M, Gray LC, Williams DC, et al. Juvenile idiopathic epilepsy in Egyptian Arabian foals: 22 cases (1985–2005). *J Vet Intern Med* 2006;20:1443–1449.

[7] Furr MO, Bender H. Cerebrospinal fluid variables in clinically normal foals from birth to 42 days of age. *Am J Vet Res* 1994;55:781–784.

[8] Lacombe VA, Podell M, Furr M, et al. Diagnostic validity of electroencephalography in equine intracranial disorders. *J Vet Intern Med* 2001;15:385–393.

[9] Redding RW. Electroencephalography. In: Oliver JE, Horlein BF, Mayhew IG, eds. *Veterinary Neurology*, 1st ed. Philadelphia, PA:W.B. Saunders;1987:111–145.

[10] Lacombe VA, Andrews M. Electrodiagnostic evaluation of the nervous system. In: Furr M, Reed S, eds. *Equine Neurology*, 1st ed. Ames, IA:Wiley Blackwell;2007:127–148.

[11] Klemm WR. Electroencephalography in the diagnosis of epilepsy. *Probl Vet Med* 1989;1:535–557.

[12] Lacombe VA, Mayes M, Mosseri S, et al. Epilepsy in horses: etiologic classification and predictive factors. *Equine Vet J* 2012;44:646–651.

[13] Lacombe VA, Robinson C, Reed S. Diagnostic utility of computed tomography of the head in horses with intracranial diseases. *Equine Vet J* 2010;42:393–399.

[14] Robinson C, Lacombe VA, Reed S, et al. Factors predictive of abnormal results for computed tomography of the head in horses affected by neurologic disorders. *J Am Vet Med Assoc* 2009;235:176–183.

[15] Podell ML. Antiepileptic drug therapy. *Clin Tech Small Anim Pract* 1998;13:185–192.

[16] Dowling PM. Drugs acting on the neurological system and behavior modification. In: Bertone JJ, Horspool LJ, eds. *Equine Clinical Pharmacology*, 1st ed. Philadelphia, PA: W.B. Saunders;2004:145–154.

[17] Norman WM, Court MH, Greenblatt DJ. Age-related changes in the pharmacokinetic disposition of diazepam in foals. *Am J Vet Res* 1997;58:878–880.

[18] Muir WW, Sams RA, Huffman R, et al. Pharmacodynamic and pharmacokinetic properties of diazepam in horses. *Am J Vet Res* 1982;43:1756–1762.

[19] Furr M. Managing seizure disorders in neonatal foals. *Vet Med* 1996;91:772–778.

[20] Wilkins PA. How to use midazolam to control equine neonatal seizures. *Proc Annu Meet Am Assoc Equine Pract* 2005;51:279–280.

[21] Magdesian KG. Intensive care medicine. In: Higgins AJ, Snyder JR, eds. *The Equine Manual*, 1st ed. Philadelphia, PA:W.B. Saunders;2006:1255–1326.

[22] Hubbell JAE, Kelly EM, Aarnes TK, et al. Pharmacokinetics of midazolam after intravenous administration to horses. *Equine Vet J* 2013;45:721–725.

[23] Andrews FM, Matthews HK. Seizures, narcolepsy and cataplexy. In: Reed SM, Bayly WM, Sellon D, eds. *Equine Internal Medicine*, 2nd ed. St. Louis, MO:W.B. Saunders; 2004:560–566.

[24] Trommer BL, Pasternak JF. NMDA receptor antagonists inhibit kindling epileptogenesis and seizure expression in developing rats. *Brain Res Dev Brain Res* 1990;53:248–252.

[25] Platt SR. The role of glutamate in neurologic diseases. Proceedings of the 19th Annual Meeting ACVIM, San Diego, CA, 2001;427–430.

[26] Borris DJ, Bertram EH, Kapur J. Ketamine controls prolonged status epilepticus. *Epilepsy Res* 2000;42:117–122.

[27] Szakacs R, Weiczner R, Mihaly A, et al. Non-competitive NMDA receptor antagonists moderate seizure-induced c-fos expression in the rat cerebral cortex. *Brain Res Bull* 2003;59:485–493.

[28] Mayhew IG. When should I start anticonvulsant therapy for a mature epileptic horse, and what medication should I use? *Compend Contin Educ Pract Vet* 1998;20:744–746.

[29] Mayhew IG Rules of thumb in managing epileptic horses. Proceedings North American Veterinary Conference, Orlando, FL, 2003;172–173.

[30] Ravis WR, Duran SH, Pedersoli WM, et al. A pharmacokinetic study of phenobarbital in mature horses after oral dosing. *J Vet Pharmacol Ther* 1987;10:283–289.

[31] Knox DA, Ravis WR, Pedersoli WM, et al. Pharmacokinetics of phenobarbital in horses after single and repeated oral administration of the drug. *Am J Vet Res* 1992;53:706–710.

[32] Duran SH, Ravis WR, Pedersoli WM, et al. Pharmacokinetics of phenobarbital in the horse. *Am J Vet Res* 1987;48: 807–810.

[33] Spehar AM, Hill MR, Mayhew IG, et al. Preliminary study on the pharmacokinetics of phenobarbital in the neonatal foal. *Equine Vet J* 1984;16:368–371.

[34] Magdesian KG. Neonatal pharmacology and therapeutics. In: Robinson NE, ed. *Current Therapy in Equine Medicine 5*. Philadelphia, PA:W.B. Saunders;2002:1–5.

[35] Podell M. Seizures in dogs. *Vet Clin North Am Small Anim Pract* 1996;26:779–809.

[36] LeBlanc PH, Brunson DB. Anesthetic management of equine head trauma: a case report. *Vet Surg* 1986;15: 279–282.

[37] Wilkins PA. Hypoxic ischemic encephalopathy: neonatal encephalopathy. In: Wilkins PA, Palmer JE, eds. *Recent Advances in Equine Neonatal Care*. Ithaca, NY:International Veterinary Information Service;2003.

[38] Mayhew IG. Seizures. In: Mayhew IG, ed. *Large Animal Neurology: A Handbook for Veterinary Clinicians*, 1st ed. Philadelphia, PA:Lea & Febiger;1989:113–125.

[39] Raidal SL, Edwards S. Pharmacokinetics of potassium bromide in adult horses. *Aust Vet J* 2005;83:425–430.

[40] Fielding CL, Magdesian KG, Elliott DA, et al. Pharmacokinetics and clinical utility of sodium bromide (NaBr) as an estimator of extracellular fluid volume in horses. *J Vet Intern Med* 2003;17:213–217.

[41] Trepanier LA, Van Schoick A, Schwark WS, et al. Therapeutic serum drug concentrations in epileptic dogs treated with potassium bromide alone or in combination with other anticonvulsants: 122 cases (1992–1996). *J Am Vet Med Assoc* 1998;213:1449–1453.

[42] Knight HD, Costner GC. Bromide intoxication of horses, goats, and cattle. *J Am Vet Med Assoc* 1977;171:446–448.

[43] Kowalczyk DF, Beech J. Pharmacokinetics of phenytoin (diphenylhydantoin) in horses. *J Vet Pharmacol Ther* 1983;6:133–140.

[44] Sihna AK, Cox JH. Diseases of the brain. In: Kobluk CN, Ames TR, Geor RJ, eds. *The Horse: Diseases and Clinical Management*, 1st ed. Philadelphia, PA:W.B. Saunders;1995:413–441.

[45] May CJ, Greenwood RE. Recurrent convulsions in a thoroughbred foal: management and treatment. *Vet Rec* 1977;101:76–77.

[46] Blakely AA. Diseases of foals. *N Z Vet J* 1962;10:79–85.

[47] Podell M. Strategies of antiepileptic drug therapy. Proceedings of the 19th Annual Meeting ACVIM, San Diego, CA, 2001;430–431.

[48] Berendt M, Høgoenhaven H, Flagstad A, et al. Electroencephalography in dogs with epilepsy: similarities between human and canine findings. *Acta Neurol Scand* 1999;99:276–283.

[49] Govendir M, Perkins M, Malik R. Improving seizure control in dogs with refractory epilepsy using gabapentin as an adjunctive agent. *Aust Vet J* 2005;83:602–608.

[50] Jaggy A, Bernardini M. Idiopathic epilepsy in 125 dogs: a long-term study. Clinical and electroencephalographic findings. *J Small Anim Pract* 1998;39:23–29.

[51] Kube SA, Aleman M, Williams DC et al. How to work up a horse with seizures. *Proc Annu Meet Am Assoc Equine Pract* 2004;50:418–424.

[52] Hubbell JA, Hinchcliff KW, Grosenbaugh DA, et al. Ureteral ligation prevents the haemodynamic effect of frusemide in pentobarbitol anaesthetised horses. *Equine Vet J* 2002;34:580–586.

[53] Mackay RJ. Brain injury after head trauma: pathophysiology, diagnosis, and treatment. *Vet Clin North Am Equine Pract* 2004;20:199–216.

[54] Hines MT. Changes in mentation, seizures and narcolepsy. In: Robinson NE, ed. *Current Therapy in Equine Medicine 5*. Philadelphia, PA:W.B. Saunders;2003:764–771.

[55] Brayton CF. Dimethyl sulfoxide (DMSO): a review. *Cornell Vet* 1986;76:61–90.

[56] Blythe LL, Craig AM, Christensen JM, et al. Pharmacokinetic disposition of dimethyl sulfoxide administered intravenously to horses. *Am J Vet Res* 1986;47:1739–1743.

[57] Del Bigio M, James HE, Camp PE, et al. Acute dimethyl sulfoxide therapy in brain edema. Part 3: effect of a 3-hour infusion. *Neurosurgery* 1982;10:86–89.

[58] Tan S, Parks DA. Preserving brain function during neonatal asphyxia. *Clin Perinatol* 1999;26:733–747.

[59] Galvin N, Collins D. Perinatal asphyxia in the foal: review and case report. *Ir Vet J* 2004;57:707–714.

[60] Slovis NM. Perinatal asphyxia syndrome (hypoxic ischemic encephalopathy). Proceedings of the 21st Annual Meeting ACVIM, 2003;250–251.

[61] Eades S, Waguespack C. The gastrointestinal and digestive system. In: Higgins AJ, Snyder JR, eds. *The Equine Manual*, 1st ed. Philadelphia, PA:W.B. Saunders;2006:529–626.

[62] Vaala WE. Perinatal asphyxia syndrome in foals. In: Robinson NE, ed. *Current Therapy in Equine Medicine 5*. Philadelphia, PA:W.B. Saunders;2002:644–649.

[63] Sheather AL. Fainting in foals. *J Comp Pathol* 1924;62:106–113.

[64] Sweeney CR, Hendricks JM, Beech J, et al. Narcolepsy in a horse. *J Am Vet Med Assoc* 1984;183:126–128.

[65] Dreifuss FE, Flynn DV. Narcolepsy in a horse. *J Am Vet Med Assoc* 1984;184:131–132. (Letter).

[66] Mayhew IG. Coma and altered states of consciousness. In: Mayhew IG, ed. *Large Animal Neurology*, 1st ed. Philadelphia, PA: Lea and Febinger;1983:133–146.

[67] Ludvikova E, Nishino S, Sakai N, et al. Familial narcolepsy in the Lipizzaner horse: a report of three fillies born to the same sire. *Vet Q* 2012;32:99–102.

[68] Lunn DP, Cuddon PA, Shaftoe S, et al. Familial occurrence of narcolepsy in Miniature horses. *Equine Vet J* 1993;25:483–487.

[69] Panula P, Nuutinen S. The histaminergic network in the brain: basic organization and role in disease. *Nat Rev Neurosci* 2013;14:472–487.

[70] Nothen-Bathen A, Heider C, Fernandez AJ, et al. Hypocretin measurement in an Icelandic foal with narcolepsy. *J Vet Intern Med* 2009;23:1299–1302.

[71] Lin L, Faraco J, Li R, et al. The sleep disorder canine narcolepsy is caused by a mutation in the hypocretin (orexin) receptor 2 gene. *Cell* 1999;98:365–376.

[72] Peyron C, Furaco J, Rogers W, et al. A mutation in a case of early onset narcolepsy and a generalized absence of hypocretin peptides in human narcoleptic brains. *Nat Med* 2000;6:991–997.

[73] Lin L, Hungs M, Mignot E. Narcolepsy and the HLA region. *J Neuroimmunol* 2001;117:9–20.

[74] Hines MT, Schott HC, Byrne BA. Adult-onset narcolepsy in the horse. *Proc Annu Meet Am Assoc Equine Pract* 1992;38:289–296.

[75] Peck KE, Hines MT, Mealey KL, et al. Pharmacokinetics of imipramine in narcoleptic horses. *Am J Vet Res* 2001;62:783–786.

8 Differential Diagnosis of Equine Spinal Ataxia

Martin Furr

Marion duPont Scott Equine Medical Center, Virginia-Maryland Regional College of Veterinary Medicine, Leesburg, USA

Spinal ataxia is a common expression of central nervous system (CNS) disease in the horse. The clinical signs that result from many conditions of the equine spinal cord are similar, making a clear-cut diagnosis difficult solely on clinical grounds. Creating order out of the myriad causes of ataxia, in the form of a differential diagnosis list and a diagnostic plan, requires a careful consideration of all pertinent information. Forming a differential diagnosis is the act of bringing together all the historical and physical examination information to construct a list of reasonable disorders that will determine the next step in the diagnostic process. Doing so requires knowledge of the various conditions that can affect the horse, as well as their most common presentations. In addition, a sound neurologic examination with neuroanatomic localization of the lesion is critical in forming the differential diagnosis list and selecting appropriate ancillary tests to make a final diagnosis. (This is further discussed in Chapter 6.) In almost all cases of spinal ataxia, a complete evaluation will include, in addition to the physical and neurologic examination, a complete blood cell count, serum biochemistry profile, radiographs of the cervical spine, and a cerebrospinal fluid evaluation. Depending upon the specific presentation, microbial or viral culture, viral antibody titers, *Sarcocystis neurona* testing, or other specific procedures may be required.

A routine physical examination is important as it will help illuminate any other physical abnormalities that may contribute to or be a part of the neurologic problem. In horses that demonstrate hind limb gait deficits, a rectal examination to assess internal iliac artery pulses may be necessary. Palpation of large muscle masses for pain or firmness, joints for distention, and digital pulses to rule out laminitis should be a part of the examination to eliminate these nonneurologic problems that can be confused with nervous system disease (Table 8.1).

Results of the physical and neurologic examination allow the clinician to answer a few important questions, which are as follows:

1 Are there conclusive signs of nervous system disease, and is it central or peripheral?
2 What is the neuroanatomic localization of the lesion?
3 Do the clinical signs arise from a single site, multifocal sites, or diffuse inflammation?
4 Are the clinical signs symmetric or asymmetric?

In animals in which spinal ataxia is the predominant clinical sign, the lesion may arise from brain, brainstem, or spinal cord. The ataxia associated with focal brain lesions (cranial to the red nucleus) is usually very mild. The ataxia arising from focal brainstem lesions results in proprioceptive deficits, variable degrees of ataxia, and some alteration of mentation. Brain and brainstem lesions should also be reflected by changes in the cranial nerve responses as detected from a neurologic examination. In cases in which the ataxia originates from the spinal cord, the mentation will be normal (see video clips demonstrating clinical signs for videos).

From the findings of the neurologic examination, a determination of whether the clinical signs arise from a single site can be made. Conditions that result in a single focus include the compressive diseases (cervical compressive myelopathy, intervertebral disc protrusion, fracture, and extradural masses), while multifocal or diffuse disease is most often associated with conditions such as equine protozoal myeloencephalitis (EPM), verminous myelitis, infectious disease, and polyneuritis equi. In addition, the presence or absence of symmetry can be useful. Cervical compressive myelopathy, equine degenerative encephalomyelopathy, neuroaxonal dystrophy, and motor neuron disease are typically symmetrical, while EPM, verminous myelitis, or neoplastic growths are more likely to be asymmetrical. These are generalizations, of course, and an individual case may differ, but they generally hold true (Tables 8.2 and 8.3).

Equine Neurology, Second Edition. Martin Furr and Stephen Reed.

The presence of systemic illness is an important finding in horses with neurologic disease. Infectious diseases such as viral encephalitis (e.g., equine encephalitis, West Nile virus encephalitis (WNV), and equine herpesvirus 1 (EHV-1) encephalitis) usually result in constitutional signs of illness such as fever, depression, and anorexia, which may precede or be coincident with the neurologic abnormalities. Vague and nonspecific neurologic signs can be seen in horses that are in circulatory shock from any cause or that have serious electrolyte disturbances. Severe pain associated with colic may make horses tremble uncontrollably and stumble when walking yet not demonstrate more classic signs of abdominal pain. Careful examination of such horses is necessary to determine the true nature and extent of their illness (see video clips demonstrating clinical signs for videos).

Signalment includes the horse's breed, age, gender, and use. Certain conditions have been demonstrated to have a breed, age, and gender association, and while this does not confirm a specific condition, it is important information in narrowing the differential diagnosis list. In one study of 100 horses with spinal ataxia, Thoroughbred horses were much more commonly affected by cervical compressive myelopathy than any other breed represented in the study [1]. Another report reviewing the cause of ataxia in 19 horses did not demonstrate a clear breed or age predisposition for cervical compressive myelopathy [2]; however, both studies were retrospective surveys and there were strong population biases. It is widely reported, however, that

Thoroughbreds and Quarter horses have a higher incidence of cervical compressive myelopathy than other breeds, and a more recent report has found that Thoroughbreds, warmbloods, and Tennessee Walking horses were overrepresented [3–5]. Cerebellar abiotrophy and atlantooccipital malformation are more commonly (but not exclusively) seen in the Arabian, and neuroaxonal dystrophy is seen as a breed-related phenomenon in Morgan horses (Tables 8.4 and 8.5).

Age is also an important factor to consider in formulating the differential diagnosis for horses with spinal ataxia. Most horses presented for ataxia are 3 years of age or less, corresponding to the high prevalence of

Table 8.1 Some nonneurologic conditions that can be confused with ataxia in the horse.

Internal iliac thrombosis
Muscle disease
Multiple limb lameness
Laminitis
Pelvic fracture
Sacroiliac subluxation
Severe dehydration/shock/hypotension

Table 8.3 Infectious, iatrogenic, idiopathic, and inflammatory conditions in which spinal ataxia is a prominent component.

Viral meningoencephalitis
   Numerous agents
Bacterial meningitis [7]
   Numerous agents
Protozoal myeloencephalitis
   Sarcocystis neurona
   Neospora hughesi
Verminous myelitis
   Numerous agents
Vertebral osteomyelitis
Discospondylitis [8]
Cauda equina neuritis
Fibrocartilagenous embolism [9, 10]
Aortic–iliac thrombosis [11]
Air embolism
Postanesthetic hemorrhagic myelopathy
Cholesterol granuloma [12, 13]
Intracarotid injection
Fourth ventricle vascular anomaly [14]
Lidocaine toxicity
Epidermoid cyst [15]
Epidural hemorrhage [16]
Neuronal intranuclear inclusion disease [17]
Systemic granulomatous disease [18]

Table 8.2 Comparative characteristics of some common causes of equine spinal ataxia.

	CVM	EHV-1	EPM	LMND	Fracture
History	Chronic, progressive	Acute, progressive	Chronic, progressive	Chronic, progressive	Acute, nonprogressive
Symmetrical (Y/N)	Yes	Yes	No	Yes	Variable
UMN/LMN	UMN predominant	Mixed	Mixed/LMN	LMN	Mixed
Muscle atrophy (Y/N)	No	Rare	Yes	Yes	No
Unifocal/multifocal	Unifocal	Multifocal	Uni- or multifocal	Diffuse	Unifocal

CVM, cervical vertebral myelopathy; LMN, lower motor neuron; LMND, lower motor neuron disease; UMN, upper motor neuron.

Table 8.4 Developmental/degenerative conditions in which spinal ataxia is a prominent component.

Cerebellar abiotrophy [19]
Atlantoaxial malformations [20]
Focal Compression
   Cervical Compressive Myelopathy [1, 2]
   Tumors (see Table 3.5)
   Intervertebral disk prolapse [8, 21]
   Cervical arthritis [22]
   Vascular malformations [23]
   Synovial cysts [24]
   Arachnoid diverticulum [25]
Cleft vertebral column [26]

Table 8.5 Selected toxic agents in which spinal ataxia is a prominent component.

Stinging nettles [27]
Onion weed (*Trachyandra divaricata*) [28]
Topical amitraz [29]
Amprolium [30]
Sorghum-associated (lolitrem B) [31, 32]
Moxidectin [33]
Ivermectin [34]
Crotalaria [35]
Propylene glycol [36, 37]
Ionophores
   Monensin [38]
   Lasalocid
   Salinomycin [39]
Pipothiazine [40]
Perphenazine [40]
Fluphenazine [41, 42]
Tremetol [43]
Heavy metals
   Lead [44]
   Arsenic [45]
Bromide [46]
Moldy corn [47]
Lathyrism
Swainsonia poisoning [48–50]
Locoism
Acute selenium toxicity [51]
Indigofera lespedezioides [52]
Rhaponticum repens (creeping knapweed) [53]
Trema micrantha [54]
Vetch (*Vicia* spp.) [18]
Sina carpinifoli-induced mannosidosis [55]

cervical compressive myelopathy in young horses that are of training age [1, 6]. Congenital abnormalities are most usually noted at a very young age. Cervical fracture

was most commonly noted in horses less than 5 years of age, while lumbar fractures and sacroiliac subluxations and fractures appeared more common in horses over 5 years of age [1].

The clinical history and progression of the illness is of particular importance in the evaluation of ataxic horses. It is important to proactively question the owner or caretaker and to probe until given precise answers. An acute or rapid onset is often associated with traumatic events; however, it is important to determine if more subtle signs of ataxia were present prior to an observed fall. Alternately, a fall or other traumatic event may worsen a preexisting but less severe condition. Cervical compressive myelopathy is most often slowly progressive and may have a mild waxing and waning course or rarely a sudden worsening. A similar history is most often observed in horses with EPM, although clinical signs in horses with EPM can progress rapidly in a small number of cases. The clinical signs associated with equine degenerative myeloencephalopathy are reported to progress moderately rapidly after they are first observed. Infectious diseases such as eastern or western encephalitis, rabies, or WNV usually are observed to have a rapid progression, with clinical signs observed to worsen quickly for a few days, then stabilize.

A history of recent medications is important to note as various anthelmintics and tranquilizers have been noted to result in CNS disease. The type of feed and forage should be noted as ataxia has been observed in horses that consumed sorghum, and a variety of ataxia syndromes have been described in horses grazing various grasses (Table 8.5).

As most horses are fastidious eaters, toxicity syndromes appear to be fairly rare in the horse, but a rather bewildering variety of toxins have been reported in the horse. While most horses will avoid toxic plants, horses that are starving on a grossly overgrazed pasture may be forced to consume plants that they would otherwise avoid. Hence, examining the horse's housing may be useful. Many intoxications of the horse lead to generalized neurologic signs (trembling, seizures, mentation changes), while few are associated with spinal ataxia alone. These include Ryegrass–associated ataxia, Dallis grass ataxia, and sorghum-associated ataxia/cystitis. Nonspecific neurologic signs noted in horses with many forms of intoxication may be related to specific neurologic damage, as well as nonspecific changes such as dehydration, alteration in blood pressure, or electrolyte disorders, underscoring the importance of a complete evaluation (Table 8.6).

Once a differential list is constructed, the clinician will use it to direct further evaluation and determine ancillary testing that may be needed. Additional testing may include imaging, clinical chemistry analysis, myelography, electrodiagnostic testing, or collection and assay of various biological fluids or feed samples.

Table 8.6 Specific neoplastic conditions reported in the horse in which spinal ataxia has been noted as a prominent component.

Plasma cell myeloma [56]
Undifferentiated sarcoma [57]
Melanoma [58]
Pheochromocytoma [59]
Squamous cell carcinoma [60]
Lymphoma/lymphosarcoma [61, 62]
Angioma [63]
Hemartomas
Ependymoma [64]
Hemangiosarcoma [65, 66]
Angiosarcoma [67]
Meningioangiomatosis [68]
Oligodendroglioma [69]
Choroid plexus papilloma [70]
Metastatic intestinal adenocarcinoma [71]

References

[1] Reed, S., Bayly, W., Traub, J.L. *et al.* (1981) Ataxia and paresis in horses. Part 1: Differential diagnosis. *Compend Contin Educ Pract Vet*, 3, S88–S98.

[2] Nappert, G., Vrins, A., Breton, L. *et al.* (1989) A retrospective study of nineteen ataxic horses. *Can Vet J*, 30, 802–806.

[3] Mayhew, I.G., DeLahunta, A. and Whitlock, R.H. (1978) History and clinical evaluation [of spinal cord disease in horses]. *Cornell Vet*, 68 (Suppl 6), 24–35.

[4] Mayhew, I.J. (1989) Neurologic Evaluation, in *Large Animal Neurology* (ed. I.G. Mayhew), Lea and Febinger, Philadelphia, pp. 15–47.

[5] Levine, J.M., Scrivani, P.V., Divers, T.J. *et al.* (2010) Multicenter cases-control study of signalment, diagnostic features, and outcome associated with cervical vertebral malformation-malarticulation in horses. *J Am Vet Med Assoc*, 237, 812–822.

[6] Smith, J.M. and Cox, J.H. (1987) Central nervous system disease in adult horses. Part II: Differential diagnosis. *Compend Contin Educ Pract Vet*, 9, 772–778.

[7] Rutten, M., Lehner, A., Pospischil, A. *et al.* (2006) Cerebral listeriosis in an adult Freilberger gelding. *J Comp Pathol*, 134, 249–253.

[8] Furr, M.O., Anver, M. and Wise, M. (1991) Intervertebral disk prolapse and diskospondylitis in a horse. *J Am Vet Med Assoc*, 198, 2095–2096.

[9] Taylor, H.W., Vandevelde, M. and Firth, E.C. (1977) Ischemic myelopathy caused by fibrocartilaginous emboli in a horse. *Vet Pathol*, 14, 479–481.

[10] Walling, B.E., Stewart, M.C. and Valli, V.E. (2011) Pathology in practice: fibrocartilaginous embolism. *J Am Vet Med Assoc*, 239, 199–201.

[11] Mayhew, I.G. and Kryger, M.D. (1975) Aortic-iliac-femoral thrombosis in a horse. *Vet Med Small Anim Clin*, 70, 1281–1284.

[12] de Lahunta, A., Jefferson, D.A., Geary, J.C. *et al.* (1969) Granuloma compressing the brain of a pony. *Cornell Vet*, 60, 622–639.

[13] Johnson, P.J., Lin, T.L. and Jennings, D.P. (1993) Diffuse cerebral encephalopathy associated with hydrocephalus and cholesterinic granulomas in a horse. *J Am Vet Med Assoc*, 203, 694–697.

[14] Miller, L.M., Reed, S.M., Gallina, A.M. *et al.* (1985) Ataxia and weakness associated with fourth ventricle vascular anomalies in two horses. *J Am Vet Med Assoc*, 186, 601–603.

[15] Kelly, D.F. and Watson, W.J. (1976) Epidermoid cyst of the brain in the horse. *Equine Vet J*, 8, 110–112.

[16] Gold, J.R., Divers, T.J., Miller, A.J. *et al.* (2008) Cervical vertebral spinal hematomas in 4 horses. *J Vet Intern Med*, 22, 481–485.

[17] Pumerola, M., Vidal, E., Trens, J.M. *et al.* (2005) Neuronal intranuclear inclusion disease in a horse. *Acta Neuropathol*, 110, 191–195.

[18] Woods, L.W., Johnson, B., Hietala, S.K. *et al.* (1992) Systemic granulomatous disease in a horse grazing pasture containing vetch (Vicia sp.). *J Vet Diagn Invest*, 4, 356–360.

[19] Baird, J.D. and Mackenzie, C.D. (1974) Cerebellar hypoplasia and degeneration in part-Arab horses. *Aust Vet J*, 50, 25–28.

[20] Mayhew, I.G., Watson, A.G. and Heissan, J.A. (1978) Congenital occipitoatlantoaxial malformations in the horse. *Equine Vet J*, 10, 103–113.

[21] Jansson, N. (2001) What is your diagnosis? Multiple cervical intervertebral disk prolapses. *J Am Vet Med Assoc*, 219, 1681–1682.

[22] von Schebitz, H. and Schulz, L.C. (1965) On the pathogenesis of spinal ataxia in horses—spondyloarthrosis, clinical findings. *Dtsch Tierarztl Wochenschr*, 72, 496–501.

[23] Gilmour, J.S. and Fraser, J.A. (1977) Ataxia in a Welsh cob filly due to a venous malformation in the thoracic spinal cord. *Equine Vet J*, 9, 40–42.

[24] Fisher, L.F., Bowman, K.F. and MacHarg, M.A. (1981) Spinal ataxia in a horse caused by a synovial cyst. *Vet Pathol*, 18, 407–410.

[25] Allison, N. and Moeller, R.B., Jr (2000) Spinal ataxia in a horse caused by an arachnoid diverticulum (cyst). *J Vet Diagn Invest*, 12, 279–281.

[26] Doige, C.E. (1996) Congenital cleft vertebral centrum and intra- and extraspinal cyst in a foal. *Vet Pathol*, 33, 87–89.

[27] Bathe, A.P. (1994) An unusual manifestation of nettle rash in three horses. *Vet Rec*, 134, 11–12.

[28] Huxtable, C.R., Chapman, H.M., Main, D.C. *et al.* (1987) Neurological disease and lipofuscinosis in horses and sheep grazing *Trachyandra divaricata* (branched onion weed) in south Western Australia. *Aust Vet J*, 64, 105–108.

[29] Auer, D.E., Seawright, A.A., Pollitt, C.C. *et al.* (1984) Illness in horses following spraying with amitraz. *Aust Vet J*, 61, 257–259.

[30] Cymbaluk, N.F., Fretz, P.B. and Loew, F.M. (1978) Amprolium-induced thiamine deficiency in horses: clinical features. *Am J Vet Res*, 39, 255–261.

[31] Adams, L.G., Dollahite, J.W., Romane, W.M. *et al.* (1969) Cystitis and ataxia associated with sorghum ingestion by horses. *J Am Vet Med Assoc*, 155, 518–524.

[32] Sloet van Oldruitenborgh-Oosterbaan, M.M., Schipper, F.C., Goehring, L.S. *et al.* (1999) Rhinopneumonia or mycotoxin intoxication? Neurologic phenomena in horses from a riding school. *Tijdschr Diergeneeskd*, 124, 679–681.

[33] Khan, S.A., Kuster, D.A. and Hansen, S.R. (2002) A review of moxidectin overdose cases in equines from 1998 through 2000. *Vet Hum Toxicol*, 44, 232–235.

[34] Hautekeete, L.A., Khan, S.A. and Hales, W.S. (1998) Ivermectin toxicosis in a zebra. *Vet Hum Toxicol*, 40, 29–31.

[35] Arzt, J. and Mount, M.E. (1999) Hepatotoxicity associated with pyrrolizidine alkaloid (*Crotalaria spp.*) ingestion in a horse on Easter Island. *Vet Hum Toxicol*, 41, 96–99.

[36] McClanahan, S., Hunter, J., Murphy, M. *et al.* (1998) Propylene glycol toxicosis in a mare. *Vet Hum Toxicol*, 40, 294–296.

[37] Dorman, D.C. and Haschek, W.M. (1991) Fatal propylene glycol toxicosis in a horse. *J Am Vet Med Assoc*, 198, 1643–1644.

[38] Matsuoka, T. (1976) Evaluation of monensin toxicity in the horse. *J Am Vet Med Assoc*, 169, 1098–1100.

[39] Rollinson, J., Taylor, F.G. and Chesney, J. (1987) Salinomycin poisoning in horses. *Vet Rec*, 121, 126–128.

[40] McCrindle, C.M., Ebedes, H. and Swan, G.E. (1989) The use of long-acting neuroleptics, perphenazine enanthate and pipothiazine palmitate in two horses. *J S Afr Vet Assoc*, 60, 208–209.

[41] Kauffman, V.G., Soma, L., Divers, T.J. *et al.* (1989) Extrapyramidal side effects caused by fluphenazine decanoate in a horse. *J Am Vet Med Assoc*, 195, 1128–1130.

[42] Brewer, B., Hines, M., Stewart, J.T. *et al.* (1990) Fluphenazine induced Parkinson-like syndrome in a horse. *Equine Vet J*, 22, 136–137.

[43] Olson, C.T., Keller, W.C., Gerken, D.F. *et al.* (1984) Suspected tremetol poisoning in horses. *J Am Vet Med Assoc*, 185, 1001–1003.

[44] Sojka, J.E., Hope, W. and Pearson, D. (1996) Lead toxicosis in 2 horses: similarity to equine degenerative lower motor neuron disease. *J Vet Intern Med*, 10, 420–423.

[45] Pace, L.W., Turnquist, S.E., Casteel, S.W. *et al.* (1997) Acute arsenic toxicosis in five horses. *Vet Pathol*, 34, 160–164.

[46] Knight, H.D. and Costner, G.C. (1977) Bromide intoxication of horses, goats, and cattle. *J Am Vet Med Assoc*, 171, 446–448.

[47] McCue, P. (1989) Equine leukoencephalomalacia. *Compend Contin Educ Pract Vet*, 11, 646–651.

[48] van Essen, G.J., Blom, M. and Fink, G.-G.J. (1995) Ryegrass cramps in horses. *Tijdschr Diergeneeskd*, 120, 710–711.

[49] Locke, K.B., McEwan, D.R. and Hamdorf, I.J. (1980) Experimental poisoning of horses and cattle with *Swainsona canescens var horniana*. *Aust Vet J*, 56, 379–383.

[50] O'Sullivan, B.M. and Goodwin, J.A. (1977) An outbreak of Swainsona poisoning in horses. *Aust Vet J*, 53, 446–447.

[51] Desta, B., Maldonado, G., Reid, H. *et al.* (2011) Acute selenium toxicosis in polo ponies. *J Vet Diagn Invest*, 23, 623–628.

[52] Lima, E.F., Riet-Correa, F., Gardner, D.R. *et al.* (2012) Poisoning by *Indigofera lespedezioides* in horses. *Toxicon*, 60, 324–328.

[53] Elliot, C.R. and McGowan, C.I. (2012) Nigropallidal encephalomalacia in horses grazing *Rhaponticum repens* (creeping knapweed). *Aust Vet J*, 90, 151–154.

[54] Banderra, P.M., Pavarini, S.P., Raymundo, D.L. *et al.* (2010) *Trema micrantha* toxicity in horses in Brazil. *Equine Vet J*, 42, 456–459.

[55] Loretti, A.P., Colodel, E.M., Gimeno, E.J. *et al.* (2003) Lysosomal storage disease in *Sida carpinifolia* toxicosis: an induced mannosidosis in horses. *Equine Vet J*, 35, 434–438.

[56] Edwards, D.F., Parker, J.W., Wilkinson, J.E. *et al.* (1993) Plasma cell myeloma in the horse. A case report and literature review. *J Vet Intern Med*, 7, 169–176.

[57] Van Biervliet, J., Alcaraz, A., Jackson, C.A. *et al.* (2004) Extradural undifferentiated sarcoma causing spinal cord compression in 2 horses. *J Vet Intern Med*, 18, 248–251.

[58] Traver, D.S., Moore, J.N., Thornburg, L.P. *et al.* (1977) Epidural melanoma causing posterior paresis in a horse. *J Am Vet Med Assoc*, 170, 1400–1403.

[59] Johnson, P.J., Goetz, T.E., Foreman, J.H. *et al.* (1995) Pheochromocytoma in two horses. *J Am Vet Med Assoc*, 206, 837–841.

[60] Patterson, L.J., May, S.A. and Baker, J.R. (1990) Skeletal metastasis of a penile squamous cell carcinoma. *Vet Rec*, 126, 579–580.

[61] Kannegieter, N.J. and Alley, M.R. (1987) Ataxia due to lymphosarcoma in a young horse. *Aust Vet J*, 64, 377–379.

[62] Shamis, L.D., Everitt, J.I. and Baker, G.J. (1984) Lymphosarcoma as the cause of ataxia in a horse. *J Am Vet Med Assoc*, 184, 1517–1518.

[63] Palmer, A.C. and Hickman, J. (1960) Ataxia in a horse due to an angioma of the spinal cord. *Vet Rec*, 72, 611–613.

[64] Huxtable, C.R. (2000) Marginal siderosis and degenerative myelopathy: a manifestation of chronic subarachnoid hemorrhage in a horse with myxopapillary ependymoma. *Vet Pathol*, 37, 483–485.

[65] Berry, S. (1999) Spinal cord compression secondary to hemangiosarcoma in a saddlebred stallion. *Can Vet J*, 40, 886–887.

[66] Ladd, S.M., Crisman, M.V., Duncan, R. *et al.* (2005) Central nervous system hemangiosarcoma in a horse. *J Vet Intern Med*, 19, 914–916.

[67] Haghdoost, I.S. and Zakarian, B. (1985) Neoplasms of equidae in Iran. *Equine Vet J*, 17, 237–239.

[68] Frazier, K., Liggett, A., Hines, M. *et al.* (2000) Mushroom toxicity in a horse with meningioangiomatosis. *Vet Hum Toxicol*, 42, 166–167.

[69] Reppas, G.P. and Harper, C.G. (1996) Sudden unexpected death in a horse due to a cerebral oligodendroglioma. *Equine Vet J*, 28, 163–165.

[70] Pirie, R.S., Mayhew, I.G., Clark, C.J. *et al.* (1998) Ultrasonographic confirmation of a space-occupying lesion in the brain of a horse: choroid plexus papilloma. *Equine Vet J*, 30, 445–448.

[71] Spoormakers, T.J.P., Ijzer, J. and van Oldruitenborgh-Oosterbaan, S. (2000) Neurologic signs in a horse due to metastases of an intestinal adenocarcinoma. *Vet Q*, 23, 49–50.

9 Differential Diagnosis and Management of Cranial Nerve Abnormalities

Robert J. MacKay

College of Veterinary Medicine, University of Florida, Gainesville, USA

Head tilt and circling

The vestibular system is responsible for the mainte-nance of balance and reflex orientation to gravity and thus controls one of the three "qualities" of proprioception [1]. Cerebellar and general proprioception are the two other qualities. The vestibular system maintains appropriate eye, trunk, and limb position in relation to movements and position of the head.

The sensory organ for the vestibular component of the vestibulocochlear system is located within the petrous temporal bone. Acceleration–deceleration movements of the head mobilize endolymph within the ducts of the membranous labyrinth of the inner ear and thereby stimulate the hair cell receptors of the crista ampulla and macula. Sensory signals pass centrally in axons of the vestibular division of the vestibulocochlear nerve (CN VIII) and enter the rostral medulla at the level of the caudal cerebellar peduncle. Most vestibular fibers termi-nate in the four ipsilateral vestibular nuclei located under the ventrolateral surface of the fourth ventricle in the pons and rostral medulla. The remaining fibers course via the direct vestibulocerebellar tract through the caudal cerebellar peduncle to the fastigial nucleus of the cere-bellar medulla and the cortex of the flocculonodular lobe. Additional input to the vestibular nuclei is provided from muscle spindles in the rostral part of the neck via the first three cervical spinal nerves and spinovestibular tracts. From the vestibular nuclei, projections go (i) to the cerebellum via the caudal peduncle, as described above for the direct vestibulocerebellar tract, (ii) rostrally in the medial longitudinal fasciculus to the nuclei of CN III, CN IV, and CN VI which are motor to the extraocular muscles; (iii) caudally in the vestibulospinal tracts to ter-minate in all spinal cord segments on interneurons that facilitate ipsilateral extensor muscles and inhibit ipsilat-eral flexors; some interneurons cross to the opposite side to inhibit contralateral extensors and facilitate flexors, and (iv) rostrally to the contralateral forebrain to provide conscious perception of balance. The overall effect is a coordinated muscle response to maintain balance and produce smooth, coordinated movements (see video clips demonstrating clinical signs for videos).

Clinical signs of acute asymmetric vestibular dysfunction include head tilt, nystagmus, falling, cir-cling, reluctance to move, and asymmetric ataxia with preservation of strength [2]. Horses with peracute severe vestibular dysfunction are often violent and dan-gerous because of sudden disorientation. A true head tilt is a consistent sign of vestibular disease (see Figure 9.1) and is characterized by rotation of the long axis of the head such that the poll tilts *toward* the affected side when the lesion is located in the peripheral or medullary parts of the vestibular system and *away* from the lesion when the vestibular components of the cerebellum are involved. The latter setting, wherein abnormal clinical signs occur on the side away from the lesion, is known as *paradoxic central vestibular syndrome*. Paradoxic central vestibular syndrome should be suspected when addi-tional abnormal neurologic signs such as facial paresis or limb weakness localize to the side opposite the head tilt (see video clips demonstrating clinical signs for videos).

Affected horses prefer to lie on the side of the head tilt and may lean against a wall on the affected side when standing. When forced to move, they take short, stag-gering, albeit accurate, steps in a circle toward the direction of the head tilt. Extensor hypotonia ipsilateral to the lesion and hypertonia and hyperreflexia of the extensor muscles of the contralateral side are respon-sible for abnormal body positions characteristic of vestibular dysfunction. The neck is turned and thoraco-lumbar spine curved so that the torso is concave and the body leans to the affected side. In severe cases, the horse falls to the affected side and rolls in the same direction as it struggles to regain its feet. With vestibular dysfunction, ataxia is often severe and righting reactions are compromised; however, strength is maintained.

Equine Neurology, Second Edition. Martin Furr and Stephen Reed.
© 2015 John Wiley & Sons, Inc. Published 2015 by John Wiley & Sons, Inc.
Companion website: www.wiley.com/go/furr/neurology

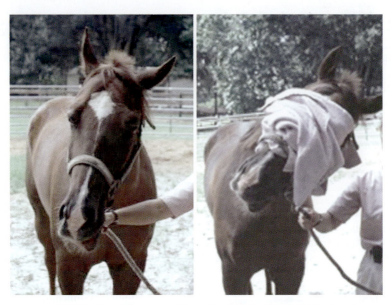

Figure 9.1 A horse demonstrating left sided head tilt worsened by application of a blindfold (Romberg's test).

Any acquired conjugate *jerk* nystagmus that occurs when the head is stationary is always pathologic and indicative of a lesion in the vestibular system. Nystagmus that occurs when the head is in a neutral position is termed *spontaneous*; when nystagmus is elicited only after the head is moved to other head positions, it is described as *positional*. Nystagmus may be horizontal, vertical, or rotatory. The direction of rotatory nystagmus is defined by the direction of movement of the limbus from the 12 o'clock position during the fast phase. Many horses blink during each fast phase, which may hinder determining the direction of the nystagmus. Peripheral vestibular lesions typically cause horizontal or rotatory nystagmus, although vertical nystagmus also is possible [1]. With central lesions, nystagmus is less likely but may be in any direction when it occurs. In the case of a peripheral or medullary vestibular lesion, the fast phase of horizontal (or rotatory) nystagmus should be away from the affected side. By contrast, in horses with involvement of the vestibular components in the cerebellum, the fast phase is toward the lesion. *Physiologic* nystagmus occurs in normal horses when the head is moved and is defined by fast phases in the direction of head movement. With asymmetric vestibular dysfunction, especially that caused by a peripheral lesion, physiologic nystagmus may be abnormal when the head is moved toward the affected side.

In horses with a vestibular head tilt, the eyeballs are positioned appropriately relative to the deviated skull; however, when the horse's head is forced into an upright position and the chin is elevated, vestibular

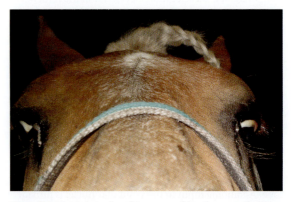

Figure 9.2 Ventrolateral strabismus resulting from vestibular disease.

strabismus is revealed such that the eye on the side toward which the head was tilted is now infraducted relative to the head position and the other eye is supraducted (see Figure 9.2).

Facial nerve (CN VII) paralysis frequently occurs concurrently with vestibular disease because of the proximity of the facial nerve to the vestibular components within the petrous bone and the position of the facial nucleus immediately ventral to the vestibular nuclei in the medulla. Paresis or paralysis of the facial nerve produces one to all of the following signs: muzzle deviation away from the affected side, absent menace response, absent palpebral reflex, ear droop, decreased nostril flare, lip droop, and accumulation of feed in the cheek because of buccinator paralysis. Keratitis and corneal ulceration occur because of inability to blink and (more importantly) decreased tear production. Tear production is affected by damage to parasympathetic fibers of the facial nerve as they travel to the lacrimal gland. About 2 weeks after facial denervation, atrophy of the parotidoauricularis muscle becomes evident as a groove parallel with and behind the vertical ramus of the mandible (see video clips demonstrating clinical signs for videos).

Differentiation of central versus peripheral vestibular disease is a critical step in establishing a list of differential diagnoses, initiating therapy, and formulating a prognosis [3]. A thorough examination may identify non-vestibular neurologic signs that provide additional information regarding lesion location. The duration of vestibular signs, rate of onset, and disease progression may aid in differentiation of central from peripheral vestibular disease. The principles relating the direction of nystagmus to the location of lesions within the vestibular system are described earlier. With central, but not with peripheral lesions, the direction of nystagmus may vary with changing head position. The onset of vestibular signs in a horse with an expanding space-occupying central lesion will not be as sudden as that due to peripheral nerve damage; adjustments by compensatory mechanisms occur during slow development of the lesion in the latter setting. Signs caused by central lesions, however, are not likely to show significant clinical improvement, as may occur after peripheral vestibular lesions. Signs of peripheral vestibular disease may improve within 2–3 weeks by visual compensation. If vestibular signs are accompanied by obtundation, limb weakness, non-vestibular ataxia, seizures, or dysfunction of cranial nerves other than the facial nerve, a central lesion should be suspected.

Blindfolding a horse with visually compensated vestibular dysfunction immediately causes recrudescence of ataxia and head tilt; this is known as the Romberg test. Because blindfolding causes anxiety in many normal horses, it is important to distinguish nonspecific signs of panic from those of vestibular dysfunction.

Vestibular disease is part of several infectious, traumatic, and noninfectious conditions of horses (Table 9.1) [3]. Temporohyoid osteoarthropathy (THO) and head trauma are common noninfectious causes; equine protozoal myeloencephalitis (EPM), West Nile virus encephalitis, alphaviral encephalitis, equine herpes myeloencephalopathy (EHM), brain abscess, otitis media-interna, mycotic encephalitis, and aberrant parasitic migration are all potential infectious causes [4–7]. Space-occupying lesions causing compression of vestibular components in the caudal fossa of the skull include neoplasia, cholinisteric granulomas of the fourth ventricle, or extramedullary abscesses. Because all components of

Table 9.1 Neurologic causes of head tilt in the horse.

Skull fractures
Temporohyoid osteoarthropathy
Equine protozoal myeloencephalitis
Eastern equine encephalitis (EEE)/western equine encephalitis (WEE)
West Nile encephalomyelitis
Equine herpes myeloencephalopathy
Otitis media/interna
Intracranial abscess
Medullary or cerebellar infarct
Choroid plexus granuloma, fourth ventricle
CNS neoplasia
Idiopathic labyrinthitis
Verminous encephalitis
Lightning strike
Listeriosis
Streptomycin
Polyneuritis equi

the vestibular system are perfused by branches of the vertebrobasilar arteries, accidental intracarotid injection should not cause signs of vestibular dysfunction; however, disintegration of a *Strongylus vulgaris*-associated thrombus in the territory of the vertebral artery could cause peracute onset of signs of central vestibular dysfunction. Idiopathic vestibular syndrome (also known as idiopathic labyrinthitis) is a diagnosis of exclusion. Affected horses have a sudden onset of signs of unilateral peripheral vestibular dysfunction which may be severe, without facial neuropathy, and without signs of any other known rule-out. After several days to weeks, the signs begin to improve and completely resolve over several days. At least at low challenge doses, the signs of lolitrem intoxication (i.e., perennial ryegrass staggers) are attributable to bilateral vestibular dysfunction [8] with general proprioceptive and cerebellar qualities of ataxia only evident at high doses. Interpretation of concurrent neurologic signs, cerebrospinal fluid (CSF) analysis, specific antibody testing, advanced imaging, and brainstem auditory-evoked response testing are used to help distinguish among the diagnostic possibilities.

Temporohyoid osteoarthropathy

THO is a progressive syndrome involving periosteal reaction, enlargement and sclerosis of the stylohyoid bone, tympanic bulla, and petrous portion of the temporal bone [9]. Ultimately, there is fusion between the skull and hyoid apparatus, stricture of the external ear canal, and obliteration of the lumen of the tympanic bulla. These changes are thought to represent a primary degenerative process in the temporohyoid joint (THJ), although it is conceivable that some cases are secondary to chronic otitis media [9–11]. Horses from 6 months to greater than 20 years of age have been affected with a mean or median age of 10–12 years reported in all studies [9, 12–16]. Quarter Horse and Quarter horse-type breeds accounted for more than 50% of cases in several, but not all, series [12–15]. Both joints are affected, albeit asymmetrically, in most horses with clinical THO [12]. In rare instances, there are associated clinical signs on both sides [13, 14]. Fusion of the THJ causes interference with the interdependent coordinated movements of the tongue, hyoid apparatus, and larynx. Particular stress is placed on the fused joint(s) during chewing, swallowing, vocalizing, and combined head and neck movements. Veterinary procedures such as dental work and passage of a nasogastric tube also put unaccustomed pressure on the THJ. Any of these mechanical forces applied to the immobilized THJ may result in fractures through the petrous temporal or proximal stylohyoid bones. In addition, THO also is likely a risk factor for fracture of the petrous temporal bone during head trauma, especially in horses that flip over backward and strike the poll. The facial nerve (CN VII), vestibulocochlear nerve (CN VIII), and membranous labyrinth are within the petrous temporal bone and can be impinged upon by bony proliferation or lacerated by fracture. After fracture of the petrous temporal bone, there also may be extension of middle/inner ear infection around the brainstem with signs of leptomeningitis or extramedullary abscess.

Clinical signs

Early in the syndrome, including the period before ankylosis of the THJ, reluctance to chew, dysphagia, head shaking, ear rubbing, sensitivity to pressure at the base of the ear, facial hyperesthesia, wild tossing of the head and neck under tack, reluctance to take a bit, dropping of feed, or even weight loss may be seen, although most horses with THO are probably subclinical until development of neurologic signs. Fracture of the proximal stylohyoid bone increases the likelihood of pain-associated clinical signs. Because of bony proliferation around the ear canal, the external ear may be unusually narrow and difficult to examine by otoscope.

After fusion of the THJ, the disease may manifest as sudden onset of asymmetric signs of CN VII and/or VIII dysfunction. Almost all affected horses have degrees of facial paresis [9, 14, 15], which may occasionally be bilateral [13]. Schirmer tear tests commonly disclose reduced tear production with values of 5–20 mm (normal >20 mm) [13], indicative of injury to the parasympathetic lacrimal branch of the facial nerve. By the time of presentation, most such horses already have a deep horizontal corneal ulcer with corneal edema and miosis. Signs of vestibular dysfunction accompany facial paresis in the majority of cases. Of 29 horses with THO that had involvement of CN VII, 23 (~80%) had vestibular signs [14]. In a study of 11 horses with THO and neurologic signs, all had electrodiagnostic evidence of partial to complete hearing loss on the affected side; five also had partial hearing loss on the contralateral side [13]. Although it is unusual, vestibular signs can occur without concurrent involvement of the facial nerve. Rarely, horses may also have difficulty eating and swallowing because of either pain (e.g., from acute stylohyoid fracture) or involvement of CN's IX and X. A few horses have seizure-like convulsions at the onset of neurologic signs. Bacterial abscess adjacent to the brainstem or meningitis may be sequels to fracture of the petrous temporal bone and result in the death of the horse.

Diagnosis

Endoscopic examination of the inside of the guttural pouches is the diagnostic imaging test of choice because of its convenience in standing horses and its high sensitivity for detection of THO [14]. Evaluation of the external contour of the THJ from within the guttural pouch can detect asymmetric enlargement and discoloration of the stylohyoid bone and THJ, and, in some cases, hyperemia, edema, and/or hemorrhage in the guttural pouch lining surrounding the joint (Figure 9.3). The joint does not move when pressure is put on the lingual process of the basihyoid bone by pushing dorsally between the horizontal rami of the mandibles [17]. Previously healed fractures of the stylohyoid bone may be evident as angulation and distortion of the bone close to the THJ. Computed tomographic (CT) imaging of the THJ allows appreciation of changes not always evident by endoscopy including bilateral involvement, enlargement of the ceratohyoid bone, fractures of the petrous temporal and stylohyoid bones, and the presence of fluid in the tympanic bullae [12, 18]. A system has been developed to quantify the remodeling changes found in THO cases [12]. The main disadvantage of CT is the expense and requirement for general anesthesia. In Europe, where standing CT units are available in some referral practices, this is less of a concern, although adequate positioning can be difficult in horses with severe vestibular dysfunction [16]. Radiographic examination of the skull using ventrodorsal, lateral, and lateral oblique views detects those cases in which the bony proliferation has progressed to cause osteitis and fusion of the THJ. Optimal images are obtained with the horse under general anesthesia and in dorsal recumbency; however, adequate views can be taken using a dorsoventral projection with the horse

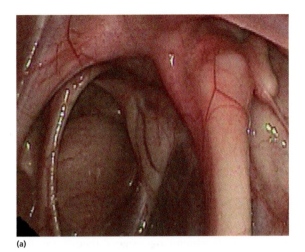

(a)

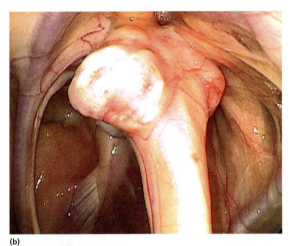

(b)

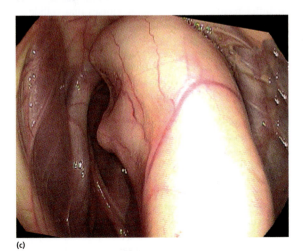

(c)

Figure 9.3a–c Endoscopic images from within the left guttural pouches of horses with temporohyoid osteoarthropathy.

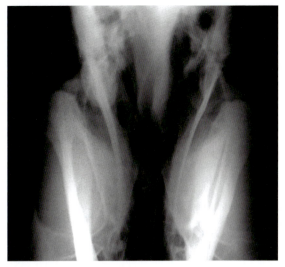

Figure 9.4 Dorsoventral radiograph of a horse's head showing enlarged temporohyoid joint, associated with temporohyoid osteoarthropathy.

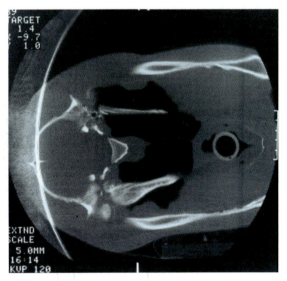

Figure 9.5 Computed tomographic image demonstrating proliferative osteitis of the stylohyoid bone (courtesy Dr. S Reed).

standing but heavily sedated. Sensitivity for detection of THO by plain radiography in one series was 20/24 (83%) [14] (Figure 9.4). Magnetic resonance imaging (MRI) and nuclear scintigraphy are imaging techniques that have been applied successfully to THO diagnosis but have not found wide application [14, 16, 19] (Figure 9.5).

Brainstem auditory-evoked response (BAER) testing of vestibulocochlear nerve function has been described for horses with THO and is the only way of evaluating auditory function in these horses [13]. It also is a sensitive method for detecting involvement of the contralateral side.

In horses with neurologic signs other than dysfunction of CN VII and VIII, CSF collection, analysis, and possible culture are recommended. Two of four horses tested in one report had increased nucleated cell counts or protein concentrations suggestive of meningitis [14]. Xanthochromia and increased RBC counts also are expected in acute cases [11].

Treatment and prognosis

Medical and surgical approaches to THO have been described [9, 11, 20]. Conservative medical therapy involves prolonged rest and treatment with NSAID (e.g., 1g phenylbutazone orally for 3 days, then once daily, or 1.1 mg/kg flunixin meglumine IV or orally twice daily for 3 days, then once daily for 1–2 weeks) and broad-spectrum antibiotics (e.g., trimethoprim-sulfa, 30 mg/kg orally twice daily for 30 days). The lever action of the hyoid apparatus on the petrous temporal bone can be eliminated surgically by complete removal of the ipsilateral ceratohyoid bone or removal of a 1- to 2-cm section from the middle of the stylohyoid bone [11, 20, 21]. Because mid-body stylohyoid ostectomies have a tendency to heal [21], the ceratohyoid procedure is now favored. If necessary, this surgery can be done bilaterally and the procedure can be performed in the standing sedated horse. With facial nerve paralysis and keratitis sicca, corneal ulcers are a medical emergency and must be treated or prevented with topical antibiotics, artificial tears, and, preferably, a multifocal partial split-thickness tarsorrhaphy [11]. The tarsorrhaphy is maintained permanently or until resumption of lacrimal and eyelid function, which may take up to 18 months.

Both medical and surgical approaches reportedly have returned most treated horses to athletic activity after a period of weeks to months, so there is not yet clear evidence to support the need for surgery in all cases [9, 14, 15]. On theoretical grounds, however, it is clear that a horse with THO will remain at risk for catastrophic relapse of neurologic signs as long as the hyoid apparatus and skull remain connected through a fused THJ. Relapse is particularly likely if there is a temporal bone fracture. In one series, 20 of 30 horses treated medically (18) or surgically (2) survived with 19/20 returning to athletic function albeit with persistent mild residual facial nerve and/or vestibular dysfunction in most cases [14]. Four horses in this series died or were euthanized because of fractures along the base of the skull, complications that should be preventable by ceratohyoidectomy.

If possible, the management of convalescent horses should be adjusted to minimize stress on the remaining THJ(s). Cribbing collars can be tried for crib biting a known risk factor for THO, bitless bridles can be used for riding, and dental work and other veterinary procedures can be minimized and done very cautiously.

Head trauma

Head injuries to horses occur from blows to the frontal-parietal area from running into stationary objects or being kicked by other horses, and from impact to the occipital protuberance (poll) or temporal areas after flipping over backward during handling or restraint accidents [22]. Specific cranial nerves may also be injured on the outside of the skull by focal trauma. In the special case of THO, fractures of the petrous temporal bone can occur suddenly without any external trauma. Detailed review of THO is covered in the previous section.

Frontal/parietal trauma

Blows to the front of the head over the dome of the calvarium directly injure the cerebral cortex adjacent to the point of impact [23]. Brain injuries are most severe when the overlying bone is fractured and pushed inward or if there is hemorrhage around or within the brain. Because of the violent distortions and movements of the cerebral hemispheres related to the impact, additional cortical injuries may occur diametrically opposite the point of collision (contrecoup) and caudally adjacent to the tentorium cerebelli. With the development of the secondary phase of cerebral injury and edema, the enlarging cerebral hemispheres herniate under the falx cerebri (asymmetric injury) and/or tentorium cerebelli to compress other parts of the brain. Horses may recover from the acute effects of calvarial fracture only to suffer recurrent seizures later. Horses that collide at speed with fixed objects are at risk for both head trauma and spinal cord injury [24].

Impact to the poll and temporal areas

When a horse flips over backward, the point of contact is either the poll or the side of the skull. Fifteen of thirty-four horses with neurologic signs due to head trauma were injured by flipping over backward [25–35]. Nine of these horses were less than a year old. The force of impact is absorbed by the occipital protuberance and/or zygomatic arch and transmitted around the skull to the petrous temporal bones. Presumably because of the asymmetry of impact, only one side is usually injured. This may be either the upper or the lower (i.e., impacted) side. There is hemorrhage into the middle and inner ear with or without fracture through the petrous temporal bone. The membranous vestibulocochlear end organs in the inner ear are vulnerable to injury by both hemorrhage and the lacerating effects of fracture. In the latter

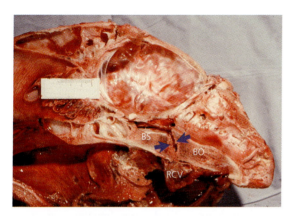

Figure 9.6 Postmortem photograph demonstrating a basisphenoid fracture. BS, basisphenoid; BO, basioccipital; RCV, rectus capitus ventralis.

case, the facial nerve may be damaged as it courses through the facial canal. When the point of impact is centered on the occipital protuberance, the basilar bones under the brainstem are subject to fracture and separation (Figure 9.6). The basioccipital and basisphenoidal bones are pulled apart at their synchondrosis connection, at least in part by the strong distracting force of the rectus capitis ventralis muscles. Fragments of bone from the basisphenoid may be displaced ventrally and caudally by muscular attachments [34]. Because the synchondrosis is beneath the midbrain and flanked by the foramina lacerum and guttural pouches, basilar fractures are clinically very serious. There may be life-threatening arterial hemorrhage between or into the guttural pouches, injury to CN IX (glossopharyngeal), X (vagus), XI (accessory), and the mandibular branch of CN V (trigeminal) as they pass through the foramen lacerum, and/or direct laceration and contusion of the midbrain and adjacent parts of the brainstem. Because the connection between the basilar bones ossifies and fuses by 2–5 years of age, basilar injuries after poll trauma are more likely in young horses. In the most serious cases, fracture lines extend laterally and dorsally through the squamous temporal and occipital bones or rostrally through the sphenoidal bones (see the following section).

Other cranial nerve injuries

The optic nerve(s) of one or both eyes can be stretched and damaged within the optic canals by the violent to-and-fro gyrations of the brain after impact to the head [32, 36] and/or by fractures through the optic canals. Sphenoidal bone fractures also may involve CNs III, IV, VI, or the ophthalmic and maxillary branches of CN V as they pass to the orbital foramen and foramen rotundum. Injury to the facial nerve proximal to the vertical

ramus of the mandible causes full facial paresis. Proximal facial nerve trauma usually is caused by fractures of the petrous temporal bone, vertical ramus of the mandible, or stylohyoid bone, or fracture of the paracondylar process related to pulling back in a tied horse [37]. Distal facial nerve damage usually is due to direct injury from a blow or lateral recumbency or strangulation by a tight-fitting halter. The nerve or its branches often are damaged as they cross the mandible and/or zygomatic arch. Facial paresis following recumbency during general anesthesia is common and usually involves only the nose and/or lips. When a horse pitches headfirst into the ground while traveling at speed, it is possible for components of a fractured atlas to be driven rostrally around the occipital condyles where they may traumatize CN XII as it exits the hypoglossal foramen.

Clinical signs

Epistaxis is common after a blow to the head of sufficient severity to cause neurologic signs [25, 29]. After frontal/parietal or poll trauma, blood may flow from either or both nostrils and typically is dark (venous) and of low to moderate volume. With poll trauma, epistaxis also may be bilateral, copious, occasionally bright red and may also issue from the mouth [34]. In such cases, the hemorrhage is from one (usually) or both guttural pouches and originates from adjacent veins and/or arteries [38]. If the tympanum is perforated, blood additionally may flow from the external ear. Profuse hemorrhage into the retropharyngeal area may cause obvious swelling behind the vertical ramus of the mandible and inspiratory dyspnea which can be life-threatening. Respiratory distress also may be associated with a poorly understood syndrome of noncardiogenic pulmonary edema that is reported to occur after serious head injury. Head trauma in humans is often complicated by systemic arterial hypotension. The cause is not completely understood but may be explained in part by brain–heart syndrome wherein myocardial damage is inflicted by the reflex actions of sympathetic nerves.

Immediately after impact to the frontal/parietal area, there often is a period of apparent concussion that may last minutes to hours. Even after recovery of consciousness, horses typically are obtunded for up to several hours. Altered behavior (i.e., dementia) is another characteristic of forebrain injury—there can be loss of affinity of a suckling foal for its dam, failure to respond to training cues, yawning, head-pressing, compulsive walking, often in circles around the inside of an enclosure (usually toward the side of the injury) or, rarely, hyperexcitability or aggression. Because of damage to the visual centers in the occipital cortex, vision and menace response(s) may be impaired in the eye contralateral to the lesion; however, pupillary light reflexes should be intact. Injury to the somesthetic centers of the parietal cortex interferes with awareness of (and thus response to) touch on the opposite side of the head and body. This is best evaluated by comparing the horse's reactions to tapping the nasal septal mucosa on either side. Seizures occurred in 7 of 34 horses with head trauma [35]. Seizures are likely to be generalized, with loss of consciousness and uncontrolled autonomic activity (e.g., salivation, urination, defecation, pupillary dilatation, and chewing movements) and abnormal motor function (e.g., muscular rigidity, followed by running and paddling movements of the limbs). In comatose horses with cerebral injury, the breathing pattern may be irregular with periods of either Cheyne-Stokes breathing or hyperventilation.

Fortunately, midbrain injury is a relatively uncommon but serious complication of head trauma of any type. It may occur immediately after the injury or be secondary to subtentorial herniation of forebrain components, rostral herniation of the cerebellum, or intra-parenchymal bleeding. Because of involvement of the ascending reticular activating system, affected horses are usually obtunded and may be comatose. There is weakness of the limbs bilaterally or on the side opposite to an asymmetric midbrain lesion. In recumbent horses with severe midbrain injury, the neck, back, and limbs may be rigidly extended in a decorticate posture. If the nucleus of CN III (oculomotor) is involved, there is ptosis, strabismus, and a dilated, unresponsive pupil. With severe diffuse midbrain injury, bilateral pupillary miosis may be seen initially, followed by gradual progression to fixed, dilated pupils. Vision is normal unless there is involvement of other parts of the brain.

Vestibular dysfunction is seen commonly in horses after poll trauma or THO. Clinical signs may arise because of injury centrally or, more commonly, because of involvement of the vestibular apparatus or vestibulocochlear nerve (CN VIII). With peripheral vestibular disease, there is head tilt, neck turn, body lean, and staggering in tight circles, all toward the side of the lesion. These signs can be revealed or exacerbated by blindfolding. With acute severe vestibular dysfunction secondary to THO, there may be sudden recumbency with flailing and thrashing movements. These signs of vestibular disease can easily be mistaken for seizures. The ipsilateral eye is usually rotated ventrally and laterally, especially when the horse's nose is elevated, and there may be horizontal or rotatory nystagmus, with the fast phase away from the side of the lesion. There also may be facial paralysis attributable to damage to CN VII as it passes close to the middle/inner ear. With central vestibular injury, signs are similar to those seen when the injury is peripheral; however, there will likely be additional signs suggestive of brainstem damage, including spontaneous vertical nystagmus, signs of other cranial nerve dysfunctions, obtundation, and limb ataxia and weakness. In horses, central lesions quite commonly result in a paradoxical central vestibular syndrome. (See Section "Head Tilt and Circling" for full discussion of vestibular disease.)

In horses with traumatic damage to the pons and medulla, there is evidence of dysfunction of multiple cranial nerves in association with obtundation and limb ataxia/weakness. There may be reduced jaw tone or deviation of the lower jaw (Vm), reduced facial sensation (CN Vs), facial paralysis (CN VII), vestibular signs (CN VIII), dysphagia and respiratory stridor (CN's IX and X), or tongue paralysis (CN XII). The gait may appear hypometric (spastic) like that seen in horses with compression of the cervical spinal cord. With severe hindbrain lesions, rapid deep breathing or other abnormal respiratory patterns are sometimes seen.

Signs of cerebellar injury occur rarely and are usually a result of poll trauma. Coarse head tremors are the most consistent sign; these are especially obvious during attempts to eat or suckle (intention tremor). The horse with cerebellar injury typically has a broad-based swaying stance and limb movements may be hypermetric or spastic, clumsy, faltering, and jerky. Infrequent signs of cerebellar trauma include absent menace response(s) with normal vision on the side of the lesion and paradoxical central vestibular syndrome.

With traumatic optic neuropathy, vision and pupillary light reflexes (PLR) are impaired or absent and pupils are dilated in one or both eyes immediately after the injury. Because the secondary phase of nerve injury continues for many hours after the initial trauma, visual function may progressively deteriorate during at least the first 24 h posttrauma. The signs of facial nerve injury depend upon the site of damage and are given earlier.

Pathophysiology

Impact to the brain causes immediate damage to intracranial vasculature, neurons, and glia [39, 40]. Neuronal depolarization initiated at the site of impact may spread centrifugally throughout the cortex to cause the transient coma characteristic of severe concussion. In axons, a dramatic rise in intracellular calcium concentration activates processes that cause interruption of axoplasmic flow and result over hours to days in death of the distal axon. Diffuse axonal injury is thought to account for many of the permanent neurologic sequelae of head trauma. These early events constitute primary brain injury. Subsequent damage occurring during the response phase is termed secondary injury.

The surface and parenchyma of the brain may be lacerated by fracture fragments pushed inward from the calvarium. Significant bleeding at any site compresses the brain against the skull thereby raising intracerebral pressure (ICP). Extravasated blood also elicits inflammatory responses in glial and other cells initiating many of the autodestructive cascades which characterize the secondary phase of traumatic brain injury. Bleeding, ischemia, and mechanical damage to tissues evoke liberation and production of vasoactive and other mediators [39, 41]. The production and action of damaging mediators is very much affected by brain temperature—adverse effects are muted when there is hypothermia and exacerbated by increased temperature.

Hemorrhage, increased permeability of damaged vasculature, and inflammatory edema all increase extravascular volume at the expense of brain volume. Exuberant swelling of the relatively mobile cerebral hemispheres may force portions under the falx cerebri (if asymmetric) or tentorium cerebelli [39, 40]. In extreme cases, the pressure of subtentorial herniation in turn pushes the caudal cerebellum through the foramen magnum. The effects of reduced systemic blood pressure and increased ICP combine to compromise oxygen and glucose supply to cells and prevent removal of cellular metabolites such as lactic acid [41]. The consequent tissue hypoxia is more severe if there also is reduced blood oxygen content as may occur after traumatic blood loss anemia or hypoxemia.

In the hypoxic environment of the traumatized brain, there is rapid depletion of neuronal ATP and collapse of energy-dependent membrane homeostatic systems [41]. Calcium and sodium ions flux into cells in response to changes in membrane ion channel function associated with energy depletion, damage by reactive oxygen species, and the actions of glutamate/aspartate. Brain damage that occurs during the primary traumatic event is irreversible; however, there is a window of minutes to days in which equally important secondary injuries theoretically can be prevented or treated.

Diagnosis

Changes in routine hemograms and chemistries are nonspecific. Collection of CSF from the atlantooccipital cistern is generally contraindicated in head trauma because of concern about inducing cerebellar herniation, but CSF can be collected via the lumbosacral space. Characteristic changes include yellow discoloration (xanthochromia), high RBC count, and protein with normal nucleated cell count.

Conventional diagnostic radiography is the best and most practical method for initial evaluation of skull trauma; however, radiographs significantly underestimate the extent of bony and soft tissue abnormality. Because the brain is not visible in plain radiographs, degrees of brain injury must be inferred from secondary changes in the skull. Fractures are visible as radiolucent lines within the calvarium, which may or may not be associated with normal suture lines. A step defect is visible when there is misalignment of the fracture fragments. Lateral views are most useful for detecting parietal/frontal and basilar fractures and for finding bone fragments originating from the basisphenoid or nuchal crest. On dorsoventral projections, a thickened stylohyoid or radiodense osseous bulla is most easily appreciated. Increased opacity of the affected bulla may reflect hemorrhage into the middle ear associated with petrous temporal bone injury or reactive thickening of the ventral bulla wall in cases of THO. Intracranial or spinal intrathecal gas shadows may be seen if there is a communication between the subarachnoid space and the skin surface, nasal cavity, paranasal sinuses, or middle ear. There may be radiographic evidence of bleeding into the paranasal sinuses, guttural pouches, or retropharyngeal area. In cases of frontal/parietal impact, it is prudent also to radiograph the cervical spine so as to detect fractures/dislocations caused by the axial compressive force of the original impact.

Characteristics of CT of brain trauma include change in ventricular size, shape or position, deviation of the falx cerebri (falx shift), and focal change in brain opacity. Administration of iodinated contrast medium intravenously causes focal enhancement of areas of brain injury or hemorrhage. CT is particularly useful for identifying fractures of the bones that surround the caudal fossa—such fractures often are not well resolved by conventional radiography [42]. These include fractures of the petrous temporal bone, basilar and sphenoid bones, occipital condyles, and squamous temporal bone [36]. Blood in the middle ears, paranasal sinuses, guttural pouches, or retropharyngeal tissues and changes associated with THO also are easily seen. The principal disadvantage of CT in North America, apart from high cost and limited availability of necessary equipment, is the need for general anesthesia. The main advantages of MRI over CT include lack of beam-hardening artifacts, ability to acquire images in any plane, and higher sensitivity for detection of early infarcts and edema. CT is more sensitive than MRI for detection of bony abnormalities, acute brain hemorrhage, and intracranial gas.

The brain is not accessible to ultrasound imaging; however, the technique sometimes is useful for assessing fractures of the skull.

Treatment

Relevant treatments for brain injury can be classified into two levels according to evidence-based support for their use. All applicable level 1 treatments should be used in every case of clinically apparent brain injury, whereas level 2 treatments are less clearly indicated and can be considered optional. Refer Chapter 31 for more detailed discussion on the treatment of central nervous system (CNS) trauma.

Level 1
Treat other injuries or diseases
The normal principles of critical care medicine apply to the brain-injured patient. An airway must be established and protected, vascular access obtained, wounds cleaned and dressed, bleeding staunched, and the horse sedated if necessary and moved to a cool, well-padded area. If necessary, a padded helmet can be used to minimize additional head trauma. A regimen of broad-spectrum antibiotics should be begun if there is an open wound or fracture.

Treat hyperthermia
Hyperthermia after head trauma results either from a resetting of the hypothalamic temperature set-point (fever) or from excessive heat production in horses with normal set-points. High brain temperature accelerates all of the destructive forces unleashed during the secondary phase of brain injury so must be detected and treated vigorously. Rectal temperature should be checked frequently and efforts at cooling should begin when the temperature exceeds 101°F. In brief, ambient temperature can be reduced, the body can be clipped, ice water or isopropyl alcohol repeatedly applied to and removed from the skin (including the head), and overhead or box fans can be placed close by. Antipyretic medication (e.g., flunixin meglumine 1.1 mg/kg IV) is particularly useful when the horse has a fever but should be tried in all cases of hyperthermia. Nonsteroidal anti-inflammatory drugs have the additional advantages of analgesic and anti-inflammatory action.

Prevent or treat hypotension
Blood pressure must be at or close to normal to sustain adequate cerebral perfusion. Blood pressure should be monitored frequently if possible and heart base-adjusted systolic blood pressure maintained above 110 mm Hg [43]. Blood volume should be maintained or expanded by IV infusion of isotonic (Normosol-R, Plasmalyte-A, Lactated Ringer's Solution) or hypertonic (hypersaline) crystalloid, colloid (plasma, hetastarch) solutions, or cross-matched whole blood. If volume resuscitation alone is inadequate to restore normal pressure, pressor/inotropic drugs may be used (e.g., dobutamine and nor-epinephrine) [43]. Remember that the effects of these drugs on cerebral vascular tone are difficult to predict.

Optimize oxygen content of blood
Oxygen is carried in blood either bound to hemoglobin (predominantly) or as free gas. Thus, it is important that both hemoglobin concentration and PaO_2 are at least in the normal range. Hypoxemia (arterial oxygen saturation <94% in this setting) [43] should be treated by establishing airway patency, treating underlying pulmonary disease, and beginning nasal or tracheal insufflation with oxygen. Foals may be intubated and manually or mechanically ventilated. At several equine hospitals, there are hyperbaric oxygen chambers that theoretically could be used to dramatically increase blood oxygen content in horses with brain injury. The efficacy and safety of this approach has not been established. Hemoglobin concentration must be kept above 7 g/dl (approximate PCV of 21%) and should probably be kept above 11 g/dl. Anemia can be treated with whole blood (preferable in the case of blood-loss anemia) or packed red blood cells.

Ensure adequate pulmonary ventilation
High pCO_2 has the potential to exacerbate CNS acidosis and cerebral edema. In foals, hypercapnia can be addressed by mechanical ventilation of the lungs. In all horses with head trauma, pulmonary ventilation must be optimized by ensuring a patent airway and treating lung disease. For example, acute pulmonary edema may be treated with furosemide (0.5–1 mg/kg every 4–8 h or equivalent constant rate infusion (CRI)).

Control pain
Alleviating pain in brain-injured horses is not only humane but also may reduce ICP [44]. A nonsteroidal anti-inflammatory drug (e.g., flunixin meglumine, 1.1 mg/kg BID) or opioid (e.g., morphine, 0.1–0.3 mg/kg IV or IM QID) can be used for this purpose. Analgesic effects of butorphanol or lidocaine CRI in this setting are questionable.

Regulate blood glucose and maintain nutrition
Experimental studies have shown that at least 140% of maintenance energy is expended by animals with severe brain injury [45]. Even during the first 24 h after injury, nutrition (enteral or parenteral) probably should be provided to anorexic horses with signs of brain trauma. Blood glucose concentration ought to be kept greater than 80 mg/dl in order to provide adequate substrate for brain cells and less than 150 mg/dl so as to prevent hyperglycemia-induced exacerbation of CNS acidosis and apoptosis of brain cells. IV infusions of dextrose and regular insulin can be used as necessary to maintain normal blood glucose concentration.

Prevent or treat brain swelling
If possible, the neck should be free of constrictive wraps and only one jugular vein should be punctured or catheterized in order to prevent obstruction of venous flow from the head. Likewise, any recumbent horse should have its head elevated 8 to 10° in order to facilitate blood flow. If the horse is significantly obtunded or has signs of worsening brain function, a hyperosmolar infusion should be given to try to reduce the extravascular volume of the brain. The solution of choice is

hypertonic saline (e.g., 1232 mmol Na/l) which is given as a continuous IV infusion of 1 ml (1.2 mmol)/kg/h for 6 h and then 0.2 ml/kg for another 12 h. Alternatively, boluses of 2 ml/kg can be given every 4 h for five infusions. Further treatment with hypertonic saline should be based on reassessment of clinical signs and plasma Na concentration (keep <150 mmol/l). Hypertonic saline has additional salutary actions including plasma volume expansion, anti-inflammatory effect, and reduction of microvascular permeability. Mannitol (20% solution) also can be used for this purpose as a series of bolus infusions of 0.25–1 g/kg every 4–6 h. Craniectomy is not used yet for this purpose in horses, although the necessary surgical approaches have been described [46].

Treat seizures

There is no justification for prophylactic anti-seizure medication. Seizures should however be treated vigorously when they occur. They may be treated with diazepam, phenobarbital, or pentobarbital. Once a horse seizes for the first time, antiseizure medication (usually phenobarbital) should be continued for at least a week. If delirious thrashing or recurrent seizures remain a problem, the horse can be anesthetized for several hours. Refer Chapters 4 and 7 for more detailed discussion on the management of seizures.

Perform emergency skull surgery

After initial stabilization of the patient, depressed fractures of the frontal/parietal area that impinge upon the cerebral cortex may be carefully elevated and reduced under general anesthesia using techniques described in standard texts [47–49]. No surgical approach to basilar fractures has been described for the horse— such an effort would be extremely difficult and risky.

Level 2

Such treatments are not supported either by strong anecdotal data from equine practice or by convincing experimental data in other species. The downside of these treatments is that they do not meet the standard of evidence-based medicine.

Treat with antioxidants

Oxidant damage is known to be an important part of the secondary phase of brain injury, yet clinical evidence supporting the therapeutic use of antioxidants is scant. Dimethyl sulfoxide is very widely used by equine practitioners for treatment of CNS trauma. The potential advantages of this drug's antioxidant and diuretic actions are obvious; however, there is virtually no evidence for effectiveness in the setting of equine brain injury. Common use suggests a protocol of 1 g/kg as a 10% solution in isotonic solution given IV or by NG tube every 12 h. Vitamin E (RRR-α-tocopherol; 50 IU/kg

PO daily), vitamin C (ascorbic acid, 20 mg/kg PO daily), mannitol, and allopurinol (5 mg/kg PO every 12 h) are all antioxidant therapies that can be used in the horse and can be rationalized as part of the overall approach to brain trauma.

Give conventional doses of corticosteroids

High-dose steroids are harmful to humans with brain trauma [50] and should not be used in horses. Traditional anti-inflammatory doses of dexamethasone (0.05–0.1 mg/kg IV or 0.1–0.2 mg/kg PO every 12–24 h) or prednisolone (1–4 mg/kg PO BID) likely inhibit the production and action of injurious mediators in the brain and may be of some value.

Give magnesium sulfate

Magnesium sulfate has the potential to inhibit several aspects of the secondary injury cascade including glutamate release, activity of the N-methyl-D-aspartate and calcium channels, and lipid peroxidation [51]. In light of these findings and its demonstrated safety in horses, it seems reasonable to give a single IV infusion of $MgSO_4$ at 50 mg/kg. This dose (25 g in a 500-kg horse) can conveniently be administered with the first 5–10 l of IV fluids.

Prognosis

In one series, horses that had basilar fractures were 7.5 times more likely to die than those that did not [35]. Nevertheless, one horse with a basilar fracture retuned to racing, and 21 of 34 horses survived to discharge. Most horses should recover completely, although residual vestibular and facial nerve signs are sometimes seen.

Facial nerve dysfunction due to neurapraxia should resolve over days to weeks. If there is morbid axonal injury (axonotmesis), the facial nerve may regrow via axonal sprouting along existing nerve sheaths. Regrowth of nerves occurs at a rate of about 1 cm/week and reinnervation may continue for at least a year.

Drug toxicities

Drug toxicities can result in unilateral or bilateral peripheral vestibular disease and deafness. Degeneration of hair cells within the peripheral receptor organs of the auditory and vestibular system occurs with prolonged administration of aminoglycoside antibiotics. Early vestibular disease may be reversible or centrally compensated, but loss of auditory function is permanent. Streptomycin preferentially affects the vestibular system, whereas dihydrostreptomycin, kanamycin, gentamicin, neomycin, and vancomycin are more toxic to the auditory system. Vincristine, a vinca alkaloid, can cause bilateral cochlear nerve damage in humans. Auditory function improves several months after discontinuation of the drug.

Lightning strike

Lightning strike is reported to cause acute vestibular disease in horses due to degeneration and necrosis of the sensory hair cells of the inner ear. The clinical signs are typically unilateral. Facial nerve paralysis may or may not accompany the vestibular signs. Additional physical findings that support a diagnosis of lightning strike include serosanguinous nasal discharge, epistaxis, anal hemorrhage, and retinal damage. Approximately 90% of lightning strike victims have burn lesions, including burnt skin at the tips of the ears, linear full thickness defects, or feathering burn lines in the hair. Histopathology may reveal hemorrhage and necrosis of the temporal bone, vestibular nerve, and adjacent tissue. Whether the mechanism of damage is electrocution or noise trauma is unknown.

Auditory/vestibular diagnostic testing

The caloric test historically has been used to aid in differentiation of central from peripheral vestibular disease. In the normal horse, irrigation of ice cold water (12°C) into the external auditory canal for 3–5 min induces horizontal nystagmus with the fast phase away from the test side. Warm water (45°C) irrigation of the external auditory canal causes nystagmus with the fast phase toward the test side. The warm water test is less reliable. Because the test is difficult to perform and not entirely reliable, it is no longer recommended.

Because diseases that damage the membranous labyrinth and sensory nerves of the vestibular system usually also affect auditory structures, auditory testing may help to differentiate central from peripheral vestibular disease. The BAER is stimulated by a series of standard clicks [52–54]. Far-field potentials of the brainstem auditory components are recorded via cutaneous electrodes and a signal averaging system that appear on the oscilloscope as a series of five waveforms. Functional damage to or loss of the cochlea or CN VIII results in the diminution or loss of waveforms on the side of injury and thus differentiates a central from a peripheral vestibular lesion. The test can be performed in sedated horses. Auditory brainstem testing is further described in Chapter 13.

Differential diagnosis and management of disorders of mastication and deglutition

Normal chewing and swallowing

Mastication is the process by which food is crushed and ground by the teeth. In herbivores, this process is particularly important in that tough long-stem fibrous feeds must be reduced to boluses that can be handled by the gastrointestinal tract. In contrast to the multiple cycles of rumination available to animals with forestomachs, horses must process feed during a single round of mastication. After ingestion, feed is reflexively positioned between the cheek teeth by the actions of the cheek and lingual muscles (CN Vs, pons, medulla oblongata, CN VII, and CN XII). The rotatory movements of the mandible during chewing are controlled by the chewing reflex, which involves proprioceptive and other sensory information relayed from the temporomandibular joint, the teeth, and muscle spindles in chewing muscles, to central pattern generators in the reticular formation of the brainstem, and the actions of the motor division of CN V on the masticatory muscles. Chewing can be modulated by conscious influences arising from areas important for taste perception in the forebrain.

Swallowing (deglutition) is a complicated process that requires the multifunctional pharynx to become transiently a food propulsion tube. Although the term dysphagia connotes difficulty with any phase of eating [55], including mastication; it is used medically to mean abnormal swallowing. The process is initiated consciously during the oral stage then continued by serial involuntary stages, pharyngeal then esophageal, which move food from the mouth to the stomach. When food is ready for swallowing, it is consciously squeezed and rolled caudally toward the pharynx by 10–20 movements of the tongue dorsally and caudally against the palate [56]. As the food bolus enters the caudal oral cavity and cranial oropharynx, it stimulates swallowing receptors around the pharyngeal opening and initiates a swallow reflex. Afferent sensory components of this reflex course principally in the glossopharyngeal nerve, with additional involvement of the trigeminal and vagus nerves. Impulses are transmitted centrally to the pons and medulla oblongata where successive stages of the swallowing process are controlled by the central pattern generating circuitry of the swallowing centers of the reticular formation of the pons and medulla. The essential mechanical components of the pharyngeal stage are closure of the larynx, opening of the esophagus, and transmission of a peristaltic wave caudally into the esophagus. These motor events are mediated by the glossopharyngeal, vagus, and hypoglossal nerves via the actions of a series of pharyngeal, hyoid, lingual, and extrinsic and intrinsic laryngeal muscles [56]. The paramount role of the vagus nerve in swallowing in the horse is illustrated by the observations that unilateral mycotic neuritis of the pharyngeal branch of the vagus nerve of a 20-year-old horse caused severe dysphagia [57], whereas bilateral anesthesia of the glossopharyngeal nerves did not affect swallowing [56]. The esophageal stage of swallowing involves aboral propulsion of a food bolus by a peristaltic wave. *Primary* peristalsis is simply a continuation of the pharyngeal peristaltic

Table 9.2 Neurologic causes of difficulty eating and swallowing in horses.

Lightning strike
Botulism
Polyneuritis equi
Tetanus
EEE/WEE
West Nile encephalomyelitis
Rabies
EPM
Verminous meningoencephalitis
Equine leukoencephalomalacia
Equine nigropallidal encephalomalacia
Chronic lead toxicity
Otitis media/interna
Guttural pouch disease with secondary peripheral neuropathy
Cholestineric granuloma (lateral ventricle)
Hydrocephalus
Skull trauma
Chronic grass sickness
Neonatal encephalopathy
Bacterial meningoencephalitis
Hepatic encephalopathy
Gastrointestinal hyperammonemia
Brainstem tumors

Table 9.3 Non-neurologic causes of dysphagia and difficulty eating.

Dental disease
Esophageal dysfunction
  Megaesophagus
  Stricture
  Intraluminal obstruction
  Diverticulum
  Persistent right aortic arch
Fractured jaw
Temporomandibular joint disease
Pharyngeal foreign bodies/masses
Mycotic granulomatous pharyngitis
Pharyngeal pythiosis
Thrush of tongue/pharynx
Foreign body in tongue
Branchial remnant cysts
Pharyngeal retention cysts
Hyoid apparatus fracture
Jugular thrombosis with secondary swelling
White muscle disease

wave. Any food that remains in the esophagus after primary peristalsis or that refluxes through the distal esophageal sphincter from the stomach dilates the esophagus and thus initiates *secondary* peristaltic waves that attempt to propel residual food distally. The musculature of the cranial third of the esophagus is striated and peristalsis is controlled only by somatic branches of the glossopharyngeal and vagus nerves. In the lower two-thirds, the smooth muscle is controlled by vagovagal reflexes acting via interactions with the myenteric nervous system. When a peristaltic wave passes down the esophagus, the lower esophageal sphincter and stomach relax in response to a wave of inhibitory impulses transmitted through myenteric neurons, thereby facilitating passage of the food bolus into the stomach.

Causes of dysphagia

Difficulties with mastication and deglutition can usefully be categorized as either oral, pharyngeal, or postpharyngeal, according to the location of the affected area. *Oral* causes include chewing disorders and dysphagia occurs because of conditions that impair transfer of food or water from the mouth to the pharynx. Horses with oral disorders may eat or drink in an anomalous way and often drool saliva and drop food or

water from the mouth. Because the oral stage of swallowing is consciously initiated, horses with forebrain dysfunction often have prepharyngeal dysphagia. Dysfunction of either the oropharynx or nasopharynx may lead to *pharyngeal* dysphagia, which is typically associated with nasal regurgitation of food, water, or saliva, coughing, and frequently the development of aspiration pneumonia. Occasionally, affected horses may be able to breathe in or out through the mouth. *Postpharyngeal* dysphagia is seen in horses that regurgitate food secondary to esophageal dysfunction. Clinically, such horses appear similar to those with pharyngeal dysphagia but seldom develop aspiration pneumonia. Disorders of the stomach and proximal intestinal tract can also cause signs of nasal regurgitation. Such diseases, although not strictly classified as dysphagia, must be considered diagnostic differentials (Tables 9.2 and 9.3).

Interference with chewing and/or swallowing may be caused by pain, structural abnormality, or movement dysfunction. Commonly, a single disease can interfere with swallowing at more than one site or by more than one mechanism.

Pain

The following may induce sufficient discomfort to affect eating or cause dysphagia: inflammation or ulceration of the mucous membranes of the upper alimentary tract, dental problems, inflammation of adjacent lymph nodes, trauma to or microbial infection of the bones and soft tissues involved in swallowing, arthritis of relevant joints, foreign bodies in or adjacent to the lumen of the mouth, pharynx, or esophagus. Important examples of painful chewing disorders or dysphagia include severe mycotic/bacterial glossitis ("thrush") in foals; glossitis/mucosal ulceration secondary to pyrimethamine toxicity, phenylbutazone toxicity, immune-mediated oral mucosal disease; vesicular stomatitis viral infection; foreign bodies (e.g., baling wire or foxtail awns in the tongue) [58–60]; bit or chain-induced injuries of the mouth; tooth root abscesses or missing teeth, otitis media/THO; fracture or luxation of the bones of the jaw or hyoid apparatus; severe ulceration or inflammation of the epiglottis or pharynx [61–63]; and reflux esophagitis in foals with gastroduodenal ulcer disease [64].

Mechanical

Blockage of the lumen of the mouth, pharynx, or esophagus may be caused by internal obstructions including soft tissue thickening due to edema (e.g., venous obstruction, anaphylaxis, and snake bite), masses (e.g., neoplastic, inflammatory), circumferential scar tissue (e.g., stricture), impacted food material, or foreign bodies. Obstructing external compression may be produced by space-occupying lesions (e.g., inflammatory, neoplastic, hemorrhagic, and edematous), "ligating" bands of scar tissue, anomalous blood vessels, or ropes or straps that tightly encircle the neck. Dysfunction of structures involved in swallowing can also be caused by nonobstructive abnormalities such as congenital cysts (usually in the pharynx), anatomic defects (either congenital or traumatic), and neoplasms or other masses. Important causes of dysphagia of mechanical origin include (in addition to many of the examples cited for pain) tumors (e.g., squamous cell carcinoma, lymphoma, and fibroma) of the structures and/or associated lymph nodes of the mouth, pharynx, or esophagus [65–67]. Obstructive inflammatory lesions (intra- or extraluminal) include granulomatous masses caused by fungi (*Conidiobolus, Basidiobolus, Aspergillus,* and *Cryptococcus* species [68–71]), *Phythium* species, *Halicephalobus gingivalis* [72], and retropharyngeal lymph node infections including strangles or other infections [73]. Enlargement of the tongue and other soft tissues sufficient to cause dysphagia may occur secondary to bilateral jugular thrombosis and external compression of the pharynx or esophagus, by air-distended guttural pouches [74], hematoma after cranial trauma or bleeding disorder [75, 76], or persistent right aortic arch [77] or epiglottic frenulum [78]. Dysphagia is likewise a feature of choke including postchoke esophageal stricture or diverticulum, esophageal fistula [79], cleft palate, epiglottic entrapment [80], and congenital subepiglottic, palatine, or esophageal cysts [81–84].

Movement disorders

In most cases, disruption of coordinated chewing and/or swallowing movements is due to neurologic, neuromuscular, or muscular dysfunction of the structures involved in eating. In some cases, dysphagia of this type is but one sign of generalized disease. For example, spastic dysphagia is a component both of tetanus and hyperkalemic periodic paralysis [85], and dysphagia due to flaccid pharyngeal paralysis is often a sign of botulism [86, 87] or nutritional myodegeneration (white muscle disease) [88, 89], and rarely a sign of tick paralysis of horses in Australia [90]. Grass sickness is caused by autonomic neuronal necrosis and results in reduced motility of the smooth muscle of the entire alimentary tract [91]. The dysphagia associated with grass sickness results from paralytic megaesophagus. Myasthenia gravis is associated with megaesophagus and dysphagia in humans and dogs, although it is yet to be reported as a cause of dysphagia in horses.

Diffuse forebrain diseases may affect motor control of and sensory perception from swallowing structures and are most likely to affect the initiation of swallowing. Examples of forebrain diseases that may induce some form of dysphagia include neonatal encephalopathy of foals [81], postseizure encephalopathy, rabies and other viral encephalitides [92], bacterial meningitis, leukoencephalomalacia, and hepatoencephalopathy [93]. Subcortical nuclei (globus pallidus and substantia nigra) are involved in coordination of the transfer of food from the mouth to the pharynx. Consumption by equids of the neurotoxin repin in several toxic plants, including yellow star thistle (*Centaurea solstitialis*), Malta star thistle (*Centaurea melitensis*), and Russian knapweed (*Rhaponticum repens*), destroys these nuclei and causes a characteristic and permanent dysphagia as the main sign of equine nigropallidal encephalomalacia [94, 95]. Less well-characterized neurologic syndromes of horses, with dysphagia as part of the clinical presentation, are caused by ingestion of *Indigofera* spp. plants (e.g., creeping indigo, Birdsville indigo) [96].

Dysphagia also frequently results from damage, either centrally or peripherally, to any of several cranial nerves involved in chewing and swallowing. The more important of these are CN Vs (mucosal sensation), CN Vm (chewing muscles), CN VII (tone of lips and cheeks), CN IX (pharyngeal, cranial esophageal function), CN X (pharyngeal, laryngeal, and esophageal function), and CN XII (motor to the tongue and pharynx). Specific causes of dysfunction of these nerves include EPM, viral (especially rabies) or parasitic encephalitis, neuroborreliosis, bacterial meningitis, lightning strike, intracranial abscesses or tumors (especially extramedullary melanoma or lymphoma) [97, 98], cranial trauma, especially that complicated by basilar fractures/

separations, guttural pouch conditions (e.g., mycosis [57], empyema, neoplasia, and fibrosis), THO, polyneuritis equi, and chronic lead poisoning. Damage to the intrinsic neural plexuses or muscle of the esophageal wall apparently occurs in rare cases of megaesophagus (other than that associated with grass sickness) or other esophageal dysfunction [99].

Diagnostic approach

The most common causes of eating disorders are not neurologic; thus, it is important to first rule out anatomic or physical causes. A thorough history, physical examination (including watching the horse eat and passing a nasogastric tube), dental examination, and one to several additional imaging examinations (e.g., endoscopy, plain radiography, ultrasonography, CT, MRI) are usually sufficient for this purpose. A full neurologic examination should be performed to identify additional signs of nervous system disease and, if indicated, further diagnostic tests for specific diseases can be performed. These may include CSF aspiration and analysis, testing for infectious diseases, imaging as described earlier, feed analyses, and inspection of pasture and environments for toxins and toxic plants.

Blindness, anisocoria, and strabismus

This section considers only neurologic causes of blindness and focuses on the steps in the neurologic examination necessary to localize a causative lesion. The reader should consult standard veterinary ophthalmology texts for a more comprehensive treatment of the subject (Table 9.4).

In horses, neurologic causes of blindness are first localized by testing menace responses and pupillary light reflexes. Additional information may be provided by obstacle tests. Accurate neuroanatomic localization then is used to generate likely differential diagnoses and diagnostic plans.

Because the afferent portion of the menace response pathway and the visual pathway are shared (Figure 9.7), it is possible to have vision but no menace in an eye but probably not menace without vision. If possible, test menace responses while standing directly in front of the horse. Use the palm of the hand to make a threatening gesture toward the eye, testing each eye from both temporal and nasal directions. Stimulate the horse just before each menace gesture by tapping the skin below the eye. For safety, always hold the noseband of the halter with one hand while using the other for testing. It is not usually necessary to cover the other eye during routine menace testing of horses. A normal menace response is blinking of the ipsilateral eyelids. There often also is retraction of the eyeball and evasive

Table 9.4 Neurogenic causes of blindness in the horse.

Traumatic optic neuropathy
Traumatic forebrain injury
Cholinisteric granuloma
Hydrocephalus
Anesthetic-associated cerebral necrosis
Bacterial meningoencephalitis
Postseizure encephalopathy
Cerebral abscess
Caudal tentorial herniation
EEE/WEE
Cryptococcal meningitis
Parasitic meningoencephalitis
Mycotic encephalitis (secondary to guttural pouch mycosis)
Equine protozoal myeloencephalitis
Thiamine deficiency
Neonatal encephalopathy
Pars intermedia adenoma
Hepatoencephalopathy
Gastrointestinal hyperammonemia
Toxicity
   Stypandra spp. toxicity
   Ivermectin toxicity
   Equine leukoencephalomalacia
Inadvertent intrarterial injection

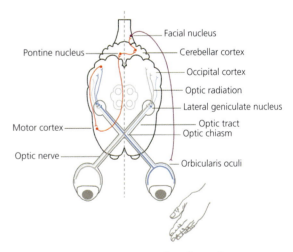

Figure 9.7 Diagram demonstrating the reflex pathways involved in the menace reflex.

movement of the head and neck but this response follows different central pathways than does the menace. Compare carefully the intensity of the menace responses elicited from each side. In this regard, menace should be considered a quantitative response. Unlike simple reflexes, which are assessed as present or absent, a menace response can be considered abnormal if it is less vigorous than that elicited from the opposite (normal) side. At least 80% of vision fibers cross at the chiasm in horses; thus, for routine clinical purposes in horses, vision in one eye is assumed to be perceived completely by the opposite visual cortex. If necessary, the small temporal portion of the retina served by the ipsilateral visual cortex can be tested by a menacing gesture from the extreme nasal aspect, performed while the opposite eye is covered. The menace response can be interrupted anywhere in its afferent pathway from the eye via the optic nerve to the contralateral optic tract, lateral geniculate nucleus, optic radiation, and occipital cortex. From the visual centers in the occipital lobe of the cortex, the menace response pathway continues via the contralateral motor cortex, then projects to the brainstem on the side being tested. Before terminating on the facial nucleus in the ipsilateral medulla oblongata, the menace pathway either passes through the ipsilateral cerebellum or receives essential input from the cerebellar cortex. If the menace response is defective in an eye, but there is no sign of cerebellar involvement and facial nerve function and pupillary light reflexes are intact, then the responsible lesion is contralateral and most likely in the forebrain. In normal neonates up to 2 weeks of age and in Arabian foals with cerebellar abiotrophy, there is no menace response, but the horse can see. In these settings, vigorous threatening gestures toward the eye may cause retraction of the eyeball and evasive movements of the head without blinking of the eyelids.

In horses with defective menace responses, there may be other signs of asymmetric forebrain disease such as compulsive walking in circles, dementia, head and neck turn, obtundation, seizures, and hypalgesia of the face on the side opposite the lesion (i.e., the same side as the defective menace). If the lesion causing a menace deficit is in the optic nerve or fundus of the eye, the PLR on the side of the defective menace should be abnormal. Head-bobbing, limb hypermetria, and ataxia are expected in horses with abnormal menace responses resulting from cerebellar dysfunction. If eyelid paralysis is preventing the menace response, the palpebral reflex should also be abnormal and there may be additional signs of facial paralysis.

If possible, examine the eyes in subdued or dim light so that the pupils are large enough to easily allow appreciation of reflex constriction. Stand in front of the horse while holding the noseband of the halter and swing the light back and forth from one side to the other so as to obliquely and briefly illuminate each eye without causing constriction of the pupils. Unequal pupillary size is termed *anisocoria*, an abnormally constricted pupil *miotic*, and a dilated pupil *mydriatic*. From this examination,

determine whether or not the pupils are of equal size and if the diameter of each pupil is appropriate for the conditions. In this way, refine the diagnosis of anisocoria to miosis or mydriasis affecting a single eye. Next, direct the beam directly into the eye. This strong light should elicit both a dazzle reflex in the ipsilateral eye and PLRs in both eyes. The dazzle reflex refers to eyelid closure in response to bright light. The full dazzle reflex also includes retraction of the eyeball and movement of the head away from the light. A normal direct PLR is immediate constriction of the illuminated pupil in response to light. Next, test the indirect (consensual) reflex. To perform the indirect reflex, watch the pupil in one eye while an assistant shines the light into the opposite eye. Alternatively, the examiner can remain in front of the horse and swing the light from eye to eye to observe both direct and indirect reflexes (swinging light test).

The dazzle reflex is mediated via afferent input through the optic nerve to regions of the midbrain distinct from those required for the PLR and by efferent impulses along the facial nerve. It is possible for a horse to be cortically blind but still have dazzle reflexes, or to have PLRs but not dazzle reflexes. For a PLR, the stimulus pathway is via the optic nerves and optic tracts to the midbrain and thence to the efferent parasympathetic fibers of the oculomotor nerve. Fibers in the afferent limb of the reflex (i.e., optic nerve, optic tracts) can either pass on the same side or decussate at the optic chiasm and again in the midbrain (Figure 9.8). Results

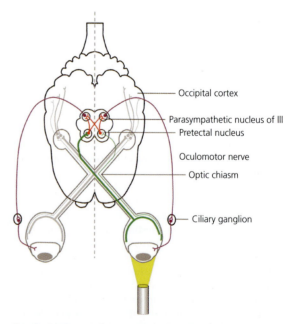

Figure 9.8 Diagram demonstrating the reflex pathways involved in the pupillary light reflex.

of testing of menace responses along with direct and consensual PLRs usually allow anatomic localization of a lesion in horses with a defective PLR. In brief, without consideration of effects on indirect PLR, a lesion in an optic nerve affects the direct PLR and the menace on the same side; a lesion in an optic tract (rostral to the lateral geniculate nucleus) affects the contralateral menace but does not affect direct PLR from either side, and a lesion in the ipsilateral midbrain or oculomotor nerve affects the ipsilateral PLR but not the menace responses.

Mydriasis is caused either by increased sympathetic dilator tone, interference with the afferent arm of the PLR, or damage to the parasympathetic oculomotor nucleus or nerve. Mydriasis caused by sympathetic overstimulation is usually bilateral and PLRs are normal. With a complete optic nerve lesion on one side, slight ipsilateral mydriasis is seen. Light directed into the opposite eye constricts the mydriatic pupil. With complete oculomotor nerve lesions, the ipsilateral pupil is fixed and dilated and unresponsive to light directed into either pupil; however, light directed into the fixed pupil causes reflex constriction of the pupil on the opposite side.

Miosis occurs because of removal of sympathetic dilator influence to the pupil or possibly because of excessive stimulation of pupillary constrictors. The sympathetic pathway can be affected anywhere along the three-neuron pathway from the midbrain to the eye. With damage anywhere along the preganglionic (second) or postganglionic (third) neurons of the sympathetic supply to the head, there are signs of Horner's syndrome in addition to ipsilateral miosis. This is considered in more detail in the next section.

Horses with abnormal PLR because of cerebral swelling have other signs of forebrain disease such as obtundation, dementia, and cortical blindness. Within 4 weeks of optic nerve injury, abnormal pigmentation of the fundus develops and there is atrophy of the vasculature of the optic disc. In addition to miosis and ptosis, interruption of the sympathetic supply to the head causes other signs of Horner's syndrome, including spontaneous facial sweating and hyperemia of mucous membranes.

While continuing to stand in front of the horse, observe the position and size of the pupils while the head is held level (i.e., a line through the center of each eyeball is parallel to the ground). While keeping the head level, lift the chin slowly. The eyeballs should remain stationary while the chin moves upward; thus, the eyes rotate ventrally relative to the long axis of the head. In horses with vestibular disease, abnormal eye positions are exaggerated by this maneuver. If the pupils are in abnormal positions, try to position the head in such a way (usually by rotation) that the pupils are normally oriented relative to the transverse axis of the head. For example, a horse with peripheral vestibular

disease often has ventral deviation of the eyeball on the side of the lesion and dorsal deviation on the opposite side. Eye position can be normalized relative to the axis of the head simply by rotating the head in the direction of the ventrally deviated eye. The abnormal position of the eyes in horses with vestibular disease is termed *vestibular strabismus*. *True strabismus* is eye deviation that cannot be corrected by repositioning the head and usually reflects mechanical interference with eye position or dysfunction of nerves to the extraocular muscles (i.e., oculomotor, trochlear, or abducens nerves). In horses with strabismus, the eyeball may be rotated medially or laterally, clockwise or counterclockwise. Newborn foals normally have slight dorsomedial rotation of the pupils compared with older horses.

For horses with vestibular strabismus, the causative lesion could be anywhere in the peripheral or central vestibular system (including connections with the cerebellum and nerves to the extraocular muscles), usually on the same side as the ventrally deviated eye. A horse exhibiting true strabismus most likely has a lesion in CN III, IV, or VI (or its roots or nucleus). These nerves exit the brainstem and pass a short distance to the oblique and rectus muscles of the eye. The roots of the nerves to the extraocular muscles are subject to dorsal pressure exerted by the cerebrum as it swells and herniates under the tentorium cerebelli. Other signs associated with cerebral swelling are obtundation, blindness, seizures, and fluctuant to dilated, fixed pupils. There may also be jerky head movements as a result of pressure on the cerebellum. As compression of the midbrain and rostral hindbrain becomes more severe, obtundation progresses to coma with decerebrate posturing. With more focal lesions of the nerves or their nuclei, mydriasis (CN III) is likely.

Determination of the portion of the visual pathways involved is helpful in determining the etiology and in planning further diagnostic testing, treatment, and establishing a prognosis. The eye should be carefully examined to ensure that it is not the source of the blindness prior to considering neurogenic causes.

Many conditions have been associated with neurogenic blindness in the horse. These include a toxic, traumatic, and infectious causes. Head trauma is common injury in the horse and may injure central pathways, especially in the visual cortex and/or unilateral or bilateral optic neuropathy (see Section "Trauma") [32]. Blindness associated with cortical injury may resolve but treatment of traumatic optic neuropathy is unrewarding and blindness is permanent. Meningoencephalitidies arising from bacterial, viral, parasitic, and mycotic agents have been reported to be associated with blindness in the horse [5, 81, 100–106]. In such cases, blindness is only a part of the clinical presentation, and profound neurologic abnormalities are usually present indicating more widespread CNS disease. Similarly, a variety of toxins may have blindness as a part of the clinical signs, but blindness is never the sole sign in such cases. Overdosage with ivermectin can result in transient blindness, and blindness is a major component of the clinical presentation of horses with leukoencephalomalacia [107, 108]. Horses with leukoencephalomalacia demonstrate diffuse signs of forebrain disease including dementia. The ingestion of *Stypandra* spp. (blindgrass), found in West and southeastern Australia and *Indigofera* species in Australia, Brazil, and the US can cause blindness and ataxia in horses. Iatrogenic causes include air embolism and intracarotid injection. Foals and, to a lesser extent, adult horses, will often demonstrate transient blindness following a generalized seizure from any cause.

The evaluation of blind horses should include a careful history and physical examination, and a complete neurologic examination to localize any lesion and detect other neurologic signs. A variety of clinicopathologic tests (PCR, immunodiagnostics of blood and CSF), imaging techniques (plain radiography, CT, MRI, ultrasound, endoscopy), and electrodiagnostic procedures (electroretinogram, electroencephalogram, evoked visual potential) are available to aid in the evaluations, and the tests selected will depend upon the history, physical, and neurologic examination findings.

Horner's syndrome

Horner's syndrome results from interruption of ocular sympathetic pathways. Sympathetic pathways to the head originate as first-order neurons (upper motor neurons) in the tectum of the midbrain. Axons descend to the first to third thoracic (T1 to T3) segments of the spinal cord, where they enter the gray matter of the intermediolateral horn, synapse on second order (preganglionic) sympathetic motor neurons, and exit in the ventral spinal nerve roots. From there, the nerves pass through the cervicothoracic and middle cervical ganglia (combined as the stellate ganglion) and ascend in the cervical sympathetic trunk (part of the vagosympathetic trunk) to the cranial cervical ganglia (CCG) where they synapse on the third-order (postganglionic) sympathetic nerve. In the horse, the CCG is part of a neurovascular bundle on the caudodorsal aspect of the guttural pouch under the petrous temporal bone. The third-order fibers are distributed with the blood supply via canals through the petrous temporal bone to the sweat glands of the head, ciliary muscles, periorbital smooth muscles, including the eyelid levator, Müller's superior tarsal muscle [109], and periarteriolar musculature. The sympathetic supply of the head thus can be damaged within the brainstem or spinal cord (first order), cranial thoracic nerve roots or spinal nerves or cervical sympathetic trunk (second order), or within the CCG, the skull or behind the eye (third order).

Specific causes of Horner's syndrome include mycotic guttural pouch infections, traumatic lesions of the basisphenoid area, otitis media, cervical trauma; abscesses, tumors, or space-occupying lesions in the anterior aspect of the thorax, periorbital abscesses or tumors; parotid duct obstruction and inflammation; esophageal rupture, inadvertent extrajugular injections of irritating substances, and complications associated with surgical ligation of the common carotid artery. Lesions involving first-order sympathetic neurons in the ipsilateral brainstem are rare but have been reported as a consequence of metastatic neoplasia or with EPM in horses [1]. Horner's syndrome also has occurred after IV injection of certain drugs, including xylazine, vitamin E or selenium, and phenylbutazone [110–112]. The sympathetic supply to the eye rarely may be involved in the inflammatory polyneuropathy characterizing horses with polyneuritis equi (cauda equina neuritis) syndrome [113, 114]. Tumors that have resulted in Horner's syndrome include sclerosing respiratory epithelial carcinoma, squamous cell carcinoma, lymphoma, mesothelioma, and melanoma [110, 115–117].

Clinical signs

The clinical signs of Horner's syndrome in horses vary but include miosis, ptosis, regional hyperthermia, excessive sweating on the ipsilateral side of the face, congested mucous membranes, inspiratory stridor, and dermatitis caused by chronic sweating. Although enophthalmos is reported to be a reliable sign of equine Horner's, many (most?) affected horses do not prolapse the nictitans and thus affected eyes are probably not enophthalmic. The presence of this sign apparently is variable among species: enophthalmos is not part of Horner's syndrome in humans and ruminants [118] but is so in cats and dogs [1]. Ptosis is caused by the combined effects of loss of the eyelid levator function of Müller's muscle and variable enophthalmos. It is most reliably detected by comparison of the eyelash angles on each side. On the affected side the eyelashes slope at a relatively downward angle. The palpebral reflex and the menace response are normal. Facial sweating may begin to decrease 6–14 days after sympathectomy [110]. If there is concomitant damage to the vertebral nerve or its cervical sympathetic branches, sweating of the skin of the neck also may be seen. Regional hyperthermia results from cutaneous and mucosal vasodilation, which results from removal of sympathetic vasomotor tone. Sweating is thought to be caused by vasodilation and increased delivery of epinephrine to sweat glands [119, 120].

Diagnosis

The level of sympathetic interruption can be determined by pharmacologic testing [1]. Hydroxyamphetamine (1% solution) instilled into the eye will result in release of norepinephrine from intact postganglionic sympathetic neurons, causing pupillary dilation, but no response when the postganglionic neurons are damaged. A positive response to this test indicates a preganglionic sympathetic lesion, and a lack of response indicates a postganglionic lesion. In animals with a postganglionic lesion, topical administration of 0.1 ml of 1:1000 epinephrine solution directly activates the iris musculature and produces mydriasis by 20 min, whereas the onset of dilation occurs at about 40 min in animals with preganglionic lesions. Similarly, 2.5–10% phenylephrine solution will produce pupillary dilation in an eye with a postganglionic sympathetic lesion, but not in a normal eye. The increased sensitivity to these direct-acting sympathomimetics in animals with postganglionic sympathetic lesions results from the phenomenon of denervation hypersensitivity, with numbers and sensitivity of norepinephrine receptors in the iris muscle increasing over days to weeks after postganglionic nerve injury. A positive response therefore is not seen until several days after the injury. Parenteral administration of 1 ml of 1:1000 epinephrine solution causes affected horses to sweat profusely over the affected side of the face [110]. However, this test does not differentiate between preganglionic and postganglionic lesions.

The guttural pouches of horses and the pharynx of all patients should be examined endoscopically to exclude the possibility of pharyngeal or laryngeal paralysis or guttural pouch disease. The jugular furrows should be palpated for swellings. Insertion of a nasogastric tube during palpation may be helpful for detecting subtle lesions on the left side of the neck. The thorax should be examined using auscultation and ultrasound and, if indicated, radiographs taken. Cranial ribs can be evaluated for lesions by scintigraphy [121]. A neurologic examination should be performed to evaluate the function of the spinal cord. The skin temperature may be measured using thermography [116, 122, 123]; on the affected side it is 1–3.5°C (33.4–37.5°F) higher than normal.

Treatment

The treatment for Horner's syndrome depends on the underlying cause of the denervation. Except for Horner's syndrome related to IV injection of xylazine, the signs often are irreversible, even if the primary cause of the condition has been eliminated. With xylazine-associated Horner's, the condition disappears spontaneously. The necrotizing effects of perivascular drug injections can be minimized by immediate dilution and/

or irrigation with large volumes of saline infiltrated into the perivascular tissues. Anti-inflammatory doses of flunixin and dexamethasone can be given systemically. Abscesses should be drained and fungal infections of the guttural pouch should be treated as appropriate.

Facial paralysis

The head should be examined carefully for symmetry of facial expression, particularly with respect to the ears, eyes, and muzzle. With complete unilateral facial paralysis, there is drooping of the ear, upper eyelid (ptosis), and lower lip, and immobility, narrowing, and lengthening of the affected external naris. The muzzle is deviated away from the affected side and saliva may drool from the mouth. Any or all of these components can be affected separately. Facial nerve function should additionally be evaluated by testing "flick" reflexes on each side of the face. Each of these reflexes requires intact trigeminal sensory branches, central connections in the pons and medulla oblongata, and functioning facial nerves. To test these reflexes, the commissure of the lips, the medial and lateral canthi of the eye and the supraorbital fossa, and the ear are touched lightly. Appropriate responses are retraction and elevation of the commissure of the lip, blinking of the eyelids, and flick of the ear, respectively. It is helpful to have the handler cover the ipsilateral eye during testing of the lip and ear.

The facial innervation of lacrimal glands can be tested by performing Schirmer tear tests. If tear production is reduced to less than 50% of normal on the side of the face that is paralyzed, there is likely to be a lesion affecting secretomotor fibers proximal (central) to the middle ear. The symmetry of facial tone can further be tested by using the thumbs or fingers to assess resistance simultaneously on both sides to retraction of lip commissures, elevation of upper eyelids, and forward extension of the ears. If there has been facial paralysis for more than 2 weeks, there usually is an obvious subcutaneous depression running ventrally from the base of the ear along the back of the vertical ramus of the mandible. This reflects atrophy of the parotidoauricularis muscle. Finally, test the cervicofacial reflex as part of the examination of long spinal reflexes. This reflex is not used as a primary test of facial nerve function but, clearly, its interpretation is affected by facial nerve paralysis.

Commonly, there is also head tilt and spontaneous nystagmus because of involvement of the vestibular system. In horses with facial paralysis caused by brain disease, there may be other signs of hindbrain disorder such as obtundation, signs of abnormal cranial nerve function, such as dysphagia or masseter atrophy, or limb ataxia and weakness on the same side as the lesion. Non-neurologic signs include exposure keratitis or keratoconjunctivitis sicca and inspiratory stridor during exercise.

Abnormalities of facial tone reflect damage to the facial nucleus in the medulla oblongata, facial nerve root, or facial nerve or its motor branches, including dorsal and ventral buccal nerves, posterior and internal auricular and auriculopalpebral nerves, and the digastric nerve. If the Schirmer tear test gives a normal result on the affected side, the lesion is most likely at or peripheral to the middle ear; if tear production is reduced more than 50%, at least one lesion is central to the middle ear.

Injury to the facial nerve proximal to the vertical ramus of the mandible causes full facial paresis. Proximal facial nerve trauma usually is caused by fractures of the vertical ramus of the mandible, the stylohyoid bone, or the petrous temporal bone (after a blow to the head or as a complication of THO). Damage within the facial canal often is associated with concurrent signs of vestibular nerve damage, such as head tilt, nystagmus, and circling. Tear production also may be reduced. Unilateral facial paralysis due to proximal facial nerve trauma must be differentiated from facial nerve damage or inflammation due to a variety of other causes. These include medullary lesions involving the facial nucleus (e.g., EPM) as well as polyneuritis equi (neuritis of the cauda equina) and idiopathic facial nerve paralysis. Hemorrhage into the middle/inner ear, otitis media/interna, guttural pouch mycosis, and parotid lymph node abscessation each can involve the adjacent facial nerve, causing ipsilateral facial paralysis. Distal facial nerve damage usually is due to direct injury from a blow or lateral recumbency or strangulation by a tight-fitting halter. The nerve or its branches often are damaged as they cross the mandible and/or zygomatic arch. Facial paresis following recumbency during general anesthesia is common and usually involves only the nose and/or lips. The prognosis for return of facial nerve function depends on the site and severity of the causative process. Large motor nerves like the facial nerve contain numerous fascicles, and each fascicle is made up of many axons within a connective tissue sheath. The functional effect of damage is seldom as straightforward as single-fiber classifications would suggest and usually reflects differing degrees of damage across a nerve.

Damage to individual axons fall into two major functional categories. Type 1 injury, also known as neurapraxia, refers to loss of function without loss of axonal continuity. Type 2 injury represents damage to axonal structures such that Wallerian degeneration of

the axon ensues distal to the site of injury; the proximal axonal segment and the cell body remain intact. Retrograde degeneration of the proximal nerve occurs if connectivity is not reestablished [124]. Type 1 lesions are characterized by a failure of conduction of the action potential across the injured axonal segment. Normal muscle action potentials are evoked by stimulation of the nerve anywhere distal to the lesion, but they are absent when the nerve is stimulated proximal to the injury. The pathologic basis for these reversible injuries could be nerve compression, damage to the myelin sheath, or alteration of the functions of the axonal cell membrane or its channel proteins. Type 2 injuries are characterized by axonal interruption, or axonotmesis. If there is disruption of components of the connective tissue sheath and axon, the process is termed neuronotmesis. Immediately after axonotmetic injury, the distal axonal segment is competent to conduct action potentials; however, within 3–8 days after injury, the distal segment degenerates and no longer responds to electrical stimulation. In this way, neurapractic (type 1) and axonotmetic (type 2) injuries of greater than 8 days' duration can be theoretically distinguished by nerve stimulation studies. Longstanding axonotmetic injuries result in retrograde degeneration of the neuronal cell body and secondary demyelination of the proximal axonal segment. After axonotmesis of motor nerves, muscle reinnervation occurs by two separate mechanisms: collateral sprouting and axonal regrowth. If there is incomplete loss of axons to a muscle, surviving motor axons generate sprouts from their nerve terminals, which can establish competent junctions with adjacent denervated muscle units. Reinnervation of muscle units by this process occurs within days to weeks. However, if the motor axons to a muscle are severed, reinnervation occurs by growth of collateral sprouts from the proximal stump. Axonal sprouts grow at a rate of 1 mm/day (~1 inch/month). Regeneration occurs under the influence of growth factors including neurotrophic growth factor, brain-derived neurotrophic factor, and ciliary neurotrophic factor. Successful reinnervation of the entire face thus may take several months. Because of progressive fibrous replacement of denervated muscle and retrograde degeneration of the proximal parts of affected motor neurons, it has been suggested that reinnervation may not be possible if more than 12 months have elapsed since the original injury. However, reinnervation surgery has been successful when performed on human patients 20 years or more after denervation. If there is skin damage with section of the nerve, the nerve ends should be identified and either immediately repaired surgically or tagged (e.g., with stainless-steel sutures) for future identification and anastomosis.

References

[1] De Lahunta A, Glass EN. *Veterinary Neuroanatomy and Clinical Neurology*. 3rd ed. St. Louis: Saunders Elsevier; 2009.

[2] Johnson PJ, Constantinescu GM, Frappier BL. The vestibular system. Part I: anatomy, physiology and clinical signs from altered vestibular function. *Equine Vet Educ* 2001; 13:105–109.

[3] Johnson PJ, Kellam LL. The vestibular system. Part II: differential diagnosis. *Equine Vet Educ* 2001;13:141–150.

[4] Johnson AL, Morrow JK, Sweeney RW. Indirect fluorescent antibody test and surface antigen ELISAs for antemortem diagnosis of equine protozoal myeloencephalitis. *J Vet Intern Med* 2013;27:596–599.

[5] Raphel CF. Brain-abscess in 3 horses. *J Am Vet Med Assoc* 1982;180:874–877.

[6] Mair TS, Pearson GR. Melanotic hamartoma of the hind brain in a riding horse. *J Comp Pathol* 1990;102:239–243.

[7] Teuscher E, Vrins A, Lemaire T. A vestibular syndrome associated with *Cryptococcus neoformans* in a horse. *Zentralbl Veterinarmed A* 1984;31:132–139.

[8] Johnstone LK, Mayhew IG, Fletcher LR. Clinical expression of lolitrem B (perennial ryegrass) intoxication in horses. *Equine Vet J* 2012;44:304–309.

[9] Blythe LL. Otitis media and interna and temporohyoid osteoarthropathy. *Vet Clin North Am Equine Pract* 1997;13: 21–42.

[10] Naylor RJ, Perkins JD, Allen S, et al. Histopathology and computed tomography of age-associated degeneration of the equine temporohyoid joint. *Equine Vet J* 2010;42:425–430.

[11] Divers TJ, Ducharme NG, De Lahunta A, et al. Temporohyoid osteoarthropathy. *Clin Tech Equine Pract* 2006;5:17–23.

[12] Hilton H, Puchalski SM, Aleman M. The computed tomographic appearance of equine temporohyoid osteoarthropathy. *Vet Radiol Ultrasound* 2009;50:151–156.

[13] Aleman M, Puchalski SM, Williams DC, et al. Brainstem auditory-evoked responses in horses with temporohyoid osteoarthropathy. *J Vet Intern Med* 2008;22:1196–1202.

[14] Walker AM, Sellon DC, Cornelisse CJ, et al. Temporohyoid osteoarthropathy in 33 horses (1993–2000). *J Vet Intern Med* 2002;16:697–703.

[15] Grenager NS, Divers TJ, Mohammed HO, et al. Epidemiological features and association with crib-biting in horses with neurological disease associated with temporohyoid osteoarthropathy (1991–2008). *Equine Vet Educ* 2010;22:467–472.

[16] Palus V, Bladon B, Brazil T, et al. Retrospective study of neurological signs and management of seven English horses with temporohyoid osteoarthropathy. *Equine Vet Educ* 2012;24:415–422.

[17] Borges AS, Watanabe MJ. Guttural pouch diseases causing neurologic dysfunction in the horse. *Vet Clin North Am Equine Pract* 2011;27:545–572.

[18] Pownder S, Scrivani PV, Bezuidenhout A, et al. Computed tomography of temporal bone fractures and temporal region anatomy in horses. *J Vet Intern Med* 2010;24:398–406.

[19] Frame EM, Riihimaki M, Berger M, et al. Scintigraphic findings in a case of temporohyoid osteoarthropathy in a horse. *Equine Vet Educ* 2005;17:11–13.

[20] Blythe LL, Watrous BJ, Shires GMH, et al. Prophylactic partial stylohyoidostectomy for horses with osteoarthropathy of the temporohyoid joint. *J Equine Vet Sci* 1994;14:32–37.

[21] Pease AP, Van Biervliet J, Dykes NL, et al. Complication of partial stylohyoidectomy for treatment of temporohyoid osteoarthropathy and an alternative surgical technique in three cases. *Equine Vet J* 2004;36:546–550.

[22] Mackay RJ. Brain injury after head trauma: pathophysiology, diagnosis, and treatment. *Vet Clin North Am Equine Pract* 2004;20:199–216.

[23] Sinha AK, Hendrickson DA, Kannegieter NJ. Head trauma in two horses. *Vet Rec* 1991;128:518–521.

[24] Ruedi M, Hagen R, Luchinger U, et al. Subluxation of C2 and C3 and fracture of C2 caused by severe head trauma in two Warmblood horses. *Pferdeheilkunde* 2011;27:522–527.

[25] Stick JA, Wilson T, Kunze D. Basilar skull fractures in three horses. *J Am Vet Med Assoc* 1980;176:228–231.

[26] Tietje S, Becker M, Bockenhoff G. Computed tomographic evaluation of head diseases in the horse: 15 cases. *Equine Vet J* 1996;28:98–9105.

[27] Rullan-Mayol AJ, Gashen L, Ramirez S, et al. What is your diagnosis? *J Am Vet Med Assoc* 2007;231:1499–1500.

[28] Mckelvey WA, Owen RR. Acquired torticollis in eleven horses. *J Am Vet Med Assoc* 1979;175:295–297.

[29] Alexander K, Baird JD, Dobson H, et al. What is your diagnosis? Displaced avulsion fracture of the basisphenoid-basioccipital bone. *J Am Vet Med Assoc* 2002;220:297–298.

[30] Darien BJ, Watrous BJ, Huber MJ, et al. What is your diagnosis? Avulsion of a portion of the attachment of the longus capitus muscle from the basisphenoid bone. *J Am Vet Med Assoc* 1991;198:1799–1800.

[31] Johnson PJ, Moore LA, Reed AL. What is your diagnosis? Trauma-induced skull fracture and bacterial meningitis. *J Am Vet Med Assoc* 1996;209:901–902.

[32] Martin L, Kaswan R, Chapman W. Four cases of traumatic optic nerve blindness in the horse. *Equine Vet J* 1986;18:133–137.

[33] Blogg JR, Stanley RG, Phillip CJ. Skull and orbital blow-out fractures in a horse. *Equine Vet J Suppl* 10;1990:5–7.

[34] Beccati F, Angeli G, Secco I, et al. Comminuted basilar skull fracture in a colt: use of computed tomography to aid the diagnosis. *Equine Vet Educ* 2011;23:327–332.

[35] Feary DJ, Magdesian KG, Aleman MA, et al. Traumatic brain injury in horses: 34 cases (1994–2004). *J Am Vet Med Assoc* 2007;231:259–266.

[36] Beccati F, Pepe M, Nannarone S, et al. Computed tomography for evaluation of some head diseases in 11 horses. *Ippologia* 2012;23:3–17.

[37] Lischer CJ, Walliser U, Witzmann P, et al. Fracture of the paracondylar process in four horses: advantages of CT imaging. *Equine Vet J* 2005;37:483–487.

[38] Sweeney CR, Freeman DE, Sweeney RW, et al. Hemorrhage into the guttural pouch (auditory tube diverticulum) associated with rupture of the longus capitis muscle in three horses. *J Am Vet Med Assoc* 1993;202:1129–1131.

[39] Finnie JW, Blumbergs PC. Traumatic brain injury. *Vet Pathol* 2002;39:679–689.

[40] Shaw NA. The neurophysiology of concussion. *Prog Neurobiol* 2002;67:281–344.

[41] Zauner A, Daugherty WP, Bullock MR, et al. Brain oxygenation and energy metabolism: Part I: biological function and pathophysiology. *Neurosurgery* 2002;51:289–301.

[42] Solano M, Brawer RS. CT of the equine head: technical considerations, anatomic guide, and selected diseases. *Clin Tech Equine Pract* 2004;3:374–388.

[43] Marik PE, Varon J, Trask T. Management of head trauma. *Chest* 2002;122:699–711.

[44] Dougherty JA, Rhoney DH. Gabapentin: a unique antiepileptic agent. *Neurol Res* 2001;23:821–829.

[45] Donaldson J, Borzatta MA, Matossian D. Nutrition strategies in neurotrauma. *Crit Care Nurs Clin North Am* 2000;12:465–475.

[46] Kramer J, Coates JR, Hoffman AG, et al. Preliminary anatomic investigation of three approaches to the equine cranium and brain for limited craniectomy procedures. *Vet Surg* 2007;36:500–508.

[47] Auer JA. Craniomaxillofacial disorders. In: Auer JA, Stick JA, eds. *Equine Surgery*. 4th ed. St. Louis: Elsevier; 2012: 1456–1482.

[48] Mcilwraith CW. Surgical repair of depression fractures of the skull. In: Mcilwraith CW, Robertson JT, eds. *Mcilwraith & Turner's Equine Surgery: Advanced Techniques*. Philadelphia: Lippincott, Williams & Wilkins; 1998:276–277.

[49] Schaaf KL, Kannegieter NJ, Lovell DK. Management of equine skull fractures using fixation with polydioxanone sutures. *Aust Vet J* 2008;86:481–485.

[50] Muzha I, Filipi N, Lede R, et al. Effect of intravenous corticosteroids on death within 14 days in 10008 adults with clinically significant head injury (MRC CRASH trial): randomised placebo-controlled trial. *Lancet* 2004;364: 1321–1328.

[51] Heath DL, Vink R. Optimization of magnesium therapy after severe diffuse axonal brain injury in rats. *J Pharmacol Exp Ther* 1999;288:1311–1316.

[52] Marshall AE, Byars TD, Whitlock RH, et al. Brain-stem auditory evoked-response in the diagnosis of inner-ear injury in the horse. *J Am Vet Med Assoc* 1981;178:282–286.

[53] Mayhew IG, Washbourne JR. A method of assessing auditory and brainstem function in horses. *Br Vet J* 1990; 146:509–518.

[54] Rolf SL, Reed SM, Melnick W, et al. Auditory brain-stem response testing in anesthetized horses. *Am J Vet Res* 1987; 48:910–914.

[55] Mackay RJ. On the true definition of dysphagia. *Compend Contin Educ Pract Vet* 2001;23:1024–1028.

[56] Klebe EA, Holcombe SJ, Rosenstein D, et al. The effect of bilateral glossopharyngeal nerve anaesthesia on swallowing in horses. *Equine Vet J* 2005;37:65–69.

[57] Eichentopf A, Snyder A, Recknagel S, et al. Dysphagia caused by focal guttural pouch mycosis: mononeuropathy of the pharyngeal ramus of the vagal nerve in a 20-year-old pony mare. *Ir Vet J* 2013;66:7.

[58] Hudson NPH, Mcgorum BC, Dixon PM. A review of 4 cases of dysphagia in the horse: buccal abscess, lingual abscess, retropharyngeal foreign body and oesophageal obstruction. *Equine Vet Educ* 2006;18:199–204.

[59] Pusterla N, Latson KM, Wilson WD, et al. Metallic foreign bodies in the tongues of 16 horses. *Vet Rec* 2006;159: 485–488.

[60] Johnson PJ, Lacarrubba AM, Messer NT, et al. Ulcerative glossitis and gingivitis associated with foxtail grass awn irritation in two horses. *Equine Vet Educ* 2012;24: 182–186.

[61] Dacre KJ, Pirie RS, Prince DR. Primary epiglottitis with associated dysphagia in a foal. *Equine Vet Educ* 2004; 16:296–298.

[62] Gille D, Lavoie JP. Review of seven cases of ulcers of the soft palate. *Equine Pract* 1996;18:9–13.

[63] Berthelon M, Rampin D. Course of an outbreak of influenza due to the A/equi 1 type of virus in a thoroughbred stud. *Rev Med Vet* 1972;123:293–304.

[64] Murray MJ, Ball MM, Parker GA. Megaesophagus and aspiration pneumonia secondary to gastric ulceration in a foal. *J Am Vet Med Assoc* 1988;192:381–383.

[65] Hudson NPH, Dixon PM, Pirie RS, et al. Dysphagia caused by squamous cell carcinoma of the tongue. *Equine Vet Educ* 2000;12:133–136.

[66] Schneider A, Tessier C, Gorgas D, et al. Magnetic resonance imaging features of a benign peripheral nerve sheath tumour with 'ancient' changes in the tongue of a horse. *Equine Vet Educ* 2010;22:346–351.

[67] Jones SL, Zimmel D, Tate LP, et al. Case presentation—dysphagia caused by squamous cell carcinoma in two horses. *Compend Contin Educ Pract Vet* 2001;23:1020–1024.

[68] Greet TRC. Nasal aspergillosis in 3 horses. *Vet Rec* 1981;109:487–489.

[69] Corrier DE, Wilson SR, Scrutchfield WL. Equine cryptococcal rhinitis. *Compend Contin Educ Pract Vet* 1984;6:S556–S558.

[70] Hanselka DV. Equine nasal phycomycosis. *Vet Med Small Anim Clin* 1977;72:251–253.

[71] Zamos DT, Schumacher J, Loy JK. Nasopharyngeal conidiobolomycosis in a horse. *J Am Vet Med Assoc* 1996;208:100–101.

[72] Teifke JP, Schmidt E, Traenckner CM, et al. *Halicephalobus* (syn. *Micronema*) *deletrix* as cause of a granulomatous gingivitis and osteomyelitis in a horse. *Tierarztl Prax Ausg G Grosstiere Nutztiere* 1998;26:157–161.

[73] Golland LC, Hodgson DR, Davis RE, et al. Retropharyngeal lymph-node infection in horses—46 cases (1977–1992). *Aust Vet J* 1995;72:161–164.

[74] Ohnesorge B, Ameer K, Hetzel U, et al. Transendoscopic laser surgery of guttural pouch tympany in foals—an endoscopic, light- and electron microscopic study. *Tierarztl Prax Ausg G Grosstiere Nutztiere* 2001;29:58–65.

[75] Henninger RW. Hemophilia A in 2 related Quarter horse colts. *J Am Vet Med Assoc* 1988;193:91–94.

[76] Knight AP. Dysphagia resulting from unilateral rupture of rectus capitis ventralis muscles in a horse. *J Am Vet Med Assoc* 1977;170:735–738.

[77] Butt TD, Macdonald DG, Crawford WH, et al. Persistent right aortic arch in a yearling horse. *Can Vet J* 1998; 39:714–715.

[78] Bertuglia A, Gandini M, Bozzini C, et al. Transoral resection of persistent epiglottis frenulum in a foal. *Ippologia* 2007;18:5–8.

[79] Schott HCI, Wheeler LC, Murnane R. Dysphagia caused by oesophageal fistulas in a thoroughbred foal. *Equine Vet Educ* 1991;3:64–67.

[80] Ohnesorge B, Deegen E. Diagnosis and minimally invasive surgery of epiglottic diseases in horses. Part 2: Epiglottic entrapment. *Tierarztl Prax Ausg G Grosstiere Nutztiere* 2003; 31:273–279.

[81] Holcombe SJ, Hurcombe SD, Barr BS, et al. Dysphagia associated with presumed pharyngeal dysfunction in 16 neonatal foals. *Equine Vet J* 2012;44:105–108.

[82] Salz RO, Ahern BJ, Lumsden JM. Subepiglottic cysts in 15 horses. *Equine Vet Educ* 2013;25:403–407.

[83] Nolen-Walston RD, Parente EJ, Madigan JE, et al. Branchial remnant cysts of mature and juvenile horses. *Equine Vet J* 2009;41:918–923.

[84] Ohnesorge B, Deegen E. Diagnosis and minimally invasive surgery of epiglottic diseases in horses. Part 1: Subepiglottic cysts. *Tierarztl Prax Ausg G Grosstiere Nutztiere* 2003;31: 215–220.

[85] Guglick MA, Macallister CG, Breazile JE. Laryngospasm, dysphagia, and emaciation associated with hyperkalemic periodic paralysis in a horse. *J Am Vet Med Assoc* 1996; 209:115–117.

[86] Johnson AL, Mcadams SC, Whitlock RH. Type A botulism in horses in the United States: a review of the past ten years (1998–2008). *J Vet Diagn Invest* 2010;22:165–173.

[87] Whitlock RH, Buckley C. Botulism. *Vet Clin North Am Equine Pract* 1997;13:107–128.

[88] Ludvikova E, Jahn P, Lukas Z. Nutritional myodegeneration as a cause of dysphagia in adult horses: three case reports. *Vet Med* 2007;52:267–272.

[89] Pearson EG, Snyder SP, Saulez MN. Masseter myodegeneration as a cause of trismus or dysphagia in adult horses. *Vet Rec* 2005;156:642–646.

[90] Ruppin M, Sullivan S, Condon F, et al. Retrospective study of 103 presumed cases of tick (*Ixodes holocyclus*) envenomation in the horse. *Aust Vet J* 2012;90:175–180.

[91] Cottrell DF, Mcgorum BC, Pearson GT. The neurology and enterology of equine grass sickness: a review of basic mechanisms. *Neurogastroenterol Motil* 1999;11:79–92.

[92] Suchy A, Weissenbock H, Waller R, et al. Evidence of Borna disease in an Austrian horse. *Wien Tierarztl Monatsschr* 1997;84:317–321.

[93] Gava A, Barros CSL. *Senecio* spp. poisoning of horses in southern Brazil. *Pesqui Vete Bras* 1997;17:36–40.

[94] Elliott CRB, Mccowan CI. Nigropallidal encephalomalacia in horses grazing *Rhaponticum repens* (creeping knapweed). *Aust Vet J* 2012;90:151–154.

[95] Robles M, Choi BH, Han B, et al. Repin-induced neurotoxicity in rodents. *Exp Neurol* 1998;152:129–136.

[96] Ossedryver SM, Baldwin GI, Stone BM, et al. *Indigofera spicata* (creeping indigo) poisoning of three ponies. *Aust Vet J* 2013;91:143–149.

[97] Covington AL, Magdesian KG, Madigan JE, et al. Recurrent esophageal obstruction and dysphagia due to a brainstem melanoma in a horse. *J Vet Intern Med* 2004;18:245–247.

[98] Mcconkey S, Lopez A, Pringle J. Extramedullary plasmacytoma in a horse with ptyalism and dysphagia. *J Vet Diagn Invest* 2000;12:282–284.

[99] Clark ES, Morris DD, Whitlock RH. Esophageal dysfunction in a weanling thoroughbred. *Cornell Vet* 1987;77:151–160.

[100] Hatfield CE, Rebhun WC, Dietze AE, et al. Endocarditis and optic neuritis in a Quarter horse mare. *Compend Contin Educ Pract Vet* 1987;9:451–454.

[101] Brault LS, Penedo MCT. The frequency of the equine cerebellar abiotrophy mutation in non-Arabian horse breeds. *Equine Vet J* 2011;43:727–731.

[102] Toth B, Aleman M, Nogradi N, et al. Meningitis and meningoencephalomyelitis in horses: 28 cases (1985–2010). *J Am Vet Med Assoc* 2012;240:580–587.

[103] Pellegrini-Masini A, Bentz AI, Johns IC, et al. Common variable immunodeficiency in three horses with presumptive bacterial meningitis. *J Am Vet Med Assoc* 2005;227:114–122.

[104] Hatziolos BC, Sass B, Albert TF, et al. Blindness in a horse probably caused by gutturomycosis. *Zentralbl Veterinarmed B* 1975;22:362–371.

[105] Lester G. Parasitic encephalomyelitis in horses. *Ippologia* 1994;5:39–42.

[106] Dubey JP, Lindsay DS, Saville WJA, et al. A review of *Sarcocystis neurona* and equine protozoal myeloencephalitis (EPM). *Vet Parasitol* 2001;95:89–131.

[107] Swor TM, Whittenburg JL, Chaffin MK. Ivermectin toxicosis in three adult horses. *J Am Vet Med Assoc* 2009; 235:558–562.

[108] Giannitti F, Diab SS, Pacin AM, et al. Equine leukoencephalomalacia (ELEM) due to fumonisins B1 and B2 in Argentina. *Pesqui Vet Bras* 2011;31:407–412.

[109] Hahn CN, Mayhew IG. Studies on the experimental induction of ptosis in horses. *Vet J* 2000;160:220–224.

[110] Firth EC. Horner's syndrome in the horse: experimental induction and a case report. *Equine Vet J* 1978;10:9–13.

[111] Sweeney RW, Sweeney CR. Transient Horner's syndrome following routine intravenous injections in two horses. *J Am Vet Med Assoc* 1984;185:802–803.

[112] Green SL, Cochrane SM, Smith-Maxie L. Horner's syndrome in ten horses. *Can Vet J* 1992;33:330–333.

[113] Mayhew IG. Horner's syndrome and lesions involving the sympathetic nervous system. *Equine Pract* 1980;2:44.

[114] White PL, Genetzky RM, Pohlenz JFL, et al. Neuritis of the cauda equina in a horse. *Compend Contin Educ Pract Vet* 1984;6:S217–S237.

[115] Muller A, Niederhofer M. Malignant mesothelioma of the pleura in a 13-year-old gelding. *Praktische Tierarzt* 2009;90:220–227.

[116] Murray MJ, Cavey DM, Feldman BF, et al. Signs of sympathetic denervation associated with a thoracic melanoma in a horse. *J Vet Intern Med* 1997;11:199–203.

[117] Bacon CL, Davidson HJ, Yvorchuk K, et al. Bilateral Horner's syndrome secondary to metastatic squamous cell carcinoma in a horse. *Equine Vet J* 1996;28: 500–503.

[118] Van Der Wiel HL, Van Gijn J. No enophthalmos in Horner's syndrome. *J Neurol Neurosurg Psychiatry* 1987;50: 498–499.

[119] Robertshaw D, Taylor CR. Sweat gland function of the donkey (*Equus asinus*). *J Physiol* 1969;205:79–89.

[120] Smith JS, Mayhew IG. Horners syndrome in large animals. *Cornell Vet* 1977;67:529–542.

[121] Dahlberg JA, Ross MW, Martin BB, et al. Clinical relevance of abnormal scintigraphic findings of adult equine ribs. *Vet Radiol Ultrasound* 2011;52:573–579.

[122] Palumbo MIP, Moreira JJ, Olivo G, et al. Right-sided laryngeal hemiplegia and Horner's syndrome in a horse. *Equine Vet Educ* 2011;23:448–452.

[123] Purohit RC, Mccoy MD, Bergfeld WA. Thermographic diagnosis of Horners syndrome in the horse. *Am J Vet Res* 1980;41:1180–1182.

[124] Sunderland S. *Nerves and Nerve Injuries*. Edinburgh: Churchill Livingstone; 1978.

10 Sleep and Sleep Disorders in Horses

Joseph J. Bertone

College of Veterinary Medicine, Western University, Pomona, USA

Sleep, in its broadest sense, is defined as a period of inactivity with an increased arousal threshold and stereotypic body position. The definition does not necessarily include unconsciousness, nor lying down, as the brain is clearly highly active in some stages of sleep, and the position associated with each stage can vary according to species [1, 2]. Interestingly, the brain of cetaceans can alternate sleep from cortical hemisphere to hemisphere. Usually the animal is either at rest on the bottom, or travels, commonly, in a clockwise direction during sleep phases [3]. Universally, disrupted sleep is at some point followed by sleep rebound. Sleep rebound is a period of increased duration of rapid eye movement (REM) sleep [3–6]. This definition is applied to a large genetically diverse group of organisms. Sleep seems to be an important indirect function. Various hypotheses for sleep have been proposed and they include the following:

1 The somatic theory—healing of the body and sleep-associated endocrine functions.

2 The cellular metabolic theory—reactive oxidative waste removal and energy recovery.

3 The brain-specific function theory—memory consolidation via synaptic plasticity and synaptic downscaling (i.e., forget what is not necessary to remember) [4].

4 The adaptive theory—one should only be awake as long as one needs to maintain reproductive capabilities by eating, avoiding being eaten, and multiplying [7]. Intriguing evidence for the adaptive theory comes from the fact that hemicellulose-ingesting herbivorous species tend to be large, based on a dietary need for long gastrointestinal transit time. They also have large offspring that need to be precocious because they are prey at birth. In fact, precocious species have brains that are closer to adult weight than non-precocious species (e.g., human beings), and there is an inverse relationship between sleep duration needs and brain size at birth. In other words, the closer the neonatal brain is to the adult brain in weight, the shorter the duration of all sleep stages [1, 3, 8].

Sleep deprivation induces cellular and organismal stress because it exceeds the physiological and genetically determined time one can maintain wakefulness. There is tremendous variation in sleep requirements across species. Assuming that restorative cellular processes required by species is conserved in the quantity of time needed for restoration, we can assume and it has also been shown that what one species accomplishes in sleep other species accomplish while awake [4].

Confusion regarding equine sleep

The literature concerning equine sleep disorders is not clear to say the least. This is likely due its "seeming" nascence as an area of veterinary concern. What has brought equine sleep medicine "closer to the light" and has increased interest is the widespread availability and use of the Internet. Isolated cases can now be seen by many individuals and dealt with using global resources rather than those limited to a single geographic local. This does not mean it is a new science, however. Dr. Andre Dallaire (Université de Montréal) and Yves Ruckebusch (Ecole nationale Vétérinaire de Toulouse) created a significant body of literature in this area from the 1960s through the 1980s which should not be lost simply because it is not digitized [9]. Much of their work is relevant and has set the groundwork for equine sleep science. In addition, we must take great care when using other species as comparisons, especially in light of horses as prey-migrating species and their ability to go long periods without full cycles of sleep.

So, what's the confusion? There is a tendency to label all horses that seem to repeatedly doze off, stumble, and recover as suffering from narcolepsy which is simply not the case. In addition, the implications, clinical signs, and impact of full-cycle sleep deprivation on performance is not well understood and may be more relevant than we know. Clearly, if other species are a model, there is an effect on performance [10, 11]. This confusion is similar to the early stages in the evolution of human sleep medicine. Terms such as hypersomnia, narcolepsy, parasomnia, for example, have specific definitions in human sleep medicine that are more clearly defined by molecular, structural information, and their associations with different stages of sleep. In addition, care must be taken with extrapolations of other findings in other species to horses and the continued propagation of confusion in the equine literature as it exists. The value of the physostigmine challenge test for narcolepsy, response of patients to imipramine, and cerebrospinal fluid concentrations of hypocretin and its relevance are examples of information that require greater scrutiny and careful evaluation.

Human sleep

Sleep generally cycles through stages. These stages are based on features recorded in the electroencephalogram (EEG), electrooculogram (EOG), electromyogram (EMG), electrocardiogram (ECG) and various respiratory parameters. Polysomnography is the medical field concerned with the interpretation of this multiparametric data [12]. Sleep stages associated with characteristic EEG features were first described in 1937 by Loomis and coworkers. They separated behavioral and EEG features of sleep into five stages (A–E) [13]. Today, the stages of sleep are described by two categories. Nonrapid eye movement (NREM) is generally considered the stages leading to REM sleep. NREM is divided into three stages, NREM 1, 2, and 3. These stages are characterized by progressively slower ocular movements, a reduction in muscle tone, and increased EEG amplitude (voltage) and decreased frequency (fewer per waves second). However, once entering REM sleep, muscle tone is nearly absent except for occasional tonic twitches, and the EEG with some respects has similar patterns as when awake and alert (i.e., low-voltage amplitude and mixed to high frequency). Non-REM 3 is commonly called "delta sleep" due to its characteristic delta wave (large and slow) EEG and usually proceeds REM [14].

Sleep in horses

Understanding sleep in horses has been much more difficult due to the likely effect of the environment on sleep patterns and the lack of need for diurnal rhythmicity. Telemetric EEG may soon provide important and improved information. Hard-wired EEG studies of horses during sleep have been performed [15–17]. At least for now, in practical clinical terms, the summarized

work by Ruckebusch and Dallaire and corroborated to a large extent by Williams [15] indicates that the EEG has a high correlation to sleep behavior. That is useful since in large part behavior predicts the EEG. These findings are summarized in the following [9]. Presented below is the progression from alert wakefulness to paradoxical sleep.

1 Alert wakefulness is the period when the brain is actively processing information and the animals are on high alert. The head is held high, lips are firm, and eye movements are rapid and irregular. The EEG is characterized by small amplitude (10–30 μV) and high frequency (25–40 cycles/s). Muscle tone in the neck is present, diffuse, and inconsistent [9].

2 Diffuse wakefulness is the next stage as the horse becomes drowsy. Large (up to 150 μV) and reduced frequency (1–4 cycles/s) begin to occur. REMs are replaced by slow, rhythmic, and to a large extent horizontal movements. Neck muscle tone is moderately high [9].

3 Drowsiness is the next phase in the progression. The EEG progressively enlarges (up to 250 μV) and remains slow in frequency (1–4 cycles/s). Eye movements are rare and when they occur, they are slow, horizontal, and rhythmic. The eyelids are often partly open. Neck muscle tone persists but is reduced and it nearly disappears if the head is supported. This is the point where especially the lower lip is completely relaxed. Horses can enter this phase while standing. However, an environmentally acclimated horse will lie down more commonly in this phase.

4 The intermediate phase then occurs. At this point, horses will hover somewhere between alert and diffuse wakefulness. What is hypothesized to occur in this phase is watchful attentiveness to the horse's environment and herd mates and to assure safety before moving to recumbency [9]. In recumbency, the horse will go through various durations of stages 1, 2, 3, and 4. Even when recumbent, horses often do not enter stage-5 paradoxical sleep directly from stage-3 slow wave sleep in 30% of the observations. This is possibly a protective mechanism to avoid entering paradoxical sleep (which requires greater arousal stimulus) without considering environmental security [9].

5 Paradoxical sleep may now follow. This term is used because the EEG findings are similar in many ways to stage-1 alert wakefulness. The EOG is characterized by intermittent bursts of REM. Muscle tone is essentially absent with small bursts of ear twitching and muscle contraction and even vocalization that may include whinnying. At this point, greater stimulation is needed to awaken the animal compared to other stages. Respiratory and cardiac frequency variability is increased more than during wakefulness. Periods of

tachycardia followed by extreme bradycardia are reported. Respiration was characterized by sudden tachypnea followed by inspiratory pauses. It is important to note that Dallaire does not call this stage "REM." It is clear that bursts of REM and periods of non-REM occur in this stage and the EEG remains fairly constant with loss of muscle tone. So in paradoxical sleep, most of the characteristics of REM stage sleep occur without consistent REM.

Importantly, as occurs in humans, each phase leads to the next, and paradoxical sleep is not achieved unless horses proceeded through stage 3. In general, horses require approximately 15 min to complete a cycle with stage-3 slow wave sleep lasting for 6–7 min and stage-5 paradoxical sleep lasting 4–5 min. Five to seven cycles occur during the night lasting 30–40 min with total cyclic sleep time averaging 3–5 h/day. Paradoxical sleep time represents approximately 45 min of the day. Stage-5 paradoxical sleep time decreases from foal (15%) to weanling (2%) age. Stabled horses tend to sleep nocturnally, but pastured horses also sleep regularly between 12:00 noon and 2:00 p.m. The level of activity in the barn, more than the position of the sun, tends to be the issue. Most paradoxical sleep does not occur in afternoon sessions. Sleep, for most horses, is distributed from 8:00 p.m. to 5:00 a.m. Importantly, complete loss of muscle tone during paradoxical sleep is consistent [9].

A horse cannot complete a sleep cycle while standing. Horses that cannot lie down will be sleep-deprived of at least the paradoxical sleep fraction of the cycle. In response, the stage-3 drowsiness fraction may increase, but this does not compensate for loss of paradoxical sleep. When the deprived horse can and chooses to lie down, there should be a rebound in paradoxical sleep [9–11].

Environmental sleep influences

Habitat

Considering that horses are prey species, it is intuitive to believe that the environment affects sleep due to the need for vigilance. Most horses require familiarity with the environment to assume recumbency. When they are moved to a new environment, sleep may be postponed for a period of time that ranges from two to several days. When horses are moved outdoors or indoors when accustomed to the opposite, it may be up to 2 days before they first lie down [9]. Habituation to the environment may be facilitated and shortened by the presence of other horses and especially familiar partners. The dominant animal is usually the first to lie down [18]. Feral Assateague Island ponies had resting behavior 40% of the nighttime hours and 16% of that was spent lying down. All the ponies were never seen down simultaneously, possibly to ensure that sentinels were in place [19].

Sleep requirements change in early life. Time in lateral recumbency progresses from 15 to 2.7% in newborn and preweaning foals, respectively [20]. Dallaire interprets these results to suggest that paradoxical sleep decreases sharply after birth, slow wave sleep decreases slightly, and drowsiness increases dramatically. As animals become older, the time allotted to slow wave sleep and paradoxical sleep is replaced by increased drowsiness [9]. Dallaire identified that in horses moved from stalls to pasture, total rest time slightly increased, but there was a decrease in sternal and lateral recumbency time. Dallaire concludes that there is a decrease in slow wave and paradoxical sleep and a concomitant increase in drowsiness when animals are moved to pasture. Ruckebush suggested that total sleep time in horses kept in stables is greater than for free-ranging horses [21].

Diet

Diet likely influences sleep. Total rest time increases when the diet is changed from hay to oats [22]. Total sleep time slows wave sleep and paradoxical sleep occupied a greater proportion of each 24-h period, but this was only for transient 3–4 days before returning to the original hay diet values. In the first 2 days of feed withdrawal, slow wave and paradoxical sleep increase 20 and 17%, respectively [22].

Environmental stimuli

Partial sensory deprivation caused ponies to have increased slow wave and paradoxical sleep. This raises some postulates concerning horses that doze, partially collapse, and catch themselves while in cross-ties for prolonged periods [23]. Many practitioners know these cases.

Disorders of sleep

It is important to use terms more specifically and definitively for the science of sleep disorders in horses to move forward. The vast majority of horses that become drowsy and "catch" themselves before falling do not have defined narcolepsy with cataplexy. Narcolepsy is a REM sleep disorder with shortened to nonexistent pre-REM periods. Affected horses could not "catch" themselves if this were the case since REM sleep is associated with near to complete conscious paralysis. In addition, the collapse would be spontaneous, rapid, and complete, not occurring over periods of time with limited stimuli as is observed in many of these cases. Some have argued that these horses suffer from narcolepsy without cataplexy, but that is based on a broad definition of narcolepsy that may not be appropriate [24]. Diagnosis of narcolepsy based on a response to imipramine as a diagnostic test or as treatment is another questionable paradigm. Historically, imipramine was used to manage human narcolepsy, but its poor success and adverse effects have voided it as a treatment option [24]. Imipramine is a tricyclic antidepressant with multiple effects throughout the central nervous system and the therapeutic window is small [25]. Regardless of these issues, imipramine still lingers as the treatment for narcolepsy in horses in several texts. However, imipramine does have effects on promoting sleep in severe depression in people [26] and sleep promotion was shown in an equine pharmacokinetic study [25]. The physostigmine challenge test in the equine literature and in the authors experience has been shown to be inconsistent and essentially useless [27, 28]. The use of this test in horses was based on the disease in dogs which is very different than the disease pathophysiology in people. In dogs, the problem is the receptor type-2 gene, and hypocretin concentrations do not change [29]. In human beings, hypocretin concentrations range from diminished to completely absent [24] (see video clips demonstrating clinical signs for videos).

Recumbent sleep-deprived behavior is characterized by drowsiness and partial collapse. There is acute awareness of the loss of posture and the horses catch themselves before completely falling (Figure 10.1). It is clear since these horses catch themselves before falling that they are in a state from which they can be easily aroused, which is not consistent with narcolepsy. Narcolepsy is a defined REM sleep disorder with a deficiency of the neuropeptide hypocretin, with episodes induced by emotions, and it is exceedingly rare in human patients.

We can logically assume therefore that it is exceedingly rare in horses as well. In addition, narcolepsy with cataplexy in people and in dogs is almost always hereditary and evident near birth, while the clinical signs in almost all horses reported in the literature purported to be suffering from narcolepsy have been acquired.

Sleep deprivation

Horses that frequently become drowsy and partially collapse and catch themselves may be suspected of recumbent sleep deprivation [30]. This author has identified clinical patterns of horses that have been identified with this behavior in a review of more than 300 cases over a 15 year period. One common feature in many of these cases is abrasions over the dorsal fetlock area (Figure 10.2). Witnessed incidences and video images have shown horses collapsing onto the dorsum before catching themselves [15, 30]. A common complaint in the chronic condition is decreased to poor performance, poor weight maintenance, and often a poor attitude. Clinical patterns identified by the author include the following:

1 **Behavior associated with pain or physical discomfort**. Horses were categorized into this group when these issues were clearly diagnosed (Figure 10.3). Disease conditions varied from severe joint disease, polysaccharide storage myopathy, other musculoskeletal disease, gastric ulcers, and abdominal adhesions, among others. Some horses responded to pain management including nonsteroidal anti-inflammatory drug administration or a response to omeprazole. Heavy late pregnancy mares were also included in this group and signs invariably resolved postparturition [15, 30]. A pain management trial may elucidate these cases.

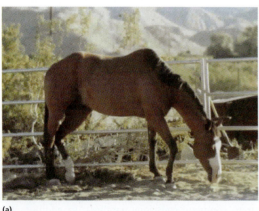
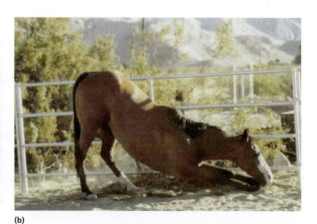

(a)   (b)

Figure 10.1 A chronically recumbent sleep-deprived horse. The image shows him as he becomes diffusely drowsy on the left (a). Rather than arousing and lying down, he ends in the position in the right image (b) for several seconds. Abruptly, the horse rises, wakes, and cycles given a lack of disturbances. This occurs over and over again. This horse has been seen recumbent and rolling, but he will not lie down to go through the entire, required sleep cycle. This was a solitary individual and the behavior ceased on introduction of other horses to the facility.

2 **Monotony-associated behavior**. Horses were categorized into this group when they manifest the signs when placed for prolonged periods in cross-ties or forced to stand quietly for prolonged periods. These

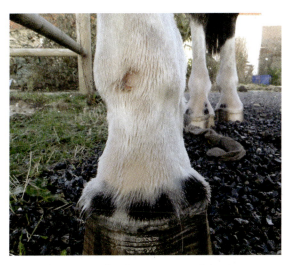

Figure 10.2 Common dorsal carpometacarpal abrasions seen in horses with sleep-deprivation behavior.

horses do not express this behavior at other times and avoidance of the low stimuli environment seems to resolve these cases. Of note is the findings of Dallaire in ponies in a stimuli-deprived environment [9].

3 **Behavior associated with environmental insecurity**. Horses were categorized into this group when issues in the environment were identified, changed, and resolution was achieved. These included stall location and/or size changes, stall relocation, loss of other horses to which the patient seemed be behaviorally attached, light bulb wattage changes, blanket issues, window coverings, weather, and many more seemingly incidental issues in the environment led to this behavior.

4 **Aggression displacement (aggressive gelding)-associated behavior**: Horses were characterized in this group when they had a history or presentation of excessive and continuous aggression toward single or all horses in a group. These horses responded to the addition of an alpha female or, more rarely, an alpha male when available. Often a period of aggression mostly by the unaffected alpha horse against the aggressive gelding was required.One issue of note is that when removing all horses for physical issues (pattern 1) and monotony behavior (pattern 2).

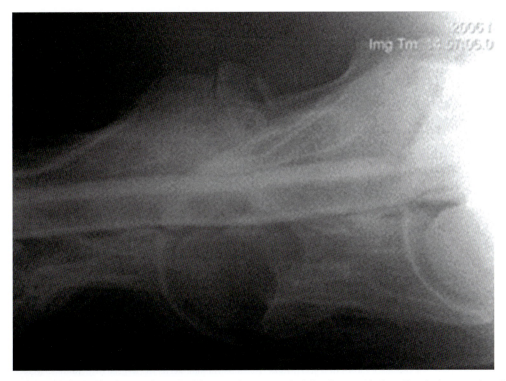

Figure 10.3 The radiograph shows a dorsal vertebral fracture that occurred while a horse with sleep disorder became pinned under a pipe rail fence.

Geldings are overrepresented in patterns 3 and 4 by 17 geldings per 1 mare. Interestingly, no stallions were presented. This leads one to hypothesize that there may be sex hormone and herd structure issues with geldings in these two patterns.

5 **Behavior associated with Lyme disease**: Horses were characterized into this group when horses were positive for Lyme disease. These horses did not show evidence of joint pain. They also responded to therapy for Lyme disease.

6 **Sleep terror-associated behavior**. Horses were characterized into this group when there was evidence of behavior similar to sleep terror behavior in human patients (see video clips demonstrating clinical signs for videos). This is a relatively new finding in the data set as all cases have been identified since January 2012. This may be at a higher incidence and we may see more of these cases since all-night videography is now more affordable and common.

The nature of internet case referrals and the evolving approach to these cases require no conclusions be drawn as to breed or geographic predilection, prevalence, or incidence information as all these data are considered by the author to be heavily biased. In addition, technical capabilities of the owners and improving video capability have also evolved through the time of this data set. As an example, a recent group of cases were characterized as manifesting sleep terrors (pattern 6). This occurred due to submitted night-time video camera files and may explain many uncategorized cases in the past. An evolving protocol may also be an issue. Until recently, a screening for Lyme disease was not requested of cases. Again that may have impacted earlier diagnoses and classification because an accurate test was not available and it was not considered likely that this behavior could be induced in Lyme disease. Yet these cases were identified following diagnosis of one serendipitous case and then further investigation. More severe and chronic clinical signs were most likely overrepresented in this group of cases. Milder behavioral signs may go unnoticed or pose little concern for owners. It is necessary to rule out recumbent sleep deprivation before considering any other sleep disorders in horses (see video clips demonstrating clinical signs for videos).

Hypersomnia

Hypersomnia is defined as excessive quantities of sleepiness. These horses seem to lack periods of REM sleep despite being seen lying down. This will result in rebound and excessive episodes of sleep. A common complaint in these horses, besides excessive sleep, is decreased or poor performance. It may be secondary to other diseases such as pituitary pars intermedia dysfunction [31], neurologic disease of any kind, and other causes to be defined [32].

Narcolepsy

Familial narcolepsy has been documented in Miniature [33] and Lipizzaner horses [27]. It is clear that many other reported cases do not fulfill the full spectrum of narcolepsy clinical signs and diagnostics. It is more likely that other reports in horses have used the term narcolepsy more loosely. In addition, there have been anecdotal accounts of foals that when removed from their mares will have episodes that appear similar to narcoleptic. These foals invariably grow out of this behavior by the time they are weaned (see video clips demonstrating clinical signs for videos).

References

[1] Zepelin H, Siegel JM, Tobler I. Mammalian sleep. In: Kryger M, Roth T, Dement W, eds. *Principles and Practice of Sleep Medicine*. Philadelphia:Elsevier Saunders; 2005:91–100.

[2] Ruckebusch Y. Etude comparée du sommeil physiologue chez les equidés, ruminants porcins et carnivores adultes. *Bull Soc Vet Lyon* 1962;64:375–390.

[3] Siegel JM. Clues to the functions of mammalian sleep. *Nature* 2005;437:1274.

[4] Crocker A, Seigal A. Genetic analysis of sleep. *Genes Dev* 2010;24:1220–1235.

[5] Huber R, Hill SL, Holladay C, et al. Sleep homeostasis in Drosophila melanogaster. *Sleep* 2004;27:628–639.

[6] Rechtschaffen A, Bergmann BM, Gilliland MA, et al. Effects of method, duration, and sleep stage on rebounds from sleep deprivation in the rat. *Sleep* 1999;1:11–31.

[7] Webb WB. Sleep an adaptive response. *Percept Mot Skills* 1974;38:1023–1027.

[8] O'Hara BF, Watson FL, Srere HK, et al. Gene expression in the brain across the hibernation cycle. *J Neurosci* 1999;19: 3781–3790.

[9] Dallaire, A. Rest behavior. *Vet Clin North Am Equine Pract* 1986;2:591–607.

[10] Bonnett, M. Acute sleep deprivation. In: Kryger M, Roth T, Dement W, eds. *Principles and Practice of Sleep Medicine*. Philadelphia:Elsevier Saunders;2005:51–66.

[11] Dinges D, Rogers N, Baynard M. Chronic sleep deprivation. In: Kryger M, Roth T, Dement W, eds. *Principles and Practice of Sleep Medicine*. Philadelphia:Elsevier Saunders; 2005:67–76.

[12] Chervin R. Use of clinical tools and tests. In: Kryger M, Roth T, Dement W, eds. *Principles and Practice of Sleep Medicine*. Philadelphia:Elsevier Saunders;2005:602–614.

[13] Loomis AL, Harvey EN, Hobart GA. Cerebral states during sleep, as studied by human brain potentials. *J Exp Psychol* 1937;21:127–144.

[14] Carskadon MA, Rechtschaffen A. Monitoring and staging human sleep. In: Kryger MH, Roth T, Dement W, eds. *Principles and Practice of Sleep Medicine*. Philadelphia:Elsevier Saunders;2005:1359–1377.

[15] Williams D, Aleman M, Holliday T, et al. Qualitative and quantitative characteristics of the electroencephalogram in normal horses during spontaneous drowsiness and sleep. *J Vet Intern Med* 2008;22:630–638.

[16] Ruckebusch Y. Etude E.E.G. et comportementale des alternances veille-sommeil chez l'ane. *CR Soc Biol (Lyon)* 1963;157:840–844.

[17] Ruckebusch Y, Barbey P, Guillemot P. Les etats de sommeil chez le cheval (Equus caballos). *CR Soc Biol (Paris)* 1970; 164:658–665.

[18] Ruckebusch Y. The relevance of drowsiness in circadian cycle of farm animals. *Anim Behav* 1972;20:637–643.

[19] Keiper R, Keenan MA. Nocturnal activity patterns of feral ponies. *J Mammal* 1980;61:116–118.

[20] Duncan P. Time-budget of Camargue horses. Part II: Time-budget of adult horses and weaned sub-adults. *Behaviour* 1980;72:26–49.

[21] Ruckebusch Y. The hypnogram as an index of adaption of farm animals to changes in their environment. *Appl Anim Ethol* 1975;2:3–18.

[22] Dallaire A, Ruckebusch Y. Sleep and wakefulness in the housed pony under different dietary conditions. *Can J Comp Med* 1974;38:65–71.

[23] Dallaire A, Ruckebusch Y. Sleep patterns in the pony with observations on partial perceptual deprivation. *Physiol Behav* 1974;12:789–796.

[24] Mignot E. Narcolepsy: pharmacology, pathophysiology, and genetics. In: Kryger M, Roth T, Dement W, eds. *Principles and Practice of Sleep Medicine*. Philadelphia:Elsevier Saunders;2005:761–779.

[25] Peck K, Hines M, Mealey K, et al. Pharmacokinetics of imipramine in narcoleptic horses. *Am J Vet Res* 2001;62:783–786.

[26] Wichniak A, Wierzbicka A, Jernajczyk W. Sleep and antidepressant treatment. *Curr Pharm Des* 2012;18: 5802–5817.

[27] Ludvikova E, Nishino S, Sakai N, et al. Familial narcolepsy in the Lipizzaner horse: a report of three fillies born to the same sire. *Vet Q* 2012;32:99–102.

[28] Lacombe V, Furr M. Differential diagnosis and management of horses with seizures or alterations of consciousness. In: Furr M, Reed S, eds. *Equine Neurology*. Ames:Blackwell;2008:77–94.

[29] Hungs M, Fan J, Lin L, et al. Identification and functional analysis of mutations in the hypocretin (orexin) genes of narcoleptic canines. *Genome Res* 2001;11:531–539.

[30] Bertone, J. Excessive drowsiness secondary to recumbent sleep deprivation in two horses. *Vet Clin North Am Equine Pract* 2006;22:157–162.

[31] McFarlane D, Maidment N, Lam H. Cerebrospinal fluid concentration of hypocretin-1 in horses with equine pituitary pars intermedia disease and its relationship to oxidative stress. *Proc Annu Meet Am Coll Vet Intern Med* 2007;25:791.

[32] Aleman M, Williams C, Holliday T. Sleep and sleep disorders in horses. *Proc Annu Meet Am Assoc Equine Pract* 2008;54:180–185.

[33] Lunn D, Cuddon P, Shaftoe S, et al. Familial occurrence of narcolepsy in miniature horses. *Equine Vet J* 1993; 25:483–487.

11 Headshaking

Monica Aleman[1] and Kirstie Pickles[2]

[1] College of Veterinary Medicine, University of California, Davis, USA
[2] Scarsdale Equine Veterinary Practice, Derby, UK

The following text includes information reviewed from multiple peer-reviewed studies including those from the authors. The text does not necessarily reflect the opinion of the authors except when stated. The section on treatment includes data of various pharmacological agents reported in the literature to manage horses with idiopathic headshaking. The authors suggest caution, since for most of the drugs used, there are no pharmacokinetic and safety studies in the horse.

Idiopathic headshaking in horses was first described in the veterinary literature over a hundred years ago [1, 2]. Despite "neurosis of the infraorbital portion of super-maxillary division of the trifacial nerve" being proposed in these initial reports, confirmation of trigeminal involvement in the pathogenesis of headshaking has only recently been definitively identified [3]. Despite this recent advancement, the disease remains poorly understood. The incidence of headshaking is reported to be 1–1.5% (UK National Equine Health Survey 2010–2013). This disorder may be a cause of substantial suffering for the horse, frustration for the owner, and therapeutic challenge for the veterinarian.

Signalment

Headshaking can occur at any age but is primarily a disease of adult horses with a reported median age of 8 years (range 4–17 years) [4], 9 years (range 1–30 years) [5], and 10 years (range 5–16 years) [6]. Mills reported that the majority of horses first developed signs of headshaking at 5 years of age or younger (41.5%) [7].

Intriguingly geldings appear to be overrepresented comprising 71.5% of US cases (OR 2.16) compared to 26.5% mares and 2% stallions [5], and 85 and 63%, respectively, in UK studies [4, 7]. All breeds are affected, although some studies have shown Thoroughbreds to be at greater risk comprising 41% (OR 3.21) of a series of 109 cases [5] while other studies show all breeds equally affected [7]. Other commonly affected breeds included Quarter Horses (24%) and Warmblood breeds (16%) [5]. Headshaking affects horses used in most equine disciplines including pleasure riding (43%), dressage (27%), hunter–jumper (17%), and eventing (7%) [5], although racehorses may be underrepresented (K. J. Pickles, pers. obs.). There have been reports of headshaking in many countries worldwide including the United States, Canada, United Kingdom, Germany, Australia, and New Zealand. Increasing awareness of this problem has likely resulted in greater numbers of horses diagnosed.

Clinical signs

Horses afflicted by this disorder are called "headshakers." Affected horses manifest uncontrollable, violent, usually downward, shakes, flicks, or jerks of the head in the absence of any apparent physical stimulus. Horses might display this headshaking behavior intermittently or continuously and progression of clinical signs has been reported [4]. The signs can be so severe that it may impair the horses' ability to eat, and affected horses may be dangerous to handle and ride (Figure 11.1).

A seasonal onset and cessation of clinical manifestations has been reported in 59% of headshaking horses compared to constant or erratic episodes with no apparent seasonality in 41% of horses [5]. The majority (91%) of these seasonal headshakers developed signs in the spring and early summer and ceased in late summer and fall, although a small proportion (4%) were symptomatic in the fall and ceased headshaking in the spring [5].

The most commonly reported headshaking behaviors are shaking or flipping the head in a vertical plane (89%), acting as if an insect had flown up the nose (88%), muzzle rubbing (75%), snorting (64%), and an

Equine Neurology, Second Edition. Martin Furr and Stephen Reed.
© 2015 John Wiley & Sons, Inc. Published 2015 by John Wiley & Sons, Inc.
Companion website: www.wiley.com/go/furr/neurology

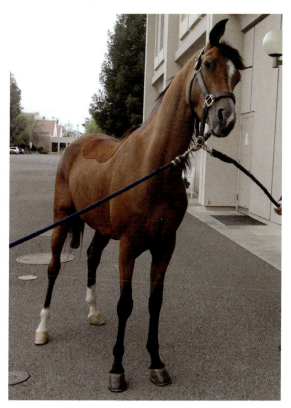

Figure 11.1 Horse headshaking that had to be handled by two people due to safety concerns as the result of violent and constant headshaking.

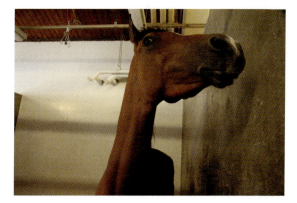

Figure 11.2 Note apparent anxious facial expression and nose rubbing.

(hard carrots, fibrous hay). Video surveillance is useful to document when headshaking occurs, how frequently, and possibly what triggers the episodes, if anything.

Etiopathogenesis

It is believed that the sharp, quick, flicking head movements/tossing, excessive snorting, rubbing of the head or nose, nose flipping, immersing the head in water, and striking at the face reflect trigeminal neuropathic pain. Trigeminal neuralgia is a common and debilitating cause of facial pain in humans [10]. Human sufferers of trigeminal neuralgia report intermittent or continuous burning, itching, tingling, tickling, or electric-like pain originating in area innervated by the trigeminal nerve [10], which appears to equate well to the observed signs displayed by horses with idiopathic headshaking. A recent study by the authors showed differences in threshold of nerve conduction between healthy horses and those with a clinical diagnosis of headshaking [3]. This study demonstrated the involvement of the trigeminal nerve in the pathophysiology of the disorder. The term "trigeminal-mediated headshaking" might therefore now be a more accurate term for this disorder than idiopathic headshaking.

The cause of the aberrant trigeminal nerve activity remains elusive. Despite its predilection for latency in the trigeminal ganglion, equine herpesvirus-1 does not appear to be involved [11]. Focal compression and demyelination of the trigeminal nerve are frequently documented in trigeminal neuralgia patients; however, the limited equine pathological studies performed to date do not demonstrate this in affected horses [3, 12]. Demyelination results in reduced trigeminal nerve conduction velocity in human sufferers of trigeminal neuralgia, which is not present in horses with headshaking [3]. The pathophysiology of headshaking and

anxious expression (61%) (see Figure 11.2) [5]. Nose rubbing can lead to abrasions or lacerations. In one study, headshaking was displayed at both rest and exercise in 55% of horses, precipitated by exercise in 41% of horses, and observed only at rest in 4%. Ten percent of the horses developed signs only when ridden.

Horses with severe clinical signs during bright sunny days and reduction of headshaking at night are termed "photic headshakers" [8]. There is some evidence to suggest that the proportion of horses with a photic component to headshaking varies geographically worldwide. Madigan and Bell reported that 52% of 109 headshakers (86% of which resided in North America) have a photic component [5], while Newton et al. reported only a 5% prevalence in a study of 20 headshakers in the United Kingdom [4]. Another study reported light stimulated behavior in 60% of affected horses [9]. Different levels of UV exposure could explain this geographical variable.

The authors have also observed horses in which headshaking is triggered by riding on windy days and associated with sound (metal sound, clap) or eating human trigeminal neuralgia might therefore differ. Nurmikko and Eldridge (2001) argue that the paroxysmal nature of trigeminal neuralgia pain is inconsistent with compression-induced ectopic impulses at the site of injury and that spontaneous discharges arising from select neurons whose threshold for firing has been altered is a more plausible explanation [10]. Studies have shown that dorsal root ganglion cells possess properties that can, in certain circumstances, lead to this type of firing activity [13]. Increase in subthreshold oscillations in the resting membrane potential of a subpopulation of A neurons leads to increased spike activity and subsequent cross-excitation of adjacent hyperexcitable C fibers [14, 15]. If sufficient neurons are recruited into this spreading cluster of discharging cells, it will lead to a pain signal [15]. The abrupt cessation of such signals (and thus pain) as occurs in trigeminal neuralgia is the result of inherent cell self-quenching mechanisms. Central sensitization or progressive damage to the central terminals of trigeminal afferents is suggested to occur in patients with continuous ectopic discharge and unrelenting trigeminal neuralgia [16].

Some headshaking horses demonstrate spontaneous remission, some after many years of headshaking. This suggests that the aberrant trigeminal nerve activity can be reversed and is not the result of permanent damage. Some horses stay in remission for years, while others recommence headshaking after only a few weeks or months. One headshaking horse in remission has been observed to exhibit clinical signs again shortly after receiving an electric shock to the muzzle (J. Madigan, pers. commun.).

The photic component to clinical signs in some headshakers has been postulated to be similar to the human photic sneeze, which results when persistent photic stimulation via the optic nerve leads to activation of the maxillary branch of the trigeminal nerve through an unknown mechanism, leading to a tickling sensation in the nasal mucosa [8, 17]; optic-trigeminal summation and a photic sneeze result. This same neural pathway could be involved in causing irritating sensations and subsequent headshaking behavior in horses in response to light stimulation [8]. The clinical signs of photic headshaking are identical to those of non-photic headshakers and suggesting that multiple triggers can activate the same end trigeminal response [4, 6].

Exercise has been described in several reports to be a stimulus for headshaking activity; however, the underlying mechanism by which onset of exercise induces headshaking is unknown [5, 8, 18, 19]. Likewise, the overrepresentation of geldings documented in several studies remains unexplained. Lack of negative feedback of the vernal rise in gonadotropins was investigated as a hypothesis for this and the seasonality of clinical signs but was not supported [20]. Fluctuations in the nutritive

Table 11.1 Causes of headshaking other than trigeminal-mediated abnormalities that should be considered in the evaluation of suspect case.

Middle and inner ear infection
Temporohyoid osteoarthropathy
Ear tick (*Otobius megnini*)
Ear mites (*Trombicula autumnalis*)
Guttural pouch disease
Periapical dental osteitis
Dental disease (e.g., wolf teeth)
Allergic rhinitis
Photic mediated
Ocular disorders (cysts, masses)
Equine protozoal myeloencephalitis
Vasomotor rhinitis
Intranasal masses
Sinusitis
Nuchal crest avulsion
Inappropriate bridle
Rider mediated
Behavioral

From References [6, 15, 18–27].

value in grasses, particularly improved grassland, might offer an alternative explanation of the seasonality of headshaking clinical signs.

Additional causes of headshaking have been determined in a small number of cases [18, 19, 21–31] (see Table 11.1). It is important to rule out any pathological disorder before a clinical diagnosis of idiopathic headshaking is made. Evaluation of cases should include appropriate examination and diagnostic techniques to eliminate these possible disorders before a diagnosis of idiopathic headshaking is made in which there should be a lack of anatomical and pathological abnormalities.

Anatomy

The trigeminal complex is formed by peripheral (trigeminal nerve, trigeminal ganglion, three main branches (ophthalmic, maxillary, mandibular; Figure 11.3), and subsequent branches) and central (spinal tract and nuclei of the trigeminal complex within the brainstem) components. The trigeminal nerve is the thickest of all cranial nerves and includes both sensory and motor components. The sensory components include the ophthalmic, maxillary, and mandibular nerves. The mandibular nerve also has motor function. The trigeminal ganglion contains sensory cell bodies for pain and temperature modalities of all three sensory branches of the trigeminal nerve [32]. The cell bodies of neurons of proprioceptive modalities are not located in the trigeminal ganglion but in nuclei within

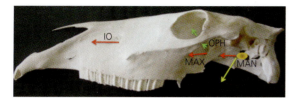

Figure 11.3 Horse skull representing the three sensory branches of the trigeminal nerve. Oval structure represents the trigeminal ganglion (not drawn to scale). IO, infraorbital nerve (red arrow) branch of maxillary nerve; MAN, mandibular nerve (yellow arrow); MAX, maxillary nerve (red arrows); OPH, ophthalmic nerve (green arrows).

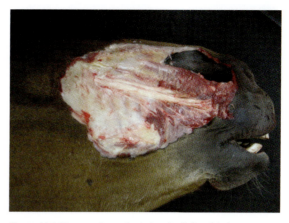

Figure 11.4 Horse cadaver depicting the infraorbital nerve as it exits the infraorbital canal through the infraorbital foramen. Note the multiple branches originating from the infraorbital nerve.

the brainstem [32]. The motor part of the mandibular nerve is ventral to the trigeminal ganglion. The ophthalmic nerve is the smallest of the three sensory nerves and runs lateral to the cavernous sinus. The ophthalmic nerve enters the orbital fissure along with the oculomotor, trochlear, and abducent nerves. The ophthalmic nerve gives the lacrimal, frontal, nasociliary, and ethmoidal nerves [33].

The maxillary nerve emerges from the round foramen and continues into the infraorbital canal as the infraorbital nerve. The maxillary nerve has several branches including zygomaticofacial, pterygopalatine, major palatine, minor palatine, caudal nasal, and infraorbital nerve [33]. The mandibular nerve gives rise to the masseteric, temporal, pterygoid, tensor tympani, tensor veli palatine, mylohyoid, auriculotemporal, buccal, lingual, and mental nerves among others [33].

The signs of apparent facial discomfort displayed by affected horses appear to be mainly localized to the muzzle/nose area. The maxillary nerve is sensory to the lower eyelid, maxillary teeth, upper lip, maxillary sinus, and nose. Therefore, attempts to diagnose the disorder have been made through local anesthesia of the infraorbital/maxillary nerve (Figure 11.4).

Diagnosis

Important information for the workup of the horse with a complaint of headshaking include the signalment of the horse, type of headshaking activity (vertical, horizontal, rotatory), frequency (how many per hour, day, week), occurrence (day vs. night, sunny vs. overcast, windy, etc.), seasonality (seasonal vs. all year round), association with exercise (yes or no, under saddle or lunge line), snorting (yes or no, association with headshaking?), nose rubbing (nose on the ground when exercised, rubbing against objects or feet), apparent distress or anxiety, any events associated or concurrent to headshaking episodes, and response to the

environment/sound. It is helpful for the attending veterinarian if the owner has kept a diary of daily weather patterns, the horse's management, exercises, and headshaking events. Additionally, it is useful to review video recordings of the horse headshaking, particularly if the behavior is associated with particular types of weather or conditions that might not be present when the horse is examined.

The evaluation of a horse with headshaking must include a general physical examination including examination of the oral cavity, nasal passages, eyes, ears, sinuses, and guttural pouches. Our routine evaluation includes ophthalmic, otoscopic, and oral exam, upper airway endoscopy including guttural pouches, and head radiography. Computed tomography and magnetic resonance imaging are useful to rule out other disorders of bone and soft tissue of the head. The authors have not observed abnormalities on CT studies of horses with idiopathic headshaking. The horse is observed with the bridle and bit if appropriate and under saddle if headshaking occurs only when ridden. It is important in these cases to rule out problems with the bridle, bit, rider skills, and behavior of the horse (acting up to avoid being ridden). However, the horse must not be ridden as part of the evaluation if headshaking is so violent that riding is unsafe).

A diagnosis of "idiopathic" headshaking is based on clinical evaluation of a specific phenotype of "headshakes" seen as a rapid downward jerk of the nose followed by upward flinging of the head, plus ruling out other diseases. Local anesthetic block of the infraorbital nerve is used by some clinicians as a diagnostic aid; however, reported success rates of this block are low. Mair (1999) found that of the 19 horses, 3 horses improved, 8 remained unchanged, and 8 were worse following infraorbital block with 12 ml mepivacaine [6], while Newton et al. reported a 50% improvement in 1 of 8 horses following 2–3 ml mepivacaine [4]. The low volumes of local anesthetic used in these studies might be partly responsible for the poor response as approximately 20 ml of local anesthetic (applied with a 20G, 2.5 cm needle) is necessary to block this large-size nerve, which usually takes approximately 20–40 min to be effective. Bilateral anesthesia of the posterior ethmoid nerve has been performed with a reported improvement in 13 of 17 and 23 of 27 headshakers [4, 34]. This block requires aseptic preparation of a 3 × 4 cm area below the zygomatic arch, subcutaneous local anesthetic injection, and then insertion of a 7 cm 19-gauge spinal needle in a rostroventral direction toward the upper sixth cheek tooth. The stilette is removed when the needle is at a depth of 5 cm and 5 ml mepivacaine injected. Headshaking should be reassessed after 20 min, 1 h, and 1.5 h [4]. The horse must be physically and chemically restrained to perform both these local anesthetic blocks safely. Video surveillance is recommended to monitor the frequency of the "shakes" before and after the block in a more objective manner. Possible complications of these procedures are common and include hematoma, worsening of the clinical signs, infection, neuritis, and painful neuroma [4, 6]. Additionally, nerve blocks will block all areas innervated by the specific nerve (e.g., will block dental pain).

Likewise there is no definitive diagnostic technique for human trigeminal neuralgia which is often diagnosed by a positive response to treatment with carbamazepine [10]. Quantitative sensory testing, which is useful in human trigeminal neuralgia sufferers to accurately map areas of altered sensory perception, appears to be an insensitive tool in the horse (K.J. Pickles, unpublished observation). More recently our neurophysiology studies, in which low thresholds of nerve activity were found in affected horses, have provided evidence of trigeminal involvement in the pathophysiology of the disorder [3]. The results of such neurophysiological study provide objective and quantitative data.

Treatment

There is no single curative treatment that works for all headshaking horses and the vast majority of horses are managed to minimize clinical signs and distress rather than cured. Such management can be challenging; however, some headshakers do respond to particular treatments. Most of the suggested treatments are aimed at reducing clinical signs rather than correcting the abnormal trigeminal neurophysiology, which likely explains their poor success rates. The fact that some horses go into remission implies that the aberrant activity of the trigeminal nerve might be reversible and invites speculation about how this could be achieved. It is the authors' opinion that such manipulation will hold the key to curative treatment of headshaking.

The number of published studies that have critically examined the efficacy of headshaking treatments is limited. It is also extremely difficult to differentiate between clinical effect, spontaneous or seasonal remission, and proxy placebo effect on owner interpretation of headshaking [35]. The following information provides a summary of the various therapies that have been attempted to treat and prevent headshaking.

Knowledge of when the episodes occur might help to address environmental factors such as light and seasonality. If light seems to be a trigger, the horse might be able to be ridden at night or in an indoor arena. For most owners however this is impractical or inconvenient, especially for competing horses.

Nose nets and face masks have been reported to be beneficial in reducing clinical signs of headshaking in over 70% of 36 seasonally affected headshaking horses [36]. Three types of nose net were evaluated, a traditional cylindrical net (full net) and two forms of larger mesh nets which cover only the nostrils and dorsorostral muzzle (half nets). Approximately 75% of owners reported some overall improvement with each net; around 60% recorded a 50% or greater improvement and 30% had a 70% or greater improvement [35]. There were few significant differences between the different net types, but the half nets were reported to be significantly better at controlling "bee up the nose" behavior. Additionally, horses greater than 10 years old were reportedly less likely to show a 50% or greater improvement in "nose flipping" and "headshaking at exercise."

Some headshaking horses that do not respond to a traditional nose net might improve with the use of soft rope plaits, or a similar device, that attaches to the noseband or dangles over the nostril and muzzle area (J. Madigan, pers. commun.). The mechanism by which these nose nets provide relief is unknown. They might act to reduce aversive stimulation of hyperesthetic areas or alternatively the constant presence of the net might work by adjacent receptor field inhibition or receptor adaptation of the contact area [37]. Perhaps, the sensory input is altered or inhibited by applying a different type of stimulus. Examples of some nose covers and beaded nose nets can be found at www.horsemask.com. Photic headshakers might obtain significant relief from the use of fly masks which provide UV blocking sun shade (e.g., Guardian Mask®, San Diego, USA; www.horsemask.com) (Figure 11.5).

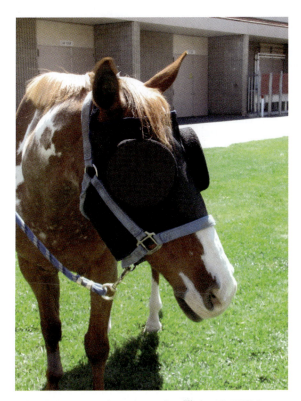

Figure 11.5 Horse wearing a Guardian mask with UV light protection.

Pharmacologic treatment

There are few published studies regarding pharmacological treatment efficacy of headshaking. Equine pharmacokinetic data for most of the medications is also lacking. The following are a few examples of drugs used. Note that all medications listed have potential adverse effects; avoid polypharmacy. The veterinarian is advised to consult with their sport federation about regulations and withdrawal times for the use of the following drugs in the competing or show horse. These drugs are detected by most antidoping detection methods.

Cyproheptadine: 0.3 mg/kg orally twice daily

Cyproheptadine (Periactin®) is a first-generation antihistamine with additional anticholinergic, antiserotonergic, calcium channel blocking, and local anesthetic activity [38]. Its use has been reported to have variable efficacy for the treatment of headshaking with 70% of 61 headshakers improved moderately to greatly, with response noted within 1 week of commencing therapy [5]. Additionally, owners who stopped using cyproheptadine treatment reported recurrence of clinical signs. In contrast, British studies found no improvement with use of cyproheptadine [4, 6]. The presence or absence of a photic component to the headshaking might be responsible for this apparent difference in response as, anecdotally, photic headshakers appear less common in the United Kingdom. There are no available data on the bioavailability or pharmacokinetics of cyproheptadine in horses. Mild lethargy and anorexia have been reported with cyproheptadine treatment of headshaking [8].

Carbamazepine: 2–8 mg/kg orally two to four times daily, alone or in combination with cyproheptadine

Carbamazepine (Tegretol®) is an anticonvulsant that acts to stabilize voltage-gated sodium channels. It is the drug of choice in treatment of human trigeminal neuralgia. Carbamazepine treatment reduced headshaking in 88% of horses in one study, although this efficacy has not been repeated in later studies [4]. Again the bioavailability or pharmacokinetics of carbamazepine in horses is unknown.

Hydroxyzine: 0.8 mg/kg orally twice daily

Hydroxyzine is a first-generation antihistamine. There are no published reports of its efficacy in the treatment of headshaking. Madigan and Bell report that 1 of 16 headshakers responded to antihistamines but the particular antihistamine is not listed [5].

Fluphenazine: 50 mg total intramuscular once, repeat as needed every 1–4 months

Always use a new fluphenazine vial. Fluphenazine is an antipsychotic drug that acts by blocking central dopamine receptors. Anecdotally, fluphenazine has improved headshaking in some horses (P. Smith, unpublished observation. University of California, Davis); however, treatment with fluphenazine should be carefully considered due to the risk of idiosyncratic toxicity reactions [39].

Clonidine: 0.0025 mg/kg orally twice daily

Clonidine is a sympatholytic drug that has been used in the treatment of trigeminal neuralgia. There are no published reports of its pharmacokinetics in horse or its use for treatment of headshaking.

Phenobarbitone: approximately 3–6 mg/kg orally twice daily

Phenobarbitone has been used with some success to treat extremely severe headshaking in horses that are very distressed by the condition (J. Madigan, pers. commun.). Mild sedation is a common effect of the treatment.

Gabapentin: 5–20 mg/kg orally twice to thrice daily

Gabapentin is an antiepileptic drug that is also used for the treatment of neuropathic pain in humans. Gabapentin's mechanism of action is unclear but it is thought to involve the subunit of voltage-gated calcium channels [40]. Anecdotally, variable success has been reported following treatment of headshaking with gabapentin. Recent pharmacokinetic studies report poor oral bioavailability (16%) in the horse [41].

Corticosteroids

Madigan and Bell report 3 of 20 horses responded to corticosteroid treatment but the particular regimen administered was not listed [5]. Dexamethasone pulse therapy has been used as a treatment for neuropathic pain in humans but its use in headshaking has not resulted in improvement.

Sodium cromoglycate eye drops: one drop per eye four times a day

Sodium cromoglycate eye drops have been used successfully in three horses with seasonal headshaking that also showed excessive tear production and photophobia [42]. Sodium cromoglycate stabilizes mast cell membranes and prevents the release of histamine and other mediators. These findings support an allergic condition in this group of horses, although these horses were previously treated with ophthalmic dexamethasone with no response.

Melatonin: 15–18 mg orally daily at 5 p.m

Manipulation of the photoperiod with melatonin has been reported to improve seasonal headshaking in 2 of 7 horses [5]. Melatonin treatment of seasonal headshakers that begin in spring and cease in late fall and winter is most successful when melatonin is started before the onset of spring. The dose must be given promptly at 5 p.m. each day. Some horses may require treatment all year round while treatment can be stopped in during winter. Due to manipulation of the photoperiod, the horse might not shed its coat and require clipping.

Nutritional supplements of various forms have been attempted to manage headshaking. Over 40% of owners have tried feed supplements for the treatment of headshaking with approximately 35% of these perceiving an improvement [7]. A strong observer placebo effect is suspected in these reports.

Magnesium increases the threshold for nerve firing and therefore increases the stimuli needed for depolarization. The authors have recommended supplementation of 10–20 g of oral magnesium once daily and anecdotally owners report some improvement in headshaking. It is recommended to measure plasma ionized magnesium before supplementation and 2 weeks after beginning supplementation and then adjust dosing to maintain ionized magnesium within reference values.

Other alternative therapies have been attempted but proved unsuccessful. Studies report that chiropractic treatment of headshaking is tried by approximately one-quarter of owners; however, over 92% of those treated show a complete lack of response [7]. Acupuncture is used by a similar percentage of owners with approximately 10% of owners considering their horse had some beneficial effect from therapy [5]. Homeopathy has been used by 38% of owners with approximately 35% of these considering their horses derived at least a partial improvement [7]. Fly-control measures are commonly utilized, with 100% application in one study; however, these yielded improvement in only 2% of headshaking horses [5].

The use of infraorbital neurectomy for the treatment of headshaking dates back to the first report of headshaking in the veterinary literature [1]. Review of this procedure determined poor response and high postsurgical complication rates [6]. Likewise posterior ethmoid nerve sclerosis has been discontinued due to the high rate of recurrence of headshaking [4]. More recently the application of platinum coils to provide compression of the caudal infraorbital nerve +/− laser cautery of the nerve has been described as a salvage procedure for headshaking horses unresponsive to medical therapy [34, 43]. The procedure was successful in approximately 50% of horses, although multiple surgeries were required in a substantial proportion of the horses due to recurrence of headshaking. Nose-rubbing was a common postoperative complication.

Idiopathic headshaking in the horse is a poorly understood disorder, in which recently, the trigeminal nerve was proved to be associated with the pathophysiology of disease. However, a definitive cause remains unknown. Detailed descriptions of morphometric and histochemical features of the trigeminal complex in affected horses have not been performed and therefore structural abnormalities have not been ruled out. It is essential to rule out other causes of headshaking before considering idiopathic headshaking.

References

[1] Williams, W.L. (1897) Involuntary twitching of the head relieved by trifacial neurectomy. *J Comp Med Vet Arch*, 18, 426–428.

[2] Williams, W.L. (1899) Involuntary shaking of the head and its treatment by trifacial neurectomy. *Am Vet Rev*, 23, 321–326.

[3] Aleman, M., Williams, D.C., Brosnan, R.J. *et al.* (2013) Sensory nerve conduction and somatosensory evoked potentials of the trigeminal nerve in horses with idiopathic headshaking. *J Vet Intern Med*, 27, 1571–1580.

[4] Newton, S.A., Knottenbelt, D.C. and Eldridge, P.R. (2000) Headshaking in horses: possible aetiopathogenesis suggested by the results of diagnostic tests and several treatment regimes used in 20 cases. *Equine Vet J*, 32, 208–216.

[5] Madigan, J.E. and Bell, S.A. (2001) Owner survey of headshaking in horses. *J Am Vet Med Assoc*, 219, 334–337.

[6] Mair, T.S. (1999) Assessment of bilateral infra-orbital nerve blockade and bilateral infra-orbital neurectomy in the investigation and treatment of idiopathic headshaking. *Equine Vet J*, 31, 262–264.

[7] Mills, D.S., Cook, S. and Jones, B. (2002) Reported response to treatment among 245 cases of equine headshaking. *Vet Rec*, 150, 311–313.

[8] Madigan, J.E., Kortz, G., Murphy, C. and Rodger, L. (1995) Photic headshaking in the horse: 7 cases. *Equine Vet J*, 27, 306–311.

[9] Madigan, J.E. and Bell, S.A. (1988) Characterisation of headshaking syndrome—31 cases. *Equine Vet J*, (Suppl 27), 28–29.

[10] Nurmikko, T.J. and Eldridge, P.R. (2001) Trigeminal neuralgia–pathophysiology, diagnosis and current treatment. *Br J Anaesth*, 87, 117–132.

[11] Aleman, M., Pickles, K.J., Simonek, G. and Madigan, J.E. (2012) Latent equine herpesvirus-1 in trigeminal ganglia and equine idiopathic headshaking. *J Vet Intern Med*, 26, 192–194.

[12] Newton SA. The functional anatomy of the trigeminal nerve in the horse. PhD thesis. University of Liverpool, Liverpool; 2001.

[13] Amir, R., Michaelis, M. and Devor, M. (1999) Membrane potential oscillations in dorsal root ganglion neurons: role in normal electrogenesis and neuropathic pain. *J Neurosci*, 19, 8589–8596.

[14] Liu, C.H., Wall, P.D., Ben-Dor, E. *et al.* (2000) Tactile allodynia in the absence of C-fiber activation: altered firing properties of DRG neurons following spinal nerve injury. *Pain*, 85, 503–521.

[15] Amir, R. and Devor, M. (2000) Functional cross-excitation between afferent A and C neurons in dorsal root ganglia. *Neuroscience*, 95, 189–195.

[16] Burchiel, K.J. and Slavin, K.V. (2000) On the natural history of trigeminal neuralgia. *Neurosurgery*, 46, 152–155.

[17] Whitman, W.W. and Packer, R.J. (1993) The photic sneeze reflex: literature review and discussion. *Neurology*, 43, 868–871.

[18] Lane, J.G. and Mair, T.S. (1987) Observations on headshaking in the horse. *Equine Vet J*, 19, 331–336.

[19] Mair, T.S. and Lane, J.G. (1990) Headshaking in horses. *In Pract*, 9, 183–186.

[20] Pickles, K.J., Berger, J., Davies, R. *et al.* (2011) Use of a gonadotrophin-releasing hormone vaccine in headshaking horses. *Vet Rec*, 168, 19.

[21] Cook, W.R. (1979) Headshaking in horses. Part 2: History and management tests. *Eq Pract*, 1, 36–39.

[22] Cook, W.R. (1980) Headshaking in horses. Part 3: Diagnostic tests. *Eq Pract*, 2, 31–40.

[23] Cook, W.R. (1992) Headshaking in horses: an afterward. *Compend Contin Educ Pract Vet*, 14, 1369–1372.

[24] Kold, S.E., Ostblom, L.C. and Philipsen, H.P. (1982) Headshaking caused by a maxillary osteoma in a horse. *Equine Vet J*, 14, 167–169.

[25] Mair, T.S. (1994) Headshaking associated with *Trombicula autumnalis* larval infestation in two horses. *Equine Vet J*, 26, 244–245.

[26] McGorum, B.C. and Dixon, P.M. (1990) Vasomotor rhinitis with headshaking in a pony. *Equine Vet J*, 22, 220–222.

[27] Moore, L.A., Johnson, P.J., Messer, N.T. *et al.* (1997) Management of headshaking in three horses by treatment for protozoal myeloencephalitis. *Vet Rec*, 141, 264–267.

[28] Berger, J.M., Bell, S.A., Holmberg, B.J. and Madigan, J.E. (2008) Successful treatment of head shaking by use of infrared diode laser deflation and coagulation of corpora nigra cysts and behavioral modification in a horse. *J Am Vet Med Assoc*, 233, 1610–1612.

[29] Voigt, A., Saulez, M.N. and Donnellan, C.M. (2009) Nuchal crest avulsion fracture in 2 horses: a cause of headshaking. *J S Afr Vet Assoc*, 80, 111–113.

[30] Fiske-Jackson, A.R., Pollock, P.J., Witte, T.H. *et al.* (2012) Fungal sinusitis resulting in suspected trigeminal neuropathy as a cause of headshaking in five horses. *Eq Vet Educ*, 24, 126–133.

[31] Stephenson, R. (2005) An unusual case of headshaking caused by a premaxillary bone cyst. *Equine Vet Educ*, 17, 79–82.

[32] de Lahunta, A.S. and Glass, E. (2009) *Veterinary Neuroanatomy and Clinical Neurology*, 3rd edn, Saunders Elsevier, St.Louis.

[33] Budras, K.D., Sack, W.O., Rock, S. *et al.* (2009) *Anatomy of the Horse*, 5th edn, Schlutersche, Hannover.

[34] Roberts, V.L., Perkins, J.D., Skärlina, E. *et al.* (2013) Caudal anaesthesia of the infraorbital nerve for diagnosis of idiopathic headshaking and caudal compression of the infraorbital nerve for its treatment, in 58 horses. *Equine Vet J*, 45, 107–110.

[35] Talbot, W.A., Pinchbeck, G.L., Knottenbelt, D.C. *et al.* (2013) A randomised, blinded, crossover study to assess the efficacy of a feed supplement in alleviating the clinical signs of headshaking in 32 horses. *Equine Vet J*, 45, 293–297.

[36] Mills, D.S. and Taylor, K. (2003) Field study of the efficacy of three types of nose net for the treatment of headshaking in horses. *Vet Rec*, 152, 41–44.

[37] Raj, S.N., Meyer, R.A., Ringkamp, M. and Campbell, J.N. (1999) Peripheral neural mechanisms of nociception, in *Pain* (eds P.D. Wall and R. Melzack), Churchill Livingstone, Edinburgh, pp. 11–57.

[38] Lowe, D.A., Matthews, E.K. and Richardson, B.P. (1981) The calcium antagonistic effects of cyproheptadine on contraction, membrane electrical events and calcium influx in the guinea-pig taenia coli. *Br J Pharmacol*, 74, 651–663.

[39] Baird, J.D., Arroyo, L.G., Vengust, M. *et al.* (2006) Adverse extrapyramidal effects in four horses given fluphenazine decanoate. *J Am Vet Med Assoc*, 229, 104–110.

[40] Manuef, Y.P., Luo, A.Z. and Lee, K. (2006) Alpha-2-delta and the mechanism of action of gabapentin in the treatment of pain. *Semin Cell Dev Biol*, 17, 565–570.

[41] Terry, R.L., McDonnell, S.M., Van Eps, A.W. *et al.* (2010) Pharmacokinetic profile and behavioral effects of gabapentin in the horse. *J Vet Pharmacol Ther*, 33, 485–494.

[42] Stalin, C.E., Boydell, I.P. and Pike, R.E. (2008) Treatment of seasonal headshaking in three horses with sodium cromoglycate eye drops. *Vet Rec*, 163, 305–306.

[43] Roberts, V.L., McKane, S.A., Williams, A. and Knottenbelt, D.C. (2009) Caudal compression of the infraorbital nerve: a novel surgical technique for treatment of idiopathic headshaking and assessment of its efficacy in 24 horses. *Equine Vet J*, 41, 165–170.

12 Differential Diagnosis of Urinary Incontinence and Cauda Equina Syndrome

Melissa Hines

College of Veterinary Medicine, University of Tennessee, Knoxville, USA

Urinary incontinence in horses

Urinary incontinence (UI), defined by the involuntary voiding of urine, appears to be a relatively uncommon clinical problem in horses [1–3]. Reported cases have been infrequent, with a 2004 review documenting 37 cases over an 8 year period [1]. However, when present, UI is often a frustrating problem as both determining the etiology and managing the condition can be difficult. There are several potential causes of UI, which can be generally categorized as non-neurogenic, neurogenic, and idiopathic or myogenic [1–4] (Table 12.1). In horses, non-neurogenic causes include developmental anomalies such as an ectopic ureter, urolithiasis, estrogen-responsive incontinence, and incontinence associated with pregnancy and parturition [1, 5, 6]. Neurogenic causes include infectious, toxic, traumatic, compressive, degenerative, and inflammatory etiologies. In addition, a syndrome of idiopathic or myogenic bladder paralysis has been described [1, 7]. While the cause of this condition is not completely understood, it may be associated with prior or subtle neurologic disease or chronic lumbosacral pain. The following discussion will focus primarily on neurogenic UI.

Innervation and neurophysiology of the lower urinary tract

The control of urination is complex, involving both the autonomic (sympathetic and parasympathetic) and somatic nervous systems [4, 8–10] (Table 12.2). Some aspects of the neurogenic control of micturition in horses remain unknown, requiring information to be extrapolated from other species, although species differences are known to exist.

The sympathetic nerve supply to the urinary tract arises from spinal segments L1–4, via the hypogastric nerve, with preganglionic fibers synapsing in the caudal mesenteric ganglia [4, 8–10]. Postganglionic fibers supply the bladder body (primarily beta 2) and also the bladder neck and proximal urethra (primarily alpha 1). The stimulation of alpha fibers causes contraction of the bladder neck and proximal urethra, while stimulation of beta fibers causes relaxation of the bladder body. Thus, sympathetic stimulation generally facilitates urine storage.

Parasympathetic fibers innervating the bladder leave the spinal cord at the level of the second, third, and fourth sacral vertebrae, forming the pelvic nerve [4, 8–10]. These same spinal cord segments innervate the external genitalia and urethra. The primary role of parasympathetic innervation of the bladder is detrusor contraction with relaxation of the internal urethral sphincter facilitating bladder emptying.

Somatic innervation is primarily to the striated muscle of the urethra via a branch of the pudendal nerve, which originates from the second, third, and fourth sacral segments [4, 8–10]. Other branches of this nerve go to the external genitalia, perineum, and anal sphincter. In addition, general somatic efferent neurons to the striated muscle of the abdomen play a role in the voluntary control of urination, initiating voluntary abdominal wall contractions that can assist in voiding.

Normal voiding is an autonomic spinal cord reflex which is modulated by the central nervous system [4, 8–10]. This reflex is influenced primarily by input from the micturition reflex center within the pontine-mesencephalic reticular formation of the brainstem. There are interconnections from this center to the frontal lobes and other areas in the cerebral cortex and subcortical areas.

Equine Neurology, Second Edition. Martin Furr and Stephen Reed.

© 2015 John Wiley & Sons, Inc. Published 2015 by John Wiley & Sons, Inc.

Companion website: www.wiley.com/go/furr/neurology

Table 12.1 Causes of urinary incontinence in horses.

Non-neurogenic causes
    Developmental anomalies (ectopic ureter, etc.)
    Urolithiasis
    Estrogen-responsive sphincter incontinence
    Pregnancy and parturition
Neurogenic causes
    Equine herpes myeloencephalopathy
    Equine protozoal myeloencephalopathy
    West Nile virus
    Toxins
        Sorghum
        Johnson grass
        Sudan grass
    Sacral trauma
    Cervical compressive myelopathy
    Equine degenerative myelopathy
    Cauda equina syndrome
        Trauma, polyneuritis equi, etc.
Idiopathic bladder paralysis syndrome

Table 12.2 Primary peripheral innervation to the lower urinary tract.

Innervation (spinal cord segment)	Nerve	Predominant action
Sympathetic (L1–4)	Hypogastric nerve	Filling and storage (relaxation of bladder body; contraction of bladder neck and proximal urethra)
Parasympathetic (S2–4)	Pelvic nerve	Emptying (contraction of bladder body; relaxation of internal urethral sphincter)
Sacral somatic pathways (S2–4)	Pudendal nerve	Contraction of external urethral sphincter

The nerves contain both sensory and motor axons.

As the bladder progressively fills (filling phase), there is a gradual increase in the tone of the muscles comprising the urethral sphincters. During filling, the detrusor muscle remains relaxed due to the influence of pelvic nerve afferents and sympathetic nerves innervating the detrusor muscle. This is due to a reflex arc that comprises bladder stretch and pressure receptors, the afferent pelvic nerve, spinal cord interneurons, and sympathetic tone in hypogastric nerve efferents. Upper motor neuron (UMN) input from higher centers can also mediate the tone of urethral sphincters. This reflex allows the bladder to accumulate large volumes of urine, with little increase in intravesicular pressure.

Once the detrusor can no longer stretch, the intravesicular pressure increases and sensory impulses are transmitted via the pelvic nerve to the pons, cerebrum, and cerebellum, giving the sensation of fullness. There is stimulation of descending UMNs in the reticulospinal tract to the sacral parasympathetic nuclei, which triggers the emptying phase of urination. From the sacral segments, impulses reach the detrusor muscle via the pelvic nerve initiating detrusor contraction. There is simultaneous inhibition of transmission from the somatic pudendal nerve and hypogastric sympathetic activity, allowing relaxation of the urethral sphincter, facilitating voiding.

There are many mechanisms by which disruption of normal micturition can originate. Traditionally, UI has been categorized into two major types: the UMN bladder (spastic or reflex bladder) and the lower motor neuron (LMN) bladder (paralytic or autonomous bladder) [1, 4, 9, 10].

UMN disease is associated with a lesion above the sacral segments in the cord, brainstem, or cortex. As a result of UMN dysfunction, there is a loss of inhibitory signals with increased tone of both the detrusor (detrusor hyperreflexia, DH) and urethral sphincter. In some cases, a lack of coordination between the detrusor and urethral sphincter, known as detrusor-external sphincter dyssynergia (DESD), may occur.

The loss of UMN inhibition of the external sphincter typically results in increased urethral resistance, so that greater intravesicular pressure is required before voiding occurs. Although there is loss of voluntary control of urination, partial voiding will occur due to the intact local reflex arc. The UI associated with UMN dysfunction is often initially manifested as intermittent short squirts of urine with incomplete emptying. Although the residual bladder volume is variable, the bladder is typically large and turgid, and it is generally difficult to express or catheterize. Over time, the chronic bladder distention associated with UMN dysfunction can result in atony and overflow incontinence.

The term automatic bladder is sometimes used synonymously with UMN bladder, but it is most appropriately used to describe a neurogenic bladder due to complete transection of the spinal cord above the sacral segments. This condition is marked by complete loss of both sensation and micturition reflexes with uncontrolled reflex emptying of the bladder. This is poorly described in horses with spinal cord trauma.

A LMN bladder results from a lesion in the sacral segments (S2–4) and associated nerve roots (cauda equina) or peripheral nerves, interrupting the local reflex arc. There is a loss of detrusor function (detrusor areflexia, DA) leading to a paralyzed, atonic bladder. As the bladder becomes overdistended, there is overflow incontinence. The urine dribbling typically appears continuous, which may help distinguish the condition from an early UMN bladder. The bladder is large and easy to manually express or catheterize. The bladder volume is generally higher than what is seen with an UMN bladder. Also, damage to sensory nerve fibers can result in overdistention of the bladder and overflow incontinence, as the transmission of stretch signals from the bladder to initiate the micturition reflex is impaired.

This traditional classification of UI into UMN and LMN bladder dysfunction can be useful in the neuroanatomical localization of the lesion but it can also be misleading. There is evidence in human medicine that a significant percentage of patients may not have the clinical signs expected for the lesion [11–13]. Similarly, in horses, signs consistent with a LMN bladder have occasionally been observed in association with cervical cord compression and equine degenerative myelopathy, conditions which would be expected to cause an UMN bladder [1, 7]. One possible explanation for this is that early signs of UMN incontinence were unrecognized until prolonged distention resulted in overflow incontinence, making the problem more evident. Also, neural lesions may actually have variable effects on lower urinary function, which is possible given the complexity of the system.

Neurogenic causes of UI

It can be difficult to determine a specific cause for UI in horses [1–3, 14, 15]. In the series of 37 cases evaluated by Schott et al., a cause was identified in 80% of cases, with 11 of 37 being neurological in origin [1]. In a series of 10 cases of bladder paralysis associated with sabulous urolithiasis, a specific cause (cauda equina neuritis) was diagnosed only in one horse [15].

Several specific neurological disorders have been identified in association with UI. Of the 11 cases with neurogenic incontinence reported by Schott et al., three were diagnosed with equine protozoal myeloencephalopathy (EPM), three with cervical cord compression, three with cauda equina syndrome (CES), one with equine degenerative myelopathy (EDM), and one with an undiagnosed neurologic disorder [1]. Disorders that have been typically associated with LMN dysfunction include sacral trauma, equine herpesvirus type 1 myeloencephalitis (EHM), cauda equina neuritis, Sudan grass toxicity, and sorghum cystitis ataxia (enzootic ataxia cystitis) [1, 16–21]. Also, iatrogenic bladder paralysis after epidural injections, particularly of alcohol in show horses, has been documented as a cause of a LMN bladder. The most frequent causes of an UMN bladder in horses include EPM, EDM, and spinal cord lesions causing compression such as trauma or cervical compressive myelopathy [1, 4]. These horses frequently

have concurrent ataxia. Also, it should be remembered that UI is not a consistent feature of these disorders. Other reported causes of UI include neoplasia, such as lymphosarcoma and melanoma, aberrant parasite migration, vertebral osteomyelitis, abscesses and epidural empyema, and cryptococcal leptomeningitis [22–26]. Clearly, any inflammatory condition of the spinal cord can result in UI. UI has been reported in mares due to iatrogenic trauma resulting in muscle and nerve damage during reproductive evaluation [26]. While the site of the lesion can affect the specific clinical signs, it is important to remember that the division between UMN and LMN dysfunction is not absolute.

Clinical approach to UI

Neurogenic UI may be recognized in horses of any gender and age, although it has been reported more frequently in adults than foals. In the 11 cases of neurogenic UI reported by Schott et al., seven were geldings and four were mares [1].

A complete history is important when evaluating UI. In some cases, the inciting cause may have occurred months to years prior to presentation for incontinence. The reproductive history of mares as well as any history of musculoskeletal injury, epidural injections, vaccinations or exposure to other horses may be of particular importance.

Both the history and physical exam findings can help to characterize the incontinence. Constant urine dribbling is typically associated with LMN dysfunction and overflow incontinence, while intermittent squirts are typically seen with UMN dysfunction, especially in the early stages. In some cases, coughing or exercise, which increases intraabdominal pressure, may worsen the signs, suggesting decreased sphincter tone. Horses with UI that continue to intermittently posture to urinate are assumed to have intact sensory input indicating fullness but have lost motor function.

A thorough examination, including a general physical, musculoskeletal, and neurologic exam, is important in the evaluation of horses with UI. The presenting complaint, especially in chronic cases, is often urine scald and depilation on the hind limbs and around the perineum of mares and ventral abdomen of males [1–4] (Figure 12.1). The urine scald can be quite painful. In some cases, the UI and resultant urine scald are the only signs, but in other cases there may be additional signs that are helpful in identifying the etiology. The presence of fever may suggest an infectious etiology. Depending on the site of the lesion, there may be additional neurologic deficits. A LMN bladder is often accompanied by other signs of LMN dysfunction, including decreased tail and anal tone, analgesia or hypalgesia of the perineum, atrophy of the muscles of the hip and hind limb, and hind limb weakness. Horses with an UMN lesion, such as

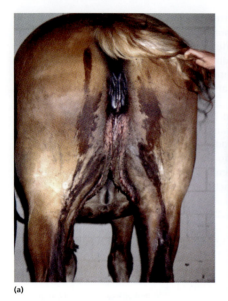

(a)

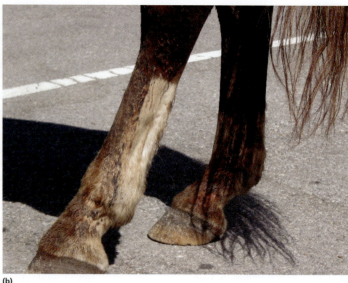

(b)

Figure 12.1 Urine scalding of the (a) perineum of a mare and (b) hind limbs of a gelding with urinary incontinence. Management of horses with urinary incontinence often requires careful attention to nursing care. (Photos courtesy of Dr. HC Schott.)

that due to EPM or EDM, often have additional neurologic deficits such as ataxia. Horses that are recumbent for any reason may have some degree of urine and/or fecal retention without having actual neurologic damage [10]. This may be due in part to the inability to posture and strain appropriately, as well as possible contusions and pain in the region. In some cases, it can be difficult to distinguish these horses from those with incontinence due to neurologic dysfunction.

Rectal palpation is recommended in the evaluation of cases of UI. Bladder tone, size, and pain should be assessed. A turgid, difficult to express bladder is suggestive of UMN disease, while an enlarged, easily expressed bladder is suggestive of LMN disease. In cases with sabulous urolithiasis, the accumulation of sediment can be palpated and should be differentiated from a cystolith (Figure 12.2). The pelvic cavity can also be evaluated for evidence of trauma or neoplasia. A transrectal ultrasonographic examination can be utilized to evaluate the bladder's content (sediment and fluid clarity), and bladder wall and pelvic soft tissues. Urethral catheterization can also be performed and may provide information about sphincter tone. In mares, a vaginal exam may provide useful information in some cases [26].

Standard clinicopathologic analyses (CBC, fibrinogen and serum chemistry profile) are often normal, but may be valuable in some cases and should be performed. Additional tests, such as serology, vitamin E assays, cerebrospinal fluid (CSF) analyses, and culture will be

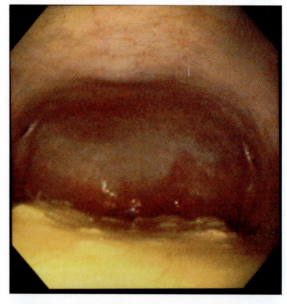

Figure 12.2 Sabulous urolithiasis is a common complication of urinary incontinence in horses. Endoscopic view of accumulated sediment in the bladder. (Photo courtesy of Dr. HC Schott.)

determined by the clinical examination and history. A urinalysis and quantitative urine culture are also indicated, as ascending urinary tract infection is one of the major complications of UI [1, 7].

Endoscopic exam of the lower urinary tract allows for evaluation of anatomical structures, urethral sphincter tone, material within the bladder, and degree of bladder mucosal damage. In chronic cases, the ureteral openings may become dilated due to chronic distention and loss of bladder compliance. Also, the patient's response to inflation of the bladder during cystoscopy may help in the assessment of sensation.

Radiographic evaluation of the pelvis and the caudal spine are challenging but potentially useful in the diagnosis of paravertebral abscesses or trauma. For example, discospondylitis of S2–4 associated with *Rhodococcus equi* was identified by radiography in a 4-month-old foal presented for UI [22]. Nuclear scintigraphy can also be useful in the identification of fractures and osteomyelitis. Advanced imaging techniques such as computed tomography (CT) and magnetic resonance imaging (MRI) are currently not practical for most cases but have some application in foals.

A variety of techniques have been utilized both in human and veterinary medicine to evaluate the dynamics of micturition in both normal and incontinent animals. These urodynamic techniques include cystometrography, urethral pressure profilometry, and simultaneous cystometry and uroflowmetry [27–30]. Cystometrography consists of pressure and volume recordings performed with the aid of fluid or gas in the bladder, during filling [14]. Bladder and urethral pressures profiles are pressure recordings obtained from the bladder and urethra using a cuffed catheter connected to a pressure transducer, and measurements are recorded as the catheter is withdrawn from the bladder through the urethra. Urinary pressure profiling has been reported in a few horses, but its value in the diagnostic evaluation of equine neurologic disease is not established [27–29].

Treatment

Goals of therapy for horses with UI are (i) to provide treatment for the specific disease causing the incontinence and (ii) to manage the incontinence itself. In many cases, therapeutic options are limited regardless of the cause. Patient management is often complicated by urine scalding, sabulous urolithiasis, and recurrent urinary tract infection. The following discussion will focus on the management of incontinence; specific treatments of inciting neurologic conditions are discussed elsewhere in the text.

There are few drugs available to treat UI in horses and these have largely been extrapolated from therapeutic protocols employed in other species. The most commonly used drug is bethanechol hydrochloride, a parasympathomimetic used primarily in cases of bladder atony [4, 31–33]. In the lower urinary tract, the primary effects of bethanechol include increased tone and contractility of the detrusor muscle [31]. The subcutaneous administration of bethanechol has been used as a diagnostic test for residual detrusor function, as rapid detrusor contraction and voiding may occur if there is residual function while no effect would be expected if the bladder is completely atonic. Bethanechol should not be used in cases of urinary outflow obstruction, due to the potential for bladder rupture. Overdosing causes excessive cholinergic stimulation with the potential for clinical signs such as arrhythmias, respiratory problems, and colic. The drug should not be given intramuscularly or intravenously as adverse effects are more common.

The recommended dosage of bethanechol in horses for treatment for detrusor muscle atony ranges from 0.025 to 0.075 mg/kg SC q8–12 h [4, 31]; however at this time, there are no commercial injectable formulations available, although compounded formulations may be available. While some anecdotal reports suggest more vigorous voiding after the subcutaneous administration of bethanechol, data supporting efficacy are lacking [33, 34]. Oral administration (0.2–0.4 mg/kg PO q6–12 h) has been employed in horses, but efficacy has not been reported. In cases where urinary outflow resistance is increased due to increased urethral tone, bethanechol has been combined with diazepam, dantrolene, or phenoxybenzamine for relaxation of the urethra [31, 35]. The utility of these drug combinations has not been determined in the horse.

The administration of α-adrenergic antagonists such as phenoxybenzamine and prazosin has been recommended in cases where dysfunction of the external urethral sphincter is suspected [31, 33, 35]. These drugs may reduce urethral resistance by blocking the α-mediated contraction of smooth muscle in both the bladder neck and the urethra. Phenoxybenzamine (0.2–0.7 mg/kg PO every 6–8 h) can decrease urethral resistance, thus facilitating emptying. For prazosin, a starting dose of 5 mg PO q8 h for an adult horse has been used. Individual titration to effect is required, due to interindividual variability, and the total dose should not exceed 10 mg due to the potential for hypotension.

Drugs that increase sphincter tone have been advocated in cases that have decreased urethral sphincter tone with normal detrusor function or DESD [31]. The most common drug used for this purpose is the α-adrenergic agonist, phenylpropanolamine (0.5–1.0 mg/kg PO every 8–24 h); however, a successful response has not been documented in horses. There have been a few reports in mares of improvement of UI following treatment with estradiol cypionate (4–10 μg/kg IM 24 every 24 h for 3 days, then every 48 h) [34–37]. While the mechanism is not fully understood, it appears that estrogen enhances the sensitivity of alpha-adrenergic receptors, improving sphincter tone.

Keys for successful management of horses with UI are limiting bladder distention and urine scalding [1, 2, 15, 38]. Especially in acute cases, bladder catheterization several times per day may be necessary to prevent bladder distention and rupture. Maintaining a small residual volume is also expected to enhance healing of the detrusor muscle and optimize the chances for recovery of the micturition reflex. Repeated catheterization may become difficult due to urethral trauma, but this can be avoided by the use of an indwelling urinary catheter, which is commercially available. Along with draining urine, lavage of the bladder to remove sabulous material may enhance the outcome in cases with sabulous urolithiasis [1, 2, 15, 38]. Antibiotics are often indicated to prevent or control urinary tract infection [1, 33, 34].

Careful attention to care of urine scalding is important [1–3, 15]. Frequent cleaning and application of soothing protective ointment (e.g., vaseline) is recommended to prevent skin excoriations. Limiting calcium in the diet or manipulation of the dietary cation–anion balance may be helpful in the management of chronic UI by reducing the development of crystals and the accumulation of sediment [7].

Prognosis

The prognosis of horses affected by UI is variable, depending to some extent on the primary cause and chronicity of the problem. If the primary cause of the UI can be corrected, as in the case of some congenital anomalies or cystolithiasis, the prognosis is good [39–42]. In the case of neurogenic UI, if the incontinence occurs with acute neurological disease which resolves, such as in some cases of EHM or EPM, the incontinence may also resolve provided appropriate care is taken to prevent prolonged bladder distention. In general, the prognosis is best when urinary function returns within 10–14 days after onset [1, 33].

In contrast, the prognosis is usually poor for chronic UI [1–3, 7, 33]. In some cases, especially those with detrusor dysfunction, the problem may be longstanding before clinical UI is recognized. Once sabulous urolithiasis becomes marked, the chances for a long-term recovery decrease considerably [1, 7, 15, 34]. Affected horses often require ongoing veterinary evaluation and treatment, including intermittent bladder lavage and antimicrobial therapy.

In the series of 37 cases of UI, 68% (25/37) were discharged from the hospital, but euthanasia due to persistent UI was performed after discharge in seven horses, making the long-term survival 49% (18/37) [1]. The UI was resolved (7) or successfully managed (1) in 8 of 37 cases, making the overall treatment success 21%. Of the horses with neurogenic UI specifically, 54% (6/11) were discharged from the hospital, but the UI was only

resolved in one horse with undiagnosed neurologic disease. One should note that limitations to long-term survival are often due to the need for continued nursing care, which requires the intervention of skillful personnel or the training of very committed owners.

Cauda equina syndrome

CES is not a specific disease but rather a constellation of clinical signs referable to disease of the cauda equina [10, 43, 44]. The cauda equina is defined as the spinal cord and nerve roots that lie caudal to the second sacral spinal cord segments [1] (Table 12.3). Due to the incongruity between the spinal cord segments and vertebral segments, the cauda equina is caudal to the lumbosacral vertebral junction. Specifically, lesions associated with CES may involve sacrococcygeal spinal cord segments, spinal nerve rootlets and roots of the cauda equina, sacral plexus and peripheral nerves to the bladder, rectum, anus, tail, and perineum [10]. This syndrome has been recognized in several species in addition to horses, including humans [45]. The predominant clinical signs that define CES include hypotonia, hypalgesia, and hyporeflexia of the tail, rectum anus, and perianal and perineal region [10, 43, 44]. There are varying degrees of urinary and fecal incontinence. The external genitalia are frequently affected as well. Pelvic limb disease, including ataxia, weakness, and muscle atrophy, may also be present, but it is not a consistent finding.

Clinical findings

The primary client complaint in horses with CES is often urine dribbling or urine scalding, which is sometimes associated with obvious tail paralysis [10, 43, 44]. In some cases, rectal impactions leading to colic may be the initial complaint. Penile protrusion in males, as well as decreased reproductive efficiency in stallions and mares, may also be reported by owners.

Table 12.3 Anatomic innervations of the nerves of the cauda equina.

Spinal cord segment	Nerve	Innervation
S1–S2	Sciatic and gluteal	Muscles of pelvic limbs
S2–S4	Pudendal	External genitalia, urethra
S2–S4	Caudal rectal	Rectum, anus, perianal and perineal skin
S2–S4	Pelvic	Pelvic plexus, parasympathetic to bladder, urethra, distal small colon, rectum, anus
	Coccygeal	Skin and muscle of tail

Findings on physical and neurologic examination typically include hypalgesia of the skin around the tail head, and perianal and perineal regions [10, 43, 44]. In some cases, there is a zone of hypersensitivity surrounding the area of reduced skin sensitivity. This hypersensitivity may be the result of either inflammation involving nerve fibers at the edge of the lesion or sprouting of sensory axons attempting repair. The tail clamp reflex is often obviously weak, and the anal reflex is weak or absent. Inability to retract the penis, associated with loss of sensation of the penis and sheath, may be present in geldings and stallions. Lack of sensation of the udder may be noted in mares. Reproductive abnormalities, including incomplete erections in males, impotence, urospermia, and urine pooling in mares, may be seen. Rear limb weakness and ataxia and muscle wasting of the rump and pelvic limbs are uncommon but can be seen if spinal cord disease extends cranial to the cauda equina.

Causes of cauda equina syndrome

As previously noted, CES is not a specific disease but a group of disorders defined by damage to the cauda equina giving rise to similar clinical signs. A variety of disorders have been shown to damage the cauda equina, including developmental, inflammatory, toxic, infectious, or traumatic etiologies (Table 12.4). Trauma to the sacrococcygeal area, particularly a fracture of S2, is the most common cause of CES in horses [10].

Table 12.4 Causes of cauda equina syndrome.

Trauma [1]
  Fracture, exuberant callus formation
  Soft tissue swelling
  Hematoma
Congenital caudal vertebral anomalies
Sorghum/sudan toxicity
Epidural abscess
Osteomyelitis [4]
Neoplasia
  Melanoma
  Lymphosarcoma
  Hemangiosarcoma
Bacterial meningitis
Cryptococcal meningitis
Verminous myelitis
Listeria monocytogenes myelitis
EHV-1
Rabies
West Nile virus
Equine protozoal myeloencephalitis
Cauda equina neuritis (polyneuritis equi)

Following a traumatic event, the signs are usually acute, but may be delayed in cases of unstable fractures or gradual hematoma development. Although uncommon, cauda equina neuritis, also known as polyneuritis equi (PNE), is another specific cause of CES that should be considered [46–49]. This is an inflammatory condition that is thought to be immune mediated and the onset is often insidious. The presence of concurrent clinical signs may help to differentiate individual causes of CES. For example, while disorders such as EHV-1, EPM, and West Nile virus may sometimes cause CES, they are usually associated with additional signs due to the multifocal or diffuse disease associated with these disorders [10, 50]. Additional information about the specific causes and management of CES can be found in appropriate sections in the text.

Diagnostic approach to CES

The accurate diagnosis of CES requires a thorough history, careful physical and neurologic examination, and the use of various ancillary diagnostic techniques. Knowledge of the regional anatomy is helpful in determining the nature and extent of specific neurologic deficits that may be detected.

Obtaining a careful history of the problem is essential, as with any disorder. Owners should be specifically questioned about the potential for trauma, as this is the most common cause. Falling over backward, breeding injuries, lifting by the tail, and other traumatic events all can result in fractures with resultant clinical signs. Ascending infection may be seen in horses that have had a tail injury, had their tails docked recently, or have had a tail block. As information regarding some of these circumstances may not be offered by the owner, specific questioning may be necessary. Information about in-contact animals should be obtained to support EHV-1 infection, and vaccination status for rabies and other encephalitides should be obtained. Access to sorghum or Sudan grass should be ascertained to rule out sorghum cystitis.

A complete physical examination will determine the presence of fever or lethargy suggesting an infectious process. Rectal palpation to determine the presence of rectal impactions and urinary bladder size and tone is important; the sacrum should be carefully palpated to determine if there are any areas of discontinuity, pain, or soft tissue swelling suggesting fracture. Also, the aorta and iliac arteries should be palpated for a pulse.

A complete neurologic evaluation should be completed to localize the neurologic signs and determine if a more widespread problem exists. Presence of cranial nerve signs, specifically wasting of the muscles of the head, would suggest PNE, or other diffuse CNS disease (often infectious). From a consideration of the origin of the nerve tracts, it is clear that spinal cord disease at the level of S2–3 should result in rectal impactions and UI, tail weakness, and hypalgesia of perineal skin. Failure to demonstrate all of these signs would suggest involvement of a nerve root or peripheral nerve, rather than the spinal cord. The presence of all of these signs associated with caudal ataxia suggests spinal cord disease that extends cranial to the limits of the cauda equina.

Routine clinicopathologic tests, including a CBC, blood biochemistry analysis, and urinalyses should be performed. These tests may reveal signs of inflammation, infection, or cystitis. A CSF evaluation is indicated in the evaluation of most cases, and when fluid is collected from the lumbosacral space it may be particularly likely to reflect any changes as it is likely to be close to the lesion. In addition to routine CSF analysis, additional testing, such as immunologic testing for EPM, may be appropriate depending on the specific differentials. Fractures caudal to the second sacral vertebra may not lead to any changes within the CSF. Also, epidural abscesses, discospondylitis, or soft tissue swelling from trauma and fractures are unlikely to result in changes in the CSF. Alternatively, trauma cranial to S2 will usually result in bloody CSF, with a minimally increased WBC count. Bacterial infections will result in an elevated CSF WBC count, while the changes with viral infections are more variable. In EHV-1 myeloencephalitis, the CSF is typically xanthochromic, with an increased protein and minimally increased WBC count. In cases of PNE, CSF protein and WBC count are typically mildly increased, consistent with a mixed nonsuppurative inflammatory response.

Various imaging modalities can be helpful in the diagnostic evaluation of CES, especially because of the common association with trauma. Both percutaneous and transrectal ultrasonography may aid in the examination and have been reported to be abnormal in some cases. Radiography is useful and can be accomplished on foals and smaller horses; more powerful equipment is necessary for adult animals, and it may not be possible even then. Pelvic radiographs taken with the horse anesthetized can be useful and should be considered on a case-by-case basis. Nuclear scintigraphy can be a more sensitive technique for the detection of fractures and infection and has become widely available. Lumbar myelography can be performed and this may delineate extradural compression from tumors, soft tissue swelling, displaced fractures, or hematomas. In smaller patients, advanced imaging such as CT or MRI may be useful.

Needle EMG may be helpful in assessing the extent of muscle denervation and in monitoring progress of the condition, sometimes indicating reinnervation [10]. Also, measurement of conduction velocity across the cauda equina can assist in monitoring progress [10]. Intravesicular and urethral pressure profiles may help in the evaluation of the UI.

Treatment and prognosis

The management of CES includes treatment of the primary cause when possible, supportive care, and in some cases empirical therapy. The specific treatment is determined by the specific etiologic cause giving rise to the clinical signs. For example, if bacterial infection or EPM is suspected or confirmed, appropriate antimicrobial therapy is indicated. Cases suffering from trauma may do well with stall rest and time. Surgical treatment including laminectomies and drainage of abscesses has been described and performed with some success. Additional information regarding treatment for specific conditions causing CES are detailed in appropriate sections throughout the text.

Nursing care is an important component of the management of horses with CES. As with any case involving UI, the incontinence should be managed by frequent drainage and intermittent lavage. Sabulous urolithiasis and urinary tract infection are common complications. Rectal impactions may require manual removal of feces at frequent intervals. Treatment with fecal softeners such as mineral oil and a low bulk diet may aid in the management of such horses. Anti-inflammatory drugs, including corticosteroids, have palliative value in some cases. The prognosis for cases of CES appears to depend primarily on the underlying cause and is hence quite variable.

References

[1] Schott, H.C., Carr, E.A., Patterson, J.S. *et al.* (2004) Urinary incontinence in 37 horses. *Proc Annu Meet Am Assoc Equine Pract*, 50, 345–347.

[2] Holt, P.E. (1997) Urinary incontinence in horses. *Equine Vet J*, 9, 81–84.

[3] Holt, P.E. (1997) Urinary incontinence in mature horses. *Equine Vet Educ*, 9, 85–88.

[4] Bayly, W.M. (2010) Urinary incontinence and bladder dysfunction, in *Equine Internal Medicine* (eds S.M. Reed, W.M. Bayly and D.C. Sellon), Saunders, Philadelphia, pp. 1224–1227.

[5] Odenkirchen, S., Huskamp, B. and Scheidemann, W. (1994) Two congenital anomalies of the urinary tract in warmblood horses: ectopia ureteris and diverticulum vesicae. *Tierarztl Prax*, 22, 462–465.

[6] Laverty, S., Pascoe, J.R., Ling, G.V. *et al.* (1992) Urolithiasis in 68 horses. *Vet Surg*, 21, 56–62.

[7] Schott, H.C. (2006) Urinary incontinence and sabulous cystitis: chicken or egg? *Equine Vet Educ*, 18, 17–19.

[8] Saper, C.B. (2002) The central autonomic nervous system: conscious visceral perception and autonomic pattern generation. *Annu Rev Neurosci*, 25, 433–469.

[9] Fowler, C.J., Griffiths, D. and deGroat, W.C. (2008) The neural control of micturition. *Nat Rev Neurosci*, 9, 453–466.

[10] Mayhew, J. (2009) Urinary bladder distention, dilated rectum and anus, and atonic tail: cauda equina syndrome, in *Large Animal Neurology* (ed. J. Mayhew), Wiley-Blackwell, Oxford, pp. 136–166.

[11] Watanabe, T., Rivas, D.A. and Chancellor, M.B. (1996) Urodynamics of spinal cord injury. *Urol Clin North Am*, 23, 459–473.

[12] Watanabe, T., Vaccaro, A.R., Kumon, H. *et al.* (1998) High incidence of occult neurogenic bladder dysfunction in neurologically intact patients with thoracolumbar spinal injuries. *J Urol*, 159, 965–968.

[13] Doherty, J.G., Burns, A.S., O'Ferrell, D.M. *et al.* (2002) Prevalence of upper motor neuron vs. lower motor neuron lesions in complete lower thoracic and lumbar spinal cord injuries. *J Spinal Cord Med*, 25, 289–292.

[14] Attenburrow, D.P. and James, E.D. (1981) Urinary incontinence in a pony mare. *Equine Vet J*, 13, 206–208.

[15] Holt, P.E. and Mair, T.S. (1990) Ten cases of bladder paralysis associated with sabulous urolithiasis in horses. *Vet Rec*, 127, 108–110.

[16] Friday, P.A., Scarratt, W.K., Elvinger, F. *et al.* (2000) Ataxia and paresis with equine herpesvirus type 1 infection in a herd of riding school horses. *J Vet Intern Med*, 14, 197–201.

[17] Reed, S.M. and Toribio, R.E. (2004) Equine herpesvirus 1 and 4. *Vet Clin North Am Equine Pract*, 20, 631–642.

[18] Wilson, W.D. (1997) Equine herpesvirus 1 myeloencephalopathy. *Vet Clin North Am Equine Pract*, 13, 53–72.

[19] Adams, L.G., Dollahite, J.W., Romane, W.M. *et al.* (1969) Cystitis and ataxia associated with sorghum ingestion by horses. *J Am Vet Med Assoc*, 155, 518–524.

[20] Van Kampen, K.R. (1970) Sudan grass and sorghum poisoning of horses: a possible lathyrogenic disease. *J Am Vet Med Assoc*, 156, 629–630.

[21] Knight, P.R. (1968) Equine cystitis and ataxia associated with grazing of pastures dominated by sorghum species. *Aust Vet J*, 44, 257.

[22] Chaffin, M.K., Honnas, C.M., Crabill, M.R. *et al.* (1995) Cauda equina syndrome, discospondylitis, and a paravertebral abscess caused by Rhodococcus equi in a foal. *J Am Vet Med Assoc*, 206, 215–219.

[23] Cudmore, L.A., Groenendyk, J.C., Hodge, P. and Church, S. (2012) Pyogranulomatous lesion causing neurological signs localized to the sacral region in a horse. *Aust Vet J*, 90, 392–394.

[24] Johnson, J.S., Hibler, C.P., Tillotson, K.M. and Mason, G.L. (2001) Radiculomeningomyelitis due to *Halicephalobus gingivalis* in a horse. *Vet Pathol*, 38, 559–561.

[25] Mayhew, I.G. (1999) The diseased spinal cord. *Proc Annu Meet Am Assoc Equine Pract*, 45, 67–84.

[26] Gehlen, H. and Klug, E. (2001) Urinary incontinence in the mare due to iatrogenic trauma. *Equine Vet Educ*, 13, 183–186.

[27] Kay, A.D. and Lavoie, J.P. (1987) Urethral pressure profilometry in mares. *J Am Vet Med Assoc*, 191, 212–216.

[28] Ronen, N. (1994) Measurements of urethral pressure profiles in the male horse. *Equine Vet J*, 26, 55–58.

[29] Clark, E.S., Semrad, S.D., Bichsel, T. *et al.* (1987) Cystometrography and urethral pressure profiles in healthy horse and pony mares. *Am J Vet Res*, 48, 552–555.

[30] Lane, I.F., Fischer, J.R., Miller, E. *et al.* (2000) Functional urethral obstruction in 3 dogs: clinical and urethral pressure profile findings. *J Vet Intern Med*, 14, 43–49.

[31] Jose-Cunilleras, E. and Hinchcliff, K.W. (1999) Renal pharmacology. *Vet Clin North Am Equine Pract*, 15, 647–664.

[32] Khanna, O.P., Heber, D. and Gonick, P. (1975) Cholinergic and adrenergic neuroreceptors in urinary tract of female dogs. Evaluation of function with pharmacodynamics. *Urology*, 5, 616–623.

[33] Schott HC Urinary incontinence: a drippy problem. Proceedings of the Central Veterinary Conference, August 28–31, Baltimore, MD; 2010.

[34] Keen, J.A. and Pirie, R.S. (2006) Urinary incontinence associated with sabulous urolithiasis: a series of 4 cases. *Equine Vet Educ*, 18, 11–19.

[35] Khanna, O.P. and Gonick, P. (1975) Effects of phenoxybenzamine hydrochloride on canine lower urinary tract: clinical implications. *Urology*, 6, 323–330.

[36] Watson, E.D., McGorum, B.C., Keeling, N. *et al.* (1997) Oestrogen responsive urinary incontinence in two mares. *Equine Vet Educ*, 9, 81–84.

[37] Madison, J.B. (1984) Estrogen responsive urinary incontinence in an aged pony mare. *Compend Contin Educ Pract Vet*, 6, S390–S392.

[38] Rendle, D.I., Durham, A.E., Hughes, K.J. *et al.* (2008) Long-term management of sabulous cystitis in five horses. *Vet Rec*, 162, 783–787.

[39] Schumacher, J. and Brink, P. (2011) Repair of an incompetent urethral sphincter in a mare. *Vet Surg*, 40, 93–96.

[40] Johnson, P.J., Goetz, T.E., Baker, G.J. *et al.* (1987) Treatment of two mares with obstructive (vaginal) urinary outflow incontinence. *J Am Vet Med Assoc*, 191, 973–975.

[41] Sullins, K.E., McIlwraith, C.W., Yovich, J.V. *et al.* (1988) Ectopic ureter managed by unilateral nephrectomy in two female horses. *Equine Vet J*, 20, 463–466.

[42] Squire, K.R. and Adams, S.B. (1992) Bilateral ureterocystostomy in a 450-kg horse with ectopic ureters. *J Am Vet Med Assoc*, 201, 1213–1215.

[43] MacKay, R.J. (1997) Cauda Equina Syndrome, in *Current Therapy in Equine Medicine* (ed. N.E. Robinson), Saunders, Philadelphia, pp. 311–314.

[44] Pirie, R.S. (2003) Bladder, Rectal, Anal, and Tail Paralysis; Perineal Hypalgesia; and Other Signs of Cauda Equina Syndrome, in *Current Therapy in Equine Medicine* (ed. N.E. Robinson), Saunders, Philadelphia, pp. 755–760.

[45] Mukherjee, S., Thakur, B. and Crocker, M. (2013) Cauda equina syndrome: a clinical review for the frontline clinician. *Br J Hosp Med (Lond)*, 4, 460–464.

[46] Wright, J.A., Fordyce, P. and Edington, N. (1987) Neuritis of the cauda equina in the horse. *J Comp Pathol*, 97, 667–675.

[47] Yvorchuk-St Jean, K. (1987) Neuritis of the cauda equina. *Vet Clin North Am Equine Pract*, 3, 421–427.

[48] Hahn, C.N. (2008) Polyneuritis equi: the role of T-lymphocytes and importance of differential clinical signs. *Equine Vet J*, 40, 100.

[49] van Galen, G., Cassart, D., Sandersen, C. *et al.* (2008) The composition of the inflammatory infiltrate in three cases of polyneuritis equi. *Equine Vet J*, 40, 185–188.

[50] Long, M.T. (2010) Flavivirus Infections, in *Equine Infectious Diseases* (eds D. Sellon and M.T. Long), Saunders/Elsevier, St. Louis, pp. 198–206.

13 Differential Diagnosis of Muscle Tremor and Paresis

Amy L. Johnson

New Bolton Center, University of Pennsylvania School of Veterinary Medicine, Kennett Square, USA

Both muscle tremors and weakness are fairly nonspecific clinical signs that can accompany a number of divergent diagnoses. When presented with a trembling horse, the clinician must first determine whether a neurologic problem is the likely cause. Eliminating nonneurologic causes of trembling and weakness can be easier than confirming a diagnosis of neurologic disease. Therefore, clinicians should begin with thorough anamnesis and physical examination to assess whether systemic disease or pain is the likely source of tremors and weakness. Relatively common nonneurologic causes include severe cachexia; visceral or musculoskeletal pain; shock; endotoxemia, systemic inflammatory response syndrome, or both; hypothermia; and various adverse drug reactions or intoxications. When available, hematological and serum biochemical results might assist in evaluation by providing an indication of the systemic health of the patient as well as revealing electrolyte abnormalities that might be contributing to weakness. While mild increases in muscle enzyme activities are often insignificant, moderate to severe increases in an ambulatory patient raise suspicion for a myopathy. However, normal or mildly increased muscle enzyme activities do not eliminate the possibility of a myopathy.

If nonneurologic problems are deemed unlikely causes of the patient's tremors and paresis, neurologic diseases should be considered. In clinical neurology, paresis is defined as "a deficiency in the generation of gait or the ability to support weight" and it has two qualities: upper motor neuron (UMN) and lower motor neuron (LMN, also known as neuromuscular) [1]. UMN paresis is almost always accompanied by general proprioceptive (GP or "spinal") ataxia and is rarely accompanied by noteworthy tremors. Conversely, LMN (neuromuscular) paresis is frequently characterized by trembling.

Neuromuscular disease occurs due to dysfunction in any part of the motor unit, including the LMN and all the muscle cells it innervates. This unit can be affected at any level: the LMN cell body within the ventral gray column of the spinal cord; the LMN axon as it courses through the ventral root, spinal nerve, and peripheral nerve; the neuromuscular junction; or the muscle cell. Clinical signs are similar regardless of whether the motor unit is affected at the level of the spinal cord or at the level of the muscle cell. Therefore, myelopathies (or neuronopathies), neuropathies, junctionopathies, and myopathies often need to be considered simultaneously in the differential diagnosis of muscle tremor and paresis.

In addition to the affected part of the motor unit, neuromuscular disease can be characterized as diffuse or focal. This determination is more clinically useful and will guide the differential list. Signs of diffuse neuromuscular disease include a short-strided gait, base-narrow stance ("elephant on a ball" or "pedestal" stance), frequent weight-shifting or restlessness, and generalized muscle atrophy. Progressive disease can lead to flaccid paralysis with loss of tone and reflexes. Low head and neck carriage is common. If cranial nerves are affected, dysphagia, dysphonia, and dyspnea might be observed, and tone might be noticeably decreased in ears, eyelids, jaw, or lips. The most common causes of diffuse neuromuscular disease in horses include botulism, equine motor neuron disease (EMND), and various myopathies. Tick paralysis is also important in Australia. Signs of focal neuromuscular disease vary depending on the peripheral nerves or muscles involved. The horse might have an abnormal gait that mimics an orthopedic lameness. The limb might tremor or collapse upon weight-bearing. Focal muscle atrophy might be observed. Common causes of focal neuromuscular disease include trauma, compressive injury, and equine protozoal myeloencephalitis (EPM).

Equine Neurology, Second Edition. Martin Furr and Stephen Reed.

© 2015 John Wiley & Sons, Inc. Published 2015 by John Wiley & Sons, Inc.

Companion website: www.wiley.com/go/furr/neurology

Differentials for diffuse neuromuscular disease

Historical details, signalment, physical examination findings, and muscle enzyme activities often allow the clinician to arrive at a presumptive diagnosis, although more specialized testing is usually necessary for confirmation (Table 13.1).

Botulism

Botulism (see Chapter 25) should immediately be considered as a potential cause of diffuse neuromuscular disease so that antitoxin treatment can be administered as soon as possible [2]. Historical details of importance include endemic region (especially mid-Atlantic region and Kentucky), vaccination status, access to large hay bales, carrion contamination of feed, and recent wounds. This disease usually has an acute onset and short clinical course in accordance with the severity of intoxication. Horses exposed to high doses of toxin can show severe generalized weakness or death due to respiratory failure within 6–12 h, whereas horses exposed to low doses might only show mild clinical signs 10–14 days later. In addition to the aforementioned signs, botulism causes decreased tongue, eyelid, tail, and anal tone; mydriasis with decreased pupillary light reflexes; dysphagia; and decreased gastrointestinal borborygmi. Two clinical tests that are used to support a diagnosis of botulism are the tongue stress test and the grain test. To assess tongue strength, the examiner should gently withdraw the tongue through the interdental space while holding the jaws closed with the other arm. Normal horses should quickly retract the tongue back into the mouth with one or two contractions; horses with botulism are unable or slow to pull the tongue into the mouth (Figure 13.1). To perform the grain test, the horse is offered 8 oz of grain in a flat feeding tub on the ground. If the horse takes longer than 2 min to consume the grain, the test is abnormal. Horses with botulism usually have normal muscle enzyme activities unless signs have progressed to frequent or prolonged recumbency. Laboratory testing includes mouse bioassay to confirm botulinum toxin in suspect feed or patient samples (gastrointestinal contents, manure, or wound discharge), as well as PCR assays to detect the botulinum toxin gene [3].

Equine motor neuron disease

EMND (see Chapter 26) is most common in the northeast United States and in horses with no access to green pasture or good-quality hay for prolonged periods [4]. EMND generally has a more protracted clinical course than botulism. Weight loss due to generalized, symmetric muscle atrophy is often present. In addition to the short-strided gait, low head and neck carriage, and base-narrow stance characteristic of neuromuscular disease (Figure 13.2), horses with EMND often have a raised tailhead and increased sweating. These horses often appear more comfortable walking than standing still due to the relative

Table 13.1 Common causes of diffuse neuromuscular disease.

Disease	Notes/common features
Botulism	Endemic region; history of exposure to round (large) bale hay or carrion; cranial nerve abnormalities especially dysphagia
EMND	Weight loss; lack of access to green pasture/hay; mild increases in muscle enzyme activities; normal cranial nerve function
Myopathies	See Table 13.2. Usually moderate to marked increases in muscle enzyme activities (with certain exceptions)
Tick paralysis	Australia; exposure to *Ixodes holocyclus* tick; smaller horse size
Viral encephalomyelitis	West Nile virus and rabies can cause polioencephalomyelitis; usually accompanied by ataxia and change in behavior

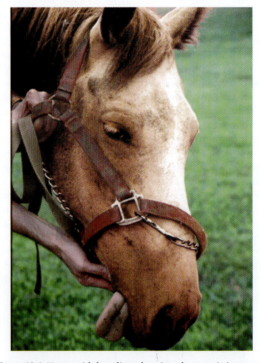

Figure 13.1 Horse with botulism showing characteristic tongue weakness with inability to retract the tongue back into the mouth.

sparing of type II muscle fibers as compared with type I muscle fibers. Notably, horses with EMND are not dysphagic and should not have any cranial nerve abnormalities. Fundic examination might reveal brown pigment deposits characteristic of lipofuscin. Mild to moderate increases in muscle enzyme activities are typical. Low serum vitamin E levels are supportive of the disease. More definitive diagnosis can be pursued through biopsy of the sacrocaudalis dorsalis medialis muscle or the ventral branch of the spinal accessory nerve.

Myopathies

Myopathies are a frequent cause of muscle tremors and paresis. Many different muscle disorders have been described in horses, and some of the more common diseases are listed in Table 13.2; for more thorough review,

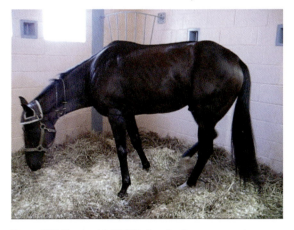

Figure 13.2 Horse with EMND showing base-narrow stance characteristic of diffuse neuromuscular disease. Note low head and neck carriage and shifting weight.

the reader is referred elsewhere [5, 6]. If a history of exercise precedes clinical signs, exertional myopathies should be considered. Sporadic causes of exertional rhabdomyolysis include dietary imbalances and overexertion, while chronic causes include recurrent exertional rhabdomyolysis (primarily in Thoroughbreds) and polysaccharide storage myopathy (PSSM; primarily in Quarter Horse-type, warmblood, and draft breeds). The most common causes of nonexertional rhabdomyolysis include nutritional myodegeneration due to selenium and vitamin E deficiency, infectious or immune-mediated myositis, or toxins such as hypoglycin A and organophosphates [7, 8]. Horses with the aforementioned myopathies generally have marked increases in muscle enzyme activities, although some horses with PSSMs only have mild or moderate increases. Biopsy of an affected muscle should allow definitive diagnosis; genetic testing is also available for type I PSSM. In contrast, muscle disorders characterized by abnormal muscle membrane conduction will not show large increases in muscle enzyme activities or histologic abnormalities. One important example is hyperkalemic periodic paralysis in Quarter Horse-type breeds, for which genetic testing is available.

Tick paralysis (Australia)

Tick paralysis is an important cause of diffuse neuromuscular disease in the eastern parts of Australia (Queensland and New South Wales) where the *Ixodes holocyclus* tick is found [9, 10]. Although *Dermacentor* spp. ticks cause tick paralysis in small animals in North America, they are generally associated with less severe disease than that caused by *Ixodes*, and equine tick paralysis has not been described in North America. Typical clinical signs of LMN dysfunction predominate and have been described as an ascending flaccid paresis to paralysis, affecting first

Table 13.2 Common myopathies.

Disease	Notes/common features
HYPP (hyperkalemic periodic paralysis)	QH-type breed; descendant "Impressive"; genetic disease—mutation in α-subunit of skeletal muscle sodium channel, *SCN4A* gene; normal muscle enzyme activities but increased potassium level
PSSM (polysaccharide storage myopathy)	QH, draft, or WB breed; type 1 is genetic disease—mutation in glycogen synthase, *GYS1* gene; muscle enzyme activities variable
RER (recurrent exertional rhabdomyolysis)	TB breed; associated with exercise; autosomal dominant with variable expression; abnormal intracellular calcium regulation
Nutritional myodegeneration	Dietary deficiency of selenium and vitamin E; usually foals; markedly increased CK and AST activities
Seasonal pasture (atypical) myopathy	Grazing equids; exposure to box elder seeds (hypoglycin A); fall season; markedly increased CK and AST activities; frequently fatal
Immune-mediated myositis	Secondary to infectious diseases (particularly *Streptococcus equi equi*)

AST, aspartate aminotransferase; CK, creatine kinase; QH, Quarter Horse; TB, Thoroughbred; WB, warmblood.

the pelvic limbs, then the thoracic limbs, and finally the respiratory muscles. Dysphagia is not a typical finding although abnormal phonation has been noted. Index of suspicion for this disease should be increased if the horse lives in a tick-endemic area, has skin lesions suggestive of prior tick attachment, or has attached ticks identified as *Ixodes holocyclus*. Smaller horses (<100 kg) appear to be at higher risk of developing disease.

Less common causes of diffuse neuromuscular disease
Infectious
Viral encephalitides such as rabies and West Nile virus (WNV) (see Chapters 19 and 20) can cause diffuse polioencephalomyelitis and therefore can cause signs compatible with diffuse neuromuscular disease [11]. WNV causes notable muscle fasciculations in approximately 50% of cases [12]. Most cases would have additional signs of neurologic disease including changes in behavior (obtundation or hyperresponsiveness) and ataxia. Antemortem diagnosis of WNV is most commonly made via serum immunoglobulin M (IgM) capture ELISA. Diagnosis of rabies can only be achieved postmortem; relatively rapid clinical deterioration is expected.

Although uncommon in horses [13], bacterial meningoencephalitis (see Chapter 21) can cause generalized paresis and trembling. Specifically, neuroborreliosis (infection due to *Borrelia burgdorferi*) is likely to cause meningitis, neuritis, and radiculoneuritis with subsequent tremors and paresis [14]. Cerebrospinal fluid (CSF) analysis is likely to be abnormal, usually with a neutrophilic pleocytosis, and positive culture or PCR results can confirm bacterial infection. Evidence of intrathecal antibody production (serum and CSF paired testing as described in Chapter 3) against *Borrelia* can also be useful for diagnosis.

Metabolic
Metabolic abnormalities including derangements in calcium, potassium, and magnesium can affect neuromuscular transmission [15, 16]. Hypocalcemia usually leads to the most severe signs, known as hypocalcemic tetany. Although horses may have diffuse tremors and difficulty rising or ambulating, the perceived weakness is due to tetany (sustained muscular contraction) as opposed to the flaccid paresis or paralysis resulting from a lesion in the neuromuscular system. Hypokalemia and hypomagnesemia can worsen signs in animals with neuromuscular problems or contribute to weakness in systemically compromised patients but would be unusual sole causes of diffuse weakness in horses.

Drug- or anesthesia-related
Several drugs commonly used in equine medicine affect neuromuscular transmission. These medications are highly unlikely to induce clinical signs in otherwise healthy patients but might worsen signs in patients with neuromuscular disease. Therefore, medications such as aminoglycosides, antiarrhythmics, metronidazole, and procaine penicillin are contraindicated in horses with neuromuscular disease. For a more complete list of drugs associated with altered neuromuscular transmission, refer to Ref. [17].

A stressful but rare scenario is the horse that peracutely shows signs of diffuse neuromuscular disease following anesthesia and is recumbent and unable to rise. The two most important differentials include a previously unrecognized myopathy and hemorrhagic myelomalacia [18]. If a myopathy is the cause, markedly increased muscle enzyme activities would be expected. Myoglobinuria might also be observed. If appropriate supportive care is provided, including the provision of a high-fat diet, intravenous lipid infusion, or both, recovery would be anticipated. If hemorrhagic poliomyelomalacia is the cause, a grave prognosis is warranted. Horses with this condition rapidly deteriorate, showing progressive loss of motor and sensory function.

Intoxications, infestations, and envenomations
Lead toxicosis is rare in horses but has been described in horses that have ingested paint, motor oil, or pasture contaminated by lead from mining or smelting operations [19]. Clinical signs are variable but might mimic those of EMND; two horses with lead toxicosis were reported to show a "camped-under" posture, spontaneous muscle fasciculations in all major muscle groups, sweating, weight loss despite a good appetite, and increased muscle enzyme activities [19]. Additional clinical signs reported with lead intoxication include laryngeal and/or pharyngeal dysfunction, rough hair coat, anorexia, seizures, and incoordination.

Not to be confused with tick paralysis, tick myotonia has been described in the United States in horses infested with *Otobius megnini* (ear tick) [20]. Signs included severe muscle cramping, tremors, and fasciculations with percussion-induced myotonia.

Snake envenomation is a very rare cause of diffuse neuromuscular disease in the horse [21]. Myasthenia gravis and polyradiculoneuritis (Coonhound paralysis) are well described in small animals but poorly described or recognized in horses.

Differentials for focal neuromuscular disease

Focal neuromuscular disease most commonly arises from damage to a nerve, plexus, or localized region of gray matter within the spinal cord. Clinical signs can be quite variable depending on the location of the lesions, ranging from facial paralysis to gait deficits mimicking orthopedic lameness to tail paralysis. Depending on severity and chronicity, marked focal muscle atrophy might be present. An important yet challenging task in assessing horses with focal neuromuscular disease is localizing the lesion to the central or peripheral nervous system (Table 13.3). Differential diagnoses for peripheral nervous system disease include trauma (common), infectious or noninfectious neuritis (less common), and neoplasia (less common). If a focal lesion within the central nervous system (spinal cord or brainstem) is responsible for signs of neuromuscular disease, the differential diagnoses list will change to include infectious diseases such as EPM or diseases that cause focal spinal cord compression. The distinction between peripheral and central disease is made through careful clinical examination and ancillary diagnostic testing. Although central diseases may be markedly asymmetric and cause obvious clinical signs in only one limb, subtle signs of similar dysfunction may be evident in the contralateral limb. Electromyography might be useful in these situations, showing mild signs of denervation such as occasional fibrillation potentials or positive sharp waves in the questionably affected limb. CSF analysis will sometimes assist in confirming a central disease process, although not all central diseases alter CSF composition.

Peripheral causes of focal neuromuscular disease

Trauma
Trauma is one of the most important causes of nerve damage and is discussed in greater detail in Chapter 33. Characteristic gait deficits develop with trauma to certain nerves. In brief, radial and femoral neuropathies result in an inability to support weight on the affected limbs, suprascapular neuropathy leads to lateral movement of the shoulder during weight-bearing, obturator neuropathy prevents adduction of the pelvic limb, and sciatic neuropathy causes dragging of the pelvic limb with extension of the stifle and hock and knuckling of the fetlock. Gluteal nerve damage can cause profound atrophy of the proximal pelvic limb

musculature without gait deficits. Damage to these nerves may occur via external trauma (blunt impact, compression, or penetrating) or internal trauma. Long bone, pelvic, or axial skeleton fractures can traumatize nerves or their roots. Diagnosis of a traumatic neuropathy is often achieved through radiographic or sonographic evidence of perineural trauma. Although nerve conduction velocity testing could assist in documenting nerve damage, this modality is rarely utilized in clinical cases.

Neuritis
Neuritis is less commonly described in horses. Infection or inflammation in structures adjacent to nerves may cause a secondary neuritis; one example is guttural pouch mycosis causing hypoglossal neuritis and lingual hemiplegia [22]. Polyneuritis equi is a rare but important cause of neuritis in horses; this disease generally causes signs of dysfunction in structures innervated by the cauda equina or cranial nerves but can also cause pelvic limb abnormalities including paresis and tremor. Presumptive diagnosis of polyneuritis equi is generally based on clinical signs and exclusion of other potential causes such as sacral fracture or EPM. However, more definitive diagnosis via muscle biopsy and transrectal sonography has been described [23].

Neoplasia
Neoplasia can cause nerve damage through compression or infiltration. Although both benign and malignant nerve sheath tumors have been described in horses, they are a much less common cause of neuropathy in horses compared with other species. Lymphoma is a more common neoplasia to affect nerves in horses [24]. Sonographic examination and biopsy can allow diagnosis in the living horse.

Diseases of the axial skeleton can affect peripheral or central parts of the nervous system to cause signs of focal neuromuscular disease. Cervical vertebral compressive myelopathy, discospondylitis, vertebral osteomyelitis, and vertebral fractures or subluxations can all

Table 13.3 Common causes of focal neuromuscular disease.

Disease	Notes/common features
Trauma	Can affect peripheral or central nervous system (nerves, nerve roots, spinal cord)
Neuritis	Due to extension of local inflammatory process or immune-mediated mechanisms (polyneuritis equi)
Neoplasia	Lymphoma, melanoma most common; can cause peripheral or central damage
Equine protozoal myeloencephalitis	Affects brainstem or spinal cord but can cause very focal deficits
Lyme neuroborreliosis	Meningitis, polyradiculoneuritis, and neuritis can cause focal or diffuse signs
Vertebral disease	Cervical vertebral compressive myelopathy, vertebral osteomyelitis, and discospondylitis can affect ventral gray column or nerve roots

impinge on nerve roots and spinal nerves, causing injury through direct compression or trauma as well as through inflammatory mechanisms. Radiography and myelography might show changes in the cervical vertebral column that are consistent with these conditions although confirmation of nerve compression is difficult with imaging studies. Limitations of conventional radiography often preclude full evaluation of the thoracolumbar vertebral column in adult horses, and nuclear scintigraphy is frequently used to evaluate this region instead. A combination of imaging abnormalities with other clinical evidence of nerve disease such as focal atrophy or electromyographic abnormalities (with ventral nerve root involvement) or focal hypalgesia (with dorsal nerve root involvement) provides the strongest evidence for diagnosis.

Central causes of focal neuromuscular disease
Infectious

The most common central nervous system disease to cause signs of focal neuromuscular disease is EPM, which is discussed in detail in Chapter 22. This disease can cause a plethora of abnormalities but most commonly causes a combination of UMN/GP and LMN signs. However, lesions confined to the gray matter can cause focal neuromuscular dysfunction in the absence of any other clinical signs. Diagnosis is generally based on clinical neurologic evaluation compatible with central nervous system disease, exclusion of other likely diagnoses, and

proof of exposure to the protozoan parasite (ideally, with evidence of intrathecal antibody production).

Although much less common than EPM, central nervous system infection with *Borrelia burgdorferi* can lead to meningoencephalomyelitis and radiculoneuritis with associated muscle tremors, atrophy, and weakness [25]. Signs can be diffuse or focal depending on the extent of infection and resulting inflammation. As with EPM, diagnosis should be based on the presence of neurologic disease, exclusion of other likely causes, and proof of exposure to the spirochete (ideally with evidence of intrathecal antibody production). In the author's experience, horses with Lyme neuroborreliosis tend to have a prolonged disease course, often having shown abnormalities for months; abnormal CSF cytology, usually a neutrophilic pleocytosis; and a combination of muscle atrophy, muscle tremors or fasciculations, and cranial nerve abnormalities (particularly CN 7–12).

Although in theory other infectious viral, bacterial, fungal, and parasitic agents could affect gray matter of the spinal cord or nerve roots and lead to signs of focal neuromuscular disease, most of these organisms tend to cause more prominent clinical signs of white matter or brain disease and so are less easily confused with diseases that cause focal neuromuscular signs.

Noninfectious

Any space-occupying mass that affects predominantly gray matter of the spinal cord could cause signs of focal neuromuscular disease. Clinical signs are most evident

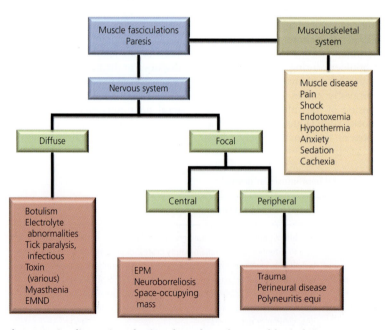

Figure 13.3 Flowchart demonstrating diagnostic evaluation of muscle weakness and fasciculations.

when either the cervical or the lumbosacral intumescence is affected. Generally, masses that affect gray matter in the cervical intumescence will also cause signs of UMN/GP dysfunction in the pelvic limbs, aiding in neurolocalization. Occasionally, lesions that are ventral to the cervical intumescence cause such mild pelvic limb signs and such severe thoracic limb signs that they mimic problems of the brachial plexuses or nerves. Masses affecting the lumbosacral intumescence cause pelvic limb problems without corresponding thoracic limb abnormalities. Although bilateral peripheral disease is possible, signs in both pelvic limbs should point the examiner toward spinal cord disease as opposed to bilateral plexus or nerve disease.

Abscesses, granulomas, cysts, and neoplasms can all cause compression of the spinal cord. Of these, neoplasms are most commonly reported in horses, including melanoma [26], undifferentiated sarcoma [27], angiosarcoma [28], hemangiosarcoma [29], plasma cell myeloma [30], and lymphoma [31].

As discussed under peripheral causes of focal neuromuscular disease, diseases of the axial skeleton can affect the spinal cord as well.

In summary, horses with signs of muscle tremor and paresis should be characterized as having diffuse or focal signs (Figure 13.3). Those with diffuse disease should immediately be evaluated for botulism, and EMND and myopathies should also be considered. Those with focal disease should be carefully evaluated for indications of central nervous system involvement. If a peripheral lesion is suspected, trauma and perineural disease (infection, inflammation, neoplasia) are likely causes. If central disease is likely, EPM should be an immediate consideration with Lyme neuroborreliosis and space-occupying masses other possibilities.

References

[1] de Lahunta, A. and Glass, E. (2009) The neurologic examination, in *Veterinary Neuroanatomy and Clinical Neurology*, 3rd edn (eds A. de Lahunta and E. Glass), W.B. Saunders, St. Louis, pp. 487–501.

[2] Whitlock, R.H. and McAdams, S. (2006) Equine botulism. *Clin Tech Equine Pract*, 5, 37–42.

[3] Johnson, A.L., Sweeney, R.W., McAdams, S.C. *et al.* (2012) Quantitative real-time PCR for detection of the neurotoxin gene of *Clostridium botulinum* type B in equine and bovine samples. *Vet J*, 194, 118–120.

[4] Divers, T.J., Mohammed, H.O., Cummings, J.F. *et al.* (1994) Equine motor neuron disease: findings in 28 horses and proposal of a pathophysiological mechanism for the disease. *Equine Vet J*, 26, 409–415.

[5] Aleman, M. (2008) A review of equine muscle disorders. *Neuromuscul Disord*, 18, 277–287.

[6] Valberg, S.J. (2009) Diseases of muscles, in *Large Animal Internal Medicine*, 4th edn (ed. B.P. Smith), Mosby, St. Louis, pp. 1388–1418.

[7] Valberg, S.J., Sponseller, B.T., Hegeman, A.D. *et al.* (2013) Seasonal pasture myopathy/atypical myopathy in North America associated with ingestion of hypoglycin A within seeds of the box elder tree. *Equine Vet J*, 45, 419–426.

[8] Myers, C.J., Aleman, M., Heidmann, P. *et al.* (2006) Myopathy in American miniature horses. *Equine Vet J*, 38, 272–276.

[9] Tee, S.Y. and Feary, D.J. (2012) Suspected tick paralysis (*Ixodes holocyclus*) in a miniature horse. *Aust Vet J*, 90, 181–185.

[10] Ruppin, M., Sullivan, S., Condon, F. *et al.* (2012) Retrospective study of 103 presumed cases of tick (*Ixodes holocyclus*) envenomation in the horse. *Aust Vet J*, 90, 175–180.

[11] Summers, B.A., Cummings, J.F. and de Lahunta, A. (1995) Inflammatory diseases of the central nervous system, in *Veterinary Neuropathology*, 1st edn (eds B.A. Summers, J.F. Cummings and A. de Lahunta), Mosby, St. Louis, pp. 95–188.

[12] Ward, M.P., Schuermann, J.A., Highfield, L.D. *et al.* (2006) Characteristics of an outbreak of West Nile virus encephalomyelitis in a previously uninfected population of horses. *Vet Microbiol*, 118, 255–259.

[13] Toth, B., Aleman, M., Nogradi, N. *et al.* (2012) Meningitis and meningoencephalomyelitis in horses: 28 cases (1985–2010). *J Am Vet Med Assoc*, 240, 580–587.

[14] James, F.M., Engiles, J.B. and Beech, J. (2010) Meningitis, cranial neuritis, and radiculoneuritis associated with Borrelia burgdorferi infection in a horse. *J Am Vet Med Assoc*, 237, 1180–1185.

[15] Toribio, R.E. (2011) Disorders of calcium and phosphate metabolism in horses. *Vet Clin North Am Equine Pract*, 27, 129–147.

[16] Stewart, A.J. (2011) Magnesium disorders in horses. *Vet Clin North Am Equine Pract*, 27, 149–163.

[17] Aleman, M. (2011) Miscellaneous neurologic or neuromuscular disorders in horses. *Vet Clin North Am Equine Pract*, 27, 481–506.

[18] Lerche, E., Laverty, S., Blais, D. *et al.* (1993) Hemorrhagic myelomalacia following general anesthesia in a horse. *Cornell Vet*, 83, 267–273.

[19] Sojka, J.E., Hope, W. and Pearson, D. (1996) Lead toxicosis in 2 horses: similarity to equine degenerative lower motor neuron disease. *J Vet Intern Med*, 10, 420–423.

[20] Madigan, J.E., Valberg, S.J., Ragle, C. and Moody, J.L. (1995) Muscle spasms associated with ear tick (*Otobius megnini*) infestations in five horses. *J Am Vet Med Assoc*, 207, 74–76.

[21] Fitzgerald, W.E. (1975) Snakebite in the horse. *Aust Vet J*, 51, 37–39.

[22] Kipar, A. and Frese, K. (1993) Hypoglossal neuritis with associated lingual hemiplegia secondary to guttural pouch mycosis. *Vet Pathol*, 30, 574–576.

[23] Aleman, M., Katzman, S.A., Vaughan, B. *et al.* (2009) Antemortem diagnosis of polyneuritis equi. *J Vet Intern Med*, 23, 665–668.

[24] de Lahunta, A. and Glass, E. (2009) Lower motor neuron: spinal nerve, general somatic efferent system, in *Veterinary Neuroanatomy and Clinical Neurology*, 3rd edn (eds A. de Lahunta and E. Glass), W.B. Saunders, St. Louis, pp. 77–133.

[25] Imai, D.M., Barr, B.C., Daft, B. *et al.* (2011) Lyme neuroborreliosis in 2 horses. *Vet Pathol*, 48, 1151–1157.

[26] Traver, D.S., Moore, J.N., Thornburg, L.P. *et al.* (1977) Epidural melanoma causing posterior paresis in a horse. *J Am Vet Med Assoc*, 170, 1400–1403.

[27] Van Biervliet, J., Alcaraz, A., Jackson, C.A. *et al.* (2004) Extradural undifferentiated sarcoma causing spinal cord compression in 2 horses. *J Vet Intern Med*, 18, 248–251.

[28] Kennedy, F.A. and Brown, C.M. (1993) Vertebral angiosarcoma in a horse. *J Vet Diagn Invest*, 5, 125–127.

[29] Newton-Clarke, M.J., Guffoy, M.R., Dykes, N.L. *et al.* (1994) Ataxia due to a vertebral haemangiosarcoma in a horse. *Vet Rec*, 135, 182–184.

[30] Drew, R.A. and Greatorex, J.C. (1974) Vertebral plasma cell myeloma causing posterior paralysis in a horse. *Equine Vet J*, 6, 131–134.

[31] Zeman, D.H., Snider, T.G., 3rd and McClure, J.J. (1989) Vertebral lymphosarcoma as the cause of hind limb paresis in a horse. *J Vet Diagn Invest*, 1, 187–188.

14 Electrodiagnostic Evaluation of the Nervous System

George M. Strain[1], Frank Andrews[1], and Veronique A. Lacombe[2]

[1] School of Veterinary Medicine, Louisiana State University, Baton Rouge, USA
[2] Center for Veterinary Health Sciences, Oklahoma State University, Stillwater, USA

Evaluation of the nervous system in horses requires a comprehensive approach that includes signalment, history, and complete physical and neurologic examinations. The overall goal of a comprehensive approach is to confirm the presence or absence of neurologic disease and to localize the lesion to a focal or multifocal area of the nervous system. Once the horse has been examined, electrodiagnostic aids can be used to further refine and localize lesions within the nervous system and to differentiate neurologic from musculoskeletal disease. Abbreviations used in this chapter are listed in Table 14.1.

Neurologic disease is characterized by altered cell electrical activity, and these changes can only be measured by specialized electronic equipment. The branch of medical science that measures this electrical activity is referred to as electrodiagnostics or clinical neurophysiology. Electromyography (EMG), brainstem auditory evoked response (BAER) testing, visual and somatosensory evoked potentials, and electroencephalography (EEG) are electrodiagnostic aids that help localize, diagnose, and aid in the prognosis of neurologic diseases. EMG (needle EMG) and nerve conduction studies (NCS) are used to evaluate lesions of the lower motor neuron or motor unit. In addition, the use of magnetic motor evoked potentials (MMEPs) can be coupled with an EMG to assess the functional integrity of motor pathways in the spinal cord [1], as can the F wave and Hofmann's reflex. The presence of disease affecting the vestibulocochlear nerve (CN VIII) and its pathways within the brainstem can be evaluated using BAER testing, while the somatosensory evoked potential (SEP) is used to assess ascending somatosensory pathways to the cortex. The electroretinogram (ERG) assesses the integrity of neural elements of the retina, while the visual evoked potential (VEP) is used to assess postretinal visual pathways. EEG is used to identify focal and diffuse cerebral lesions. These diagnostic aids, separately or collectively, should always be used in conjunction with a complete neurologic examination and can provide valuable information about the function of the neurologic system. These techniques are relatively noninvasive and, in many cases, can be done with mild sedation in the standing horse. Even when these techniques do not provide the information necessary to arrive at a diagnosis, they provide a more complete understanding of the disease process and with serial examinations can help monitor disease progression, inform treatment options, and determine prognosis. All of these techniques are utilized extensively in human neurology, and officially accepted standards for their use have been developed and promulgated by the International Federation of Clinical Neurophysiology [2]. This document provides a valuable resource for the use of these electrodiagnostic tests in veterinary applications.

Nerve cell responses to injury can include (i) Schwann cell damage, resulting in segmental demyelination and slowed or blocked conduction; (ii) axon damage, leading in Wallerian degeneration of the distal portion of the axon; or (iii) dying-back neuropathies, where there is a diminished response to nerve stimulation. Nerve injury can be (i) neurapraxia, with paralysis followed by rapid (minutes to weeks) recovery of function, and conduction loss without axon structural change; (ii) axonotmesis, with break in axon continuity without loss of support cells, and possible regeneration at 1–2 mm/day, taking months to years for full regeneration; or (iii) neurotmesis, where there is complete transection of axon and support structures and little chance of regeneration without surgical intervention.

Muscle responses to injury can be either (i) shorter-duration and smaller-amplitude muscle motor unit action potentials (MUAPs) when muscle is damaged or (ii) denervation hypersensitivity with denervation. Processes affecting the neuromuscular junction result in diminished or absent responses to nerve stimulation.

Equine Neurology, Second Edition. Martin Furr and Stephen Reed.
© 2015 John Wiley & Sons, Inc. Published 2015 by John Wiley & Sons, Inc.
Companion website: www.wiley.com/go/furr/neurology

Table 14.1 Abbreviations.

BAER	Brainstem auditory evoked response
CRD	Complex repetitive discharge
EEG	Electroencephalogram
EMG	Electromyography, electromyogram
ERG	Electroretinogram
MEPP	Miniature end-plate potential
MMEP	Magnetic motor evoked potential
MNCV	Motor nerve conduction velocity
MUAP	Motor unit action potential
NCS	Nerve conduction studies
NCV	Nerve conduction velocity
QEMG	Quantitative electromyography
SEP	Somatosensory evoked potential
SNCV	Sensory nerve conduction velocity
VEP	Visual evoked potential

Electromyography

Needle EMG is the graphic recording of muscle cell electrical activity—during contraction or at rest—from a recording electrode placed in the muscle and does not involve muscle or nerve stimulation. The electrical activity of the muscle is amplified and converted into a digital and audio signal for capture by a computer. NCS, on the other hand, involve stimulating peripheral nerves with electrical current and recording the resultant physiologic electrical activity from other segments of the nerve or from the muscles innervated by that nerve. Together, EMG and NCS aid in the localization, diagnosis, and prognosis of diseases of the motor unit, which consists of the ventral horn motor neuron cell body (located in the ventral horn of the spinal cord or brainstem), its axon (ventral root), peripheral nerve, myoneural junction, and the muscle fibers it innervates [3–7]. The innervated muscle fibers can be classified as either slow-twitch or fast-twitch. Slow-twitch (tonic, type I) motor units fire in the frequency range of 70–125 Hz, while fast-twitch (phasic, type II) motor units fire in the frequency range of 126–250 Hz [8]. An anatomic knowledge of the major muscles, nerves, and nerve roots is important for optimizing the clinical information that can be gleaned from an EMG examination (Table 14.2).

Instrumentation

Commercially available electromyographs are appropriate for examination of horses. The essential components of electromyographs are needle electrodes for recording electrical activity arising from muscles, a preamplifier and amplifier to amplify the small-voltage signal in the muscle fibers, and a computer

monitor with attached speakers for viewing and hearing the high-frequency muscle electrical potentials. Auditory output is essential since electromyographic potentials produce characteristic sounds that help to identify the visual signal. Also included are image and auditory capture systems for storage on a hard drive or portable media.

Several types of electrodes are available for use in recording the EMG: adhesive surface disc electrodes, monopolar needle electrodes, concentric needle electrodes, and single-fiber electrodes. In all configurations, three electrodes are used: an active (exploring) electrode, a reference electrode, and a ground electrode to minimize electrical interference. Self-adhesive surface electrodes designed for human use have been utilized in horses but may be restricted to recording electrical activity from superficial muscles and usually require shaving hair for adequate adhesion [9]. Standard disposable monopolar and concentric needle electrodes, ranging from 25 to 100 mm in length with diameters of 0.45–0.8 mm, are most commonly used for electromyographic examination in horses. These electrodes provide a sampling area of approximately 0.068 mm², which corresponds to approximately 30–50 muscle fibers.

Active, or exploring, electrodes can either be monopolar or be concentric (coaxial) bipolar needles. Concentric electrodes typically consist of an outer 26-gauge needle (reference) that is insulated except at its tip, with a central 0.1 mm wire serving as the active electrode. The exposed tip area measures $150 \times 600\,\mu m$. This limits the explored area. The ground electrode is inserted in the subcutaneous tissue, often over or near a bony prominence (wing of atlas, spine of scapula, tuber coxae, or tuber ischii). The concentric electrode is inserted into the muscle of interest, and muscle electrical activity is recorded. Approximately 50 muscle fibers, an area with a 0.5-mm radius around the needle electrode, contribute to the majority of the observed electrical potential [10]. Concentric needle electrodes with two contained wires are also available where the needle serves as the ground and the wires in the needle are the active and reference electrodes. These electrodes are larger in diameter (23-gauge) but permit sampling of a much smaller area of muscle tissue. Concentric needle electrodes have high electrical impedance due to the limited areas of uninsulated metal.

Electromyographic examination can also be done using three monopolar electrodes: the uninsulated ground electrode (typically 12 mm, 30-gauge), which is placed in the subcutaneous tissue; an identical reference electrode placed in the subcutaneous tissue between the ground electrode and muscle to be explored; and the exploring electrode (25–100 mm, 28-gauge, insulated except for the distal 0.2–0.4 mm), which is inserted in the muscle of interest. The recorded signal reflects all

Table 14.2 Muscles, nerves, and nerve roots evaluated during a routine electromyographic examination.

Muscle	Peripheral nerve	Spinal nerve root
Rear limb		
Long digital extensor	Peroneal	L6 to S1
Gastrocnemius	Tibial	S1 to S2
Deep digital flexor	Tibial	S1 to S2
Semimembranosus	Ischiatic	L5 to S2
Vastus lateralis	Femoral	L4 to L6
Biceps femoris	Caudal gluteal, ischiatic, peroneal	L6 to S2
Middle gluteal	Cranial and caudal gluteal	L5 to S2
Paravertebral		
Paravertebral muscle (segmentally)	Dorsal branches of ventral spinal	L6 to C1
Forelimb		
Subclavian	Pectoral	C6, C7 (T1)
Supraspinatus and infraspinatus	Suprascapular	C6, C7, C8
Deltoideus	Axillary	C6, C7, C8
Biceps brachii	Musculocutaneous	C6, C7, C8
Triceps brachii	Radial	C7, C8, T1
Extensor carpi radialis	Radial	C7, C8, T1
Superficial digital flexor	Ulnar	C8, T1, T2
Deep digital flexor	Ulnar and median	C7, C8, T1, T2

activity between the active and reference electrodes, so localization is less precise than with concentric needles, but the likelihood of identifying abnormal activity is increased. The needle electrodes should be kept in close proximity to reduce electrical interference. Different electrodes, the distance between electrodes, and types of patient ground will affect the size and duration of recorded potentials [11]. Electromyographic recordings are typically made with bandpass filter settings of 30 Hz to 10 kHz.

Single-fiber electrodes are designed to record from single muscle fibers instead of motor units to provide a finer discrimination of extracellular activity. A wire 25 μm in diameter is attached to the side of a needle or inserted inside the needle with the tip bent back a few millimeters behind the needle tip. The wire and the needle are insulated except at the tip and the needle serves as the reference electrode. Single-fiber EMG recordings are infrequently utilized in clinical veterinary applications.

Nerve conduction studies

The evaluation of nerve conduction velocities (NCVs) requires knowledge of the topographic anatomy of nerves and muscles. Instrumentation requires a stimulator capable of delivering up to 150 V at durations of 0.1–3 ms. However, typically supramaximal stimulus can be obtained at 70–90 V for 0.1 s. Newer systems use a constant-current stimulator, where the voltage is varied to produce a desired current. This is safer for both the subject and the examiner by preventing inadvertent excess current; maximum current is limited to 100 mA. Most standard electromyographs have built-in stimulators with adequate parameters to do NCVs.

Two electrodes attach to the stimulator. A needle attached to the cathode (negative pole, black, attracts cations) depolarizes the neuron; this typically is a monopolar EMG needle electrode (25–100 mm, 28-gauge) stripped of its insulation at its tip. The return electrode connects to the anode (positive pole, red, attracts anions) and is typically a short subcutaneous needle electrode. If the deep electrode is connected to the anode instead of the cathode, the neuron is hyperpolarized; an action potential may still be triggered when the stimulus pulse ends, but a greater stimulus amplitude is required. The ground electrode must be positioned between the stimulating and recording electrodes to minimize stimulus artifact in the recording.

Motor NCV measurement

Standard EMG recording electrodes are positioned in a distal muscle innervated by the nerve to be assessed. The nerve is located either by palpation or by using anatomic landmarks, and two well-separated locations along the nerve are identified for stimulation. The distance (Δl) between the stimulation sites is measured on the skin in millimeters, assuming that the nerve's course under the skin is linear. Muscle contractions resulting from stimulation can be palpated and observed, and the evoked muscle action potential, which has a thumping sound once fed through an auditory amplifier, can be viewed on the computer monitor. The response recorded from the muscle is called the M wave. Once the nerve is stimulated at two different sites along the nerve, the arrival times of the muscle response from the stimulus artifact to the onset of the M response are measured in ms and the latency difference is designated ΔT. The NCV is calculated as $NCV = \Delta l$ (mm)$/\Delta T$ (ms) (Figure 14.1), expressed in meters per second (m/s). The motor nerve conduction velocity (MNCV) measurement is for the length of nerve between the distal and the proximal stimulation sites; both responses include the time for conduction of the nerve impulse from the distal electrode to the neuromuscular junction and across the synapse to the muscle. This is known as the indirect MNCV technique, since recordings are not made directly from the nerve. NCV values for the horse are shown in Table 14.3. In practice, any value greater than 50 m/s is considered to be within the reference range.

Measurements of NCV are affected by body temperature, typically decreasing by 1.8 m/s/°C with decreasing body temperature. However, except in extreme situations, the difference is not of clinical significance. Most EMG machines have the ability to correct the NCV based on an entered value for environmental temperature.

Sensory NCV measurement

Recording the conduction velocity of sensory nerves differs from the MNCV in that no muscle contraction is recorded. A sensory nerve is stimulated distally—often confirmed by a contraction of a distal muscle if the nerve is mixed motor and sensory—and the evoked nerve action potential is recorded from the sensory nerve at two more proximal locations. Sensory nerve conduction velocity (SNCV) is calculated by dividing the distance between recording sites by the latency differences from the two nerve recordings. The SNCV is more difficult to measure than the MNCV because positioning electrodes close to deep nerves is more of a challenge

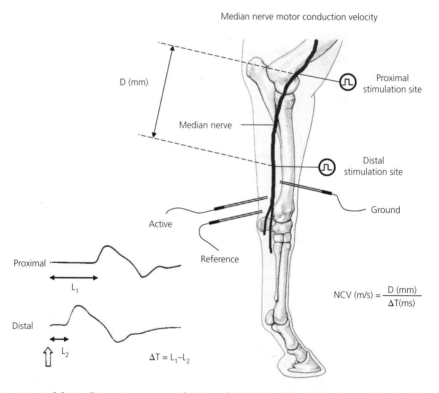

$$NCV \ (m/s) = \frac{D \ (mm)}{\Delta T (ms)}$$

$$\Delta T = L_1 - L_2$$

Figure 14.1 Measurement of the median motor nerve conduction velocity. Stimulating electrodes are placed at the median nerve where it crosses over the medial epicondylar crest of the humerus (proximal) and in the mid-antebrachium as the nerve passes to the radial head of the deep digital flexor muscle (distal). The active recording electrode is placed in the radial head of the deep digital flexor muscle. The reference electrode is placed subcutaneously adjacent to the active electrode, and the ground electrode is positioned subcutaneously between stimulating electrode and the recording electrode [12]. Forelimb, medial aspect.

Table 14.3 Reported motor and sensory nerve conduction velocities in horses and ponies.

Species	Nerve function	Nerve conduction velocity (m/s)									
		Radial	Median	Ulnar	Tibial	Peroneal	Facial	Palmar	Sural	Antebrachial	Trigeminal
Horse [13]	Motor	79	73	71	90	90					
Horse and pony [12]	Motor	81–87	72–78								
Horse [14]	Motor	98	88								
Horse [3]	Motor						60–70				
Pony [15]	Sensory		79	71							
Horse [16]	Sensory		65	54							
Pony [17]	Sensory							62–68			
Horse [17]	Sensory							58–62			
Horse [18]	Sensory								63	56	
Horse [19]	Sensory										78–86

than recording from a muscle and the response is smaller and may be obscured by larger muscle potentials. The SNCV, like the MNCV, decreases with decreasing temperature [20] and changes with age: It increases during the first year of life, then declines with age [21]. SNCV values are faster in ponies than in horses [17]. SNCVs for horses and/or ponies have been reported for the median, ulnar, palmar, caudal cutaneous sural, medial cutaneous antebrachial, and trigeminal nerves (Table 14.3). They have been used to evaluate the effects of extracorporeal shock wave therapy in horses [22], to assess continuous peripheral nerve block [16], and to determine function of the dorsal penile nerve in the bull [23].

F wave and H reflex measurement

Recording of F waves and H (Hofmann's) waves or reflexes, which are considered late responses, uses the same stimulation and recoding placements as those for the MNCV (Figure 14.2). The F wave is recorded from motor or mixed motor and sensory nerves, while the H reflex is only measured from mixed motor and sensory nerves. The latency of the M wave depends on the distance between the stimulating electrodes and the recording electrodes; F waves and H waves always occur after the M wave.

The F wave is a second action potential recorded from the muscle from supramaximal stimulation of the nerve and is a result of antidromic activation of the motor neuron cell body [24]. F wave amplitudes are only 1–5% of M wave amplitudes, so a higher display gain is required to see them, and they only occur with about 20% of stimuli. The latency is variable due to variable processing times in the soma. A MNCV can be estimated from the F wave recording.

The H reflex relies on the fact that sensory fibers in mixed nerves, mostly type Ia afferents from muscle spindles, have a larger diameter than most motor neuron axons; [25] as a result of the larger diameter, the sensory fibers have a lower stimulus threshold. Using a submaximal intensity stimulus, it is possible to stimulate sensory fibers but few if any motor fibers. The activated sensory fibers ascend to the spinal cord and synapse on motor neurons, eliciting an action potential in the neuron that produces a subsequent response in the muscle called the H wave, the classical monosynaptic reflex. The H reflex is only elicited in extensor muscles. With increasing stimulus intensity, the H wave is suppressed and the M wave amplitude increases. H waves have smaller amplitudes than M waves and a more consistent latency than F waves.

Repetitive nerve stimulation

The motor unit is able to fire repeatedly in response to short bursts of stimuli without fatigue. Once fatigue sets in, the evoked response (M wave) decreases in amplitude with repetitive stimulation. Normal motor units respond to 5 s of 2–5 Hz stimulation without a decrementing response, but in certain diseases such as myasthenia gravis, myasthenic syndrome, botulism, and tick paralysis [26], the successive responses decrease, due to either reduced acetylcholine release or reduced muscle responses. EMG equipment has the ability to apply the desired burst of stimuli and to calculate any amplitude decrement, typically in the third, fifth, and tenth responses, which are then compared with the first [27]. When normal muscles are stimulated at 2–3 Hz, a decrement of up to 5–8% can be present [28]. Decrements in excess of 10% are considered

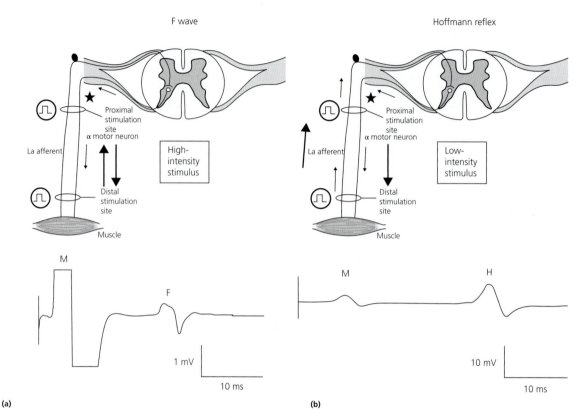

Figure 14.2 Diagram of the recording of the F wave and Hofmann's reflex (a) The F wave is elicited by a high-intensity stimulus. The resulting action potential proceeds to the muscle, producing the M wave, and back to the spinal cord, followed by an action potential in the same neuron and the muscle F wave. The F wave results from antidromic activation of motor neurons and both action potentials are in the same neuron. The F wave amplitude is only 1–5% of the M wave and is variable in latency. Simultaneous stimulation at both distal and proximal sites can block the response by collision (star) of action potentials traveling in opposite directions. (b) Hofmann's reflex is elicited by a low-intensity stimulus, activating Ia sensory afferents to the spinal cord, followed by synaptic activation of the alpha motor neuron and production of the muscle H wave. Little or no M wave is produced, but with increasing stimulus the M wave increases and the H wave decreases. Two neurons and their connecting synapse are involved in the prototype monosynaptic reflex. Note amplitude scale differences.

abnormal [29]. Stimulation at high frequencies (50 Hz) is avoided since it can actually produce an incrementing response.

Electromyographic examination

A history, physical, and neurological examination should always precede the electromyographic examination. This aids in localization of the lesion, shortens examination time, and minimizes trauma to the horse. Initially, electromyographic examination is performed under mild sedation while the horse is restrained in stocks. Tranquilization with xylazine (0.2–0.6 mg/kg, IV), xylazine–butorphanol (0.2–0.6 mg/kg, IV and 0.01–0.02 mg/kg, IV, respectively), or detomidine (0.01–0.02 mg/kg, IV) can be used. Examination of the animal prior to sedation aids in evaluating individual MUAPs,

summated MUAPs, and the interference pattern. An interference pattern is a sustained burst of MUAPs associated with a voluntary or induced contraction of the muscle from which recordings are being taken; increasing muscle contraction is associated with increasing MUAP frequency and amplitude. Normal and abnormal MUAPs can be evaluated with respect to amplitude and duration. Many MUAPs or an interference pattern can sometimes obscure low-amplitude abnormal potentials on the monitor and may require further examination under general anesthesia.

The exploring electrode should be thrust briskly into the muscle and held until the animal completely relaxes. To assist relaxation, the animal can be forced to bear weight on the opposite limb. Once relaxation has occurred, the resting activity or any postinsertional activity of the muscle can be evaluated. At least four areas and depths of smaller skeletal muscles and six to eight areas and depths of large skeletal muscles should be evaluated when possible [3].

A neurologic examination should be done on each case to localize any lesion so that the electromyographic examination can be performed in a systematic fashion to save time and limit pain to the patient. In cases of generalized muscle weakness or a suspected neuropathy, a comprehensive needle EMG examination should be done that includes the major extrinsic muscles of the pelvic limb, including the long digital extensor, gastrocnemius, deep digital flexor, semimembranosus, vastus lateralis, biceps femoris, and middle and superficial gluteal muscles; the epaxial or paravertebral muscles, segmentally from the sixth lumbar to the first cervical vertebrae; and finally, the extrinsic muscles of the forelimb, including the subclavius, infraspinatus, supraspinatus, deltoideus, biceps brachii, triceps brachii, extensor carpi radialis, superficial digital flexor, and deep digital flexor muscles. Other muscles may be included such as facial, laryngeal, esophageal, pectoral, coccygeal, and external anal sphincter if indicated by the neurologic examination. NCS and/or muscle biopsies can be done to further isolate and characterize suspected lesions or confirm a diagnosis. Muscle-produced creatine kinase can be increased for up to 6 h following an EMG examination, but the increase does not exceed the normal reference range [30], so samples can be collected immediately after an EMG if desired, as artifactually increased values will not be seen from needle penetrations.

Quantitative EMG studies can be performed by examining the patterns of individual MUAPs and assessing amplitudes, durations, number of phases, and number of turns [31–33]. These analyses have been applied in studies of grass sickness, myogenic disorders, lower motor neuron disease, and lesion localization [34, 35].

Conduct of NCS

NCS are difficult to perform in the horse; consequently, they are not done routinely. The techniques for assessing radial, median, ulnar, tibial, peroneal, facial, palmar, sural, antebrachial, recurrent laryngeal, and trigeminal NCVs in the horse have been reported [3, 12–15, 17–19]. Motor nerve conduction testing is used to evaluate the speed of conduction of large myelinated motor nerve axons. Nerve stimulation is painful, so NCS are performed with the horse under general anesthesia and positioned in lateral recumbency with the tested side up [3]. The appropriate motor nerve is stimulated by monopolar needle electrodes inserted at or near the nerve, and an evoked M wave from an innervated

muscle is recorded by electrodes placed in a muscle innervated by this nerve. Contraction of appropriate muscles can be visualized or palpated and needle electrodes repositioned until a repeatable response is obtained. The normal limb can be used as a control. In the horse, radial nerve recordings can be taken from the extensor carpi radialis and abductor digiti longus (extensor carpi obliquus) muscles [12, 14]. Median nerve recordings can be obtained from the humeral and radial heads of the deep digital flexor muscle [12, 14]. Facial NCVs can be taken from the levator nasolabialis by stimulating the buccal branch of the facial nerve just ventral to the facial crest [3].

Normal electromyographic potentials

Muscles can be examined at rest, under submaximal contraction, and under maximal contraction in the awake horse. Recordings in awake horses are frequently used in studies of locomotion, in both the normal and the diseased state [36–39]. However, muscle contraction is absent in the anesthetized horse, so only resting activity is examined in this state. NCS can only be done under general anesthesia. Normal muscle responses include insertion activity, MUAPs, end-plate potentials, and recruitment/interference pattern.

Insertional activity

Insertional activity is a short burst of positive or negative high-amplitude, moderate- to high-frequency (<200 Hz) electrical spikes following insertion or movement of the exploring needle electrode in the muscle. In normal skeletal muscle, this activity lasts up to 300 ms after cessation of needle movement [40]. Insertional activity is likely caused by damage, mechanical irritation of muscle cells, or depolarization of muscle fibers directly adjacent to the EMG needle. Insertional activity response depends on the magnitude and speed of needle movement and is considered semiquantitative [40]. Positive sharp waves and fibrillation potentials may occur during or associated with needle insertion but in normal muscle should stop after cessation of needle movement. Damage of muscle fibers due to insertion of the needle is probably the source of these abnormal spikes. However, persistent positive sharp waves (>2) and fibrillation potentials after needle insertion are considered abnormal and may suggest early muscle denervation [40]. Insertional activity has been reported to vary from 120 ms to 2 s in horses [41, 42]. Mean (SD) insertional activity in the subclavius muscle of warmblood horses was 472 (103) ms or 561 (200) ms, which was significantly different than insertional activity in the triceps and vastus lateralis muscles, which was 519 (133) ms and 497 (114) ms, respectively [43]. The authors also found that the mean duration of insertional activity was significantly shorter in younger

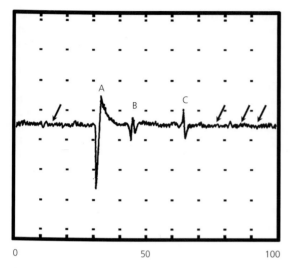

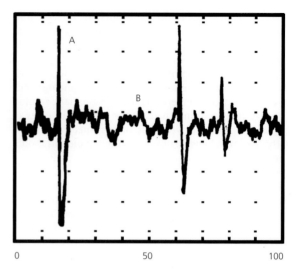

Figure 14.3 Electromyogram from the right middle gluteal muscle of a horse showing resting activity (postinsertional baseline, arrows), positive sharp wave (A), fibrillation potential (B), and a small motor unit action potential (MUAP) (C) with early denervation atrophy due to equine protozoal myeloencephalitis.

Figure 14.4 Electromyogram from the semitendinosus muscle showing end-plate spikes (A) and end-plate noise (B).

horses (13–18 months of age) when compared with older horses (18–21 years of age) [43]. The clinical significance of this difference was not apparent, and because the range was similar to those published in other horses, these values appear to be suitable for use as normals in horses.

Resting and spontaneous activity

Resting activity (postinsertional baseline) in a totally relaxed muscle is characterized by electrical silence and a flat baseline (see Figure 14.3). However, if the needle comes to rest near a nerve twig or end plate, the needle may irritate small intramuscular nerve terminals, resulting in the production of spontaneous activity that is referred to as spontaneous miniature end-plate potentials (MEPPs) and end-plate spikes. MEPPs in horses are approximately 25–100 μV in amplitude and 5–10 ms in duration and produce a low-pitched continuous noise [43]. These potentials are caused by the spontaneous quantal release of acetylcholine from nerve terminals in the area near the needle electrode (see Figure 14.4). End-plate spikes, on the other hand, are high-amplitude (100–200 μV), short-duration (3–4 ms) intermittent spikes that make a popping sound [44]. End-plate spikes are thought to be single muscle fiber contractions secondary to needle electrode irritation of the nerve terminals. In humans, these potentials are associated with dull pain, and repositioning the needle often eliminates their activity.

Motor unit action potentials

MUAPs are from voluntary or reflex muscle contractions that occur after insertion of the needle electrode. They represent the sum of a number of single muscle fiber potentials belonging to the same motor unit. MUAPs are described based on duration, amplitude, phases, turns, and recruitment pattern [43]. The MUAP duration is defined as the time from initial deflection to the final return to baseline. Amplitude is defined as the peak-to-peak measurement (see Figure 14.3). A phase is defined as the unit between departure from and return to baseline and can be counted as the number of baseline crossings plus one (see Figure 14.3). Number of turns is defined as a change in the direction of the signal independent of crossing the baseline (see Figure 14.3). Generally, normal MUAPs are potentials that are mono-, bi-, and triphasic, 3–10 ms in duration, and have an amplitude of approximately 1500 μV (range 500–3000 μV) [3]. Normal values for various muscles in the horse have been previously reported and differ between muscles explored [43]. A few polyphasic potentials (more than four phases) can be seen in normal skeletal muscle but should not exceed 5–15% of the total MUAPs observed during the examination [3]. The MUAPs can be observed when the horse is forced to bear weight on or retract a limb, resulting in contraction of that explored muscle. In lightly stimulated muscle, a single MUAP can be seen as a single motor unit is recruited (see Figure 14.3). As the muscle contraction becomes more intense, more motor units are recruited (see Figure 14.5), and the greater frequency of MUAPs appears on the computer monitor until the screen is

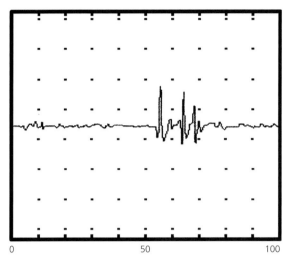

Figure 14.5 Electromyogram from the supraspinatus muscle showing three recruited motor unit action potentials (MUAPs).

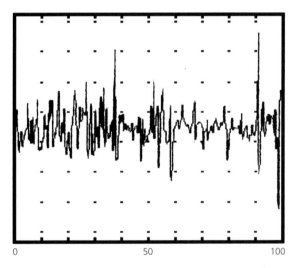

Figure 14.6 Electromyogram from the supraspinatus muscle showing an interference pattern due to strong recruitment of MUAPs due to muscle contraction from weight bearing.

filled, which results in an interference pattern (see Figure 14.6) [3, 31, 45]. An interference pattern can obscure low-amplitude fibrillation or positive sharp wave potentials or polyphasic MUAPs; thus general anesthesia may be necessary [46]. Clinically, the number of phases and the duration of MUAPs are of greater importance than amplitude because amplitude is influenced by muscles, age, and electrode position [47]. MUAP analyses are not routinely performed in clinical practice.

Abnormal electromyographic potentials

Spontaneous activity in a relaxed muscle after cessation of needle movement may be clinically significant. Diseases affecting the lower motor unit (or final common path) can lead to altered muscle electrical activity, such as prolonged or decreased insertional activity, postinsertional activity, altered waveforms, and complex repetitive discharges (CRDs). Some abnormal electromyographic potentials are described in the following sections, including prolonged insertion activity, fibrillation potentials, positive sharp waves, CRDs, and myotonic discharges.

Prolonged or decreased insertional activity

Prolonged electrical activity continuing 1–10 ms or more after insertion of the needle and its placement in the muscle is considered abnormal and is probably due to hyperirritability and instability of the muscle fiber membrane [47]. This activity is most prominent 4–5 days after denervation in dogs [48] and 12–16 days in horses, reflecting differences in axon length between species. Increased or prolonged insertional activity usually precedes the onset of other denervation potentials (fibrillation potentials and positive sharp waves) and may suggest early denervation atrophy [47] but can also be seen in myotonic disorders and myositis [49]. Decreased insertional activity (decreased amplitude, duration, or both) may be associated with a decreased number of functioning muscle fibers and may suggest a long-standing neuropathy and/or myopathy. Infiltration of the muscle by connective tissue and fat can lead to a decreased number of muscle fibers, which in turn decreases insertional activity. Complete muscle fibrosis may result in loss of all insertional activity although fibrillation potentials and positive sharp waves may remain. Insertional activity may also be absent when muscle fibers are not functionally excitable, as occurs during attacks of familial periodic paralysis, when a faulty needle electrode is used, or when the needle is introduced into normal resting muscle [40].

Polyphasic or myopathic action potentials

Myopathic MUAPs have a frequency of greater than four phases and decreased amplitude and duration compared with normal MUAPs.

Polyphasic MUAPs are observed during submaximal muscle contraction and result from an increased number of action potentials for a given strength of contraction. Myopathic potentials result from a diffuse loss of muscle fibers and indicate the need for extra motor units to perform the work normally done by fewer motor units [50]. Myopathic MUAPs are polyphasic and are most often seen in humans with primary myopathies such as myotonia-like syndromes, periodic paralysis, myositis, botulism, and myasthenia-like syndrome [47] and sometimes in early and incomplete denervation [51]. Myopathic potentials have also been reported in steroid-induced myopathies resulting from equine Cushing's syndrome and membrane-defect myopathies [47]. Very limited data exist in horses with muscle pathology, but polyphasic MUAPs have been recorded in horses with hypocalcemic and hypomagnesemic states [45].

Neuropathic or neurogenic spontaneous activity
Neuropathic potentials are MUAPs of decreased frequency and longer duration than myopathic potentials and may be seen during minimal and maximal muscle contraction. Fewer MUAPs of increased amplitude are observed than expected for the strength of contraction. This is more noticeable during maximal contraction and produces a "sputtering" or "motor boat" sound. These potentials were most often present in primary neuropathies, such as suprascapular and radial nerve paralysis, in which collateral reinnervation has occurred. Neurogenic spontaneous activity has been recorded from the long head of the triceps muscle in horses with hypocalcemia and hypomagnesemia [45].

Fibrillation potentials
Fibrillation potentials, or "fibs," are the most commonly observed abnormal spontaneous potentials on electromyographic examination. These spontaneous discharges often sound like frying eggs, crinkling cellophane, frying bacon, or rain on a tin roof and have an initial positive deflection of 100–300 μV in amplitude, are smaller than MUAPs, and are 2–4 ms in duration in humans (see Figure 14.3). They are bi- or triphasic and strongly suggest muscle denervation but have also been observed in polymyositis, muscular dystrophy, and botulism. They may occur spontaneously or in response to needle movement. The exact origin of these potentials is unproven, but they are thought to be spontaneous discharges resulting from the release of acetylcholine onto hypersensitive denervated muscle fibers. Following denervation, numerous additional acetylcholine receptors appear on the denervated muscle, making it more sensitive to the random release of the transmitter. Fibrillation potentials may also be secondary to muscle necrosis, muscle inflammation, and focal muscle degeneration. Fibrillation potentials have been observed in normal healthy muscle, but they are usually not reproducible in other areas of the muscle. The onset of fibrillation potentials following denervation depends upon the size of the animal (i.e., the larger the animal, the later the onset of fibrillation potentials). They have been reported to occur in 5 days after denervation in dogs and 16 days in humans. We have observed fibrillation potentials 4–10 days after nerve injury in the horse, but the expected time window is 12–16 days. The presence of fibrillation potentials can be enhanced by heat, passive stretching, or neostigmine. A recent report showed the presence of

fibrillation potentials in horses with hypocalcemia and hypomagnesemia [45]. These fibrillation potentials ranged from 12 to 155 μV in amplitude and 1–10 ms in duration, which is shorter in duration than those reported in humans [44]. Fibrillation potentials are most often seen in conjunction with positive sharp waves and are indicators of denervation. They increase, then decrease in amplitude as the muscle atrophies; they may cease upon complete muscle atrophy, once fibrous connective tissue and fat have totally infiltrated the muscles but in some cases may still persist. Fibrillation potentials are helpful in diagnosing and evaluating the length of the time muscle denervation has been present, and serial examinations are useful in assessing clinical prognosis of muscle atrophy. A decrease in amplitude and duration over time carries a poor prognosis, whereas a decrease in the presence of fibrillation potentials followed by the recording of MUAPs suggests reinnervation, which carries a favorable prognosis.

Positive sharp waves
Positive sharp waves are potentials in which the primary deflection is in the downward direction and is followed by a lower-amplitude longer-duration negative deflection (see Figure 14.3). This waveform has been described as resembling a saw tooth. Positive sharp waves occur with muscle denervation and muscular diseases such as myositis, exertional rhabdomyolysis (tying-up syndrome), and spinal shock in humans. Sometimes, positive sharp waves are observed in association coincident with or shortly after insertional activity and persist after electrode placement. If more than two positive sharp waves are observed after insertional activity, it may indicate early denervation. We have observed positive sharp waves in denervated muscle secondary to chronic exertional rhabdomyolysis, myotonia, protozoal myeloencephalitis, laryngeal hemiplegia, suprascapular nerve injury, and compressive myelopathies. One recent report quantified positive sharp waves in horses with hypocalcemia and hypomagnesemia [45]. Positive sharp waves in that study ranged from 13 to 261 μV in amplitude and 1.46–12.78 ms in duration, which was shorter than those recorded in humans [44]. These potentials can be observed singly or in trains and may sound like machine gun fire, a musical tone, an idling motor, or a diving airplane. Their origin is uncertain but may be associated with hyperexcitable muscle cell membranes and may be identical to fibrillation potentials recorded from a closer distance.

CRDs and myotonic potentials
CRDs (bizarre high-frequency potentials) and myotonic potentials are observed less frequently in the horse than in other domestic species. Both of these potentials are repetitive MUAPs induced by insertion of the needle electrode or percussion of muscle. The CRDs are shorter in duration and end abruptly, with a uniform frequency (5–100 Hz),

shape, and amplitude (100 μV to 1 mV), compared with myotonic potentials, which wax and wane in amplitude (50–300 μV) and duration (4–5 s) and sound like a dive bomber due to changing frequency (20–80 Hz) (see Figure 14.7). Both CRDs and myotonic potentials are associated with hyperexcitable muscle membranes. CRDs have a fixed amplitude and frequency, and the initial deflection can be either positive or negative. The CRDs are seen in amyotrophic lateral sclerosis, spinal muscle atrophy, myotonic syndromes, and polymyositis [51]. In horses, CRDs have been recorded in rhabdomyolysis and myotonia [52], hypocalcemia and hypomagnesemia [45], laryngeal hemiplegia [53], hyperkalemic periodic paralysis [54, 55], equine motor neuron disease [46, 56], and only rarely in normal horses [31]. Myotonic potentials are repetitive discharges with an initial positive deflection. Warming up or cooling down of muscles influences the occurrence of myotonic discharges [45]. They have been recorded in horses with myotonia congenita [52, 57], myotonia dystrophia [58], and hyperkalemic periodic paralysis; [42, 54, 55, 59] they may reflect hyperexcitability due to abnormal electrolyte transport in the muscle.

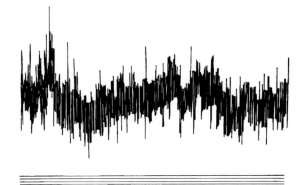

Figure 14.7 Electromyographic recording from the middle gluteal muscle from a foal with myotonia congenita. Note the repetitive waxing and waning discharges or myotonic potentials.

A summary of the sounds associated with normal and abnormal EMG activity is shown in Table 14.4.

Table 14.4 Sounds associated with normal and abnormal EMG activity.

EMG activity	Sound
Normal muscle	
Resting	
Electrode insertion	No added sounds when electrode is released
Non–end-plate region	Electric "silence" (background low-level hissing; amplifier noise)
End-plate region	Moderately loud hissing
Nerve activity	High-pitched hissing
Contracting (maximal effort)	
Many motor unit potentials	Sharp, single cracking or popping that ceases with relaxation
Abnormal muscle	
Resting (denervation >12–16 days)	
Insertion activity	Loud crackling that decreases after one to several minutes
Fibrillation potential	Rain on a tin roof or frying eggs
Positive sharp waves	Varies from a musical tone or a sound like an idling outboard motor to roar of diving airplane
Complex repetitive discharge	Banjo-like twang
Contracting (immediate postdenervation effort)	
Complete denervation	
No motor unit potentials	No change with effort
Partial denervation	
A few motor unit potentials	Response similar to normal minimal effort pattern even though a maximal effort is attempted
Reinnervation	
Miniature motor unit potentials	Rough rasping, crackling, or popping sound that has a higher pitch than normal motor unit potentials sound
Myotonia (tap electrode)	Diving airplane or revving motorcycle (sound may wax and wane)
Interference	
ECG	Dull thumping that follows pulse rate
60 Hz	Hum or buzz

Magnetic motor evoked potentials

It is often useful to be able to assess the integrity of descending motor pathways—primarily the cortico-spinal tracts—in trauma cases and other conditions with diminished or absent motor function. MMEPs are recorded from distal muscles in a manner similar to repetitive nerve stimulation. The potentials are evoked by stimulation of the contralateral motor cortex, a technique first reported clinically in humans with transcranial electrical stimulation by Merton and Morton [61] and with transcranial magnetic stimulation by Barker et al. [62]. When the magnetic stimulating coil is placed over the motor cortex, electrical current in the coils of the electromagnet induces a current in the tissues below the skull, primarily the cerebral cortex. This synchronously activates neurons in the corticospinal tract, which in turn activate alpha motor neurons to muscles of the extremities [63]. The primary application is cortical stimulation because activation of the spinal cord and nerve roots is difficult to achieve from inadequate penetration of the magnetic field. Anesthesia is required when electrical stimuli are used because passage of sufficient electrical current is painful [64], but magnetic stimulation is not uncomfortable and has been used in both anesthetized and awake horses [65–68]. MMEPs have been used to study cervical spinal cord disease in horses [1] and to differentiate between motor neural pathway lesions and other causes of recumbent horses [69]. MMEPs may also be used for intraoperative monitoring of procedures potentially impinging on descending motor pathways [70]. A separate high-powered magnetic stimulator is required in addition to EMG recording equipment, which is expensive and not affordable for most clinical settings.

Sensory evoked potentials

The integrity of pathways for the various sensory systems can be assessed by recording potentials evoked by appropriate stimulation of sensory receptors; these differ from the electroencephalogram in being evoked rather than spontaneous. The amplitude of many of these responses is small when compared with other biological and nonbiological signals that may be present, so the responses to multiple stimuli are typically averaged to reinforce the evoked (and presumably relatively invariant) responses and minimize the unrelated signal activity, which is not time-locked to the stimuli and thus tends to cancel out. The most commonly used sensory evoked potentials are the BAER, the ERG and VEP, and the SEP. Other sensory evoked potentials have been described for vestibular, olfactory, and pain systems, but they are not being used clinically. Of the earlier described

potentials, the BAER and the ERG are the most commonly utilized tests in clinical veterinary medicine. Clinical EMG machines usually have the capacity to perform sensory evoked potential testing, but the acquisition of appropriate additional stimulators may be necessary.

BAER testing

BAERs are electric potentials arising from the eighth cranial nerve and its projections along the brainstem. These potentials are measured using platinum or stainless steel subdermal needle electrodes placed in the subcutaneous tissue of the head of the horse in response to acoustic stimulation (a click stimulator placed in the ear or headphones over the ear). These evoked potentials appear as waves arising within the first 10 ms after the delivery of an acoustic stimulus. In horses, five to seven peaks are recognized and designated as Roman numerals I through VII; of these, peaks I through V are the most commonly seen in horses, and peaks IV and V are often merged. Each peak corresponds to different anatomic generator sites along CN VIII and the brainstem auditory pathway [71, 72]. Peaks I to III are generated by the eighth cranial nerve, cochlear nucleus, and superior olivary complex, respectively. Peaks IV through VII are thought to be generated by the lateral lemniscus, inferior colliculus, and medial geniculate nucleus of the thalamus. However, it is argued that later peaks may have multiple generator sites and there is less certainty about their origins. Peaks VI and VII are rarely present in horse. The latencies of the peaks have been established and reported and are highly repeatable within a species. Information about intracranial disorders can be inferred based on increases in interpeak latencies or frank absence of late peaks. Increased latencies of all peaks suggest a peripheral disorder. Increases in interpeak latencies can suggest decreased conduction velocity and a possible demyelinating disorder in the region(s) associated with those peaks. The absence of a peak (and by necessity those following it) suggests a lesion in the auditory pathway at the point of the first missing peak. Horses are a precocious species, and there is negligible postnatal maturation of the brainstem, so maturational changes are not seen in equine BAER recordings.

A wide range of clinical applications of BAER testing in human beings have been described. The clinical use of BAER testing in horses has been limited but is an ancillary method of assessing auditory function and neurologic disorders involving the brainstem. Since the state of arousal of the patient does not affect BAERs, testing can be done on sedated and anesthetized patients without degradation of the response. However, testing is typically performed on awake or slightly sedated horses.

Instrumentation

Commercially available electromyographs have settings and components available to do BAER testing. The general equipment and procedure includes a click stimulus produced by a square wave generator (rarefaction polarity at a rate of 11.3 clicks per second, avoiding submultiples of the 60 Hz mains frequency) delivered to the ears by a pair of insert earphones or headphones with a frequency response of 100–6000 Hz [71, 73]. The earphones can be inserted into the horse's external auditory canals or held outside the ear canal opening. In the case of possible conductive deafness, a bone stimulation transducer can be applied against the skull caudal to the pinna so that the acoustic stimulus travels as a vibration through the skull to the inner ear, bypassing the outer and middle ears; [74] however, the use of a bone stimulus transducer has not been validated in the horse.

Platinum or stainless steel needle EEG electrodes (12 mm in length) are inserted subcutaneously with the active electrode placed over the ipsilateral (to the stimulus) zygomatic process of the temporal bone near the base of the pinna and the reference electrode inserted at the vertex over the parietal suture just rostral to the site where the temporalis muscles diverge from the midline and the ground positioned over the bony part of the caudal aspect of the external occipital protuberance or wing of the atlas [75, 76]. A ground electrode is placed over an electrically inactive area such as the neck. An upward deflection is produced on the computer screen in response to electrical activity at the vertex. Electrode impedance should be less than 10 000 Ω. The BAERs are recorded with a high-pass filter set at 1 000 Hz and a low-pass filter set at 3 kHz. Display gain is varied to produce the best record. The differential voltage is sampled for 10 ms after each click, digitized, and multiple responses summed for approximately 500–1 000 stimuli to produce the desired evoked waveform. BAERs can usually be recorded over a 70-dB range (30–90 dB nHL), with the best response seen between 60 and 90 dB nHL. Horses can be examined while awake, with or without mild sedation (xylazine hydrochloride (0.4 mg/kg, IV), detomidine hydrochloride (0.013 mg/kg, IV)) [76], or while anesthetized [75]. Each ear is stimulated, and resultant waveforms are recorded independently [75]. It is good practice to repeat tests of each ear to confirm that the results are physiologic and not affected by some type of artifact. BAER testing is used as a screening test for deafness and for the presence of intracranial disease. Hearing threshold determination is rarely performed due to the time required and the need for anesthesia.

Interpretation of BAER

Five peaks are commonly observed and are considered analogous to the waves I through V seen in humans. Mean latencies have been reported in the literature for normal horses [75, 77, 78]. A variety of extrinsic and intrinsic factors can affect the recorded BAER, separate from any existing pathology. These include the electrodes used, the electrode montage, the stimulus transducer used, stimulus parameters, recording parameters, age, head size, body temperature, drugs, and artifacts [73].

Clinical uses of the BAER include both audiologic and neurologic applications. BAER testing can be used clinically in horses with a head tilt to evaluate brainstem or peripheral nerve injury in horses with trauma [79], to verify the presence of hearing loss especially in horses with congenital hearing deficits [3, 80], particularly horses with large areas of white pigmentation and heterochromia iridis or blue eyes [81, 82], age-related hearing loss [83], middle or inner ear infections, inner ear injury [84], toxicology studies [85, 86], and stylohyoid osteomyelitis [87]. It may also be helpful in the diagnosis and prognosis of traumatic, infectious, or inflammatory brainstem lesions such as vascular infarcts or anomalies, ischemic fibrocartilaginous emboli, basisphenoid–basioccipital bone fracture, and equine protozoal myeloencephalitis. Persistent prolonged latencies suggest retrocochlear or nerve conductive pathologies. Interaural latency differences of wave V may suggest unilateral brainstem disease, except when cochlear disease is present. Qualitative BAER changes are of greater use in equine medicine because quantitative measures of normal and abnormal horses are limited. Peak amplitude differences between ears or in comparison with species norms are not usually informative since many nonpathologic factors can affect amplitudes. In human beings, qualitative changes such as peak presence, waveform morphologic characteristic, and response stability are of greater use in the diagnosis of central disorders, particularly acoustic neuromas and demyelinating diseases, which are not well characterized in horses. Limitations of BAER testing include a dependence on cochlear function, susceptibility to extraneous noise that may affect waveform morphology, and limits of the machinery in excluding 60-cycle interference. The BAER has been used to confirm congenital deafness in blue-eyed, sorrel, white overo American Paint horses [80, 88] and to show a subtle left-to-right interaural latency difference of waves I, III, and V in a pony that was suspected to have been struck by lightning [80].

Electroretinography

Although the ERG is traditionally performed by ophthalmologists, the retina is the first structure examined when there is a visual disturbance. Standardized guidelines for ERG testing in the dog have been published [89], and guidelines for the horse have been derived from dogs [90, 91]. Horses are sedated (0.015 mg/kg detomidine hydrochloride, IV) and the pupil dilated with topical tropicamide (0.2 ml, 1% solution) and a topical anesthetic applied (0.2 ml of 0.5% proparacaine). An auriculopalpebral nerve block may be required to immobilize eyelid muscles. A contact lens monopolar electrode is applied to the axial cornea with methylcellulose to assist with adherence. The reference electrode is placed lateral to the lateral canthus of the eye and ground is placed over the vertex, typically using subdermal needle electrodes. Dark adaptation is observed for approximately 20 min before stimulation is initiated. Responses are recorded with a bandpass of 0.3–300 Hz.

Stimuli for the ERG can be either a flash or an alternating pattern of stripes or a checkerboard, but since the latter requires the subject to focus on the middle of the pattern, only flashes are typically used. If a variable-intensity photostimulator is available, the response to low-intensity flashes is tested first to obtain a rod (scotopic) response, then at higher intensities to get a combined rod and cone response. Finally, responses to a 30-Hz flicker stimulus are obtained in a lighted setting for a cone (scotopic) response. If desired, colored lenses are available for the photostimulator to produce red or blue light. Because the ERG amplitude is larger than that of other sensory responses, only small numbers of responses are averaged and in some cases responses to single flashes are used. Rapidly repeated stimuli result in photobleaching and reduced amplitudes in the response.

The ERG waveform in a dark-adapted eye consists of a corneal-negative "a" wave followed by a positive "b" wave; a later "c" wave may also be observed (Figure 14.8). The "a" wave, or late receptor potential, is generated by rods and cones, while the "b" wave is generated in the inner nuclear layer of the retina, from either bipolar cells or Müeller glial cells. The "c" wave, only seen with dark adaptation, results from pigmented epithelial cells hyperpolarized in response to decreased extracellular potassium around the photoreceptor cells. No component of the ERG results from retinal ganglion cells or the optic nerve, so it is theoretically possible to have a normal ERG with optic nerve pathology.

The clinically relevant measurements taken from the ERG are the amplitude from baseline to the "a" wave trough, the peak-to-peak amplitude between the "a" wave trough and the "b" wave peak, and the latencies (implicit times) to the "a" wave trough and the "b" wave peak.

The ERG is used clinically to assess retinal function prior to cataract surgery, in the diagnosis of congenital stationary night blindness [92], recurrent uveitis, glaucoma, ocular trauma, acute blindness [93, 94] and equine motor neuron disease, which results in reduced vitamin E [95].

Visual evoked potentials

Electrodiagnostic testing of the postretinal visual system is performed with the VEP. A monocular flash stimulus is applied while the opposite eye is covered, and responses are recorded and averaged between electrodes on the midline of the nuchal crest (O_z) and interorbital line (F_{pz}), with ground on the vertex. The response duration is 100–200 ms and consists of a series of positive and negative waveform peaks. VEP recordings have not been reported in horses but have been used in cattle, sheep, and miniature potbellied pigs and in studies of polioencephalomalacia, central blindness from a brain abscess, and scrapie [96–103].

Somatosensory evoked potentials

Electrodiagnostic testing of the somatosensory system is performed with the SEP. Electrical (or less commonly mechanical) stimulation of peripheral nerves activates sensory afferent nerves, and the response can be monitored at various points along the neuraxis, which with hind limb stimulation may include behind the stifle, over spinal cord roots at L4/5, over lumbar spinal cord, and over the contralateral somatosensory cortex and with forelimb stimulation, behind the knee, over spinal cord roots at C6/7, over cervical spinal cord, and over the contralateral somatosensory cortex. Cortical recordings are from electrodes at the midpoint of the interorbital line (active electrode, F_{pz}), ground over an inactive site, and the negative electrode over the vertex for hind limb recordings and approximately 2 cm lateral to the vertex, contralateral to the stimulated side, for forelimb recordings. The negative electrode placements are intended to overlie locations on the somatosensory cortex for forelimb

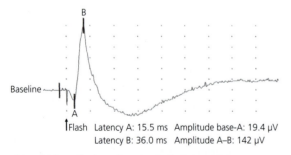

Flash   Latency A: 15.5 ms   Amplitude base-A: 19.4 µV
         Latency B: 36.0 ms   Amplitude A–B: 142 µV

Figure 14.8 Dark-adapted equine flash electroretinogram resulting from the average of 20 responses at 0.5 Hz. Recordings are taken between a contact lens electrode and a subdermal needle electrode at the lateral canthus of the eye. The negative A wave is produced by rods and cones in the retina, while the B wave is produced by cells in the inner nuclear layer of the retina.

and hind limb. Recordings last approximately 100 ms and consist of a series of positive and negative waveform peaks [104].

Thoracic limb stimulation is applied to the lateral palmar nerve, a branch of the ulnar nerve, at the level of the metacarpophalangeal joint, and pelvic limb stimulation is applied to the lateral plantar nerve, a branch of the tibial nerve, at the level of the metatarsophalangeal joint. Electrical stimulation is applied with paired subdermal needle electrodes separated by 2 cm over the appropriate nerve with the anodal electrode distal to the cathodal electrode. Stimuli are 0.2-ms square wave pulses at 2.7/s at amplitudes of 2–20 mA. Stimulus intensity is gradually increased until there is an aversive hoof withdrawal response, at which point the intensity is reduced until there is no further aversive response. Normal ulnar and tibial SEPs have been reported for unsedated horses [104]. SEPs have been used to study equine headshaking [19, 105] and in studies of local anesthetic drug effects [106, 107].

Electroencephalography

EEG is a graphic recording of spontaneous electrical activity originating predominately from the cerebral cortex and measured by subcutaneous electrodes. It is a relatively simple and noninvasive neurophysiological technique used extensively in humans and small animals [108–118] and increasingly in horses for monitoring central nervous system (CNS) effects and antinociceptive efficacy of anesthetic agents and depth of general anesthesia [119–133] and in clinical applications [134–149].

With the introduction of MRI and CT, EEG is not done routinely in small animals except in those patients with epilepsy. In contrast, MRI is not routinely available for most equine patients and CT is less sensitive than MRI to image soft tissue structures like the brain. An EEG should be considered as part of the diagnostic workup for patients presented with abnormal behavior, collapse, or seizure-like activity. The EEG is a good tool to diagnose intracranial disorders in horses presented with a history of seizure-like activity, with a specificity of 70% and sensitivity of 100% and with a positive neuroanatomic correlation in 70% of cases [142]. However, EEG is a complementary test, rather than an alternative to other diagnostic tests, and may allow the clinician to determine differential diagnoses that help identify the cause of the seizures in the light of history, neurological examinations, and other diagnostic tests. The main limitations of this electrodiagnostic test are related to the facts that (i) the recorded electrical activity arises primarily from the superficial part of the cerebral cortex; (ii) it requires extensive expertise from the clinician to interpret the reading; and (iii) it is mostly limited to neurology referral institutions.

Electrophysiological basis of EEG

The complete description of the electrophysiological process underlying the generation of EEG signals is beyond the scope of this chapter, and the reader can refer to a detailed review on this topic [150]. If two electrodes are placed on the scalp where the cerebral hemisphere is close to the surface, spontaneous (without any stimulation) electrical activity from the cerebral cortex can be recorded with the use of appropriate recording systems. These activities are primarily the algebraic summation of excitatory and inhibitory postsynaptic potentials from a large population ($>10^5$) of cortical neurons [151]. It is thought that the potentials recorded by the surface electrode originate mostly from pyramidal cell apical dendrites located within a 2-mm depth of the cerebral cortex [152]. This electrical activity may also contain contributions from deeper structures such as the brainstem, reticular activating system, and thalamus. Summation of large numbers of postsynaptic potentials will result in the generation of the EEG signal, with a typical voltage ranging from 3 to 300 μV, recurring at frequencies of 0.5–40 Hz.

Equipment and montage

The EEG machine consists of inputs for multiple electrodes, amplifiers, filters, and a paper or electronic display. Electrodes may be platinum alloy or stainless steel needle electrodes placed subcutaneously in the scalp or small disk electrodes applied to the skin surface of the head. Electroencephalograph recordings are differential: the activity from one electrode is subtracted from the activity of a second. This reduces or eliminates signals common at both electrodes, such as 60- or 50-Hz mains artifacts, muscle artifacts, and other undesired signals. The electrodes are placed symmetrically in the scalp over frontal, central, occipital, parietal, and occasionally temporal cortical areas, with an additional ground electrode. The difference of potential detected between pairs of electrodes (or between an electrode and a reference) is amplified and filtered. EEGs may be recorded with ink on continuously moving paper or displayed and stored electronically. The direction of the movement of the signal is determined by the polarity of the electrodes relative to each other [152].

Montages are various patterns for pairing recording electrodes on the scalp. The montage is the arrangement of reference and recording electrodes placed over the brain. The two main montages are reference and bipolar (see Figure 14.9). The reference montage contains the reference electrode that is placed over the vertex or alternately over some electrically "inactive" site, allowing the determination of absolute voltage

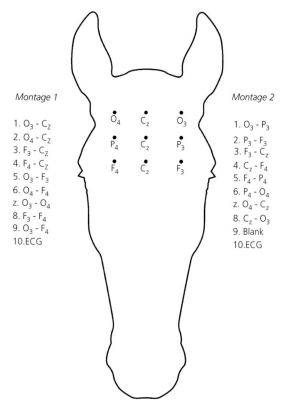

Montage 1

1. O_3 - C_z
2. O_4 - C_z
3. F_3 - C_z
4. F_4 - C_z
5. O_3 - F_3
6. O_4 - F_4
z. O_3 - O_4
8. F_3 - F_4
9. O_3 - F_4
10. ECG

Montage 2

1. O_3 - P_3
2. P_3 - F_3
3. F_3 - C_z
4. C_z - F_4
5. F_4 - P_4
6. P_4 - O_4
z. O_4 - C_z
8. C_z - O_3
9. Blank
10. ECG

Figure 14.9 Drawing of the forehead of a horse illustrating electroencephalographic electrode placements and the two montages used: bipolar left-to-right, back-to-front montage (1) and bipolar circular montage (2). C, central; F, frontal; O, occipital; P, parietal. (Reprinted with permission from Ref. [142].)

and polarity. However, the common reference site is never completely inactive and thus contributes to the output signal and can become contaminated [151]. A bipolar montage links a serial pair of active electrodes in the transverse or coronal direction (Figure 14.9). Since each electrode records electrical activity from a small localized area underneath it, the electrodes can be configured in several bipolar arrangements, which aids in the localization of epileptic foci. With such a montage, one can compare the potentials generated by the left occipital region with those of the right occipital cortex, the potentials generated by the left frontal cortex region with those of the right frontal area, and the potentials generated by the left side with those of the right side [3]. Localization of discrete focal abnormalities in bipolar montages is usually accomplished by locating the common electrode of two adjacent pairs, at which the pen deflection shows a reversal of polarity (phase reversal). Other advantages of

bipolar recording include elimination of the possibility of a contaminated reference and prevention of problems that can arise from unbalanced amplifier input with a common reference. On the other hand, widely distributed potentials may be distorted, and voltage and polarity determinations are always relative to electrode placement [151]. Since the two types of montages provide complimentary information, the use of multiple montages including bipolar and referential types and a combination of both may be used during EEG recordings.

The EEG examination should be performed in a quiet, relatively dark environment. The duration of recording depends on the condition of restraint of the patient and the level of cooperation, but a minimum of 20-min recording is recommended.

Patient restraint

The EEG exam may be performed on awake, sedated, or anesthetized horses, and the condition of recording greatly depends on the preference of the clinician. General anesthesia will significantly reduce artifacts caused by head, ear, and eye movements of the patient and those caused by auditory and visual stimuli but will also alter the EEG from that of the awake state [153]. To easily identify bioelectrical artifacts on awake or lightly sedated horses, electrooculographic, electromyographic, and electrocardiographic activities and behavior can also be recorded; EEG segments can then be separated from artifacts [144]. Even with recording artifacts, interpretation of EEG findings can be challenging, so sedation or general anesthesia can be used to decrease muscle contraction artifact. In any event, a standardized protocol should be used, and cautious interpretation of the EEG recording obtained under such condition is crucial to avoid overinterpretation.

Interpretation of the EEG

Simple visual inspection or automated computerized analysis can be utilized for interpretation. The quantitative computerized method analyses the EEG signal in the frequency domain and provides power spectrum, bispectral analyses, and cortical mapping capabilities [154]. This quantitative analysis has been used in equine anesthesiology to evaluate the anesthetic depth [129, 131, 132, 155] and to study sleep and sedation [149, 156], but artifacts or paroxysmal discharges may be missed during this global analysis.

Visual inspection is useful for many clinical applications, but it requires experience due to the subjective nature of its interpretation. The principal goal of visual inspection is to assess the dominant frequency and amplitude of the signals and the presence or absence of asymmetrical patterns, of paroxysmal activity, and of artifacts. Frequency is defined as the number of observed

Table 14.5 Scoring system for semiquantitative analysis of the equine EEG performed under general anesthesia.

Measurement		Low	Moderate	High
Frequency	Score	2	0	1
		<8 Hz	8–13 Hz	>13 Hz
Voltage	Score	1	0	2
		<25 μV	25–50 μV	>50 μV
Asymmetry	Score	0	1	2
Paroxysmal	Score	0	1	2
activity		<25%	25–50%	>50%

Reprinted with permission from Ref. [142].

events (changes in the direction of voltage) per second, and amplitude of the wave refers to the magnitude of changes between peaks. Alternatively, a semiquantitative visual analysis may be used to remove some of the subjectivity [142, 157]. In each category (frequency, voltage, asymmetry, and paroxysmal activity), a score of 0 or 2 can be assigned when normal or the most abnormal activity is observed, respectively. By default, intermediate-range activity between normal and most abnormal is then given the intermediate value (score of 1) (see Table 14.5).

Computerized analysis of the EEG permits detection of subtle changes in the EEG and quantification of the frequency distribution of the signal. The dominant frequency of the EEG can be classified into four or more frequency ranges, each of which has different characteristics and is associated with different physiological states or diseases. The most commonly recognized frequency ranges are named with Greek letters: beta, alpha, theta, and delta, ranked in order of decreasing frequency. Beta is high frequency (14–50 Hz) and low amplitude (2–20 μV) and is associated with an awake, alert state or during REM, the dreaming stage of sleep. Alpha is slower frequency (8–13 Hz) and higher amplitude (5–100 μV) and is associated with an awake, relaxed state, especially with the eyes closed. The delta and theta ranges have increasingly lower frequencies (4–7 Hz, 0.5–3 Hz) and higher amplitudes (5–100 μV, 20–400 μV) and are associated with deeper stages of sleep, anesthesia, or coma. Seizure activity is typically high frequency and high amplitude, while deep coma is low frequency and low amplitude. Computerized analysis of the EEG most commonly is used to determine the relative amount of power in these frequency ranges (Figure 14.10), which changes with behavioral or disease state, or the overall total power, comparing treatment effects or different animals.

Normal EEG patterns: background, artifact, and normal values

The establishment of universally recognized normal values is difficult because frequency and amplitudes are consciousness state–dependent (e.g., awake, drowsy, sleeping, sedated, or anesthetized). Furthermore, cortical activity is also influenced by physiological states. For instance, interpretation of EEG in foals is difficult because large variations on EEG recording may be observed dependent on the stage of maturation of the brain. Furthermore, the age at which cerebral maturation occurs is unknown in horses, although they are a precocial species. In most mammalian species, alpha rhythm (electrical activity with a frequency of 8–13 Hz) has been considered the most predominant pattern observed in a mature brain [146]. In neonatal foals, the normal patterns include high-voltage, slow-wave activity [142, 146]. As brain maturation occurs with an increased complexity and divergence of the dendritic network, faster and lower-voltage activity becomes more predominant on EEG recordings. Therefore, it is critical to take into consideration the state of awareness and age of the patient and to know what is considered a normal EEG tracing under such condition.

In order to accurately interpret the EEG pattern and to recognize possible pathological changes, one must first evaluate the background for frequency, amplitude, and symmetry and identify normal transients and potential artifacts. Frequently encountered artifacts include muscle potential artifacts, movement artifacts, and respiratory artifacts. Early identification of artifacts is critical for obtaining a high-quality recording of the baseline and possibly eliminating them. Artifacts such as ocular movements and facial muscle twitches produce symmetric and asymmetric low-voltage, slow-wave activity, respectively [3]. When muscle potential artifacts are detected during the recording, the skin and muscle underlying the electrodes can be desensitized with 2% mepivacaine by subdermal injection. Normal waveforms that may be misleading include spindles and burst suppression, which are normal transient events observed during sedation or anesthesia. Spindles are repetitive sinusoidal waves, and burst suppression refers to intervals of high-amplitude activity interrupted by brief relatively isoelectric periods, usually only observed during deep anesthesia [154]. Vertex waves are observed in response to stimulation and do not have a spike component, which allow them to be differentiated from paroxysmal waveforms [152].

Normal EEG background in the awake alert horse, which was first described in 1968, consists of a dominant waveform of low-voltage (8–15 μV) and fast-wave activity (18–30 Hz) (Table 14.6) [143, 146]. Usually, this activity is superimposed over a low- to medium-voltage

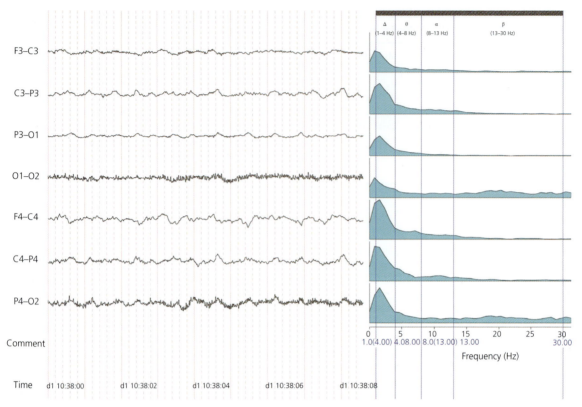

Figure 14.10 Electroencephalogram and power spectrum recorded from an awake horse with reported seizure activity, displayed using a hatband montage. The power spectrum in microvolts for the 10 s of EEG on the left is shown to the right, with frequencies split into Δ (1–4 Hz), θ (4–8 Hz), α (8–13 Hz), and β (13–30 Hz) frequency bands. Note that β activity is greater in the O_1–O_2 and P_4–O_2 channels, localizing the higher-frequency activity to the right occipital (O_2) electrode location. The greatest power in all channels is in the Δ frequency range.

(10–40 μV) and slow-wave activity (5–10 Hz). Normal values have also been established in adult horses under general anesthesia and include a frequency of 8–13 Hz and a voltage of 25–50 μV (see Figure 14.11 and Table 14.6) [142]. In sedated foals, the observed pattern includes high-voltage (50–200 μV) and slow-wave activities (1–2 Hz) [142, 146].

It is also important to recognize normal EEG patterns during various states of sleep, although there is limited information in horses [149, 158–160]. As in other species, slow-wave sleep is characterized by synchronized high-voltage (100 μV) and slow-wave activities (2–4 Hz) in normal adult horses, which is similar to the pattern in tranquilized horses. Paradoxical (REM) sleep is characterized by desynchronized low-voltage and fast-wave activity, which resembles the patterns of alert wakefulness. During this period, the horse is recumbent; eye movements, frequently accompanied by ear and leg movements and even by vocalization, are observed [149, 156, 161].

Abnormal EEG patterns associated with disease

EEG has been used to investigate horses presenting with a history of seizures, abnormal behavior, collapse, and narcolepsy and also horses affected with cerebellar disease and encephalitis. Accurate interpretation of the EEG recording can provide usual information in regard to the presence (or absence) of cerebral disease and its nature (acute vs. chronic; focal vs. diffuse; inflammatory vs. degenerative). One should assess the background for abnormal frequency and amplitude, for the presence of asymmetrical patterns between regions, and for the presence of paroxysmal activity. The most common abnormalities associated with cerebral diseases are a change in either amplitude or frequency, or both; and the following general principles can be applied: [162]

1 Low-voltage, fast-wave activity along with paroxysmal spikes may occur with ongoing irritative processes such as seizures or inflammation (see Figure 14.12).

2 High-voltage, slow-wave activity may indicate death of neurons in diseases such as brain abscess, neoplasia,

Table 14.6 Amplitudes and frequencies observed in normal electroencephalographic patterns from awake and sedated adult horses.

		Normal patterns	
		Voltage (µV)	Frequency (Hz)
Awake	Primary pattern	8–15	18–30
	Secondary pattern	10–40	5–10
Sedated with xylazine	Dominant	10–70	1–3 [84]
		10–80	10–15
		10–90	0.5–4
		5–30	25–40
Sedated with acetylpromazine	Primary pattern	5–40	25–40
	Secondary pattern	5–10	1–4

Reprinted with permission from Refs. [133, 146].

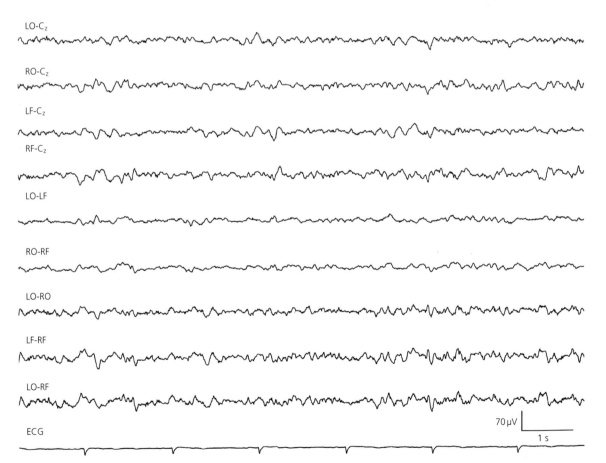

Figure 14.11 A normal adult equine electroencephalographic recording made under general anesthesia with a bipolar left-to-right, back-to-front montage. A moderate-voltage (25–50 mV) and moderate-frequency (8–13 Hz) pattern, without any asymmetry or paroxysmal activity, was present. ECG, electrocardiogram; F, frontal; L, left; O, occipital; R, right. (Reprinted with permission from Ref. [142]. © Wiley.)

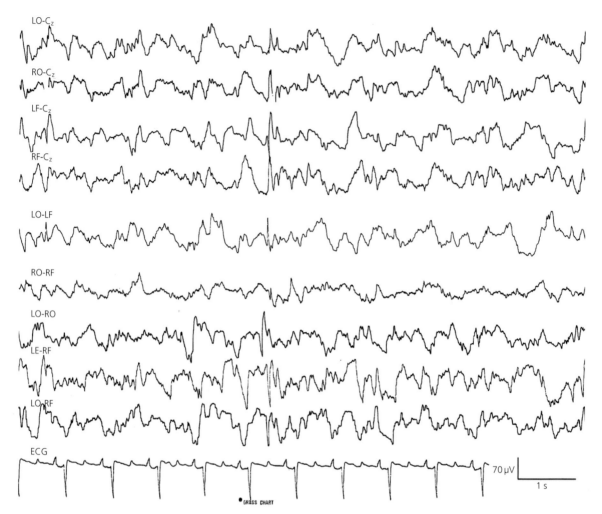

Figure 14.12 Electroencephalographic recording made under general anesthesia from a 1-day-old filly that presented for lack of nursing and intermittent tremors. The recording contained diffuse high-voltage slow waves and focal discrete paroxysmal discharge activity. Multifocal paroxysmal activity was seen on the remaining EEG recording. (Reprinted with permission from Ref. [142]. © Wiley.)

and cerebrocortical necrosis. For example, such pattern was observed in sheep and cattle with experimental cerebrocortical necrosis and in foals with hypoxic ischemic encephalopathy [142, 163, 164]. However, neither change is pathognomonic of a particular disease but rather reflects the nature of the pathologic process occurring (e.g., inflammation or degeneration).

3 Localized EEG changes may indicate focal cortical disease such as infarcts, hemorrhage, early tumor, or abscessation (see Figure 14.13).

4 Generalized EEG changes may indicate a diffuse cortical or subcortical disease such as infection, trauma, space-occupying lesions (hydrocephalus, tumor), idiopathic epilepsy, or a systemic metabolic illness (hepatic encephalopathy or hypocalcemia). For example, generalized slower activity with a high voltage (100–200 μV) has been reported in dogs and calves with hydrocephalus [165, 166].

5 EEG can reflect ongoing pathological changes; thus, serial recording may be helpful as a prognostic indicator for following the response to therapy and disease progression.

One of the most common indications for performing an EEG is to confirm the clinical diagnosis of a seizure disorder or epilepsy, which is defined as a clinical manifestation of excessive and/or hypersynchronous abnormal neuronal activity in the cerebral cortex, and to potentially determine etiology [167]. The EEG is the

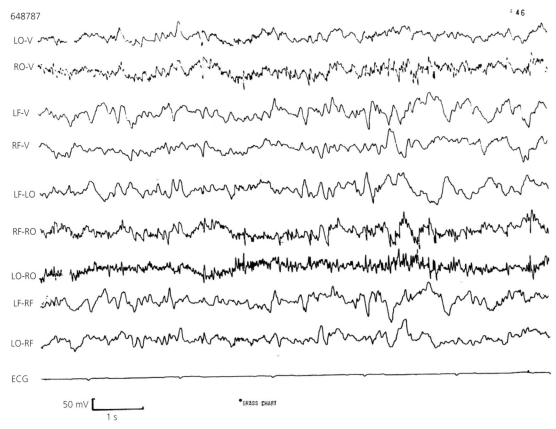

Figure 14.13 Electroencephalogram from a horse with a space-occupying mass in the left frontal area of the brain under general anesthesia. The generalized high-voltage, low-frequency waves and asymmetry of the left cortex are notable. ECG, electrocardiogram; F, frontal; L, left; O, occipital; R, right; V, vertex.

most important paraclinical test in humans suffering from epilepsy, and this diagnostic test has also been shown to be useful in dogs and horses with seizures [142, 168, 169]. In epileptic patients, an increase toward low-voltage, fast-wave activity or high-voltage, slow-wave activity may be seen [113]. In addition, epileptiform paroxysmal activity appears on the majority (40–90%) of EEGs recorded on epileptic patients [142, 169, 170]. The proximity in time of a seizure to the EEG examination may also influence the amount of epileptiform activity present in the EEG [168]. These activities are defined as abnormal paroxysmal transient events, consisting of spikes or sharp waves, isolated or followed by a wave; spike and wave; or polyspike and wave complexes [168, 170]. Both generalized and focal epileptiform activity have been recorded in epileptic horses [142]. Although epileptiform paroxysmal activity has been associated with the pathophysiology of seizures, it is important to realize that failure to record seizure activity does not automatically rule out epilepsy, since

the use of tranquilizers may increase the threshold for seizures and the window of recording may not have been long enough to record interictal paroxysmal epileptiform discharges. To avoid this, frequent and prolonged sophisticated EEG monitoring is routinely performed in humans, but it is not practical in large animals. Therefore, one should consider repeating EEG examination in an animal suspected of having epilepsy and for which the first EEG recording was normal. As an alternative, ambulatory EEG may be employed, where long-term EEG recordings are collected with the animal in a relatively unrestrained state [137, 171].

Electroencephalographic recording could be used in the investigation of other neurologic disorders such as in cases of suspected cerebral inflammatory processes. The EEG has proven to be a very useful tool in the diagnosis of encephalitis and meningitis. For instance, serial EEG recording in horses with experimental West Nile virus encephalitis revealed a generalized abnormal electrical activity before the development of any clinical sign [143]. An acute case of encephalitis is characterized by high-voltage activities, whereas a late stage is characterized by slow-voltage (1–5 μV) and slow-wave (3–4 Hz) activities in the awake horse. The EEG in an 11-month-old filly infected by equine encephalitis was characterized by periodic episodes of generalized synchronous high-voltage, slow-wave activity with generalized seizure activity [141]. In a few cases of equine protozoal myeloencephalitis presenting with seizures, EEG demonstrated a higher generalized voltage than normal and was used to establish the neurophysiologic and anatomic basis for the seizure activity [135]. Brain abscesses frequently show localized slow-wave activity superimposed by some sharp waves. In a case of sinonasal adenocarcinoma extending into the right cranial vault and causing CNS disease, the EEG pattern included low-voltage irregular delta waves (e.g., activity <4 Hz), which is characteristic of asymmetric space-occupying mass [140]. Although EEG is helpful in localizing structural abnormalities, in some instances, the EEG pattern of horses with intracranial masses, such as abscesses, includes generalized continuous high-voltage, slow-wave activity and is not specific for localization [140, 142]. Similar observations have been reported in other species [112].

Finally, horses suffering from extracranial diseases may have an abnormal EEG recording associated with metabolic disease. For instance, it has been reported in other species that hypothyroidism may produce symmetric low-voltage, medium-frequency activity and that hepatoencephalopathy is characterized by fast frequencies (5–20 Hz) and medium voltages (15–50 μV). The EEG patterns of hypocalcemia-induced seizures in a foal included diffuse and symmetric slow-wave activity associated with discrete epileptiform activity [142]. Finally, an abnormal EEG pattern, including beta activity (e.g., frequency >13 Hz) and numerous triphasic waves, was recorded in a horse suffering from ongoing malignant hyperthermia episodes [172].

References

[1] Nollet, H., Deprez, P., Van Ham, L. et al. (2002) The use of magnetic motor evoked potential in horses with cervical spinal cord disease. Equine Vet J, 34, 156–163.

[2] International Federation of Clinical Neurophysiology (1999) Recommendations for the practice of clinical neurophysiology: guidelines of the International Federation of Clinical Neurophysiology, in Electroencephalography and Clinical Neurophysiology (eds G. Deuschl and A. Eisen), Elsevier, New York, p. 304.

[3] Andrews, F.M. and Fenner, W.R. (1987) Indications and use of electrodiagnostic aids in neurologic disease. Vet Clin North Am Equine Pract, 3, 293–322.

[4] van Wessum, R., Sloet van Oldruitenborgh-Oosterbaan, M.M. and Clayton, H.M. (1999) Electromyography in the horse in veterinary medicine and in veterinary research—a review. Vet Q, 21, 3–7.

[5] Wijnberg, I.D., van der Kolk, J.H., Franssen, H. et al. (2003) Needle electromyography in the horse compared with its principles in man: a review. Equine Vet J, 35, 9–17.

[6] Wijnberg, I.D., Back, W., de Jong, M. et al. (2004) The role of electromyography in clinical diagnosis of neuromuscular locomotor problems in the horse. Equine Vet J, 36, 718–722.

[7] Wijnberg, I.D. (2005) A review of the use of electromyography in equine neurological diseases. Equine Vet Educ, 17, 123–127.

[8] DeLuca, C.J. (1984) Myoelectric manifestations of localized muscular fatigue in humans. Crit Rev Biomed Eng, 11, 251–279.

[9] Robert, C., Valette, J.P., Degueurce, C. et al. (1999) Correlation between surface electromyography and kinematics of the hindlimb of horses at trot on a treadmill. Cells Tissues Organs, 165, 113–122.

[10] Stewart, C.R., Nanedkar, S.D., Massey, J.M. et al. (1989) Evaluation of an automatic method of measuring features of motor unit action potentials. Muscle Nerve, 12, 141–148.

[11] Guld, C., Rosenfalck, A. and Willison, R.G. (1971) Technical factors in recording, in Electrodiagnostics and Electromyography (ed. S.L. Licht), Waverly Press Inc., Baltimore, pp. 452–478.

[12] Henry, W.H., Diesem, C.D. and Wiechers, M.D. (1979) Evaluation of equine radial and median nerve conduction velocities. Am J Vet Res, 40, 1406–1410.

[13] Sprinkle FP. 1977. Nerve Conduction Velocities in the Horse. M.S. thesis, Auburn University, Auburn.

[14] Henry, R.W. and Diesem, C.D. (1981) Proximal equine radial and median motor nerve conduction velocity. Am J Vet Res, 42, 1819–1822.

[15] Blythe, L.L., Kitchell, R.L., Holliday, T.A. et al. (1983) Sensory nerve conduction velocities in forelimb of ponies. Am J Vet Res, 44, 1419–1426.

[16] Zarucco, L., Driessen, B., Scandella, M. et al. (2010) Sensory nerve conduction and nociception in the equine lower forelimb during perineural bupivacaine infusion along the palmar nerves. Can J Vet Res, 74, 305–313.

[17] Blythe, L.L., Engel, H.N., Jr and Rowe, K.E. (1988) Comparison of sensory nerve conduction velocities in horses versus ponies. Am J Vet Res, 49, 2138–2142.

[18] Whalen, L.R., Wheeler, S.J., LeCouteur, R.A. et al. (1994) Sensory nerve conduction velocity of the caudal cutaneous sural and medial cutaneous antebrachial nerves of adult horses. Am J Vet Res, 55, 892–897.

[19] Aleman, M., Williams, D.C., Brosnan, R.J. et al. (2013) Sensory nerve conduction and somatosensory evoked potentials of the trigeminal nerve in horses with idiopathic headshaking. J Vet Intern Med, 27, 1571–1580.

[20] Wheeler, S.J. (1989) Influence of limb temperature on sensory nerve conduction velocity in horses. *Am J Vet Res*, 50, 1817–1819.

[21] Wheeler, S.J. (1990) Effect of age on sensory nerve conduction velocity in the horse. *Res Vet Sci*, 48, 141–144.

[22] Bolt, D.M., Burba, D.J., Hubert, J.D. *et al.* (2004) Functional and morphological changes in palmar digital nerves after non-focused extracorporeal shock wave therapy in horses. *Am J Vet Res*, 65, 1714–1718.

[23] Mysinger, P.W., Wolfe, D.F., Redding, R.W. *et al.* (1994) Sensory nerve conduction velocity of the dorsal penile nerves of bulls. *Am J Vet Res*, 5, 898–900.

[24] Kimura, J. (2013) The F wave and the A wave, in *Electrodiagnosis in Diseases of Nerve and Muscle: Principles and Practice*, 4th edn (ed. J. Kimura), Oxford University Press, New York, pp. 149–179.

[25] Kimura, J. (2013) H, T, and the masseter reflexes and the silent period, in *Electrodiagnosis in Diseases of Nerve and Muscle: Principles and Practice*, 4th edn (ed. J. Kimura), Oxford University Press, New York, pp. 208–234.

[26] Aleman, M., Williams, D.C., Jorge, N.E. *et al.* (2011) Repetitive stimulation of the common peroneal nerve as a diagnostic aid for botulism in foals. *J Vet Intern Med*, 25, 365–372.

[27] Sims, M.H. and McLean, R.A. (1990) Use of repetitive nerve stimulation to assess neuromuscular function in dogs. A test protocol for suspected myasthenia gravis. *Progr Vet Neurol*, 1, 311–319.

[28] Slomić, A., Rosenfalck, A. and Buchthal, F. (1968) Electrical and mechanical responses of normal and myasthenic muscle. *Brain Res*, 10, 1–78.

[29] Keesey, J.C. (1989) AAEE minimonograph #33: electrodiagnostic approach to defects of neuromuscular transmission. *Muscle Nerve*, 12, 613–626.

[30] Strain, G.M., Kerwin, S.C., Tedford, B.L. *et al.* (1998) Creatine kinase level changes following electromyography in the normal anesthetized dog. *Vet J*, 156, 231–233.

[31] Wijnberg, I.D., Franssen, H., van der Kolk, J.H. *et al.* (2002) Quantitative motor unit action potential analysis of skeletal muscles in the Warmblood horse. *Equine Vet J*, 34, 556–562.

[32] Wijnberg, I.D., Graubner, C., Auriemma, E. *et al.* (2011) Quantitative motor unit action potential analysis in 2 paraspinal neck muscles in adult Royal Dutch Sport horses. *J Vet Intern Med*, 25, 592–597.

[33] Ciminaghi, B., Albertini, M., Costanzi, M. *et al.* (2004) Quantitative motor unit action potential analysis in skeletal muscles in horses and ponies. *Vet Res Commun*, 28, 177–179.

[34] Wijnberg, I.D., Frassen, H., Jansen, G.H. *et al.* (2003) Quantitative electromyographic examination in myogenic disorders of 6 horses. *J Vet Intern Med*, 17, 185–193.

[35] Wijnberg, I.D., Franssen, H., Jansen, G.H. *et al.* (2006) The role of quantitative electromyography (EMG) in horses suspected of acute and chronic grass sickness. *Equine Vet J*, 38, 230–237.

[36] Harrison, S.M., Whitton, R.C., King, M. *et al.* (2012) Forelimb muscle activity during equine locomotion. *J Exp Biol*, 215, 2980–2991.

[37] Zsoldos, R.R., Kotschwar, A.B., Kotschwar, A. *et al.* (2010) Electromyography activity of the equine splenius muscle and neck kinematics during walk and trot on the treadmill. *Equine Vet J*, 42 (Supp 38), 455–461.

[38] Zaneb, H., Kaufmann, V., Stanek, C. *et al.* (2009) Quantitative differences in activities of back and pelvic limb muscles during walking and trotting between chronically lame and nonlame horses. *Am J Vet Res*, 70, 1129–1134.

[39] Lesimple, C., Fureix, C., De Margerie, E. *et al.* (2012) Towards a postural indicator of back pain in horses (Equus caballus). *PLoS One*, 7, e44604.

[40] Kimura, J. (2013) Electromyography and other measures of muscle function, in *Electrodiagnosis in Diseases of Nerve and Muscle: Principles and Practice*, 4th edn (ed. J. Kimura), Oxford University Press, New York, pp. 333–360.

[41] Mayhew, I.G., Whitlock, R.H. and de Lahunta, A. (1978) Spinal cord disease of the horse, electromyographic and radiographic studies. *Cornell Vet Suppl*, 68, 44–62.

[42] Robinson, J.A., Naylor, J.M. and Crichlow, E.C. (1990) Use of electromyography for the diagnosis of equine hyperkalemic periodic paresis. *Can J Vet Res*, 54, 495–500.

[43] Wijnberg, I.D., Franssen, H., van der Kolk, J.H. *et al.* (2001) Quantitative analysis of motor unit action potentials in the subclavian muscle of healthy horses. *Am J Vet Res*, 63, 198–203.

[44] Oh, S.J. (1998) Needle electromyographic study, in *Principles of Clinical Electromyography: Case Studies* (ed. S.J. Oh), Williams and Wilkins, Baltimore, pp. 78–120.

[45] Wijnberg, I.D., van der Kolk, J.H., Franssen, H. *et al.* (2002) Electromyographic changes of motor unit activity in horses with induced hypocalcemia and hypomagnesemia. *Am J Vet Res*, 63, 849–856.

[46] Podell, M., Valentine, B.A., Cummings, J.F. *et al.* (1995) Electromyography in acquired equine motor neuron disease. *Progr Vet Neurol*, 6, 128–134.

[47] Bowen, J.M. (1976) Electromyography, in *Applied Electronics for Veterinary Medicine and Small Animal Physiology* (ed. W.R. Klemm), Charles C. Thomas Publisher, Springfield, pp. 188–276.

[48] Kugelberg, E. and Petersen, L. (1949) Insertion activity in electromyography with notes on denervation muscle response to constant current. *J Neurol Neurosurg Psychiatry*, 12, 268–273.

[49] Kornegay, J.N., Gorgacz, E.J., Dawe, D.L. *et al.* (1980) Polymyositis in dogs. *J Am Vet Med Assoc*, 176, 431.

[50] Warmolts, J.R. and Engel, W.K. (1970) A critique of the "myopathic" electromyogram. *Trans Am Neurol Assoc*, 95, 173–177.

[51] Daube, J.R. (1985) Electrophysiologic studies in diagnosis and prognosis of motor neuron disease. *Neurol Clin*, 3, 540–541.

[52] Beech, J., Fletcher, J.E., Lizzo, F. *et al.* (1988) Effect of phenytoin on clinical signs and in vitro muscle twitch in horses with chronic intermittent rhabdomyolysis and myotonia. *Am J Vet Res*, 49, 2130–2133.

[53] Moore, M.P., Andrews, F.M., Reed, S.M. *et al.* (1988) Electromyographic evaluation of horses with laryngeal hemiplegia. *Equine Vet Sci*, 8, 424–427.

[54] Naylor, J.M., Robinson, J.A., Crichlow, E.C. *et al.* (1992) Inheritance of the myotonic discharges in American Quarter horses and the relationship to hyperkalemic periodic paralysis. *Can J Vet Res*, 56, 62–66.

[55] Naylor, J.M., Jones, V. and Berry, S.L. (1993) Clinical syndromes and diagnosis of hyperkalemic periodic paralysis in Quarter horses. *Equine Vet J*, 25, 227–232.

[56] Divers, T.J., Mohammed, H.O., Cummings, J.F. *et al.* (1994) Equine motor neuron disease: findings in 28 horses and proposal of pathological mechanism for the disease. *Equine Vet J*, 26, 409–415.

[57] Andrews, F.M., Spurgeon, T.L. and Reed, S.M. (1986) Histochemical changes in skeletal muscle of four male horses with neuromuscular disease. *Am J Vet Res*, 47, 2078–2083.

[58] Hegreberg, G.A. and Reed, S.M. (1990) Skeletal muscle changes associated with equine myotonic dystrophy. *Acta Neuropathol*, 80, 426–431.

[59] Spier, S.J., Carlson, G.P., Holiday, T.A. *et al.* (1990) Hyperkalemic periodic paralysis in horses. *J Am Vet Med Assoc*, 197, 1009–1017.

[60] Bowen, J.M. (1978) Peripheral nerve electrodiagnostics, electromyography, and nerve conduction, in *Canine Neurology*, 3rd edn (ed. B.F. Hoerlein), Saunders, Philadelphia, p. 262.

[61] Merton, P.A. and Morton, H.B. (1980) Stimulation of the cerebral cortex in the intact human subject. *Nature*, 285, 227.

[62] Barker, A.T., Jalinous, R. and Freeston, I.L. (1985) Non-invasive magnetic stimulation of human motor cortex [letter]. *Lancet*, 1, 1106–1107.

[63] Chawla J. 2012 n. Medscape Reference; http://emedicine. medscape.com/article/1139085-overview [accessed November 28, 2014].

[64] Strain, G.M., Prescott-Mathews, J.S. and Tedford, B.L. (1990) Motor potentials evoked by transcranial stimulation of the canine motor cortex. *Progr Vet Neurol*, 1, 321–331.

[65] Mayhew, I.G. and Washbourne, J.R. (1996) Magnetic motor evoked potentials in ponies. *J Vet Intern Med*, 10, 326–329.

[66] Nollet, H., Van Ham, L., Deprez, P. *et al.* (2003) Transcranial magnetic stimulation: review of the technique, basic principles and applications. *Vet J*, 166, 28–42.

[67] Nollet, H., Van Ham, L., Dewulf, J. *et al.* (2003) Standardization of transcranial magnetic stimulation in the horse. *Vet J*, 166, 244–520.

[68] Nollet, H., Deprez, P., van Ham, L. *et al.* (2004) Transcranial magnetic stimulation: normal values of magnetic motor evoked potentials in 84 normal horses and influence of height, weight, age and sex. *Equine Vet J*, 36, 51–57.

[69] Nollet, H., Vanschandevijl, K., Van Ham, L. *et al.* (2005) Role of transcranial magnetic stimulation in differentiating motor nervous tract disorders from other causes of recumbency in four horses and one donkey. *Vet Rec*, 157, 656–658.

[70] MacDonald, D.B., Skinner, S., Shils, J. *et al.* (2013) Intraoperative motor evoked potential monitoring—a position statement by the American Society of Neurophysiological Monitoring. *Clin Neurophysiol*, 124, 2291–2316.

[71] Wilson, W.J. and Mills, P.C. (2005) Brainstem auditory-evoked response in dogs. *Am J Vet Res*, 66, 2177–2187.

[72] Chiappa, K.H. and Hill, R.A. (1997) Brain stem auditory evoked potentials: interpretation, in *Evoked Potentials in Clinical Medicine*, 3rd edn (ed. K.H. Chiappa), Lippincott-Raven Press, Philadelphia, pp. 199–268.

[73] Strain, G.M. (2011) Brainstem auditory evoked response (BAER), in *Deafness in Dogs and Cats* (ed. G.M. Strain), CABI, Oxfordshire, pp. 83–107.

[74] Strain, G.M., Green, K.D., Twedt, A.C. *et al.* (1993) Brain stem auditory evoked potentials from bone stimulation in dogs. *Am J Vet Res*, 54, 1817–1821.

[75] Rolf, S.L., Reed, S.M., Melnick, W. *et al.* (1987) Auditory brainstem response testing in anesthetized horses. *Am J Vet Res*, 48, 910–914.

[76] Mayhew, I.G. and Washbourne, J.R. (1997) Brainstem auditory evoked potentials in horses and ponies. *Vet J*, 153, 107–113.

[77] Marshall, A.E. (1985) Brain stem auditory-evoked response in the nonanesthetized horse and pony. *Am J Vet Res*, 46, 1445–1450.

[78] Mayhew, I.G. and Washbourne, J.R. (1990) A method of assessing auditory and brainstem function in horses. *Br Vet J*, 146, 509–518.

[79] Bedenice, D., Hoffman, A.M., Parrott, B. *et al.* (2001) Vestibular signs associated with suspected lighting strik e in two horses. *Vet Rec*, 149, 519–522.

[80] Harland, M.M., Stewart, A.J., Marshall, A.E. *et al.* (2006) Diagnosis of deafness in a horse by brainstem auditory evoked potential. *Can Vet J*, 47, 151–154.

[81] Sponenberg, D.P. (2009) *Equine Color Genetics*, 3rd edn, Wiley-Blackwell, Ames.

[82] Hauswirth, R., Haase, B., Blatter, M. *et al.* (2012) Mutations in MITF and PAX3 cause "splashed white" and other white spotting phenotypes in horses. *PLoS Genet*, 8, e1002653.

[83] Wilson, W.J., Mills, P.C. and Dzulkarnain, A.A. (2011) Use of BAER to identify loss of auditory function in older horses. *Aust Vet J*, 89, 73–76.

[84] Marshall, A.E., Byars, T.D., Whitlock, R.H. *et al.* (1981) Brainstem auditory evoked response in the diagnosis of inner ear injury in the horse. *J Am Vet Med Assoc*, 178, 282–286.

[85] Nostrandt, A.D., Pedersoli, W.M., Marshall, A.E. *et al.* (1981) Ototoxic potential of gentamicin in ponies. *Am J Vet Res*, 52, 494–498.

[86] Steiss, J.E., Storrs, D.P., Brendemuehl, J.P. *et al.* (1991) Nerve conduction velocities and brain stem auditory evoked responses in clinically normal neonatal foals, with comparison to foals from mares grazed on endophyte-infected fescue. *Progr Vet Neurol*, 2, 252–260.

[87] Aleman, M., Puchalski, S.M., Williams, D.C. *et al.* (2008) Brainstem auditory-evoked responses in horses with temporohyoid osteoarthropathy. *J Vet Intern Med*, 22, 1196–1202.

[88] Magdesian, K.G., Williams, D.C., Aleman, M. *et al.* (2009) Evaluation of deafness in American Paint Horses by phenotype, brainstem auditory-evoked responses, and endothelin receptor B genotype. *J Am Vet Med Assoc*, 235, 1204–1211.

[89] Narfstrom, K., Ekesten, B., Rosolen, S. *et al.* (2002) Guidelines for clinical electroretinography in the dog. *Doc Ophthalmol*, 105, 83–92.

[90] Church, M.L. and Norman, J.C. (2012) Electroretinogram responses of the normal thoroughbred horse sedated with detomidine hydrochloride. *Vet Ophthalmol*, 15 (Supp 2), 77–83.

[91] Ben-Shlomo, G., Plummer, C., Barrie, K. *et al.* (2012) Characterization of the normal dark adaptation curve of the horse. *Vet Ophthalmol*, 15, 42–45.

[92] Sandmeyer, L.S., Breaux, C.B., Archer, S. *et al.* (2007) Clinical and electroretinographic characteristics of congenital stationary night blindness in the Appaloosa and the association with the leopard complex. *Vet Ophthalmol*, 10, 368–375.

[93] Komáromy, A.M. (2009) Electrodiagnostic testing for retinal disease, in *Current Therapy in Equine Medicine*, 6th edn (eds N.E. Robinson and K.A. Sprayberry), Saunders, Philadelphia, pp. 668–671.

[94] Gilger, B.C. (2011) Equine ocular examination: routine and advanced diagnostic techniques, in *Equine Ophthalmology*, 2nd edn (ed. B.C. Gilger), Saunders, Philadelphia, pp. 1–50.

[95] Riis, R.C., Jackson, C., Rebhun, W. *et al.* (1999) Ocular manifestations of equine motor neuron disease. *Equine Vet J*, 31, 99–110.

[96] Strain, G.M., Olcott, B.M. and Braun, W.F., Jr (1986) Electroencephalogram and evoked potentials in naturally occurring scrapie in sheep. *Am J Vet Res*, 47, 828–836.

[97] Strain, G.M., Olcott, B.M. and Hokett, L.D. (1986) Electroretinogram and visual-evoked potential measurements in Holstein cows. *Am J Vet Res*, 47, 1079–1081.

[98] Strain, G.M., Claxton, M.S., Turnquist, S.E. *et al.* (1987) Evoked potential and electroencephalographic assessment of central blindness due to brain abscesses in a steer. *Cornell Vet*, 77, 374–382.

[99] Strain, G.M., Graham, M.C., Claxton, M.S. *et al.* (1989) Postnatal development of brainstem auditory-evoked potentials, electroretinograms, and visual-evoked potentials in the calf. *J Vet Intern Med*, 3, 231–237.

[100] Strain, G.M., Claxton, M.S., Olcott, B.M. *et al.* (1990) Visual-evoked potentials and electroretinograms in ruminants with thiamine responsive polioencephalomalacia and suspected listeriosis. *Am J Vet Res*, 51, 1513–1517.

[101] Strain, G.M., Claxton, M.S., Prescott-Mathews, J.S. *et al.* (1991) Electroretinogram and visual-evoked potential measurements in sheep. *Can J Vet Res*, 55, 1–4.

[102] Strain, G.M., Claxton-Gill, M.S., Prescott-Mathews, J.S. *et al.* (1992) Visual evoked potentials in amprolium-induced experimental polioencephalomalacia. *Progr Vet Neurol*, 3, 65–71.

[103] Strain, G.M., Tedford, B.L. and Gill, M.S. (2006) Brainstem auditory evoked potentials and flash visual evoked potentials in Vietnamese miniature pot-bellied pigs. *Res Vet Sci*, 80, 91–95.

[104] Strain, G.M., Taylor, D.S., Graham, M.C. *et al.* (1988) Cortical somatosensory-evoked potentials in the horse. *Am J Vet Res*, 49, 1869–1872.

[105] Pickles, K.J., Gibson, T.J., Johnson, C.B. *et al.* (2011) Preliminary investigation of somatosensory evoked potentials in equine headshaking. *Vet Rec*, 168, 511–515.

[106] van Loon, J.P.A.M., van Oostrom, H., Doornenbal, A. *et al.* (2010) Lumbosacral spinal cord somatosensory evoked potentials for quantification of nociception in horses. *Equine Vet J*, 42, 255–260.

[107] van Loon, J.P.A.M., Menke, E.S., Doornebal, A. *et al.* (2012) Antinociceptive effects of low dose lumbosacral epidural ropivacaine in healthy ponies. *Vet J*, 193, 240–245.

[108] Aminoff, M.J. (1986) Electroencephalography: general principles and clinical applications, in *Electrodiagnosis in Clinical Neurology* (ed. M.J. Aminoff), Churchill Livingstone, New York, pp. 21–75.

[109] Croft, P.G. (1964) The EEG as an aid to diagnoses of nervous diseases in the dog and cat. *J Small Anim Pract*, 5, 540–541.

[110] Holliday, T.A., Cunningham, J.G. and Gutnick, M.J. (1970) Comparative clinical and electroencephalographic studies of canine epilepsy. *Epilepsia*, 11, 281–292.

[111] Steiss JE. Electrodiagnostic evaluation. In: Braund KG, ed. *Clinical Neurology in Small Animals: Localization, Diagnosis and Treatment*. Ithaca:International Veterinary Information Service;2003. http://www.ivis.org/advances/Vite/steiss1/chapter_frm.asp?LA=1 [accessed November 28, 2014].

[112] Steiss, J.E., Cox, N.R. and Knecht, C.D. (1990) Electroencephalographic and histopathologic correlations in eight dogs with intracranial mass lesions. *Am J Vet Res*, 51, 1286–1291.

[113] Klemm, W.R. (1989) Electroencephalography in the diagnosis of epilepsy. *Probl Vet Med*, 1, 535–557.

[114] Niedermeyer, E. and Lopes da Silva, F. (2005) *Electroencephalography: Basic Principles, Clinical Applications, and Related Fields*, Lippincott Williams & Wilkins, Philadelphia.

[115] Redding, R.W. (1964) A simple technique for obtaining an electroencephalogram of the dog. *Am J Vet Res*, 25, 854–857.

[116] Redding, R.W. (1987) Electroencephalography, in *Veterinary Neurology* (eds J.E. Oliver, B.F. Hoerlein and I.G. Mayhew), W.B. Saunders Co, Philadelphia, pp. 111–145.

[117] Redding, R.W. and Knecht, C.E. (1984) Breed and species differences, in *Atlas of Electroencephalography in the Dog and Cat* (eds R.W. Redding and C.E. Knecht), Praeger, New York, pp. 149–197.

[118] Usenick, M.W., Kitchell, R.L., Herschler, R.G. *et al.* (1962) A surgical technique for permanent implantation of electrocorticographic electrodes in the burro and pigs. *Am J Vet Res*, 23, 70–73.

[119] Auer, J.A., Amend, J.F., Garner, H.E. *et al.* (1979) Electroencephalographic responses during volatile anesthesia in domestic ponies: a comparative study of isofluorane, enflurane, methoxyflurane, and halothane. *J Equine Med Surg*, 3, 130–134.

[120] Ekström, P.M., Short, C.E. and Geimer, T.R. (1993) Electroencephalography of detomidine-ketamine-halothane and detomidine-ketamine-isoflurane anesthetized horses during orthopedic surgery. *Vet Surg*, 22, 414–418.

[121] Johnson, C.B., Bloomfield, M. and Taylor, P.M. (1999) Effects of ketamine on the equine electroencephalogram during anesthesia with halothane in oxygen. *Vet Surg*, 28, 380–385.

[122] Johnson, C.B., Bloomfield, M. and Taylor, P.M. (2000) Effects of guaiphenesin on the equine electroencephalogram during anaesthesia with halothane in oxygen. *Vet Anaesth Analg*, 27, 6–12.

[123] Johnson, C.B., Bloomfield, M. and Taylor, P.M. (2000) Effects of thiopentone on the equine electroencephalogram during anaesthesia with halothane in oxygen. *Vet Anaesth Analg*, 27, 82–88.

[124] Johnson, C.B., Bloomfield, M. and Taylor, P.M. (2003) Effects of midazolam and sarmazenil on the equine electroencephalogram during anaesthesia with halothane in oxygen. *J Vet Pharmacol Ther*, 26, 105–112.

[125] Johnson, C.B. and Taylor, P.M. (1998) Comparison of the effects of halothane, isoflurane and methoxyflurane on the electroencephalogram of the horse. *Br J Anaesth*, 81, 748–753.

[126] Johnson, C.B., Young, S.S. and Taylor, P.M. (1994) Analysis of the frequency spectrum of the equine electroencephalogram during halothane anaesthesia. *Res Vet Sci*, 56, 373–378.

[127] Murrell, J.C., Johnson, C.B., White, K.L. *et al.* (2003) Changes in the EEG during castration in horses and ponies anaesthetized with halothane. *Vet Anaesth Analg*, 30, 138–146.

[128] Murrell, J.C., White, K.L., Johnson, C.B. *et al.* (2005) Investigation of the EEG effects of intravenous lidocaine during halothane anaesthesia in ponies. *Vet Anaesth Analg*, 32, 212–221.

[129] Otto, K.A., Voigt, S., Piepenbrock, S. *et al.* (1996) Differences in quantitated electroencephalographic variables during surgical stimulation of horses anesthetized with isoflurane. *Vet Surg*, 25, 249–255.

[130] Otto, K.A. and Mally, P. (2003) Noxious stimulation during orthopaedic surgery results in EEG "arousal" or "paradoxical arousal" reaction in isoflurane-anaesthetised sheep. *Res Vet Sci*, 75, 103–112.

[131] Otto, K. and Short, C.E. (1991) Electroencephalographic power spectrum analysis as a monitor of anesthetic depth in horses. *Vet Surg*, 20, 362–371.

[132] Haga, H.A. and Dolvik, N.I. (2002) Evaluation of the bispectral index as an indicator of degree of central nervous system depression in isoflurane anesthetized horses. *Am J Vet Res*, 63, 438–442.

[133] Purohit, R.C., Mysinger, P.W. and Redding, R.W. (1981) Effects of xylazine and ketamine hydrochloride on the electroencephalogram and the electrocardiogram in the horse. *Am J Vet Res*, 42, 615–619.

[134] Andrews, F.M. (2004) Electrodiagnostic aids and selected neurologic diseases, in *Equine Internal Medicine*, 3rd edn (eds S.M. Reed, W.M. Bayly and D.C. Sellon), Saunders, St. Louis, pp. 546–549.

[135] Dunigan, C.E., Oglesbee, M.J., Podell, M. *et al.* (1995) Seizure activity associated with equine protozoal myeloencephalitis. *Progr Vet Neurol*, 6, 50–54.

[136] Garner, H.E., Amend, J.F., Rosborough, J.P. *et al.* (1972) Electrodes for recording cortical electroencephalograms in ponies. *Lab Anim Sci*, 22, 262–265.

[137] Giovagnoli, G., de Feo, M.R., Frascarelli, M. *et al.* (1996) The use of EEG and ECG ambulatory technique in horses: preliminary observations. *Pferdeheilkunde*, 12, 446–449.

[138] Grabow, J.D., Anslow, R.O. and Spalatin, J. (1969) Electroencephalographic recordings with multicontact depth probes in a horse. *Am J Vet Res*, 30, 239–243.

[139] Haga, H.A. and Dolvik, N.I. (2005) Electroencephalographic and cardiovascular variables as nociceptive indicators in isoflurane-anaesthetized horses. *Vet Anaesth Analg*, 32, 128–135.

[140] Hepburn, R.J. and Furr, M.O. (2004) Sinonasal adenocarcinoma causing central nervous system disease in a horse. *J Vet Intern Med*, 18, 125–131.

[141] Heath, S.E., Artsob, H., Bell, R.J. *et al.* (1989) Equine encephalitis caused by snowshoe hare (California serogroup) virus. *Can Vet J*, 30, 669–671.

[142] Lacombe, V.A., Podell, M., Furr, M. *et al.* (2001) Diagnostic validity of electroencephalography in equine intracranial disorders. *J Vet Intern Med*, 15, 385–393.

[143] Lapras, M., Florio, R., Joubert, L. *et al.* (1968) Normal electroencephalogram in the horse. Its pathological variations in West Nile viral meningoencephalomyelitis. Relations to clinical findings, virology and histopathology. *Rev Méd Vét*, 119, 673–693.

[144] Lewin, W. and Tînhardt, H. (1998) Non-invasive EEG of the conscious standing horse. *Pferdeheilkunde*, 14, 285–294.

[145] Lunn, D.P., Cuddon, P.A., Shaftoe, S. *et al.* (1991) Familial occurrence of narcolepsy in Miniature horses. *Equine Vet J*, 25, 483–487.

[146] Mysinger, P.W., Redding, R.W., Vaughan, J.T. *et al.* (1985) Electroencephalographic patterns of clinically normal, sedated, and tranquilized newborn foals and adult horses. *Am J Vet Res*, 46, 36–41.

[147] Stromberg, M.W., Kitchell, R.L., Unsenik, F.A. *et al.* (1962) Electrocorticographic patterns in normal burros and pigs. *Am J Vet Res*, 23, 737–743.

[148] Usenick, M.W., Kitchell, R.L., Herschler, R.G. *et al.* (1962) The EEG as an aid to diagnosis of nervous diseases in the dog and cat. *J Small Anim Pract*, 3, 205–208.

[149] Williams, D.C., Aleman, M., Holliday, T.A. *et al.* (2008) Qualitative and quantitative characteristics of the electroencephalogram in normal horses during spontaneous drowsiness and sleep. *J Vet Intern Med*, 22, 630–638.

[150] Speckmann, E.J. and Elger, C.E. (2005) Introduction to neurophysiological basis of the EEG and DC potentials, in *Electroencephalography* (eds E. Niedermeyer and F. Lopes Da Silva), Lippincott Williams & Wilkins, Philadelphia, pp. 17–30.

[151] Sharbrough, F.W. (1990) Electrical fields and recording techniques, in *Current Practice of Clinical Electroencephalography* (eds D.D. Daly and T.A. Pedley), Raven Press, New York, pp. 29–49.

[152] Holliday, T.A. and Williams, D.C. (1999) Clinical electroencephalography in dogs. *Vet Neurol Neurosurg*, 1, 1–6.

[153] Engel, J. and Pedley, T.A. (1998) *Epilepsy*, Lippincott-Raven, Philadelphia.

[154] March, P.A. and Muir, W.W. (2005) Bispectral analysis of the electroencephalogram: a review of its development and use in anesthesia. *Vet Anaesth Analg*, 32, 241–255.

[155] Miller, S.M., Short, C.E. and Ekström, P.M. (1995) Quantitative electroencephalographic evaluation to determine the quantity of analgesia during anesthesia of horses for arthroscopic surgery. *Am J Vet Res*, 56, 374–379.

[156] Williams, D.C., Aleman, M., Tharp, B. *et al.* (2012) Qualitative and quantitative characteristics of the electroencephalogram in normal horses after sedation. *J Vet Intern Med*, 26, 645–653.

[157] MacLean, A.W., Lue, F. and Moldofksy, H. (1995) The reliability of visual scoring of alpha EEG activity during sleep. *Sleep*, 18, 565–569.

[158] Ruckebusch, Y. (1970) Loss of consciousness during sleep in the horse and cow. *Canadian Mèd Vet*, 39, 210–225.

[159] Ruckebush, Y. (1972) The relevance of drowsiness in the circadian cycle of farm animals. *Anim Behav*, 20, 637–643.

[160] Houpt, K.A. (1980) The characteristics of equine sleep. *Equine Pract*, 2–4, 8–17.

[161] Ruckebush, Y., Barbey, P. and Guillemot, P. (1970) Les états de sommeil chez le cheval. *C R Seances Soc Biol*, 164, 638–665.

[162] Klemm, W.R. and Hall, C.L. (1974) Current status and trends in veterinary encephalography. *J Am Vet Med Assoc*, 164, 529.

[163] Itabisashi, T., Horino, R., Hirano, K. *et al.* (1990) Electroencephalographic observation on sheep and cattle with experimental cerebrocortical necrosis. *Jpn J Vet Sci*, 52, 551–558.

[164] Suzuki, M., Sitizyo, K., Takeuchi, T. *et al.* (1990) Electroencephalogram of Japanese black calves affected with cerebrocortical necrosis. *Jpn J Vet Sci*, 52, 1077–1087.

[165] Suzuki, M., Sitizyo, K., Takeuchi, T. *et al.* (1990) Electroencephalograms of three Japanese Black calves with hydranencephaly. *J Jpn Vet Med Assoc*, 43, 723–727.

[166] DeLahunta, A. and Cummings, J.F. (1965) The clinical and electroencephalographic features of hydrocephalus in three dogs. *J Am Vet Med Assoc*, 146, 954.

[167] Engel, J. (2013) *Seizures and Epilepsy*, 2nd edn, Oxford, New York.

[168] Berendt, M., Høgoenhaven, H., Flagstad, A. *et al.* (1999) Electroencephalography in dogs with epilepsy: similarities between human and canine findings. *Acta Neurol Scand*, 99, 276–283.

[169] Jaggy, A. and Bernardini, M. (1998) Idiopathic epilepsy in 125 dogs: a long-term study. Clinical and electroencephalographic findings. *J Small Anim Pract*, 39, 23–29.

[170] Holliday, T.A. and Williams, D.C. (1998) Interictal paroxysmal discharges in the electroencephalograms of epileptic dogs. *Clin Tech Small Anim Pract*, 13, 132–143.

[171] van der Ree, M. and Wijnberg, I. (2012) A review on epilepsy in the horse and the potential of ambulatory EEG as a diagnostic tool. *Vet Q*, 32, 159–167.

[172] Aleman, M., Brosnan, R.J., Williams, D.C. *et al.* (2005) Malignant hyperthermia in a horse anesthetized with halothane. *J Vet Intern Med*, 19, 363–366.

15 Anesthetic Considerations for Horses with Neurologic Disorders

Adriana G. Silva

Faculty of Veterinary Medicine, University of Montreal, Saint Hyacinthe, Canada

This chapter was adapted from a chapter originally written by Dr. Allison Smith, *Equine Neurology*, First edition. Neurologic disease can present a variety of challenges for the anesthetist. The unique anatomical features of the brain limit its ability to respond to inflammatory, traumatic, and neoplastic challenges. Furthermore, horses presenting with spinal cord or peripheral neuropathies can be challenging to the anesthetist due to the increased danger of a large, ataxic patient. The goal of neurologic anesthesia is to maintain adequate nourishment and blood delivery to the brain, minimize the development of seizures, minimize the effects of ataxia on the patient's safety, and prevent further deterioration of neurologic status.

An understanding of the anatomy and physiology of the nervous system and how it relates to anesthesia is important in understanding how best to maximize patient safety and minimize morbidity and mortality. The brain is housed entirely within a boney cavity. This rigid structure does not allow for an increase in volume when faced with a traumatic, an inflammatory, or a neoplastic insult. Minor changes in cerebral blood flow (CBF), cerebrospinal fluid (CSF), or tissue volume (i.e., mass) can quickly result in a moderate to severe increase in intracranial pressure (ICP). Elevated ICP can cause regional and global cerebral ischemia and hypoxia due to a reduction in cerebral perfusion pressure (CPP) and CBF and ultimately lead to potentially fatal displacement of brain and neuronal tissue, including brainstem herniation [1]. CBF is directly proportional to CPP and indirectly proportional to cerebral vascular resistance (CVR). Of these components, only CBF can be easily influenced by the anesthetist and thus is of particular interest.

In a normal horse, CBF is under metabolic (chemical), myogenic (autoregulation), and neurogenic control [2]. This control ensures consistent, high flow of blood to the brain over a range of arterial blood pressures. The mean arterial pressure (MAP) range within which CBF remains under autoregulatory control has not been defined in horses; however, in humans, the CBF remains relatively consistent from 70 to 140 mmHg, and animals may have better regulation of flow at lower arterial pressures [2]. Horses, due to their large size, undergo large orthostatic shifts when positioned in lateral or dorsal recumbency for general anesthesia [3]. These fluid shifts can alter MAP and thus have an effect on CPP.

Chemical or metabolic factors that influence CBF include cerebral metabolic rate (CMR), the partial pressure of arterial carbon dioxide ($PaCO_2$), the partial pressure of arterial oxygen (PaO_2) and temperature. An increase in CMR will lead to an increase in CBF [2]. Anesthetics, both injectable and inhaled, can alter CMR and therefore influence CBF. Likewise, an increase in the temperature of the brain causes an increase in CBF.

There is a directly proportionate relationship between CBF and $PaCO_2$. These changes are due to intra- and extracellular pH alterations. Hypocapnia and alkalemia lead to a decrease in CBF due to vasoconstriction, resulting in an increase in CVR. Conversely, hypercapnia and acidemia result in an increase in CBF, due to vasodilation [4]. Hypoxemia, that is, a PaO_2 less than 60 mmHg, causes an increase in CBF, resulting from vasodilation. Hyperoxia may mildly decrease CBF [2].

Brosnan and colleagues directly measured the ICP of awake horses and horses undergoing isoflurane anesthesia. A transducer was surgically implanted at the level of the subarachnoid space. Measurements of awake, standing horses revealed ICP values in the range of 2 ± 4 mmHg, which are consistent with that of other animals [5]. In contrast, anesthesia and recumbency affect the body's ability to maintain normal CBF, CPP, and ICP. When horses are placed in head-dependent positions, both ICP and CPP increase 10-fold over values in awake, standing horses [6]. The clinical significance of this observation is unclear. A marked increase in ICP and CPP in normal, anesthetized, recumbent horses suggests that horses with preexisting elevations of ICP and CPP may be at a greater risk for catastrophic brain

Equine Neurology, Second Edition. Martin Furr and Stephen Reed.
© 2015 John Wiley & Sons, Inc. Published 2015 by John Wiley & Sons, Inc.
Companion website: www.wiley.com/go/furr/neurology

herniation. Additionally, normal horses may experience mild to marked cerebral hypoxia and ischemia while receiving general anesthesia.

Premedication of neurologic patients is generally recommended and can be quite helpful in maximizing the safety of the anesthetic event. Since premedications help to decrease anxiety, provide smoother induction, aid maintenance and recovery phases of anesthesia, decrease the required doses of both induction and maintenance drugs required for anesthesia, and can provide analgesia to the patient, they should generally be included in an anesthetic protocol. Exceptions to this may include severely obtunded patients in whom further central nervous system (CNS) depression is not warranted.

Alpha-2 agonists are commonly used for sedation of horses with neurologic disease. Examples of commonly used alpha-2 agonists include xylazine, detomidine, medetomidine, and romifidine. Advantages to the use of this class of sedatives include good to profound sedation that is fairly reliable, muscle relaxation, and analgesia. This class of drugs can also cause hypotension, respiratory depression, decreased cardiac output, and bradycardia [7–9].

Some controversy exists regarding the use of acepromazine, a phenothiazine tranquilizer, in animals with neurologic disease and especially in patients with a history of seizures or undergoing a procedure that can potentially induce seizures. The belief is that acepromazine lowers the seizure threshold and therefore could potentiate seizures. Retrospective studies in dogs with a history of seizures found no association between clinical administration of acepromazine and incidence or recurrence of seizures. Additionally, in dogs with active seizures, acepromazine administration was associated with a decrease in seizure activity and prevention of short-term recurrence [10, 11]. Administration of acepromazine results in mild tranquilization and anxiolysis. Johnson et al., in the confidential enquiry of perioperative equine fatalities, demonstrated that premedication with acepromazine is related to increased survival [12]. It can also cause mild to profound systemic vasodilation, resulting in hypotension, although in normovolemic patients, this may not be clinically significant [13]. Acepromazine should be avoided in shocky, dehydrated, or hypovolemic patients or in patients undergoing procedures that may result in excessive hemorrhage. The decision to use acepromazine in the neurologic horse should be based on the individual patient. Horses that are especially nervous and difficult to sedate using alpha-2 agonists may benefit from the inclusion of acepromazine in the sedation protocol.

The benzodiazepine class of tranquilizers can also be used as part of the preanesthetic protocol in horses with neurologic disease. Both diazepam and midazolam may be appropriate. These drugs are especially beneficial in patients that are exhibiting seizures as they have anticonvulsant capabilities. The benzodiazepine class of drugs functions by increasing activity of gamma-amino-butyric acid (GABA) and thus causes depression of the CNS [14]. The benzodiazepines also decrease CBF [15]. Diazepam and midazolam can also provide muscle relaxation, and mild tranquilization, especially at higher doses [16]. These last two effects are important considerations, as an excited horse may not become sedate enough for induction and yet may become profoundly ataxic, especially if ataxia is a component of the horse's presenting clinical signs. This ataxia may further excite the horse, precluding a safe and controlled induction of general anesthesia. In an already ataxic horse, benzodiazepines should not be the first-choice drug for sedation but can be safely used as an adjunct for the induction of general anesthesia or to control seizures.

Opioid analgesics can be included in the premedication protocol. Butorphanol is commonly administered to horses as a premedicant. As a mu antagonist–kappa agonist opioid, butorphanol provides minor sedation and analgesia with few side effects. When given concurrently with an alpha-2 agonist or phenothiazine tranquilizer, the sedative and analgesic effects of both drugs are synergistically enhanced. This effect can be beneficial for a neurologic patient. Side effects of butorphanol are usually mild and can include respiratory depression, decreased heart rate, and ataxia. Butorphanol is much less likely to cause increased locomotion compared with morphine or other pure mu opioid agonists [17].

Other opioids can likewise be administered to horses as part of a premedication protocol. These can include pure mu agonist opioids like morphine and fentanyl or a partial mu agonist like buprenorphine. Morphine and fentanyl provide potent analgesia, but their sedative effects can vary in horses. Horses may exhibit mild to profound sedation, but excitation and increased locomotion can also occur [18]. Morphine remains an option for providing analgesia to horses undergoing potentially painful procedures [19]; however, the degree of analgesia can vary from profound to none, and increased excitation may occur.

Barbiturates are most frequently used for induction of anesthesia in patients with neurologic disease. Barbiturates decrease CMR and ICP, and are neuroprotective via prevention of free radical formation, enhancement of GABA activity and inhibition of calcium ion influx [20, 21]. Thiopental is the induction drug of choice in horses with suspected or confirmed traumatic brain injury. Side effects of thiopental administration include hypotension and prolonged, disordered recoveries, even in neurologically normal patients [22, 23]. An ataxic horse that receives thiopental may have a rough recovery with multiple unsuccessful, uncoordinated attempts to stand; however, the beneficial cerebral effects make thiopental an excellent choice for patients with central neurologic disease.

Propofol is commonly used alone and combined with thiopental for induction of humans and dogs undergoing anesthesia for neurologic disease [21]. Horses have a variable response to propofol, ranging from excellent induction to general anesthesia to mild sedation. The degree of anesthesia achieved is dose-dependent and is improved with premedication [24, 25]. The cost associated with the larger dose required for more reliable anesthesia may preclude routine use of propofol in clinical practice.

Human neuroanesthesia has embraced the use of propofol infusions for total intravenous anesthesia in patients at higher risk for elevated ICP as propofol is better at reducing ICP than is inhalant anesthesia [26]. Propofol is generally inadequate for total intravenous anesthesia as a sole agent and is generally combined with either an alpha-2 agonist or ketamine. Recovery from propofol anesthesia is generally excellent, although hypoxemia and hypercapnia may occur [24, 27].

Use of ketamine in horses with suspected or confirmed traumatic brain injury should be undertaken cautiously. Ketamine, as a dissociative anesthetic, raises CMR, increases CBF and ICP, and can cause seizure-like activity on an electroencephalogram [15, 28]. Ketamine may be a viable choice for induction in patients with peripheral neurologic disease and in whom seizures and an increase in ICP are unlikely. Ketamine should not be used alone as the potential for seizures and excessive muscle rigidity may result. The negative CNS effects can be attenuated with concomitant administration of a benzodiazepine [15]. Muscle relaxation can also be provided by an alpha-2 agonist or guaifenesin.

Inhalants are recommended for maintenance of anesthesia in horses. Halothane, isoflurane, and sevoflurane can all be used successfully in patients with neurologic disease. The inhalants can cause a reduction in CPP due to vasodilation-induced reduction in MAP [29, 30]. There is a risk that use of an inhalant can increase CBF. Volatile anesthetics have dose-dependent effects on CBF. In doses larger than the minimal alveolar concentration (MAC), CBF is not significantly altered compared with that while being awake. Beyond doses of 1 MAC, direct cerebral vasodilation results in an increase in CBF and cerebral blood volume [31].

All of the inhalants, especially isoflurane, are respiratory depressants and hypoventilation and hypercapnia may result [32]. This could lead to an increase in ICP [33]. Intermittent positive pressure ventilation (IPPV) can reduce or prevent hypoventilation.

Hypocapnic hyperventilation has long been a cornerstone of therapy in patients with suspected or confirmed increase in ICP [4, 34]. Although a method of direct measurement of ICP in horses is possible, it is not feasible in most clinical patients [5]. Elevated ICP can be indirectly inferred from MAP: in order to maintain CPP, MAP will increase in response to increased ICP. This phenomenon is the Cushing's effect [2]. Hypercapnic, spontaneously ventilated horses anesthetized with isoflurane have elevated ICP when compared with normocapnic horses receiving controlled ventilation [3]. The goal of hyperventilation therapy is to maintain $PaCO_2$ between 30 and 40 mmHg. Excessive hypocapnia (<25 mmHg) reduces CBF excessively and should be avoided. Hypoxemia should likewise be avoided. Providing an enriched oxygen supply and maintaining the horse on mechanical ventilation should be utilized as necessary to maintain PaO_2 greater than 80 mmHg.

An elevated ICP that cannot be managed by hyperventilation alone may benefit from hyperosmotic solutions. Mannitol is frequently used to decrease cerebral volume by drawing fluid out of neuronal tissue. Hypertonic saline can also be administered for this purpose [1].

Hypotension should be avoided in the healthy horse, and the neurologic horse is no exception. As CPP is a function of MAP(CPP = MAP − ICP), ensuring adequate systemic blood pressures will help to ensure that cerebral perfusion is maintained. The diseased brain may lose its ability to autoregulate, so cerebral perfusion becomes flow-dependant. Fluids should be administered in order to help maintain MAP and CPP. Any balanced salt electrolyte solution is acceptable; these fluids should not contain glucose or glucose precursors, including lactate as hyperglycemia is associated with increased morbidity [21]. Vasopressors such as phenylephrine, norepinephrine, ephedrine, and dopamine do not have significant direct effects on the cerebral circulation. Their effect on CBF is dependent on their effect on systemic blood pressure. When MAP is below the lower limit of autoregulation, vasopressors increase systemic pressure and thereby increase CBF. If systemic pressure is within the limits of autoregulation, vasopressor-induced increases in systemic pressure have little effect on CBF. Cardiovascular-supportive drugs, including dobutamine and ephedrine, should be used as needed to maintain acceptable MAP [35].

Monitoring a neurologic horse under general anesthesia is similar to monitoring a healthy horse anesthetized with an inhalant. Direct arterial blood pressure should be monitored, as blood pressure can change very quickly, and maintaining adequate MAP is essential in limiting morbidity [36]. An end-tidal CO_2 ($EtCO_2$) monitor is helpful to noninvasively gauge ventilation trends [37]. However, the difference between $EtCO_2$ and $PaCO_2$ can be large, so an arterial blood gas should be evaluated to ensure that the hyperventilated horse is in fact hypocapnic [38]. An arterial blood gas will also ensure that the patient is not hypoxemic. An electrocardiogram should also be utilized to ensure that the horse does not have any cardiac arrhythmias that would interfere with maintenance of CBF. Although not essential, a pulse oximeter to measure oxygen saturation can provide additional information about the stability of the patient [39].

Recovery from anesthesia can be dangerous with normal horses; horses suffering from neurologic disease are often ataxic, which can increase the difficulty of recovery. Brosnan et al. speculates that some of the difficult and delayed recoveries from anesthesia may in fact be due to increased ICP and its sequelae, and horses with preexisting neurologic conditions are certainly susceptible [6]. Horses should be placed in a recovery area that is free of obstructions and preferably well-padded. Oxygen should be supplemented via an endotracheal tube, nasotracheal tube, or nasopharyngeal tube to ensure adequate oxygenation during the recovery period. Horses that had myelography and received contrast solution can be placed with their head elevated, to encourage the contrast solution to drain away from the brain. When elevating the head, be sure to use objects that will not injure the horse nor be in the way during recovery. Assistance, in the form of head and/or tail ropes, and physical restraint by trained personnel can also increase the safety of recovery for the horse. If a horse has a cervical injury or underwent cervical surgery, the use of a head rope may cause more harm than good, however. In these situations, a tail rope alone may provide enough assistance without further risking trauma to the horse's neck. The recovery stall should be as quiet as possible so as to not disturb the horse. Diazepam or midazolam should be available during the recovery phase in the event of seizures. Additional sedation—frequently a lower dose of the sedative used for premedication—can also be given to the horse to smooth the recovery period. Alpha-2 agonists provide analgesia and tranquilization during the anesthetic recovery, which prolongs recovery time, allowing for sufficient time for anesthetic washout and improves the quality of recovery from inhalation anesthesia. Romifidine may provide a better option for additional sedation in the recovery period compared with xylazine. Romifidine is 10 times as potent and has a longer duration of clinical effect than xylazine and, most importantly, produces less ataxia at doses that similarly reduce responses to stimulation. A dose of 20 μg/kg of romifidine for postanesthetic sedation improves recovery quality compared with lower romifidine doses or xylazine [40].

Neurologic complications of general anesthesia

Neurologic complications can result in patients that have preexisting neurologic complications or in horses anesthetized for other reasons. Peripheral neuropathies can result from improper positioning of the horse. These neuropathies can include trauma to the radial and peroneal nerves and less commonly the femoral nerve.

Femoral nerve injury occurs from caudal extension of the limb, stretching the femoral nerve as it passes over the psoas muscle. Horses should be positioned on thickly padded tables devoid of pressure points. All limbs should be independently supported and in a neutral position. When the horse is in lateral recumbency, the dependent thoracic limb should be pulled forward to relieve pressure from the radial nerve. Postanesthetic neuropathy may closely resemble postanesthetic myopathy. Treatment for both is largely supportive and includes intravenous fluids, physical support of the horse, analgesics, and sedatives.

Postanesthetic cerebral necrosis is a rare complication associated with general anesthesia in horses. Clinical signs can occur minutes to hours after anesthesia and include bilateral blindness with normal papillary light reflex, abnormal behaviors including pacing and head pressing, lethargy, and seizures. In a case report of five horses that were euthanized following the development of postanesthetic cerebral necrosis, McKay et al. reported that these horses' brains displayed neuronal necrosis consistent with cerebral ischemia [41]. Thus, any horse that undergoes a period of hypoperfusion and or hypoxemia is at risk for the development of postanesthetic cerebral necrosis. Horses that are anesthetized for colic may be at increased risk of developing cerebral ischemia as they often have circulatory compromise. Ensuring proper blood pressure and oxygenation should minimize the risk of this complication.

Postanesthetic myelopathy or myelomalacia is another uncommon complication of general anesthesia in horses. There are occasional reports in the literature of horses developing the complication following inhalation anesthesia. Affected animals were unable to stand in recovery, had an inability to use their hind limbs and had loss of deep pain perception, while tail tone and anal tone were normal or hypertonic. The horses affected were typically young (1–2 years) and rapidly growing, positioned in dorsal recumbency and underwent a short duration of anesthesia [42, 43]. The etiology is unknown but is hypothesized to involve poorly developed blood supply or poor venous drainage in combination with reduced arterial blood pressure during anesthesia [44]. This may be very difficult to distinguish from femoral paralysis. Because the exact cause is unknown, the only recommendation for prevention is to avoid deep anesthesia and low arterial blood pressure.

Anesthesia for myelography

Horses requiring general anesthesia for myelography likely constitute the bulk of neurologic anesthetic cases. There are three components that contribute to the challenge facing the anesthetist: (1) injection of volume of fluid into the CSF, which could alter cerebral fluid balance; (2) introduction of a potentially noxious substance into the CSF; and (3) the patient's preexisting neurologic status. Injection of contrast solution into the CSF can change the volume of fluid housed within the cranial vault and lead to an increase in ICP. Frequently, a volume of CSF is removed from the horse before injection of contrast media. While this practice decreases the chance for elevated ICP, the fluid balance within the brain may be temporarily altered. The choice of contrast solution can influence the risk of complications. Iohexol cervical myelography had fewer complications than metrizamide in a clinical study. Side effects included seizures, prolongation of anesthetic recovery, and worsening of the horse's presenting neurologic signs [45]. The horse's neurologic status must also be taken into consideration. Most horses requiring myelography are ataxic and thus pose a challenge for safe recovery from anesthesia.

Myelography can be performed effectively and with few complications in less than 1 h. In the author's experience, the majority of the procedures are completed within 30–45 min of induction of anesthesia. Since the procedure is relatively short, maintenance of anesthesia with a combination of injectable drugs instead of inhalants is beneficial. Recoveries of horses from short-term (20–30 min) and long-term (up to 60 min) injectable anesthesia are generally smooth, controlled, and predictable, whereas recoveries from inhalation anesthesia may be complicated by dysphoria or excitement that resembles emergence delirium in humans. These complications are likely a result of inhaled anesthetic still present in horses during attempts to stand in substantial quantity sufficient to adversely affect neurologic and motor function [46].

For procedures lasting up to an hour in which total intravenous anesthesia is used, an infusion of combined drugs, including an alpha-2 agonist, ketamine, and guaifenesin, is often used. It is important to recognize that the infusion rates that are required to maintain anesthesia may vary with individual horses. Frequent monitoring of patient status and adjustment of infusion rate accordingly is essential.

Anesthesia for cervical surgery

Cervical vertebral surgery can present a few challenges to the anesthetist. These patients are generally ataxic both before and after surgery. Analgesia is an important consideration for these cases as the procedures can be quite painful. Recovery is also a very critical time for these patients as it is easy for them to traumatize their neck as they emerge from anesthesia and attempt to stand. The use of a head rope can be both a help and a hindrance. Guidance of the head may allow the horse to

stand with minimal scrambling, but it can also place undue torque and strain on the neck and worsen the cervical trauma. Only very careful use of a head rope by an experienced individual should be allowed. Sedation in recovery, generally with alpha-2 agonists, can limit the development of emergence delirium.

Anesthesia for head trauma or cranial mass

The main goal in a patient with head trauma or a cranial mass is to prevent an increase in ICP and to keep the CMR low. Minimal sedation may be needed as these patients can be quite obtunded prior to anesthesia. If additional sedation is required, alpha-2 agonists are appropriate. If the horse is recumbent, benzodiazepines may also be administered. Thiopental should be used for

Table 15.1 Key points for anesthesia of horses with neurologic disease.

Physiology	Elevated ICP can lead to cerebral ischemia and hypoxia
	ICP influenced by MAP, CBF
	CBF proportional to $PaCO_2$
	ICP may be elevated in normal, anesthetized horses
Anesthetic drugs	Alpha-2 agonists most commonly used for sedation
	BZD is an anticonvulsant, may exacerbate ataxia
	Thiopental is neuroprotective, first choice for induction of anesthesia
	Propofol is neuro-friendly but anesthetic effects are unpredictable
	Ketamine increases CBF and ICP and can potentiate seizures
	Inhalants recommended for maintenance of anesthesia
Maintenance	IPPV to prevent hypercapnia
	Maintain with less than 1 MAC inhalant
	Hyperosmolar solutions can help decrease ICP
	MAP measured and maintained greater than 70 mmHg
	Glucose- and lactate-free IV fluids
	Arterial blood gases
Recovery	Supplemental oxygen
	Additional sedation with romifidine as necessary
	Assisted recovery, head and tail ropes
	Area free from distractions

BZD, benzodiazepine; CBF, cerebral blood flow; ICP, intracranial pressure; IPPV, intermittent positive pressure ventilation; IV, intravenous; MAP, mean arterial pressure.

the induction of general anesthesia and the horse maintained on an inhalant. IPPV is essential to keep the $PaCO_2$ low enough to decrease CBF and therefore limit any increase in ICP. IPPV, by use of a demand vale, should likewise be continued during recovery, until the horse is conscious enough to maintain appropriate ventilation. Recovery may be prolonged, and a patient recumbent prior to anesthesia may remain recumbent after anesthesia.

Conclusions

Providing safe anesthesia for a patient with neurologic disease does not differ greatly from the protocol for a healthy horse. Regardless of the patient's status, careful monitoring and early recognition and treatment of abnormalities and complications will decrease the incidence of morbidity and mortality (Table 15.1).

References

[1] Mayer, S. and Chong, J. (2002) Critical care management of intracranial pressure. *J Intensive Care Med*, 17, 55–67.

[2] Drummond, J. and Patel, P. (2000) Cerebral physiology and the effects of anesthetics and techniques, in *Anesthesia* (ed. R. Miller), Churchill Livingstone, Philadelphia, pp. 695–733.

[3] Brosnan, R.J., Steffey, E.P., LeCouteur, R.A. *et al.* (2003) Effects of ventilation and isoflurane end-tidal concentration on intracranial and cerebral perfusion pressures in horses. *Am J Vet Res*, 64, 21–25.

[4] Raichle, M. and Plum, F. (1972) Hyperventilation and cerebral blood flow. *Stroke*, 3, 566–575.

[5] Brosnan, R.J., LeCouteur, R.A., Steffey, E.P. *et al.* (2002) Direct measurement of intracranial pressure in adult horses. *Am J Vet Res*, 63, 1252–1256.

[6] Brosnan, R.J., Steffey, E.P., LeCouteur, R.A. *et al.* (2002) Effects of body position on intracranial and cerebral perfusion pressures in isoflurane-anesthetized horses. *J Appl Physiol*, 92, 2542–2546.

[7] Bueno, A., Cornick-Seahorn, J., Seahorn, T.L. *et al.* (1999) Cardiopulmonary and sedative effects of intravenous administration of low doses of medetomidine and xylazine to adult horses. *Am J Vet Res*, 60, 1371–1376.

[8] Taylor, P., Bennett, R., Brearley, J.C. *et al.* (2001) Comparison of detomidine and romifidine as premedicants before ketamine and halothane anesthesia in horses undergoing elective surgery. *Am J Vet Res*, 62, 359–363.

[9] Yamashita, K., Muir, W., Tsubakishita, S. *et al.* (2002) Clinical comparison of xylazine and medetomidine for premedication of horses. *J Am Vet Med Assoc*, 221, 1144–1149.

[10] Tobias, K.M., Marioni-Henry, K. and Wagner, R. (2006) A retrospective study on the use of acepromazine maleate in dogs with seizures. *J Am Anim Hosp Assoc*, 42, 283–289.

[11] McConnell, J., Kirby, R. and Rudloff, E. (2007) Administration of acepromazine maleate to 31 dogs with a history of seizures. *J Vet Emerg Crit Care*, 17, 262–267.

[12] Johnston, G., Eastment, J., Wood, J.L.N. *et al.* (2002) The confidential enquiry into perioperative equine fatalities (CEPEF): mortality results of Phases 1 and 2. *Vet Anaesth Analg*, 29, 159–170.

[13] Murison, P., Clutton, R., Blissitt, K.J. *et al.* (2003) Blood pressure and electrocardiographic effects of acepromazine in anesthetized horses. *Vet Anaesth Analg*, 30, 94–95.

[14] Plumb, D. (2002) *Veterinary Drug Handbook*, Iowa State Press, Ames.

[15] Reves, J., Glass, P. and Lubarsky, D.A. (2000) Nonbarbiturate intravenous anesthetics, in *Anesthesia* (ed. R. Miller), Churchill Livingstone, Philadelphia, pp. 228–272.

[16] Muir, W., Sams, R., Huffman, R.H. *et al.* (1982) Pharmacodynamic and pharmacokinetic properties of diazepam in horses. *Am J Vet Res*, 43, 1756–1762.

[17] Sellon, D., Monroe, V., Roberts, M.C. *et al.* (2001) Pharmacokinetics and adverse effects of butorphanol administered by single intravenous injection or continuous intravenous infusion in horses. *Am J Vet Res*, 62, 183–189.

[18] Bennett, R. and Steffey, E. (2002) Use of opioids for pain and anesthetic management in horses. *Vet Clin North Am Equine Pract*, 18, 47–60.

[19] Mirica, E., Clutton, R. *et al.* (2003) Problems associated with perioperative morphine in horses: a retrospective case analysis. *Vet Anaesth Analg*, 30, 147–155.

[20] Fragen, R. and Avram, M. (2000) Barbiturates, in *Anesthesia* (ed. R. Miller), Churchill Livingstone, Philadelphia, pp. 209–227.

[21] Hirsch, N. (2003) State of the art: advances in neuroanaesthesia. *Anaesthesia*, 58, 1162–1165.

[22] Hubbell, J., Hinchcliff, K., Schmall, L.M. *et al.* (2000) Anesthetic, cardiorespiratory, and metabolic effects of four intravenous regimens induced in horses immediately after maximal exercise. *Am J Vet Res*, 61, 1545–1552.

[23] Wagner, A., Mama, K., Steffey, E.P. *et al.* (2002) Behavioral responses following eight anesthetic induction protocols in horses. *Vet Anaesth Analg*, 29, 207–211.

[24] Mama, K., Steffey, E.P., Pascoe, P.J. *et al.* (1995) Evaluation of propofol as a general anesthetic for horses. *Vet Surg*, 24, 188–194.

[25] Frias, A., Marsico, F., Gomez de Segura, I.A. *et al.* (2003) Evaluation of different doses of propofol in xylazine premedicated horses. *Vet Anaesth Analg*, 30, 193–201.

[26] Peterson, K., Landsfeldt, U., Cold, G.E. *et al.* (2002) ICP is lower during propofol anaesthesia compared to isoflurane and sevoflurane. *Acta Neurochir Suppl*, 81, 89–91.

[27] Bettschart-Wolfensberger, R., Freeman, S., Jäggin-Schmucker, N. *et al.* (2001) Infusion of a combination of

propofol and medetomidine for long-term anesthesia in ponies. *Am J Vet Res*, 62, 500–507.

[28] Albanese, J., Arnaud, S., Rey, M. *et al.* (1997) Ketamine decreases intracranial pressure and electroencephalographic activity in traumatic brain injury patients during propofol sedation. *Anesthesiology*, 87, 1328–1334.

[29] Bundgaard, H., von Oettingen, G., Larsen, K.M. *et al.* (1998) Effects of sevoflurane on intracranial pressure, cerebral blood flow and cerebral metabolism. A dose-response study in patients subjected to craniotomy for cerebral tumours. *Acta Anaesthesiol Scand*, 42, 621–627.

[30] Sponhein, S., Skraastad, O., Helseth, E. *et al.* (2003) Effects of 0.5 and 1.0 MAC isoflurane, sevoflurane and desflurane on intracranial and cerebral perfusion pressures in children. *Acta Anaesthesiol Scand*, 47, 932–938.

[31] Brosnan, R.J., Steffey, E.P., LeCouteur, R.A. *et al.* (2011) Effects of isoflurane anesthesia on cerebovascular autoregulation in horses. *Am J Vet Res*, 72, 18–24.

[32] Grosenbaugh, D. and Muir, W. (1998) Cardiorespiratory effects of sevoflurane, isoflurane, and halothane anesthesia in horses. *Am J Vet Res*, 59, 101–106.

[33] Cold, G.E., Bundgaard, H., von Oettingen, G. *et al.* (1998) ICP during anaesthesia with sevoflurane: a dose-response study. Effect of hypocapnia. *Acta Neurochir Suppl*, 71, 279–281.

[34] Stocchetti, N., Maas, A.I., Chieregato, A. *et al.* (2005) Hyperventilation in head injury: a review. *Chest*, 127, 1812–1827.

[35] Moppett, I., Wild, M., Sherman, R.W. *et al.* (1992) Effects of ephedrine, dobutamine and dopexamine on cerebral haemodynamics: transcranial Doppler studies in healthy volunteers. *Br J Anaesth*, 92, 39–44.

[36] Duke, T., Filzek, U., Read, M.R. *et al.* (2006) Clinical observations surrounding an increased incidence of postanesthetic myopathy in halothane-anesthetized horses. *Vet Anaesth Analg*, 33, 122–127.

[37] Palmer, J. (2005) Ventilatory support of the critically ill foal. *Vet Clin North Am Equine Pract*, 21, 457–486.

[38] Teixeira Neto, F., Luna, S., Massone, F. *et al.* (2000) The effect of changing the mode of ventilation on the arterial-to-end-tidal CO_2 difference and physiological dead space in laterally and dorsally recumbent horses during halothane anesthesia. *Vet Surg*, 29, 200–205.

[39] Matthews, N., Hartke, S., Allen, J.C., Jr *et al.* (2003) An evaluation of pulse oximeters in dogs, cats and horses. *Vet Anaesth Analg*, 30, 3–14.

[40] Woodhouse, K.J., Brosnan, R.J., Nguyen, K.Q. *et al.* (2013) Effects of postanesthetic sedation with romifidine or xylazine on quality of recovery from isoflurane anesthesia in horses. *J Am Vet Med Assoc*, 242, 533–539.

[41] McKay, J.S., Forest, T.W., Senior, M. *et al.* (2002) Postanaesthetic cerebral necrosis in five horses. *Vet Rec*, 150, 70–74.

[42] Trim, C.M. (1997) Postanesthetic hemorrhagic myelopathy or myelomalacia. *Vet Clin North Am Equine Pract*, 13, 73–77.

[43] Zink, M.C. (1985) Postanesthetic poliomyelomalacia in a horse. *Can Vet J*, 26, 275–277.

[44] Wagner, A.E. (2008) Complications in equine anesthesia. *Vet Clin North Am Equine Pract*, 24, 735–752.

[45] Widmer, W., Blevins, W., Jakovljevic, S. *et al.* (1998) A prospective clinical trial comparing metrizamide and iohexol for equine myelography. *Vet Radiol Ultrasound*, 39, 106–109.

[46] Wiese, A.J., Brosnan, R.J. and Barter, L.S. (2014) Effects of acetylcholinesterase inhibition on quality of recovery from isoflurane-induced anesthesia in horses. *Am J Vet Res*, 75, 223–230.

16 The Basics of Equine Neuropathology

Fabio Del Piero[1] and John L. Robertson[2]

[1] *School of Veterinary Medicine, Louisiana State University, Baton Rouge, USA*
[2] *Virginia Tech, Virginia-Maryland Regional College of Veterinary Medicine, Leesburg, USA*

The most important issue for veterinarians when seeing a horse with neurologic signs is determining the site of disease. Often, the veterinarian must determine if disease is primarily localized in the central nervous system (CNS) and peripheral nerves or whether it is a nonneurologic disease simply presenting as neurologic disease. This determination, which is sometimes difficult, will be based on the analysis of history, physical examination findings, neurologic evaluation, and laboratory tests. Arriving at an accurate diagnosis of neurologic disease is the subject of other chapters found in this book and in other reference texts [1–3]. This chapter focuses on procedures for dealing with pathologic evaluation of horses with suspected neurologic disease.

The pathologic examination of the nervous system

Common presentations and problems

Common presentations confronting the veterinary practitioner and pathologist in horses with suspected neurologic diseases are as follows:

- Horses with primary musculoskeletal problems and injuries, in which there is clearly some degree of neurologic dysfunction (alterations in coordination and gait, abnormal neurologic examination) and in which there may be secondary neurologic lesions (e.g., the neurodegeneration associated with suprascapular nerve paralysis) [2]
- Horses of any age (the young and old alike), in which there is altered mentation and coordination
- Horses in which there are vague or nonspecific neurologic signs, suggestive of primary neurologic disease, but for which there can be many causes (toxic, traumatic, metabolic, neoplastic, infectious)
- Horses with signs characteristic of a specific type of neurologic disease (e.g., the hirsutism associated with hyperplastic or neoplastic pituitary disease)

- Horses suspected of having a neurologic disease that may be infectious in nature, and for which there is a valid concern for the health of other horses, animals, and people (many of the viral encephalitides are in this category)

Horses that appear healthy but which die unexpectedly or which are found dead present unique problems for both the practitioner and the pathologist. The postmortem examination of these horses may not clearly determine a cause of death, and neurologic and cardiovascular diseases are frequently considered as part of the differential diagnosis that must be pursued.

Postmortem evaluation of the nervous system of horses

The most important point in this chapter can be made by stating the obvious: if the nervous system is not examined grossly and microscopically, it is impossible to find lesions and to determine their importance in the death of horses. By far, the most common error made by practitioners *and by pathologists* who examine dead horses is a failure to actually examine the brain, spinal cord, and peripheral nerves and to collect tissues for microscopic evaluation. There are many excuses given for avoiding a postmortem evaluation of the nervous system including the belief that special equipment, techniques, or fixatives are required; none of these are valid reasons for not doing a neurologic postmortem examination.

While it is true that horses are large animals and it is physically demanding to deal with their bodies and tissues, most veterinarians are quite capable of doing so, especially if they seek some assistance (which does not have to be skilled). Virtually all postmortem examinations, including that of the CNS, can be performed with common tools available at most hardware stores. Veterinarians in equine specialty practices or mixed practices would do well to invest roughly $150 in equipment and keep it for postmortem examinations.

Equine Neurology, Second Edition. Martin Furr and Stephen Reed.
© 2015 John Wiley & Sons, Inc. Published 2015 by John Wiley & Sons, Inc.
Companion website: www.wiley.com/go/furr/neurology

Following a systematic approach to dissection allows all practitioners to adequately sample tissues in the nervous system. The very first step in arriving at a definitive diagnosis is tissue collection and preservation. Once this is done, tissues can be transferred to a veterinary pathologist for further processing and evaluation. Pathologists will trim fixed tissue into pieces suitable for histologic sectioning and examination and have access to specialized tissue processing equipment needed for this work. However, if the practitioner does not collect and preserve tissue, the pathologist has nothing to work with. It is important to remember that just like any other learned skill "practice makes perfect." The more postmortem exams done, the easier they become. Likewise, the more postmortem exams you have done, the better the outcome in terms of tissue collection and disease diagnosis.

Concern about the rapidity of autolysis of the nervous system is often given as a reason for not doing a neurologic postmortem, the assumption being that autolysis will preclude the collection of useful information. Of course, it is always better to collect and preserve fresh tissue, but autolysis begins at the moment of death in all tissues, not just those of the nervous system. It is possible to make meaningful gross and microscopic observations, even in tissues observed and collected 12–36 h after the death of a horse. Cooling carcasses immediately after death (below 45°F, but above 32°F, if possible) slows the process of autolysis and helps preserve tissue morphology. Horses that are febrile when they die, or carcasses kept at temperatures above 70°F, will inevitably show more signs of autolysis the longer they remain warm. Patients with autolysis of abdominal viscera may still have the nervous tissue in adequate condition for microscopic examination.

For most diagnostic purposes, specialized fixatives are not necessary. Tissues immersed in 10% neutral buffered formalin solution are adequately preserved for most histologic evaluations. The most important thing for the practitioner to remember when collecting and preserving tissue is that adequate amounts of formalin fixative have to be used or tissue will not fix properly. The usual guideline followed is to use 10 volumes of formalin fixative to one volume of tissue. Practically, this means a horse brain needs to be completely immersed in a large plastic pail of buffered formalin solution and then the pail covered or sealed (to prevent leakage and vaporization of fixative). The spinal cord should go in a separate pail filled with formalin. There is a strong temptation to attempt fixation of an entire equine brain in one- to two-quart containers. This is pointless and tissue will not fix properly—precluding accurate evaluation later. Small pieces of tissue (roughly the size of a 25-cent piece) must be fixed at least 24 h before they can be processed. Larger pieces, like whole brains, are generally fixed intact for at least 48 h and then trimmed carefully to allow further penetration of fixative, before final trimming and processing.

At times, it may be important to collect and freeze portions of the brain, especially the brainstem. This may be done when viral disease is suspected and when fluorescent antibody (FA) stains, virus isolation (VI), and molecular techniques will be used on frozen tissue. In many state diagnostic laboratories, this is the method commonly used for rapid determination of rabies virus infection. When nervous tissue is collected for these evaluations, the practitioner should cut the brain in half, double-bag in a properly labeled plastic freezer bag (which is then placed in a second labeled freezer bag) and place in a freezer. The nonfrozen portion of the brain should be immediately placed, as aforementioned, in 10% neutral buffered formalin solution. Arrangements should be made to ship this material to a diagnostic laboratory as soon as possible. At times, diagnostic laboratories may prefer to work with cold (nonfrozen) tissue and the practitioner should be aware of tissue preferences of their local diagnostic laboratories. Regulations may vary and should be always followed (e.g., in some European countries, the legislation indicates that the whole head should be submitted to the state laboratory for rabies testing, and in the United States, the recommended areas of sampling of the brain for rabies testing has changed several times during the last 20 years).

Special fixatives, such as Bouin's solution, are sometimes used by veterinary pathologists to fix nervous system tissues. Bouin's solution penetrates and fixes tissue more quickly than 10% neutral buffered formalin (which penetrates roughly 1–2 mm of tissue per hour at 70°F). However, special fixatives are not readily available to practitioners or needed for most pathologic studies. For some research studies, mixtures containing buffered glutaraldehyde are perfused into nervous system tissues in order to preserve them for electron microscopy. Again, this is for special work, not routine diagnostics. We believe that 10% buffered formalin does a great job and do not use other fixatives.

A concern about the possibility of infectious or zoonotic disease of the nervous system can be given as a reason not to perform a postmortem examination of the nervous system. A number of simple steps should **ALWAYS** be taken if rabies or other potentially zoonotic diseases are suspected.

First, it is absolutely mandatory to know what to do, how to do it, and who to call if rabies/zoonotic disease is suspected. Veterinarians should know what zoonotic diseases are present in their practice area and should know who to contact if exposure is suspected. This will very likely be a state veterinarian, state diagnostic laboratory, and the local department of public (human) health. It is highly advisable to know requirements for tissue submission (fresh tissue, refrigerated tissue, multiple serum samples, frozen tissue, formalin-fixed tissue) to diagnostic laboratories—well before there is a potential exposure or illness that is creating a public health crisis.

Second, it is absolutely mandatory to keep careful track of the names of all people potentially exposed to a suspect animal, including owners, family, farm personnel, veterinarians, veterinary technicians, laboratory personnel who handle fresh tissue/blood samples, or casual contacts. Collecting addresses and telephone numbers for these people will be important if the presence of a significant disease, such as rabies, is confirmed in a horse displaying neurologic signs. Third, it is absolutely mandatory to collect tissues and submit them for diagnostic evaluation. Some precautions are necessary to do this safely, however.

It is important to limit exposure of all personnel to a potentially infectious animal. The animal should be segregated from other animals and from people. As soon as is practical, if the animal is not already dead, it should be euthanized and moved to an area where an adequate post mortem evaluation can take place. In many cases, this will occur on the farm and be done by a veterinary practitioner.

Arrangements should be made in advance for carcass disposal, preferably by burying deeply after postmortem evaluation. Potentially infected carcasses should NOT be transported for rendering as this increases the risk of inadvertent exposure for anyone handling the carcass. Carcasses may be transported for incineration or digestion, but only by qualified personnel and with explicit warnings regarding potential exposure to infectious agents.

The veterinarian and personnel who will assist the veterinarian in performing the postmortem examination ALWAYS must minimize their potential for exposure to infectious agents. While it is relatively common for both horses and veterinarians to be vaccinated against rabies, at least in the United States, one should never presume that either the horse or the veterinarian is immune. There are significant individual variations in the length of immunity following vaccination and in the actual antibody titer for each individual. Veterinarians who were routinely vaccinated and titered while in veterinary school may allow years to elapse before having their titer checked or being revaccinated. Some veterinarians will not keep their personal rabies vaccinations up to date—and will be susceptible to disease if exposed.

Some veterinarians wrongly presume that horse owners are diligent in maintaining vaccinations of their horses against common, and potentially zoonotic, infectious agents. Some horse owners do not believe in or understand the necessity of regular vaccination against infectious diseases. Given the surge in popularity of herbal and holistic medical approaches, and some lay literature regarding potential "harm" of vaccinations in people and animals, including the fear of Theiler's disease, some owners may not vaccinate for any disease. This has resulted in the death of horses due to preventable diseases. Other owners will attempt to save costs on husbandry and veterinary care by vaccinating their own animals. This is unfortunately an all too common practice. The quality of some vaccines from nonpractitioner sources can be quite variable, due to conditions of storage, length of storage, lot-to-lot variation, and manufacturer. Owners performing their own vaccination procedures may not administer vaccines correctly (giving a vaccination in the subcutis, for example, when intramuscular administration is required). Rabies vaccinations, and records of these vaccinations, may not be up to date—and these animals will be susceptible to disease if exposed. Without records of adequate vaccination against rabies, most public health officials will require vaccination of exposed humans. This is costly, can be medically complicated (in the event of vaccine reactions), and can be modestly painful, especially for small children.

As a rule, when encountering an animal with a history of neurologic signs that may have an infectious (and potentially zoonotic) origin, it is best to assume there is a risk of exposure and to use personal protections. It is mandatory to completely prepare all tools and solutions before beginning the postmortem examination. Labeled containers with fixative, and bags for specimens, should be prepared ahead of time. This saves time, ensures proper labeling, and minimizes contamination of the containers. If at all possible, the carcass should be placed either on a surface that can be sanitized or on a disposable tarpaulin (to contain fluids and tissues). The veterinarian should do the following:

- Be wearing rubber gloves without holes (double-glove with standard latex examination gloves or use examination gloves and standard kitchen gloves)
- Be wearing face protection to prevent exposure of mucous membranes to spattering fluids and bone chips (this absolutely will happen!). This should include wrap-around eye shield, disposable mask covering both nose and mouth, or full face shield.
- Be wearing coveralls or scrub clothes that can be removed at the end of the dissection, bagged, and then properly sanitized or incinerated (Tyvek disposable coveralls are relatively inexpensive, relatively fluid-resistant, and work very well for this; they can be found in many larger hardware stores).
- Be wearing rubber boots that can be sanitized at the end of the postmortem.

- Have detergent and disinfectants available to clean all surfaces, equipment, and themselves. Disinfectants MUST be effective against viruses, bacteria, fungi, and protozoa. An excellent guide on disinfectants is found in the *Merck Veterinary Manual* [3]. A further discussion of disinfection procedures is found later.
- Have tools, pails, and brushes available for cleanup and to hold solutions. A supply of plastic bags to hold contaminated clothing such as coveralls and masks should be available. Very tough biohazard bags are available from most veterinary supply houses and are ideal for holding contaminated items. These bags are puncture-resistant, leak-resistant, highly visible (red or orange are common and bear the label "BIOHAZARD"), and much more durable than standard trash bags.

Methods for postmortem examination: a practical approach

There are three common elements in all good postmortem examinations. These are preparation, developing and following a system for examination, and finalizing the case (gross and microscopic pathology reports, communication with clients and colleagues). First, and as noted earlier, is preparation. The veterinarian should have done the following:

- Taken a good medical history of the animal to be dissected, be aware of the clinical presentation and previous medical/surgical therapy, and have formulated a list of potential problems and differential diagnoses
- Collected any antemortem clinical pathology samples needed to help make the diagnosis
- If possible, taken diagnostic radiographs of head, neck, and limbs to aid with case analysis and arriving at a meaningful final diagnosis
- Be ready to document any abnormalities, both in writing and with photographs
- Prepared the environment for the postmortem examination (see aforementioned)
- Secured any help needed for dealing with a large animal carcass and pieces of this animal
- Have the equipment, clothing, and solutions needed (see aforementioned)
- Secured adequate lighting to work safely, to be able to see abnormalities, and for photographic documentation
- Be prepared to disinfect the premises at the end of the examination and to properly dispose of the remains.

Second, develop and follow a system. Do every postmortem the same way, using your system. There are two possible systems. A practical procedure for field necropsy is presented here, and other methods are presented elsewhere [4].

Most veterinarians who conduct a postmortem examination on a horse will do so "in the field." In many cases, this may literally be at a farm or boarding facility where the horse has died unexpectedly or has been humanely destroyed. Some veterinarians may be conducting the postmortem at their practice. When doing a "field necropsy," most veterinarians will be working with a horse lying on its side. Personal preference by the veterinarian usually dictates which side is up and which side is down. Most right-handed people prefer to work with the left side of the horse on the ground. A very brief description is given later of the major elements of the necropsy, and this is followed by a more detailed description of the neurologic portion of the necropsy.

Here are some simple steps to follow:

1 Perform a thorough external examination, noting any gross abnormalities, including discharges from nose, mouth, eyes, anus, and urethra. Note the condition of the coat and any lacerations, bruises, areas of alopecia, and gross abnormalities of trunk and limbs. Examine the feet for wear and symmetry, noting whether the animal has been shod or not. Record coat color, markings, any tattoos or identification, and gender or neutering.

2 Skin the carcass, carefully, from the tip of the chin to the anus and coronary bands. Yes, this seems like a lot of tedious work and in fact, it is. However, many lesions not easily seen from the haired side of the skin are easily visualized from the subcutis. Penetrating but nonbleeding puncture wounds (such as bullet holes) are a good example of lesions visualized more easily from the subcuticular side of the skin. Evaluation of the skin from the subcutis also will provide information on position (postmortem hypostatic congestion is more prominent on the "down" side), duration of recumbency (areas of bruising and pressure sores), and peripheral vascular congestion (sometimes seen with heat exhaustion and shock) and occasionally be useful in finding "burn tracks" associated with lightning strikes. In horses that are insured or that die unexpectedly, it is important to meticulously examine the subcutis for puncture wounds and bruising that may indicate injection sites.

3 After examining the external musculature and body walls, dissect around and remove the front and hind limbs on the "up" side. When the limbs are reflected and removed, note the condition of the brachial plexus under the front leg and collect samples of nerve. Place this in a labeled container with fixative. Note the condition of the hip joint and sciatic nerve when removing the hind leg and collect a small (2-cm) section of the sciatic nerve. Place this in a labeled container with fixative. Then, beginning at the juncture of the last rib and the backbone, dissect CAREFULLY down the wall of the abdominal cavity, following the curve of the last rib. We find that

holding the knife by the handle, placing my hand and handle in the abdominal cavity, with the blade up (like a shark cutting the surface of the ocean) and gently pushing the knife forward, usually will prevent accidentally cutting abdominal viscera. Put the limbs aside for later evaluation.

4 Allow the abdominal organs to push out of the opening. Collect any fluid samples, such as bacterial cultures, from inside the cavity, in areas not contaminated by the knife or hands. Note any fluid present (type, amount, position, consistency, color). At this point, note the condition of the diaphragm. Unless inadvertently punctured during dissection or injured before death, this should be concave in respect to the thoracic cavity.

5 Examine the abdominal organs and note/photograph any abnormalities. We believe it is important to open the entire gastrointestinal tract on every horse, to evaluate contents, to look for lesions, and, like the skin/subcutis, to get the view "from the inside."

6 Incise the top portion of the diaphragm, adjacent to the top of the last rib. Loss of negative intrathoracic pressure will allow air to enter. Look inside the thoracic cavity for any gross abnormalities and collect samples needed for later evaluation, including samples for bacterial culture. Note any fluid present (type, amount, position, consistency, color).

7 Incise the base of the tongue at the mandible, penetrating into the oral cavity, and then strip back, using sharp and blunt dissection, the tongue, trachea, esophagus, thyroids (collect these and place immediately in fixative—they tend to get lost easily), to the thoracic inlet. Using rib cutters (heavy duty pruning shears), cut the ribs in two places—at the junction with the spine and at the junction with the sternum. Remove this side of the rib cage; examine it and the viscera in the thoracic cavity. Remove these tissues ("the pluck") that includes the tongue, upper airway and esophagus, lungs, heart, thymus, and mediastinum. Note and photograph gross lesions. Continue dissection of heart and lungs.

8 This is a good point to stop and take a break to reflect on whether the lesions seen to this point help explain the clinical signs noted in this horse prior to death. Make notes, take additional photographs for documentation (include labels of time, date, animal identification), and collect tissue samples and place them in fixative (see aforementioned). As a rule, it is always a reasonable idea to collect small samples of major organs, even if there are no visible lesions, for later diagnostics. These will include liver, kidney, spleen, adrenals, lung, heart, skeletal muscle, tongue, representative sections of the gastrointestinal tract, and pancreas. Dispose of tissue safely before proceeding.

9 Turn the carcass over, finish skinning and evaluation of skin, subcutis and body wall, remove legs (set aside), and rib cage.

10 At this point, specific attention is directed to dissection of the CNS. Trim muscle and connective tissue from the spinal column, from the base of the neck to the cauda equina. Carefully dissect around the cauda equina at the base of the spinal column.

11 Disarticulate the head from the spinal column at the atlantooccipital junction.

12 Skin the head, note any gross abnormalities, and carefully remove the eyes; place these in fixative.

13 With a saw, cut the skull around the brain.

14 Using a large screw driver or pry bar, peel back the skull cap, revealing the brain. Note, record or photograph any abnormalities of the meninges, and collect fluid samples for bacterial culture, if indicated.

15 Tip the head nose up, allowing the brain to pull backward and down under its own weight, and then tease/cut the brain out, severing the cranial nerves. It is likely the pituitary will remain lodged in the *sella turcica*, having pulled loose from the stalk of the pituitary. Gently dissect around the pituitary, remove it intact, examine it, and place it in a labeled container with fixative. Place the appropriate portion(s) of the brain in fixative (see aforementioned). If fresh or frozen tissue is to be submitted for diagnostic evaluation, collect these samples prior to immersion in fixative. Put them in labeled, sealed double plastic bags, with identification of horse, time, and date noted (Figure 16.1 a–g).

16 Examine the oral cavity, guttural pouches, and other portions of the skull for lesions. Note and record or photograph these.

17 There are two common approaches for examining the spinal cord. Each has merits and shortcomings but all are better than not examining the spinal cord. Any of the following methods are made more easy by suspending the carcass, such as from a tree, overhead beam, or front-end loader.

Strategy #1: The spinal column is sawed in cross-section at several locations. This sawing will cut the spinal cord. Typical points of sawing are between C2–C3, T1–T2, T4–T5, T10–T11, L1–L2, L4–L5 and at the L–S junction. The cut ends of the cord are examined and any abnormalities noted. At the points of sawing, the cord is gently pulled by the meninges and cut with scalpel approximately 1–2 cm in back of the sawed edge (the morphology of which is damaged by sawing). These sections are placed in separately labeled containers, by anatomic site, with fixative. This is the most common, and acceptable, method used by practitioners during field necropsies. This method is very useful for tissue collection but

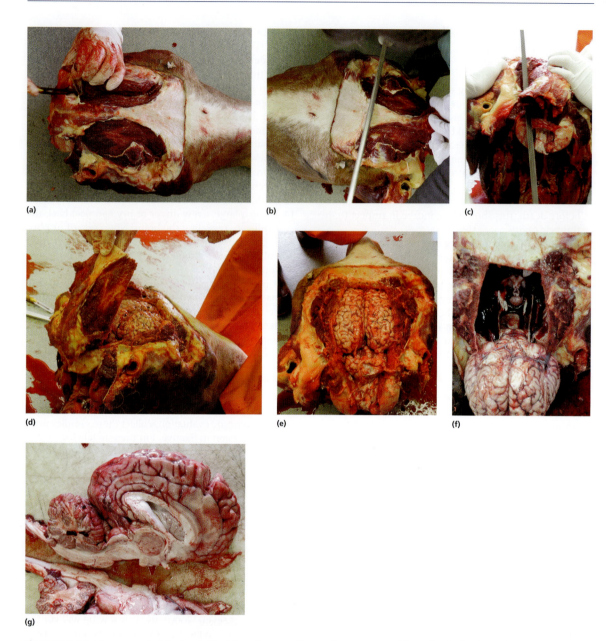

Figure 16.1 (a) After removal of the head, the skin and temporalis muscles are removed from the skull—this makes sawing the skull much easier; (b) after trimming, make the first cut across the skull as shown, and angle the saw after passing through the skull to avoid cutting too deeply into the brain tissue; (c) after the first cut is completed, the second and third cuts are angled as shown through the temporal region (just above the top of the mandible) and into the center of the spinal canal on each side—again—be careful to avoid cutting too deep and going into the brain; (d) the skull flap that has been created is lifted up (sometimes a tool to pry with is needed); (e) this allows the brain to be examined in situ, and swelling, discoloration, and displacements can be seen; (f) the skull is then tipped up and gently "banged" on the floor to loosen the brain, which will come partially out allowing the underside to be observed and revealing the pituitary—the brain is then physically removed; (g) after removal, the brain is sagittally sectioned for examination of the cut surface.

does not sample the entire cord, allow for focal lesions to be detected and sampled, and may damage tissue for morphologic evaluation.

Strategy #2: The spinal column can be sawed into pieces, as aforementioned; these pieces can be cooled (just above freezing) and packed in a cooler and transported IMMEDIATELY to a diagnostic facility with a band saw, where the spinal column sections can be longitudinally sawed, the cord collected intact, and after examination can be placed in fixative prior to further trimming. This strategy requires communication with the laboratory and arrival of specimens within 6 h of postmortem for best results.

This method is used by diagnostic pathologists in many laboratories. It requires special equipment and skill. It allows anatomic orientation of the cord to be preserved, facilitates detection of abnormalities, and allows exhaustive trimming and sectioning when looking for lesions. The author has used this method and has at times prepared and examined over 100 cross-sections of spinal cord looking for minute lesions associated with equine protozoal myeloencephalitis (EPM). Tissues from horses suspected of having rabies should not be sawed with a band saw, due to potential aeresolation of virus, rather sawed by hand and tissue removed using a cord puller, as described in Chapter 19.

18 Examination of peripheral nerves requires careful dissection along the length of the nerve. These nerves frequently run through muscle and fascia and it may be time-consuming (*but rewarding*) to follow them from a point of origin near the trunk of the body to the nerve endings at the distal limb and tip of the tail. Prior to dissection, it is important to consider if there are any injuries or musculoskeletal lesions surrounding the peripheral nerves that need to be examined during the course of dissection. Nerve dissection requires a gentle touch, handling of the connective tissue around nerves (not the nerve itself), and attention to obvious abnormalities. Photographs documenting suspected areas of injury are immensely helpful in later discussions with pathologists, with horse owners, and with insurance agents.

19 Finally, dissect and examine the limbs, including opening the joints. In some cases, this is simple, requiring splitting of the joint capsule and major ligaments. In other joints, like the tarsus, this is both time-consuming and difficult, given the complex bony articulations. Again, it is important to continue to focus on determining all contributions to presumed neurologic signs, including those due to bone, tendon/ligament, and muscle injury.

20 When working with foals, several additional points should be considered in conjunction with the postmortem examination:

- Is there a history or observations of dystocia with the birth of this foal?
- Were there any exposures to vaccines, infectious agents, or toxicants, such as fungal feed contaminants or toxic pasture plants, at any time during gestation?
- Was the foaling abnormal in any way?
- Is the placenta available for evaluation and is it normal or abnormal?
- If the placenta is available, portions should be saved for microbial culture and also fixed for histologic evaluation?
- Did the mare have an uneventful pregnancy (fevers, illness, or vaginal discharge)?
- Have any foals born to the mare or stallion previously had birth defects, including neonatal maladaptation?
- Did the foal suckle normally or was there evidence of failure of passive transfer of colostral antibodies?
- If there is gross evidence of one type of birth defects (such as limb or facial deformities), it is very worthwhile to search for others during the post mortem examination
- Microscopic lesions associated with neonatal hypoxia may be difficult to find histologically.
- Evaluation of joints and umbilicus for the presence of sepsis are a mandatory part of the postmortem examination.

Many of these additional points are addressed by questioning of the owner before the dissection. Answers to these questions help the practitioner and pathologist when interpreting lesions and preparing reports. Postmortem examinations of foals are done in the same manner as adult horses.

The third element of the postmortem examination is as important as the first two. You MUST document gross lesions. Gross lesions of the nervous system can be simply and adequately described by noting (in writing—on the medical record) size (in comparison with normal), shape, color, gross consistency (soft, firm, gelatinous, crumbly, clot-like), and anatomic position (spinal cord segment, etc.). Nothing elaborate is needed and this is the basis for all gross pathologic description. Noting the extent of a lesion in terms like *focal* (in a single small (<1 cm) spot in diameter), *focally extensive* (in a single spot exceeding 1 cm diameter), *multifocal* (lesions scattered about in tissue), or *diffuse* (affecting the entire tissue). An example of a gross description of a lesion might be as follows: "There is a focally extensive area of grey, brown, and red discoloration in the cerebral cortex and extending into the middle of the brain." Note that taking a photograph of this lesion, at the time it was fresh, will help the pathologist and other specialists who might eventually work on this case understand the nature, position, and extent of the lesion.

Gross abnormalities of the nervous system—some working generalizations

It is important to know normal anatomy and morphology of tissues in the CNS so that one can adequately detect and describe abnormalities. Gross abnormalities found during the postmortem examination can be very helpful in determining causes of sickness and death in horses; the definitive diagnosis of many cases relies on both gross and microscopic evaluations, hence the practitioner should never "guess" on diagnosis based only on gross appearance of lesions. A few generalizations about disease, based on gross appearance, may be useful.

Changes in color of the brain or spinal cord can indicate trauma, hemorrhage, degeneration, or inflammation. Normally, the color of fresh equine brain and spinal cord is pearly white to tan. Brains and cords that are undergoing autolysis may become grayer with advancing time (and also become much softer as degradative enzymes break down tissue). Diffuse vascular congestion, due to hyperthermia (inflammatory disease or heat stroke), may cause the meninges of the brain and cord to be red-purple. Red or purple foci may indicate areas of vascular disruption and hemorrhage, and there are many causes of this, ranging from trauma to vascular leakage associated with coagulopathies. Foci with dark red, brown, or gray discoloration, in which there is also softening of brain or spinal cord tissue, may indicate hemorrhage, malacia, infarction, or even the presence of a neoplasm. Many diseases can be expressed by the same changes in color, and these areas sampled for further histopathologic evaluation.

Normal, fresh brain and spinal cord have a soft but spongy/rubbery consistency. The longer brains and spinal cords remain between 25 and 38°C (ambient room temperature to physiologic temperature) after death, the more they will undergo autolysis and soften. The brains of animals that have suffered from hyperthermia may be soft, to the point of liquefaction, even when collected within 1–2 h of death. In some diseases, changes in consistency are very important clues to the final diagnosis. A classic example of this is the gelatinous liquefaction of areas of the brain in horses exposed to the toxin fumonisin (moldy corn poisoning). Foci of necrosis, which can be caused by many things (e.g., infarction, trauma, and infections), are soft and

discolored due to the release of enzymes from brain and cord tissue and infiltrating inflammatory cells, if present.

Notable changes in symmetry and position also can be useful in finding lesions. Both the brain and spinal cord display a high degree of bilateral symmetry. This also applies to the morphology of the ventricular system that circulates fluid in the brain and to the vertebral bodies surrounding the spinal cord. Deviations from symmetry, or malpositioning (as might be seen with atlantooccipital malformations in Arabian horses or cervical vertebral instability), are good indicators of lesions/disease at those sites.

Changes in normal size matter. Dilation of the ventricles of the brain may be indicators of some lesion or disease process that has interfered with fluid production and flow. Many veterinarians understand that dilated ventricles (hydrocephalus) compress surrounding brain tissue into the noncompressible bones of the skull and spinal cord, leading to atrophy and degeneration of brain tissue. It is not uncommon to see subtle to very remarkable enlargements of the pituitary gland in horses with equine Cushing's disease.

Another generalization about size and position is important to consider. In general, the larger the lesion, the more significant and serious the disease and clinical signs are. Minor cases of hydrocephalus or small meningeal cysts may be incidental findings in horses without overt signs of nervous system disease. Diffuse inflammation and hyperthermia associated with infection by encephalitic viruses (herpesvirus, equine encephalitis arboviruses, and rabies) produce profound signs and lesions. Of course, the position of lesions may dictate clinical signs (blindness due to pressure on the optic chiasm from the growth of a large pituitary adenoma is an example). Localizing lesions, based on antemortem clinical signs, is an important part of analyzing cases and performing diagnostic postmortem exams.

A final generalization is one we are all familiar with. The brain and spinal cord are encased in protective bone. Space-occupying lesions (such as abscesses and neoplasms) and processes that result in brain/cord swelling (edema, inflammation, and neoplastic disease) readily produce neurologic signs and tissue damage.

Working with the neuropathologist

Most practitioners are going to rely on the services of a pathologist in helping to sort out lesions seen in horses with neurologic disease and in helping to finalize cases. The practitioner and pathologist form an important team in diagnosing, treating, and, in some cases, preventing disease. Both parties need to cultivate this relationship and foster good communication.

Once pathologists receive tissues and observations from practitioners, it is common for them to call to discuss the results of the gross postmortem examination with the practitioner and to review points raised in the history and antemortem examination.

Well-fixed tissue specimens are carefully trimmed by pathologists and then prepared for histologic evaluation. This trimming and preparation may take several days after tissue is received. If fresh or frozen tissue is submitted, especially for priority evaluation of rabies or other agents, FA testing on frozen sections is generally completed within 24–48 h.

Most routine sections are stained with hematoxylin–eosin, a general-purpose set of stains that will stain nuclei purple/blue and proteins (cytoplasm) pink/orange. This stain is usually adequate for diagnostic evaluation of most cases.

Several types of special stains are used in neuropathology. Stains containing silver and gold have an affinity for nerve tissue and can be used for contrasting neurons and axons from surrounding connective tissues. A host of antibody-based stains (FA and immunohistochemical stains) are used to show localization of proteins or infectious agents in brain and spinal cord. These stains typically contain an antibody directed against some organism (e.g., equine herpesvirus 1 (EHV-1), West Nile flavivirus, Eastern equine encephalitis (EEE) alphavirus, and rabies rhabdovirus) or cell component (such as epidermal growth factor receptor or glial fibrillary acidic protein (GFAP)) and a chromogen that either fluoresces or develops a long-lasting pigment that can be viewed microscopically. These stains are extremely helpful in definitive diagnosis of infectious diseases of the nervous system or to differentiate specific types of tumors.

Interpreting the pathologist's report

Pathologists typically report findings as a series of morphologic diagnoses and final summary statements that relate the diagnoses with clinical signs, history, and gross lesions. There is a rather consistent "language" and sentence structure of most pathology reports, since many veterinary pathologists are trained in diagnostic terminology originally developed through the Armed Forces Institute of Pathology (now The Joint Pathology Center) and adopted both by veterinary pathology training programs and the American College of Veterinary Pathologists. At times, pathology reports may be difficult to "decode" and it is wise to ask for a more descriptive summary that contains less overt "pathologese."

Some terms used by pathologists are common. "**Malacia**" typically refers to necrosis and degeneration of brain tissue and morphology. Terms containing the suffix "itis" indicate inflammation. "**Encephalo-**" refers to brain and "**Myelo-**" "to spinal cord." The term "**leuko-**" refers to the white matter (myelin-containing portions of the nervous system) and "**polio-**" to gray matter (neurons, neuropil).

Most neuropathologists will send a report to the referring veterinarian that gives a brief review of the clinical and gross pathology findings, as well as a more extensive description of microscopic lesions. Pathologists vary widely in the style and content of these reports. Some may prefer to simply list the tissues and enter short morphologic diagnosis, containing the elements of lesion type, severity, distribution, and an indication of chronicity. An example of this type of reporting might be as follows:

> "Spinal cord: Acute, severe, diffuse suppurative meningitis." One translation of this into more common terminology is "there is severe, diffuse acute inflammation of the meninges and this is manifested by the presence of neutrophils, perhaps other inflammatory cells, and necrotic cell debris (things that make "purulent" material, i.e., "pus")." Other pathologists may prefer to write reports as a narrative, using more common language (the translation aforementioned is an example of this style).

A number of terms commonly are used by all pathologists, especially when describing changes in the morphology of nerve cells. It may be necessary to review the basic organization of the nervous system in order to understand common pathology terms indicating the presence of disease. A few of the common pathology terms used frequently by pathologists are included here. A few simple working definitions and an indication of significance of the terms are included.

Neuropathy—this can refer to the gross and histologic changes seen in nerve tissue or more specifically may indicate lesions in nerve cells. The term neuropathy says something is wrong but lacks precision in indicating what and where the problem is.

Axonopathy—here there are morphologic changes in the shapes of axons. Two very typical axonopathies are seen in horses. In one, there is shrinkage of the axon within the axon sheath. This may be indicative of damage to nerve cell bodies upstream or overall nutrient availability for nerve cells and axons. Another common axonopathy is swelling of the axon within the sheath. This gives the appearance of enlarged axon spaces. In reality, this swelling may be the result of fluid accumulation within and around axons, but the fluid is not easily visualized (low protein content) or is leached during histologic processing.

Myelinopathy—this is the loss of integrity of the myelin sheath surrounding axons. This can be the result of nerve cell body and axon damage or may be a primary lesion specific to a disease. In dogs, for example, canine distemper virus produces a myelinopathy resulting in dissolution of myelin. Similarly, multiple sclerosis in people has a myelinopathy as one important disease component. Since myelin protects axons and regulates nerve impulse conduction integrity, a loss of myelin has significant consequences for affected cells.

Wallerian degeneration—this term refers to degeneration of axons and myelin distal to an injury.

Perivascular cuffing—this indicates the presence usually of inflammatory cells around blood vessels in the brain and spinal cord substance. Many pathologists believe this lesion probably represents a loss of integrity of the blood–brain barrier at these sites. A number of viral and bacterial infections of the CNS have foci of perivascular cuffing as primary lesions.

Perivascular edema—this is seen fairly commonly, both as an indicator of the presence of disease and also as an artifact of fixation. One must interpret this with caution. The lesion described usually refers to clear spaces surrounding blood vessels and nerves.

In this age of widely available electronic communication, there is no reason that anyone receiving a pathology report should hesitate, even for an instant, to call the pathologist who wrote it to get a better understanding of the contents of the report. Translation: you need to pick up the phone!

Primary and secondary diseases affecting the nervous system of horses are common causes of morbidity and mortality. Every practitioner can become competent in diagnosing these diseases with clinical and pathologic evaluations. However, if one does not look, one does not find. Practitioners are strongly encouraged to hone skills for examining the tissues making up the nervous system and for developing good working relationships with pathologists and diagnostic laboratories. Together, this team will find the answers to many problems and help many horses and their owners.

Systemic neuropathology

This section will concisely describe the diseases affecting the nervous system of equines: causes, lesions, agent distribution, and diagnostic tests [5].

Malformations
Hydrocephalus
Hydrocephalus is the excessive accumulation of cerebrospinal fluid (CSF) in ventricles resulting in compression atrophy of the neuropil [6, 7]. This condition can be primary or secondary. The primary form generally occurs in young animals and is idiopathic, while the secondary hydrocephalus manifests in older animals and is caused by other diseases. Mechanisms include obstruction or, rarely, fluid overproduction. The obstruction can be congenital or acquired. In horses, hydrocephalus tends to be rare. Arab newborn foals present

with a naturally domed cranium, and this should not be mistaken for a deformity associated with hydrocephalus. Hydrocephalus seems to be more frequent in Friesian horses. Affected Friesian foals present tetraventricular and venous dilatations with malformation of the petrosal bone and, as a result, narrowing of the jugular foramen. These observations suggest a communicative hydrocephalus with a diminished absorption of CSF into the systemic circulation at the venous sinuses due to a distorted, nonfunctional jugular foramen. This type of hydrocephalus is also recognized in humans and dogs and has been linked genetically to chondrodysplasia. This has been also recognized in dwarfism, which is another monogenetic defect in Friesian horses.

Chiari malformation
This malformation sometimes is also called Arnold–Chiari malformation [8]. The scale of severity is rated I–IV, with IV being the most severe. Types III and IV are very rare. It consists of a downward displacement of the cerebellar tonsils through the foramen magnum, sometimes causing noncommunicating hydrocephalus as a result of obstruction of CSF outflow. This malformation is very rarely seen in horses.

Meningocele
Meningocele is the hernial protrusion of the meninges through a defect in the cranium (cranial meningocele) or vertebral column (spinal meningocele) [9]. They are both presentations of *spina bifida manifesta*. This is very rare in horses.

Spina bifida
Spina bifida is the incomplete closing of the embryonic neural tube [10]. Some vertebrae overlying the spinal cord are not fully formed and remain unfused and open. If the opening is large enough, this allows a portion of the spinal cord to protrude through the opening in the bones. There may or may not be a fluid-filled sac surrounding the spinal cord. Spina bifida is classified as *spina bifida aperta* (or *cystica*), defined by a protrusion of spinal tissue through the cleft vertebrae, or as *spina bifida occulta*, where the spinal cord tissue remains in place. Depending on the protruding tissue, a *spina bifida aperta* can result in a meningocele, myelomeningocele, and myeloschisis. These conditions are very rare in the horse.

Perosomus elumbis (with cerebral aplasia and spina bifida)
Perosomus elumbis represents a rare congenital anomaly characterized by aplasia of the lumbosacral spinal cord and vertebrae [10]. This anomaly is often associated with arthrogryposis and malformations of the urogenital and intestinal tract. A Thoroughbred aborted

fetus with perosomus elumbis, cerebral aplasia, and spina bifida has been described.

Microphthalmia

This is a rare malformation in horses [11]. In severe microphthalmia, no internal structures, such as lens and retina, are apparent and a cystic malformed globe that consists solely of a scleral sheet and some pigmentary differentiation, typical of persistence of the primary optic vesicle, may be observed. In mild cases of microphthalmia, there is a reduction in size of the main structures only. Treatment with griseofulvin for dermatomycosis in the second month of pregnancy may cause bilateral microphthalmia, severe brachygnathia superior, and palatocheiloschisis.

Retinal dysplasia

Retinal dysplasia is an uncommon developmental lesion characterized histologically by retinal folds and rosettes [12]. It may occur in association with other ocular anomalies in animals with anterior segment dysgenesis. Retinal detachments are generally secondary to posterior segment inflammation of equine recurrent uveitis, head trauma, perforating globe wounds, and tumors. Nonetheless, they may also be congenital, possibly associated with other ocular abnormalities.

Vascular malformations

Vascular hamartomas are considered developmental lesions [13]. They consist of nonneoplastic proliferation of thin-walled vessels with caliber variation. These vessels are generally elastin-negative, with varying amounts of collagen and no muscular component. A clinically significant prominent vascular hamartoma was identified in the cerebellum of an old mule also affected by a pinealoma.

Arachnoid diverticula

These very rare lesions are intra-arachnoid membrane accumulations of CSF that may occur in any location along the cerebral spinal fluid axis [14]. Spinal arachnoid diverticula have also been referred to as arachnoid cysts, meningeal cysts, leptomeningeal cysts, intraarachnoid cysts, and subarachnoid cysts. True cysts are lined by epithelium; hence, cavitations or diverticula are more accurate descriptions of these lesions. Animals may exhibit clinical signs at young age, but diverticula have been also reported in adults.

Degenerative diseases
Leukoencephalomalacia

This disease is caused by the consumption of moldy corn or hay contaminated by the microscopic fungus *Fusarium verticillioides* (formerly *F. moniliforme*) [15, 16]. Fumonisins B1, B2, A1, and A2 are a structurally closely related group of mycotoxins resembling the structure of natural sphingolipids. The major toxin involved in leukoencephalomalacia is fumonisin B1. Fumonisins are heat-stable compounds that survive under most conditions. Fumonisin inhibits the enzyme ceramide synthase and interferes with the synthesis of sphingolipids. The resulting lesion is bilateral, asymmetrical, liquefaction necrosis of the cerebral white matter involving frontal and parietal lobes, and sometimes also the brainstem and spinal cord grey matter. Histologically, there are varying degree of necrosis; hemorrhages; and infiltration of neutrophils, lymphocytes, and sometimes eosinophils. Gross and histologic lesions are diagnostic. The toxins can be detected in the feedstuff via enzyme immunoassays.

Nigropallidal encephalomalacia

This is a disease caused by the consumption of yellow star thistle (*Centaurea solstitialis*) and Russian knapweed (*Rhaponticum repens*) [17, 18]. The toxic compounds are lactones and pyrones, effective in 30–90 days of eating the plant on a daily basis. This is a regional disease in the Northwestern states of the United States, especially North California, Washington, Montana, Idaho, Oregon, and Colorado. Repin, a sesquiterpene isolated from *R. repens*, has cytotoxic effect associated with depletion of glutathione, increase in reactive oxygen species, and cell membrane damage. High concentrations of monoamine oxidase in the dopaminergic striatonigral tract likely render these areas more susceptible to oxidative damage. Other potential toxins are the excitotoxic amino acids aspartate and glutamate isolated from *C. solstitialis*. Bilateral symmetric malacia, often with yellow-tan discoloration, in the substantia nigra and anterior globus pallidus are observed. Occasionally, lesions involve other brainstem nuclei as well. Sometimes the lesion is not bilateral. A detailed study revealed that lesions are located in the substantia nigra pars reticulata, sparing the cell bodies of the dopaminergic neurons in the substantia nigra pars compacta and in the rostral portion of the globus pallidus, with partial disruption of dopaminergic (tyrosine hydroxylase–positive) fibers passing through the globus pallidus. Changes are similar to human Parkinsonism, but Lewy bodies are not present. Gross and histologic lesions are diagnostic. Toxins can be identified via spectrometry.

Cerebellar abiotrophy

Abiotrophy means the loss of a vital nutritive factor [19]. The exact cause of cerebellar abiotrophy is not known, but it is thought to be due to an intrinsic metabolic defect. This condition is characterized by loss of organization of the cerebellum during fetal life and up to 6 months of age leading to progressive symmetric atrophy. It occurs primarily in Arabian horses and can also be observed in miniature horses, Gotland Pony, Eriskay Pony, and Oldenburg. There is bilateral symmetrical cerebellar abiotrophy with homogeneously decreased cerebellar volume, prominent sulci separating the vermis, deranged orientation of Purkinje cells, and loss of granular cells. Gross and histologic lesions are diagnostic.

Equine motor neuron disease

Equine motor neuron disease (EMND) occurs sporadically in individual animals or rarely in outbreaks affecting the motor neurons in the ventral horns of the spinal cord [20, 21]. This is a proposed vitamin E–responsive disease. Neuronal degeneration affects the facial nucleus and the motor nucleus of the trigeminal nerve. Primary lesions are found in the motor neurons of spinal cord ventral horn cells; in the brainstem nuclei V, VII, and XII; and the nucleus ambiguous. More specifically, CNS lesions include lipofuscinosis, lower motor neuron chromatolysis (sometimes with intracytoplasmic acidophilic inclusion bodies), glial scar formation, peripheral nerve Wallerian degeneration with digestion chambers, and retinopathy with endothelial lipofuscinosis. Coccygeal, triceps brachii, and femoral muscles may display a macroscopic pale gelatinous appearance that microscopically corresponds to neurogenic small angular atrophy, affecting predominantly the type 2 fibers. Hepatocellular lipofuscinosis and hepatocellular and Kupffer cell hemosiderosis may be also observed in some cases. Gross lesions affecting the aforementioned muscular groups and histologic lesions are diagnostic. Histologic examination of the sacrocaudalis dorsalis muscle is an in vivo diagnostic tool for the identification of this disease.

Equine degenerative myeloencephalopathy and equine neuroaxonal dystrophy

Equine degenerative myeloencephalopathy (EDME) is a vitamin E–responsive disease with familial predisposition [22, 23]. Equine neuroaxonal dystrophy (NAD) is considered the underlying basis of EDME and clinically, the two diseases are indistinguishable. EDME can be considered a more severe variant of NAD. NAD/EDME appears to be an inherited disorder, and it may be that vitamin E acts as a modifier to determine the overall severity of the disease in horses affected with NAD/EDME. Age of onset ranges from birth up to 3 years of age, although most affected animals demonstrate clinical signs by 6–12 months of age. Breeds that appear to have a hereditary basis include Appaloosa, Standardbred, Paso Fino, Norwegian Fjord, Arabian, Quarter Horse, Welsh Pony, and Haflinger as well as Burchell's zebras. Lesions involve the spinal cord and medulla oblongata. The spinocerebellar and ventromedian tracts of thoracic segments, the lateral cuneate

nuclei, and thoracic nuclei are particularly affected with severe NAD. Neuronal fiber degeneration, spheroids, neuronal loss, astrogliosis, and lipofuscinosis are observed in these areas. NAD in Quarter Horses is clinically indistinguishable from EDME but has a different lesion distribution. Similar conditions include the spinal ataxia in Captive Grant zebras and the myelopathy of Przewalskii Horses. The diagnosis is based on the observation of the histologic findings. Age and topography of the lesions differ from animals affected by EMND.

Myoclonus of the Peruvian Paso horse

Purebred Peruvian Paso horses can present with a specific deficiency in the density of [3H]strychnine binding to inhibitory glycine receptor sites in the spinal cord [24]. Specificity of the deficit can be confirmed by the demonstration of changes in the density of several other receptor types in affected spinal cord, including muscarinic receptors and γ-aminobutyric acid (GABA)/benzodiazepine receptors. No lesions have been described.

Equine dysautonomia (grass sickness)

Equine dysautonomia causes marked reduction of gastrointestinal motility due to widespread degeneration within the autonomic nervous system [25–28]. The etiology is unknown. It is observed throughout northern Europe, where it is epidemiologically associated with leporine dysautonomia, and a few cases have recently been diagnosed in the United States in the Midwest, where canine dysautonomia has been also observed. In acute and subacute cases, the stomach and small intestine are severely distended with fluid, which can result in gastric rupture, and the large intestine is impacted. The digesta tend to be viscous proximally, and the impacted digesta are attached to the mucosa. In chronic cases, the gastrointestinal tract is usually empty. Linear ulceration of the esophagus and hard, tarry fecal balls are generally observed. Neuronal degeneration, characterized by chromatolysis, is common in pre- and postganglionic sympathetic and parasympathetic neurons. Chromatolytic autonomic and somatic lower motor neurons can be observed in the brainstem and spinal cord. Aspiration pneumonia is a frequent complication. Biopsies of ileal and rectal tissue can confirm the clinical presumptive diagnosis. Histopathologic examination of autonomic ganglia, in particular the celiac mesenteric ganglion, is diagnostic. Other causes of emaciation should be considered in the chronic form, including EMND.

Colonic aganglionosis (Hirschsprung disease)

Breeding for color results in the occasional production of a foal suffering from overo lethal white syndrome (OLWS) [29, 30]. This is most common among overo paint crosses but does not exclusively occur from overo crosses, and in many overo-to-overo crosses this condition does not result. Some horses are heterozygotes and do not express the classic phenotype of heavy white pattern (calico, splash white, or frame). On the other hand, some horses have a lot of white such as a frame overo yet are not heterozygotes. Therefore, allele-specific genotyping of DNA must be performed to accurately determine an individual horse's potential to produce a foal affected by OLWS. The Ile118Lys endothelin receptor B mutation is responsible for the lack of migration of melanocyte and colonic ganglia cell precursors from the neural crests. These foals appear normal at birth but within a few hours develop symptoms of colic. They have white hair and pink skin with the exception of occasional pigmented foci about the muzzle, ventral abdomen, and hindquarters. Gross lesions include severe meconium impaction often associated with enterocolitis. Histologic lesions are an almost complete absence of mural ganglia within the sections of colon and sometimes enterocolitis with bacterial colonies and morphologic evidence of sepsis in other organs. Although the histologic lesion is readily identifiable, immunohistochemistry (IHC) for the detection of S-100 protein will highlight the distribution and morphology of the myenteric plexi and ganglia. The postmortem diagnosis is based on the identification of a depigmented neonate with impaction and colitis, followed by histologic examination of the colon.

Laryngeal hemiplegia

Left recurrent laryngeal hemiplegia is characterized by paresis or paralysis of the left arytenoid cartilage and vocal fold [31, 32]. It manifests clinically as exercise intolerance and inspiratory respiratory noise ("roaring") during exercise. Right-sided hemiplegia and bilateral (paraplegia) arytenoid dysfunction are uncommon. All breeds are affected, but prevalence is higher in males and long-necked and larger breeds. It may be a heritable disease. There is progressive loss of the large myelinated fibers in the distal portion of the recurrent laryngeal nerves with neurogenic atrophy of the intrinsic laryngeal musculature, the most crucial of which is the cricoarytenoideus dorsalis muscle. The left recurrent nerve is more commonly affected. Its extended length around the base of the heart may be a predisposing factor. Trauma to the recurrent laryngeal nerve, perivascular injection of irritating substances, prior neck surgery, esophageal rupture, guttural pouch mycosis, organophosphate intoxication, lead poisoning, toxic plants, strangles, degenerative CNS diseases, and thiamine deficiency are possible causes. Plants include chick peas (*Cicer arietinum*) and *Lathyrus* spp. Lead toxicity causes bilateral laryngeal paralysis. The postmortem diagnosis is based on the observation of various degrees of atrophy characterized by pallor and size reduction of the left cricoarytenoideus dorsalis muscle and muscle atrophy at the microscope. Arytenoid chondritis can be confused with this condition. In arytenoid chondritis, there are degenerative changes and calcification of the arytenoid cartilages.

Stringhalt

Classical and Australian stringhalts have been described [33, 34]. Australian stringhalt is differentiated from classical stringhalt by the severity, occurrence of outbreaks, distinct seasonal pattern, and the ability of affected horses to recover spontaneously. There is sudden exaggerated flexion of either one or both hocks. It tends to occur in the summer and fall while horses are out on pasture and epidemics are observed in dry conditions. This distal axonopathy is associated with atrophy of long and lateral digital extensor and lateral deep digital flexor muscle atrophy. Nerve fibers with thin myelin sheaths are more common in the proximal parts of affected nerves. The cause of this distal axonopathy remains unknown. Common plant species that have been found and identified in pastures where affected horses were located include flatweed (*Hypochaeris radicata*), sheep's sorrel (*Rumex acetosella*), and couch grass (*Elymus repens*). Mycotoxins are also a possible cause. Unlike Australian stringhalt, classic stringhalt does not typically occur in outbreaks and usually has no obvious cause. Clinical signs are similar, although classic stringhalt frequently has stronger effects in a single leg. Lesions may be observed in the peripheral nerves but also in the cervical or cranial thoracic area.

Cervical compressive stenotic myelopathy

This condition, also called by clinicians "wobbler syndrome," is a disorder of young fast-growing Thoroughbred and Standardbred horses associated with dysplasia of the vertebrae of the cervical spinal cord [35, 36]. It is believed that the syndrome is caused by several factors such as genetic predisposition, nutritional imbalances, rapid growth, trauma, or a combination of these. It has been suggested that this condition may be related to neck length, implying the longer the neck, the more likely the horse is to develop the syndrome. Surveys have shown that males outnumber females three to one. There is compression of the cervical spinal cord from either narrowing of the epidural space or instability. There are two forms: the static form affecting C5–C6 vertebrae and the dynamic stenotic form affecting C3–C4 vertebrae. Osteochondrosis of the articular facets is another differential cause as are healed fractures of vertebral facets. Thorough evaluation for vertebral malformation predisposing the compression may necessitate the disarticulation of affected vertebrae. Lesions include the identification of the cervical compressive stenotic myelopathy site, the vertebral dysplasia and the neuroaxonal degeneration (Wallerian degeneration) of ascending (cranial to the lesion) and descending (caudal to the lesion) nervous spinal tracts with digestion chambers containing myelomacrophages, spheroids, hemosiderosis, and perivascular fibrosis in more chronic cases. The diagnosis is based on the identification of gross and histologic lesions. (Figures 16.2 and 16.3)

Inflammatory diseases
Viral diseases
Rabies

This zoonotic disease affecting the CNS of many mammalian species is caused by a neurotropic RNA rhabdovirus [37]. Both vicious and paralytic forms may occur. The virus reaches the CNS by retrograde axonal transport from bite wounds. Rabies can be prevented by vaccination. Grossly a few hemorrhagic areas may be observed within the brainstem and spinal cord. Histologically, there is polioencephalomyelitis and trigeminal ganglionitis with perivascular lymphocytic cuffs, ring hemorrhage, and intracytoplasmic acidophilic viral inclusions (Negri bodies). FA tissue evaluation is the official mandatory test. In infected animals, there are so many viruses within the target areas of the CNS that FA direct IHC is still the most convenient technique to use even in the era of indirect IHC and molecular diagnostics. Cervical spinal cord and adjacent brainstem are optimal tissue regions for rabies testing in the horse. Virus abounds in the cytoplasm of CNS and trigeminal neurons and fibers; viral antigens are also visible within retinal ganglion cells, cornea, and salivary glands. A few cases may be characterized by absence of Negri bodies.

American equine encephalitides caused by alphaviruses

EEE, Western equine encephalitis (WEE), and Venezuelan equine encephalitis (VEE) strains have been described for this family of alphaviruses *Togaviridae*, all arthropod-borne viruses. EEE is prevalent in the north-east, east, and south-east of the United States, and cases are observed every year [38, 39]. WEE has been rarely detected within the last few decades. VEE is a notifiable disease that is not present in North America, but its vector is present. The agents have affinity to neurons, glial cells, cardiocytes, smooth muscle cells, and antigen-presenting cells of the renal interstitium. EEE can be controlled by vaccination. Alphaviruses are a public health consideration in that they are transmitted to people via mosquitoes (e.g., *Culiseta* sp. and *Culex* sp.), and EEE is listed as a category B bioterrorism agent. They can affect not only birds (pheasants are particularly sensitive) but also mammals. In addition to equines, camelids; deer; and rarely cattle, pigs, and seals may be also affected. Primates can become infected, and lesions in humans are severe. Lesions include polioencephalomyelitis with perivascular lymphocytic cuffs, neuronal necrosis and neutrophil infiltration, and cardiocyte and smooth muscle multifocal necrosis. Although the virus can be immunohistochemically detected also in nonneural tissues, the CNS with lesions remains the choice for diagnostic testing, which includes histopathology, IHC, PCR, and VI.

Ross River fever

Ross River virus is a small encapsulated single-stranded RNA zoonotic alphavirus endemic to Australia, Papua New Guinea, and other islands in the South Pacific [40]. It is responsible for a type of mosquito-borne nonlethal but debilitating tropical disease known as Ross River fever, previously termed "epidemic polyarthritis." The virus is suspected to be enzootic in populations of various

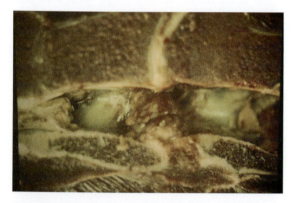

Figure 16.2 Spinal cord compression arising from a boney proliferation.

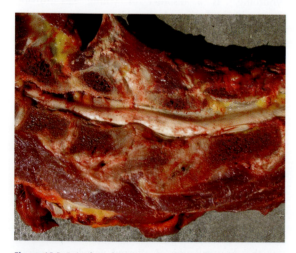

Figure 16.3 Spinal cord compression arising from impingement from bone proliferation associated with spondylosis.

native Australian mammals and has been occasionally detected in horses. Diagnostic testing includes histopathology, IHC, PCR, and VI.

West Nile fever

This is an acute to subacute encephalomyelitis caused by a single-stranded RNA flavivirus [41, 42]. A chronic relapsing form has been occasionally identified. Outbreaks were described in Africa, Europe, and North and South America. The distribution of this disease, as all arthropod vector–related diseases, depends on season and vector activity. Potential reservoirs and hosts include catholic feeding mosquitoes and multiple avian species. This disease has been described in birds (some species, such as craws, are very sensitive, others, like poultry, very resistant), camelids, seals, primates, sheep (rare), dogs (rare), alligators, and some amphibians. Gross lesions may include multifocal to confluent hemorrhages mainly through gray segments of the spinal cord. Brainstem and rhombencephalon are affected by hemorrhage to a lesser degree. Microscopically, there is mild to severe polioencephalomyelitis with perivascular small T lymphocytes, a few macrophages, multifocal glial nodules, occasional neutrophils and neuronal necrosis, spheroids, and ring hemorrhage. In mammals, the virus colonizes the cytoplasm of a few neurons, fibers, and clustering glial cells. In birds, abundant virus can be observed in any tissue and cell type, particularly within intestine, pancreas, lymphoid tissues and bone marrow, kidney, and brain. The diagnosis in mammals is based on the observation of the histologic lesions, PCR, and IHC on multiple CNS tissue sections with lesions (glial nodules). VI and IHC are not very sensitive for the detection of West Nile virus (WNV) in mammals, and PCR should be preferred.

Japanese encephalitis

Japanese encephalitis is caused by a flavivirus closely related to WNV and other encephalitic flaviviruses [43]. The first clinical reports in humans date from 1870, but the virus appears to have evolved in the mid-1500s. The disease is widely distributed in Asia, including countries such as Japan, Korea, Thailand, Malaysia, India, southeast part of Russia, and some parts of Oceania. It has been occasionally detected in birds in Europe. An inactivated vaccine against the disease used in Japan since 1948 has significantly reduced mortality among horses over the years. Transplacental infection followed by abortion occurs in humans, and this is also the most serious expression of the disease in pigs, the most importantly infected domestic species. The disease is transmitted mainly by the mosquito *Culex*, but *Aedes* and *Armigeres* seem to play a role as well. Many animals and birds are susceptible. Among animals infected naturally with the virus, only horses and donkeys develop clinical encephalitis. Lesions in equines are more prevalent in the cerebral hemispheres. Lesions are similar to WNV infection but often more severe. Plasma cells are described within the perivascular cuffs. The diagnosis can be achieved via the identification of the lesions and the use of IHC, PCR, and VI.

Louping-ill

This is an acute viral tick-transmitted disease primarily of sheep, also called ovine encephalomyelitis, infectious encephalomyelitis of sheep, and trembling-ill [44]. The occurrence of the disease is closely related to the distribution of the primary vector, the sheep tick *Ixodes ricinus*. This flavivirus also causes disease in the red grouse and can affect humans and horses. The name "louping-ill" is derived from an old Scottish word describing the effect of the disease in sheep whereby they "loup" or spring into the air. Lesions are similar to those of WNV and several other encephalitic flaviviruses. Additionally, the cerebellum may be involved with striking necrosis of Purkinje cells. The diagnosis is based on the observation of the histologic lesions, PCR and IHC on multiple sections with lesions, and VI.

Tick-borne encephalitis

Tick-borne encephalitis (TBE) is the most important viral tick-borne zoonosis in Europe [45, 46]. Many human cases are reported every year. The flavivirus that causes TBE circulates between ticks and hosts and is in the majority of cases transmitted by tick bite. In veterinary medicine, TBE cases are infrequent, but infections with neurological signs have been reported in dogs, monkeys, and horses. Lesions and diagnostic procedures are very similar to these of the other encephalitogenic flaviviruses.

Kunjin virus encephalomyelitis

Kunjin flavivirus (KV) is closely related to WNV and is present in Australia [47]. Kunjin virus can occasionally cause disease in humans, but illness is usually mild. Disease due to KV has not been recognized in birds in Australia, though it is possible that it does occasionally occur. A few horses develop clinically significant disease, and about 10% of horses may die during outbreaks. Lesions and diagnostic procedures are very similar to those of other encephalitogenic flaviviruses.

Murray valley encephalitis

Murray Valley encephalitis (MVE) virus is a flavivirus spread by mosquitoes, and antibodies against MVE virus can be demonstrated in a wide range of animals, including horses, pigs, marsupials, poultry and wild birds [48]. It has the capacity to cause severe illness in humans and horses. The principal vector is the freshwater mosquito *Culex annulirostris*. The virus is considered to be endemic in northern Australia and is periodically reactivated or reintroduced into southern and eastern Australia, but the epidemiology is complex, involving the interplay of vertebrate host, vector, and environmental factors. Although infections occur in a variety of vertebrate hosts, amplification of the virus is thought to occur principally in wild birds (waders), especially the Nankeen night heron (*Nycticorax caledonicus*). Lesions and diagnostic procedures are very similar to these of the other encephalitogenic flaviviruses. Identification of histologic lesions and PCR should be performed. IHC should be performed on multiple sections with lesions since the infection seems to be characterized by small quantity of viral antigen.

EHV-1 myeloencephalopathy

A member of the Alphaherpesvirinae subfamily, EHV-1 is highly contagious and potentially fatal when causing neurologic disease in horses [49–51]. Horses can contract EHV-1 from sneeze droplets of infected animals and from aborted fetuses, but also water, fences, and contaminated equipment. Mortality rates may range from 10 to 75%. Vaccination has been so far unprotective against the neurologic form of EHV-1. A single nucleotide polymorphism in the viral DNA polymerase gene (ORF30) at a 752 (N→D) is associated with the neurovirulent potential of EHV-1, leading to enhanced viremia. There may be gross evidence of linear perivascular hemorrhage in the spinal cord. Multifocal necrotizing vasculitis with thrombosis is a key histologic feature associated to malacia and hemorrhage in the gray matter substance. Viral inclusions should not be expected. This virus is not neurotropic like many other herpesviruses. Instead EHV-1 replicates within the nucleus and cytoplasm of endothelial cells, as well as of vascular myocytes and pericytes. The diagnosis is achieved via the combination of gross lesions, microscopic lesions and PCR in the areas with lesions. IHC may be useful on serial sections. FA and VI are not very sensitive. Evaluation of the seroconversion (four folds increase expected) is also helpful, but may not be observed in all cases.

Pseudorabies

This disease has been also called Aujeszky's disease, Mad Itch, and Bulbar Paralysis [52]. Although horses do not appear to be very susceptible to Suid herpesvirus 1, Aujeszky's disease should be included in the differential diagnosis of horses with transient or fatal neurological disease in areas where the virus is endemic. In horses, lesions are florid, microscopic characterized by lymphocytic meningoencephalitis with perivascular cuffing and neuronal necrosis involving a gray and white matter. The virus colonizes neurons and nerve fibers and can be identified via in situ histochemistry (IHC), ISH, PCR, and VI.

Borna disease

This single-stranded RNA virus of undetermined classification is exotic to the United States [53–56]. It is of focal geographic distribution in Western and Eastern Europe. The virus is transmitted by ticks and principally infects sheep, cats, and rabbits. The European shrews are able to carry large amounts of the virus in numerous organs and cell types with no evidence of clinical signs and lesions. Gross lesions may include meningeal petechiae. Microscopic features include perivascular, often prominent lymphocytic cuffing, neuronal necrosis, and sometimes glial nodules. Occasional neuronal intranuclear or intra-cytoplasmic inclusion bodies known as Joest–Degen bodies are conclusive for the diagnosis of Borna disease. Ganglionitis, optic neuritis and retinal disease can also occur. The neuron-to-Müller cell ratio for the whole retina is significantly smaller in diseased animals. Spinal cord involvement seems to be infrequent. The virus infects neurons and nerve fibers, including the retina. Diagnostic tools include histopathology, IHC, and PCR.

Equine infectious anemia (swamp fever)

This equine disease, also known by horsemen as "swamp fever," is caused by a lentivirus, and transmitted by bloodsucking insects [57]. The virus is endemic in the Americas, parts of Europe, the Middle and Far East, Russia, and South Africa. EIA can be transmitted through blood, saliva, milk, and body secretions. Transmission is primarily through biting flies, such as the horse fly and deer fly. The virus survives up to 4 h in the carrier. Contaminated surgical equipment, recycled needles and syringes, and bits can transmit the disease. Mares can transmit the disease to their fetuses. The risk of transmitting the disease is greatest when an infected horse is ill, as the blood levels of the virus are then highest. Acute to subacute changes include hemolysis and icterus. Chronic lesions include emaciation, lymphade-nomegaly, splenomegaly and hepatomegaly associated with lymphoid hyperplasia and hemosiderosis, hepatic hemosiderosis and lymphocytic hepatitis, and bone marrow erythroid hypoplasia or aplasia. CNS lesions are uncommon and vary from mild lymphocytic to severe histiocytic encephalitis with malacia and giant cells. The infection is pauciviral with viral localization within lymphocytes, macrophages and endothelial cells, demonstrated via ISH. The diagnosis is based on serology, PCR and identification of the lesions.

Hendra disease

Henipavirus is a genus of the family Paramyxoviridae, order Mononegavirales containing three established species: Hendra virus, Nipah virus and Cedar Virus [58]. The henipaviruses are naturally harbored by pteropid fruit bats (flying foxes) and some microbat species. Henipavirus has a wide host range, and emerged as zoonotic pathogens capable of causing illness and death in domestic animals and humans. The virus colonizes endothelia and vascular myocytes causing a widespread fibrinoid necrosis of small blood vessels in many organs, including lungs, heart, kidneys, spleen, lymph nodes, meninges, alimentary tract, skeletal muscle, and bladder. When respiratory disease is predominant, the principal macroscopic lesions are severe edema and congestion of the lungs and marked dilatation of the subpleural lymphatics. The airways are filled with thick froth, which is often blood-tinged. Additional lesions seen in some affected horses include increased pleural and pericardial fluids, congestion of lymph nodes, hemorrhages in various organs, and slight jaundice. Microscopically, the primary lesions are those of an acute interstitial pneumonia. Severe vascular damage, with serofibrinous alveolar edema, hemorrhage, thrombosis of capillaries, necrosis of alveolar walls, and alveolar macrophages are evident in the lungs. Endothelial syncytia can be observed and are considered almost pathognomonic for this disease. If neurologic disease is predominant, lesions of meningitis or meningoencephalitis, including perivascular lymphocytic cuffing, neuronal necrosis, and focal gliosis, have been observed. Intracytoplasmic viral inclusion bodies can be seen in infected endothelial cells by electron microscopy, but not light microscopy. The diagnosis is achieved following the identification of the lesions and of the virus via histopathology, IHC, PCR, and VI.

Equine encephalosis

The equine encephalosis virus (EEV) is an orbivirus related to the African Horse Sickness Virus and the Blue Tongue Virus. EEV was first described in South Africa more than hundred years ago by Arnold Theiler [59]. EEV is the causative agent of equine encephalosis, an arthropod-borne disease transmitted by the *Culicoides* spp. midges affecting all equids. Serological studies estimated the presence of anti-EEV antibodies in over 75% of all South African horses. EEV has been identified also in an outbreak in Israel. The name equine encephalosis is misleading as the disease is not primarily a neurological disorder. Postmortem findings include pulmonary edema, hydropericardium, mild hepatomegaly and splenomegaly, petechia on serosal surfaces, mainly intestines, hyperemia of the glandular part of the stomach and in some cases congestion and edema of the brain. Lesions are attributable to severe endothelial damage. There is no encephalitis. EEV can be identified via PCR.

Protozoal diseases

Equine protozoal myeloencephalitis

This important neurologic disease of horses is caused by the apicomplexan protozoa *Sarcocystis neurona*, although occasional cases caused by *Neospora hughesi* have been seen [60–62]. The horse is a dead-end host for *S. neurona*; the opossum is considered the definitive host, and a variety of species including raccoons, skunks and armadillos serve as intermediate hosts. Lesions may be symmetric or focally asymmetric, may be limited to a single or few spinal cord segments, hence the former descriptive term "segmental myelitis." Encephalitic lesions are most common in the medulla and pons. Microscopic changes consist of mixed inflammatory infiltrates composed of lymphocytes, plasma cells, eosinophils, macrophages, and multinucleate giant cells in the neuropil and around blood vessels. Neutrophils are sometimes present in areas of severe necrosis. The presence of eosinophils is suggestive of this condition. Differential etiologic diagnosis should include the neurotropic form of equine infectious anemia retrovirus, which may induce a nonsuppurative histiocytic encephalomyelitis. In untreated cases, intralesional protozoa can be demonstrated in neurons or in the neuropil especially via IHC. Treated cases, which are very common, often do not contain protozoa, and the inflammation can be reduced to mild perivascular lymphocytic infiltration. In these cases the final diagnosis is obtained by ruling out the other infectious diseases of the equine CNS. Testing for EPM is described in detail in Chapter 22.

Equine trypanosomiasis

Trypanosoma evansi is a flagellate protozoan parasite that causes disease in several mammalian species [63]. The hind limb weakness of equine trypanosomiasis gave rise to the disease name *mal das cadeiras* in Brazil or *mal de caderas* in the Spanish-speaking countries of South America. Both terms translate as "sickness of the hips." The disease is called *murrina* in Panama and *surra* in many Asian countries. In the past, *T. evansi* was designated as *T. equinum*, *T. hippicum*, and *T. venezuelense*. In South America, capybaras (*Hydrochoerus hydrochaeris*), coatis (*Nasua nasua*), small marsupials (e.g., *Monodelphis* spp.), and armadillos (*Dasypus* spp.) may serve as reservoirs for *T. evansi*. Unlike the African *Trypanosoma* species that cause "nagana" in animals and "sleeping sickness" in human beings, *T. evansi* does not require the biologic cycle in *Glossina* spp. flies, and it is mechanically transmitted by biting insects, especially tabanids and stomoxids, by vampire bats (*Desmodus rotundus*) and, possibly, by ticks. In Brazil, *T. evansi* is enzootic in horses from the midwestern part of the country, specifically in the Pantanal region, where the disease has great economic importance because of the large equine population. Neurologic disease has been described occasionally in the terminal phase of the natural infection by *T. evansi* in horses, cattle, deer, and buffaloes but has not been well documented in horses. Macroscopic lesions include asymmetric leukoencephalomalacia with yellowish discoloration of white matter and flattening of the gyri.

Histologically, there is necrotizing encephalitis that is most severe in the white matter, with edema, demyelination, and lymphoplasmacytic perivascular cuffs. Mild to moderate lesions can be also observed in the spinal cord. *T. evansi* can be detected immunohistochemically in the perivascular spaces and neuropil.

Amebic meningoencephalitis

Amebic encephalitis in humans and animals is caused by several species of free-living amoebas belonging to the genera *Acanthamoeba*, *Naegleria*, and *Balamuthia* [64]. In humans free-living amebas cause three type of diseases: primary amebic meningoencephalitis (PAM) caused by *Naegleria fowleri*, granulomatous amebic encephalitis (GAE) caused by *Acanthamoeba* spp. and *Balamuthia mandrillaris*, and chronic amebic keratitis (AK) caused by *Acanthamoeba* spp. Both PAM and chronic AK occur in healthy individuals while GAE is often associated with patients having acquired immunodeficiency. Humans and animals acquire the infection via the ethmoidal lamina cribrosa when they inhale stagnant water containing the organisms. Gross lesions appear as yellowish areas that tend to be slightly friable.

Horses are affected by necrotizing and pyogranulomatous meningoencephalitis with lymphoplasmacytic cuffs and neutrophils. The organisms can be identified in histologic section with conventional stain, but histochemistry (Gridley's and periodic acid Schiff (PAS) stains) and IHC are more rewarding techniques. PCR allows precise species identification.

Bacterial diseases

Bacteria to be considered for meningoencephalitis or cerebral abscesses are *Streptococcus equi* subsp. *equi* and *S. zooepidemicus*, *Klebsiella pneumoniae*, and *Rhodococcus equi*, *Salmonella* spp., *Pseudomonas* spp., and *Escherichia coli*. *Listeria monocytogenes* infections are rare and *Borrelia burgdorferi* infections are very rare. *Clostridium tetani* and *Clostridium botulinum* cause clinical neurologic disease, but they do not induce pathologic changes. Bacterial suppurative meningoencephalitis is sporadic in foals and rare in adults.

Mycotic encephalitis

Aspergillus spp. causes random angiotropic and necrohemorrhagic embolic pneumonia with thrombosis and hyphae predisposed by *Salmonella enterica* necrotizing colitis [65]. In some of these cases encephalic fungal colonization can be observed. The infection is diagnosed by observing the pathognomonic histologic lesions characterized by hemorrhagic necrosis with angiotropic intralesional fungal hyphae causing thrombosis. IHC and PCR can be used to identify this fungus. Histochemistry (PAS and Gomori-methanamine silver (GMS) stains) will also help to detect the organisms in the tissues. *Cryptococcus*

neoformans is saprophytic yeast able to infect animals. It is found chiefly in pigeon feces, and is most frequently acquired through airborne transmission by inhalation, which may lead to opportunistic infection in animals and humans. It causes a systemic fungal disease affecting various organs, mainly of the respiratory system and CNS. Gross lesions in horses are characterized by foamy exudate involving the meninges and small cavitations in cross section. Histologically pyogranulomatous meningoencephalitis is observed. The infection is diagnosed based on the suggestive gross lesions and the pathognomonic histologic lesions. IHC and PCR can be used to identify this yeast. Histochemistry (e.g., Mayer's mucicarmine stain) will also help to detect the organisms in the tissues. *Blastomyces dermatitides*, *Coccidioides immitis*, *Histoplasma capsulatum* and *Paracoccidioides* spp may also cause systemic granulomatous disease, ophthalmitis and meningoencephalitis.

Algal encephalitis

Prototheca spp., is an achlorophyllous alga able to cause random pyogranulomatous systemic infection and meningoencephalitis with perivascular lymphoplasmacytic cuffs and intralesional algal organisms often characterized by radial appearance [66]. It is mainly a disease of cattle, dogs, cats, and rodents. This algal infection is very rare in the horse, but should be considered in the differential diagnosis of meningoencephalitis. Histochemistry (e.g., Mayer's mucicarmine stain, GMS, and PAS) is very helpful to detect the organisms in the tissues. IHC and PCR can be used to identify this alga.

Cerebral nematodiasis (verminous encephalitis)

Strongylus vulgaris is the most pathogenic of the large strongyles because of the prolonged (at least 4 months) and extensive migrations through the mesenteric arterial system and its branches before returning to mature in the cecum and colon [67]. Larval migrations cause damage to the arterial endothelium predisposing to thrombosis and the formation of fibrinoparasitic emboli able to cause infarcts. Chronic mesenteric endarteritis with aneurysm is a common complication. Occasionally the parasite causes the formation of granulomas at the base of the aorta. When a granuloma ruptures, the necrotic debris may produce obstruction of the carotid artery with cerebral infarction. Erratic cerebral migration is also observed. The widespread use of effective anthelmintic drugs has greatly reduced *Strongylus* infestation and its complications. The diagnosis is based on the identification of the suggestive gross and histologic lesions and the identification of the morphology of the parasite, which is generally present as larva.

Parelaphostrongylus tenuis is a white-tailed deer metastrongylid nematode that colonizes the meninges. Adult worms lay eggs in the meningeal tissues which then reach the lungs via the circulation, where they hatch. The larvae are then coughed up, swallowed, and proceed through the gastrointestinal tract. Snails and slugs serve as intermediate hosts, which are later ingested by ungulates allowing the cycle to continue. Other wild ungulates such as moose, elk, mule deer and caribou are also susceptible. This parasite can cause significant lesion in paratenic hosts such as small ruminants, camelids and horses. Migration tracts with malacia and eosinophilic meningoencephalomyelitis are the histologic lesions. Ocular colonization is also described. The diagnosis is based on the identification of the suggestive histologic lesions, the identification of the parasite in cross section and confirmation via PCR [68–70].

Halicephalobus gingivalis is a free-living rhabditid nematode of the order. Females are able to penetrate the skin of horses and humans and during their migration produce severe and fatal lesions including pyogranulomatous and eosinophilic nephritis, meningoencephalitis, and ophthalmitis. Stomatitis, dermatitis and mastitis are also observed, and direct transmission to foal via the infested mammary gland has been described. Gross lesions, especially if severe, are suggestive and the final diagnosis is based on the identification of the histologic lesions and parasites in cross section. Centrifugation of the formalin used to store the tissues to recover and identify the nematodes has been successful [71, 72].

Angiostrongylus cantonensis is a nematode that commonly resides in the pulmonary arteries of rats. Snails are the primary intermediate hosts, in which larvae develop until they are infective. The ingested larvae are able to colonize the CNS causing multifocal lymphoplasmacytic and eosinophilic meningoencephalomyelitis in several mammals including humans and horses. The diagnosis is based on the identification of the suggestive gross and histologic lesions and the identification of the morphology of the larvae [73].

Cerebral myiasis

Larvae of the dipteran flies *Hypoderma lineatum* and *H. diana* are able to colonize CNS of horses causing severe focal necrosis and hemorrhage [74]. Sporadic reports mention lesions within midbrain and pons. More frequently only the skin is affected.

Neoplasia

Primary CNS tumors are extremely rare in horses. Occasional ependymomas, choroid plexus tumors, and meningiomas have been described [75, 76]. Metastasizing tumors include malignant melanomas and hemangiosarcomas. Tumors within the epidural space of the spinal cord may be peripheral nerve sheath tumors (benign and malignant schwannomas, and very rare neurofibromas and neurofibrosarcoma), lymphomas, hemangiomas,

hemangiosarcomas, or plasma cell tumors, with a compressing effect on the overriding spinal cord. Hemangiosarcomas and melanomas often extend from the vertebral bodies, and tumors of other types can involve the CNS by direct expansion. Lymphoma often induces meningeal infiltration sometimes followed by intraparenchymal and intraneural infiltration. Lymphoma of the leptomeninges resembling lymphocytic meningoencephalitis can be sporadically observed. If primary, the identification of the neoplasm can be difficult. The very frequent pituitary adenomas of the pars intermedia may cause compressive atrophy of the hypothalamus and optic chiasma (Figure 16.4).

We observed a lymphoma arising from the pituitary gland and progressively invading the cerebrum. The diagnosis of these neoplasms is always histological and sometimes via IHC.

Cutaneous schwannomas are solitary cutaneous masses generally identified in the skin of the head, neck, shoulder, hip, thorax, abdomen, rump, extremities, or tail. When dermal, they tend to be well demarcated and expansive. They may be nodular or multinodular. Antoni A areas are observed in all tumors; some contain

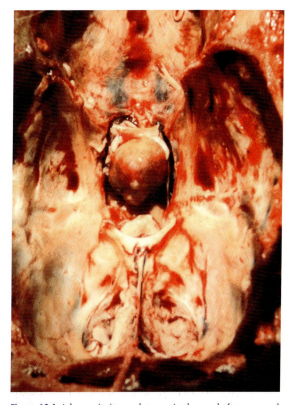

Figure 16.4 A large pituitary adenoma is observed after removal of the brain.

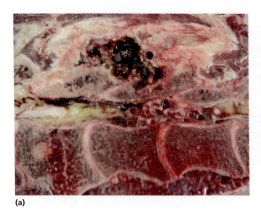 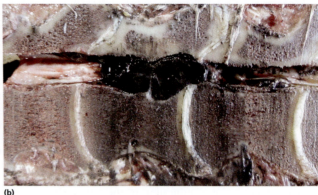

(a)   (b)

Figure 16.5 (a, b) Sagittal sectioning of the spine reveals invasive melanoma also forming large masses within the spinal canal.

also Antoni B areas. In Antoni A areas, the densely packed spindle-shaped neoplastic cells are arranged in short fascicles with nuclear palisading. In the hypocellular Antoni B areas, neoplastic cells are separated by abundant myxomatous stroma. Tumors commonly have hyalinization of the stroma and vessel walls and ancient change. Cellular vacuolation is frequently observed. Schwannomas express S100 protein, laminin and GFAP. Ultrastructurally neoplastic cells have branched cytoplasmic processes and are surrounded by an external lamina. Surgical excision of the tumor is generally curative. The histologic differentiation from the equine sarcoid is important (Figure 16.5a and b).

Trauma, ischemia, edema, hemorrhage

Trauma
Traumatic injuries and their consequences to the brain and spinal cord depend on three factors: severity, speed, and duration. Trauma to the skull may result in fractures of basilar bones resulting in hemorrhage and laceration of the adjacent brain tissue. Penetrating foreign bodies can cause severe encephalic inflammatory septic lesions. Trauma to the spinal column can lead to vertebral fractures, spinal cord contusion, or laceration. Compound fractures of a vertebral body often occur between T5 and T12 but can occur also in other locations. They may result in compression of the overriding spinal cord. Lightning should be considered as cause of unexpected fractures of well-protected vertebrae in otherwise healthy horses. Also malicious electrocution needs to be considered as a cause.

Hypoxic ischemic neonatal encephalopathy (neonatal maladjustment syndrome)
The primary causes of this condition are systemic hypoxemia and/or reduced cerebral blood flow [77, 78]. Lesions include cerebrocortical necrosis with hemorrhage and sometimes edema. Necrosis in the diencephalon and brain stem is sometimes observed. Some foals also present brain edema. Histologically there is laminar cortical necrosis with ischemic shrunken red neurons, white matter vacuolization with axonal and myelin loss and Gitter cells accumulation, astrocytic hypertrophy with gemistocyte formation, and endothelial hypertrophy. The diagnosis is based on the identification of the cortical necrosis in affected neonates (Figure 16.6).

Fibrocartilaginous embolic myelopathy
This is a sporadic condition predisposed by disk nucleus pulposus degeneration and trauma [79]. The embolic disk fragments cause infarctive and ischemic malacia; lesions are characterized by segmental malacia. Some of these areas are wedge-shaped ventral spinal infarction, sometimes with the apex directed towards the ventral horns. The nerve fibers in the white tracts are dilated and contain spheroids, and there are neutrophils, gliosis, and hemorrhage. Blood vessels near the areas of infarction contain fibrocartilaginous material and fibrin. The diagnosis is based on the observation of the gross and histologic lesions. Alcian blue stain helps the visualization of the emboli.

Hepatic encephalopathy, intestinal encephalopathy and renal encephalopathy
Hepatic encephalopathy is characterized by suggestive neurologic clinical signs and subtle but reliable histologic lesions secondary to severe hepatopathy such as hepatic necrosis and, very rarely in horses, vascular portosystemic shunt [80–83]. The same clinical signs and brain lesions can be observed in some cases characterized by bacterial enterocolitis, where there may be excessive production of ammonia in the intestine with or without liver disease. Renal encephalopathy has been also described in large animals and occasionally observed

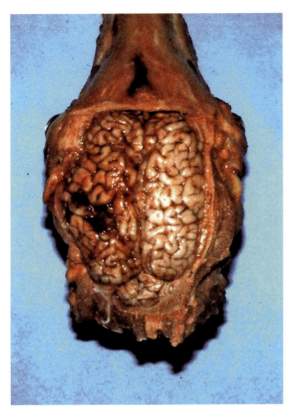

Figure 16.6 Cerebral infarct in a foal with neonatal encephalopathy, left cerebral hemisphere.

in horses. The pathogenesis is still uncertain and seems to gravitate around hyperammonemia. Astrocytes use ammonia when synthesizing glutamine from glutamate. The increased levels of glutamine seem to lead to an increase in osmotic pressure in the astrocytes, resulting in intracellular cytotoxic edema. There may be increased activity of the inhibitory GABA system, and the energy supply to other brain cells seems to be decreased. Other catabolites implicated in hepatic encephalopathy may include mercaptans short-chain fatty acids and phenol. Other abnormalities that have been investigated include the detection of benzodiazepine-like compounds, abnormalities in the GABA neurotransmission system, an imbalance between aromatic amino acids (phenylalanine, tryptophan and tyrosine) and branched-chain amino acids (leucine, isoleucine and valine). The latter can lead to generation of false neurotransmitters, such as octopamine and 2-hydroxyphenethylamine. Dysregulation of the serotonin system has been also reported. Depletion of zinc and accumulation of manganese may play a role. Inflammation of other organs may precipitate encephalopathy through the action of cytokines and bacterial lipopolysaccharide on

astrocytes. There are no gross lesions in the CNS. Histologically there is brain edema with pallor, increase of Virchow–Robin spaces, astrocyte hypertrophy and hyperplasia, and Alzheimer type 2 cells forming couples, triplets and even quadruplets. These lesions are mainly visible in the neocortex and are always observed in Theiler's disease characterized by massive hepatic necrosis. The identification of the brain lesion is therefore very helpful in cases in which the liver is severely autolyzed and not useful for histologic examination.

Grove poisoning

The plant *Indigofera spicata* (creeping indigo) produces indospicine [84, 85]. Indospicine is a hepatic and nervous tissue single peptide toxin that inhibits protein synthesis as an antagonist to the amino acid arginine. When consumed by horses, the toxin induces hepatic necrosis and consequent encephalopathy with brain edema (pallor, increase of perivascular spaces) and astrocytosis. Histologic lesions combined with evidence of ingestion of the plant are necessary to diagnose this disease. *Cassia* spp. is able to cause hepatic necrosis and hepatic encephalopathy in horses as well.

Miscellaneous
Choroid plexus cholesteatoma
(cholesterol granuloma)

These granular growth commonly occurs within the lateral or fourth ventricles. They are incidental findings with no neurologic impact and only rarely are larger than 1 cm. Histologically they are comprised of foamy macrophages, cholesterol and sometimes hemosiderophages. The pathogenesis has been discussed for many years and is still unknown.

Epidural synovial cyst

This lesion often appears as a gelatinous gray folded tissue in a collar-like fashion next to the spinal nerves [86]. It is considered the result of synovial membrane detachment from degenerative facet joint disease. The proliferating tissue may compress spinal nerves.

Polyneuritis equi, polyradiculitis
and cauda equine neuritis

This disease of adult horses progressively involves the sacrocaudal nerves to produce clinical signs of hind leg paresis and urinary bladder paralysis with secondary rupture and uroperitoneum [87]. The exact cause of this disease is unknown. An immune-mediated antimyelin basic protein disorder is postulated. Recently numerous agents were investigated via IHC and PCR testing from fixed tissue with no positive results. Equine adenovirus 1 was isolated from two cases, but no viral antigen was visualized within the lesions via FA. The nerve roots are diffusely and severely thickened by granulomatous or pyogranulomatous perineuritis and ganglioneuritis, with disruption of the morphology of the fibers. The diagnosis is reached via identification of the pathognomonic gross and histologic lesions.

Cerebral vascular mineralization

Cerebral vascular mineralization can be a sporadic incidental finding during histologic examination of the horse brain [88]. It is a nonsignificant lesion. It is variable in degree and occurs mostly in the pallidal arteries. It is characterized by small globoid bodies along capillaries, and amorphous deposits in the wall of arterioles, small- or medium-sized arteries and veins. Both patterns of mineralization are strongly positive for periodic acid-Schiff reaction, and weakly positive for von Kossa's and Berlin blue stains. Elemental analysis of the deposits indicated the presence of large amounts of aluminum, moderate amounts of phosphorus, zinc, calcium and iron, and small amount of sodium.

References

[1] Robertson, J.L. (1996) Nervous System, in *Equine Pathology* (eds J.R. Rooney and J.L. Robertson), Iowa State University Press, Ames, pp. 308–343.

[2] Rooney, J.R. (1998) *The Lame Horse*, Russell Meerdink Co Ltd, Neenah.

[3] Kahn, C.M. (ed.) (2010) Nervous System, in *Merck Veterinary Manual*, 10th edn, National Publishing, Inc, Philadelphia, pp. 2153–2158.

[4] Rooney, J.R. (1996) Autopsy Method, in *Equine Pathology* (eds J.R. Rooney and J.L. Robertson), Iowa State University Press, Ames, pp. 367–377.

[5] Buergelt, C. and Del Piero, F. (2014) *Color Atlas of Equine Pathology*, Wiley Blackwell, Ames.

[6] Sipma, K.D., Cornillie, P., Saulez, M.N. *et al.* (2013) Phenotypic characteristics of hydrocephalus in stillborn Friesian foals. *Vet Pathol*, 50, 1037–1042.

[7] Crowe, M.W. and Swerczek, T.W. (1985) Equine congenital defects. *Am J Vet Res*, 46, 353–358.

[8] Lempe, A., Heine, M., Bosch, B. *et al.* (2012) Imaging diagnosis and clinical presentation of a Chiari malformation in a Thoroughbred foal. *Equine Vet Educ*, 24, 618–623.

[9] Rivas, L.J., Hinchcliff, K.W. and Robertson, J.T. (1996) Cervical meningomyelocele associated with spina bifida in a hydrocephalic miniature colt. *J Am Vet Med Assoc*, 209, 950–953.

[10] Gerhauser, I., Geburek, F. and Wohlsein, P. (2012) Perosomus elumbis, cerebral aplasia, and spina bifida in an aborted thoroughbred foal. *Res Vet Sci*, 92, 266–268.

[11] van Schutte, J.G. and den Ingh, T.S. (1997) Microphthalmia, brachygnathia superior, and palatocheiloschisis in a foal associated with griseofulvin administration to the mare during early pregnancy. *Vet Q*, 19, 58–60.

[12] Munroe, G.A. and Barnett, K.C. (1984) Congenital ocular disease in the foal. *Vet Clin North Am Large Anim Pract*, 6, 519–537.

[13] Miller, L.M., Reed, S.M., Gallina, A.M. and Palmer, G.H. (1985) Ataxia and weakness associated with fourth ventricle vascular anomalies in two horses. *J Am Vet Med Assoc*, 186, 601–603.

[14] Allison, N. and Moeller, R.B., Jr (2000) Spinal ataxia in a horse caused by an arachnoid diverticulum (cyst). *J Vet Diagn Invest*, 12, 279–281.

[15] Wilkins, P.A., Vaala, W.E., Zivotofsky, D. and Twitchell, E.D. (1994) A herd outbreak of equine leukoencephalomalacia. *Cornell Vet*, 84, 53–59.

[16] Marasas, W.F. (2001) Discovery and occurrence of the fumonisins: a historical perspective. *Environ Health Perspect*, 109 (Suppl 2), 239–243.

[17] Cordy, D.R. (1954) Nigropallidal encephalomalacia in horses associated with ingestion of yellow star thistle. *J Neuropathol Exp Neurol*, 13, 330–342.

[18] Chang, H.T., Rumbeiha, W.K., Patterson, J.S. *et al.* (2012) Toxic equine parkinsonism: an immunohistochemical study of 10 horses with nigropallidal encephalomalacia. *Vet Pathol*, 49, 398–402.

[19] de Lahunta, A. (1990) Abiotrophy in domestic animals: a review. *Can J Vet Res*, 54, 65–76.

[20] Cummings, J.F., de Lahunta, A., George, C. *et al.* (1990) Equine motor neuron disease; a preliminary report. *Cornell Vet*, 80, 357–379.

[21] Valentine, B.A., de Lahunta, A., George, C. *et al.* (1994) Acquired equine motor neuron disease. *Vet Pathol*, 31, 130–138.

[22] Mayhew, I.G., de Lahunta, A., Whitlock, R.W. and Geary, J.C. (1977) Equine degenerative myeloencephalopathy. *J Am Vet Med Assoc*, 170, 195–201.

[23] Mayhew, I.G., deLahunta, A., Whitlock, R.H. *et al.* (1978) Spinal cord disease in the horse. *Cornell Vet*, 68 (Suppl 6), 1–207.

[24] Gundlach, A.L., Kortz, G., Burazin, T.C. *et al.* (1993) Deficit of inhibitory glycine receptors in spinal cord from Peruvian Pasos: evidence for an equine form of inherited myoclonus. *Brain Res*, 628, 263–270.

[25] Hahn CN. Grass sickness, equine motor neuron disease and related disorders. Proceedings of the First International Workshop, October 26–27, 1995, Bern, Switzerland. Newmarket, Suffolk: Equine Veterinary Journal, Ltd;1997.

[26] Hahn, C.N., Mayhew, I.G. and de Lahunta, A. (2001) Central neuropathology of equine grass sickness. *Acta Neuropathol*, 102, 153–159.

[27] Hudson, N., Mayhew, I. and Pearson, G. (2001) A reduction in intestinal cells of Cajal in horses with equine dysautonomia (grass sickness). *Auton Neurosci*, 92, 37–44.

[28] Shotton, H.R., Lincoln, J. and McGorum, B.C. (2011) Effects of equine grass sickness on sympathetic neurons in prevertebral and paravertebral ganglia. *J Comp Pathol*, 145, 35–44.

[29] Vonderfecht, S.L., Bowling, A.T. and Cohen, M. (1983) Congenital intestinal aganglionosis in white foals. *Vet Pathol*, 20, 65–70.

[30] McCabe, L., Griffin, L.D., Kinzer, A. *et al.* (1990) Overo lethal white foal syndrome: equine model of aganglionic megacolon (Hirschsprung disease). *Am J Med Genet*, 36, 336–340.

[31] Duncan, I.D., Amundson, J., Cuddon, P.A. *et al.* (1991) Preferential denervation of the adductor muscles of the equine larynx. I: muscle pathology. *Equine Vet J*, 23, 94–98.

[32] Duncan, I.D., Reifenrath, P., Jackson, K.F. and Clayton, M. (1991) Preferential denervation of the adductor muscles of the equine larynx. II: nerve pathology. *Equine Vet J*, 23, 99–103.

[33] Locombe, R.F., Huntington, P.J., Friend, S.C. *et al.* (1992) Pathological aspects of Australian stringhalt. *Equine Vet J*, 24, 174–183.

[34] Cahill, J.I., Goulden, B.E. and Jolly, R.D. (1986) Stringhalt in horses: a distal axonopathy. *Neuropathol Appl Neurobiol*, 12, 459–475.

[35] Rooney, J.R. (1969) Disorders of the Nervous System, in *Biomechanics of Lameness in Horses* (ed. J.R. Rooney), Williams & Wilkins, Baltimore, pp. 219–233.

[36] Mayhew, I.G. (2009) *Large Animal Neurology*, 2nd edn, Wiley–Blackwell, Oxford.

[37] Del Piero, F., Wilkins, P.A., DeLahunta, A., et al. Rabies in horses in New York State: clinical, pathological, immunohistochemical and virological findings. Proceedings of the Eighth International Conference on Equine Infectious Diseases. Equine Veterinary Journal, 2010;42(Suppl. 38):291–296.

[38] Del Piero, F., Wilkins, P.A., Dubovi, E.J. *et al.* (2001) Clinical, pathologic, immunohistochemical, and virologic findings of eastern equine encephalomyelitis in two horses. *Vet Pathol*, 38, 451–456.

[39] Nolen-Walston, R., Bedenice, D., Rodriguez, C. *et al.* (2007) Eastern equine encephalitis in 9 South American camelids. *J Vet Intern Med*, 21, 846–852.

[40] Zacks, M.A. and Paessler, S. (2010) Encephalitic alphaviruses. *Vet Microbiol*, 140, 281–286.

[41] Cantile, C., Del Piero, F., Di Guardo, G. and Arispici, M. (2001) Pathologic and immunohistochemical findings in naturally occurring West Nile virus infection in horses. *Vet Pathol*, 38, 414–421.

[42] Wilkins, P.A. and Del Piero, F. (2004) West Nile virus: lessons from the 21st century. *J Vet Emerg Crit Care*, 14, 2–14.

[43] Miyake, M. (1964) The pathology of Japanese encephalitis. *Bull World Health Organ*, 30, 153–160.

[44] Timoney, P.J., Donnelly, W.J., Clements, L.O. and Fenlon, M. (1976) Encephalitis caused by louping ill virus in a group of horses in Ireland. *Equine Vet J*, 8, 113–117.

[45] Rushton, J.O., Lecollinet, S., Hubálek, Z. *et al.* (2013) Tick-borne encephalitis virus in horses, Austria, 2011. *Emerg Infect Dis*, 19, 635–646.

[46] Bagó, Z., Bauder, B., Kolodziejek, J. *et al.* (2002) Tickborne encephalitis in a mouflon (*Ovis ammon musimon*). *Vet Rec*, 150, 218–220.

[47] Prow, N.A. (2013) The changing epidemiology of kunjin virus in Australia. *Int J Environ Res Public Health*, 25, 6255–6272.

[48] Holmes, J.M., Gilkerson, J.R., El Hage, C.M. *et al.* (2012) Murray valley encephalomyelitis in a horse. *Aust Vet J*, 90, 252–254.

[49] Jackson, T.A., Osburn, B.I., Cordy, D.R. *et al.* (1977) Equine herpesvirus 1 infection of horses: studies on the experimentally induced neurologic disease. *Am J Vet Res*, 38, 709–719.

[50] Wilkins, P.A., Del Piero, F., deLahunta, A., et al. Paralytic equine herpes virus type 1: a retrospective study of 34 cases from 1978–1997. Proceedings of the International Equine Neurology Conference. Ithaca, NY. Cornell:Cornell University, College of Veterinary Medicine;1997.

[51] Del Piero, F., Wilkins, P.A., Timoney, P.J. *et al.* (2000) Fatal non-neurological EHV-1 infection in a yearling filly. *Vet Pathol*, 37, 672–676.

[52] Kimman, T.G., Binkhorst, G.J., van den Ingh, T.S. *et al.* (1991) Aujeszky's disease in horses fulfills Koch's postulates. *Vet Rec*, 128, 103–106.

[53] Gosztony, G. and Ludwig, H. (1984) Borna disease of horses: an immunohistological and virological study of naturally infected animals. *Acta Neuropathol*, 64, 213–221.

[54] Dürrwald, R. and Ludwig, H. (1997) Borna disease virus (BDV), a (zoonotic?) worldwide pathogen. A review of the history of the disease and the virus infection with comprehensive bibliography. *J Vet Med Ser B*, 44, 147–184.

[55] Dietzel, J., Kuhrt, H., Stahl, T. *et al.* (2007) Morphometric analysis of the retina from horses infected with the Borna disease virus. *Vet Pathol*, 44, 57–63.

[56] Puorger, M.E., Hilbe, M., Müller, J.P. *et al.* (2010) Distribution of Borna disease virus antigen and RNA in tissues of naturally infected bicolored white-toothed shrews, *Crocidura leucodon*, supporting their role as reservoir host species. *Vet Pathol*, 47, 236–244.

[57] Oaks, J.L., Long, M.T. and Baszler, T.V. (2004) Leukoencephalitis associated with selective viral replication in the brain of a pony with experimental chronic equine infectious anemia virus infection. *Vet Pathol*, 41, 527–532.

[58] Hooper, P.T., Ketterer, P.J., Hyatt, A.D. *et al.* (1997) Lesions of experimental equine morbillivirus pneumonia in horses. *Vet Pathol*, 34, 312–322.

[59] Aharonson-Raz, K., Steinman, A., Bumbarov, V. *et al.* (2011) Isolation and phylogenetic grouping of equine encephalosis virus in Israel. *Emerg Infect Dis*, 17, 1883–1886.

[60] Rooney, J.R., Prickett, M.E., Delaney, F.M. *et al.* (1970) Focal myelitis-encephalitis in horses. *Cornell Vet*, 60, 494–501.

[61] Mayhew, I.G., Dellers, R.W., Timoney, J.F. *et al.* (1978) Spinal cord disease in the horse. VII. Microbiology and serology. *Cornell Vet*, 68 (Suppl 6), 148–160.

[62] Mayhew, I.G. and de Lahunta, A. (1978) Spinal cord disease in the horse. VI. Neuropathology. *Cornell Vet*, 68 (Suppl 6), 106–147.

[63] Rodrigues, A., Fighera, R.A., Souza, T.M. *et al.* (2009) Neuropathology of naturally occurring *Trypanosoma evansi* infection of horses. *Vet Pathol*, 46, 251–258.

[64] Kinde, H., Read, D.H., Daft, B.M. *et al.* (2007) Infections caused by pathogenic free-living amebas (*Balamuthia mandrillaris* and *Acanthamoeba* sp.) in horses. *J Vet Diagn Invest*, 19, 317–322.

[65] Barclay, W.P. and deLahunta, A. (1979) Cryptococcal meningitis in a horse. *J Am Vet Med Assoc*, 174, 1236–1238.

[66] Taniyama, H., Okamoto, F., Kurosawa, T. *et al.* (1994) Disseminated protothecosis caused by *Prototheca zopfii* in a cow. *Vet Pathol*, 31, 123.

[67] Little, P.B., Lwin, U.S. and Fretz, P. (1974) Verminous encephalitis of horses: experimental induction with *Strongylus vulgaris* larvae. *Am J Vet Res*, 35, 1501–1510.

[68] Reinstein, S.L., Lucio-Forster, A., Bowman, D.D. *et al.* (2010) Surgical extraction of an intraocular infection of *Parelaphostrongylus tenuis* in a horse. *J Am Vet Med Assoc*, 237, 196–169.

[69] Tanabe, M., Gerhold, R.W., Beckstead, R.B. *et al.* (2010) Molecular confirmation of *Parelaphostrongylus tenuis* infection in a horse with verminous encephalitis. *Vet Pathol*, 47, 759.

[70] Tanabe, M., Kelly, R., de Lahunta, A. *et al.* (2007) Verminous encephalitis in a horse produced by nematodes in the family protostrongylidae. *Vet Pathol*, 44, 119–122.

[71] Wilkins, P.A., Wacholder, S., Nolan, T.J. *et al.* (2001) Evidence for transmission of *Halicephalobus deletrix* (*H. gingivalis*) from dam to foal. *J Vet Intern Med*, 15, 412–417.

[72] Cantile, C., Rossi, G., Braca, G. *et al.* (1997) A horse with *Helicephalobus deletrix* encephalitis in Italy. *Eur J Vet Pathol*, 3, 29–33.

[73] Wright, J.D., Kelly, W.R., Waddell, A.H. *et al.* (1991) Equine neural angiostrongylosis. *Aust Vet J*, 68, 58–60.

[74] Hadlow, W.J., Ward, J.K. and Krinsky, W.L. (1977) Intracranial myiasis by Hypoderma bovis (Linnaeus) in a horse. *Cornell Vet*, 67, 272–281.

[75] Schöniger, S., Valentine, B.A., Fernandez, C.J. *et al.* (2011) Cutaneous schwannomas in 22 horses. *Vet Pathol*, 48, 433–442.

[76] Bogaert, L., Heerden, M.V., Ceck, H.E. *et al.* (2011) Molecular and immunohistochemical distinction of equine sarcoid from schwannoma. *Vet Pathol*, 48, 737–741.

[77] Palmer, A.C. and Rossdale, P.D. (1975) Neuropathology of the convulsive foal syndrome. *J Reprod Fertil Suppl*, 1, 691–694.

[78] Palmer, A.C. and Rossdale, P.D. (1976) Neuropathological changes associated with the neonatal maladjustment syndrome in the thoroughbred foal. *Res Vet Sci*, 20, 267–275.

[79] Sebastian, M.M. and Giles, R.C. (2004) Fibrocartilaginous embolic myelopathy in a horse. *J Vet Med A Physiol Pathol Clin Med*, 51, 341–343.

[80] Panciera, R.J. (1969) Serum hepatitis in the horse. *J Am Vet Med Assoc*, 155, 408–410.

[81] Vicente, F. (2013) Hepatic encephalopathy: effects of liver failure on brain function. *Nat Rev Neurosci*, 14, 851–858.

[82] Peek, S.F., Divers, T.J. and Jackson, C.J. (1997) Hyperammonaemia associated with encephalopathy and abdominal pain without evidence of liver disease in four mature horses. *Equine Vet J*, 29, 70–74.

[83] Chandriani, S., Skewes-Cox, P., Zhong, W. *et al.* (2013) Identification of a previously undescribed divergent virus from the Flaviviridae family in an outbreak of equine serum hepatitis. *Proc Natl Acad Sci U S A*, 110, 15.

[84] Ossedryver, S.M., Baldwin, G.I., Stone, B.M. *et al.* (2013) *Indigofera spicata* (creeping indigo) poisoning of three ponies. *Aust Vet J*, 91, 143–149.

[85] Oliveira-Filho, J.P., Cagnini, D.Q., Badial, P.R. *et al.* (2013) Hepatoencephalopathy syndrome due to *Cassia occidentalis* (Leguminosae, Caesalpinioideae) seed ingestion in horses. *Equine Vet J*, 45, 240–244.

[86] Gerber, H., Fankhauser, R. and Straub, R. (1980) Spinal ataxia in the horse, caused by synovial cysts in the cervical spinal cord. *Schweiz Arch Tierheilkd*, 122, 95–106.

[87] Fankhauser, R., Gerber, H. and Cravero, G.C. (1975) Clinical aspects and pathology of neuritis caudae equina (NCE) in the horse. *Schweiz Arch Tierheilkd*, 117, 675–699.

[88] Yanai, T., Masegi, T., Ishikawa, K. *et al.* (1996) Spontaneous vascular mineralization in the brain of horses. *J Vet Med Sci*, 58, 35–40.

17 Diagnostic Imaging of the Equine Nervous System

Katherine Garrett

Rood and Riddle Equine Hospital, Lexington, USA

Radiography

Technique and equipment

Excellent quality radiographic images of the cervical spinal column can be obtained using portable x-ray generators in the field. The increasing use of portable digital radiographic equipment has further increased diagnostic yield in an ambulatory setting. For the thoracic and lumbar regions, portable x-ray generators are often not powerful enough to obtain diagnostic quality images, so the use of a more powerful stationary x-ray generator in a clinic or hospital setting may be required to image these thicker body parts in adult horses.

Regardless of the type of x-ray generator used, proper positioning is critical for diagnostic-quality radiographic images, especially if lateral–lateral images will be used for sagittal ratio calculation in the cervical spine region. Many clinic-based tube stands have mechanisms to simplify the process of aligning the x-ray generator and the x-ray detector. In the field, utilizing a person standing in front of the horse to assist in aligning the x-ray generator and x-ray detector can greatly increase efficiency. The use of an antiscatter grid can also improve image quality but requires that the x-ray detector and the x-ray generator be positioned exactly parallel to one another to avoid artifact from grid cutoff. The use of oblique or ventrodorsal views of the cervical spine can provide additional information, including assisting if a radiographic finding is on the left or right side of the horse [1]. This assists with correlating radiographic findings with clinical signs and is especially helpful in cases of traumatic injury if surgical intervention is undertaken.

Most horses require light sedation in order to remain motionless and cooperative during standing radiography, but sedation protocols should be chosen with the clinical condition of the patient and personnel safety in mind. The use of a larger (14×17 in.) x-ray detector permits capture of more vertebrae per image as compared to a smaller x-ray detector. This makes determination of exact vertebral location easier, as landmarks such as the distinctive shape of C2 or the prominent transverse processes of C6 can be located. Alternatively, external radioopaque markers (e.g., barium paste, lead markers) can be applied to the horse's neck to assist with precise anatomic location determination. In a typical adult horse, the entire cervical spine can be captured in three images using a 14×17 in. x-ray detector. Generally, the cranial image consists of the occipital condyles of the skull and C1–C2, the middle image consists of C3–C5, and the caudal image consists of C6–T1. However, there should be overlap between images, so partial images of adjacent vertebrae are included.

Myelography

Although standing myelography via a lumbosacral approach has been described, it carries additional risks to the horse and personnel and may result in an incomplete study [2]. More commonly, myelograms are performed under short-term general anesthesia utilizing the atlantooccipital approach. Myelography performed under general anesthesia requires appropriate facilities to induce and recover the horse. This is particularly important when faced with horses with neurologic abnormalities as recovery from anesthesia may be more difficult and some horses may experience a worsening of their neurologic signs following the procedure.

The horse is anesthetized routinely and placed in lateral recumbency. Iodinated radiographic contrast material (nonionic) is instilled slowly, over 5 min, in the subarachnoid space via the atlantooccipital space and allowed to flow caudally. Elevation of the head can assist with the caudal flow of the contrast material. After the contrast has distributed (typically about 5 min), radiographic images of the cervical vertebral column are obtained in the neutral, flexed, and extended head positions, as some horses may have dynamic lesions that compress the spinal cord only in certain head positions. In some situations, ventrodorsal myelographic images may be possible and useful.

Positioning of the horse for a myelographic study and obtaining true lateral–lateral radiographic images can be challenging. Depending upon the robustness of the x-ray detector, it may be placed under the horse with a minimal amount of protection. However, the use of a table with a radiolucent top for the horse to lie on with slots beneath that allow insertion of the x-ray detector safely can both protect the equipment and make positioning substantially easier.

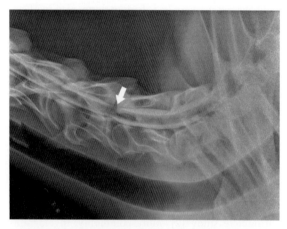

Figure 17.1 Lateral myelographic image demonstrating complete attenuation of the dorsal contrast column at C6–C7 (arrow). Cranial is to the left of the image.

Vertebral column

Standing lateral–lateral cervical spinal radiographs are an important part of the diagnostic plan to investigate horses with cervical disease, including compression and trauma. Substantial work has been done investigating measurement of various vertebral canal parameters from standing lateral–lateral radiographs and relationships between various intra- and intervertebral sagittal ratios and cervical vertebral myelopathy (CVM) [3, 4]. Although helpful, this approach has some drawbacks. These ratios only allow assessment of the vertebrae in the sagittal plane, but the spinal canal and spinal cord compression involve interactions in a three-dimensional sense. Additionally, sagittal ratios do not show spinal cord compression (as a myelogram does); they serve as an indirect measure that attempts to predict the likelihood of cord compression [5].

Myelography allows assessment of spinal cord compression by assessing attenuation of the contrast column in the subarachnoid space surrounding the spinal cord (Figure 17.1). As with sagittal ratios, there are a variety of methods used to determine if spinal cord compression is present, including use of a threshold of a 50% attenuation of the dorsal contrast column, narrowing of the dorsal contrast column to less than 2 mm, and reduction of the total dural diameter [6]. The limitation of myelography to only assess spinal cord compression in the sagittal plane is similar to that of lateral–lateral radiographs; a two-dimensional measurement is being used to assess a three-dimensional disease.

As in other body regions, radiography is excellent for assessment of fractures, other types of bony trauma, osteoarthritis, osteochondrosis, or malformations to the vertebral column (Figures 17.2 and 17.3). Depending upon the power of the available x-ray generator, the

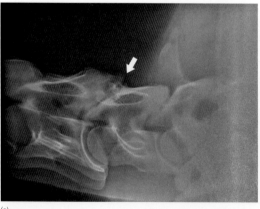

(a)

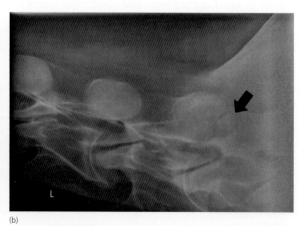

(b)

Figure 17.2 Lateral (a) and oblique (b) radiographic images of osteochondrosis dissecans (arrows) of the caudal cervical articular process of C6. Cranial is to the left of the images.

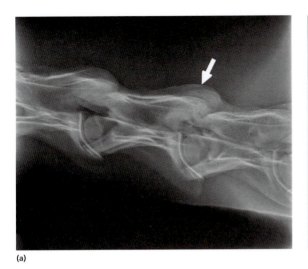

(a)

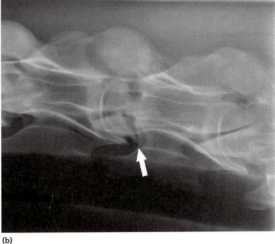

(b)

Figure 17.3 Lateral (a) and oblique (b) radiographic images of a horse with a fracture of the cranial articular process of C5 following a fall (arrows). Cranial is to the left of the images.

thoracic and lumbar regions can be evaluated in adult horses, and portable machines are generally adequate for foals or weanlings. With increasing sensitivity of digital radiography detectors, standing ventrodorsal pelvic radiographs may be obtained in many adults.

If contemplating surgical procedures involving the cervical vertebral canal, radiographic guidance can be extremely valuable during the surgical approach as well as assisting with implant placement for cervical vertebral stabilization or internal fixation of fracture in cases of trauma. Portable digital radiography can be easily incorporated into the surgical plan as radiographic images are immediately available to the surgeon.

Skull

Radiographs of the skull can be difficult to interpret, but yield valuable information in many types of neurologic disease, particularly those involving the cranial nerves or brain. The extent of fractures in cases of trauma can be appreciated (Figure 17.4). Masses involving the paranasal sinuses or guttural pouches may impinge upon peripheral nerves or invade the calvarium. Enlarged stylohyoid bones are indicative of temporohyoid osteoarthropathy and may prompt additional diagnostic testing, such as upper airway endoscopy and cross-sectional imaging.

Ultrasound

Technique and equipment

Use of ultrasonography is becoming increasingly common in the diagnosis of neurologic disease. More superficial areas, such as the cervical spine, can be imaged using a

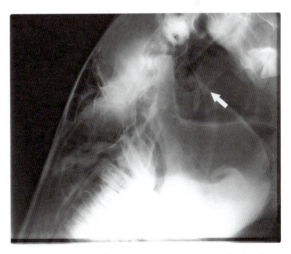

Figure 17.4 Lateral radiographic image showing a displaced basisphenoid bone fracture (arrow). Cranial is to the left of the image.

higher frequency linear or microconvex transducer at 6–10 MHz, while deeper areas such as the lumbar spine and pelvis often require a lower frequency (2–5 MHz) curvilinear transducer.

Vertebral column

The bony margins of the articular processes, joint capsule, and synovium of the cervical synovial joints can be assessed ultrasonographically, providing complementary information to radiographic findings. Subtle osteophytosis may be more apparent ultrasonographically, and joint capsule thickening and the presence of increased synovial fluid can be determined in cases of osteoarthritis. Ultrasound-guided injection of the cervical vertebral synovial articulations allows precise needle placement for therapeutic purposes [7]. Although similar resolution cannot be obtained for the thoracolumbar intervertebral synovial joints due to their depth, injection of these joints using ultrasound guidance has also been described [8, 9].

Ultrasound-guided collection of cerebrospinal fluid from the atlantooccipital and lumbosacral spaces has been previously described [10, 11]. More recently, a technique for ultrasound-guided collection of cerebrospinal fluid from between the first and second cervical vertebrae in the standing horse has been published and involves a ventrolateral approach to the space [12]. The spinal cord can be imaged at this level as well, allowing positioning of the needle to obtain fluid while avoiding the spinal cord. The authors note that the use of morphine as part of the sedation protocol helps to prevent horse movement after needle penetration of the dura.

Although uncommon in adults, in foals ultrasonography can be used to document the presence of osteomyelitis, physitis, and/or septic synovitis of the vertebral column and its articulations resulting in neurologic signs (Figure 17.5). Ultrasonographic imaging can be used to guide needle placement to obtain samples for cytology and culture or for joint lavage. If debridement or drain placement are required, ultrasonography can be very useful intraoperatively, especially if the affected structure is not located superficially.

Peripheral neuropathies

Ultrasound can also be useful in the diagnosis of peripheral neuropathies. Ultrasound can be used to document increases in echogenicity in the muscles innervated by the recurrent laryngeal nerve in cases of recurrent laryngeal neuropathy [13, 14]. Images of the cricoarytenoideus dorsalis, cricoarytenoideus lateralis, and vocalis muscles are obtained and compared to the contralateral side. The increase in echogenicity is thought to represent infiltration of the muscle with fibrous tissue and fat secondary to denervation atrophy. Similar changes have been documented in denervated muscles of both humans with naturally occurring disease as well as in experimental animal models [15, 16]. It is possible that this technique could be used to monitor denervation in other muscles.

Rectal ultrasound has been used as a diagnostic aid in horses with polyneuritis equi by detecting thickening of the nerve roots as they exit the ventral sacrum.

Magnetic resonance imaging/ computed tomography

Technique and equipment

Cross-sectional imaging represents the gold standard for diagnostic imaging in many situations. However, there are obvious challenges when considering either computed tomography (CT) or magnetic resonance imaging (MRI) for horses. General anesthesia is nearly always necessary, but there are a few CT installations that allow imaging of the head and cranial cervical spine of the standing, sedated adult horse. Proper positioning can be logistically challenging, but should be a priority to obtain high-quality images. Since CT images are obtained perpendicular to the bore of the scanner, having the head positioned as straight as possible is imperative. For MRI, the region to be scanned should be positioned as close to isocenter of the magnet as possible. In adults, imaging is generally limited to the head and cranial cervical spine, but the entire vertebral column can be evaluated in foals, depending upon the size of the bore of the scanner. Foals can be imaged on the human patient table, but specialized tables are

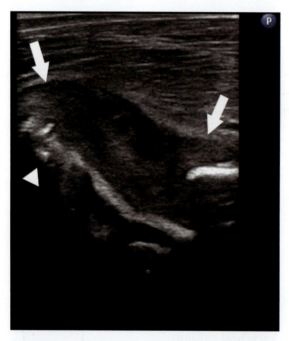

Figure 17.5 Ultrasound image of the left atlantoaxial joint demonstrating echogenic synovial effusion within the joint (arrows) and irregularity of the cranial aspect of C2 consistent with osteomyelitis (arrowhead) in a foal. *Rhodococcus equi* was cultured from the synovial fluid. Cranial is to the right of the image.

required for patients greater than 300–400 lbs. The other major drawbacks for both CT and MRI are availability, expense, and staff training.

CT images are initially acquired perpendicular to the bore of the scanner but can be reformatted into any desired plane and reconstructed into three-dimensional representations. Intravenous contrast is often used, with scans performed before and after contrast administration. As CT scanners use ionizing radiation, appropriate technique settings and attention to principles of radiation safety are important considerations. MR images are acquired in any plane using a variety of different sequences which highlight different types of pathology. For example, T1-weighted sequences have excellent anatomic detail and are commonly used before and after intravenous contrast administration to assess areas of increased or decreased blood flow. T2-weighted sequences highlight locations containing fluid, while FLAIR sequences null out signal from cerebrospinal fluid, allowing further assessment of areas of edema. A body coil can be used for MRI, but superior image quality can be obtained by using a flexible surface coil or spine coil. Since MR scanners utilize very strong magnetic fields, precautions must be taken to exclude ferromagnetic items from the vicinity, and individuals with certain types of implants or pacemakers that may be affected by the magnetic field should not be permitted in the area.

Although both MRI and CT are cross-sectional imaging techniques, they rely upon different physical principles. MRI imaging depends upon the chemical composition of tissues, while CT assesses x-ray beam attenuation of tissues. As such, they each have their strengths and weaknesses. CT has superior spatial resolution, allowing for very thin slices, excellent bony detail, and superb reconstruction capability as compared to MRI. Scan times for CT are also quite short, often less than 10–15 min, while most brain MRI studies take approximately 1 h. However, MRI has superior contrast resolution, allowing better assessment of the brain and spinal cord parenchyma than CT.

Brain

Some lesions localized to the brain have typical findings in MRI or CT examination [17–19]. Intracranial masses, including neoplasia, hematoma, granuloma, or abscess, are generally readily identified on both CT and MRI examination and may involve any structure (Figure 17.6). Similarly, the enlarged ventricles typical of hydrocephalus are apparent using both modalities (Figure 17.7), as are changes typical of temporohyoid osteoarthropathy [20]. Horses with equine protozoal myeloencephalitis may have areas of increased signal on T2W images in the brainstem on MRI (Figure 17.8)

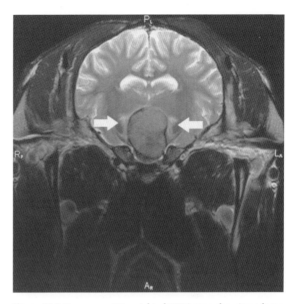

Figure 17.6 Transverse T2-weighted MR image showing a large pituitary adenoma (confirmed histopathologically at necropsy) with increased T2W signal in the surrounding brain parenchyma (arrows).

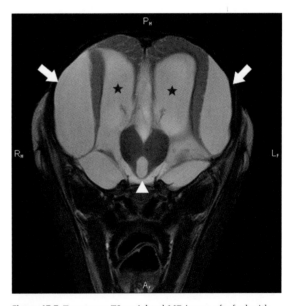

Figure 17.7 Transverse T2-weighted MR image of a foal with hydrocephalus demonstrating severe dilation of the lateral (stars) and third (arrowhead) ventricles with accumulation of cerebrospinal fluid surrounding the brain (arrows).

[21]. In the author's experience, most horses presenting with seizures have normal MRI and CT examinations. Bony lesions in cases of trauma are generally better seen

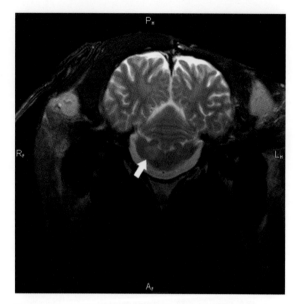

Figure 17.8 Transverse T2-weighted MR image of the brainstem showing focally increased T2W signal (arrow). Protozoal organisms consistent with *Sarcocystis neurona* were identified in this region during necropsy examination.

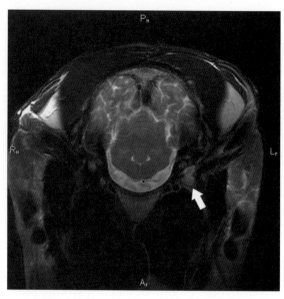

Figure 17.10 Transverse T2-weighted MR image showing increased heterogeneous signal intensity in the left tympanic bulla (arrow). Purulent material was obtained following fenestration of the tympanic membrane.

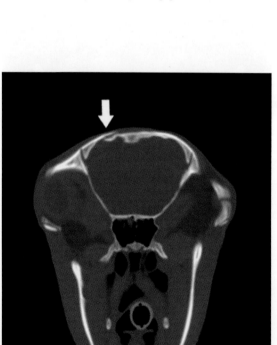

Figure 17.9 Transverse CT image showing a frontal bone fracture following head trauma (arrow).

on CT scans, while pathology affecting the brain is better assessed on MR images (Figure 17.9). The presence of otitis leading to peripheral neuropathies can be confirmed as well (Figure 17.10).

Vertebral column

Although MRI of the entire cervical spinal canal is not currently possible in clinical cases, some early work with cadaver specimens has shown that MRI is superior to radiography for the diagnosis of cervical stenotic myelopathy [22]. This is unsurprising, since three-dimensional imaging of the spinal canal allows assessment of the vertebral canal area in all directions, not simply in the dorsal–ventral direction. As one of the parameters associated with disease status in this study was cross-sectional area of the spinal canal, it is likely that this parameter could be assessed using CT as well. This is encouraging, as it is more likely that a CT scanner capable of imaging the entire equine cervical spinal cord will be a reality in the near future. However, additional work needs to be done to confirm its use in clinical cases.

Currently, clinical use of MRI or CT in adults does not allow imaging caudal to the cervical spine, but the entire spine and pelvis can be imaged in smaller foals. This is particularly useful in cases of trauma or suspected orthopedic sepsis involving the vertebral canal or pelvis where a definitive diagnosis has not been made using more traditional modalities (Figures 17.11 and 17.12).

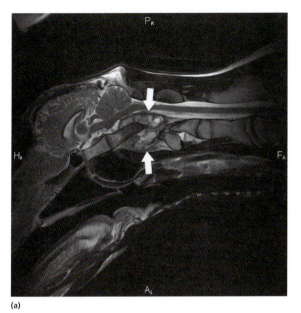

(a)

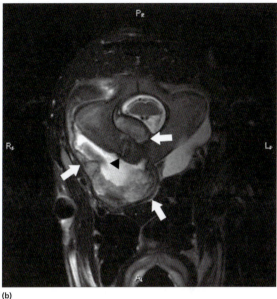

(b)

Figure 17.11 Sagittal (a) and transverse (b) T2-weighted MR images of a foal with septic synovitis and osteomyelitis at the atlantooccipital joint. Note the effusion of the joint (arrows) and abnormal signal intensity within the bone (arrowheads). *Rhodococcus equi* was cultured from the synovial fluid and osteomyelitis was confirmed at necropsy. Cranial is to the left of the sagittal image.

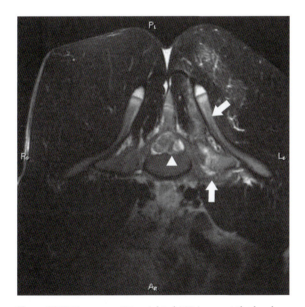

Figure 17.12 Transverse T2-weighted MR image at the level of the sacrum. There is heterogeneous increased signal in and surrounding the left sacral wing (arrows) as well as lateral to the spinal cord, resulting in compression of the spinal cord (arrowhead). Purulent material was obtained from a more superficial component of this lesion and *Salmonella* was cultured.

References

[1] Withers, J.M., Voûte, L.C., Hammond, G. and Lischer, C.J. (2009) Radiographic anatomy of the articular process joints of the caudal cervical vertebrae in the horse on lateral and oblique projections. *Equine Vet J*, 41, 895–902.

[2] Rose, P.L., Abutarbush, S.M. and Duckett, W. (2007) Standing myelography in the horse using a nonionic contrast agent. *Vet Radiol Ultrasound*, 48, 535–538.

[3] Hahn, C.N., Handel, I., Green, S.L. *et al.* (2008) Assessment of the utility of using intra- and intervertebral minimum sagittal diameter ratios in the diagnosis of cervical vertebral malformation in horses. *Vet Radiol Ultrasound*, 49, 1–6.

[4] Rush Moore, B., Reed, S., Biller, D.S. *et al.* (1994) Assessment of vertebral canal diameter and bony malformations of the cervical part of the spine in horses with cervical stenotic myelopathy. *Am J Vet Res*, 55, 5–13.

[5] Papageorges, M., Gavin, P.R., Sande, R.D. *et al.* (1990) Survey radiography and myelography of the cervical vertebral column. *Vet Radiol Ultrasound*, 28, 53–59.

[6] van Biervliet, J., Scrivani, P.V., Divers, T.J. *et al.* (2004) Evaluation of decision criteria for detection of spinal cord compression based on cervical myelography in horses: 38 cases (1981–2001). *Equine Vet J*, 36, 14–20.

[7] Mattoon, J.S., Drost, W.T., Grguric, M.R. *et al.* (2004) Technique for equine cervical articular process joint injection. *Vet Radiol Ultrasound*, 45, 238–240.

[8] Cousty, M., Firidolfi, C., Geffroy, O. and David, F. (2011) Comparison of medial and lateral ultrasound-guided approaches for periarticular injection of the thoracolumbar intervertebral facet joints in horses. *Vet Surg*, 40, 494–499.

[9] Fuglbjerg, V., Nielsen, J.V., Thomsen, P.D. and Berg, L.C. (2010) Accuracy of ultrasound-guided injections of thoracolumbar articular process joints in horses: a cadaveric study. *Equine Vet J*, 42, 18–22.

[10] Aleman, M., Borchers, A., Kass, P.H. and Puchalski, S.M. (2007) Ultrasound-assisted collection of cerebrospinal fluid from the lumbosacral space in equids. *J Am Vet Med Assoc*, 230, 378–384.

[11] Audigie, F., Tapprest, J., Didierlaurent, D. and Denoix, J.M. (2004) Ultrasound-guided atlanto-occipital puncture for myelography in the horse. *Vet Radiol Ultrasound*, 45, 340–344.

[12] Pease, A., Behan, A. and Bohart, G. (2012) Ultrasound-guided cervical centesis to obtain cerebrospinal fluid in the standing horse. *Vet Radiol Ultrasound*, 53, 92–95.

[13] Garrett, K.S., Woodie, J.B. and Embertson, R.M. (2011) Association of treadmill upper airway endoscopic evaluation with results of ultrasonography and resting upper airway endoscopic evaluation. *Equine Vet J*, 43, 365–371.

[14] Chalmers, H.J., Yeager, A.E., Cheetham, J. and Ducharme, N. (2012) Diagnostic sensitivity of subjective and quantitative laryngeal ultrasonography for recurrent laryngeal neuropathy in horses. *Vet Radiol Ultrasound*, 53, 660–666.

[15] Küllmer, K., Sievers, K.W., Reimers, C.D. *et al.* (1998) Changes of sonographic, magnetic resonance tomographic, electromyographic, and histopathologic findings within a 2-month period of examinations after experimental muscle denervation. *Arch Orthop Trauma Surg*, 117, 228–234.

[16] Bargfrede, M., Schwennicke, A., Tumani, H. and Reimers, C.D. (1999) Quantitative ultrasonography in focal neuropathies as compared to clinical and EMG findings. *Eur J Ultrasound*, 10, 21–29.

[17] Ferrell, E.A., Gavin, P.R., Tucker, R.L. *et al.* (2002) Magnetic resonance for evaluation of neurologic disease in 12 horses. *Vet Radiol Ultrasound*, 43, 510–516.

[18] Lacombe, V.A., Sogaro-Robinson, C. and Reed, S.M. (2010) Diagnostic utility of computed tomography imaging in equine intracranial conditions. *Equine Vet J*, 42, 393–399.

[19] Sogaro-Robinson, C., Lacombe, V.A., Reed, S.M. and Balkrishnan, R. (2009) Factors predictive of abnormal results for computed tomography of the head in horses affected by neurologic disorders: 57 cases (2001–2007). *J Am Vet Med Assoc*, 235, 176–183.

[20] Hilton, H., Puchalski, S.M. and Aleman, M. (2009) The computed tomographic appearance of equine temporohyoid osteoarthropathy. *Vet Radiol Ultrasound*, 50, 151–156.

[21] Stieler, A.L., Reuss, S.M., Werpy, N.M. and MacKay, R.J. (2013) What is your diagnosis. *J Am Vet Med Assoc*, 243, 779–781.

[22] Janes, J.G., Garrett, K.S., McQuerry, K.J. *et al.* (2014) Comparison of magnetic resonance imaging to standing cervical radiographs for evaluation of vertebral canal stenosis in equine cervical stenotic myelopathy. *Equine Vet J*, 46, 681–686.

Specific Disease Syndromes

SECTION 3

Specific Disease Syndromes

18 Equid Herpesvirus-Associated Myeloencephalopathy

Lutz S. Goehring

College of Veterinary Medicine, Ludwig Maximillians University, Munich, Germany

Equid herpesvirus-associated myeloencephalopathy (EHM) is an infrequent but serious outcome of common equid herpesvirus type 1 (EHV-1) infection in horses. Although many questions on the pathogenesis of this disease are still unanswered, it is commonly believed that EHM is the result of multiple, vascular, stroke-like insults to the central nervous system (CNS). Progress in EHM research has been slow, due to the lack of a model that effectively reproduces EHM and that allows ethical and cost-conscientious hypothesis testing. Furthermore, EHM is a rare disease that presents under local outbreak conditions. While awareness during an actual outbreak peaks due to concurrent reporting and media attention, horse owners, farm managers and the equine industry may not perceive this disease as a real threat despite the fact that the virus, EHV-1, is presumed endemic in horses worldwide—with few exceptions.

History of equine herpesvirus myeloencephalopathy

In 1966, the link between a rare syndrome of paralysis among horses and a concurrent infection with an equine herpesvirus was demonstrated by Saxegaard et al. in Scandinavia. Since then, outbreaks of variable magnitude mainly in Northern Europe and North America and a single report from Australia have been described in the scientific literature. Additional outbreaks in Southern Europe (Italy and Spain), Israel, Japan, and South Africa have been reported but as of yet remain unpublished. While the first large-scale outbreaks during the 1980s were reported from stud farms and Standardbred training facilities, recent reports more commonly describe outbreaks on large boarding facilities, facilities that specialize in sport horse training and showing, and equine hospitals after admission of a neurological horse. There is a general impression that outbreaks of EHM have occurred more frequently over the past 15 years. Whether this is a true increase in outbreak incidence, the result of a higher attack rate, or due to increased reporting is still a topic of discussion [1].

The virus

Basic information on the virus that is associated with EHM is deemed necessary as it aids our understanding of virus-specific strategy and virus–host interaction. EHV-1 is a member of the alpha-herpesvirinae and shares general characteristics with many other herpesviruses which include being an enveloped DNA virus that is species-specific and typically causes life-long infections in the host. This life-long infection is maintained through immunologically inconspicuous phases of latency switching with brief periods of lytic, replicative cycles. Herpesviruses contain double-stranded DNA and thus are not prone to mutation as is common with RNA viruses. The intact viral envelope, which has a structure similar to the mammalian cell membrane, contains glycoproteins that are essential for viral entry into host cells. Disruption of this envelope by a number of environmental conditions (e.g., freezing, UV-light, desiccation) or detergents renders the virus noninfective. Species specificity allows "close contact" transmission; however, it also limits the number of suitable hosts of viral infection. If an infection would lead to severe disease or death in the species affected, it would rapidly become extinct. Therefore, to maintain endemically within the equine population, clinical disease needs to be mild. EHV-1 is well adapted to the equine population; infections resulting in EHM seem to offer little if any advantage for this virus' survival in a population. Equine herpesvirus myeloencephalopathy may be more the result of a circumstantial, aberrant immune-mediated phenomenon [2].

Equine Neurology, Second Edition. Martin Furr and Stephen Reed.
© 2015 John Wiley & Sons, Inc. Published 2015 by John Wiley & Sons, Inc.
Companion website: www.wiley.com/go/furr/neurology

Interestingly, a single-point mutation in the polymerase gene causes an amino acid switch in the polymerase enzyme, with the result that EHV-1 strains can be distinguished into either a D-phenotype (containing an aspartic acid) or an N-phenotype (containing an asparagine). The D-phenotype seems to occur more often but is not exclusively associated with EHM outbreaks when compared to the N-phenotype. It has been proposed that the D-phenotype causes the virus to replicate faster, resulting in a more robust viremia and a more aggressive course of infection. As there are distinct differences among EHM outbreaks, that is, the numbers of neurologically affected horses in a herd, an infection with the D- or N-phenotype is likely to be one of many risk factors that determine the course and the fatality rate of an outbreak [3, 4].

Pathogenesis

Equine herpesvirus myeloencephalopathy is caused by a multifocal, stroke-like disease in the vasculature of the CNS, mainly in the spinal cord. Disease develops at or near sites of endothelial cell (EC) infection with EHV-1. The infection of ECs follows the phase of primary viral replication in the respiratory tract and subsequent viremia that is cell-associated in lymphocytes and monocytes (peripheral blood mononuclear cells or PBMC). Infection of EC occurs not only in the CNS but also in the gonads and at the fetal–maternal interface resulting in abortion [5].

Neurological disease is attributed to spinal cord damage; however, upon careful histopathological examination, lesions can be detected in many vascular structures associated with the CNS including choroid of the eye, spinal cord, brain stem, and cortex. Histological characteristics of EHM are typically multifocal vasculitis, thrombosis, hemorrhage, and perivascular cuffing of mononuclear cells. A gliosis and Wallerian degeneration of axons in spinal cord or brain can be seen depending on the time between onset of clinical signs and tissue specimen collection. Lesions can range from very extensive, being macroscopically visible, to only being noted on microscopic examination [6].

Knowledge on the pathogenesis of EHM has improved especially as it relates to the initial stages of CNS EC infection. EHV-1 viremia is "cell-associated" within PBMCs [7]. This phase follows within a few days after viral replication in the respiratory tract and is typically associated with a fever of several days duration. *In vitro* studies have shown that EC infection is likely only possible if EHV-1 infected subclasses of PBMC make physical contact with the EC via presumed upregulated adhesion molecules on both cell surfaces to facilitate this contact [8]. What follows the EC infection remains elusive; it is possible that viral replication in ECs could lead to an activation of the coagulation cascade either directly through EC lysis and exposure of subendothelial collagen or indirectly through a combination of surface changes and micro-particle activation leading to Tissue Factor release [9, 10]. This area is particularly difficult to access for hypothesis-driven research and progress has slowed. One strategy of possible intervention is to slow down the rate of EC infection at the CNS, which seems possible to accomplish by reducing viral burden during viremia or by blocking PBMC–EC interaction.

Clinical signs

Clinical signs typical of EHM are those attributed to spinal cord damage. While we assume that damage to the choroidal vasculature might have a wider distribution among infected and viremic horses, clinical signs of blepharospasm and photophobia may not become apparent. Spinal cord signs depend on lesion frequency, location, and dissemination and can best be described as cumulative. Hence, degrees of ataxia and weakness can be mild to severe, asymmetrical or symmetrical, culminating toward tetraparalysis [11]. Dog-sitting is an often mentioned, although not pathognomonic, finding with EHM. Whether this is due to a more severely affected thoracolumbar versus cervical cord, whether a horse has greater difficulties in lifting the hind in an equally affected cord, or whether in a situation of random spinal cord damage the tracts of the hind limbs are at greater risk to become damaged due to their increased length remains up for debate.

The pathway for micturition and bladder sphincter control runs from the cortex caudad to the bladder sphincter as an uninterrupted tract, running the entire length of the spinal cord. Due to its length, it is likely the most vulnerable tract in the spinal cord for multifocal damage. Thus, it is very common that horses, even with only mild to moderate EHM, will show signs of dysuria due to bladder sphincter spasm (i.e., a bladder that is filled up to its limits which will not empty when manual pressure is applied or "upper motor neuron bladder"[UMN]). A paralyzed or "lower motor neuron bladder" can occur with moderate to severe forms of EHM where, in addition to the micturition tract, the pudendal nerve became severely damaged. In this situation, the bladder will appear fluid-filled yet flaccid on palpation per rectum, and manual pressure will allow urine to escape through the urethra. It is, however, the UMN bladder that needs immediate attention with (indwelling) catheterization.

Although somewhat subjective, tail tone of EHM horses can also be decreased. In addition, there can be hypothermia due to a decreased anal sphincter tone. Brain stem deficits are rare, but most likely will present with signs of vestibular syndrome including head-tilt, nystagmus, ipsilateral weakness, and contralateral hypermetria. Although clinical signs of an encephalopathy are rare, histological lesions in the cortex can be found after careful sampling and examination. Clinical signs of EHM usually develop rapidly within 24–48 h after cessation of a fever and will be worst 24–48 h after onset of clinical signs. Thereafter, a relatively fast improvement might be seen within the next 5–7 days. Full bladder sphincter control of a UMN bladder usually returns at that time unless there has been permanent damage to the detrusor muscle, but full recovery might take several more days. The horse should be reevaluated in several weeks to months for chronic-persistent signs of EHM. Horses can return to full function, but this is more likely if the initial damage has been mild to moderate. There have been anecdotal reports of horses returning to full function after having severe signs including tetraplegia. In severe cases, intense nursing care including sling applications are necessary, and success largely depends upon the demeanor of the horse— that is, how well it tolerates being recumbent [12]. (Figure 18.1)

Diagnosis

A diagnosis of EHM is easy to establish when several horses are febrile, some of them with clinical signs of spinal cord disease. The diagnosis is more challenging when one is confronted with the index case (IC). This horse might have a suspicious history, such as "been to a show," the horse possibly has had a fever recently, and the clinical signs of ataxia and weakness with seemingly undisturbed mentation suggest spinal cord damage. At this stage, isolation of this horse should be prompt. A laboratory diagnosis, antemortem, can be made quickly with high sensitivity using (real-time, quantitative) PCR [13]. At a stage when neurological signs just developed, it is likely that the horse is still nasal swab positive and viremic. While the viral load in nasal swabs is typically higher than the viremic load, nasal swabs are the better choice for a diagnosis; however, there is a risk that nasal shedding has already stopped leading to false-negative results. Therefore, a combination of nasal swabs and EDTA venous blood sample should always be submitted from a suspect IC to an accredited laboratory for EHV-1-specific PCR diagnostics.

A cerebrospinal fluid (CSF) sample collected at the lumbosacral junction might further aid in the EHM diagnosis, but results are supportive only. With acute

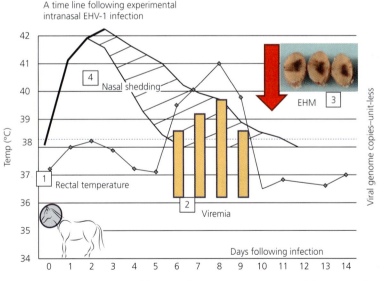

Figure 18.1 This figure illustrates findings of nasal shedding, rectal temperature, viremia, and the (potential) occurrence of EHM following an experimental intranasal infection with EHV-1. X-axis represents time in days, with infection occurring on day = 0; Y-axis represents rectal temperature in degrees Celsius; alternative Y-axis is a unitless scale for viral genome quantities; dotted line indicates fever cut-off (38.3°C–101.3°F). 1- rectal temperature curve is often biphasic. Secondary fever is associated with "cell-associated viremia." 2- cell-associated viremia, duration 3–5 days as determined by PCR. 3-clinical EHM usually follows viremia. 4-nasal shedding is high during the first 3 days and may be associated with a primary fever. Duration of nasal shedding varies significantly between horses, which is represented by the shaded area between the two lines of nasal shedding.

onset of EHM, the sample collected can be xanthochromic (pink or yellow discoloration) in absence of a pleocytosis (<5 cells/µl), but with an increased protein concentration (>800 mg/l), all are indicative of a vasculitis with erythrocyte leakage and lysis in the CNS [14]. Whether CSF carries sufficient viral DNA for a PCR diagnosis is yet to be verified; however, viral genome copies are considered low in CSF and may be below detection limits of many PCR assays [15]. Complement fixation assays will show titers of recently produced (complement binding) antibody. This assay is diagnostic in the circumstances of a recent infection (within <14 days) with EHV-1 when nasal shedding and viremia may have already ceased. However, only few laboratories, mainly in the UK, Ireland, and Australia, offer this test [16].

A horse and possible IC that requires euthanasia during the early stages of a suspected EHM outbreak should undergo a complete nervous system necropsy to confirm the diagnosis. Spinal cord tissue sections should be submitted for EHV-1—specific PCR as a rapid (and sensitive) testing method. Immunohistochemistry on spinal cord sections is another more time-consuming method to establish a diagnosis.

Other horses in the vicinity of the IC should be carefully evaluated for fevers, and, if detected, a representative number of nasal swabs and EDTA blood should be included for a herd diagnosis. Generally, once a herd diagnosis has been made, subsequent cases with similar clinical signs, including fever, are assumed to have an EHV-1 infection (Figure 18.2).

Once a definitive diagnosis of EHV-1 infection has been made, the premises should be quarantined. In some countries, EHM is a reportable disease that requires prompt notification of regulatory authorities. However, a voluntary notification of authorities and quarantine of the premises are highly recommended as movement of horses away from an affected property is a major risk factor of disease spread. Serum samples should be banked for virus neutralization-testing which is usually based on paired samples to detect a three- to fourfold titer increase between acute and convalescent samples collected 3 weeks apart. Serum neutralization tests do not distinguish between EHV-1 and EHV-4 antibodies. An EHV-1-specific ELISA is available; however, the test is currently only licensed as a diagnostic tool in a select number of countries. Virus isolation and paired serology are currently done less frequently but are still invaluable samples for research and in those situations where initial PCR results are negative [17].

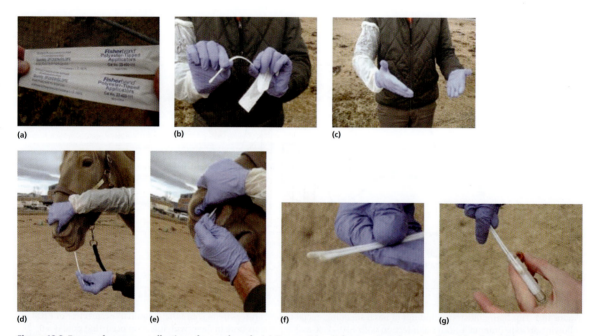

Figure 18.2 Process for proper collection of a nasal swab. (a) Dacron™ or Polyester-tipped swabs; (b) with a bendable, plastic shaft; (c) disposable gloves and change between horses; (d) place your thumb against the nasal septum and grasp with your fingers across the nasal plane; (e) quickly insert both swabs in the nasal passage. Go in and out for at least three to four times and make sure there is contact with the nasal mucosa; (f) swabs show some signs of cellular debris; (g) swabs should go into an empty transport container for PCR analysis; (g) label appropriately.

Therapeutic recommendations for horses with EHM

Currently, therapeutic recommendations target different aspects of EHM pathogenesis, including decreasing overall viral load in the body of an infected horse, blocking viral transfer from infected PBMC into EC during viremia, and palliative drugs treating secondary complications associated with viral replication and EC infection such as vasculitis and tissue inflammation.

Drugs inhibiting viral load

Robust replication of virus in the respiratory tract is assumed to contribute to a higher magnitude and duration of viremia. It is currently believed that this more extensive viremia will result in a more widespread EC infection of the spinal cord vasculature. Antiviral agents such as thymidine kinase inhibitors like valaciclovir, famciclovir, or ganciclovir, are effective against herpesviruses in general. They are administered during EHV-1 infection in the effort to reduce viral replication in the respiratory tract, reduce the magnitude of viremia in PBMCs, and limit the extent of EC infection [18, 19]. Oral valaciclovir will reach effective plasma concentrations when administered at 30 mg/kg body weight (bw) PO three times daily for the first 48 h, then the dose can be decreased to 20 mg/kg bw PO twice daily [20]. Intravenously administered ganciclovir, which is more potent, may be advantageous, but is currently cost-prohibitive in many cases, and its efficacy is still under investigation [21, 22]. Although virustatics have been shown to decrease viral replication *in vitro*, *in vivo* efficacy has not been demonstrated conclusively. Despite results of prospective studies being equivocal, the general recommendation is to start antiviral therapy as early as possible and preferably within the first hours of detecting a fever. Once neurological signs have occurred in the horse, it is likely too late to start antiviral therapy.

Drugs blocking viral transfer

Anti-inflammatory drugs have been shown experimentally to prevent infected PBMC adhesion to EC of CNS vasculature. Specifically, *in vitro* studies, conducted by the author's laboratory, have shown a decreased EC infection with EHV-1 when infected PBMCs are allowed contact with EC in the presence of a variety of anti-inflammatory drugs. This effect was most notably seen with nonsteroidal anti-inflammatory (NSAID) drugs, by a lidocaine constant rate infusion and least consistently with dexamethasone. Anti-inflammatory drugs are assumed to downregulate the expression of cellular adhesion molecules on both EC and PBMC, thereby decreasing the frequency of contact between cells and thus the rate of EC infection. As the risk of EC infection is highest in viremic horses and these horses typically develop a concurrent fever, an important therapeutic intervention may include treating febrile horses with anti-inflammatory drugs starting on the first day of fever detection. As the effects of dexamethasone are inconsistent, and the use of a lidocaine CRI is impractical under field conditions, we recommend treatment with an NSAID. Currently, our drug of choice is firocoxib due to its gastrointestinal mucosa sparing effect and its once daily administration. While the latter is convenient, it also limits caretaker contact with a potentially virus-shedding animal. The author recommends treating with firocoxib beginning at the first detection of a fever and continuing an additional 3–5 days once the fever has ceased [8].

Drugs targeting secondary complications

Many different therapeutic options such as dimethyl sulfoxide (DMSO), heparin, and low-dose aspirin are used empirically to prevent secondary complications at different stages of this disease despite a lack of evidence of efficacy. Therefore, these drugs should be used with caution, especially as interactions with other drugs have not been evaluated. However, oral vitamin E is likely to be safe and may be administered to combat the propagation of inflammation associated with a lack of tissue antioxidant capacity. Specific efficacy for this is currently lacking, however.

When clinical signs of EHM become apparent, the therapeutic focus must shift to controlling damage to the CNS. However, one should not forget that horses with clinical signs are likely to still shed virus through nasal/respiratory secretions. As mentioned previously, the efficacy of antivirals at this stage is questionable. In the face of vasculitis, there is a need for anti-inflammatory therapy. At this stage, dexamethasone is likely to be more efficacious and should be preferred over NSAIDs. Dexamethasone should be used at a judicious dose (≤0.05 mg/kg once to twice daily) and not in combination with an NSAID. As horses with EHM frequently show dysuria due to a spastic bladder sphincter, catheterization of the bladder is extremely important. While this should always be a sterile procedure, it is nonetheless recommended to treat a horse with a broad-spectrum antimicrobial to prevent the occurrence of urinary tract infection.

Epidemiology

Epidemiology of EHM, and the occurrence of an outbreak, is intricately linked to fixed risk factors of heightened susceptibility to develop EHM and (dynamic) risk factors that influence the dynamics of transmission including how many horses will become infected, and of those, how many will develop neurological disease or

EHM. At the beginning of an outbreak on a particular farm or, rarely, during a competitive event, there is a "Case 0" or IC. The IC is either the one that reactivated latent virus or became infected by an unrecognized shedder through horizontal transmission. Further transmission occurs by direct nose-to-nose contact with other horses or through indirect transmission via fomites [17].

In retrospect, the IC of an EHM outbreak is often a horse that recently attended a show or competition, was newly introduced to the herd, or recently returned from a veterinary hospital. On occasion, an abortion attributed to EHV-1 has been associated with the onset of an EHM outbreak. Recrudescence of latent virus is assumed to be associated with "stress." However, detecting virus in nasal secretions under many different stressful conditions including long-distance transportation, colic surgery or developing a fever in an equine hospital, yearling sales, or following administration of immune-suppressive doses of a corticosteroid, is uncommon [1, 23, 24]. EHV-1 recrudescence may therefore be an extremely rare event, which could explain the relatively low number of EHM outbreaks per year worldwide. Outbreaks of EHM are reported more frequently during the cooler season of the year, when horses are more likely to be housed indoors. While an indoor environment might facilitate transmission, lower temperatures, higher humidity, and less UV-light during the winter might also enhance viral survival compared to summer months [1].

Humoral and cellular immunity against EHV-1 will differ between horses based on age, genetics, general health, environmental factors, previous infection with EHV-1, whether previous vaccination has been done and which vaccine product was used, and the time that has gone by between vaccination and an encounter with the pathogen. Viremia is the second stage of an EHV-1 infection and a variable proportion of infected horses will become viremic, depending on their immune status [25, 26]. However, based on data from several natural and experimental infections, only a proportion of viremic horses will subsequently develop EHM. Typically, horses less than 3 years of age are least likely to develop EHM with the likelihood of occurrence increasing with age. This has led to an "old horse-infection model" that is utilized when the anticipated outcome of an infection study is EHM. Breed has also been found to be associated with the development of EHM. Robust small pony breeds are less likely to develop EHM when compared to the tall breeds (the standardbred, thoroughbred, various warmblood breeds, quarter and draft horses) despite both groups becoming viremic [1]. The EHM attack rate appears to depend on a number of fixed and dynamic risk factors. The sum of risk-contributing and risk-minimizing factors determines the number of

EHM cases during an outbreak. Early outbreak mitigation will focus on dynamic factors, such as creating distance between horses, early detection of shedders, and implementation of biosecurity measures, with the intent of minimizing the proportion of horses developing EHM during an outbreak.

Outbreak prevention and mitigation

Outbreak prevention of a contagious disease can only be achieved on well-managed horse operations where animals are routinely monitored for clinical signs, where immunization and biosecurity protocols are in place, and where animals are strategically grouped according to age and use. Naturally, the farm management plays a pivotal role in this process as does education on biosecurity strategies.

Equine herpesvirus myeloencephalitis outbreak prevention requires a stringent immunization protocol according to the manufacturer's or industry recommendations, and both horses and ponies should be included. A horse that relocates to the property should be inspected by a veterinarian prior to moving; the horse should not have a recent history of fever and should not relocate from a farm with (recent) fever cases or unexplained cases of neurologic disease. As relocation may cause circumstances for latency recrudescence, a horse should be quarantined for up to 14 days with daily recording of body temperature. While vaccination against EHV-1 is strongly recommended, a recent paper found evidence that horses vaccinated within the 5-week-period prior to attending an event where EHM occurred were more likely to develop EHM compared to those vaccinated more than 5 weeks prior to the event [27]. This observation highlights the fact that any vaccination is a challenge to any horse's immune system, and vaccinations should be carefully planned.

Preventing outbreaks of EHM further requires daily data collection of body temperature of all horses, immediate isolation of febrile horses, and investigations into the causes of fevers. Horses should be grouped such that the competitive or traveling horses are separated from horses that never leave the farm or facility. In-foal mares and yearlings should be housed in separate buildings as two independent groups. If this is not possible, horses upon return from a competition should be housed separately for a minimum of 4 days, while body temperature and signs of respiratory disease are monitored and any fever is investigated as to its cause.

Outbreak mitigation combines all efforts to reduce infection transmission and requires cooperation of all involved personnel and horse owners. Key strategies are to provide information to personnel, owners, and visitors; to quickly identify newly infected (and likely shedding) horses; to create distance between horses; and to recognize sources of fomite transmission. Although EHV-1 is not a reportable disease everywhere in the world, veterinary regulatory authorities should be involved as early as possible as they can play a significant advisory role. Horses should not enter or leave an affected farm or facility without proper authorization. Information on the disease for horse owners is pivotal to avoid panic and a sudden exodus of seemingly unaffected horses with the risk of disease spread to other operations. It might be advantageous, and certainly only after approval by regulatory authorities, that owners move their horses from an affected facility or farm into total solitude for a minimum of 3 weeks. While this decreases animal density on affected premises, it needs to be carefully planned to prevent spread of the infection. Sampling and nasal swab PCR analysis can be helpful during decision-making processes; however, one has to be aware of the risk of false-negative swab results. A horse should still be stabled in isolation and not be moved with less than three negative nasal swabs collected one per day.

An ovine parapoxvirus-based immunomodulator (Zylexis™) targeting the innate immune response of horses is often administered to horses on premises with an acute EHM outbreak or to horses attending a sport event. A publication by Traub et al. provided evidence that recent vaccination (<3 weeks) prior to an EHM outbreak increases the risk to develop neurological disease upon infection. Although no explanation was provided for this observation, the stress of vaccination could be reason for this greater risk. A nonspecific immunomodulator administered in the face of an infection might have similar effects and could be counterproductive. In a placebo-controlled infection experiment with equine influenza virus, the protective properties of this ovine parapox-based immunomodulator were evaluated and no differences between groups were observed [28]. Hence, the value of the parapoxvirus-based immunomodulator in the treatment of EHM is unknown at this time.

During a confirmed EHM-outbreak, the most cost-efficient method to identify newly infected horses is to obtain rectal temperatures. Fevers that occur during the early phase of a respiratory tract infection are more likely to be high normal (37.9–38.3°C/101.0–101.3°F), while fever associated with viremia is typically higher (>38.0°C/101.0°F). Any horse with a fever should be isolated and nose-to-nose contact between all horses should be prevented. If space to isolate is sparse, an effective measure to isolate is to seal or to close the side walls between two adjacent stalls (boxes). A horse should only be approached in disposable or horse-individual gear (coat, gloves, shoe and head cover for

the person who enters), and only a horse's own tack and head collar should be used. A footbath or foot mat containing disinfectants at the entrance of a stall (box) should be installed. As virus remains infective for more than 48h under optimal conditions (smooth surfaces, constant temperature conditions), regular disinfection of strategic high traffic or activity areas (wash racks) is necessary. Horse activity should be kept to a minimum, and, if unavoidable, should be done in a thoughtfully planned way avoiding unnecessary "crossing of lines," and without moments of direct contact. Vaccination of horses on an affected premise during an outbreak remains controversial and is in general not recommended. Also, benefits of using various immunity inducers of the innate immune system have not been demonstrated for EHM.

In conclusion, there are still many unanswered questions on EHV-1 infection and the pathogenesis of EHM. This is mainly due to the lack of a suitable and ethical model to reproduce this disease. While effective strategies for the prevention of viremia or recrudescence from latency are highly desired, science moves slowly. Outbreak prevention has to focus on increasing the awareness of this constant threat to all aspects of the horse industry and on early recognition of disease with immediate implementation of mitigation. The risk of transmission and infection increases with growing horse densities and on premises with increased horse mobility and trafficking. A combination of immunization and management, which includes a basic understanding of biosecurity measures and owner education, needs to be promoted to prevent outbreaks in the future. Additionally, vaccine efficacy needs further improvement. In the meantime, some success has been accomplished with strategic use of therapeutics decreasing viral load and virus–host interactions during the primary infection and viremia. This area of research needs to be continued.

References

[1] Goehring, L.S., van Winden, S.C., van Maanen, C. *et al.* (2006) Equine herpesvirus type 1-associated myeloencephalopathy in the Netherlands: a four-year retrospective study (1999–2003). *J Vet Intern Med*, 20, 601–607.

[2] Henle, W. and Henle, G. (1982) Immunology of Epstein-Barr Virus, in *The Herpesviruses* (ed. B. Roizman), Plenum Press, New York, pp. 209–252.

[3] Nugent, J., Birch-Machin, I., Smith, K.C. *et al.* (2006) Analysis of equid herpesvirus 1 strain variation reveals a point mutation of the DNA polymerase strongly associated with neuropathogenic versus nonneuropathogenic disease outbreaks. *J Virol*, 80, 4047–4060.

[4] Perkins, G.A., Goodman, L.B., Tsujimura, K. *et al.* (2009) Investigation of the prevalence of neurologic equine herpes virus type 1 (EHV-1) in a 23-year retrospective analysis (1984–2007). *Vet Microbiol*, 139, 375–378.

[5] Edington, N., Bridges, C.G. and Patel, J.R. (1986) Endothelial cell infection and thrombosis in paralysis caused by equid herpesvirus-1: equine stroke. *Arch Virol*, 90, 111–124.

[6] Whitwell, K.E. and Blunden, A.S. (1992) Pathological findings in horses dying during an outbreak of the paralytic form of Equid herpesvirus type 1 (EHV-1) infection. *Equine Vet J*, 24, 13–19.

[7] Wilsterman, S., Soboll-Hussey, G., Lunn, D.P. *et al.* (2011) Equine herpesvirus-1 infected peripheral blood mononuclear cell subpopulations during viremia. *Vet Microbiol*, 149, 40–47.

[8] Goehring LS, Brandes KM, Wittenburg L, et al. In vitro effect of anti-inflammatory drugs on endothelial cell infection with equid herpesvirus-1. Proceedings of the ninth Equine Infectious Disease Conference, October 21–26, Lexington, KY;2013.

[9] Yeo, W.M., Osterrieder, N. and Stokol, T. (2013) Equine herpesvirus type 1 infection induces procoagulant activity in equine monocytes. *Vet Res*, 44, 16.

[10] Morris, D.D. (2009) Hemostatic Dysfunction, in *Large Animal Internal Medicine*, 4th edn (ed. B.P. Smith), Mosby Elsevier, St. Louis, pp. 1146–1147.

[11] Henninger, R.W., Reed, S.M., Saville, W.J. *et al.* (2007) Outbreak of neurologic disease caused by equine herpesvirus-1 at a university equestrian center. *J Vet Intern Med*, 21, 157–165.

[12] van Maanen, C., Sloet van Oldruitenborgh-Oosterbaan, M.M., Damen, E.A. *et al.* (2001) Neurological disease associated with EHV-1-infection in a riding school: clinical and virological characteristics. *Equine Vet J*, 33, 191–196.

[13] Pusterla, N., Hussey, S.B., Mapes, S. *et al.* (2009) Comparison of four methods to quantify Equid herpesvirus 1 load by real-time polymerase chain reaction in nasal secretions of experimentally and naturally infected horses. *J Vet Diagn Invest*, 21, 836–840.

[14] Donaldson, M.T. and Sweeney, C.R. (1998) Herpesvirus myeloencephalopathy in horses: 11 cases (1982–1996). *J Am Vet Med Assoc*, 213, 671–675.

[15] Goodman, L.B., Wagner, B., Flaminio, M.J. *et al.* (2006) Comparison of the efficacy of inactivated combination and modified-live virus vaccines against challenge infection with neuropathogenic equine herpesvirus type 1 (EHV-1). *Vaccine*, 24, 3636–3645.

[16] Crabb, B.S., MacPherson, C.M., Reubel, G.H. *et al.* (1995) A type-specific serological test to distinguish antibodies to equine herpesviruses 4 and 1. *Arch Virol*, 140, 245–258.

[17] Lunn, D.P., Davis-Poynter, N., Flaminio, M.J. *et al.* (2009) Equine herpesvirus-1 consensus statement. *J Vet Intern Med*, 23, 450–461.

[18] Garre, B., Gryspeerdt, A., Croubels, S. *et al.* (2009) Evaluation of orally administered valacyclovir in experimentally EHV1-infected ponies. *Vet Microbiol*, 135, 214–221.

[19] Garre, B., van der Meulen, K., Nugent, J. *et al.* (2007) In vitro susceptibility of six isolates of equine herpesvirus 1 to acyclovir, ganciclovir, cidofovir, adefovir, PMEDAP and foscarnet. *Vet Microbiol*, 122, 43–51.

[20] Bentz, B.G., Maxwell, L.K., Bourne, D.W.A. and Erkert, R.S. (2007) Pharmacokinetics of valacyclovir in the adult horse. *J Vet Intern Med*, 21, 601–602.

[21] Carmichael, R.J., Whitfield, C. and Maxwell, L.K. (2013) Pharmacokinetics of ganciclovir and valganciclovir in the adult horse. *J Vet Pharmacol Ther*, 36, 441–449.

[22] Maxwell, L. (2011) *Efficacy of Delayed Antiviral Therapy Against EHV-1 Challenge*, Forum ACVIM, Denver.

[23] Carr, E., Schott, H. and Pusterla, N. (2011) Absence of equid herpesvirus-1 reactivation and viremia in hospitalized critically ill horses. *J Vet Intern Med*, 25, 1190–1193.

[24] Pusterla, N., Mapes, S., Madigan, J.E. *et al.* (2009) Prevalence of EHV-1 in adult horses transported over long distances. *Vet Rec*, 165, 473–475.

[25] Kydd, J.H., Townsend, H.G. and Hannant, D. (2006) The equine immune response to equine herpesvirus-1: the virus and its vaccines. *Vet Immunol Immunopathol*, 111, 15–30.

[26] Allen, G.P. (2008) Risk factors for development of neurologic disease after experimental exposure to equine herpesvirus-1 in horses. *Am J Vet Res*, 69, 1595–1600.

[27] Traub-Dagartz, J.L., Pelzel-McCluskey, A.M., Creekmore, L.H. *et al.* (2013) Case-control study of a multistate equine herpesvirus myeloencephalopathy outbreak. *J Vet Intern Med*, 27, 339–346.

[28] Lunn, D.P. and Rush, B.R. (2004) Immunomodulation: principles and mechanisms. *Proc Ann Meet Am Assoc Equine Pract*, 50, 447–453.

19

Mosquito-Borne Infections Affecting the Central Nervous System

Maureen T. Long

College of Veterinary Medicine, University of Florida, Gainesville, USA

Worldwide, there are many arthropod-borne viruses that can cause significant outbreaks, most of which are alphaviruses and flaviviruses (Table 19.1). In the Americas, the alphaviruses and flaviviruses are the most common causes of viral neurological disease and death in horses on an annual basis even though the vaccines are highly protective [1]. There are many different arthropod-borne encephalitides worldwide that affect equids, some of which are likely not as yet identified as an equine pathogen. The reporting of these diseases (or the suspicion of such) is required of all veterinarians usually at the state level to ensure the health and safety of humans and horses. Vaccination against alphaviruses and flaviviruses are considered the core component of immunoprophylaxis for all horses in the United States by the American Association of Equine Practitioners. In addition to the flaviviruses and alphaviruses, the bunyaviruses are also endemic in the United States. Unfortunately, the true incidence of the Bunyaviruses are unknown because testing for these is uncommon in many state veterinary diagnostic laboratories; the sporadic reports result most frequently from postmortem isolation of virus [1].

History and signalment

History, signalment, and environment are key factors of arbovirus-induced neurologic disease. Of primary importance is vaccine history since immunization is highly effective. Most horses with eastern equine encephalitis virus (EEEV) are either not vaccinated or are incompletely vaccinated. In the latter, these are either young horses (<3 years of age) or recent arrivals to endemic locales with no or minimal EEEV vaccination. Regarding West Nile virus (WNV) infection, current flavivirus vaccines have excellent immunogenicity, and even an annual vaccination that follows a full primary immunization series is greater than 90% protective irrespective of vaccine formulation.

Arthropods are seasonal except where environmental temperatures are not sustained below temperatures associated with cessation of adult mosquito feeding (<50°F or 10°C). In the southeastern United States, when lack of sustained frost occurs preceeded by late fall rains, EEEV can be reported in horses commonly along the Florida–Georgia border in January. Unless drought-like conditions prevail for the spring, cases will continue to accrue throughout the whole year. Thus, because of the unpredictability of local weather activity, new regional arrivals are always at risk for disease if incompletely vaccinated. The occurrence of EEEV in horses and people is also highly associated with the same locales year after year because the habitat is usually where pastureland borders the edge of a hardwood swamp. Flavivirus disease is harder to predict since the virus is essentially endemic in all of North America. The recent reemergence of WNV in the UnitedStates in 2012 indicates that the interplay of available reservoir hosts, high seasonal temperature, and drought coupled with polluted standing water are important for occurrence of mammalian disease. Given the complexity of arthropod-borne diseases, the use of disease-specific reporting is critical as a diagnostic aid. The CDC Division of Vector-Borne Diseases maintains a real-time site in conjuction with the United States Geological Survey (USGS) for state-and county-level (ArboNET) arboviral activity (http://www.cdc.gov/westnile/statsMaps/index.html).

Physical examination

Both systemic and neurological examinations are important for antemortem identification of a viral infection of the central nervous system (CNS). Viral infection can affect a specific brain or spinal cord region, but most

Equine Neurology, Second Edition. Martin Furr and Stephen Reed.
© 2015 John Wiley & Sons, Inc. Published 2015 by John Wiley & Sons, Inc.
Companion website: www.wiley.com/go/furr/neurology

Table 19.1 Common alphaviruses and flaviviruses that cause encephalomyelitis in horses.

Virus group	Virus species	Geographic location	Reservoir species	Equine syndrome
Alphavirus	Eastern equine encephalitis	North, South, and Central America, Carribean	Birds, rodents, snakes?	Encephalomyelitis
	Western equine encephalitis	North and South America	Birds, rodents, snakes	Encephalomyelitis
	Venezualen equine encephalitis	Central and South America, Carribean	Cotton rat	Encephalomyelitis
	Ross River	Australia, Papua New Guinea	Marsupial and placental mammals	Systemic: hemolymphatic Neurologic: ataxia
	Semliki Forest	East and West Africa	Unknown	Encephalomyelitis
Flavivirus Japanese encephalitis	Japanese encephalitis	Asia, India, Russia, Western Pacific	Birds, swine	Encephalomyelitis
	Murray valley	Australia, Papua New Guinea	Birds, horses, cattle, marsupials, and foxes	Encephalomyelitis
	Kunjin virus	Australia	Water birds: herons and ibis	Encephalomyelitis
	St. Louis encephalitis	North, Central, and South America	Birds	Serological only recorded
	Usutu	Europe, Africa	Birds	Serological only recorded
	West Nile	Africa, Middle East, Europe, North, Central, and South America, Australia	Passerine birds (crows, sparrows, robins)	Encephalomyelitis
Tick-borne encephalitis	Louping Ill	Iberian Peninsula, United Kingdom	Sheep, grouse	Encephalomyelitis
	Powassan	North America, Russia	Lagomorphs, rodents, mice, skunks, dogs, birds	Encephalomyelitis
	Tick-borne encephalitis	Asia, Europe, Finland, Russia	Small rodents	Encephalomyelitis

infections include some encephalitis that results in generalized change in body temperature, behavior or activity, and locomotor signs. Under experimental infection, all clinically affected animals demonstrate a rise in rectal temperature at the onset of clinical signs between 102 and 104°F (38.8–40.0°C). For many pastured horses, a significant change in body temperature is often missed. Change in behavior can be mild and demonstrated by lack of activity and moderate depression or, depending on lesion localization, may reflect profound mentation abnormalities. Inappetance or decreased feed intake is a common manifestation. Most viral CNS diseases are acute, and thus gait abnormality without significant muscle loss is a hallmark. Neurological examination should include evaluation of gait and cranial nerve function and most arboviruses are characterized by sudden, progressive ataxia and weakness. If the horse is recumbent, determination of any possible traumatic cause or laminitis is also important. Attempting to hoist and assist in standing is therapeutic as well as part of the diagnostic evaluation. Ability to defecate and urinate is also important; diseases of the cauda equina as well as herpesvirus infection are important differentials for horses with fecal and urinary retention.

Ancillary testing

The major differential diagnoses for arboviruses include rabies, equine protozoal myeloencephalitisn (EPM), equine herpesvirus (EHV-1), verminous encephalitis (VE), hepatoencephalopathy, moldy corn poisoning, botulism, trauma, cervical vertebral myelopathy (CVM), neoplasia, and laminitis. Where present geographically, neuroborelliosis should be considered. Ancillary testing can be either antemortem or postmortem. Frequently, identification of a viral etiology is based on the exclusion of other agents and causes. A complete blood count (CBC), serum biochemistry, and blood ammonia should be performed. If available, radiographs of the cervical spine can assist in ruling out CVM.

One of the most useful diagnostic tools is cerebrospinal fluid (CSF) analysis (Table 19.2). Although frequently normal in many diseases such as rabies and EPM, the

Table 19.2 Summary of cerebrospinal fluid findings for arbovirus diseases.

	Protein	Cells	Cell types	Color
EEEV	▲▲	▲▲	Neutrophils Mononuclear	Normal to mildly turbid
WEEV	▲	▲	Mononuclear	Normal
WNV	N to ▲	N to ▲▲	Mononuclear	Mildly Xanthochromic
KV	▲	N to ▲▲	Mononuclear (some neutrophils)	Mildly Xanthochromic

▲, mild increase; ▲▲, major increase; EEEV, Eastern equine encephalitis virus; KV, Kunjin virus; WEEV, Western equine encephalitis virus; WNV, West Nile virus.

CSF in diseases such as EEEV, WNV, EHV-1, and VE is frequently abnormal and the index of suspicion for an infectious etiology can be raised before any other confirmatory test results are available. Testing of nasal swabs and EDTA-treated whole blood should be performed to eliminate EHV-1. Antemortem confirmatory diagnostic testing now relies on the identification of immunoglobulin M (IgM) antibody at a single dilution of 1:400. Control antigen must be concurrently run to detect false-positive results that some horses have due to high nonspecific background. Neutralization testing can be performed but paired sera must be used for interpretation; the hemaglutination inhibition formats are not reliable for confirmatory diagnostic testing. Interpretation of both IgM and neutralization formats must be performed in the light of vaccination history.

Postmortem examination of nonsurviving horses should be performed for confirmatory testing. With the regionalization of many diagnostic services, the availabilty of necropsy testing can be limited and a frustrating experience for many field practitioners. Safety is the primary concern; if the whole carcass cannot be transported, alternatives remain. The first and most rewarding alternative is to disarticulate the head from the cervical spine, enclose it in a leak-proof wrapping, pack on ice, and transport to a diagnostic laboratory. This is safer than removal of the brain in the field and allows a full examination of the brain and coordinated testing for rabies, EEEV, and WNV antigen testing and histopathological examination. Alternatively, the head can be disarticulated and a piece of the pons/medulla can be removed through the foramen magnum; however, if there is very little virus in the pons/medulla, false negatives can result. When performing a necropsy on a encephalitis suspect, personal protection should consist of double gloves, an N95 mask with full face mask or eye protection, and water-proof gowns (Tyvek®,

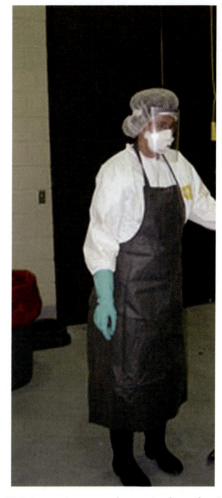

Figure 19.1 Appropriate personal protection for performing a necropsy on a horse suspected of an arbovirus infection. Personal protection includes waterproof gown, boots, gloves, N-95 or N-99 mask, face shield, and hair covering.

DuPont, Richmond/Chesterfield, VA or plastic) and foot protection (Figure 19.1). The spinal cord should never be removed via band saw which will aerosalize virus. Human spinal cord pullers are quite efficient at removing spinal cord from sections of precut cervical, thoracic, and lumbar vertebrae (Figure 19.2). See Chapter 16 for more detailed description of neurologic postmortem technique.

The gold standard for alphavirus and flavivirus identification is still viral isolation. For EEEV, a variety of antigen detection methods on fresh and fixed tissues have a high yield of reliable results and these include reverse transcription polymerase chain reaction (rt-PCR), immunohistochemistry (IHC), and viral isolation. Since

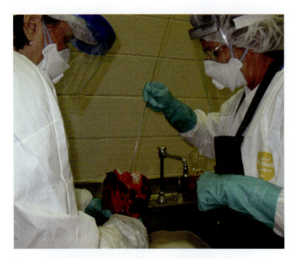

Figure 19.2 Method for pulling equine spinal cord without using a motorized saw. The metal instrument is a human spinal cord puller. The instrument is placed between the dura and the spinal cord and the nerve roots are cut. The spinal cord is then removed intact via forceps.

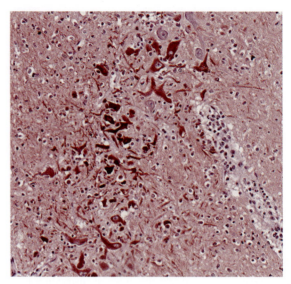

Figure 19.3 Photomicrograph of immunohistochemistry of a clinically affected horse with EEEV. The dark red staining is EEEV. Note the intense amount of antigen indicating the high viral load within the cytoplasm of neurons. (Image courtesy of Gretchen Delcambre, University of Florida.)

WNV encephalitis is associated with low viral load, care must be taken to test multiple sections of brain and spinal cord using any of the antigen formats including virus isolation, IHC, and rt-PCR. (Figure 19.3)

Zoonotic potential and environmental control

Alphaviruses and flaviviruses are considered zoonotic diseases. Reservoir hosts maintain the viruses in an endemic life cycle in the environment, allowing for transmission by mosquitoes to humans. There is little risk of disease by direct contact with an infected horse, except during postmortem examination with inappropriate handling of infected tissues. Postmortem handling of tissues should be performed with personal protection similar to that for rabies suspect cases.

The ecology of horse pastures and stables with standing water, a high degree of biologic debris, and "bridge" vectors between birds and mammals likely increase the risk of exposure in that environment. The same types of management tactics for prevention of disease in horses are important for people, except that there are no vaccines. Personal mosquito protection with a DEET-based product is recommended in areas with endemic disease. Veterinarians and horse owners should institute personal protection with appropriate clothing, gloves, and eye protection when coming into contact with animal tissues during the arbovirus season.

During outbreaks, owners should use fly sprays frequently and reapply spray repellents after rain. If fans are used, they should generate sufficient air movement to prevent landing of mosquitoes. Remove all standing water and stock water tanks and ponds with mosquito-feeding fish. If ponds are present, stock with mosquito-feeding fish. For heavy mosquito infestations, consider fogging and seek expertise from the local mosquito control department if available. Cover pools and remove all equipment, yard, and pool toys in which standing water will develop.

Equine alphaviruses

Eastern equine encephalitis
The genus Alphavirus belongs to the family Togaviridae and includes several viruses that have been isolated from horses with neurologic disease. Of these alphaviruses, EEEV, Western equine encephalitis (WEEV), and Venezuelan equine encephalitis viruses (VEEV) are the most frequently isolated from epidemics of encephalitis in horses and humans in the Western Hemisphere; however, there are others throughout the world that either are known to cause disease in horses or have only been described as pathogenic to humans (Table 19.1) [2–7]. The Togaviruses are single-stranded, enveloped, linear positive-sense ribonucleic acid (RNA) viruses measuring 60–70 nm in diameter [8–12]. Within the

envelope, there is a nucleocapsid with icosahedral symmetry composed of peplomers arranged as trimers. Each peplomer is a heterodimer composed of two glyco-proteins, E1 and E2 [13]. The glycoproteins E1 and E2 are immunodominant proteins that induce neutralizing antibody [9, 10, 13–15]. The E2 glycoprotein induces the strongest neutralizing antibody response (both poly-clonal and monoclonal), possesses hemagglutinating properties, and the activity is pH dependent [14, 16–22]. Both hemagglutination inhibition activity and neutral-izing specificity have historically been used to differen-tiate viral species and their antigenic types.

Etiology and epidemiology

The first recorded epidemic of EEEV in horses likely occurred in Massachusetts in 1831 and this virus was isolated from a horse 2 years later [23]. The first recorded human case occurred in that state in 1838 [24]. There is only one known species of EEEV, but in reality EEEV exists as separate North (NA) and South American (SA) variants [25]. Extensive work has been performed regarding the field ecology of EEEV in North America [26–31]. In North America, EEEV is perpetuated in a sylvatic cycle between primarily asymptomatic avian hosts (passerine birds) and mosquitoes such as *Culiseta melanura* that primarily feed on birds [32–36]. Recent work in Alabama indicates that the northern cardinal is the primary target for *C. melanura* feeding, but that other mosquitoes (*Culex erraticus*) are capable of feeding on a wider variety of birds, including robins, chickadees, owls, and mockingbirds in addition to bridging to mam-mals [37–39]. In Central and South Americas, the principal vectors of EEEV belong to the *Culex* (Melanoconion) spp. [40–42] These vectors feed on birds, rodents, marsupials, and reptiles. As such, SA EEEV has higher viral loads in cotton rats compared to NA EEEV [43]. Before 2000, comparatively few epi-demics of EEEV in horses were recorded in South America, with minimal disease reported in humans [44, 45]. Furthermore, there are notable differences in viru-lence between SA EEEV strains. More recently, in 2008 and 2009, larger outbreaks have occurred in Central and South America [46–51]. In Northeastern Brazil, 229 horses were affected with a case fatality rate of 73% with similar severity of disease as that of NA EEEV [49]. Enzootics of EEEV are capable of causing outbreaks of disease in multiple species besides horses, including alpacas, llamas, cattle, swine, cats, and dogs [52–59]. Exotic birds are especially susceptible including emus, the ring-necked pheasant, Pekin ducks, and Chukar partridges [60–63]. Recently, snakes have been identi-fied as a possible reservoir [64–66].

Habitat type is also associated with propensity for EEEV reemergence in Northern latitudes and the unin-terrupted transmission in Southern US latitudes [67–69].

Freshwater hardwood swamps are the most associated ecological niche for EEEV and, in the South, disease within mammalian hosts occurs in "tree farms" that are associated with these Florida's inland freshwater swamps. These cultivated swamp edges have the oppor-tunity for comingling of susceptible domesticated species and humans with infected mosquitos. Because alphavi-ruses are transmitted by arthropod vectors, clinical dis-ease occurs during the arbovirus season of late summer and early fall in temperate zones, with year-round transmission possible in the tropics and subtropics.

In the UnitedStates the highest reported infection rate is in the southeastern states but has been detected in all states east of the Mississippi River and some western states [70]. In the South, the most activity is found in Florida [71]. In recent years, intense focal activity has been reported in Michigan, Wisconsin, Ohio, Massachusetts, and New Hampshire [70, 72–75]. In 2005, Massachusetts experienced a human case affect rate over five times the preceeding 10 years. Ensuing work by the CDC indicates people affected during this time period resided with one-half mile of a cranberry bog or swamp associated with forest habitat. During this time, enzootic activity was also detected in clinically affected horses (9), alpacas (4), emus (2) and llamas (1) [72, 74, 76].

Clinical findings

Eastern equine encephalitis virus is one of the most pathological neurotropic viruses of man and horses. In Florida, many horses that succumb to EEEV are not vac-cinated, are less than 3 years of age, and are stock-type horses (Long, unpublished data) [1, 3, 77–80]. There is no gender predilection. After experimental inoculation, there is a short febrile response at 2–3 days (likely corresponding to viremia) [81]. The time to onset of neurological disease of EEEV is generally 7 days to 2 weeks (some reports indicate as short as 3 days, but this cannot be verified). In clinical cases, pyrexia is the first clinical manifestation of infection and can be as high as 104°F (40°C); in partially vaccinated horses, this may be significantly lower [82]. Clinical signs are pro-gressive in nature but variable with common systemic signs of depression and anorexia. Changes in mentation manifest frequently as severe forebrain disease including obtunded mentation (Figure 19.4), blindness, head pressing, and teeth grinding. Early hyperexcitability quickly changes to stupor, and when standing, the head hangs low with drooping ears, the eyelids become slightly swollen and partly closed, the lips become flac-cid, and the tongue protrudes from the mouth. Early signs of severe ataxia generally progresses to full paral-ysis and recumbency. Cranial nerve signs include dys-phagia and tongue weakness. The length of clinical disease in severely affected horses varies between 2 and

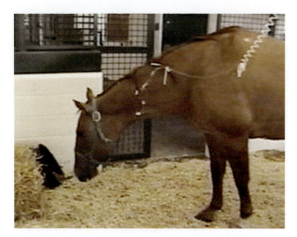

Figure 19.4 Photograph of a horse with West Nile virus (WNV) encephalomyelitis. Horse had obtunded mentation for over 3 weeks. The horse remained standing but was somnolent and stood with his head lowered in one position of the stall unless forcibly moved. The photomicrograph in Figure 19.4 is that of WNV immunohistochemistry performed on the brain of the horse after euthanasia.

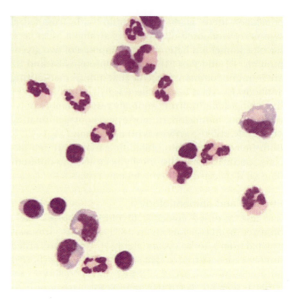

Figure 19.5 Photomicrograph of cerebrospinal fluid (CSF) from horse with eastern equine encephalitis (EEE). This horse was not vaccinated and exhibited clinical signs consistent with EEEV hours when the CSF was obtained. The CSF contains more than 70% nondegenerate neutrophils.

14 days, the former being most common in the nonvaccinated horses. Nearly all horses with NA EEEV die, and in the latest published data, it has been shown that most horses with SA EEEV die. Survivors are usually at least partially vaccinated equines [49] (Figure 19.5).

Diagnosis

Clinical signs and antemortem clinical pathologic findings are not specific for alphavirus infection. Viral encephalitides can cause abnormal CSF, but EEEV is unique in that acute infection frequently results in a neutrophilic pleocytosis (Figure 19.5). The neutrophils in the CSF are not toxic and frequently are hypersegmented. In more chronic or in partially vaccinated horses, the cellular component may be mononuclear. Because high mortality is associated with this disease, identification of a neutrophilic pleocytosis indicates probable EEE infection and offers the veterinarian a chance to prognosticate regarding the horse's survival.

The demonstration of specific IgM antibody (dilution of 1:400) is a highly specific and sensitive method for diagnosis [83]. The detection of IgM antibody in CSF (if available) is even more conclusive but this author has not found this as consistent as the detection of serum IgM. Rising antibody titers to EEEV, WEEV, or VEEV in the sera of horses that survive can be detected by testing of acute-phase and convalescent-phase sera, but the opportunity to collect a second sample is curtailed by the high death loss. Even in endemic areas, it is not possible to diagnose or differentiate EEEV, WEEV, or VEEV in the horse with any certainty based on clinical signs and epidemiologic circumstances; definitive testing is required.

Rapid rt-PCR to be performed on clinical specimens has been developed that differentiate between the alphaviruses and flaviviruses [82, 84–92]. For alphaviruses, the CDC protocol utilizes two primer sets which also detects virus in formalin-fixed tissues.

Pathologic findings

In horses, brain lesions are thought to be the direct result of viral replication and are characterized by necrotizing encephalitis with neuronal dysfunction [54, 81, 86, 87, 93–95]. No consistent gross lesions are found in horses that die of EEEV except that the meninges are frequently congested. This congestion is usually quite pronounced with EEEV infection. In addition, frequent, focal areas of dark discoloration are found in brain slices and are most prominent in gray matter of the cerebrum at the level of the corona radiata. Histologically, neuronal necrosis with neurophagia, marked perivascular cuffing with both mononuclear and polymorphonuclear leukocytes, and focal and diffuse microglial proliferation are evident. The lesions are more pronounced in the gray matter than in the white matter of the brain. Lesions are most marked in the cerebral cortex, thalamus, and hypothalamus, whereas the spinal cord is mildly affected. Severe lesions usually occur more often in the cervical spinal cord than in lumbar cord segments.

Therapy

No known antiviral medications demonstrate reliable activity against alphaviruses, and treatment of disease in affected horses is supportive. The survival rate for EEEV infection is low compared with other infectious encephalitides. Some clinicians advocate the use of corticosteroids as a component of therapy for horses with neurologic signs consistent with viral encephalitis and neutrophilic CSF. If administered early, corticosteroids (to reduce brain edema) and intravenous (IV) fluids may aid recovery. In human patients, treatment with methylprednisolone (1000 mg/100-kg patient) is often recommended. Administration of flunixin meglumine (1.1 mg/kg q12 h IV) or other anti-inflammatory medications to horses with EEEV does not often result in the dramatic response frequently observed in horses with WNV. Mannitol (0.25–2.0 g/kg q24 h IV) may assist in the control of brain edema. Detomidine hydrochloride (0.02–0.04 mg/kg IV or IM) is effective for prolonged tranquilization.

IV immunoglobin therapy has been used in humans for both its proposed neutralization of virus and immunomodulatory effects [96]. Interferon-α (IFN-α) is a relatively common therapy; its recommendation is based on anecdotal reports in the human and veterinary literature [97–100]. More data is supporting suppression of type-I interferons in the pathogenesis of EEEV infection. Limited information regarding the efficacy of IFN-α in the horse is available.

Prevention

Eastern equine encephalomyelitis is 100% preventable with proper vaccination [101, 102]. All of the vaccines are formalin-inactivated preparations, consist of the same virus seed stock, and are multivalent containing either EEEV and WEEV or EEEV, WEEV, and VEEV antigens. These preparations can also now be purchased with WNV antigen. In the states most affected by EEEV, adult horses must be vaccinated a minimum of two times per year. Veterinarians should monitor surveillance data and be aware of areas where EEEV occurs year after year.

Horses that reside in endemic areas and are aged 4 years or less should receive alphavirus vaccines three times per year. It is essential that all broodmares be vaccinated 1 month before foaling to ensure adequate passive transfer to foals. All foals should be tested for adequate passive transfer 24 h after birth. In foals from vaccinated dams, vaccination should be performed at 6, 7, and 9 months. In foals where that dam has not been adequately vaccinated, vaccination should be performed at 4, 5, and 7 months. All yearlings must be vaccinated between January and March within the year after birth and receive at least two more injections 4 months apart. This vaccination schedule should continue until horses

are 4 years of age. All horses arriving in the south from northern states should be vaccinated 30 days before arrival. Imported horses that ship directly to southern states from countries where the vaccine cannot be obtained before arrival are at risk for EEEV throughout the first 2 years of their arrival. It is imperative that these horses receive three intial injections and then continue three times a year for at least 2 years after arriving in the southern United States.

Western equine encephalomyelitis
Etiology and epidemiology

WEE virus is also an alphavirus of the family Togaviridae and classified as a group-IV positive sense single-stranded RNA virus. WEE virus is most closely related to EEEV and it is theorized that WEEV evolved from EEEV. Phylogenetic analyses indicate that North and South American WEE lineages appear to have evolved independently over several decades [103–106]. Variant WEEV virus has been reported in several countries in South America (Argentina, Guyana, Ecuador, Brazil, Uruguay), but only in Argentina has it been associated with human disease and significant enzootics in horses [107–110]. There are two primary antigenic subtypes of NA WEEV virus and these include WEEV and Highlands J (HJ) viruses [103, 104, 110–114]. Although generally considered less pathogenic for mammals than WEEV variant virus, the HJ variant virus has caused natural cases of encephalitis in horses and is pathogenic for domestic turkeys, pheasants, and exotic species of birds [103, 112, 113]. Other subtypes of WEEV that may cause disease in North American horses include Fort Morgan and Buggy Creek viruses [115]. One WEEV variant, Y62-WEEV, has been identified in Russia [116]. Over the last decade, reports of WEEV in horses have been limited and sporadic, likely reflecting vaccination and protective immunity gained by subclinical exposure [117, 118].

In North America, *Culex tarsalis* is the primary vector that maintains WEEV in an enzootic cycle with birds, especially nestling passerines [119, 120]. *C. tarsalis* population abundance is favored by a rapid increase in temperature following a cool, wet spring, resulting in the rapid melting of snow and flooding of rivers [102, 121, 122]. This species of mosquito also has a predilection for irrigated lands as breeding sites [123]. In South America, where *C. tarsalis* does not occur, antibody prevalence rates in birds are lower than in North America, and the species (vertebrate and invertebrate) responsible for maintaining the virus on that continent have not been identified [124, 125]. *Aedes albasfaciatus* has experimentally transmitted WEEV to chickens in Argentina [124, 125].

Reservoir hosts for WEEV may be variable but the classic life cycle proposed is cycling of virus between a mosquito vector and avian reservoirs. Birds, snakes, and squirrels have all been experimentally infected [126–134]. Garter snakes became infected, were asymptomatic, and sustained viremia for an average of 10–12 days. Frogs were also found to be readily susceptible to infection. Both snakes and frogs could be inoculated orally. Birds in general do not have high sustained viremias in WEEV infection and also show limited disease [61, 108, 111, 123, 135–139]. Upon intranasal infection with WEEV, squirrels develop disease and also high levels of viremia before death [140–142]. Infection with WEEV in six species of rodents has been performed and several of these species were susceptible to the virus with some having high and sustained viremias [143]. Although this was dependent upon the strain of WEEV used, small ground mammals may be important reservoirs for WEEV [123]. Like EEEV infections in emus, these animals are susceptible to disease and have been part of epizootics as recently as the mid-1990s. Vaccination is recommended for these species. Horses, even those that are obviously clinically affected, do not produce an adequate viremia to infect mosquitoes [144].

Clinical signs

Although WEEV causes less severe signs than either EEEV or VEEV, this virus is neuroinvasive across strains and neurological signs of disease in horses are similar to alphaviruses [1, 145]. Like its other neurotropic relatives, children and young animals of all susceptible species are more likely than adults to develop clinical CNS disease. After experimental inoculation, there is a short febrile response at 2–3 days (likely corresponding to viremia) [81]. The time to onset of neurological disease of WEEV is generally 7 days to 2 weeks (some reports indicate as short as 3 days, but this cannot be verified). Inapparent infections in horses are common. In clinical cases, pyrexia is the first clinical manifestation of infection. Temperature has usually abated or is only moderately elevated by the time signs of encephalitis become evident. The course of disease in severely affected horses varies between 2 and 14 days. Most horses fully recover from WEEV and the mortality rate (case-fatality rate) is 20–30%.

Diagnosis

CSF has a mononuclear cell population primarily consisting of lymphocytes. Protein concentration within the CSF may or may not be elevated and the average white blood cell count is 100–200 cells/μl. As stated earlier, most of the reliable antemortem testing is based on detection of antibody responses to WEEV. Since horses frequently survive infection, virus neutralization testing can demonstrate a rising (fourfold minimum change) titer that is confirmatory. If a horse succumbs to infection, then a postmortem examination with antigen detection consisting of either IHC, rt-PCR, or viral isolation

should be performed, especially for public and animal health purposes.

Treatment

Like EEEV, treatment of WEEV infection is supportive. In a 1933 publication, it was reported that treatment of horses with plasma from surviving (hyperimmunized) horses was therapeutic [146]. There is experimental evidence in a hamster model of WEEV that treatment with interferon increased survival [99]. Other novel antiviral agents may be on the horizon [147, 148].

Prevention

Western equine encephalomyelitis is 100% preventable with the standard protocols indicated in Section "Prevention" for EEEV [101, 102]. Because the incidence of WEEV has dramatically declined in the United States, even in sentinel and mosquito testing, it has been recommended by some clinicians that WEEV be removed from the multivalent preparations for immunization. This is inadvisable because WEEV disease in humans and horses still occurs in South America; the last reported outbreak was in Brazil in 2006 [51].

Venezuelan equine encephalitis
Etiology and epidemiology

VEEV is one of the most important human and veterinary pathogens in the New World [6, 149–152]. The VEEV complex is composed of six distinct subtypes (I–VI) with several strains within subtypes designated by letter [153]. The "epidemic or epizootic type" of VEEV (types IAB, IC, and IE) has been isolated during outbreaks of encephalitis in horses in the Western Hemisphere in the past 20 years. The "endemic or enzootic" types of VEEV are considered to be of low pathogenicity for equids under most circumstances and are isolated from reservoir hosts [81, 154, 155]. These include ID and IF variants from Central America and Brazil, respectively [150, 153]. Type II (Everglades) virus is found in Florida. Three known variants exist of type III (Mucambo) virus and these viruses have been isolated in Trinidad, French Guiana, Western North America, and Peru. The others are type IV (Pixuna) virus, type V (Cabassou) virus, and type VI virus [153, 156]. The Pixuna subtype of VEEV is associated with febrile illness in horses in Brazil [153].

Epidemics reveal the potential for VEEV to spread rapidly within an equine population, with a case-fatality rate approaching 90% in some areas and this is confirmed in more recent outbreaks [79, 157, 158]. The availability of vaccines and active surveillance throughout the Americas since the early 1970s have reduced the overall impact of the disease [155]. However, outbreaks of VEEV continue to occur in Chiapas and Oaxaca, Mexico, and in Venezuela and Colombia [155, 159–162].

Key to understanding the epidemiology of VEEV is recognition of the differences in the basic biology of two transmission cycles, enzootic and epizootic, of this virus [6]. Three basic changes occur in the enzootic–epizootic cycling: (i) the virus mutates closer to the more pathogenic IAB and IC strains, (ii) there is a change in reservoir host from the spiny rat to the equine, and (iii) there is a change in mosquito vector [163–167]. The enzootic cycle centers around sylvatic rodents such as spiny and cotton rats, which have high natural infection rates, and can develop viremia high enough to transmit VEEV to mosquitoes [156, 167–171]. Even opossums, bats, and shore birds likely are important in dispersal of enzootic virus [78, 172, 173]. The importance of equine infection in maintenance of epizootic VEEV is evidenced by the observation that human disease has never been demonstrated in the absence of equine disease [81, 174, 175]. All mammalian hosts are capable of developing a high-titer viremia of approximately 10^5–10^7 pfu/ml for up to 5 days [81, 155, 164]. In contrast to EEEV and WEEV, where horses are not considered to be a major source of virus for the vector, in VEEV epidemics, horses are the most important amplifiers of virus activity.

Humans usually develop a flu-like illness, with only 4–14% exhibiting neurologic signs and symptoms [78]. Case-fatality rate for humans is approximately 1%. Several other species of mammals, including domestic rabbits, small ruminants, and dogs, develop potentially fatal clinical disease after VEEV virus infection [176]. During an epizootic, dogs regularly become infected and may be capable of virus amplification [177–179]. Cattle and swine also seroconvert [178]. More than 100 species of birds have been either virologically or serologically associated with the transmission of epidemic VEEV virus, and shore birds and herons appear to be amplifier hosts [180]. Birds may develop viremia as high as 10^8 TCID$_{50}$/ml of blood.

The subgenus Melanoconion (*Culex cedecci*) is likely to be the most important vector of enzootic VEEV [181]. This vector resides in tropical forests and swamps and feeds on small forest mammals at night. Several species of mosquitoes from at least 11 genera have been determined to be naturally infected with epidemic strains of VEEV [109, 167, 175, 182–185]. Virus has also been isolated from *Culicoides* spp. (Ceratopogonidae) and black flies (Simuliidae), but it is not known whether insects in these families are capable of biologic transmission of VEEV [109]. In addition, ticks, including the species *Amblyomma cajennense* and *Hyalomma truncatum*, may be capable of viral transmission [132, 186–188].

Clinical findings
The clinical findings are similar to EEEV except that there can be a wider variation in mortality in horses ranging from 40 to 90%. Diagnosis and pathological findings are also similar to EEEV and WEEV.

Prevention
Immunization of horses has proved highly effective as an adjunct to other control measures, particularly in epidemics of VEEV because horses serve as a source of infection for mosquitoes [189–191]. The 1969–1971 VEEV epidemic in Central America and the southern United States was controlled partially by immunizing large numbers of horses with an attenuated VEEV virus strain, TC-83 [189–191]. This vaccine strain was produced by serial passages of an epidemic variant in guinea pig cell cultures. Because of concerns over the presence of low-level viremia in some horses and the possible transmission of vaccine virus between horses by mosquitoes and reversion to virulence, inactivated vaccines against VEEV are now available for use in horses. These vaccines are not widely used in North America because they compromise the international movement of horses for competition and breeding.

The distinct possibility exists that epidemic VEEV could be completely prevented if sustained and widespread vaccination was performed in Central and South America [192]. The use of the formalin inactivated vaccine (usually marketed as a multivalent antigen) in the face of outbreaks is likely not as effective in VEEV epidemics because of the need for multiple vaccinations (and thus delayed onset of protection) [192]. Formalinized vaccines generally induce short-lived immunity to VEEV and this results in a lack of long-term compliance by owners and agricultural officials. In the long run, more rural economies cannot sustain multiple annual vaccination protocols. Thus, development of safe vaccines that induce long-term protection in equids that is reasonable for agrarian economies is essential for controlling epizootics.

Surveillance for encroachment of alphaviruses in new geographic locales is also paramount to control. As a foreign animal disease, USDA has subsidized testing for horses with suspected viral encephalitis; however, with regionalization of testing and enhanced status as a biological threat, the surveillance testing has actually decreased in some states.

Miscellaneous alphaviruses

Semliki Forest virus
Etiology, epidemiology, clinical findings, diagnosis, pathology, and prevention
Semliki Forest virus is the type species of several viruses that infect horses and is a cause of encephalitis in horses [193, 194]. Getah virus and Ross River virus (RRV) are two other viruses that cause disease in horses. Getah causes mainly hemolymphatic disease and is not discussed in this chapter [195]. This virus is found mainly in central, eastern, southern Africa, and serologically in Europe [194]. Because of its neurotropism, most of what is known

about the virus comes from its biological manipulations as a vector and model in rodents. The pathogenesis in people appears to be relatively limited. In general, the disease causes flu-like symptoms with myalgia and weakness in people. Encephalitis has been reported in horses [193].

Ross river virus
Etiology and epidemiology
Continental Australia, Tasmania, West Papua and Papua New Guinea, New Caledonia, Fiji, Samoa, and the Cook Islands have all reported the presence of RRV [196–208]. The virus infects a variety of vertebrate hosts including a large number of placental, marsupial, and monotreme mammals and birds [209, 210]. Kangaroos and wallabies likely are the natural reservoir host [211–214]. Disease in horses occurs annually in Australia with endemic foci with year-round activity in areas. Outbreaks of encephalitis in Australian equids can have mulitple etiologies concurrently and can consist of all three encephalitides encountered including either RRV, Murray Valley encephalitis virus (MVEV), or Kunjin Virus (KV) [215].

Clinical findings
Systemic clincial signs include increased rectal temperature, anorexia, petechial hemorrhages of the mucous membranes, submandibular lymphadenopathy, and mild colic [215, 216]. Gait abnormalities include lameness, stiff gait, swollen joints, distal limbs edema, reluctance to move, and ataxia [91, 217]. Horses are often described as being ataxic, although the neurologic basis of this sign is unclear [215, 217]. The signs of debilitation and pain have been reported to persist for months.

Diagnosis
Limited data exists regarding the clinicopatholocal changes; only elevated fibrinogen and globulins in plasma were reported in three horses with the apparent disease [91, 215, 217]. Confirmation of RRV includes virus isolation from serum or heparinized blood samples or detecion of virus in blood and synovial fluid using rt-PCR [91]. Like other alphaviruses, the IgM-capture ELISA is consistent with recent infection or exposure. Neutralizing antibody develops within 2–3 weeks and paired serum is appropriate [215]. Usually once horses develop IgG, virus isolation is unrewarding [215]. Interpretation of a horse with RRV infection should be made in the light of clinical signs and lack of identification of other causes of clinical signs and/or other arboviruses that coexist geographically with RRV.

Therapy and prevention
Treatment of affected horse is supportive and mostly should consist of anti-inflammatory medications. No vaccine is currently available. Control methods reflect those previously mentioned in the overview.

Flavivirus infections

Japanese encephalitis serogroup: WNV, Japanese encephalitis virus, KV, MVEV
Among the 53 species of *Flavivirus*, there are a number of historically significant and pathologically active viruses responsible for disease in horses including Japanese encephalitis (JE), West Nile encephalitis (WNE), KV, and MVEV [194, 218–221]. Overall, the diseases caused by the JE serogroup are similar and thus will be discussed as a group except where differences are notable. All of these viruses are transmitted by a mosquito vector, with *Culex* spp. usually the most efficient transmitter [222–231]. KV is actually a strain of WNV. Disease in horses caused by MVEV, known as Murray Valley fever, is geographically restricted to the South Pacific and is sporadic in occurrence [232–235]. Several other members of the flaviviruses genus have also been detected serologically in horses but with limited reports of clinical disease (Table 19.1).

Flaviviruses are positive-sense, single-stranded RNA viruses measuring approximately 50 nm in external diameter [219]. The virions are spherical, enveloped, and contain a nucleocapsid composed of a capsid protein approximately 120 amino acids in length [236–241]. Electron microscopy reveals an icosahedral symmetry of the envelope and capsid. An approximately 11-kilobase (kb) genome contains a single open reading frame that is translated in its entirety and cleaved into 10 viral proteins by both cell and viral proteases [242]. There are three structural proteins, including capsid (C), premembrane (prM) and membrane (M), envelope (E), and seven nonstructural (NS) proteins [243, 244]. The NS proteins are cleaved after translation into NS1, NS2A, NS2B, NS3, NS4A, NS4B, and NS5 and are required for viral replication and assembly.

The C, M, and E proteins are important in virulence for the JE group [245–252]. Although not understood entirely, the C protein is essential in viron assembly and large deletions in its sequence render the WNV virus nonvirulent [253]. The E-protein of WNV has been shown to be the major antigen that elicits neutralizing antibodies [254, 255]. Thus, this antigen is of key interest for therapeutic, vaccine, and diagnostic development. The E-protein has three structural domains including domain I (DI) that is involved in E-protein structural rearrangements necessary for fusion, DII that is involved in the pH-dependent fusion of virion and host cell, and DIII that is involved in the receptor binding domain. The M protein is formed from a precursor protein (prM protein), which is modified as immature virions are secreted through the Golgi network of the cell, leaving the C-terminal portion of the protein inserted in the envelope of the mature virion.

Among other things, M protein may play a role in viral replication [256–258]. The glycoprotein NS1 is essential for virus function, appears to be important for cell activation as part of viral synthesis, and interacts with complement proteins [259–264]. NS2A and NS2B are formed by cleavage of full-length NS2 with NS2A important in viral replication and NS2B exhibiting protease activity [265–268]. The NS3 protein is highly conserved between flaviviruses and, at the N-terminal, encodes a serine protease. The C-terminal of this protein has sequences typical of RNA helicases and triphosphatases [240, 266, 269, 270]. The NS4B protein appears to block antiviral cytokines. The NS5 protein is essential for viral replication by forming the "cap" at the $5'$ end of a genome [271, 272]. In addition, this is the site of the viral RNA-dependent RNA polymerase (RdRp), an essential protein for formation of negative-strand RNA from the genome of the positive-strand "parent" RNA virus.

Japanese encephalitis serogroup viruses are vector-borne diseases, with transmission occurring to avian and mammalian hosts from blood meal–seeking mosquitoes [222–231]. Although *Culex* is important in the epidemiology and spread of these flaviviruses, relatively little is known regarding the actual vector of transmission to the horse as some of these species are limited to avian feeding [273]. Reservior hosts are required for amplification and maintenance of the virus year-round and all of these have avian reservoirs. There may be additional birds such as passerines or a mammal involved (Table 19.1). Horses and humans are "dead-end" hosts and do not amplify the virus in quantities sufficient to infect mosquitoes [273, 274]. Swine are a notable reservoir host for JE. Horses do develop virus levels of 10^1–10^3 pfu/ml after experimental exposure to WNV-positive mosquitoes, similar to other flaviviruses [275]. Additional modes of transmission have been identified in the recent North American WNV outbreak. First, transmission through oral ingestion has been proven in both avian and mammalian hosts, and oral and cloacal shedding has been demonstrated in birds [276–278]. Second, WNV may be transmitted through contaminated blood transfusion or organ transplantation if donors are viremic [279]. Third, vertical transmission through placenta and milk has been demonstrated in equids and people with WNV and in sows with JE with the primary clinical manifestation being abortion, birth of weak pigs, and neonatal mortality.

The largest documented outbreak of equine neurologic disease caused by a flavivirus began in 1999 with WNV encroachment into the United States emerging in the New York City, New York [280]. In 2002, an epizootic resulted in 14 571 cases of WNEE [281]. Between 1999 and 2006, nearly 25 000 cases of equine WNV

cases were reported in the United States with an estimated 30–40% case-fatality rate. Positive equine case reporting fell to an average of 300 a year from 2007 to 2010. In 2012, a very large epizootic occurred with 5 674 human and 690 horse cases reported [282]. Japanese encephalitis virus (JEV) causes 30 000–50 000 human encephalitis cases annually worldwide, with endemic areas including China, the southeast region of the Russian Federation, South and Southeast Asia, and Australia [283, 284]. Exact numbers of horses with clinical JE are difficult to ascertain; however, there are reports of JE isolation from horses in Taiwan, China, Pakistan, and Australia in the literature since the 1980s [1, 285–289]. Seroprevalence studies in Japan indicate that the natural exposure rate has been stable in several provences, around 15–20% and in some locations has increased as high as 50–70% [290, 291]. Outbreaks in horses have also been reported in India, Nepal, the Philippines, Sri Lanka, and Northern Thailand [292–296].

Occurrence of flaviviral disease in horses and people reflects vector activity, seasonal in temperate regions, and year-round in subtropical and tropical regions [219, 276, 297]. Intense virus activity in the United States begins in July, with a peak incidence in September and October. The appearance of disease from JE is actually highly variable depending on the locale. Seasonal occurrence of disease in specific locales should be considered to facilitate timing of equine athletic events and to tailor vaccination regimens appropriately. In 2011, Australia experienced the largest epidemic of arboviral disease in history affecting around 900 horses. Although multiple pathogens were detected including KV, MVEV, and RRV, there was emergence of a new strain of KV [216].

No sex or breed disposition is evident. Older people appear more susceptible to neuroinvasive disease from both JEV and WNV [298] and this age bias in reporting appears true, at least for WNV, in horses [299]. In one study of horses with WNV encephalomyelitis, female horses were 2.9 times more likely to die than male horses with neurologic signs.

Pathogenesis

In general, mammalian disease caused by infection with the JE serogroup viruses reflects a predilection for nervous tissue. Neurologic disease in the horse consists of changes in mentation, signs consistent with spinal cord abnormalities, and defects of cranial nerves of the hindbrain [274, 300–303]. Change in behavior likely results from viral infection and pathology induced in the neurons of the thalamus, medulla, and pons, with limited viral load in the cerebrum [304–307]. Although the thalamus integrates all sensory input to higher centers, lesions within the midbrain and rostral pons may affect the reticular formation, which has an important role in regulation of consciousness. The reticular formation projects to the thalamus, which in turn sends diffuse projections to the entire cortex. Disturbances of the reticular formation and the midbrain may induce behavioral changes ranging from severe aggression to somnolence and even coma. Flavivirus-induced motor deficits are multifocal, asymmetric, and primarily characterized by weakness and ataxia [300–303]. These two clinical signs are likely a reflection of brain and spinal cord disease through direct infection of the spinal cord, interruption of motor tracts in the hindbrain, and loss of fine motor control through infection of the large nuclei of the thalamus and the basal ganglia. Lower motor neuron disease characterized by weakness would be a common clinical sign associated with these spinal cord lesions. Involuntary skin and muscle fasciculations, tremors, and hyperesthesia are extremely common in WNV disease and have been described in horses with JE and KV, and likely result from loss of fine motor control, which is regulated mainly by the basal ganglia [197, 308, 309]. Infection in the pons and medulla oblongata can explain clinical deficits of cranial nerves VII, XII, and IX [304–307].

Like humans, horses also develop signs of flaccid paralysis which in the quadripedal movement of the horse reflects lower motor neuron disease. These clinical signs likely reflect focal invasion of the lower motor neuron. Two routes of neuroinvasion are proposed for WNV and likely other flavivirus infections. In the first, WNV causes a low-level viremia, followed by replication in the lymph nodes and entry into the CNS across the blood–brain barrier (BBB) [310]. The second proposes transaxonal transmission [311, 312]. In the first theory, it is hypothesized that systemic viral infection results in local cytokine responses that increase the permeability of the BBB to viral invasion. In particular, tumor necrosis factor alpha (TNF-α) increases vascular permeability and allows infection of peripheral nerves [313]. Evidence indicates that toll-like receptors are crucial for entry of WNV into the CNS, whether by neuronal or vascular route [310, 314, 315].

Clinical findings

Flaviviruses produce similar clinical signs, except that fatal JEV infection in horses usually results in blindness, coma, and death, whereas these signs are relatively limited in WNV in horses [274, 300–303]. For MVEV and KV, these diseases are more similar to WNV; MVEV is more pathogenic while KV appears less severe [197, 216, 316]. For all of these infections, there is evidence of widespread subclinical infection in both people and horses. Horses and people also exhibit the same disease course based on lineage of virus; clinical neurological disease develops when infected with the neurally invasive lineage type-I WNV, whereas infection with the

African lineage type-II viruses is universally subclinical in nature [317]. Infection with JEV may result in severe clinical disease in naive horses, but great variation in virulence is actually seen.

When clinically apparent disease occurs, both systemic and neurologic abnormalities are observed in horses with these infections. A mild to moderate increase in rectal temperature (38.6–39.4°C (102–103°F)), anorexia, and depression are the most common initial systemic signs [301, 318]. Abdominal pain or a colic episode may be the first clinical presentation [299, 301]. Gait abnormalities, including overt lameness or dragging of a limb, before development of an obvious neurologic syndrome have also been reported. Both spinal cord disease and moderate mental aberrations occur. Onset of neurologic signs is frequently sudden and progressive, and the exact course of disease in any one animal is unpredictable.

One of the initial signs of motor abnormality is a short, slow, stilted gait, described by observers as "lameness," with laminitis being a frequent differential diagnosis at this stage. In human patients, however, bradykinesia or slow, deliberate movement is frequently described, and this may be the equine corollary. Spinal abnormalities are characterized by ataxia and paresis that can be highly asymmetric or may involve only one or two of the forelimbs or hindlimbs and is usually characterized by a flaccid paresis that is localized to one or more limbs. This state may be of short duration, or horses may become suddenly recumbent and either die or require prolonged treatment.

The major hallmarks of equine flavivirus encephalomyelitis are muscle fasciculations and changes in personality [197, 274, 301, 308, 309]. Fine and coarse fasciculations of the muscles of the face and neck are common. Fasciculations can be severe and can involve all four limbs and the trunk, affecting normal activities such as walking, eating, and interactions with handlers and other horses. The fasciculations are most notable in the muzzle and eyelids. Eyelid activity during this period is enhanced with light, and at times horses appear photophobic. Many horses have periods of hyperexcitability and apprehension, sometimes to the point of aggression. Frequently, a quiet horse will become hyperexcitable, and an abnormally aggressive horse will become compliant. Interspersed during periods of hyperexcitability, some horses appear to have abnormalities of sudden sleeplike activity resembling narcolepsy. This can occur to the point of cataplexy, and horses may partially or completely collapse for a short period. Some horses show a persistent change of mentation, and a state of nonresponsiveness, resembling coma, results (Figure 19.6).

Cranial nerves are frequently abnormal for short periods; weakness of the tongue, muzzle deviation, and

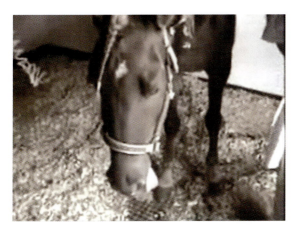

Figure 19.6 Photograph of a horse with West Nile virus encephalomyelitis. Horse would eat hay but would dribble grain. Cranial nerve examination reveals weak tongue; horse could not retract tongue back into her mouth once it was pulled to the left.

head tilt are the most common abnormalities reported (Figure 19.7). Dysphagia has been reported, with esophageal obstruction, a possible sequela. Autonomic nervous system dysfunction likely accounts for the respiratory failure and gastrointestinal distrubances [319]. A cauda equine syndrome consisting of stranguria and rectal impaction is infrequently reported.

Overall, the combination, severity, and duration of clinical signs can be highly variable. After initial clinical signs abate, about 30% of WNV horses experience a recrudescence in signs within the first 7–10 days of apparent recovery. Overall, about 30% of affected horses progress to complete paralysis of one or more limbs overall. Most of these horses are euthanized for humane reasons or die spontaneously. The overall mortality rate for JE is 10–30%, WNV is 35–45%, MVEV is 10%, and KJ is 8–10% [197, 211, 216, 299, 301, 316, 320].

Many horses with WNV will improve within 3–7 days of displaying clinical signs. If the horse demonstrates significant improvement, full recovery within 1–6 months can be expected in 90% of patients [321]. Residual weakness and ataxia appear common, with long-term loss of the use of one or more limbs infrequently described. Mild to moderate, persistent fatigue on exercise has been observed.

Diagnosis

Ancillary diagnostic testing for horses with suspected flavivirus infection should include CBC, serum biochemistry analysis, and CSF analysis [322]. CBC and serum biochemistry profiles of flavivirus-infected horses are usually normal, but basic clinical chemistry analysis

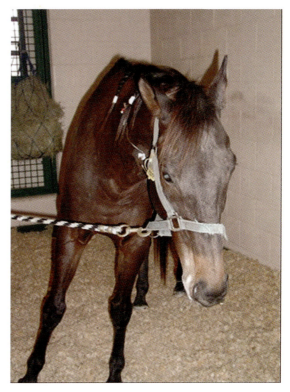

Figure 19.7 Photograph of a horse with West Nile virus encephalomyelitis. Horse is exhibiting a muzzle deviation to left consistent with right sided facial paralysis while at the same time leaning circling to the right (handler is pulling lead to left in order to keep the horse from leaning against the wall.

can rule out systemic causes of CNS abnormalities such as liver failure. In general, flavivirus-infected horses can have increased muscle enzymes secondary to trauma and prolonged periods of recumbency [301]. A frequent finding is hyponatremia, which has also been described in humans with encephalitis, potentially caused by inappropriate release of antidiuretic hormone [301, 323, 324].

CSF cell counts and protein concentration may be increased [274, 322, 325]. Differential cell counts in CSF of flavivirus-infected horses primarily have increased mononuclear cell populations (Figure 19.8). Protein concentrations in the CSF are frequently elevated (N <70 mg/dl) and the color of the fluid can be mildly xanthochromic.

No pathognomonic signs distinguish flavivirus infection in horses from other CNS diseases, and a full diagnostic evaluation should be pursued. Confirmation of flavivirus infection with encephalitis in horses begins with assessment of (i) whether the horse meets the case definition based on clinical signs and (ii) whether or not the horse resides in an area in which flavivirus has been confirmed in the current calendar year in mosquito, bird, human, or horse. Serologic testing is based on detection of the IgM antibody response that uniformly occurs in acutely infected horses and this has been found for most arboviruses [300, 326]. Horses develop a very intense IgM response on exposure to flavivirus that lasts approximately 6 weeks. This immunologic reaction is much more reliable than in human infection, where a more persistent IgM response is common. Most diagnostic laboratories utilize a flavivirus IgM-capture ELISA (MAC) for actual confirmation of disease; this may be confounded by recent vaccination [327–330]. In the nonvaccinated horse, a fourfold change in paired neutralizing antibody titers is confirmatory of a diagnosis of flavivirus infection. The most common neutralizing antibody test formats are the classic plaque reduction neutralization test (PRNT) for detecting antibody response and a more recently developed microwell format [331, 332]. Since the marketing of equine WNV vaccines in 2001 and common vaccination for JE, reliance on the PRNT for serologic confirmatory diagnosis of flaviviruses in horses has diminished. ELISA and microsphere immunoassy utilizing recombinant NS1 protein may be useful in detecting antibody response due to natural infection of vaccination [333–335].

Other methods of confirmation for a diagnosis of WNV include postmortem detection of WNV by PCR, culture, and IHC in CNS tissues [336–338]. Several methods for the detection of flavivirus nucleic acids and antigens in equine tissue have been described with caveats previously described including proper selection of tissues and relatively low virus load in tissues.

Pathologic findings

Flaviviruses cause polioencephalomyelitis (inflammation of the gray matter) with lesions that increase in number from the diencephalon through the hindbrain and frequently increase in severity caudally through the spinal cord [95, 197, 274, 305, 309]. The location of the histologic changes within the brain, including inflammatory foci and detectable virus in the thalamus, medulla, and pons, are consistent with changes in behavior. Gross pathologic findings are limited in flavivirus infection in the horse. The meninges may be congested and small to moderately sized foci of hemorrhagic discoloration may be observed in the brain and spinal cord. These areas occur most often in the basal ganglia, rostral colliculus, pons, medulla, and lumbar spinal cord. Edema and softening of tissues are also common findings.

Histopathologic changes secondary to flavivirus infection are consistent with viral infection and neural cell death (Figure 19.9) [95, 197, 274, 303–305, 309]. The basal ganglia, thalamus, pons, and medulla have the highest numbers of lesions, with two to several cell layers of predominantly mononuclear perivascular cuffing. Predominantly confined to the gray matter, glial nodules are present in the brain parenchyma. By contrast, these lesions are limited in number in the cortex and cerebellum compared to mid- and hindbrains. Neuronal damage includes chromatolytic neurons and neuronophagia. Horses with long-standing disease may have areas of neuronal dropout. In the spinal cord, there is perivascular cuffing, glial nodule formation, and damaged neurons. It is still unknown if these cellular changes are attributable to viral damage or resulting inflammation.

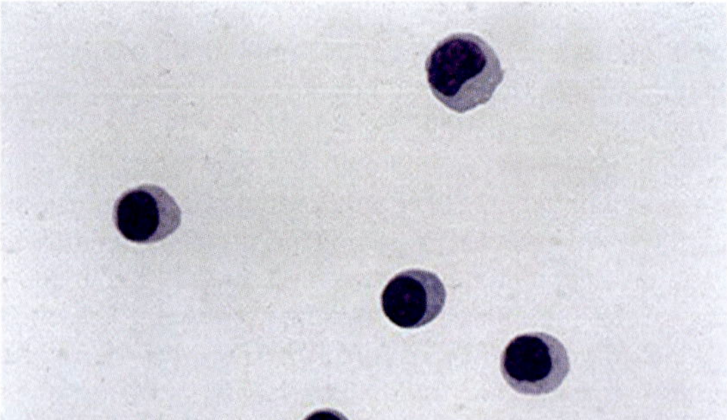

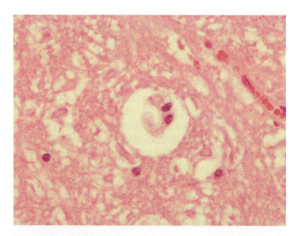

Figure 19.8 Photomicrograph of cerebrospinal fluid (CSF) from horse with WNV encephalomyelitis. The CSF contains more than 90% macrophages and lymphocytes.

Figure 19.9 Photomicrograph demonstrating an extremely dilated axon sheath from a horse with West Nile virus encephalomyelitis.

Therapy

No known antiviral medications are marketed that demonstrate reliable activity against flaviviruses, and thus treatment of disease is supportive [301]. In horses, the survival rate for WNV encephalitis is high compared with other infectious encephalitides, but WNV is more pathogenic than MVEV. Most horses appear to begin recovery 3–5 days after onset of signs, which makes it difficult to assess any pharmacologic intervention accurately, when a feature of analysis is resolving clinical disease. Flunixin meglumine, 1.1 mg/kg every 12 h (q12 h) intravenously, early in the course of the disease appears to decrease the severity of muscle tremors and fasciculations within a few hours of administration.

To date, much of the mortality in WNV horses results from euthanasia of recumbent horses for humane reasons, yet with little intervention the spontaneous death rate is 35%, while for MVEV and KV, the the case-fatality rate appears to be 10%. Therapy of recumbent horses is generally more aggressive and may include dexamethasone sodium (0.05–0.1 mg/kg q24 h IV) and mannitol (0.25–2.0 g/kg q24 h IV). Controversy remains as to whether or not corticosteroids enhance peripheral and CNS viral load, and in a canine model of WNV, viremia was increased 40–50× with methylprednisolone therapy [339]. Detomidine hydrochloride (0.02–0.04 mg/ kg IV or intramuscularly [IM]) is effective for prolonged tranquilization. Low doses of acepromazine (0.02 mg/kg IV or 0.05 mg/kg IM) provide excellent relief from anxiety in both recumbent and standing horses. In the United States, until EPM is ruled out or WNV is confirmed, therapy with antiprotozoal medications is recommended for horses in geographic areas where *Sarcocystis neurona* infection is prevalent. Other supportive measures may include oral and IV fluids and antibiotics for treatment of infections that frequently occur in recumbent horses (wounds, cellulitis, and pneumonia).

Recommendation for IFN-α therapy is based on anecdotal reports in the human and veterinary literature [340–342]. Limited information regarding efficacy in the horse is available. In a blinded study in which children with encephalitis caused by JEV were treated with IFN-α, survival was not enhanced. In fact, length of hospitalization was increased in the IFN-α-treated group.

Therapy with WNV-specific recombinant immunoglobulin has also been recommended and therapy with a monoclonal antibody is under clinical trials [343]. In a blinded placebo-controlled trial with low numbers of animals, the risk for development of recumbency was less in horses receiving plasma from horses immunized against WNV (Long, unpublished data). However, plasma treatment did not change the outcome and severity of WNV disease. For an excellent review in experimental and future treatments of viral encephalitis, see Nath and Tylor [344].

Prevention

Currently, several whole virion, one recombinant-inactivated vaccine, and a canary pox vectored vaccine are licensed for prevention of WNV viremia in the United States, and an inactived virus vaccine is readily available against JE [290, 327, 331, 345–352]. Vaccination before the mosquito season is critical. The manufacturer's labeling instructions must be followed for induction of immunity with initial immunization. More frequent vaccination in areas with year-round mosquito seasons is highly recommended. Limited information is available regarding long-term immunity after vaccination. However, it is not expected that the initial vaccine series will provide long-term protection; antibody levels rapidly decrease after 4–6 months. Where these viruses are endemic, vaccination schedules should be maintained even with a decrease in the incidence of overt disease. This is evidenced by the reports of JE disease in naive horses after introduction into endemic areas. Horses that have recovered from clinical disease have long-term immunity and should not require annual boosters.

Miscellaneous flaviviruses

Powassan virus

The Powassan virus, a flavivirus, is found in Ontario and the eastern United States and produces a nonsuppurative, focal necrotizing meningoencephalitis in horses [353–355]. There have not been any large serosurveys in the equid to Powassan since the late 1980s, and recent surveillance indicates that Powassan is still active in Canada and the United States [282, 356, 357]. Many of the clinical signs described in experimental intracerebral inoculation of the Powassan virus during the 1980s were similar to the intracerebral challenges of WNV recently performed [353–355]. Within 8 days, horses developed reluctance to move, tremors of the head and neck, hyperesthesia, continuous chewing and increased salivation leading to foamy saliva, gait abnormalities, and recumbency. Pathologically, there is a nonsuppurative encephalomyelitis, neuronal necrosis, and focal parenchymal necrosis with a predilection for the gray matter as is seen with other flaviviruses. The virus was recovered from the brain of infected ponies and horses.

Tick-borne encephalitis complex: tick-borne encephalitis and louping ill

There are three subtypes of the tick-borne encephalitis (TBE) complex including European, Far Eastern, and Siberian [358]. This type of virus was described in 1931 and isolated in 1937 [359–365]. Most of these viruses are primarily distributed throughout north central Eurasia. Transmission is predominantly via ticks including

Ixodes, *Dermacentor*, and *Haemaphysalis* species. Ruminants are more frequently infected than horses and small mammals are likely important reservoirs. Transmission can occur through milk. Serosurveys in horses conducted in Germany demonstrated that 2.9% of tested horses (240) were positive [366].

Louping ill, subtype TBE, is primarily a disease of ruminants but can infect horses, and equine infections have been described in Europe [367–370]. In particular, an outbreak in Ireland was described in the 1970s. Extensive work demonstrated that horses were susceptible to experimental challenge and developed viremia for several days after challenge. Serological surveys at that time indicated a 10% seropositivity rate in horses.

Bunyaviridae

Bunyaviridae are negative sense and antisense RNA viruses that comprise the largest group of arthropod-borne viruses found throughout the world [371]. The life cycle of this group of viruses is much more complex than alphaviruses and flaviviruses, demonstrating a tri-partite genome that has three segments (creatively named large (L), medium (M), and small (S)) that create a helical nucleic acid structure once they form a pseudocircular structure. The S segment encodes the nucleocapsid structural protein, while the M protein encodes for a polyprotein that eventually forms a protein that mediates virus assembly, formation of virus particles, and cellular attachment. The L protein primarily encodes for the RdRp, important in RNA transcription and replication. Multiple rodent and lagomorph species are reservoirs.

Most Bunyaviridae demonstrate a predilection for the nervous system including infected fetal tissues resulting in congenital malformation and postgestational infection causing mainly encephalitis. The group contains one of the important emerging zoonoses, Rift Valley fever [372]. For equids, several strains of the orthobunyavirus family have been isolated out of horses worldwide [373–380]. In the United States, most of the cases have been reported along the eastern half of the continent with focal areas of higher incidence along the Appalachian mountain range and the upper Mississippi basin; however, horses in California have demonstrated up to 60% seropositivity to the California serogroup virus, Jamestown Canyon virus. The viruses are transmitted by mosquitoes; a number of notable Bunyaviruses such as Rift Valley fever are transmitted by *Culicoides* spp.

Most information in the literature of equine Bunyavirus-mediated disease consists of serosurveys of normal horses. Regarding the disease, the Bunyamwera serogroup, Snowshoe hare virus, California serogroup, Cache Valley virus, Main Drain, Santa Cruz, and Shuni viruses have all been isolated from horses with acute encephalitis [194, 375, 381, 382]. Systemic clinical findings have included tachycardia, fever, and anorexia. Neurological abnormalities have included proprioceptive deficits, ataxia, and cranial nerve deficits consisting mostly of dysphagia. Some horses have had cortical signs including head-pressing.

Diagnosis and prevention

As there are no serological tests for Bunyaviruses commonly performed in any veterinary diagnostic laboratories, antibodies to Bunyaviruses are only rarely reported. The most common method of detection in the clinical case is virus isolation from the brain of an infected horse. Horses are not routinely screened by rt-PCR for Bunyaviruses except for some notable US states and country laboratories where these viruses are considered endemic. There is likely under-identification of these viruses in horses. There are no vaccines available.

References

[1] Gibbs, E.P. (1976) Equine viral encephalitis. *Equine Vet J*, 8, 66–71.

[2] Weaver, S.C., Scott, T.W. and Rico-Hesse, R. (1991) Molecular evolution of eastern equine encephalomyelitis virus in North America. *Virology*, 182, 774–784.

[3] Gibbs, E.P.J. (2004) Equine encephalitides caused by alphaviruses, in *Infectious Diseases of Livestock* (eds J.A.W. Coetzer and R.C. Tustin), Oxford University Press, Oxford, pp. 1014–1026.

[4] Powers, A.M. and Roehrig, J.T. (2011) Alphaviruses. *Methods Mol Biol*, 665, 17–38.

[5] Jacups, S.P., Whelan, P.I. and Currie, B.J. (2008) Ross River virus and Barmah Forest virus infections: a review of history, ecology, and predictive models, with implications for tropical northern Australia. *Vector Borne Zoonotic Dis*, 8, 283–297.

[6] Weaver, S.C. and Barrett, A.D. (2004) Transmission cycles, host range, evolution and emergence of arboviral disease. *Nat Rev Microbiol*, 2, 789–801.

[7] Weaver, S.C. (2005) Host range, amplification and arboviral disease emergence. *Arch Virol Suppl*, 19, 33–44.

[8] Gorelkin, L. (1973) Venezuelan equine encephalomyelitis in an adult animal host. An electron microscopic study. *Am J Pathol*, 73, 425–442.

[9] Pletnev, S.V., Zhang, W., Mukhopadhyay, S. *et al.* (2001) Locations of carbohydrate sites on alphavirus glycoproteins show that E1 forms an icosahedral scaffold. *Cell*, 105, 127–136.

[10] Zhang, W., Mukhopadhyay, S., Pletnev, S.V. *et al.* (2002) Placement of the structural proteins in Sindbis virus. *J Virol*, 76, 11645–11658.

[11] Mukhopadhyay, S., Chipman, P.R., Hong, E.M. *et al.* (2002) In vitro-assembled alphavirus core-like particles

maintain a structure similar to that of nucleocapsid cores in mature virus. *J Virol*, 76, 11128–11132.

[12] Wu, S.R., Haag, L., Hammar, L. *et al.* (2007) The dynamic envelope of a fusion class II virus. Perfusion stages of Semliki Forest virus revealed by electron cryomicroscopy. *J Biol Chem*, 282, 6752–6762.

[13] Mukhopadhyay, S., Zhang, W., Gabler, S. *et al.* (2006) Mapping the structure and function of the E1 and E2 glycoproteins in alphaviruses. *Structure*, 14, 63–73.

[14] Roehrig, J.T. (1993) Immunogens of encephalitis viruses. *Vet Microbiol*, 37, 273–284.

[15] Brault, A.C., Powers, A.M., Holmes, E.C. *et al.* (2002) Positively charged amino acid substitutions in the e2 envelope glycoprotein are associated with the emergence of Venezuelan equine encephalitis virus. *J Virol*, 76, 1718–1730.

[16] Calisher, C.H. and Maness, K.S. (1975) Laboratory studies of Venezuelan equine encephalitis virus in equines, Texas, 1971. *J Clin Microbiol*, 2, 198–205.

[17] Calisher, C.H., Emerson, J.K., Muth, D.J. *et al.* (1983) Serodiagnosis of western equine encephalitis virus infections: relationships of antibody titer and test to observed onset of clinical illness. *J Am Vet Med Assoc*, 183, 438–440.

[18] Calisher, C.H., el-Kafrawi, A.O., Al-Deen Mahmud, M.I. *et al.* (1986) Complex-specific immunoglobulin M antibody patterns in humans infected with alphaviruses. *J Clin Microbiol*, 23, 155–159.

[19] Calisher, C.H., Mahmud, M.I., el-Kafrawi, A.O. *et al.* (1986) Rapid and specific serodiagnosis of western equine encephalitis virus infection in horses. *Am J Vet Res*, 47, 1296–1299.

[20] Hunt, A.R., Short, W.A., Johnson, A.J. *et al.* (1991) Synthetic peptides of the E2 glycoprotein of Venezuelan equine encephalomyelitis virus. II. Antibody to the amino terminus protects animals by limiting viral replication. *Virology*, 185, 281–290.

[21] Roehrig, J.T. and Bolin, R.A. (1997) Monoclonal antibodies capable of distinguishing epizootic from enzootic varieties of subtype 1 Venezuelan equine encephalitis viruses in a rapid indirect immunofluorescence assay. *J Clin Microbiol*, 35, 1887–1890.

[22] Thibodeaux, B.A., Liss, N.M., Panella, A.N. and Roehrig, J.T. (2011) Development of a human-murine chimeric immunoglobulin M for use in the serological detection of human alphavirus antibodies. *Clin Vaccine Immunol*, 18, 2181–2182.

[23] Tenbroeck, C., Hurst, E.W. and Traub, E. (1935) Epidemiology of equine encephalomyelitis in the Eastern United States. *J Exp Med*, 62, 677–685.

[24] Webster, L.T. and Wright, F.H. (1938) Recovery of eastern equine encephalomyelitis virus from brain tissue of human cases of encephalitis in Massachusetts. *Science*, 88, 305–306.

[25] Weaver, S.C., Powers, A.M., Brault, A.C. and Barrett, A.D. (1999) Molecular epidemiological studies of veterinary arboviral encephalitides. *Vet J*, 157, 123–138.

[26] Bertram, D.S. (1971) Mosquitoes of British Honduras, with some comments on malaria, and on arbovirus antibodies in man and equines. *Trans R Soc Trop Med Hyg*, 65, 742–762.

[27] Reisen, W.K., Lothrop, H.D., Presser, S.B. *et al.* (1995) Landscape ecology of arboviruses in southern California: temporal and spatial patterns of vector and virus activity in Coachella Valley, 1990–1992. *J Med Entomol*, 32, 255–266.

[28] Reisen, W.K., Hardy, J.L., Chiles, R.E. *et al.* (1996) Ecology of mosquitoes and lack of arbovirus activity at Morro Bay, San Luis Obispo County, California. *J Am Mosq Control Assoc*, 12, 679–687.

[29] Reisen, W.K., Lothrop, H.D., Presser, S.B. *et al.* (1997) Landscape ecology of arboviruses in southeastern California: temporal and spatial patterns of enzootic activity in Imperial Valley, 1991–1994. *J Med Entomol*, 34, 179–188.

[30] Passler, S. and Pfeffer, M. (2003) Detection of antibodies to alphaviruses and discrimination between antibodies to eastern and western equine encephalitis viruses in rabbit sera using a recombinant antigen and virus-specific monoclonal antibodies. *J Vet Med B Infect Dis Vet Public Health*, 50, 265–269.

[31] Weaver, S.C., Winegar, R., Manger, I.D. and Forrester, N.L. (2012) Alphaviruses: population genetics and determinants of emergence. *Antiviral Res*, 94, 242–257.

[32] Morris, C.D. and Srihongse, S. (1978) An evaluation of the hypothesis of transovarial transmission of eastern equine encephalomyelitis virus by *Culiseta melanura*. *Am J Trop Med Hyg*, 27, 1246–1250.

[33] Scott, T.W., Hildreth, S.W. and Beaty, B.J. (1984) The distribution and development of eastern equine encephalitis virus in its enzootic mosquito vector, *Culiseta melanura*. *Am J Trop Med Hyg*, 33, 300–310.

[34] Weaver, S.C., Scott, T.W. and Lorenz, L.H. (1990) Patterns of eastern equine encephalomyelitis virus infection in *Culiseta melanura (Diptera: Culicidae)*. *J Med Entomol*, 27, 878–891.

[35] Weaver, S.C., Scott, T.W., Lorenz, L.H. and Repik, P.M. (1991) Detection of eastern equine encephalomyelitis virus deposition in *Culiseta melanura* following ingestion of radiolabeled virus in blood meals. *Am J Trop Med Hyg*, 44, 250–259.

[36] Molaei, G., Oliver, J., Andreadis, T.G., Armstrong, P.M. and Howard, J.J. (2006) Molecular identification of blood-meal sources in *Culiseta melanura* and *Culiseta morsitans* from an endemic focus of eastern equine encephalitis virus in New York. *Am J Trop Med Hyg*, 75, 1140–1147.

[37] Estep, L.K., McClure, C.J., Burkett-Cadena, N.D. *et al.* (2011) A multi-year study of mosquito feeding patterns on avian hosts in a southeastern focus of eastern equine encephalitis virus. *Am J Trop Med Hyg*, 84, 718–726.

[38] Oliveira, A., Katholi, C.R., Burkett-Cadena, N. *et al.* (2011) Temporal analysis of feeding patterns of *Culex erraticus* in central Alabama. *Vector Borne Zoonotic Dis*, 11, 413–421.

[39] Estep, L.K., McClure, C.J., Vander, K.P. *et al.* (2013) Risk of exposure to eastern equine encephalomyelitis virus increases with the density of northern cardinals. *PLoS One*, 8, e57879.

[40] Walder, R. and Suarez, O.M. (1976) Studies of arboviruses in Southwestern Venezuela: I. Isolations of Venezuelan and eastern equine encephalitis viruses from sentinel hamsters in the Catatumbo region. *Int J Epidemiol*, 5, 375–378.

[41] Walder, R., Rosato, R.R. and Eddy, G.A. (1981) Virion polypeptide heterogeneity among virulent and avirulent strains of eastern equine encephalitis (EEE) virus. *Arch Virol*, 68, 229–237.

[42] Walder, R., Suarez, O.M. and Calisher, C.H. (1984) Arbovirus studies in the Guajira region of Venezuela: activities of eastern equine encephalitis and Venezuelan equine encephalitis viruses during an interepizootic period. *Am J Trop Med Hyg*, 33, 699–707.

[43] Arrigo, N.C., Adams, A.P., Watts, D.M. *et al.* (2010) Cotton rats and house sparrows as hosts for North and South American strains of eastern equine encephalitis virus. *Emerg Infect Dis*, 16, 1373–1380.

[44] Brault, A.C., Powers, A.M., Chavez, C.L. *et al.* (1999) Genetic and antigenic diversity among eastern equine encephalitis viruses from North, Central, and South America. *Am J Trop Med Hyg*, 61, 579–586.

[45] Weaver, S.C., Hagenbaugh, A., Bellew, L.A. *et al.* (1994) Evolution of alphaviruses in the eastern equine encephalomyelitis complex. *J Virol*, 68, 158–169.

[46] Forshey, B.M., Guevara, C., Laguna-Torres, V.A. *et al.* (2010) Arboviral etiologies of acute febrile illnesses in Western South America, 2000–2007. *PLoS Negl Trop Dis*, 4, e787.

[47] Turell, M.J., O'Guinn, M.L., Dohm, D. *et al.* (2008) Susceptibility of Peruvian mosquitoes to eastern equine encephalitis virus. *J Med Entomol*, 45, 720–725.

[48] Aguilar, P.V., Robich, R.M., Turell, M.J. *et al.* (2007) Endemic eastern equine encephalitis in the Amazon region of Peru. *Am J Trop Med Hyg*, 76, 293–298.

[49] Silva, M.L., Galiza, G.J., Dantas, A.F. *et al.* (2011) Outbreaks of eastern equine encephalitis in northeastern Brazil. *J Vet Diagn Invest*, 23, 570–575.

[50] Mendoza, L.P., Bronzoni, R.V., Takayanagui, O.M. *et al.* (2007) Viral infections of the central nervous system in Brazil. *J Infect*, 54, 589–596.

[51] Figueiredo, L.T. (2007) Emergent arboviruses in Brazil. *Rev Soc Bras Med Trop*, 40, 224–229.

[52] Bedenice, D., Bright, A., Pedersen, D.D. and Dibb, J. (2009) Humoral response to an equine encephalitis vaccine in healthy alpacas. *J Am Vet Med Assoc*, 234, 530–534.

[53] Pursell, A.R., Mitchell, F.E. and Seibold, H.R. (1976) Naturally occurring and experimentally induced eastern encephalomyelitis in calves. *J Am Vet Med Assoc*, 169, 1101–1103.

[54] McGee, E.D., Littleton, C.H., Mapp, J.B. and Brown, R.J. (1992) Eastern equine encephalomyelitis in an adult cow. *Vet Pathol*, 29, 361–363.

[55] Elvinger, F., Liggett, A.D., Tang, K.N. *et al.* (1994) Eastern equine encephalomyelitis virus infection in swine. *J Am Vet Med Assoc*, 205, 1014–1016.

[56] Elvinger, F., Baldwin, C.A., Liggett, A.D. *et al.* (1996) Prevalence of exposure to eastern equine encephalomyelitis virus in domestic and feral swine in Georgia. *J Vet Diagn Invest*, 8, 481–484.

[57] Veazey, R.S., Vice, C.C., Cho, D.Y. *et al.* (1994) Pathology of eastern equine encephalitis in emus (*Dromaius novaehollandiae*). *Vet Pathol*, 31, 109–111.

[58] Bauer, R.W., Gill, M.S., Poston, R.P. and Kim, D.Y. (2005) Naturally occurring eastern equine encephalitis in a Hampshire weather. *J Vet Diagn Invest*, 17, 281–285.

[59] Tate, C.M., Howerth, E.W., Stallknecht, D.E. *et al.* (2005) Eastern equine encephalitis in a free-ranging white-tailed deer (*Odocoileus virginianus*). *J Wildl Dis*, 41, 241–245.

[60] Tully, T.N., Jr, Shane, S.M., Poston, R.P. *et al.* (1992) Eastern equine encephalitis in a flock of emus (*Dromaius novaehollandiae*). *Avian Dis*, 36, 808–812.

[61] Snoeyenbos, G.H., Weinack, O.M. and Rosenau, B.J. (1978) Immunization of pheasants for eastern encephalitis. *Avian Dis*, 22, 386–390.

[62] Faddou, G.P. and Fellows, G.W. (1965) Clinical manifestations of eastern equine encephalitis in pheasants. *Avian Dis*, 9, 530–535.

[63] Day, J.F. and Stark, L.M. (1996) Eastern equine encephalitis transmission to emus (*Dromaius novaehollandiae*) in Volusia County, Florida: 1992 through 1994. *J Am Mosq Control Assoc*, 12, 429–436.

[64] Bingham, A.M., Graham, S.P., Burkett-Cadena, N.D. *et al.* (2012) Detection of eastern equine encephalomyelitis virus RNA in North American snakes. *Am J Trop Med Hyg*, 87, 1140–1144.

[65] Graham, S.P., Hassan, H.K., Chapman, T. *et al.* (2012) Serosurveillance of eastern equine encephalitis virus in amphibians and reptiles from Alabama, USA. *Am J Trop Med Hyg*, 86, 540–544.

[66] White, G., Ottendorfer, C., Graham, S. and Unnasch, T.R. (2011) Competency of reptiles and amphibians for eastern equine encephalitis virus. *Am J Trop Med Hyg*, 85, 421–425.

[67] Kelen, P.T., Downs, J.A., Burkett-Cadena, N.D. *et al.* (2012) Habitat associations of eastern equine encephalitis transmission in Walton County Florida. *J Med Entomol*, 49, 746–756.

[68] Lubelczyk, C., Mutebi, J.P., Robinson, S. *et al.* (2013) An epizootic of eastern equine encephalitis virus, Maine, USA in 2009: outbreak description and entomological studies. *Am J Trop Med Hyg*, 88, 95–102.

[69] Moncayo, A.C., Edman, J.D. and Finn, J.T. (2000) Application of geographic information technology in determining risk of eastern equine encephalomyelitis virus transmission. *J Am Mosq Control Assoc*, 16, 28–35.

[70] Centers for Disease Control and Prevention (CDC) (2012) West Nile virus disease and other arboviral diseases—United States, 2011. *MMWR Morb Mortal Wkly Rep*, 61, 510–514.

[71] Goldrick BA. Emerging infections. *Am J Nurs* 2003; 103:25–27.

[72] CDC (2006) Eastern equine encephalitis—New Hampshire and Massachusetts, August–September 2005. *MMWR Morb Mortal Wkly Rep*, 55, 697–700.

[73] CDC (2011) West Nile virus disease and other arboviral diseases—United States, 2010. *MMWR Morb Mortal Wkly Rep*, 60, 1009–1013.

[74] Silverman, M.A., Misasi, J., Smole, S. *et al.* (2013) Eastern equine encephalitis in children, Massachusetts and New Hampshire, USA, 1970–2010. *Emerg Infect Dis*, 19, 194–201.

[75] Armstrong, P.M., Andreadis, T.G., Anderson, J.F. *et al.* (2008) Tracking eastern equine encephalitis virus perpetuation in the northeastern United States by phylogenetic analysis. *Am J Trop Med Hyg*, 79, 291–296.

[76] Molaei, G., Andreadis, T.G., Armstrong, P.M. *et al.* (2013) Vector-host interactions and epizootiology of Eastern equine encephalitis virus in Massachusetts. *Vector Borne Zoonotic Dis*, 13, 312–323.

[77] Gibbs, E.P.J. and Tsai, T.F. (1994) Eastern equine encephalitis, in *Handbook of Zoonoses* (ed. G.W. Beran), CRC Press Inc., Boca Raton, pp. 11–24.

[78] Scherer, W.F., Ordonez, J.V., Jahrling, P.B. *et al.* (1972) Observations of equines, humans and domestic and wild vertebrates during the 1969 equine epizootic and epidemic of Venezuelan encephalitis in Guatemala. *Am J Epidemiol*, 95, 255–266.

[79] Letson, G.W., Bailey, R.E., Pearson, J. and Tsai, T.F. (1993) Eastern equine encephalitis (EEE): a description of the 1989 outbreak, recent epidemiologic trends, and the association of rainfall with EEE occurrence. *Am J Trop Med Hyg*, 49, 677–685.

[80] Wilson, J.H., Rubin, H.L., Lane, T.J. and Gibbs, E.P.J. (2006) Eastern equine encephalitis in Florida horses: prevalence, economic impact, and management practices, 1982–1983. *Prev Vet Med*, 4, 261–271.

[81] Miller, L.D., Pearson, J.E. and Muhm, R.L. (1973) A comparison of clinical manifestations and pathology of the equine encephalitides: VEE, WEE, EEE. *Proc Annu Meet U.S. Anim Health Assoc*, 629–631.

[82] Scott, T.W., Olson, J.G., All, B.P., III and Gibbs, E.P. (1988) Detection of eastern equine encephalomyelitis virus antigen in equine brain tissue by enzyme-linked immunosorbent assay. *Am J Vet Res*, 49, 1716–1718.

[83] Sahu, S.P., Alstad, A.D., Pedersen, D.D. and Pearson, J.E. (1994) Diagnosis of eastern equine encephalomyelitis virus infection in horses by immunoglobulin M and G capture enzyme-linked immunosorbent assay. *J Vet Diagn Invest*, 6, 34–38.

[84] 1976) Arbovirus encephalitis-diagnostic considerations. *J Iowa Med Soc*, 66, 333–334.

[85] Monath, T.P., McLean, R.G., Cropp, C.B. *et al.* (1981) Diagnosis of eastern equine encephalomyelitis by immunofluorescent staining of brain tissue. *Am J Vet Res*, 42, 1418–1421.

[86] Gregory, C.R., Latimer, K.S., Niagro, F.D. *et al.* (1996) Detection of eastern equine encephalomyelitis virus RNA in formalin-fixed, paraffin-embedded tissues using DNA in situ hybridization. *J Vet Diagn Invest*, 8, 151–155.

[87] Patterson, J.S., Maes, R.K., Mullaney, T.P. and Benson, C.L. (1996) Immunohistochemical diagnosis of eastern equine encephalomyelitis. *J Vet Diagn Invest*, 8, 156–160.

[88] Linssen, B., Kinney, R.M., Aguilar, P. *et al.* (2000) Development of reverse transcription-PCR assays specific for detection of equine encephalitis viruses. *J Clin Microbiol*, 38, 1527–1535.

[89] Brown, T.M., Mitchell, C.J., Nasci, R.S. *et al.* (2001) Detection of eastern equine encephalitis virus in infected mosquitoes using a monoclonal antibody-based antigen-capture enzyme-linked immunosorbent assay. *Am J Trop Med Hyg*, 65, 208–213.

[90] Franklin, R.P., Kinde, H., Jay, M.T. *et al.* (2002) Eastern equine encephalomyelitis virus infection in a horse from California. *Emerg Infect Dis*, 8, 283–288.

[91] Studdert, M.J., Azuolas, J.K., Vasey, J.R. *et al.* (2003) Polymerase chain reaction tests for the identification of Ross River, Kunjin and Murray Valley encephalitis virus infections in horses. *Aust Vet J*, 81, 76–80.

[92] Wang, E., Paessler, S., Aguilar, P.V. *et al.* (2006) Reverse transcription-PCR-enzyme-linked immunosorbent assay for rapid detection and differentiation of alphavirus infections. *J Clin Microbiol*, 44, 4000–4008.

[93] Bastian, F.O., Wende, R.D., Singer, D.B. and Zeller, R.S. (1975) Eastern equine encephalomyelitis. Histopathologic and ultrastructural changes with isolation of the virus in a human case. *Am J Clin Pathol*, 64, 10–13.

[94] Poonacha, K.B., Gregory, C.R. and Vickers, M.L. (1998) Intestinal lesions in a horse associated with eastern equine encephalomyelitis virus infection. *Vet Pathol*, 35, 535–538.

[95] del Piero, F., Wilkins, P.A., Dubovi, E.J. *et al.* (2001) Clinical, pathologic, immunohistochemical, and virologic findings of eastern equine encephalomyelitis in two horses. *Vet Pathol*, 38, 451–456.

[96] Hunt, A.R., Frederickson, S., Hinkel, C. *et al.* (2006) A humanized murine monoclonal antibody protects mice either before or after challenge with virulent Venezuelan equine encephalitis virus. *J Gen Virol*, 87, 2467–2476.

[97] Lukaszewski, R.A. and Brooks, T.J. (2000) Pegylated alpha interferon is an effective treatment for virulent Venezuelan equine encephalitis virus and has profound effects on the host immune response to infection. *J Virol*, 74, 5006–5015.

[98] Chikkanna-Gowda, C.P., McNally, S., Sheahan, B.J. *et al.* (2006) Inhibition of murine K-BALB and CT26 tumour growth using a Semliki Forest virus vector with enhanced expression of IL-18. *Oncol Rep*, 16, 713–719.

[99] Julander, J.G., Siddharthan, V., Blatt, L.M. *et al.* (2007) Effect of exogenous interferon and an interferon inducer on western equine encephalitis virus disease in a hamster model. *Virology*, 360, 454–460.

[100] Sentsui, H., Wu, D., Murakami, K. *et al.* (2010) Antiviral effect of recombinant equine interferon-gamma on several equine viruses. *Vet Immunol Immunopathol*, 135, 93–99.

[101] Jochim, M.M. and Barber, T.L. (1974) Immune response of horses after simultaneous or sequential vaccination against eastern, western, and Venezuelan equine encephalomyelitis. *J Am Vet Med Assoc*, 165, 621–625.

[102] Barber, T.L., Walton, T.E. and Lewis, K.J. (1978) Efficacy of trivalent inactivated encephalomyelitis virus vaccine in horses. *Am J Vet Res*, 39, 621–625.

[103] Cilnis, M.J., Kang, W. and Weaver, S.C. (1996) Genetic conservation of Highlands J viruses. *Virology*, 218, 343–351.

[104] Weaver, S.C., Rico-Hesse, R. and Scott, T.W. (1992) Genetic diversity and slow rates of evolution in New World alphaviruses. *Curr Top Microbiol Immunol*, 176, 99–117.

[105] Bell, J.R., Bond, M.W., Hunkapiller, M.W. *et al.* (1983) Structural proteins of Western equine encephalitis virus: amino acid compositions and N-terminal sequences. *J Virol*, 45, 708–714.

[106] Powers, A.M., Brault, A.C., Shirako, Y. *et al.* (2001) Evolutionary relationships and systematics of the alphaviruses. *J Virol*, 75, 10118–10131.

[107] Sabattini, M.S., Monath, T.P., Mitchell, C.J. *et al.* (1985) Arbovirus investigations in Argentina, 1977–1980. I. Historical aspects and description of study sites. *Am J Trop Med Hyg*, 34, 937–944.

[108] Monath, T.P., Sabattini, M.S., Pauli, R. *et al.* (1985) Arbovirus investigations in Argentina, 1977–1980. IV. Serologic surveys and sentinel equine program. *Am J Trop Med Hyg*, 34, 966–975.

[109] Mitchell, C.J., Monath, T.P., Sabattini, M.S. *et al.* (1985) Arbovirus investigations in Argentina, 1977–1980. II. Arthropod collections and virus isolations from Argentine mosquitoes. *Am J Trop Med Hyg*, 34, 945–955.

[110] Weaver, S.C., Kang, W., Shirako, Y. *et al.* (1997) Recombinational history and molecular evolution of western equine encephalomyelitis complex alphaviruses. *J Virol*, 71, 613–623.

[111] Hoff, G.L., Bigler, W.J., Buff, E.E. and Beck, E. (1978) Occurrence and distribution of western equine encephalomyelitis in Florida. *J Am Vet Med Assoc*, 172, 351–352.

[112] Karabatsos, N., Lewis, A.L., Calisher, C.H. *et al.* (1988) Identification of Highlands J virus from a Florida horse. *Am J Trop Med Hyg*, 39, 603–606.

[113] Hildreth, S.W. and Beaty, B.J. (1984) Detection of eastern equine encephalomyelitis virus and Highlands J virus antigens within mosquito pools by enzyme immunoassay (EIA). I. A laboratory study. *Am J Trop Med Hyg*, 33, 965–972.

[114] Andreadis, T.G., Anderson, J.F. and Tirrell-Peck, S.J. (1998) Multiple isolations of eastern equine encephalitis and highlands J viruses from mosquitoes (*Diptera: Culicidae*) during a 1996 epizootic in southeastern Connecticut. *J Med Entomol*, 35, 296–302.

[115] Calisher, C.H., Monath, T.P., Muth, D.J. *et al.* (1980) Characterization of Fort Morgan virus, an alphavirus of the western equine encephalitis virus complex in an unusual ecosystem. *Am J Trop Med Hyg*, 29, 1428–1440.

[116] Agafonov, V.I., Gol'din, R.B., Lev, M.I. *et al.* (1974) Detection of the degree of infection of mosquitoes in the Far East with group A arboviruses antigenically close to the Semliki forest virus. *Voen Med Zh*, 52–54.

[117] Wagstaff, K.H., Dickson, S.L. and Bailey, A. (1986) Western equine encephalitis surveillance in Utah. *J Am Mosq Control Assoc*, 2, 201–203.

[118] Janousek, T.E. and Kramer, W.L. (1998) Surveillance for arthropod-borne viral activity in Nebraska, 1994–1995. *J Med Entomol*, 35, 758–762.

[119] Reisen, W.K., Meyer, R.P., Presser, S.B. and Hardy, J.L. (1993) Effect of temperature on the transmission of western equine encephalomyelitis and St. Louis encephalitis viruses by *Culex tarsalis (Diptera: Culicidae)*. *J Med Entomol*, 30, 151–160.

[120] Weaver, S.C., Hagenbaugh, A., Bellew, L.A. *et al.* (1993) A comparison of the nucleotide sequences of eastern and western equine encephalomyelitis viruses with those of other alphaviruses and related RNA viruses. *Virology*, 197, 375–390.

[121] Walton, W.E., Schreiber, E.T. and Mulla, M.S. (1990) Distribution of *Culex tarsalis* larvae in a freshwater marsh in Orange County, California. *J Am Mosq Control Assoc*, 6, 539–543.

[122] Walton, W.E., Tietze, N.S. and Mulla, M.S. (1990) Ecology of *Culex tarsalis (Diptera: Culicidae)*: factors influencing larval abundance in mesocosms in southern California. *J Med Entomol*, 27, 57–67.

[123] Hardy, J.L. (1987) The ecology of western equine encephalomyelitis virus in the Central Valley of California, 1945–1985. *Am J Trop Med Hyg*, 37 (Suppl 3), 18S–32S.

[124] Bianchi, T.I., Aviles, G. and Sabattini, M.S. (1997) Biological characteristics of an enzootic subtype of western equine encephalomyelitis virus from Argentina. *Acta Virol*, 41, 13–20.

[125] Aviles, G., Bianchi, T.I., Daffner, J.F. and Sabattini, M.S. (1993) Post-epizootic activity of Western equine encephalitis virus in Argentina. *Rev Argent Microbiol*, 25, 88–99.

[126] Thomas, L.A., Eklund, C.M. and Rush, W.A. (1958) Susceptibility of garter snakes (*Thamnophis spp.*) to western equine encephalomyelitis virus. *Proc Soc Exp Biol Med*, 99, 698–700.

[127] Thomas, L.A. and Eklund, C.M. (1960) Overwintering of western equine encephalomyelitis virus in experimentally infected garter snakes and transmission to mosquitoes. *Proc Soc Exp Biol Med*, 105, 52–55.

[128] Thomas, L.A. and Eklund, C.M. (1962) Overwintering of western equine encephalomyelitis virus in garter snakes experimentally infected by *Culex tarsalis*. *Proc Soc Exp Biol Med*, 109, 421–424.

[129] Gebhardt, L.P., Stanton, G.J., Hill, D.W. and Collett, G.C. (1964) Natural overwintering hosts of the virus of western equine encephalitis. *N Engl J Med*, 271, 172–177.

[130] Spalatin, J., Connell, R., Burton, A.N. and Gollop, B.J. (1964) Western equine encephalitis in Saskatchewan reptiles and amphibians, 1961–1963. *Can J Comp Med Vet Sci*, 28, 131–142.

[131] Burton, A.N., McLintock, J. and Rempel, J.G. (1966) Western equine encephalitis virus in Saskatchewan garter snakes and leopard frogs. *Science*, 154, 1029–1031.

[132] Bast, T.F., Whitney, E. and Benach, J.L. (1973) Considerations on the ecology of several arboviruses in eastern Long Island. *Am J Trop Med Hyg*, 22, 109–115.

[133] Gebhardt, L.P., Jeor, S.C., Stanton, G.J. and Stringfellow, D.A. (1973) Ecology of Western encephalitis virus. *Proc Soc Exp Biol Med*, 142, 731–733.

[134] Thomas, L.A., Patzer, E.R., Cory, J.C. and Coe, J.E. (1980) Antibody development in garter snakes (*Thamnophis spp.*) experimentally infected with western equine encephalitis virus. *Am J Trop Med Hyg*, 29, 112–117.

[135] Reisen, W.K., Presser, S.B., Lin, J. *et al.* (1994) Viremia and serological responses in adult chickens infected with western equine encephalomyelitis and St. Louis encephalitis viruses. *J Am Mosq Control Assoc*, 10, 549–555.

[136] Reisen, W.K., Martinez, V.M., Fang, Y. *et al.* (2006) Role of California (*Callipepla californica*) and Gambel's (*Callipepla gambelii*) quail in the ecology of mosquito-borne encephalitis viruses in California, USA. *Vector Borne Zoonotic Dis*, 6, 248–260.

[137] Huyvaert, K.P., Moore, A.T., Panella, N.A. *et al.* (2008) Experimental inoculation of house sparrows (*Passer domesticus*) with buggy creek virus. *J Wildl Dis*, 44, 331–340.

[138] O'Brien, V.A., Meteyer, C.U., Ip, H.S. *et al.* (2010) Pathology and virus detection in tissues of nestling house sparrows naturally infected with Buggy Creek virus (Togaviridae). *J Wildl Dis*, 46, 23–32.

[139] Zhang, M., Fang, Y., Brault, A.C. and Reisen, W.K. (2011) Variation in western equine encephalomyelitis viral strain growth in mammalian, avian, and mosquito cells fails to explain temporal changes in enzootic and epidemic activity in California. *Vector Borne Zoonotic Dis*, 11, 269–275.

[140] Leung, M.K., Burton, A. and Iversoen, J. (1975) Natural infections of Richardson's ground squirrels with western equine encephalomyelitis virus, Saskatchewan, Canada, 1964–1973. *Can J Microbiol*, 21, 954–958.

[141] Leung, M.K., Iversen, J., McLintock, J. and Saunders, J.R. (1976) Subcutaneous exposure of the Richardson's ground squirrel (*Spermophilus richardsonii Sabine*) to western equine encephalomyelitis virus. *J Wildl Dis*, 12, 237–246.

[142] Leung, M.K., McLintock, J. and Iversen, J. (1978) Intranasal exposure of the Richardson's ground squirrel to Western equine encephalomyelitis virus. *Can J Comp Med*, 42, 184–191.

[143] Hardy, J.L., Reeves, W.C., Rush, W.A. and Nir, Y.D. (1974) Experimental infection with western equine encephalomyelitis virus in wild rodents indigenous to Kern County, California. *Infect Immun*, 10, 553–564.

[144] Meyer, K.F., Larsell, O. and Haring, C.M. (1930) The etiology of epizootic encephalomyelitis of horses in the San Joaquin Valley. *Science*, 72, 227–228.

[145] Lillie, L.E., Wong, F.C. and Drysdale, R.A. (1976) Equine epizootic of western encephalomyelitis in Manitoba-1975. *Can J Public Health*, 67 (Suppl 1), 21–27.

[146] Meyer, K.F., Larsell, O. and Haring, C.M. (1933) Susceptibility of nonimmune, hyperimmunized horses and goats to Eastern, Western and Argentine virus of equine encephalomyelitis. *Proc Soc Exp Biol Med*, 32, 56–58.

[147] Julander, J.G., Smee, D.F., Morrey, J.D. and Furuta, Y. (2009) Effect of T-705 treatment on western equine encephalitis in a mouse model. *Antiviral Res*, 82, 169–171.

[148] Sindac, J.A., Yestrepsky, B.D., Barraza, S.J. *et al.* (2012) Novel inhibitors of neurotropic alphavirus replication that improve host survival in a mouse model of acute viral encephalitis. *J Med Chem*, 55, 3535–3545.

[149] Zehmer, R.B., Dean, P.B., Sudia, W.D. *et al.* (1974) Venezuelan equine encephalitis epidemic in Texas, 1971. *Health Serv Rep*, 89, 278–282.

[150] Calisher, C.H., Sasso, D.R. and Sather, G.E. (1973) Possible evidence for interference with Venezuelan equine encephalitis virus vaccination of equines by preexisting antibody to Eastern or Western Equine encephalitis virus, or both. *Appl Microbiol*, 26, 485–488.

[151] Calisher, C.H. and Maness, K.C. (1974) Virulence of Venezuelan equine encephalomyelitis virus subtypes for various laboratory hosts. *Appl Microbiol*, 28, 881–884.

[152] Weaver, S.C., Pfeffer, M., Marriott, K. *et al.* (1999) Genetic evidence for the origins of Venezuelan equine encephalitis virus subtype IAB outbreaks. *Am J Trop Med Hyg*, 60, 441–448.

[153] Shope, R.E., Causey, O.R. and de Andrade, A.H. (1964) The venezuelan equine encephalomyelitis complex of group A arthropod-borne viruses, including Mucambo and Pixuna from the Amazon region of Brazil. *Am J Trop Med Hyg*, 13, 723–727.

[154] Kinney, R.M., Tsuchiya, K.R., Sneider, J.M. and Trent, D.W. (1992) Genetic evidence that epizootic Venezuelan equine encephalitis (VEE) viruses may have evolved from enzootic VEE subtype I–D virus. *Virology*, 191, 569–580.

[155] Weaver, S.C., Salas, R., Rico-Hesse, R. *et al.* (1996) Re-emergence of epidemic Venezuelan equine encephalomyelitis in South America. VEE study group. *Lancet*, 348, 436–440.

[156] Young, N.A. (1972) Origin of epidemics of Venezuelan equine encephalitis. *J Infect Dis*, 125, 565–567.

[157] Mackenzie, R.M., de Siger, J. and Parra, D. (1976) Venezuelan equine encephalitis virus: comparison of infectivity and virulence of strains V-38 and P676 in donkeys. *Am J Trop Med Hyg*, 25, 494–499.

[158] Steele, K.E., Davis, K.J., Stephan, K. *et al.* (1998) Comparative neurovirulence and tissue tropism of wild-type and attenuated strains of Venezuelan equine encephalitis virus administered by aerosol in C3H/HeN and BALB/c mice. *Vet Pathol*, 35, 386–397.

[159] Oberste, M.S., Weaver, S.C., Watts, D.M. and Smith, J.F. (1998) Identification and genetic analysis of Panama-genotype Venezuelan equine encephalitis virus subtype ID in Peru. *Am J Trop Med Hyg*, 58, 41–46.

[160] Oberste, M.S., Schmura, S.M., Weaver, S.C. and Smith, J.F. (1999) Geographic distribution of Venezuelan equine encephalitis virus subtype IE genotypes in Central America and Mexico. *Am J Trop Med Hyg*, 60, 630–634.

[161] Rico-Hesse, R., Weaver, S.C., Medina, G. *et al.* (1995) Emergence of a new epidemic/epizootic Venezuelan equine encephalitis virus in South America. *Proc Natl Acad Sci U S A*, 92, 5278–5281.

[162] Estrada-Franco, J.G., Navarro-Lopez, R., Freier, J.E. *et al.* (2004) Venezuelan equine encephalitis virus, southern Mexico. *Emerg Infect Dis*, 10, 2113–2121.

[163] Fernandez, Z., Moncayo, A.C., Carrara, A.S. *et al.* (2003) Vector competence of rural and urban strains of *Aedes (Stegomyia) albopictus (Diptera: Culicidae)* from Sao Paulo State, Brazil for IC, ID, and IF subtypes of Venezuelan equine encephalitis virus. *J Med Entomol*, 40, 522–527.

[164] Weaver, S.C., Anishchenko, M., Bowen, R. *et al.* (2004) Genetic determinants of Venezuelan equine encephalitis emergence. Arch Virol Suppl, 43–64.

[165] Brault, A.C., Powers, A.M., Ortiz, D. *et al.* (2004) Venezuelan equine encephalitis emergence: enhanced vector infection from a single amino acid substitution in the envelope glycoprotein. *Proc Natl Acad Sci U S A*, 101, 11344–11349.

[166] Greene, I.P., Paessler, S., Austgen, L. *et al.* (2005) Envelope glycoprotein mutations mediate equine amplification and virulence of epizootic Venezuelan equine encephalitis virus. *J Virol*, 79, 9128–9133.

[167] Smith, D.R., Carrara, A.S., Aguilar, P.V. and Weaver, S.C. (2005) Evaluation of methods to assess transmission potential of Venezuelan equine encephalitis virus by mosquitoes and estimation of mosquito saliva titers. *Am J Trop Med Hyg*, 73, 33–39.

[168] Young, N.A., Johnson, K.M. and Gauld, L.W. (1969) Viruses of the Venezuelan equine encephalomyelitis complex. Experimental infection of Panamanian rodents. *Am J Trop Med Hyg*, 18, 290–296.

[169] Young, N.A. and Johnson, K.M. (1969) Viruses of the Venezuelan equine encephalomyelitis complex. Infection and cross-challenge of rodents with VEE, Mucambo, and Pixuna viruses. *Am J Trop Med Hyg*, 18, 280–289.

[170] Carrara, A.S., Gonzales, G., Ferro, C. *et al.* (2005) Venezuelan equine encephalitis virus infection of spiny rats. *Emerg Infect Dis*, 11, 663–669.

[171] Carrara, A.S., Coffey, L.L., Aguilar, P.V. *et al.* (2007) Venezuelan equine encephalitis virus infection of cotton rats. *Emerg Infect Dis*, 13, 1158–1165.

[172] Scherer, W.F., Reeves, W.C., Hardy, J.L. and Miura, T. (1972) Inhibitors of Western and Venezuelan equine encephalitis viruses in cattle sera from Hawaii. *Am J Trop Med Hyg*, 21, 189–193.

[173] Scherer, W.F., Campillo-Sainz, C., de Mucha-Macias, J. *et al.* (1972) Ecologic studies of Venezuelan encephalitis virus in southeastern Mexico. VII. Infection of man. *Am J Trop Med Hyg*, 21, 79–85.

[174] Kissling, R.E., Chamberlain, R.W., Eidson, M.E. *et al.* (1954) Studies on the North American arthropod-borne encephalitides. II. Eastern equine encephalitis in horses. *Am J Hyg*, 60, 237–250.

[175] Chamberlain, R.W., Kissling, R.E., Stamm, D.D. and Sudia, W.D. (1956) Transmission of eastern equine encephalitis to horses by *Aedes sollicitans* mosquitoes. *Am J Trop Med Hyg*, 5, 802–808.

[176] Sudia, W.D., Newhouse, V.F. and Henderson, B.E. (1971) Experimental infection of horses with three strains of Venezuelan equine encephalomyelitis virus. II. Experimental vector studies. *Am J Epidemiol*, 93, 206–211.

[177] Nichols, J.B., Lassing, E.B., Bigler, W.J. and Hoff, G.L. (1975) An evaluation of military sentry dogs as a sentinel system to everglades virus (Venezuelan equine encephalitis Fe3-7C strain). *Mil Med*, 140, 710–712.

[178] Dickerman, R.W., Baker, G.J., Ordonez, J.V. and Scherer, W.F. (1973) Venezuelan equine encephalomyelitis viremia and antibody responses of pigs and cattle. *Am J Vet Res*, 34, 357–361.

[179] Dickerman, R.W., Scherer, W.F., Navarro, E. *et al.* (1973) The involvement of dogs in endemic cycles of Venezuelan encephalitis virus. *Am J Epidemiol*, 98, 311–314.

[180] Bowen, G.S. and McLean, R.G. (1977) Experimental infection of birds with epidemic Venezuelan encephalitis virus. *Am J Trop Med Hyg*, 26, 808–814.

[181] Weaver, S.C., Scherer, W.F., Taylor, C.A. *et al.* (1986) Laboratory vector competence of *Culex (Melanoconion) cedecei* for sympatric and allopatric Venezuelan equine encephalomyelitis viruses. *Am J Trop Med Hyg*, 35, 619–623.

[182] Turell, M.J., Barth, J. and Coleman, R.E. (1999) Potential for Central American mosquitoes to transmit epizootic and enzootic strains of Venezuelan equine encephalitis virus. *J Am Mosq Control Assoc*, 15, 295–298.

[183] Turell, M.J. (1999) Vector competence of three Venezuelan mosquitoes (*Diptera: Culicidae*) for an epizootic IC strain of Venezuelan equine encephalitis virus. *J Med Entomol*, 36, 407–409.

[184] Mitchell, C.J., Monath, T.P., Sabattini, M.S. *et al.* (1987) Host-feeding patterns of Argentine mosquitoes (*Diptera: Culicidae*) collected during and after an epizootic of western equine encephalitis. *J Med Entomol*, 24, 260–267.

[185] Mendez, W., Liria, J., Navarro, J.C. *et al.* (2001) Spatial dispersion of adult mosquitoes (*Diptera: Culicidae*) in a sylvatic focus of Venezuelan equine encephalitis virus. *J Med Entomol*, 38, 813–821.

[186] Linthicum, K.J., Logan, T.M., Bailey, C.L. *et al.* (1991) Venezuelan equine encephalomyelitis virus infection in and transmission by the tick *Amblyomma cajennense (Arachnida: Ixodidae)*. *J Med Entomol*, 28, 405–409.

[187] Linthicum, K.J., Dickson, D.L. and Logan, T.M. (1992) Feeding efficiency of larval *Hyalomma truncatum (Acari: Ixodidae)* on hosts previously exposed to ticks. *J Med Entomol*, 29, 310–313.

[188] Linthicum, K.J. and Logan, T.M. (1994) Laboratory transmission of Venezuelan equine encephalomyelitis virus by the tick *Hyalomma truncatum*. *Trans R Soc Trop Med Hyg*, 88, 126.

[189] Walton, T.E. and Johnson, K.M. (1972) Epizootiology of Venezuelan equine encephalomyelitis in the Americas. *J Am Vet Med Assoc*, 161, 1509–1515.

[190] Walton, T.E. and Johnson, K.M. (1972) Persistence of neutralizing antibody in Equidae vaccinated with Venezuelan equine encephalomyelitis vaccine strain TC-83. *J Am Vet Med Assoc*, 161, 916–918.

[191] Walton, T.E., Alvarez, O., Jr, Buckwalter, R.M. and Johnson, K.M. (1972) Experimental infection of horses with an attenuated Venezuelan equine encephalomyelitis vaccine (strain TC-83). *Infect Immun*, 5, 750–756.

[192] Weaver, S.C., Ferro, C., Barrera, R. *et al.* (2004) Venezuelan equine encephalitis. *Annu Rev Entomol*, 49, 141–174.

[193] Robin, Y., Bourdin, P., Le, G.G. and Heme, G. (1974) Semliki forest virus and equine encephalomyelitis in Senegal (author's transl). *Ann Microbiol (Paris)*, 125A, 235–241.

[194] Lundstrom, J.O. (1999) Mosquito-borne viruses in western Europe: a review. *J Vector Ecol*, 24, 1–39.

[195] Kamada, M., Kumanomido, T., Wada, R. *et al.* (1991) Intranasal infection of Getah virus in experimental horses. *J Vet Med Sci*, 53, 855–858.

[196] Tesh, R.B., Gajdusek, D.C., Garruto, R.M. *et al.* (1975) The distribution and prevalence of group A arbovirus neutralizing antibodies among human populations in Southeast Asia and the Pacific islands. *Am J Trop Med Hyg*, 24, 664–675.

[197] Gard, G.P., Marshall, I.D., Walker, K.H. *et al.* (1977) Association of Australian arboviruses with nervous disease in horses. *Aust Vet J*, 53, 61–66.

[198] Gard, G.P., Giles, J.R., Dwyer-Grey, R.J. and Woodroofe, G.M. (1976) Serological evidence of inter-epidemic infection of feral pigs in New South Wales with Murray Valley encephalitis virus. *Aust J Exp Biol Med Sci*, 54, 297–302.

[199] Woodroofe, G., Marshall, I.D. and Taylor, W.P. (1977) Antigenically distinct strains of Ross River virus from north Queensland and coastal New South Wales. *Aust J Exp Biol Med Sci*, 55, 79–97.

[200] Le, G.G. and Fauran, P. (1981) Arboviral diseases in South-West Pacific islands (author's transl). *Méd Trop (Mars)*, 41, 85–92.

[201] Cloonan, M.J., O'Neill, B.J., Vale, T.G. *et al.* (1982) Ross River virus activity along the south coast of New South Wales. *Aust J Exp Biol Med Sci*, 60, 701–706.

[202] Hawkes, R.A., Boughton, C.R., Naim, H.M. *et al.* (1985) Arbovirus infections of humans in New South Wales. Seroepidemiology of the flavivirus group of togaviruses. *Med J Aust*, 143, 555–561.

[203] Broom, A.K., Wright, A.E., Mackenzie, J.S. *et al.* (1989) Isolation of Murray Valley encephalitis and Ross River viruses from *Aedes normanensis (Diptera: Culicidae)* in Western Australia. *J Med Entomol*, 26, 100–103.

[204] Beaman, M.H. (1997) Emerging infections in Australia. *Ann Acad Med Singapore*, 26, 609–615.

[205] Johansen, C.A., Nisbet, D.J., Zborowski, P. *et al.* (2003) Flavivirus isolations from mosquitoes collected from Western Cape York Peninsula, Australia, 1999–2000. *J Am Mosq Control Assoc*, 19, 392–396.

[206] Spokes, P.J., Doggett, S.L. and Webb, C.E. (2007) Bug breakfast in the bulletin: Ross River virus. *N S W Public Health Bull*, 18, 63–64.

[207] Liu, C., Johansen, C., Kurucz, N. and Whelan, P. (2006) Communicable Diseases Network Australia National Arbovirus and Malaria Advisory Committee annual report, 2005–06. *Commun Dis Intell Q Rep*, 30, 411–429.

[208] McFadden, A.M., McFadden, B.D., Mackereth, G.F. *et al.* (2009) A serological survey of cattle in the Thames—Coromandel district of New Zealand for antibodies to Ross River virus. *N Z Vet J*, 57, 116–120.

[209] Boyd, A.M., Hall, R.A., Gemmell, R.T. and Kay, B.H. (2001) Experimental infection of Australian brushtail possums, *Trichosurus vulpecula (Phalangeridae: Marsupialia)*, with Ross River and Barmah Forest viruses by use of a natural mosquito vector system. *Am J Trop Med Hyg*, 65, 777–782.

[210] Old, J.M. and Deane, E.M. (2005) Antibodies to the Ross River virus in captive marsupials in urban areas of eastern New South Wales, Australia. *J Wildl Dis*, 41, 611–614.

[211] Miles, J.A. (1964) Some ecological aspects of the problem of arthropod-borne animal viruses in the Western Pacific and Southeast Asia regions. *Bull World Health Organ*, 30, 197–210.

[212] Wright, A.E., Anderson, S., Stanley, N.F. *et al.* (1981) A preliminary investigation of the ecology of arboviruses in the Derby area of the Kimberley region, Western Australia. *Aust J Exp Biol Med Sci*, 59, 357–367.

[213] Marshall, I.D., Woodroofe, G.M. and Hirsch, S. (1982) Viruses recovered from mosquitoes and wildlife serum collected in the Murray Valley of South-eastern Australia, February 1974, during an epidemic of encephalitis. *Aust J Exp Biol Med Sci*, 60, 457–470.

[214] Russell, R.C. (2002) Ross River virus: ecology and distribution. *Annu Rev Entomol*, 47, 1–31.

[215] El-Hage, C.M., McCluskey, M.J. and Azuolas, J.K. (2008) Disease suspected to be caused by Ross River virus infection of horses. *Aust Vet J*, 86, 367–370.

[216] Roche, S.E., Wicks, R., Garner, M.G. *et al.* (2013) Descriptive overview of the 2011 epidemic of arboviral disease in horses in Australia. *Aust Vet J*, 91, 5–13.

[217] Azuolas, J.K., Wishart, E., Bibby, S. and Ainsworth, C. (2003) Isolation of Ross River virus from mosquitoes and from horses with signs of musculo-skeletal disease. *Aust Vet J*, 81, 344–347.

[218] Schmidt, J.R. (1965) West Nile fever. A review of its clinical, epidemiologic and ecologic features. *East Afr Med J*, 42, 207–212.

[219] Petersen, L.R., Brault, A.C. and Nasci, R.S. (2013) West Nile virus: review of the literature. *JAMA*, 310, 308–315.

[220] Gould, E.A. and Solomon, T. (2008) Pathogenic flaviviruses. *Lancet*, 371, 500–509.

[221] Gould, E.A., de Lamballerie, X., Zanotto, P.M. and Holmes, E.C. (2001) Evolution, epidemiology, and dispersal of flaviviruses revealed by molecular phylogenies. *Adv Virus Res*, 57, 71–103.

[222] Communicable Diseases Program, PAHO's Division of Disease Prevention and Control (HCP/HCT) (2002) Guidelines for surveillance, prevention and control of West Nile virus. *Epidemiol Bull*, 23, 12–14.

[223] Altma, R.M. (1963) The behavior of Murray Valley Encephalitis virus in *Culex triaeniorhynchus giles* and *Culex pipiens qluinquefasciatus say*. *Am J Trop Med Hyg*, 12, 425–434.

[224] Amraoui, F., Krida, G., Bouattour, A. *et al.* (2012) *Culex pipiens*, an experimental efficient vector of West Nile and Rift Valley fever viruses in the Maghreb region. *PLoS One*, 7, e36757.

[225] Andreadis, T.G., Anderson, J.F., Vossbrinck, C.R. and Main, A.J. (2004) Epidemiology of West Nile virus in Connecticut: a five-year analysis of mosquito data 1999–2003. *Vector Borne Zoonotic Dis*, 4, 360–378.

[226] Andreadis, T.G. (2012) The contribution of *Culex pipiens* complex mosquitoes to transmission and persistence of West Nile virus in North America. *J Am Mosq Control Assoc*, 28 (Suppl 4), 137–151.

[227] Balenghien, T., Fouque, F., Sabatier, P. and Bicout, D.J. (2011) Theoretical formulation for mosquito host-feeding patterns: application to a West Nile virus focus of southern France. *J Med Entomol*, 48, 1076–1090.

[228] Ching, C.Y., Casals, J., Bowen, E.T. *et al.* (1970) Arbovirus infections in Sarawak: the isolation of Kunjin virus from mosquitoes of the *Culex pseudovishnui* group. *Ann Trop Med Parasitol*, 64, 263–268.

[229] Dauphin, G., Zientara, S., Zeller, H. and Murgue, B. (2004) West Nile: worldwide current situation in animals and humans. *Comp Immunol Microbiol Infect Dis*, 27, 343–355.

[230] Reisen, W.K., Milby, M.M., Reeves, W.C. *et al.* (1985) Aerial adulticiding for the suppression of *Culex tarsalis* in Kern County, California, using low volume propoxur: 2. Impact on natural populations in foothill and valley habitats. *J Am Mosq Control Assoc*, 1, 154–163.

[231] Wegbreit, J. and Reisen, W.K. (2000) Relationships among weather, mosquito abundance, and encephalitis virus activity in California: Kern County 1990–98. *J Am Mosq Control Assoc*, 16, 22–27.

[232] Macdonald, F. (1952) Haemagglutination with the virus of Murray Valley encephalitis. *Br J Exp Pathol*, 33, 537–542.

[233] Evans, I.A., Hueston, L. and Doggett, S.L. (2009) Murray Valley encephalitis virus. *N S W Public Health Bull*, 20, 195–196.

[234] Williams, C.R., Fricker, S.R. and Kokkinn, M.J. (2009) Environmental and entomological factors determining Ross River virus activity in the River Murray Valley of South Australia. *Aust N Z J Public Health*, 33, 284–288.

[235] 2010) Factsheet: Murray Valley encephalitis. *N S W Public Health Bull*, 21, 148–149.

[236] Ng, M.L. (1987) Ultrastructural studies of Kunjin virus-infected *Aedes albopictus* cells. *J Gen Virol*, 68, 577–582.

[237] Ng, M.L. and Hong, S.S. (1989) Flavivirus infection: essential ultrastructural changes and association of Kunjin virus NS3 protein with microtubules. *Arch Virol*, 106, 103–120.

[238] Westaway, E.G., Mackenzie, J.M., Kenney, M.T. *et al.* (1997) Ultrastructure of Kunjin virus-infected cells: colocalization of NS1 and NS3 with double-stranded RNA, and of NS2B with NS3, in virus-induced membrane structures. *J Virol*, 71, 6650–6661.

[239] Deubel, V., Fiette, L., Gounon, P. *et al.* (2001) Variations in biological features of West Nile viruses. *Ann N.Y Acad Sci*, 951, 195–206.

[240] Roosendaal, J., Westaway, E.G., Khromykh, A. and Mackenzie, J.M. (2006) Regulated cleavages at the West Nile virus NS4A-2K-NS4B junctions play a major role in rearranging cytoplasmic membranes and Golgi trafficking of the NS4A protein. *J Virol*, 80, 4623–4632.

[241] Heinz, F.X. and Stiasny, K. (2012) Flaviviruses and their antigenic structure. *J Clin Virol*, 55, 289–295.

[242] Rice, C.M. (1990) Overview of flavivirus molecular biology and future vaccine development via recombinant DNA. *Southeast Asian J Trop Med Public Health*, 21, 670–677.

[243] Mukhopadhyay, S., Kuhn, R.J. and Rossmann, M.G. (2005) A structural perspective of the flavivirus life cycle. *Nat Rev Microbiol*, 3, 13–22.

[244] Mukhopadhyay, S., Kim, B.S., Chipman, P.R. *et al.* (2003) Structure of West Nile virus. *Science*, 302, 248.

[245] Wengler, G., Wengler, G. and Gross, H.J. (1978) Studies on virus-specific nucleic acids synthesized in vertebrate and mosquito cells infected with flaviviruses. *Virology*, 89, 423–437.

[246] Wengler, G., Castle, E., Leidner, U. *et al.* (1985) Sequence analysis of the membrane protein V3 of the flavivirus West Nile virus and of its gene. *Virology*, 147, 264–274.

[247] Castle, E., Nowak, T., Leidner, U. *et al.* (1985) Sequence analysis of the viral core protein and the membrane-

associated proteins V1 and NV2 of the flavivirus West Nile virus and of the genome sequence for these proteins. *Virology*, 145, 227–236.

[248] Castle, E., Leidner, U., Nowak, T. *et al.* (1986) Primary structure of the West Nile flavivirus genome region coding for all nonstructural proteins. *Virology*, 149, 10–26.

[249] Nowak, T. and Wengler, G. (1987) Analysis of disulfides present in the membrane proteins of the West Nile flavivirus. *Virology*, 156, 127–137.

[250] Wengler, G. and Wengler, G. (1989) Cell-associated West Nile flavivirus is covered with E+pre-M protein heterodimers which are destroyed and reorganized by proteolytic cleavage during virus release. *J Virol*, 63, 2521–2526.

[251] Wengler, G. and Wengler, G. (1989) An analysis of the antibody response against West Nile virus E protein purified by SDS-PAGE indicates that this protein does not contain sequential epitopes for efficient induction of neutralizing antibodies. *J Gen Virol*, 70, 987–992.

[252] Wengler, G. and Wengler, G. (1993) The NS 3 nonstructural protein of flaviviruses contains an RNA triphosphatase activity. *Virology*, 197, 265–273.

[253] Colpitts, T.M., Conway, M.J., Montgomery, R.R. and Fikrig, E. (2012) West Nile virus: biology, transmission, and human infection. *Clin Microbiol Rev*, 25, 635–648.

[254] Diamond, M.S., Shrestha, B., Mehlhop, E. *et al.* (2003) Innate and adaptive immune responses determine protection against disseminated infection by West Nile encephalitis virus. *Viral Immunol*, 16, 259–278.

[255] Diamond, M.S., Shrestha, B., Marri, A. *et al.* (2003) B cells and antibody play critical roles in the immediate defense of disseminated infection by West Nile encephalitis virus. *J Virol*, 77 (4), 2578–2586.

[256] Guirakhoo, F., Bolin, R.A. and Roehrig, J.T. (1992) The Murray Valley encephalitis virus prM protein confers acid resistance to virus particles and alters the expression of epitopes within the R2 domain of E glycoprotein. *Virology*, 191, 921–931.

[257] Colombage, G., Hall, R., Pavy, M. and Lobigs, M. (1998) DNA-based and alphavirus-vectored immunisation with prM and E proteins elicits long-lived and protective immunity against the flavivirus, Murray Valley encephalitis virus. *Virology*, 250, 151–163.

[258] Mukherjee, S., Lin, T.Y., Dowd, K.A. *et al.* (2011) The infectivity of prM-containing partially mature West Nile virus does not require the activity of cellular furin-like proteases. *J Virol*, 85, 12067–12072.

[259] Hall, R.A., Coelen, R.J. and Mackenzie, J.S. (1991) Immunoaffinity purification of the NS1 protein of Murray Valley encephalitis virus: selection of the appropriate ligand and optimal conditions for elution. *J Virol Methods*, 32, 11–20.

[260] Chung, K.M., Liszewski, M.K., Nybakken, G. *et al.* (2006) West Nile virus nonstructural protein NS1 inhibits complement activation by binding the regulatory protein factor H. *Proc Natl Acad Sci U S A*, 103, 19111–19116.

[261] Chung, K.M., Nybakken, G.E., Thompson, B.S. *et al.* (2006) Antibodies against West Nile virus nonstructural protein NS1 prevent lethal infection through Fc gamma receptor-dependent and -independent mechanisms. *J Virol*, 80, 1340–1351.

[262] Chung, K.M., Thompson, B.S., Fremont, D.H. and Diamond, M.S. (2007) Antibody recognition of cell surface-associated NS1 triggers Fc-gamma receptor-mediated phagocytosis and clearance of West Nile virus-infected cells. *J Virol*, 81, 9551–9555.

[263] Avirutnan, P., Hauhart, R.E., Somnuke, P. *et al.* (2011) Binding of flavivirus nonstructural protein NS1 to C4b binding protein modulates complement activation. *J Immunol*, 187, 424–433.

[264] Youn, S., Li, T., McCune, B.T. *et al.* (2012) Evidence for a genetic and physical interaction between nonstructural proteins NS1 and NS4B that modulates replication of West Nile virus. *J Virol*, 86, 7360–7371.

[265] Stocks, C.E. and Lobigs, M. (1998) Signal peptidase cleavage at the flavivirus C-prM junction: dependence on the viral NS2B-3 protease for efficient processing requires determinants in C, the signal peptide, and prM. *J Virol*, 72, 2141–2149.

[266] Mackenzie, J.M., Khromykh, A.A., Jones, M.K. and Westaway, E.G. (1998) Subcellular localization and some biochemical properties of the flavivirus Kunjin nonstructural proteins NS2A and NS4A. *Virology*, 245, 203–215.

[267] Liu, W.J., Chen, H.B. and Khromykh, A.A. (2003) Molecular and functional analyses of Kunjin virus infectious cDNA clones demonstrate the essential roles for NS2A in virus assembly and for a nonconservative residue in NS3 in RNA replication. *J Virol*, 77, 7804–7813.

[268] Leung, J.Y., Pijlman, G.P., Kondratieva, N. *et al.* (2008) Role of nonstructural protein NS2A in flavivirus assembly. *J Virol*, 82, 4731–4741.

[269] Speight, G. and Westaway, E.G. (1989) Positive identification of NS4A, the last of the hypothetical nonstructural proteins of flaviviruses. *Virology*, 170, 299–301.

[270] Ambrose, R.L. and Mackenzie, J.M. (2011) A conserved peptide in West Nile virus NS4A protein contributes to proteolytic processing and is essential for replication. *J Virol*, 85, 11274–11282.

[271] Grun, J.B. and Brinton, M.A. (1986) Characterization of West Nile virus RNA-dependent RNA polymerase and cellular terminal adenylyl and uridylyl transferases in cell-free extracts. *J Virol*, 60, 1113–1124.

[272] Grun, J.B. and Brinton, M.A. (1987) Dissociation of NS5 from cell fractions containing West Nile virus-specific polymerase activity. *J Virol*, 61, 3641–3644.

[273] Gould, D.J., Barnett, H.C. and Suyemoto, W. (1962) Transmission of Japanese encephalitis virus by *Culex gelidus* Theobald. *Trans R Soc Trop Med Hyg*, 56, 429–435.

[274] Gould, D.J., Byrne, R.J. and Hayes, D.E. (1964) Experimental infection of horses with Japanese encephalitis

virus by mosquito bites. *Am J Trop Med Hyg*, 13, 742–746.

[275] Bunning, M.L., Bowen, R.A., Cropp, B. *et al.* (2001) Experimental infection of horses with West Nile virus and their potential to infect mosquitoes and serve as amplifying hosts. *Ann N Y Acad Sci*, 951, 338–339.

[276] Komar, N. (2003) West Nile virus: epidemiology and ecology in North America. *Adv Virus Res*, 61, 185–234.

[277] Komar, N., Panella, N.A. and Boyce, E. (2001) Exposure of domestic mammals to West Nile virus during an outbreak of human encephalitis, New York City, 1999. *Emerg Infect Dis*, 7, 736–738.

[278] McLean, R.G., Ubico, S.R., Bourne, D. and Komar, N. (2002) West Nile virus in livestock and wildlife. *Curr Top Microbiol Immunol*, 267, 271–308.

[279] Centers for Disease Control and Prevention (CDC) (2002) West Nile virus activity—United States, October 10–16, 2002, and update on West Nile virus infections in recipients of blood transfusions. *MMWR Morb Mortal Wkly Rep*, 51, 929–931.

[280] Trock, S.C., Meade, B.J., Glaser, A.L. *et al.* (2001) West Nile virus outbreak among horses in New York State, 1999 and 2000. *Emerg Infect Dis*, 7, 745–747.

[281] Centers for Disease Control and Prevention (CDC) (2002) Provisional surveillance summary of the West Nile virus epidemic—United States, January–November 2002. *MMWR Morb Mortal Wkly Rep*, 51, 1129–1133.

[282] Centers for Disease Control and Prevention (CDC) (2013) West Nile virus and other arboviral diseases—United States, 2012. *MMWR Morb Mortal Wkly Rep*, 62, 513–517.

[283] Ellis, P.M., Daniels, P.W. and Banks, D.J. (2000) Japanese encephalitis. *Vet Clin North Am Equine Pract*, 16, 565–572.

[284] Endy, T.P. and Nisalak, A. (2002) Japanese encephalitis virus: ecology and epidemiology. *Curr Top Microbiol Immunol*, 267, 11–48.

[285] Grossman, R.A., Edelman, R. and Gould, D.J. (1974) Study of Japanese encephalitis virus in Chiangmai Valley, Thailand. VI. Summary and conclusions. *Am J Epidemiol*, 100, 69–76.

[286] Johnsen, D.O., Edelman, R., Grossman, R.A. *et al.* (1974) Study of Japanese encephalitis virus in Chiangmai Valley, Thailand. V. Animal infections. *Am J Epidemiol*, 100, 57–68.

[287] Gould, D.J., Edelman, R., Grossman, R.A. *et al.* (1974) Study of Japanese encephalitis virus in Chiangmai Valley, Thailand. IV. Vector studies. *Am J Epidemiol*, 100, 49–56.

[288] Gulati, B.R., Singha, H., Singh, B.K. *et al.* (2012) Isolation and genetic characterization of Japanese encephalitis virus from equines in India. *J Vet Sci*, 13, 111–118.

[289] Shimojima, M., Nagao, Y., Shimoda, H. *et al.* (2011) Full genome sequence and virulence analyses of the recent equine isolate of Japanese encephalitis virus. *J Vet Med Sci*, 73, 813–816.

[290] Konishi, E., Shoda, M. and Kondo, T. (2006) Analysis of yearly changes in levels of antibodies to Japanese encephalitis virus nonstructural 1 protein in racehorses in central Japan shows high levels of natural virus activity still exist. *Vaccine*, 24, 516–524.

[291] Konishi, E., Shoda, M. and Kondo, T. (2004) Prevalence of antibody to Japanese encephalitis virus nonstructural 1 protein among racehorses in Japan: indication of natural infection and need for continuous vaccination. *Vaccine*, 22, 1097–1103.

[292] Singha, H., Gulati, B.R., Kumar, P. *et al.* (2013) Complete genome sequence analysis of Japanese encephalitis virus isolated from a horse in India. *Arch Virol*, 158, 113–122.

[293] Pant, G.R., Lunt, R.A., Rootes, C.L. and Daniels, P.W. (2006) Serological evidence for Japanese encephalitis and West Nile viruses in domestic animals of Nepal. *Comp Immunol Microbiol Infect Dis*, 29, 166–175.

[294] Pant, G.R. (2006) A serological survey of pigs, horses, and ducks in Nepal for evidence of infection with Japanese encephalitis virus. *Ann N Y Acad Sci*, 1081, 124–129.

[295] Igarashi, A., Ogata, T., Fujita, N. *et al.* (1983) Flavivirus infections in Chiang Mai area, Thailand, in 1982. *Southeast Asian J Trop Med Public Health*, 14, 470–480.

[296] Yamada, T., Rojanasuphot, S., Takagi, M. *et al.* (1971) Studies on an epidemic of Japanese encephalitis in the northern region of Thailand in 1969 and 1970. *Biken J*, 14, 267–296.

[297] Hall, R.A., Broom, A.K., Smith, D.W. and Mackenzie, J.S. (2002) The ecology and epidemiology of Kunjin virus. *Curr Top Microbiol Immunol*, 267, 253–269.

[298] Hayes, C.G. (2001) West Nile virus: Uganda, 1937, to New York City, 1999. *Ann N Y Acad Sci*, 951, 25–37.

[299] Schuler, L.A., Khaitsa, M.L., Dyer, N.W. and Stoltenow, C.L. (2004) Evaluation of an outbreak of West Nile virus infection in horses: 569 cases (2002). *J Am Vet Med Assoc*, 225, 1084–1089.

[300] Ostlund, E.N., Crom, R.L., Pedersen, D.D. *et al.* (2001) Equine West Nile encephalitis, United States. *Emerg Infect Dis*, 7, 665–669.

[301] Porter, M.B., Long, M.T., Getman, L.M. *et al.* (2003) West Nile virus encephalomyelitis in horses: 46 cases (2001). *J Am Vet Med Assoc*, 222, 1241–1247.

[302] Snook, C.S., Hyman, S.S., Del, P.F. *et al.* (2001) West Nile virus encephalomyelitis in eight horses. *J Am Vet Med Assoc*, 218, 1576–1579.

[303] Cantile, C., Di, G.G., Eleni, C. and Arispici, M. (2000) Clinical and neuropathological features of West Nile virus equine encephalomyelitis in Italy. *Equine Vet J*, 32, 31–35.

[304] Cantile, C., Del, P.F., Di, G.G. and Arispici, M. (2001) Pathologic and immunohistochemical findings in naturally occurring West Nile virus infection in horses. *Vet Pathol*, 38, 414–421.

[305] Joubert, L., Oudar, J., Hannoun, C. and Chippaux, M. (1971) Experimental reproduction of meningo-encephalomyelitis of horses with West Nile arbovirus. 3. Relations between virology, serology, and anatomo-clinical evolution. Epidemiological and prophylactic consequences. *Bull Acad Vet Fr*, 44, 159–167.

[306] Oudar, J., Joubert, L., Lapras, M. and Guillon, J.C. (1971) Experimental reproduction of meningo-encephalomyelitis of horses with West Nile arbovirus. II. Anatomo-clinical study. *Bull Acad Vet Fr*, 44, 147–158.

[307] Guillon, J.C., Oudar, J., Joubert, L. and Hannoun, C. (1968) Histological lesions of the nervous system in West Nile virus infection in horses. *Ann Institut Pasteur (Paris)*, 114, 539–550.

[308] Wang, Y.J., Gu, P.W. and Liu, P.S. (1982) Japanese B encephalitis virus infection of horses during the first epidemic season following entry into an infected area. *Chin Med J (Engl)*, 95, 63–66.

[309] Kay, B.H., Pollitt, C.C., Fanning, I.D. and Hall, R.A. (1987) The experimental infection of horses with Murray Valley encephalitis and Ross River viruses. *Aust Vet J*, 64, 52–55.

[310] Diamond, M.S. and Klein, R.S. (2004) West Nile virus: crossing the blood-brain barrier. *Nat Med*, 10, 1294–1295.

[311] Samuel, M.A., Wang, H., Siddharthan, V. *et al.* (2007) Axonal transport mediates West Nile virus entry into the central nervous system and induces acute flaccid paralysis. *Proc Natl Acad Sci U S A*, 104, 17140–17145.

[312] Wang, H., Siddharthan, V., Hall, J.O. and Morrey, J.D. (2009) West Nile virus preferentially transports along motor neuron axons after sciatic nerve injection of hamsters. *J Neurovirol*, 15, 293–299.

[313] Zhang, B., Patel, J., Croyle, M. *et al.* (2010) TNF-alpha-dependent regulation of CXCR3 expression modulates neuronal survival during West Nile virus encephalitis. *J Neuroimmunol*, 224, 28–38.

[314] Daffis, S., Samuel, M.A., Suthar, M.S. *et al.* (2008) Toll-like receptor 3 has a protective role against West Nile virus infection. *J Virol*, 82, 10349–10358.

[315] Klein, R.S., Lin, E., Zhang, B. *et al.* (2005) Neuronal CXCL10 directs CD8+ T-cell recruitment and control of West Nile virus encephalitis. *J Virol*, 79, 11457–11466.

[316] Mackenzie, J.S. and Broom, A.K. (1995) Australian X disease, Murray Valley encephalitis and the French connection. *Vet Microbiol*, 46, 79–90.

[317] Guthrie, A.J., Howell, P.G., Gardner, I.A. *et al.* (2003) West Nile virus infection of Thoroughbred horses in South Africa (2000–2001). *Equine Vet J*, 35, 601–605.

[318] Bunning, M.L., Bowen, R.A., Cropp, C.B. *et al.* (2002) Experimental infection of horses with West Nile virus. *Emerg Infect Dis*, 8, 380–386.

[319] Wang, H., Siddharthan, V., Hall, J.O. and Morrey, J.D. (2011) Autonomic nervous dysfunction in hamsters infected with West Nile virus. *PLoS One*, 6, e19575.

[320] Epp, T., Waldner, C., West, K. and Townsend, H. (2007) Factors associated with West Nile virus disease fatalities in horses. *Can Vet J*, 48, 1137–1145.

[321] Salazar, P., Traub-Dargatz, J.L., Morley, P.S. *et al.* (2004) Outcome of equids with clinical signs of West Nile virus infection and factors associated with death. *J Am Vet Med Assoc*, 225, 267–274.

[322] Wamsley, H.L., Alleman, A.R., Porter, M.B. and Long, M.T. (2002) Findings in cerebrospinal fluids of horses infected with West Nile virus: 30 cases (2001). *J Am Vet Med Assoc*, 221, 1303–1305.

[323] Jeha, L.E., Sila, C.A., Lederman, R.J. *et al.* (2003) West Nile virus infection: a new acute paralytic illness. *Neurology*, 61, 55–59.

[324] Cernescu, C., Ruta, S.M., Tardei, G. *et al.* (1997) A high number of severe neurologic clinical forms during an epidemic of West Nile virus infection. *Rom J Virol*, 48, 13–25.

[325] Tee, S.Y., Horadagoda, N. and Mogg, T.D. (2012) Kunjin flaviviral encephalomyelitis in an Arabian gelding in New South Wales, Australia. *Aust Vet J*, 90, 321–324.

[326] Long, M.T., Jeter, W., Hernandez, J. *et al.* (2006) Diagnostic performance of the equine IgM capture ELISA for serodiagnosis of West Nile virus infection. *J Vet Intern Med*, 20, 608–613.

[327] Kitai, Y., Shirafuji, H., Kanehira, K. *et al.* (2011) Specific antibody responses to West Nile virus infections in horses preimmunized with inactivated Japanese encephalitis vaccine: evaluation of blocking enzyme-linked immunosorbent assay and complement-dependent cytotoxicity assay. *Vector Borne Zoonotic Dis*, 11, 1093–1098.

[328] Yeh, J.Y., Lee, J.H., Park, J.Y. *et al.* (2012) A diagnostic algorithm to serologically differentiate West Nile virus from Japanese encephalitis virus infections and its validation in field surveillance of poultry and horses. *Vector Borne Zoonotic Dis*, 12, 372–379.

[329] Walton, G.A. (1967) Relative status in Britain and Ireland of louping ill encephalitis virus. *J Med Entomol*, 4, 161–167.

[330] De, F.M., Ulbert, S., Diamond, M. and Sanders, N.N. (2012) Recent progress in West Nile virus diagnosis and vaccination. *Vet Res*, 43, 16.

[331] Davidson, A.H., Traub-Dargatz, J.L., Rodeheaver, R.M. *et al.* (2005) Immunologic responses to West Nile virus in vaccinated and clinically affected horses. *J Am Vet Med Assoc*, 226, 240–245.

[332] Ostlund, E.N., Andresen, J.E. and Andresen, M. (2000) West Nile encephalitis. *Vet Clin North Am Equine Pract*, 16, 427–441.

[333] Wang, T., Magnarelli, L.A., Anderson, J.F. *et al.* (2002) A recombinant envelope protein-based enzyme-linked immunosorbent assay for West Nile virus serodiagnosis. *Vector Borne Zoonotic Dis*, 2, 105–109.

[334] Hall, R.A., Broom, A.K., Hartnett, A.C. *et al.* (1995) Immunodominant epitopes on the NS1 protein of MVE

and KUN viruses serve as targets for a blocking ELISA to detect virus-specific antibodies in sentinel animal serum. *J Virol Methods*, 51, 201–210.

[335] Kitai, Y., Kondo, T. and Konishi, E. (2011) Non-structural protein 1 (NS1) antibody-based assays to differentiate West Nile (WN) virus from Japanese encephalitis virus infections in horses: effects of WN virus NS1 antibodies induced by inactivated WN vaccine. *J Virol Methods*, 171, 123–128.

[336] Pyke, A.T., Smith, I.L., van den Hurk, A.F. *et al.* (2004) Detection of Australasian flavivirus encephalitic viruses using rapid fluorogenic TaqMan RT-PCR assays. *J Virol Methods*, 117, 161–167.

[337] Shirato, K., Mizutani, T., Kariwa, H. and Takashima, I. (2003) Discrimination of West Nile virus and Japanese encephalitis virus strains using RT-PCR RFLP analysis. *Microbiol Immunol*, 47, 439–445.

[338] Tewari, D., Kim, H., Feria, W. *et al.* (2004) Detection of West Nile virus using formalin fixed paraffin embedded tissues in crows and horses: quantification of viral transcripts by real-time RT-PCR. *J Clin Virol*, 30, 320–325.

[339] Bowen, R.A., Rouge, M.M., Siger, L. *et al.* (2006) Pathogenesis of West Nile virus infection in dogs treated with glucocorticoids. *Am J Trop Med Hyg*, 74, 670–673.

[340] Lewis, M. and Amsden, J.R. (2007) Successful treatment of West Nile virus infection after approximately 3 weeks into the disease course. *Pharmacotherapy*, 27, 455–458.

[341] Chan-Tack, K.M. and Forrest, G. (2005) Failure of interferon alpha-2b in a patient with West Nile virus meningoencephalitis and acute flaccid paralysis. *Scand J Infect Dis*, 37, 944–946.

[342] Chan-Tack, K.M. and Forrest, G. (2006) West Nile virus meningoencephalitis and acute flaccid paralysis after infliximab treatment. *J Rheumatol*, 33, 191–192.

[343] Diamond, M.S. (2005) Development of effective therapies against West Nile virus infection. *Expert Rev Anti Infect Ther*, 3, 931–944.

[344] Nath, A. and Tyler, K.L. (2013) Novel approaches and challenges to treatment of CNS viral infections. *Ann Neurol*, 74, 412–422.

[345] Ng, T., Hathaway, D., Jennings, N. *et al.* (2003) Equine vaccine for West Nile virus. *Dev Biol (Basel)*, 114, 221–227.

[346] Minke, J.M., Siger, L., Karaca, K. *et al.* (2004) Recombinant canarypoxvirus vaccine carrying the prM/E genes of West Nile virus protects horses against a West Nile virus-mosquito challenge. *Arch Virol Suppl*, 18, 221–230.

[347] Siger, L., Bowen, R., Karaca, K. *et al.* (2006) Evaluation of the efficacy provided by a Recombinant Canarypox-Vectored Equine West Nile virus vaccine against an experimental West Nile virus intrathecal challenge in horses. *Vet Ther*, 7, 249–256.

[348] Long, M.T., Gibbs, E.P., Mellencamp, M.W. *et al.* (2007) Efficacy, duration, and onset of immunogenicity of a West Nile virus vaccine, live Flavivirus chimera, in horses with a clinical disease challenge model. *Equine Vet J*, 39, 491–497.

[349] El, G.H., Minke, J.M., Rehder, J. *et al.* (2008) A West Nile virus (WNV) recombinant canarypox virus vaccine elicits WNV-specific neutralizing antibodies and cell-mediated immune responses in the horse. *Vet Immunol Immunopathol*, 123, 230–239.

[350] Goto, H. (1976) Efficacy of Japanese encephalitis vaccine in horses. *Equine Vet J*, 8, 126–127.

[351] Lam, K.H., Ellis, T.M., Williams, D.T. *et al.* (2005) Japanese encephalitis in a racing thoroughbred gelding in Hong Kong. *Vet Rec*, 157, 168–173.

[352] Satou, K. and Nishiura, H. (2007) Evidence of the partial effects of inactivated Japanese encephalitis vaccination: analysis of previous outbreaks in Japan from 1953 to 1960. *Ann Epidemiol*, 17, 271–277.

[353] Little, P.B., Thorsen, J., Moore, W. and Weninger, N. (1985) Powassan viral encephalitis: a review and experimental studies in the horse and rabbit. *Vet Pathol*, 22, 500–507.

[354] Keane, D.P. and Little, P.B. (1987) Equine viral encephalomyelitis in Canada: a review of known and potential causes. *Can Vet J*, 28, 497–504.

[355] Keane, D.P., Little, P.B., Wilkie, B.N. *et al.* (1988) Agents of equine viral encephalomyelitis: correlation of serum and cerebrospinal fluid antibodies. *Can J Vet Res*, 52, 229–235.

[356] Birge, J. and Sonnesyn, S. (2012) Powassan virus encephalitis, Minnesota, USA. *Emerg Infect Dis*, 18, 1669–1671.

[357] Anderson, J.F. and Armstrong, P.M. (2012) Prevalence and genetic characterization of Powassan virus strains infecting *Ixodes scapularis* in Connecticut. *Am J Trop Med Hyg*, 87, 754–759.

[358] Ernek, E., Kozuch, O. and Nosek, J. (1968) Isolation of tick-borne encephalitis virus from blood and milk of goats grazing in the Tribec focus zone. *J Hyg Epidemiol Microbiol Immunol*, 12, 32–36.

[359] Martianova, L.I. and Rodin, I.M. (1956) Result of industrial preparation of hyperimmune horse therapeutic serum for tick-borne and Japanese encephalitis. I. Dynamics of the increase of virus-neutralizing antibodies in serum of horses hyperimmunized by viruses of tick-borne and Japanese encephalitis. *Vopr Virusol*, 1, 17–22.

[360] Naumov, R.L. and Gutova, V.P. (1977) Geographical and annual variability in the infection rate of ixoid ticks with tick-borne encephalitis virus (review of the literature). *Meditsinskaia parazitologiia i parazitarnye bolezni (Mosk)*, 46, 346–355.

[361] Heinz, F.X. and Kunz, C. (1982) Molecular epidemiology of tick-borne encephalitis virus: peptide mapping of large non-structural proteins of European isolates and comparison with other flaviviruses. *J Gen Virol*, 62 (Pt 2), 271–285.

[362] Naumov, R.L., Gutova, V.P. and Chunikhin, S.P. (1983) Experimental study of the interrelations of the tick-borne encephalitis virus and vertebrates. 1. Large and medium-sized mammals (a review of the literature). *Meditsinskaia parazitologiia i parazitarnye bolezni (Mosk)*, 52, 78–83.

[363] Vesenjak-Hirjan, J., Punda-Polic, V. and Dobe, M. (1991) Geographical distribution of arboviruses in Yugoslavia. *J Hyg Epidemiol Microbiol Immunol*, 35, 129–140.

[364] Heinz, F.X. and Mandl, C.W. (1993) The molecular biology of tick-borne encephalitis virus. Review article. *APMIS*, 101, 735–745.

[365] Gresikova, M. and Kaluzova, M. (1997) Biology of tick-borne encephalitis virus. *Acta Virol*, 41, 115–124.

[366] Muller, K., Konig, M. and Thiel, H.J. (2006) Tick-borne encephalitis (TBE) with special emphasis on infection in horses. *Dtsch Tierarztl Wochenschr*, 113, 147–151.

[367] Hyde, J., Nettleton, P., Marriott, L. and Willoughby, K. (2007) Louping ill in horses. *Vet Rec*, 160, 532.

[368] Timoney, P.J. (1980) Susceptibility of the horse to experimental inoculation with louping ill virus. *J Comp Pathol*, 90, 73–86.

[369] Timoney, P.J., Donnelly, W.J., Clements, L.O. and Fenlon, M. (1976) Encephalitis caused by louping ill virus in a group of horses in Ireland. *Equine Vet J*, 8, 113–117.

[370] Timoney, P.J. (1976) Louping ill: a serological survey of horses in Ireland. *Vet Rec*, 41, 303.

[371] Guu, T.S., Zheng, W. and Tao, Y.J. (2012) Bunyavirus: structure and replication. *Adv Exp Med Biol*, 726, 245–266.

[372] Flick, R. and Bouloy, M. (2005) Rift Valley fever virus. *Curr Mol Med*, 5, 827–834.

[373] Blitvich, B.J., Saiyasombat, R., Travassos da, R.A. *et al.* (2012) Orthobunyaviruses, a common cause of infection of livestock in the Yucatan peninsula of Mexico. *Am J Trop Med Hyg*, 87, 1132–1139.

[374] Goff, G., Whitney, H. and Drebot, M.A. (2012) Roles of host species, geographic separation, and isolation in the seroprevalence of Jamestown Canyon and snowshoe hare viruses in Newfoundland. *Appl Environ Microbiol*, 78, 6734–6740.

[375] van Eeden, C., Williams, J.H., Gerdes, T.G. *et al.* (2012) Shuni virus as cause of neurologic disease in horses. *Emerg Infect Dis*, 18, 318–321.

[376] Yang, D.K., Kim, B.H., Kweon, C.H. *et al.* (2008) Serosurveillance for Japanese encephalitis, Akabane, and Aino viruses for Thoroughbred horses in Korea. *J Vet Sci*, 9, 381–385.

[377] Nelson, D.M., Gardner, I.A., Chiles, R.F. *et al.* (2004) Prevalence of antibodies against Saint Louis encephalitis and Jamestown Canyon viruses in California horses. *Comp Immunol Microbiol Infect Dis*, 27, 209–215.

[378] Calisher, C.H., Oro, J.G., Lord, R.D. *et al.* (1988) Kairi virus identified from a febrile horse in Argentina. *Am J Trop Med Hyg*, 39, 519–521.

[379] Calisher, C.H., Francy, D.B., Smith, G.C. *et al.* (1986) Distribution of Bunyamwera serogroup viruses in North America, 1956–1984. *Am J Trop Med Hyg*, 35, 429–443.

[380] McLean, R.G., Calisher, C.H. and Parham, G.L. (1987) Isolation of Cache Valley virus and detection of antibody for selected arboviruses in Michigan horses in 1980. *Am J Vet Res*, 48, 1039–1041.

[381] Godsey, M.S., Jr, Amoo, F., Yuill, T.M. and Defoliart, G.R. (1988) California serogroup virus infections in Wisconsin domestic animals. *Am J Trop Med Hyg*, 39, 409–416.

[382] Lynch, J.A., Binnington, B.D. and Artsob, H. (1985) California serogroup virus infection in a horse with encephalitis. *J Am Vet Med Assoc*, 186, 389.

Contagious Neurological Diseases

Maureen T. Long

College of Veterinary Medicine, University of Florida, Gainesville, USA

Mononegavirales is an order composed of several viruses that can infect horses from the bite of an infected animal or via direct transmission [1]. The several different orders of these viruses that cause central nervous system (CNS) disease include Rhabdoviridae (Lyssavirus—rabies and various bat viruses), Bornaviridae (Bornavirus), and Paramyxoviridae (Henipaviruses including Hendra (HeV) and Nipah virus (NiV)) [1].

The Mononegavirales are single stranded (mono) negative-sense (nega) viruses that vary from 9 to 29 kb and are fairly heterogeneous in morphology ranging from the pleomorphic paramyxoviruses to the bullet-shaped rabies virus [1]. Nonetheless, there are similarities in the life cycle of these viruses that account for their similarities across animal and plant hosts and the associated pathogenesis of these diseases. These viruses bind to cell surface receptors and fuse with the host cell membrane. The internalized virus particle enters the cytoplasm and is uncoated, leaving a negative-sense RNA strand and an accompanying protein RNA-dependent RNA polymerase (RDRP) [1]. This protein is necessary because a negative-sense RNA virus cannot be transcribed. The proteins necessary for structure and function are transcribed as single mRNAs. Upon transcription, the virus commandeers the cell to translate the viral messages into protein. When virus structures are created, the RDRP stops transcribing separate viral messages and begins creating full-length mRNA to become a template for creation of negative strand viral. Upon self-assembly in the cytoplasm, the virus buds from the cell.

All of these diseases, depending on the geographic locale, have several other equally important differentials to consider, many of which are also zoonotic. Of the viral etiologies, these include alphaviruses, flaviviruses, and herpesviruses. Parasitic infections are also important and include protozoal agents such as *Sarcocystis neurona* and *Neospora hughesii*. Several verminous infections also may exhibit similar clinical signs and these include *Halicephalobus gingivalis*, *Setaria* spp., and *Strongylus*

vulgaris. In addition, there are many noninfectious causes of CNS diseases and these include hepatoencephalopathy, toxicities (tremorgens and leukoencephalomalacia), and electrolyte abnormalities.

No known antiviral medications demonstrate reliable activity against CNS viral diseases, and thus therapy in affected horses is supportive. The clinical course of most of the diseases discussed in this chapter are fatal. Since most confirmatory testing is postmortem, horses receive a variety of medications. Some clinicians advocate the use of corticosteroids as a component of therapy for horses with neurologic signs consistent with viral encephalitis. In human patients, treatment with methylprednisolone (1000 mg/100-kg patient) is often recommended. Administration of flunixin meglumine (1.1 mg/kg q12 h IV) or other antiinflammatory medications to horses may help alleviate signs of discomfort. Mannitol (0.25–2.0 g/kg q24 h IV) may assist in the control of brain edema. Detomidine hydrochloride (0.02–0.04 mg/kg IV or IM) is effective for prolonged tranquilization. Other sedatives include the use of acepromazine, chloral hydrate, or benzodiazepam derivatives depending on clinical signs. Promazines can lower the threshold to seizure and should be avoided in hroses with cortical signs. Benzodiazepam derivatives can increase tremors. Generally, morphine derivatives should be avoided because of possible mania, increased hyperaesthesia, and loss of coordination initially. Intravenous fluids should be instituted in horses that are not eating for whatever reason, and with prolonged lack of food intake nutritional support is indicated.

Rabies

Etiology and epidemiology

Rabies virus is a Lyssavirus and there are two main genotypes with several geographic variants. The "classic" genotype is that of the canid variant (mainly

---

isolated from wild canids, fox, raccoons, and skunks) and the bat variant [1, 2]. Rabies is present throughout the world except island and isolated countries. In the latter half of the 20th century, rabies in the US changed from an infection primarily affecting domestic animals to that of one affecting mainly wildlife [2–33]. From 1957 to 2008 [2, 8–12, 18–33], the domestic animal infection rate dropped from over 3000 annual cases and has stayed under 1000 annual cases (several years this has been under 500) with a steady rise to over 7000 cases of US wildlife cases. In the United States, cases of human rabies have dropped to 1–2 year reflecting the success of postexposure prophylaxis (PEX) [5]. However, in 2011, six human cases were reported to the CDC [5]. In other countries, the primary source of rabies exposure is rabid dogs and this reflects the limited implementation of canine vaccination in areas of inadequate public health resources [34–36].

Although direct transmission of rabies from the bite of an infected horse has not been reported, horses do sometimes become aggressive with rabies. Green reported that as of 1993 there was no documented report of rabies transmission to a human by an equine and, to the author's knowledge, there has been no documentation in the 20 years since that publication [37]. Nonetheless, infected equine tissue is a threat to human safety [37, 39]. In the carnivorous species, rabies virus is shed in the saliva, urine, milk, and placental fluids; it can also be present in the cerebrospinal fluid (CSF) [40–44]. Less is known regarding body fluid analysis in the horse. Because in other species most body fluids are positive, personal protection should be maintained when handling horses that are suspected of rabies.

Identification of rabies in any host is of extreme importance because these animals serve as sentinels of rabies activity and signify an environmental threat to other domestic species and people. In 2007, the American Association of Equine Practitioners (AAEP) recommended, as a standard of preventative care, rabies prophylaxis of all horses yearly. The 10-year average from 2001 to 2011 has been 46 equine cases in the United States annually, and this is a 50 year low, declining from 80 to 100 cases annually [2, 5–10, 12, 14–17]. The 6-year average between 2001 and 2006, which was 51.3 cases per year, dropped significantly to 42 cases per year [11, 13–16]. While data is difficult to access, PEX for horses also occurs. In a report from Texas, 72 horses were treated during a 10-year period. There were no failures of PEX in any of these animals [45, 46]. While single horse infections are the usual presentation for United States, outbreaks of rabies do occur in equids in other parts of the world. At a camp in Bhutan, India, 12 mules died in a 3-month period in 2006; the source of exposure was the wild jackal (*Canis aureus*) [47]. No mule residing at the camp during this period that was vaccinated developed rabies. No history of vaccination, 100% pasture management, and residence in focally active (endemic) areas have all been associated with risk for cases of equine rabies [37]. For labeling of a rabies vaccine for prevention against rabies disease, 100% efficacy after one dose of vaccine must be demonstrated in the buccal mucosa model where challenge results in 100% of the horse developing fatal encephalitis [48].

Examination of the literature describes diagnosis of rabies in at least six horses that had been previously vaccinated; however, little detail is provided regarding actual vaccination methods or products [37, 49–51]. In a retrospective study of horses with rabies identified at postmortem, one horse out of four had a history of vaccination, although the frequency, route, and product were not described. In another clinical study, 5 of 21 horses had a history of vaccination [49]. These reports must be interpreted with caution, due to the lack of detail regarding the actual regimen followed for prevention of rabies.

While in some reports, season is a risk factor, with warmer months associated with rabies, the activity of rabid carnivores may dictate occurrences of winter activity in livestock [37, 52–54]. Bats do hibernate when temperatures reach 50°C; thus, this route of transmission likely ceases during the winter months.

Clinical findings

Clinical cases of rabies in horse are difficult to identify antemortem based solely on clinical signs [37, 48, 49, 51, 55–59]. The incubation period of rabies virus is variable; in clinical cases, it is reported as 2–6 weeks, but in experimentally induced rabies, wherein horses are injected with rabies virus in the buccal mucosa, onset was 12 days [48]. Historically, disease caused by rabies is described with three classical presentations: dumb, furious, and paralytic [37]. Onset of clinical signs is insidious and often presents similar to other systemic and neurological clinical disease [37, 38, 48, 49, 51, 55–59]. Systemic clinical signs include abdominal pain, tenesmus, lameness, increased rectal temperature, anorexia, depression, and dyspnea [37, 48, 49, 51, 55–59] due to airway obstruction caused by laryngeal and/or pharyngeal paralysis. Disease course in the horse is exceptionally variable with horses even progressing through short episodes proceeding from dumb-furious-paralytic in about half of experimentally challenged horses [48]. In published reports of naturally infected horses, the furious form has been reported in about 20% of horses, although in the author's experience, most of the horses observed are actually self-mutilators [49, 51]. These horses are frequently violent and attempts to interrupt this behavior increase the handlers' exposure to oral secretions and uncontrolled biting behavior. Brain signs include hyperesthesia, tremors (most frequently reported), obtundation, or somnolence, head tilt, circling, teeth grinding, blindness, drooling, recumbency, seizures, blindness, head pressing, and vocalization [37, 48, 49, 54–59]. Horses may sweat uncontrollably and roar due to the laryngeal paralysis [37, 48, 49, 51, 55–59]. There can also be photophobia and hydrophobia [37, 48, 49, 51, 58, 59]. Spinal signs are most commonly described as ascending ataxia with decreased anal tone, and loss of hind- and then front-limb proprioception and then withdrawal reflexes [37, 48, 49, 51, 55–59]. These signs can be extremely variable; some horses will remain alert and eat and drink until sudden death once recumbent [37, 49]. Rabies virus is 100% fatal in horses and horses usually die within a week [37, 48, 49].

Diagnosis

There are no pathognomonic clinicopathologic changes in horses with rabies. Complete blood counts and serum biochemical profiles are generally normal and there may a mild mononuclear pleocytosis with or without increased total protein in the CSF; some texts describe xanthochromia [48]. There is no recognized antemortem antigen-based diagnostic test for rabies virus in horses. Until postmortem diagnostic testing is performed, all attempts at identification on the live horse have no utility. In addition, attempts at identification of rabies virus via antigen-detection techniques such as immunofluorescent antibody (IFA) on CSF have a high rate of false positives. Many antemortem tests are performed on humans, but CDC guidelines indicate that there is no reliable single test that exists. These tests vary from body fluid testing to brain biopsy [60–62]. Detection of antigen includes IFA, reverse-transcription PCR, and viral isolation [43, 63–65].

The gold standard for postmortem diagnosis is direct fluorescent antibody (DFA) testing performed on fresh brain samples. The DFA is based on the "Protocol for Postmortem Diagnosis of Rabies in Animals by Direct Fluorescent Antibody Testing" and provides the minimum standard for rabies diagnosis in the United States [67]. The strict protocol in this guideline was established in 1999 to ensure that there was one protocol that allowed for validation of laboratories and other diagnostic procedures [67]. Under this standard cross-section of brainstem from horses is the section of choice. While "examination" may be made at the level of the pons, medulla, or hindbrain, the guide also states that cerebellar tissue should be included. Samples are best shipped within 48h to a CDC-validated laboratory and the sample must be fresh (unfixed). Repeated freezing and thawing decreases the sensitivity of the DFA. Mailing and transport of samples should be shipped consistent for containment of infectious samples. If

rabies is suspected based on routine microscopic analysis and there is no fresh tissue, four to five unstained sections of brain mounted on slides should be sent to the Rabies Laboratory, CDC, Atlanta, GA (http://www.cdc.gov/rabies/specific_groups/laboratories/index.html). These sections must include brainstem, hippocampous, cerbellum, and any other CNS tissues with lesions.

Pathogenesis and pathology

Upon inoculation of saliva containing rabies virus via a bite from an infected animal, there is initial replication of the virus in muscle [68–71]. Infection of peripheral nerves occurs via nicotine acetylcholine recepters located at the neuromuscular junction [72, 73]. The virus ascends to the brain or spinal cord via cranial or peripheral nerves. If through a peripheral nerve, the virus also ascends to the brain from the spinal cord. In the CNS, there is rapid spread and movement to fluids of the body via efferent dissimination. Gross evaluation reveals multifocal hemorrhages most associated with gray matter. Depending on the stage of infection and the movement of virus, the degree of pathology and presence of intracytoplasmic viral inclusions (negri bodies) can be variable in the horse [49, 51, 60, 71, 74–77]. Like most RNA viruses, the primary lesion is nonsuppurative meningoencephalitis composed of a mononuclear perivascular infiltrations, focal giosis, moderate to extensive congestion. A classic lesion of rabies virus is a mononuclear ganglioneuritis that is most associated with the fifth cranial nerve (gasserion ganglioneuritis) [77]. There can be hemorrhage associated with lesions which can be focally extensive and primarily located in the gray matter. Overall, a moderately increased cellularity associated with increased numbers of glial cells can be present in the neuropil. In the spinal cord, there can be extensive areas of hemorrhage and inflammation mostly associated with the dorsal gray matter. Detection of negri bodies in the horse and large animals overall can be challenging. While distribution in humans and canine rabies usually emphasizes the hippocampus, examination of the Purkinje cell layers of the cerebellum can be more rewarding in the equine and, in particular, areas without inflammation can provide clearer visualization.

Therapy and post-exposure prophylaxis

There is no known therapy for rabies and suspected horses should be confined, handled with personal protection equipment, and observed for a minimum of 10 days. Upon euthanasia or spontaneous death, a postmortem should be performed and appropriate sections of the brain removed and sent to a CDC validated laboratory for testing.

For horses exposed to a confirmed rabid animal, the course of action is dependent upon the vaccination history of the horse [49]. If the horse has been annually vaccinated, then the horse should receive an immediate booster vaccine composed of one of the vaccines licensed for use in the horse; a veterinarian must administer the vaccine. An observation period of 45 days is recommended by the CDC and according to the 2012 AAEP vaccination guidelines. In the nonvaccinated horse, the procedures of the state veterinarian will take precedence. Three options are the most common scenarios: (i) immediate euthanasia, (ii) postexposure vaccination with isolation and observation for a prolonged period, (iii) no vaccination, isolation, and observation for a minimum of 6 months.

Vaccination, zoonotic potential and environmental control

As of 2012, three vaccines consisting of five available preparations are currently licensed for the prevention of rabies in horses. Dose of the vaccine must be followed according to the vacine label as two of the three require a 2-ml dose. The AAEP guidelines for core vaccination recommend annual revaccination for all adult horses. One vaccine is labeled for 2 years; however, adherence to the annual schedule is highly recommended especially in rabies-endemic locales. In broodmares, to ensure adequate colostral protection, annual vaccination before breeding is recommended. If a broodmare is already pregnant and has an unknown history, it should be vaccinated 4–6 weeks before foaling. In foals that are born to vaccinated mares, vaccination should commence at 6 weeks followed by a second dose 4–6 weeks later. In foals that are born to mares with no vaccination history, vaccination can commence at 3–4 months with a second dose 4–6 weeks later. All foals should be revaccinated at 12 months.

It is recommended that all veterinary personnel that handle horses and livestock in either an antemortem or postmortem occupational setting receive preexposure vaccination [78]. Since rabies is a zoonotic disease, several guidelines should be followed regarding the handling of all suspect rabies horses both antemortem and postmortem. The number of persons coming in contact with the animal antemortem should be minimized and should only consist of trained personnel and only those persons with preexposure vaccination should be used. For organizational purposes, exposure of all individuals should be recorded immediately. All specimens for any testing should be labeled "rabies suspect." Laboratory personel should work with these materials under a biological safety hood and any type of centrifugation should be performed in a closed container within a closed rotor bucket to prevent aerosolization of fluids. Gloves, eyes protections, and face shields should be worn at all times when handling suspected horses and specimens. During a postmortem of a suspected horses,

protective gear should consist of rubber boots, waterproof coveralls over hospital scrubs, an N95 mask, eye protection, and double gloves. Brain and spinal cord should be removed without the use of electrical saws to minimize aerosolization. No other testing or work should be performed on the necropsy materials until rabies testing is complete and the horse is confirmed negative.

Rabies does not persist in the environment outside the host [79]. Nonetheless, bedding should be treated as a biohazard. All instruments and farm implements should be sanitized before use or discard. All clothings contaminated with body fluid and medical waste should be treated as a biohazard. Stalls, fencing, and any restraint devices should be sanitized. Rabies is susceptible to detergent washing of debris followed by disinfection with any virocidal soap, bleach, and/or autoclaving.

Borna disease virus

Borna disease virus (BDV) infection has many pseudonyms such as "hot-headed disease," "brain fever," and "hypersomnia" due to the encephalitis that can lead to many behavioral abnormalities and an intractable increased rectal temperature [1, 80–83].

Etiology and epidemiology

BDV is an enveloped, single-stranded RNA virus that causes polioencephalomyelitis in horses [84]. Transmission most likely occurs through contact with infected nasal, lacrimal, and/or salivary secretions with viral ascent through the olfactory (and possibly trigeminal) nerve [73, 76, 80, 82, 85–88]. The incubation period is extended and infection appears to be restricted to the nervous system [81]. The prevalence and incidence of the disease worldwide are unknown [89]. There is no species or sex predilection. Age and genetics may be a factor in clinical disease, as there is a high rate of seroprevalence but low rate of disease in endemic areas [66, 84, 89–92]. Clinical BDV has been recognized in horses in Germany, Switzerland, Liechtenstein, and Austria [89]. Seroprevalence studies in Germany reveal that there is a large discrepancy between incidence of disease (low) and prevalence of BDV-specific antibodies [83]. New occurrences of disease can occur anywhere from 2 months to several years after the initial outbreak. There is no seasonal trend to the virus. Recent work reveals that BDV may be more widespread in the Middle East and East; however, these reports are controversial as to whether or not there have been outbreaks of BDV in horses outside of Europe [70, 73, 89, 92–94]. Horses and sheep are primarily affected, but clinical signs reflecting BDV infection have also been reported for cattle, goats, and rabbits [73, 80, 82, 84, 89, 90, 92, 93, 95, 96].

Clinical findings

The incubation period of BDV is quite variable ranging from 2 weeks to several months. Initial clinical signs involve changes in personality and sensorium [76, 81–84, 90, 91, 97]. Movements are deliberate and slow and include general hypokinesia, postural unawareness, and slow eating or chewing with no food in the mouth. Many horses demonstrate rhythmic/repetitive movements and often yawn frequently and head press. Changes in personality and mental status can also occur, including hyperexcitability, fear, aggression, lethargy, somnolence, and stupor. Loss of the cutaneous trunci reflex may also be noted early in the disease. A fever that is refractory to nonsteroidal anti-inflammatory medications may also occur. As the disease progresses, neurological deficits increase. Cranial nerve abnormalities are often seen, including strabismus, miosis, bruxism, trismus, nystagmus, head tilt, dysphagia, pharyngeal paralysis, and tongue paralysis. Spinal cord abnormalities are also present, including ataxia, imbalance, abnormal postures, hyporeflexia of spinal reflexes, and proprioceptive deficits. Changes in personality may progress. In the latter, end stages of BDV, horses appear extremely unbalanced and often stop eating or drinking. Neurogenic torticollis accompanied by dystonia of the neck muscles with or without constant circular walking is often present. Head tremors, convulsions, head pressing, loss of the pupillary light reflex, and coma occur as end-stage events.

Diagnosis, pathology, and prevention

Clinicopathologic assays on infected horses are basically normal. The CSF may have a mononuclear pleocytosis. There are several antemortem serological tests; however, there is no correlation between severity and antibody titer [76, 83, 84, 87, 90, 97]. BDV antigen can be identified postmortem in tissues using immunohistochemistry for proteins and PCR for nucleic acids [73, 84, 93, 94].

BDV appears to be restricted to the CNS and may invade nervous tissue through olfactory or trigeminal nerves resulting in transaxonal migration to the nerve cell bodies and then throughout the nervous system by cell-to-cell movement or through glial cells [73, 76, 80, 88]. Then, the virus transmigrates back through peripheral neurons including the optic nerve to the retina. The virus causes a polioencephalomyelitis with involvement of meninges. Histopathologically, there is mononuclear pervascular cuffing, gliosis, astrocytosis, and distinct loss of pyramidal cells.

The route of transmission of BDV is unknown. The virus has been detected in nasal, lacrimal, and salivary secretions of affected animals, so it is postulated that direct and indirect contact with infected horses can spread the virus [80, 82, 88, 89]. Whether BDV is a zoonotic agent that causes overt illness in humans is unknown. It does appear that people can be affected by either the Borna virus or a Borna-like virus. Seroprevalence studies have revealed BDV antibodies in people with psychiatric disorders and in people without the disease [98–101]. However, the exact pathology of the virus in people, whether it is transmitted to humans from horses, and whether it is a causative agent of disease in people is unknown at this time [98–101]. Veterinarians should take universal precautions when handling and/or performing necropsies on horses with any neurological disease.

Hendra and Nipah viruses

Etiology and epidemiology

HeV and NiV were first recognized in 1994 and 1998 as the causative agent of diseases in horses and pigs, respectively [102, 103]. The focus of this discussion will pertain mainly to HeV in horses; however, experimentally horses are susceptible to NiV and there is one reported (but unpublished) case in the horse [104]. These viruses are zoonotic and have resulted in many human deaths [102, 105–111]. Outbreaks of the viruses have been restricted to Oceania and Asia [105, 106]. Pteropid fruit bats (flying fox) and other microbat species are reservoirs for these viruses [112–114]. Horses and humans contract the disease through direct contact. In horses, there is no known breed, age, or sex predisposition. The major risk factor is proximity to fruit bats (genus Pteropus, order Chiroptera, suborder Megachiroptera) [105, 113–115]. In general, fruit bats are attracted to fruiting trees including figs, melaleucas, eucalypts, date palms, mulberries, guava, and citrus fruits [105, 113–115]. Specifically, contact with secretions from bats, including urine, aborted fetuses, and reproductive secretions increase the likelihood of disease. This includes housing horses in buildings where bats roost or standing under trees where bats are present. Also, cats were identified as the only other species capable of transmitting disease to horses.

As of this writing, there have been several outbreaks of HeV in horses in Australia, the most recent in September, 2013 [116]. Four horses and one dog have been affected involving four separate properties. Before this, the most notable was in 2011 where eight different properties were involved during July and August and 10 affected horses died. The occurrence of infection in eastern Australia and the latest are confined to New South Wales.

Clinical findings

A pneumotropic and neurotropic form of the HeV disease exists and in NiV this disease is biased toward the neurotropic form [107, 109, 117, 118]. In HeV, horses most commonly present with a high fever, followed by a bloody, frothy nasal discharge that progresses to neurological signs. Death occurs within 36 h of the onset of clinical signs. Horses present with the rapid onset of a high fever (106°F), anorexia, tachypnea, tachycardia, and paroxysmal coughing. Severe dyspnea follows, with a blood tinged, foamy discharge from the mouth and nose. In one outbreak, neurological signs predominated, which included ataxia, head pressing, muscular spasms involving the neck and hindlimbs, and collapse. Other signs described include head tilt with leaning to one side, unilateral facial nerve paralysis, circling, and bladder paralysis. The incubation period is approximately a week, with horses dying within 12–36 h of the onset of clinical signs.

Diagnosis
In affected horses, there are basically no major abnormalities detected via complete blood count and serum biochemistry analysis. HeV and NiV are biosafety level-4 pathogens owing to their exceptional pathogenesis in humans. As paramyxoviruses, these can be readily detected by viral cell culture or PCR of secretions and tissues [104, 117, 119–122]. In regards to HeV, once clinical signs include increased respiratory secretions, high levels of virus are shed, and horses may even shed virus up to 48 h before these signs begin. Virus is detected in lung and most internal organs as well as the endothelium of the brain. In NiV infections, virus can be detected within neurons, and in the horse, within endothelial cells in the brain [105, 117, 122]. Several serological tests have been developed and these include serum neutralization and ELISA [121]. Other diseases should be considered given the variety of clinical syndromes that may be observed and these include African horse sickness, equine encephalosis, piroplasmosis, pleuropneumonia, interstitial pneumonia, any infectious neurological disease such as Japanese encephalitis, and primary cardiac disease.

Prevention, zoonotic potential, and environmental control
A vaccine (Zoetis Animal Health) that aids in the protection against HeV in healthy horses was introduced in November 2012 [121, 123, 124]. This is a killed vaccine and the initial immunization consists of two doses administered 21 days apart. At present, the vaccine is labeled for 6 months. Use of the vaccine may affect exportation requirements to several countries such as in China, Singapore, Malaysia, Indonesia, and the United Arab Emirates. Currently, export to Great Britain, Europe, and America should not be compromised by vaccination.

Exposure to flying foxes by feeding horses under fruit trees should be minimized to limit exposure to secretions [106, 112, 114, 121, 125]. Also, efforts to keep food secure from rodents should reduce feed and water source contamination. In pastures, removing debris found under trees that could contain viral secretions and blocking access to trees are also recommended for environmental control.

HeV is considered a zoonotic pathogen [102, 108, 111]. Humans contract the disease from direct (and possibly indirect) contact with the infected equine. Veterinarians should take appropriate precautions when performing necropsies on horses suspected of having HeV.

Miscellaneous central nervous system infections

Aujeszkey's disease (pseudorabies virus)
Pseudorabies is caused by porcine herpesvirus (PHV) 1 in which swine are the primary reservoir [126]. Many species are at risk of infection with PHV from direct contact with PHV infectious pigs, and these include dogs, cats, horses, cattle, sheep, and goats.

Etiology and epidemiology
Pseudorabies is endemic in swine throughout the world and feral swine are a common source of infection in domestic species because of the success of vaccination in domestic swine controlling shedding of virus [126]. Nonetheless infected swine shed virus in saliva, nasal secretions, and aborted material. Transmission to other hosts is via ingestion, inhalation, or via bites. Rats may be a source of contamination of feed. Pseudorabies is a relatively rare disease in horses, and some texts and reviews still maintain that they do not develop clinical disease following infection. However, Koch's postulates were fulfilled in 1991 in horses, wherein the virus from a clinically affected horse was inoculated via nasal and conjunctival exposure back into two horses [127, 128]. In one of the ponies that developed neurological signs, the course of infection was fatal. Virus was recovered from the brains of both ponies. In a few published reports, horses likely contracted disease from exposure to liquid pig manure (used as fertilizer) and transmission on a farm with breeding sows.

Clinical findings
Horses become febrile around 1 week postinoculation [127, 128]. There are limited descriptions of horses with Aujeszkey's disease but in general horses appear to develop frenzy as a primary behavioral change. In addition, horses become severely ataxic with progress to recumbency. Like other species, horses develop anorexia, depression, muscle tremors, hyperexcitability, chewing, hypersalivation, pruritus and self-mutilation. Severe cortical signs develop and include head pressing, nystagmus, iridocyclitis, and blindness.

Diagnosis, pathology, and control

Because of the rareness of the disease, limited information exists regarding hematological and serum biochemical profiles of PHV-infected horses [127, 128]. Although there are many serological and antigen tests for antemortem and outbreak identification of swine, most testing will be performed postmortem in the horse. A variety of methods of antigen detection in brain tissues includes isolation of virus, immunohistochemical detection for PHV protein, and PCR for detection of viral nucleic acids.

Infection with PHV results in oro- and nasopharyngeal replication followed by infection of the cranial nerves and transaxonal spread [129]. The virus causes a ganlioneuritis with a nonsuppurative meningoencephalitis. There is marked cuffing of mononuclear cells around vessels, often several cell layers thick. In the neuropil, there is focal gliosis, with necrosis of neurons and glial cells.

There is no vaccine for the horse and the limited occurrence of this disease in horses obviates the need for a vaccine. In swine-intensive operations, control of the virus relies on good biosecurity and vaccination [126]. Feral swine are a common source of infection for domestic animals, and measures to control the feral swine population should be pursued throughout the United States. Humans are considered relatively resistant to the virus; however, precautions should be utilized to limit exposure to PHV-infected tissues and high levels of virus-laden secretions when handling suspected swine.

Equine infectious anemia virus

Rarely, and sometimes independent of any other signs, equine infectious anemia virus (EIAV) has been reported as a primary cause of neurological disease [130–132]. In areas or on farms with endemic EIAV horses, the neurotropic form of this disease is important. EIAV is transmitted mechanically via the bite of an infected horse fly and iatrogenically.

Horses with EIAV may have weight loss, cyclic anemia and thrombocytopenia, fever, and hypergammaglobulinemia. However, CNS disease may be the only clinical syndrome noted since in most EIAV-infected horses, there is chronic subclinical infection [131, 132]. While solid organs become infiltrated with chronic inflammatory cells leading to organ failure, it is thought that EIAV CNS infections result from the development of a neurotropic variant. There is intrathecal viral replication resulting in the sudden onset of neurological signs. Disease has been described in the acute and chronic stages of infection [131, 132]. Clinical signs can be both brain and/or spinal manifestations consisting of blindness, seizures, sudden death, and ataxia [131, 132].

Clinically infected horses can have high concentrations of protein with mononuclear pleocytosis upon CSF analysis [130, 131]. Antemortem diagnosis is by serology consisting of either the agar gel immunodiffusion assay or ELISA. These must be performed by an accredited laboratory.

Horses with neurological disease due to EIAV present at postmortem with a nonsuppurpative granulomatous ependymitis, meningitis, and encephalomyelitis [130–132]. There are focal to locally extensive infiltrations of lymphocytes, plasma cells, and macrophages.

EIAV has no known zoonotic potential and does not persist in the environment. However, infected herds or single horses must be destroyed or quarantined for life with permanent identification. Equine infectious anemia is an Office International des Epizooties (World Organization for Animal Health) (OIE)-listed disease and is reportable in the United States. All reported EIAV-infected horses with neurological signs have been fatal.

References

[1] Lamb, R.A. (2013) Mononegaviroles, in *Fields Virology*, 6th edn (eds D.M. Knipe and P.M. Howley), Wolters Kluwer, Philadelphia, pp. 2944–3065.

[2] Krebs, J.W., Mondul, A.M., Rupprecht, C.E. and Childs, J.E. (2001) Rabies surveillance in the United States during 2000. *J Am Vet Med Assoc*, 219, 1687–1699.

[3] Schatz, J., Fooks, A.R., McElhinney, L. *et al.* (2013) Bat rabies surveillance in Europe. *Zoonoses Public Health*, 60, 22–34.

[4] Nokireki, T., Huovilainen, A., Lilley, T. *et al.* (2013) Bat rabies surveillance in Finland. *BMC Vet Res*, 9, 174.

[5] Blanton, J.D., Dyer, J., McBrayer, J. and Rupprecht, C.E. (2012) Rabies surveillance in the United States during 2011. *J Am Vet Med Assoc*, 241, 712–722.

[6] Blanton, J.D., Palmer, D., Dyer, J. and Rupprecht, C.E. (2011) Rabies surveillance in the United States during 2010. *J Am Vet Med Assoc*, 239, 773–783.

[7] Blanton, J.D., Palmer, D. and Rupprecht, C.E. (2010) Rabies surveillance in the United States during 2009. *J Am Vet Med Assoc*, 237, 646–657.

[8] Blanton, J.D., Robertson, K., Palmer, D. and Rupprecht, C.E. (2009) Rabies surveillance in the United States during 2008. *J Am Vet Med Assoc*, 235, 676–689.

[9] Blanton, J.D., Palmer, D., Christian, K.A. and Rupprecht, C.E. (2008) Rabies surveillance in the United States during 2007. *J Am Vet Med Assoc*, 233, 884–897.

[10] Blanton, J.D., Hanlon, C.A. and Rupprecht, C.E. (2007) Rabies surveillance in the United States during 2006. *J Am Vet Med Assoc*, 231, 540–556.

[11] Picard-Meyer, E., Barrat, J., Tissot, E. *et al.* (2006) Bat rabies surveillance in France, from 1989 through May 2005. *Dev Biol (Basel)*, 125, 283–288.

[12] Blanton, J.D., Krebs, J.W., Hanlon, C.A. and Rupprecht, C.E. (2006) Rabies surveillance in the United States during 2005. *J Am Vet Med Assoc,* 229, 1897–1911.

[13] Sadkowska-Todys, M., Rosinska, M., Smreczak, M. *et al.* (2005) Rabies surveillance, trends in animal rabies and human post-exposure treatment in Poland, 1990–2004. *Euro Surveill,* 10, 226–228.

[14] Krebs, J.W., Mandel, E.J., Swerdlow, D.L. and Rupprecht, C.E. (2005) Rabies surveillance in the United States during 2004. *J Am Vet Med Assoc,* 227, 1912–1925.

[15] Krebs, J.W., Mandel, E.J., Swerdlow, D.L. and Rupprecht, C.E. (2004) Rabies surveillance in the United States during 2003. *J Am Vet Med Assoc,* 225, 1837–1849.

[16] Krebs, J.W., Wheeling, J.T. and Childs, J.E. (2003) Rabies surveillance in the United States during 2002. *J Am Vet Med Assoc,* 223, 1736–1748.

[17] Krebs, J.W., Noll, H.R., Rupprecht, C.E. and Childs, J.E. (2002) Rabies surveillance in the United States during 2001. *J Am Vet Med Assoc,* 221, 1690–1701.

[18] Krebs, J.W., Rupprecht, C.E. and Childs, J.E. (2000) Rabies surveillance in the United States during 1999. *J Am Vet Med Assoc,* 217, 1799–1811.

[19] Krebs, J.W., Smith, J.S., Rupprecht, C.E. and Childs, J.E. (1999) Rabies surveillance in the United States during 1998. *J Am Vet Med Assoc,* 215, 1786–1798.

[20] Krebs, J.W., Smith, J.S., Rupprecht, C.E. and Childs, J.E. (1998) Rabies surveillance in the United States during 1997. *J Am Vet Med Assoc,* 213, 1713–1728.

[21] Krebs, J.W., Smith, J.S., Rupprecht, C.E. and Childs, J.E. (1997) Rabies surveillance in the United States during 1996. *J Am Vet Med Assoc,* 211, 1525–1539.

[22] Krebs, J.W., Strine, T.W., Smith, J.S. *et al.* (1996) Rabies surveillance in the United States during 1995. *J Am Vet Med Assoc,* 209, 2031–2044.

[23] Krebs, J.W., Strine, T.W., Smith, J.S. *et al.* (1995) Rabies surveillance in the United States during 1994. *J Am Vet Med Assoc,* 207, 1562–1575.

[24] Krebs, J.W., Strine, T.W., Smith, J.S. *et al.* (1994) Rabies surveillance in the United States during 1993. *J Am Vet Med Assoc,* 205, 1695–1709.

[25] Krebs, J.W., Strine, T.W. and Childs, J.E. (1993) Rabies surveillance in the United States during 1992. *J Am Vet Med Assoc,* 203, 1718–1731.

[26] Krebs, J.W., Holman, R.C., Hines, U. *et al.* (1992) Rabies surveillance in the United States during 1991. *J Am Vet Med Assoc,* 201, 1836–1848.

[27] Uhaa, I.J., Mandel, E.J., Whiteway, R. and Fishbein, D.B. (1992) Rabies surveillance in the United States during 1990. *J Am Vet Med Assoc,* 200, 920–929.

[28] Reid-Sanden, F.L., Dobbins, J.G., Smith, J.S. *et al.* (1990) Rabies surveillance in the United States during 1989. *J Am Vet Med Assoc,* 197, 1571–1583.

[29] 1990) Rabies surveillance in 1988. *Wkly Epidemiol Rec,* 65, 114–145.

[30] Eng, T.R., Hamaker, T.A., Dobbins, J.G. *et al.* (1989) Rabies surveillance, United States, 1988. *MMWR CDC Surveill Summ,* 38, 1–21.

[31] Fishbein, D.B., Dobbins, J.G., Bryson, J.H. *et al.* (1988) Rabies surveillance, United States, 1987. *MMWR CDC Surveill Summ,* 37, 1–19.

[32] 1987) Rabies surveillance 1986. *MMWR Morb Mortal Wkly Rep,* 36 (Suppl 3), 1S–27S.

[33] Varughese, P. (1986) Rabies surveillance in Canada. *CMAJ,* 134, 617–618.

[34] Anderson A, Shwiff SA. The cost of canine rabies on four continents. Transbound Emerg Dis 2013 doi:10.1111/tbed.12168.

[35] Shwiff, S., Hampson, K. and Anderson, A. (2013) Potential economic benefits of eliminating canine rabies. *Antiviral Res,* 98, 352–356.

[36] Anderson, A., Shwiff, S., Gebhardt, K. *et al.* (2014) Economic evaluation of vampire bat (*Desmodus rotundus*) rabies prevention in Mexico. *Transbound Emerg Dis,* 61, 140–146.

[37] Green, S.L. (1993) Equine rabies. *Vet Clin North Am Equine Pract,* 9, 337–347.

[38] Afshar, A. (1979) A review of non-bite transmission of rabies virus infection. *Br Vet J,* 135, 142–148.

[39] Bingham, J. and van der Merwe, M. (2002) Distribution of rabies antigen in infected brain material: determining the reliability of different regions of the brain for the rabies fluorescent antibody test. *J Virol Methods,* 101, 85–94.

[40] Dacheux, L., Reynes, J.M., Buchy, P. *et al.* (2008) A reliable diagnosis of human rabies based on analysis of skin biopsy specimens. *Clin Infect Dis,* 47, 1410–1417.

[41] Liu, C. (1975) Rapid diagnosis of viral infections. *South Med J,* 68, 679–680.

[42] Sitprija, V., Sriaroon, C., Lumlertdaecha, B. *et al.* (2003) Does contact with urine and blood from a rabid dog represent a rabies risk? *Clin Infect Dis,* 37, 1399–1400.

[43] Saengseesom, W., Mitmoonpitak, C., Kasempimolporn, S. and Sitprija, V. (2007) Real-time PCR analysis of dog cerebrospinal fluid and saliva samples for ante-mortem diagnosis of rabies. *Southeast Asian J Trop Med Public Health,* 38, 53–57.

[44] Hemachudha, T. and Wacharapluesadee, S. (2004) Antemortem diagnosis of human rabies. *Clin Infect Dis,* 39, 1085–1086.

[45] Mayes, B.C., Wilson, P.J., Oertli, E.H. *et al.* (2013) Epidemiology of rabies in bats in Texas (2001–2010). *J Am Vet Med Assoc,* 243, 1129–1137.

[46] Clark, K.A. and Wilson, P.J. (1996) Postexposure rabies prophylaxis and preexposure rabies vaccination failure in domestic animals. *J Am Vet Med Assoc,* 208, 1827–1830.

[47] Numan, M., Qureshi, Z.A., Shauket, M. *et al.* (2011) Rabies out-break in mules at Mansehra, Pakistan. *Res Vet Sci,* 90, 160–162.

[48] Hudson, L.C., Weinstock, D., Jordan, T. and Bold-Fletcher, N.O. (1996) Clinical presentation of experimentally induced rabies in horses. *Zentralbl Veterinarmed B*, 43, 277–285.

[49] Green, S.L., Smith, L.L., Vernau, W. and Beacock, S.M. (1992) Rabies in horses: 21 cases (1970–1990). *J Am Vet Med Assoc*, 200, 1133–1137.

[50] Martinez, J., Montgomery, D.L. and Uzal, F.A. (2012) Vascular mineralization in the brain of horses. *J Vet Diagn Invest*, 24, 612–617.

[51] Hamir, A.N., Moser, G. and Rupprecht, C.E. (1992) A five year (1985–1989) retrospective study of equine neurological diseases with special reference to rabies. *J Comp Pathol*, 106, 411–421.

[52] Tenzin and Ward, M.P. (2012) Review of rabies epidemiology and control in South, South East and East Asia: past, present and prospects for elimination. *Zoonoses Public Health*, 59, 451–467.

[53] Tenzin, Dhand, N.K. and Ward, M.P. (2011) Patterns of rabies occurrence in Bhutan between 1996 and 2009. *Zoonoses Public Health*, 58, 463–471.

[54] Macedo, C.I., Carnieli, J.P., Fahl, W.O. *et al.* (2010) Genetic characterization of rabies virus isolated from bovines and equines between 2007 and 2008, in the States of Sao Paulo and Minas Gerais. *Rev Soc Bras Med Trop*, 43, 116–120.

[55] Feder, H.M., Nelson, R.S., Cartter, M.L. and Sadre, I. (1998) Rabies prophylaxis following the feeding of a rabid pony. *Clin Pediatr*, 37, 477–481.

[56] West, G.P. (1985) Equine rabies. *Equine Vet J*, 17, 280–282.

[57] Fuller, J.E., Jr (1984) A case of equine rabies. *N Engl J Med*, 310, 525–526.

[58] Smith, L.L. and Clare, D.A. (1972) A clinical note on equine rabies. *Can Vet J*, 13, 193.

[59] Badiali, L. and Ferris, D.H. (1966) A preliminary report on rabies in suspected equine encephalomyelitis cases in the United Arab Republic. *Bull World Health Organ*, 34, 797–798.

[60] Boone, A.C., Susta, L., Rech, R.R. *et al.* (2010) Pathology in practice. Diagnosis: poliomyelitis with intraneuronal Negri bodies. *J Am Vet Med Assoc*, 237, 277–279.

[61] Marler, R.J., Howard, D.R., Morris, P.G. and Johnson, J.L. (1979) Rabies in a horse. *J Am Vet Med Assoc*, 175, 293–294.

[62] Suwansrinon, K., Wilde, H., Benjavongkulchai, M. *et al.* (2006) Survival of neutralizing antibody in previously rabies vaccinated subjects: a prospective study showing long lasting immunity. *Vaccine*, 24, 3878–3880.

[63] Wacharapluesadee, S., Phumesin, P., Supavonwong, P. *et al.* (2011) Comparative detection of rabies RNA by NASBA, real-time PCR and conventional PCR. *J Virol Methods*, 175, 278–282.

[64] Wacharapluesadee, S., Tepsumethanon, V., Supavonwong, P. *et al.* (2012) Detection of rabies viral RNA by TaqMan real-time RT-PCR using non-neural specimens from dogs infected with rabies virus. *J Virol Methods*, 184, 109–112.

[65] Wacharapluesadee, S., Sutipanya, J., Damrongwatanapokin, S. *et al.* (2008) Development of a TaqMan real-time RT-PCR assay for the detection of rabies virus. *J Virol Methods*, 151, 317–320.

[66] Bahmani, M.K., Nowrouzian, I., Nakaya, T. *et al.* (1996) Varied prevalence of Borna disease virus infection in Arabic, thoroughbred and their cross-bred horses in Iran. *Virus Res*, 45, 1–13.

[67] Anon. *Protocol for postmortem diagnosis of rabies in animals by direct fluorescent antibody testing: a minimum standard for rabies diagnosis in the United States.* http://www.cdc.gov/rabies/pdf/rabiesdfaspv2.pdf [accessed December 5, 2014].

[68] Jackson, A.C. (1991) Biological basis of rabies virus neurovirulence in mice: comparative pathogenesis study using the immunoperoxidase technique. *J Virol*, 65, 537–540.

[69] Jackson, A.C. and Reimer, D.L. (1989) Pathogenesis of experimental rabies in mice: an immunohistochemical study. *Acta Neuropathol*, 78, 159–165.

[70] Jackson, A.C. (2006) Rabies: new insights into pathogenesis and treatment. *Curr Opin Neurol*, 19, 267–270.

[71] Jackson, A.C. (2002) Rabies pathogenesis. *J Neurovirol*, 8, 267–269.

[72] Adams, R. and Mayhew, I.G. (1985) Neurologic diseases. *Vet Clin North Am Equine Pract*, 1, 209–234.

[73] Faber, H.K., Silverberg, R.J. and Dong, L. (1953) Studies on entry and egress of poliomyelitic infection. VI. Centrifugal spread of the virus into peripheral nerve with notes on its possible implications. *J Exp Med*, 97, 455–465.

[74] Lapi, A., Davis, C.L. and Anderson, W.A. (1952) The gasserian ganglion in animals dead of rabies. *J Am Vet Med Assoc*, 120, 379–384.

[75] Jenson, A.B., Rabin, E.R., Bentinck, D.C. and Melnick, J.L. (1969) Rabiesvirus neuronitis. *J Virol*, 3, 265–269.

[76] Gosztonyi, G., Dietzschold, B., Kao, M. *et al.* (1993) Rabies and borna disease. A comparative pathogenetic study of two neurovirulent agents. *Lab Invest*, 68, 285–295.

[77] O'Toole, D., Mills, K., Ellis, J. *et al.* (1993) Poliomyelomalacia and ganglioneuritis in a horse with paralytic rabies. *J Vet Diagn Invest*, 5, 94–97.

[78] Wilde, H., Wacharapluesadee, S. and Hemachudha, T. (2012) Currently approved post-exposure rabies prophylaxis regimens. *Travel Med Infect Dis*, 10, 162–163.

[79] Lyles, D.S., Kuzmin, I.V. and Rupprecht, C.E. (2013) Rhabdoviridae, in *Fields Virology*, 6th edn (eds D.M. Knipe and P.M. Howley), Wolters Kluwer, Philadelphia, pp. 64–153.

[80] Mayr, A. and Danner, K. (1978) Borna—a slow virus disease. *Comp Immunol Microbiol Infect Dis*, 1, 3–14.

[81] Gosztonyi, G. and Ludwig, H. (1984) Borna disease of horses. An immunohistological and virological study of naturally infected animals. *Acta Neuropathol*, 64, 213–221.

[82] Ludwig, H., Kraft, W., Kao, M. *et al.* (1985) Borna virus infection (Borna disease) in naturally and experimentally infected animals: its significance for research and practice. *Tierarztl Prax*, 13, 421–453.

[83] Grabner, A. and Fischer, A. (1991) Symptomatology and diagnosis of Borna encephalitis of horses. A case analysis of the last 13 years. *Tierarztl Prax*, 19, 68–73.

[84] Richt, J.A., Grabner, A. and Herzog, S. (2000) Borna disease in horses. *Vet Clin North Am Equine Pract*, 16, 579–595.

[85] Richt, J.A., Herzog, S., Haberzettl, K. and Rott, R. (1993) Demonstration of Borna disease virus-specific RNA in secretions of naturally infected horses by the polymerase chain reaction. *Med Microbiol Immunol*, 182, 293–304.

[86] Kao, M., Hamir, A.N., Rupprecht, C.E. *et al.* (1993) Detection of antibodies against Borna disease virus in sera and cerebrospinal fluid of horses in the USA. *Vet Rec*, 132, 241–244.

[87] Ludwig H, Furuya K, Bode L, et al. . Biology and neurobiology of Borna disease viruses (BDV), defined by antibodies, neutralizability and their pathogenic potential. *Arch Virol Suppl* 1993;7:111–133.

[88] Gosztonyi, G. and Ludwig, H. (1995) Borna disease—neuropathology and pathogenesis. *Curr Top Microbiol Immunol*, 190, 39–73.

[89] Kinnunen, P.M., Palva, A., Vaheri, A. and Vapalahti, O. (2013) Epidemiology and host spectrum of Borna disease virus infections. *J Gen Virol*, 94, 247–262.

[90] Katz, J.B., Alstad, D., Jenny, A.L. *et al.* (1998) Clinical, serologic, and histopathologic characterization of experimental Borna disease in ponies. *J Vet Diagn Invest*, 10, 338–343.

[91] Berg, A.L., Dorries, R. and Berg, M. (1999) Borna disease virus infection in racing horses with behavioral and movement disorders. *Arch Virol*, 144, 547–559.

[92] Hagiwara, K., Asakawa, M., Liao, L. *et al.* (2001) Seroprevalence of Borna disease virus in domestic animals in Xinjiang, China. *Vet Microbiol*, 80, 383–389.

[93] Zimmermann, W., Durrwald, R. and Ludwig, H. (1994) Detection of Borna disease virus RNA in naturally infected animals by a nested polymerase chain reaction. *J Virol Methods*, 46, 133–143.

[94] Nowotny, N., Kolodziejek, J., Jehle, C.O. *et al.* (2000) Isolation and characterization of a new subtype of Borna disease virus. *J Virol*, 74, 5655–5658.

[95] Hilbe, M., Herrsche, R., Kolodziejek, J. *et al.* (2006) Shrews as reservoir hosts of borna disease virus. *Emerg Infect Dis*, 12, 675–677.

[96] Payne, S.L., Delnatte, P., Guo, J. *et al.* (2012) Birds and bornaviruses. *Anim Health Res Rev*, 13, 145–156.

[97] Ludwig, H. and Thein, P. (1977) Demonstration of specific antibodies in the central nervous system of horses naturally infected with Borna disease virus. *Med Microbiol Immunol*, 163, 215–226.

[98] Na, K.S., Tae, S.H., Song, J.W. and Kim, Y.K. (2009) Failure to detect borna disease virus antibody and RNA from peripheral blood mononuclear cells of psychiatric patients. *Psychiatry Investig*, 6, 306–312.

[99] Heinrich, A. and Adamaszek, M. (2010) Anti-Borna disease virus antibody responses in psychiatric patients: long-term follow up. *Psychiatry Clin Neurosci*, 64, 255–261.

[100] Oldstone, M.B. (2012) The game's afoot: seeking viruses that cause chronic and degenerative neurologic and psychiatric disorder. *Mol Psychiatry*, 17, 472–473.

[101] Hornig, M., Briese, T., Licinio, J. *et al.* (2012) Absence of evidence for bornavirus infection in schizophrenia, bipolar disorder and major depressive disorder. *Mol Psychiatry*, 17, 486–493.

[102] Murray, K., Rogers, R., Selvey, L. *et al.* (1995) A novel morbillivirus pneumonia of horses and its transmission to humans. *Emerg Infect Dis*, 1, 31–33.

[103] Murray, P.K. (1996) The evolving story of the equine morbillivirus. *Aust Vet J*, 74, 214.

[104] Geisbert, T.W., Feldmann, H. and Broder, C.C. (2012) Animal challenge models of henipavirus infection and pathogenesis. *Curr Top Microbiol Immunol*, 359, 153–177.

[105] Eaton, B.T., Broder, C.C. and Wang, L.F. (2005) Hendra and Nipah viruses: pathogenesis and therapeutics. *Curr Mol Med*, 5, 805–816.

[106] Luby, S.P. and Gurley, E.S. (2012) Epidemiology of henipavirus disease in humans. *Curr Top Microbiol Immunol*, 359, 25–40.

[107] Selvey, L.A., Wells, R.M., McCormack, J.G. *et al.* (1995) Infection of humans and horses by a newly described morbillivirus. *Med J Aust*, 162, 642–645.

[108] Gust, I.D. (1995) Of viruses, horses and men. *Med J Aust*, 162, 621.

[109] Murray, K., Selleck, P., Hooper, P. *et al.* (1995) A morbillivirus that caused fatal disease in horses and humans. *Science*, 268, 94–97.

[110] 1996) Zoonoses control. Equine morbillivirus in Queensland. *Wkly Epidemiol Rec*, 71, 208–210.

[111] McCormack, J.G., Allworth, A.M., Selvey, L.A. and Selleck, P.W. (1999) Transmissibility from horses to humans of a novel paramyxovirus, equine morbillivirus (EMV). *J Infect*, 38, 22–23.

[112] Field, H.E., Breed, A.C., Shield, J. *et al.* (2007) Epidemiological perspectives on Hendra virus infection in horses and flying foxes. *Aust Vet J*, 85, 268–270.

[113] Field, H., Crameri, G., Kung, N.Y. and Wang, L.F. (2012) Ecological aspects of hendra virus. *Curr Top Microbiol Immunol*, 359, 11–23.

[114] Hazelton, B., Ba, A.F., Kok, J. and Dwyer, D.E. (2013) Hendra virus: a one health tale of flying foxes, horses and humans. *Future Microbiol*, 8, 461–474.

[115] Middleton, D.J. and Weingartl, H.M. (2012) Henipaviruses in their natural animal hosts. *Curr Top Microbiol Immunol*, 359, 105–121.

[116] Anon. *Hendra virus outbreaks 2013*. Australian Veterinary Association. http://www.ava.com.au/news/media-centre/hot-topics/hendra-virus/hendra-virus-outbreaks [accessed December 5, 2014].

[117] Westbury, H.A. (2000) Hendra virus disease in horses. *Rev Sci Tech*, 19, 151–159.

[118] Field, H.E., Barratt, P.C., Hughes, R.J. *et al.* (2000) A fatal case of Hendra virus infection in a horse in north Queensland: clinical and epidemiological features. *Aust Vet J*, 78, 279–280.

[119] Hooper, P.T., Russell, G.M., Selleck, P.W. *et al.* (1999) Immunohistochemistry in the identification of a number of new diseases in Australia. *Vet Microbiol*, 68, 89–93.

[120] Halpin, K., Young, P.L., Field, H.E. and Mackenzie, J.S. (2000) Isolation of Hendra virus from pteropid bats: a natural reservoir of Hendra virus. *J Gen Virol*, 81, 1927–1932.

[121] Mahalingam, S., Herrero, L.J., Playford, E.G. *et al.* (2012) Hendra virus: an emerging paramyxovirus in Australia. *Lancet Infect Dis*, 12, 799–807.

[122] Rota, P.A. and Lo, M.K. (2012) Molecular virology of the henipaviruses. *Curr Top Microbiol Immunol*, 359, 41–58.

[123] Richmond, R. (2012) The Hendra vaccine has arrived. *Aust Vet J*, 90, N2.

[124] Balzer, M. (2012) Insight into vet response to Hendra. *Aust Vet J*, 90, N4.

[125] Croser, E.L. and Marsh, G.A. (2013) The changing face of the henipaviruses. *Vet Microbiol*, 167, 151–158.

[126] Murphy, F.A., Gibbs, E.P.J., Horzinek, M.C. and Studdert, M.J. (2013) Herpesviridae, in *Veterinary Virology* (eds F.A. Murphy, E.P.J. Gibbs, M.C. Horzinek, M.J. Studdert and P.M. Howley), Academic Press, San Diego, pp. 301–326.

[127] van den Ingh, T.S., Binkhorst, G.J., Kimman, T.G. *et al.* (1990) Aujeszky's disease in a horse. *Zentralbl Veterinarmed B*, 37, 532–538.

[128] Kimman, T.G., Binkhorst, G.J., van den Ingh, T.S. *et al.* (1991) Aujeszky's disease in horses fulfills Koch's postulates. *Vet Rec*, 128, 103–106.

[129] Inch, C. (1998) An overview of pseudorabies (Aujeszky's disease) and vesicular stomatitis from the Canadian Animal Health Network. *Can Vet J*, 39, 23–32.

[130] Tajima, M., Nakajima, H. and Ito, Y. (1969) Electron microscopy of equine infectious anemia virus. *J Virol*, 4, 521–527.

[131] McClure, J.J., Lindsay, W.A., Taylor, W. *et al.* (1982) Ataxia in four horses with equine infectious anemia. *J Am Vet Med Assoc*, 180, 279–283.

[132] Oaks, J.L., Long, M.T. and Baszler, T.V. (2004) Leukoencephalitis associated with selective viral replication in the brain of a pony with experimental chronic equine infectious anemia virus infection. *Vet Pathol*, 41, 527–532.

21 Bacterial Infections of the Central Nervous System

Martin Furr

Marion duPont Scott Equine Medical Center, Virginia-Maryland Regional College of Veterinary Medicine, Leesburg, USA

Bacterial infection of the equine central nervous system (CNS), including meningitis, abscesses, and meningoencephalitis, is fairly uncommon, affecting approximately 2.5% of 450 horses with any type of neurologic disease in one survey [1]. If horses with peripheral neuropathies and laryngeal hemiplegia are excluded, then 3.4% of horses with CNS disease had bacterial meningitis [1]. Baker and Ellis reported a total of 4.0% of horses examined for neurologic disease to have a form of CNS infection [2]. In another report, 5.7% of horses with complications from a strangles outbreak had CNS involvement [3]. One large-scale postmortem study found 543 of 4319 horses to have neurologic disease, of which 9.6% (52/543), ranging in age from 2 days to 18 years of age, had bacterial meningoencephalitis and meningitis [4]. In this study, it was reported that approximately 50% of the cases were in foals less than 6 months of age, making the adult infection rate approximately 4.5% of neurologic horses in which a postmortem was performed [4]. A recent study has reported a much lower occurrence in clinical patients, with a prevalence of meningitis (bacterial, fungal, parasitic, and chemical) in adults of 0.04% (28/70 000) of all equine admissions and 0.2% (28/14 000) for horses presented for neurologic disease [5]. Hence, it appears from several reports that the frequency of bacterial infection of the CNS of adult horses is quite low.

Bacterial meningitis is reported to be more common among neonatal foals than adults. Bacterial meningitis was seen in 8–10% of neonatal foals in two different retrospective reports [6, 7], while an overall incidence of 13% was reported in another study of neonatal sepsis in 61 foals [8]. Sanchez et al reported bacterial meningitis in 11 of 423 (2.6%) septic foals [9], while 5.2% of septic foals developed meningitis in another study [10]. These findings are in contrast to a recent report in which a prevalence rate of 0.5% of foals with septicemia was found [5]. The reasons for this substantial difference in infection rates is not readily apparent from review of the manuscripts; however, increasing experience with management of septic foals, early recognition, and changes in clinical practice as well as study design may explain the differences.

It is possible that these numbers underreport the true incidence of illness in either foals or adults, due to the difficulties of diagnosis and the lack of complete evaluations of the CNS at postmortem or clinically. It certainly appears, from a clinical perspective, that bacterial meningitis is being more commonly recognized in clinical patients. This is likely due to the increased recognition of CNS disease, as well as increased familiarity and comfort with diagnostic techniques such as cerebrospinal fluid (CSF) collection.

Agents

Infectious agents documented in CNS infections of horses vary. Infections in neonates are most commonly associated with the agents that result in bacterial septicemia. Hence, Gram-negative bacteria predominate. In a report of 61 foals with septicemia, *E. coli*-mediated meningitis was most common, with meningitis seen in 7 of 21 foals with *E. coli*-mediated septicemia [8]. In one series of 10 foals with meningitis, *E. coli* was recovered from the CSF in two of five foals in which culture was performed [10]. The remaining three cases had no bacterial growth. Uncommon pathogens can also be seen, such as osteomyelitis due to *Rhodococcus equi*, with secondary encroachment into the CNS [11].

In adult horses, streptococcal species appear to predominate [1, 3, 12–17] although infections with a wide variety of other organisms have been reported, including *Staphylococcus aureus* [18], *Actinomyces* sp. [19], *Actinobacillus* sp. [20, 21], *Listeria* sp. [22], *E. coli* [1], *Pseudomonas aeruginosa* and *P. pseudomallei* (melioidosis) [23], *Klebsiella* sp. [1, 24], *Salmonella* sp. [1], *Peptostreptococcus* sp. [5], *Proteus* sp. [5], *Fusobacterium* sp. [5], *Bacteroides* sp. [5], and *Corynebacteria pseudotuberculosis* [25, 26] (Figure 21.1).

Equine Neurology, Second Edition. Martin Furr and Stephen Reed.
© 2015 John Wiley & Sons, Inc. Published 2015 by John Wiley & Sons, Inc.
Companion website: www.wiley.com/go/furr/neurology

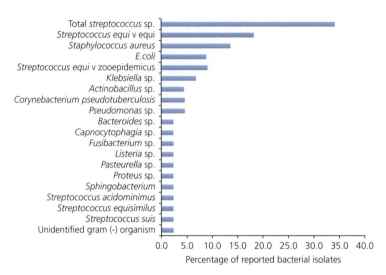

Figure 21.1 Relative frequency of bacterial isolates from adult horses with bacterial meningitis, summarized from published reports in the primary literature.

Pathophysiology

In humans, the most common pathogens causing bacterial meningitis are *Streptococcus pneumoniae* and *Neisseria meningitidis*. These organisms colonize the mucosa of the nasopharynx, then cross into the bloodstream, eventually reaching the choroid plexus [27]. In *E. coli*-induced meningitis, it has been demonstrated that multiple factors are necessary for invasion of the CNS across the blood–brain barrier (BBB) [28]. Specific factors necessary include a threshold level of bacteremia (>10 [3] cfu/ml blood) and invasion of host brain microvascular endothelial cells (BMEC), followed by replication within the subarachnoid space (SAS) [28]. Numerous specific surface proteins (OmpA, Ibe proteins, and cytotoxic necrotizing factor-1) are required for BMEC invasion [28]. The role of these compounds in equine meningitis, if any, is not known.

Interestingly, *E. coli* invasion and transcytosis of BMEC occur without damage to the BBB or endothelial cells [29]. Bacteria are then transported through the cell and into the CSF alive, with subsequent proliferation. Some *E. coli* strains (i.e., *E. coli* K1) can traverse the BMEC but do not survive, suggesting that additional capsular factors are needed to preserve viability [28]. Other bacteria that are known to result in bacterial meningitis in humans (i.e., *Listeria monocytogenes* and group B streptococcus) utilize different signaling mechanisms to achieve the same result and are less fully characterized. It is unknown if similar mechanisms exist for equine pathogens, but it is reasonable to assume that there are.

In horses, a variety of mechanisms are incriminated in bacterial colonization of the CNS. Penetrating wounds with traumatic implantation of bacteria and/or contamination of tissues is one way, and is seen in horses with fractures of the head, and which have been reported [1, 17]. Hematogenous implantation arising during bacteremia is commonly believed to be a major mechanism and as noted earlier requires a significant bacteremia. The observation that this is a common pathogenesis is supported by the distribution of the CNS lesions in many cases, as well as the well-documented association of meningitis in horses with multiple extra-nervous system abscesses and endocarditis [2, 15, 20, 24, 30, 31]. Smith and colleagues describe a search of records of two University hospitals as well as the Livestock Disease Diagnostic Center in Lexington Kentucky in which 16 of 21 horses over 1 year of age with bacterial meningitis had "systemic disease" [31]. The nature of the systemic illness in these cases was not described.

Immunosuppression is presumed to play a role in predisposing a horse to bacterial spread. In humans, there is an increased risk of bacterial meningitis in people with HIV and cancer; hence it is likely that similar factors are operative in horses. Foals, which have a higher incidence of bacterial meningitis than adult horses, may be immunosuppressed due to the presence of failure of passive transfer with suboptimal IgG concentrations. In addition, bacteremia, which is known to be a prerequisite for bacterial meningitis, has been frequently documented in neonatal foals. Hence, the importance of immune factors is not truly known and has not been carefully examined. It seems intuitively correct that there is some role, however.

Immunodeficiency in adults with bacterial meningitis has also been reported [32]. Three horses with bacterial meningitis were found to also have common variable immunodeficiency, which was considered to have a significant role in the infection [32]. Meningoencephalitis was also reported in an Arabian foal with combined immunodeficiency [22]. The presence of an "immature" BBB, with greater permeability to bacteria, has been postulated for foals [33]. The hypothesis that the BBB of immature animals is more easily colonized and traversed than adults has been tested in juvenile rats and humans, and it has been demonstrated that there is no difference in the ability of bacteria to colonize or traverse the BMEC of juvenile animals [34]. This hypothesis has not been evaluated in horses; however it is likely to be similar as foals are more precocious at birth than either humans or laboratory rodents.

A further mechanism of CNS infection is by extension of suppurative infections of the head. While the dura is considered highly resistant to bacterial translocation, it is susceptible at the points of penetration of nerve trunks. Smith et al described seven cases of bacterial meningitis that were associated with infectious processes of the head; four of the seven horses had sinusitis [31]. Thrombophlebitis was observed in the vessels of the sinuses, and it was proposed that hematogenous dissemination of bacteria from vascular connections to the venous sinuses at the base of the skull occurred. This should result in basilar empyema and pituitary abscessation, which was seen in four horses from another report in which three animals had suppurative infections of the head [35]. A similar presentation was found in a pony, and it was proposed that extension of infection via the vessels draining the venous sinuses ("emissary vessels") represented a common pathophysiology for cases of basilar empyema [36]. Infection of these vessels can lead to abscess formation with subsequent exophthalmos [36]. Migration along the optic nerve was considered to have occurred in some horses [31], and direct invasion through the thin bones of the sphenopalatine sinuses (following necrosis) may also occur.

Once bacteria gain access to the CNS or SAS, they are able to proliferate readily, due to the reduced endogenous and innate host response mechanisms present. As discussed in Chapter 3, the CSF has a low concentration of WBCs, immunoglobulins, and complement compared with serum. These are critical components necessary for efficient phagocytosis and early nonspecific bacterial clearance.

Following bacterial entry and proliferation in the CNS/SAS, a critical event in the pathophysiology of bacterial meningitis is the subsequent inflammatory reaction that ensues. It is widely considered that many of the neurologic signs and sequelae of bacterial meningitis result from inflammatory-mediated damage to the CNS, rather than the direct effects of the bacteria themselves [27, 37–39]. As such, it is important to realize that neurologic injury can progress even after the CNS has been sterilized by antibiotic therapy [27].

Bacterial cell wall components induce meningeal inflammation by stimulating the production of inflammatory cytokines from microglia, astrocytes, monocytes, CSF leukocytes, and microglial cells [27]. Important inflammatory mediators proposed include peptidoglycan, lipopolysaccharide, and lipoteichoic acid; these compounds interact with the pattern recognition receptor mCD14 and toll-like receptor-2. This results in upregulation of the nuclear factor (NF)-κB signaling pathway with subsequent production of inflammatory mediators and leukocyte infiltration [37]. The primary response is the production of tumor necrosis factor (TNF) and interleukin (IL)-1, which can appear within the CSF within 1 h after experimental inoculation of LPS in the CSF. In addition, bacterial DNA appears to initiate CNS inflammation by stimulation of macrophages and production of proinflammatory cytokines [40]. Additional proinflammatory cytokines (IL-1, IL-6), chemokines, and adhesion factors are also upregulated and help to initiate and maintain meningeal inflammation.

The cytokines act synergistically to increase the permeability of the BBB, which results in vasogenic edema and protein transudation into the CSF. The exudation of proteinaceous material and leukocytes obstructs the flow of CSF, with secondary interstitial edema. The presence of inflammatory cytokines also leads to increased leukocyte migration into the CSF. Neutrophil activation with subsequent release of inflammatory proteins leads to cytotoxic edema, cell injury, and death.

In early meningitis, there is an increase in cerebral blood flow, which is followed by decreased blood flow and a loss of cerebrovascular autoregulation. Presence of vasculitis contributes to decreased blood flow and can result in infarction and thrombosis. The combination of interstitial, vasogenic, and cytotoxic edema results in increased intracranial pressure (ICP), with further deleterious effects upon blood flow. Clinical signs result from a combination of cellular (neuronal) dysfunction due to inflammation, neuronal cell death, and increased ICP, which are mediated by circulatory and inflammatory mediator events.

Matrix metalloproteinases (MMPs) are a family of zinc-dependent endopeptidases that are responsible for tissue remodeling via degradation of extracellular matrix components [37]. MMPs have been demonstrated to be present in the CSF of human patients with bacterial meningitis, with higher concentrations associated with poorer outcomes [41]. Further, the MMPs have been demonstrated to disrupt the integrity of the

BBB during both experimental and naturally occurring meningitis [41, 42].

In addition to proteolytic enzymes and inflammatory cytokines, reactive oxygen and nitrogen species are produced during meningeal inflammation. Nitric oxide (NO) concentrations are elevated in human patients with naturally occurring bacterial meningitis as well as experimental-induced meningitis [37]. The role of this compound in bacterial meningitis is not clearly understood at this time, but it is clear that inducible NO magnifies the production of various inflammatory mediators such as IL1-b and TNF, as well as increases meningitis-induced BBB damage [43]. In contrast, endothelial nitric oxide synthase (NOS)-derived NO may downregulate meningeal inflammation [37]. The potent oxidant compound peroxynitrite also appears to have a central role in mediating neuronal damage in bacterial meningitis. Surrogates for peroxynitrite are increased in the CSF of patients with bacterial meningitis [44], and treatment with a peroxynitrite scavenger, uric acid, significantly attenuates meningeal inflammation [37]. Peroxynitrite contributes to CNS damage and edema by a number of mechanisms. Peroxynitrite leads to lipid peroxidation of cell membranes as well as induces DNA strand breakage. This results in an energy-consuming cytosolic repair mechanism that ultimately results in cellular energy depletion and death [45, 46].

A second crucial effect of the cytokines is the activation of phospholipase A2 and stimulation of the AA cascade, with subsequent production of prostaglandins and leukotrienes [47, 48]. Prostaglandin E2 is a predominate prostaglandin produced during bacterial neuroinflammation and has deleterious effects upon the BBB, leading to white blood cell pleocytosis and increased CSF protein concentrations [49, 50]. In addition, it has been demonstrated that the prostaglandins interrupt cerebral autoregulation [51] (Figures 21.2 and 21.3).

Clinical signs

Constitutional signs of illness in horses with meningitis are variable. Fever was reported in only 15% (4/28) of adult horses with meningitis in one study [5], while another case series reported that all cases (5/5) had fever [18]. Presence of dehydration, tachycardia, or tachypnea is inconsistently reported in the primary literature; however, it appears to vary considerably depending upon the severity of the nervous system abnormalities, duration of illness, and presence of infection in other tissues. Clearly, the absence of a fever or other signs of infection does not rule out meningitis in a suspect case.

Clinical signs and syndromes associated with bacterial infection of the CNS can vary widely, depending upon

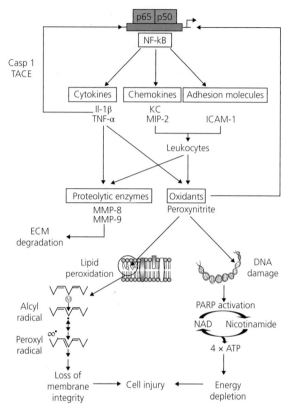

Figure 21.2 Mechanism of damage in experimental pneumococcal meningitis. NF-κB, a transcriptional activator of many genes involved in the pathogenesis of bacterial meningitis, encodes host factors including proinflammatory cytokines, chemokines (e.g., interleukin (IL)-8), and adhesion molecules. The proinflammatory cytokines IL-1b and tumor necrosis factor (TNF)-α are synthesized as inactive precursors that are processed to mature active forms by proteases (caspase 1 (Casp1), also known as IL-1b–converting enzyme, and TNF-α–converting enzyme (TACE)). IL-1b and TNF-α are potent activators of NF-κB. This process may lead to the uncontrolled expression of proinflammatory mediators and the increased expression of adhesion molecules both on the endothelium (e.g., intercellular adhesion molecules (ICAM)-1) and on neutrophils, leading to subsequent massive influx of leukocytes into the subarachnoid space. Once present, active leukocytes release a complex variety of potentially cytotoxic agents including oxidants and proteolytic enzymes (e.g., matrix metalloproteinases (MMPs)) that may contribute to tissue destruction. Also, peroxynitrite may cause brain damage via a variety of independent mechanisms. The best studies are attack of polyunsaturated fatty acids, leading to lipid peroxidation, and an alternative pathway that involves oxidant-induced DNA strand breakage and subsequent poly(ADP ribose) polymerase (PARP) activation, which initiates an energy-consuming cycle that ultimately results in cellular energy depletion and cell death. Both mechanisms likely contribute to cell injury during pneumococcal meningitis. ECM, extracellular matrix; MIP, macrophage inflammatory protein. (Reprinted with permission from Ref. [37].)

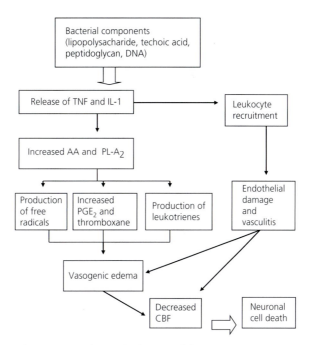

Figure 21.3 Mechanisms leading to brain injury in bacterial infections of the CNS.

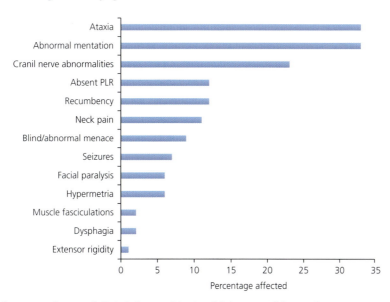

Figure 21.4 Relative frequency of reported clinical abnormalities in adult horses with bacterial meningitis, summarized from published reports in the primary literature.

the neuroanatomic localization of the lesion or lesions, as well as the presence or absence of other infectious processes. Summary of the neurologic findings reported in a large number of published case reports finds that abnormal mentation and ataxia are the most common clinical signs seen (see Figure 21.4). The ataxia in adults

with meningitis is typically symmetrical and of moderate to severe severity [5, 18, 31]. Various cranial nerve abnormalities including head tilt, strabismus, nystagmus, blindness, altered pupillary light reflexes, and facial paralysis are fairly common as well. In contrast, neck pain is rarely reported (11% of cases) and seizures were reported in only 7% of adult cases. Abscesses lead to signs of a focal, space-occupying lesion, which can result in head pressing, circling, or head tilt. In neonatal foals, early signs include depression, disorientation, and loss of the suckle reflex. Recumbency and seizures usually follow fairly quickly. Papilledema may be present due to increased ICP.

Diagnosis

Diagnosis of bacterial meningitis can be difficult, as clinical signs can be vague and nonspecific, as noted earlier. A history of a wound in the region of the head; previous sinus infections, umbilical disease, or diarrhea in a foal; or abscessing disease is suggestive. Additional signs of infectious disease, such as fever and increased white blood cell count and fibrinogen, are supportive but not universally noted. In some reported and confirmed cases in adults, the horse had a normal peripheral white blood cell count [12, 52]. Combining the results from several published papers in which these data were consistently reported, only 50% of horses with meningitis had a leukocytosis and only 56% had a neutrophilia [5, 14, 18, 24, 32]. While this does not represent an exhaustive analysis or summary, it is clear that horses with meningitis can have an unremarkable complete cell count. Interpretation of the complete blood cell count is more challenging and less definitive in neonatal foals, in which leucopenia associated with sepsis is very common [6, 53]. Clinical chemistry evaluation is also quite variable in horses with meningitis and usually reflects secondary changes associated with depression, dehydration, anorexia, or muscle enzyme increases due to seizures or recumbency.

The most useful and definitive diagnostic test for bacterial meningitis is the CSF evaluation. Collection from either the atlantooccipital (AO) or the lumbosacral (LS) sites are acceptable, and the clinician should determine which site is preferred in the context of the entire clinical case. CSF should be collected early in the course of the disease and submitted for a full examination, preferably before antibiotic therapy has begun. It has been demonstrated in human pediatric bacterial meningitis that pretreatment with antibiotics alters the clinical presentation and decreases the occurrence of positive results of the CSF culture [54]. In that report, pretreatment with antibiotics did not, however, alter CSF nucleated cell count, glucose, or protein concentration [54]. Most commonly, the CSF will be turbid and discolored and will have an increased nucleated cell count, that is predominately neutrophils, as well as an increased CSF total protein. Total protein concentrations can range widely and are typically

several 100 mg/dl, but cases have been reported with normal or very modestly increased total protein concentrations (98–121 mg/dl) [12, 32, 35]. CSF nucleated cell counts can also vary widely, being normally grossly elevated, but sometimes only very modestly increased or even normal (17–22 cells/µl) [12, 18, 32]. Such results make interpretation of the CSF difficult. An increased CSF RBC count is common in horses with meningitis, and the increased nucleated cells may be interpreted as due simply to blood contamination. However, blood contamination does not appear to influence CSF nucleated cell counts, at least up to an RBC count of less than 2000 cells/ml (see Chapter 2). In such cases, the differential cell count is very helpful, and the presence of any neutrophils, even in the presence of a normal or modestly increased nucleated cell count, suggests early meningitis. In questionable cases, the prudent clinical course is to treat such cases as if bacterial meningitis is confirmed. Repeat CSF collection in such cases is warranted and may often demonstrate a more definitive result as the condition progresses (Table 21.1).

In horses, the CSF glucose concentration is reported to be from 35 to 77% of corresponding blood concentrations [55]. Decreased CSF glucose concentrations (hypoglycorrhachia) are often observed in bacterial meningitis, and values of "0" can be seen in humans [27]. This is presumed to be due to increased glucose consumption by neurons and infiltrating inflammatory cells. Bacteria may also utilize glucose but have been considered to be present in too small a number to play a significant role [56]. CSF glucose concentrations are rarely reported in the literature; however, in one series of two cases the CSF glucose was normal [52], while in another series of cases the CSF glucose was low in four of six horses in which it was assayed [5]. Interpretation of CSF glucose concentrations in neonatal foals is quite problematic, as these patients are often hypoglycemic, but the CSF glucose/blood glucose should remain about 0.6 (normal). CSF lactate concentrations increase in bacterial meningitis [57]; however, this appears to be a nonspecific increase and has little value in diagnosis of bacterial meningitis in humans [58]. Lactate has been reported to increase in horses with brain trauma, cerebral abscess, and eastern encephalitis [59] and was increased in one case of bacterial meningitis [5]. It has not, however, been found to be of particular value in the diagnosis of bacterial meningitis.

CSF from any cases suspected of having bacterial meningitis should be cultured and an antibacterial sensitivity determined. Culture of organisms from CSF (collected antemortem) was positive in only 17% of adult horses with meningitis in one study, while postmortem culture was positive in 56% of cases [5]. The presence of any bacteria as determined by cytologic evaluation of

Table 21.1 Cerebrospinal fluid results in horses with bacterial infections of the CNS.

Diagnosis	N	CSF collection site	Color/clarity	WBC (#/µl)			RBC (#/µl)			Total protein[a] (mg/dl)			Comments
				mean	median	range	mean	median	range				
Meningitis	23	Variable	—	20991	1224	0–240000	27959	280	0–245000	697	282	45–3900	94.6% mortality [5]
Meningitis	5	LS	Variable	713	348	1–2448	10579	2763	5–46656	592.5	173	51–2000	0% mortality [18]
Brain abscess	1	AO	NR	NR			NR			98			Died [12]
Brain abscess	1	LS	Xanthochromic	22			NR			300			Died [12]
Optic neuritis	1	LS	Cloudy	760			1590			93			Died [20]
Meningitis	1	AO	Cloudy yellow	500			NR			170			Survived [52]
Meningitis	1	AO	Clear yellow	500						290			Survived [52]
Meningitis	1	NR	Cloudy yellow	>990			690			884			Died [19]
Cerebral abscess	1	AO	Xanthochromic	366000			NR			NR			Survived [14]
Basilar empyema	1	AO	Cloudy yellow	31400			NR			84			Died [35]
Basilar empyema	1	LS	Xanthochromic	11			770			119			Died [35]
Meningitis	1	LS		810			10			121			Survived [32]
Meningitis	1	LS	Xanthochromic	17			NR			209			Survived [32]
Meningitis	1	LS	Xanthochromic	223			NR			1600			Survived [32]

[a] Data converted to mg/dl units for purposes of comparison in this table.

NR, not reported.

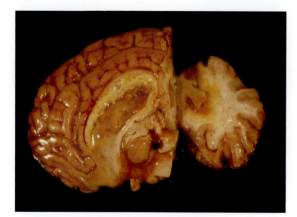

Figure 21.5 Suppurative ventriculitis in a foal.

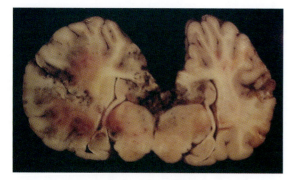

Figure 21.6 Cross-section taken through the cerebrum of an adult horse with diffuse bacterial encephalitis. Note the enlargement of the left cerebral hemisphere with necrosis.

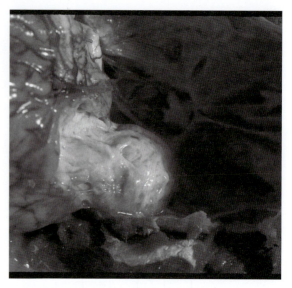

Figure 21.7 Postmortem photograph of a dissected cerebral abscess during removal of the brain. The abscess has opened and the cavitary necrosis and pus-filled cavity are demonstrated.

Treatment

The objectives for the treatment of bacterial meningitis include (i) sterilization of the CNS/CSF, (ii) control of inflammation, and (iii) management of sequelae and complications.

The optimum antibacterial should be determined by culture and sensitivity testing of a CSF sample. However, antimicrobial treatment must begin before final culture results are determined. A Gram stain of CSF is valuable in making an empiric antimicrobial choice. Table 21.2 lists recommended antimicrobials for equine bacterial meningitis. Please refer to Chapter 4 for a more thorough discussion of antibiotics for CNS infections. Chloramphenicol is a common choice, as it demonstrates a good spectrum of activity against many equine pathogens and achieves good CSF concentrations [63]. Enrofloxacin also achieves good concentrations within the CSF, but it has poor efficacy against *Streptococci* and anaerobic bacteria, hence should not be used if these organisms are suspected [64, 65]. Specific third-generation cephalosporins (cefotaxime, ceftazidime, cefepime, and ceftriaxone) are documented to achieve good CSF concentrations [66–68] and are good empiric choices, although expense may limit their use. Ceftiofur, a commonly used equine antimicrobial of the same class, has been shown not to enter the CSF, and its use in bacterial meningitis is not supported [69]. The "potentiated" sulfonamides (trimethoprim/sulfadiazine and ormetoprim/sulfadimethoxine) do achieve significant

the CSF is strong supportive evidence, even in the absence of positive culture results.

Standard radiographs of the head or cervical spine are warranted if clinical examination and neuroanatomic localization dictates. Signs of osteomyelitis or trauma may be observed, but radiographs will be negative in many cases. Advanced imaging techniques, such as computed tomography (CT) or magnetic resonance imaging (MRI), are becoming more available and are ideal modalities to confirm and provide precise localization of purulent intracranial or cervical disease. The diagnosis of brain abscesses by CT examination in living horses has been described and has been used to guide therapy [14, 60, 61]. MRI of intracranial abscessation of the horses has been described and appears to be a very useful diagnostic aid [30, 62]. Nuclear scintigraphy using labeled autologous white blood cells can also be attempted and may provide definitive evidence (Figures 21.5, 21.6, and 21.7).

Table 21.2 Recommended antimicrobials for the treatment of equine bacterial meningitis.

Drug	Dose	Comments
Ceftazidime [65]	50 mg/kg IV q6 h	Extrapolated from human dose
Cefotaxime [67, 53]	40 mg/kg IV q4–6 h	
Cefepime [66]	11 mg/kg IV q8 h	Kinetics determined in neonatal foals
Ceftriaxone [68]	50 mg/kg IV	
Chloramphenicol [63]	25–50 mg/kg PO	
TMS/SMZ [65]	2.4/12.5 mg/kg PO	Use only with appropriate documented sensitivity
OMP/SDM [65]	9.2/45.8 mg/kg (loading) 4.6/22.9 mg/kg PO q24 h (maintenance)	
Enrofloxacin [64]	5.5 mg/kg IV q24 h 7.5 mg/kg PO q24 h	Significant arthropathy in foals
Minocycline [70]	4 mg/kg PO 12 h	
Rifampin [65]	10 mg/kg PO q12 h	Must be used in combination due to resistance
Metronidazole [65]	15–25 mg/kg PO q6 h	Limited spectrum to anaerobes

CSF concentrations after routine dosing; however, the presence of resistance to these drug combinations may make them less attractive, particularly if used empirically. Oxytetracycline, doxycycline, and the aminoglycosides do not achieve significant concentrations within the CSF and should not be used [65]. The concentration of minocycline in the CSF following dosing at 4 mg/kg q12 h was 0.38 μg/ml, which exceeds the MIC$_{50}$ for several organisms known to cause meningitis in horses, and may have value in treating equine meningitis [70].

In cases of infection with resistant bacteria, intrathecal therapy can be considered. Anecdotal reports of seizures after the use of intrathecal penicillin exists; however, it is difficult to assess their validity. Aminoglycoside antibiotics are used in humans (intracerebroventricularly) and are described as well-tolerated. Dosages of 5 mg are used, once per day in human adults [71]. Intraventricular vancomycin has also been used in humans at a dosage of 10–20 mg per day [71]. These treatments should be combined with systemic administration of the antibiotic.

The duration of treatment with antibiotics in horses with bacterial meningitis is difficult to assess. A total treatment duration of at least 3 weeks is advisable. Specific guidelines do not exist for the horse, but continuing treatment for at least 10 days beyond the resolution of clinical signs is advisable, as recrudescence has been noted in human patients. Repeat CSF analysis is indicated after antimicrobial treatment has been discontinued. In cases of cerebral abscess, longer treatment times are probably indicated, and follow-up CT or MRI studies are warranted to ensure resolution of the infection.

Neuroinflammation should be controlled aggressively to minimize the development of increased ICP, potential brain herniation, or exacerbation of clinical signs. The use of corticosteroids is controversial; however, a number of large-scale analyses have demonstrated that the use of dexamethasone in humans with bacterial meningitis is associated with a decreased risk of mortality and serious neurologic sequelae [72, 73]. The risk of laminitis is of particular concern in horses, however, and corticosteroids should be used for as short a period of time as possible to minimize this concern. Nonsteroidal anti-inflammatory drugs should be employed to minimize edema associated with inflammation. Intravenous dimethyl sulfoxide (DMSO) (0.5–1 g/kg IV, q12–24 h) is widely used as an anti-inflammatory and is commonly used by the author for neuroinflammation for the first 3 days of treatment. Other means of minimizing inflammation, such as MMP inhibitors and peroxynitrite scavengers (such as uric acid), show promise but currently remain research tools only.

Focal cerebral abscessation has been successfully treated surgically in several cases; however, CT or MRI localization appears to be important in planning surgery [60, 61]. One mare was successfully treated and was recovering from the neurologic disease; however, the horse developed laminitis, which necessitated its destruction after about 2 months [14]. Surgical drainage via craniotomy and aspiration of the abscess appears to be a viable modality in the horse, at least in select cases.

Ancillary treatments are determined by the specific needs of each individual patient. Horses that cannot eat or drink will require nutritional support and fluids, either provided via a nasogastric tube or intravenously. Horses with seizures require anticonvulsant medication and associated care. Cranial nerve deficits may lead to failure to blink, resulting in corneal trauma. This can be managed with such compounds as artificial tears or by performing a tarsorrhaphy. Depression may lead to a low head carriage, with secondary dependent edema of the head. If infections of the head are present, they will need appropriate care. Horses that are recumbent need to be managed to minimize trauma.

The prognosis for horses with meningitis must be considered guarded to poor. Successful treatment in both adults and foals has been reported, and overall outcome clearly depends upon severity of condition at the beginning of treatment and the presence of primary complicating lesions. One study reported a 95% mortality; however, other case series have reported good success rates [5, 18].

References

[1] Tyler, C.M., Davis, R.E., Begg, A.P. *et al.* (1993) A survey of neurological diseases in horses. *Aust Vet J*, 70, 445–449.

[2] Baker, J.R. and Ellis, C.E. (1981) A survey of post mortem findings in 480 horses from 1958 to 1980: (1) causes of death. *Equine Vet J*, 13, 43–46.

[3] Sweeney, C.R., Benson, C.E., Whitlock, R.H. *et al.* (1987) *Streptococcus equi* infection in horses—part II. *Comp Contin Ed Pract Vet*, 9, 845–851.

[4] Laugier, C., Tapprest, J., Foucher, N. *et al.* (2009) A necropsy survey of neurologic disease in 4,319 horses examined in Normandy (France) from 1986 to 2006. *J Equine Vet Sci*, 29, 561–568.

[5] Toth, B., Aleman, M., Nogradi, N. *et al.* (2012) Meningitis and meningoencephalomyelitis in horses: 28 cases (1985–2010). *J Am Vet Med Assoc*, 240, 580–587.

[6] Koterba, A.M., Brewer, B.D. and Tarplee, F.A. (1984) Clinical and clinicopathological characteristics of the septicemic neonatal foal: review of 38 cases. *Equine Vet J*, 16, 376–382.

[7] Brewer, B.D. and Koterba, A.M. (1990) Bacterial isolates and susceptability patterns in foals in a neonatal intensive care unit. *Comp Cont Ed for the Pract Vet*, 12, 1773–1781.

[8] Platt, H. (1973) Septicaemia in the foal. A review of 61 cases. *Br Vet J*, 129, 221–229.

[9] Sanchez, L.C., Giguere, S. and Lester, G.D. (2008) Factors associated with survival of neonatal foals with bacteremia and racing performance of surviving thoroughbreds: 423 cases (1982–2007). *J Am Vet Med Assoc*, 233, 1446–1452.

[10] Viu, J., Monreal, L., Jose-Cunilleras, E. *et al.* (2012) Clinical findings in 10 foals with bacterial meningoencephalitis. *Equine Vet J* Suppl 41, 44, 100–104.

[11] Morresey, P.R., Garrett, K.S. and Carter, D. (2011) *Rhodococcus equi* occipital osteomyelitis, septic arthritis, and meningitis in a neurologic foal. *Equine Vet Ed*, 23, 398–402.

[12] Raphel, C. (1982) Brain abscess in three horses. *J Am Vet Med Assoc*, 180, 874–877.

[13] Devriese, L.A., Sustronck, B., Maenhout, T. *et al.* (1990) *Streptococcus suis* meningitis in a horse. *Vet Rec*, 127, 68.

[14] Allen, J.R., Barbee, D.D., Boulton, C.R. *et al.* (1987) Brain abscess in a horse: diagnosis by computed tomography and successful surgical treatment. *Equine Vet J*, 19, 552–555.

[15] Kaplan, N.A. and Moore, B.R. (1996) *Streptococcus equi* endocarditis, meningitis and panopthalmitis in a mature horse. *Equine Vet Ed*, 8, 313–316.

[16] Pusterla, N., Luff, J.A., Myers, C.J. *et al.* (2007) Disseminated intravascular coagulation in a horse with *Streptococcus equi* subspecies zooepidemicus meningoencephalitis and interstitial pneumonia. *J Vet Intern Med*, 21, 344–347.

[17] Atherton, R.P., Mitchell, E., McKenzie, H. *et al.* (2007) Traumatic fracture of the basisphenoid and secondary bacterial meningitis in a thoroughbred gelding. *Equine Vet Ed*, 19, 359–364.

[18] Mitchell, E., Furr, M.O. and McKenzie, H.C. (2006) Bacterial meningitis in five mature horses. *Equine Vet Ed*, 18, 249–255.

[19] Rumbaugh, G.E. (1977) Disseminated septic meningitis in a mare. *J Am Vet Med Assoc*, 171, 452–454.

[20] Hatfield, C.E., Rebhun, W.C., Dietz, A.E. *et al.* (1987) Endocarditis and optic neuritis in a Quarter horse mare. *Comp Contin Ed Pract Vet*, 9, 451–454.

[21] Chladek, D.W. and Ruth, G.R. (1976) Isolation of *Actinobacillus lignieresi* from an epidural abscess in a horse with progressive paralysis. *J Am Vet Med Assoc*, 168, 64–66.

[22] Clark, E.G., Turner, A.S., Boysen, B.G. *et al.* (1978) Listeriosis in an Arabian foal with combined immunodeficiency. *J Am Vet Med Assoc*, 172, 363–366.

[23] Ladds, P.W., Thomas, A.D. and Pott, B. (1981) Meliodosis with acute meningoencephalomyelitis in a horse. *Aust Vet J*, 57, 36–38.

[24] Timoney, P.J., McArdle, J.F. and Bryne, M.J. (1983) Abortion and meningitis in a thoroughbred mare associated with *Klebsiella pneumoniae*, type 1. *Equine Vet J*, 15, 64–65.

[25] Aleman, M., SPier, S.J., Wilson, W.D. *et al.* (1996) Corynebacterium pseudotuberculosis infection in horses: 538 cases (1982–1993). *J Am Vet Med Assoc*, 209, 804–809.

[26] Rand, C.L., Hall, T.L., Aleman, M. *et al.* (2012) Otitis media-interna and secondary meningitis associated with *Corynebacterium pseudotuberculosis* infection in a horse. *Equine Vet Ed*, 24, 271–275.

[27] Roos, K.L. and Tyler, K.L. (2005) Meningitis, encephalitis, brain abscess, and empyema, in *Harrisons Principles of Internal Medicine*, 16 edn (eds D.L. Kasper, A.S. Fauci, D.L. Longo, E. Braunwald, S.L. Hauser and J.L. Jameson), McGraw-Hill, New York, pp. 2471–2490.

[28] Kim, K.S. (2002) Strategy of *Eschericia coli* for crossing the blood-brain barrier. *J Infect Dis*, 186, S220–S224.

[29] Stins, M.F., Badger, J.L. and Kim, K.S. (2001) Bacterial invasion and transcytosis in transfected human brain microvascular endothelial cells. *Microb Pathog*, 30, 19–28.

[30] Spoormakers, T.J.P., Ensink, J.M., Goehring, L.S. *et al.* (2003) Brain abscess as a metastatic manifestation of strangles: symptomatology and the use of magnetic resonance imaging as a diagnostic aid. *Equine Vet J*, 35, 146–151.

[31] Smith, J.J., Provost, P.J. and Paradis, M.R. (2004) Bacterial meningitis and brain abscesses secondary to infectious disease processes involving the head in horses: seven cases (1980–2001). *J Am Vet Med Assoc*, 224, 739–742.

[32] Pellegrini-Masini, A., Bentz, A.I., Johns, I.C. *et al.* (2005) Common variable immunodeficiency in three horses with presumptive bacterial meningitis. *J Am Vet Med Assoc*, 227, 114–122.

[33] Santschi, E.M. and Foreman, J.H. (1989) Equine bacterial meningitis—part 1. *Compend on Contin Ed Pract Vet*, 11, 479–483.

[34] Stins, M.F., Nemani, P.V., Wass, C. *et al.* (1999) *Escherichia coli* binding to and invasion of brain microvascular endothelial cells derived from humans and rats of different ages. *Infect Immun*, 67, 5522–5525.

[35] Reilly, L., Habecker, P., Beech, J. *et al.* (1994) Pituitary abscess and basilar empyema in 4 horses. *Equine Vet J*, 26, 424–426.

[36] Gough, M.R., Mayhew, I.G., Munroe, G.A. *et al.* (1998) Purulent basilar empyema and meningitis associated with exophthalmus in a pony. *Equine Vet ed*, 10, 58–62.

[37] Scheld, W.M., Koedel, U., Nathan, B. *et al.* (2002) Pathophysiology of bacterial meningitis: mechanism(s) of neuronal injury. *J Infect Dis*, 186, S225–S233.

[38] Tauber, M.G., Borschberg, U. and Sande, M.A. (1988) Influence of granulocytes on brain edema, intracranial pressure, and cerebrospinal fluid concentrations of lactate and protein in experimental meningitis. *J Infect Dis*, 157, 456–464.

[39] van Furth, A.M., Roord, J.J. and van Furth, R. (1996) Roles of proinflammatory and anti-inflammatory cytokines in pathophysiology of bacterial meningitis and effect of adjunctive therapy. *Infect Immun*, 64, 4883–4890.

[40] Deng, G.M., Liu, Z.Q. and Tarkowski, A. (2001) Intracisternally localized bacterial DNA containing DNA CpG motifs induces meningitis. *J Immunol*, 167, 4616–4626.

[41] Leppert, D., Grygar, C., Miller, K.M. *et al.* (2000) Matrix metalloproteinase (MMP)-8 and MMP-9 in cerebrospinal fluid during bacterial meningitis: association with blood-brain barrier damage and neurological sequelae. *Clin Infect Dis*, 31, 80–84.

[42] Lukes, A., Mun-Bryce, S., Lukes, M. *et al.* (1999) Extracellular matrix degradation by metalloproteinases and central nervous system diseases. *Mol Neurobiol*, 19, 267–284.

[43] Winkler, F., Koedel, U., Kastenbauer, S. *et al.* (2001) Differential expression of nitric oxide synthetases in bacterial meningitis: a role of the inducible isoform for blood-brain barrier breakdown. *J Infect Dis*, 183, 1749–1759.

[44] Kastenbauer, S., Koedel, U., Becker, B.F. *et al.* (2002) Oxidative stress in bacterial meningitis in humans. *Neurology*, 58, 186–191.

[45] Ha, H.C. and Snyder, S.H. (2000) Poly (ADP-ribose) polymerase-1 in the nervous system. *Neurobiol Dis*, 7, 225–239.

[46] Shall, S. and DeMurcia, G. (2000) Poly (ADP-ribose) polymerase-1: what have we learned from the deficient mouse model? *Mutat Res*, 460, 1–15.

[47] de Vries, H.E., Kuiper, J., De Boer, A.G. *et al.* (1997) The blood-brain barrier in neuroinflammatory disease. *Pharmacol Rev*, 49, 143–155.

[48] Misko, T.P., Trotter, J.L. and Cross, A.H. (1995) Mediation of inflammation by encephalitogenic cells: interferon gamma induction of nitric oxide synthase and cyclooxygenase 2. *J Neuroimmunol*, 61, 195–204.

[49] Kadurugamuwa, J.L., Hengstler, B., Bray, M.A. *et al.* (1989) Inhibition of complement-factor-5a-induced inflammatory reactions by prostaglandin E2 in experimental meningitis. *J Infect Dis*, 160, 715–719.

[50] McGeer, P.L. and McGeer, E.G. (1995) The inflammatory response system of the brain: implication for therapy of Alzheimer and other neurodegenerative diseases. *Brain Res Rev*, 21, 195–218.

[51] Mertineit, C., Samlalsingh-Parker, J., Glibetic, M. *et al.* (2000) Nitric oxide, prostaglandins, and impaired cerebral blood flow autoregulation in group B streptococcal neonatal meningitis. *Can J Physiol Pharmacol*, 78, 217–227.

[52] Newton, S.A. (1998) Suspected bacterial meningoencephalitis in two adult horses. *Vet Rec*, 142, 665–669.

[53] Morris, D.D., Rutkowski, J. and Kent Lloyd, K.C. (1987) Therapy in two cases of neonatal foal septicemia and meningitis with cefotaxime. *Equine Vet J*, 19, 151–154.

[54] Rothrock, S.G., Green, S.M., Wren, J. *et al.* (1992) Pediatric bacterial meningitis: is prior antibiotic therapy associated with an altered clinical presentation? *Ann Emerg Med*, 21, 146–152.

[55] Mayhew, I.G., Whitlock, R.H. and Tasker, J.B. (1977) Equine cerebrospinal fluid: reference values of normal horses. *Am J Vet Res*, 38, 1271–1274.

[56] Baltch, A. and Osborne, W. (1957) Inquiry into causes of lowered spinal fluid sugar content: *In vivo* and *in vitro* observations. *J Lab Clin Med*, 49, 882–889.

[57] Knight, J.A., Dudek, S.M. and Haymond, R.E. (1981) Early (chemical) diagnosis of bacterial meningitis-cerebrospinal fluid glucose, lactate, and lactate dehydrogenase compared. *Clin Chem*, 27, 1431–1434.

[58] Jordan, G.W., Statland, B. and Halsted, C. (1983) CSF lactate in disease of the CNS. *Arch Intern Med*, 143, 85–87.

[59] Green EM, Green SL. Cerebrospinal fluid lactic acid concentrations: reference values and diagnostic implications of abnormal concentrations in adult horses. Proceedings of the 8th Annual Meeting ACVIM, May 10, 1990, Washington, DC; 1990:495–499.

[60] Cornelisse, C.J., Schott, H.C., Lowrie, C.T. *et al.* (2001) Successful treatment of intracranial abscesses in 2 horses. *J Vet Intern Med*, 15, 494–500.

[61] Janicek, J.C., Kramer, J., Coates, J.R. *et al.* (2006) Intracranial abscess caused by *Rhodococcus equi* infection in a foal. *J Am Vet Med Assoc*, 228, 251–253.

[62] Audigie, F., Tapprest, J., George, C. *et al.* (2004) Magnetic resonance imaging of a brain abscess in a 10-month-old filly. *Vet Radiol*, 45, 210–215.

[63] Gronwall, R., Brown, M.P., Merritt, A.M. *et al.* (1986) Body fluid concentrations and pharmacokinetics of chloramphenicol given to mares intravenously or by repeated gavage. *Am J Vet Res*, 47, 2591–2595.

[64] Giguere, S., Sweeney, R.W. and Belanger, M. (1996) Pharmacokinetics of enrofloxacin in adult horses and concentration of the drug in serum, body fluids, and endometrial tissues after repeated intragastrically administered doses. *Am J Vet Res*, 57, 1025–1030.

[65] Dowling, P.M. (1999) Clinical pharmacology of nervous system disease. *Vet Clin North Am Equine Pract*, 15, 575–588.

[66] Gardner, S.Y. and Papich, M.G. (2001) Comparison of cefepime pharmacokinetics in neonatal foals and adult dogs. *J Vet Pharmacol Ther*, 24, 187–192.

[67] Gardner, S.Y., Sweeney, R.W. and Divers, T.J. (1993) Pharmacokinetics of cefotaxime in neonatal pony foals. *Am J Vet Res*, 54, 576–579.

[68] Ringger, N.C., Brown, M.P., Kohlep, S.J. *et al.* (1998) Pharmacokinetics of ceftriaxone in neonatal foals. *Equine Vet J*, 30, 163–165.

[69] Cervantes, C.C., Brown, M.P., Gronawall, R. *et al.* (1993) Pharmacokinetics and concentrations of ceftiofur sodium in body fluids and endometrium after repeated intramuscular injections in mares. *Am J Vet Res*, 54, 573–575.

[70] Schnabel, L.V., Papich, M.G., Divers, T.J. *et al.* (2012) Pharmacokinetics and distribution of minocycline in mature horses after oral administration of multiple doses and comparison with minimum inhibitory concentrations. *Equine Vet J*, 44, 453–458.

[71] Nau, R., Sorge, F. and Prange, H. (1998) Pharmacokinetic optimisation of the treatment of bacterial central nervous system infections. *Clin Pharmacokinet*, 35, 223–246.

[72] Lebel, M.H., Freij, B.J., Syrogiannopoulos, G.A. *et al.* (1988) Dexamethasone therapy for bacterial meningitis. Results of two double-blind, placebo-controlled trials. *N Engl J Med*, 319, 964–971.

[73] de Gans, J. and van de Beek, D. (2002) Dexamethasone in adults with bacterial meningitis. *N Engl J Med*, 347, 1549–1556.

22 Equine Protozoal Myeloencephalitis

Martin Furr[1] and Daniel K. Howe[2]

[1] Marion duPont Scott Equine Medical Center, Virginia-Maryland Regional College of Veterinary Medicine, Leesburg, USA
[2] Gluck Equine Center, University of Kentucky, Lexington, USA

Equine protozoal myeloencephalitis (EPM) is a commonly diagnosed neurologic condition of the horse that was originally described in 1964 by J. Rooney as "segmental myelitis." Later descriptions used the terminology "focal myelitis encephalitis" or "toxoplasma-like encephalitis" when protozoan parasites were found in the central nervous system (CNS) of ataxic horses [1, 2]. The observed organism was determined to be a member of the genus *Sarcocystis* in 1976, and an organism was cultured from an affected horse in 1991 and named *Sarcocystis neurona* due to its association with neurons [3, 4]. Since that time, a variety of parasite strains from other ataxic horses have been isolated and described [5–12]. In addition, infection with *S. neurona* or an *S. neurona*-like organism has been observed in a number of other species including the zebra [13], domestic cat [14], Canadian lynx [15], domestic dog [16–18], sea otter [19, 20], seal [21], straw-necked ibis [22], mink, fisher, ferret, raccoon, and skunk [23–27].

Experimental inoculation of horses with *S. neurona* has been shown to induce a syndrome of neurologic disease consistent with field cases, and it is clear that *S. neurona* is the major cause of EPM [28–31]. In addition to *S. neurona*, however, the related protozoan parasite *Neospora hughesi* has been recovered from a small number of horses with EPM-like illness [32–35]. Consequently, *N. hughesi* must also be considered a cause of EPM, although much less common. *Toxoplasma gondii* was reported as a cause of EPM [36], but it is likely that the organisms were misidentified and were truly *S. neurona* [37, 38].

Biology of *Sarcocystis neurona* and *Neospora hughesi*

Both *S. neurona* and *N. hughesi* are classified in the phylum Apicomplexa [39], which encompasses a very broad and important group of obligate intracellular parasites that cause significant disease in humans and animals. The phylum includes the mosquito-transmitted *Plasmodium* spp., the causative agents of malaria, *T. gondii*, which is one of the most prevalent zoonotic pathogens worldwide, and the waterborne pathogen *Cryptosporidium* spp. In addition, there are multiple members of this phylum that cause significant disease in both wildlife and domestic animals. Greater than 4500 species of Apicomplexa have been described [40], and it is reasonable to speculate that this phylogenetic group is collectively one of the most prominent causes of infectious disease worldwide.

Although there are multiple variations on the theme, the typical apicomplexan cell contains a variety of structures and virulence factors that have evolved to allow these parasites the ability to enter and survive within their host cells. At the forward end of the crescent-shaped apicomplexan cell, termed a zoite, is a distinct collection of specialized structures called the apical complex [39, 40]. The apical complex typically comprises several cytoskeletal features, such as a polar ring and a conoid, and secretory organelles called micronemes and rhoptries [41–45]. An additional set of secretory organelles called dense granules are also found in some species of Apicomplexa [46]. Most apicomplexan zoites use actin- and myosin-based motility to actively invade into their host cell [47–50]. The components of the apical complex are generally believed to aid in this process of host cell invasion as well as the establishment of an intracellular environment that is conducive to survival [43, 46, 51–54]. Also involved in host cell invasion and parasite survival in some of the Apicomplexa are related surface antigens (SAGs). Originally described in *T. gondii* [55], SAG homologues have also been identified in *Neospora* spp. [56, 57] and *Sarcocystis* spp. [58, 59], including *S. neurona* [60, 61]. Given their importance for parasite survival, all of these unique structures and proteins of the Apicomplexa are excellent candidates for both immune and chemotherapeutic intervention during infection.

Equine Neurology, Second Edition. Martin Furr and Stephen Reed.
© 2015 John Wiley & Sons, Inc. Published 2015 by John Wiley & Sons, Inc.
Companion website: www.wiley.com/go/furr/neurology

Intermediate hosts

Raccoon *(procyon lotor)*
Skunk *(mephitis mephitis)*
Armadillo *(dasypus novemcinctus)*
Cats *(felis domesticus)*
Others?

Predation scavenging

Definitive hosts

Opossums
Didelphis virginiana
Didelphis albiventris

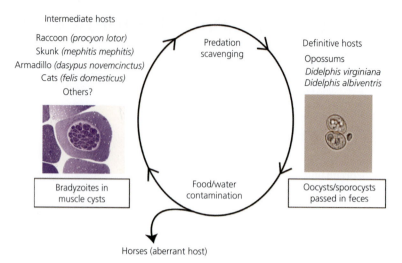

Bradyzoites in muscle cysts

Food/water contamination

Oocysts/sporocysts passed in feces

Horses (aberrant host)

Figure 22.1 Obligatory two-host life cycle of *Sarcocystis neurona*. The opossum is the definitive host, while several small mammals can serve as intermediate hosts. Horses are considered aberrant hosts since *S. neurona* typically does not form cysts in the muscle tissue of equids.

With the one exception being *Cryptosporidium* [62], most apicomplexans contain a plastid-like organelle called the apicoplast, which was likely obtained from a photosynthetic organism (green algae) by secondary endosymbiosis [63–66]. Despite its origin, this organelle does not function in photosynthesis. However, the apicoplast is indispensable for parasite survival [67] and appears to be involved in biosynthesis of fatty acids, heme, and isoprenoids [68–70]. Since this organelle's function is required by the parasite and it is not present in mammalian cells, the apicoplast is an appealing target for anti-protozoal drugs.

Many members of the Apicomplexa have complex life cycles. The obligatory heteroxenous (i.e., two hosts) life cycle of *S. neurona* is shown in Figure 22.1. The opossum (*Didelphis virginiana*) serves as the definitive host for *S. neurona* in North America [71]. In addition, South American opossums are capable of serving as the definitive host for *S. neurona* [72]. In the infected opossum, the parasites undergo sexual reproduction in the intestinal epithelium, which culminates in the production of sporozoite-containing oocysts/sporocysts that are passed in the feces of the opossum. Oocysts from the family Sarcocystidae each contains two bean-shaped sporocysts, each of which contains four crescent-shaped sporozoites [73, 74]. The *S. neurona* oocyst is fully sporulated when passed, and the oocyst wall is highly fragile so free sporocysts are most often found in the feces. When sporocysts are ingested by one of the intermediate hosts, the sporozoites initiate an acute infection that is predominated by the rapidly growing merozoite/schizont stage of the parasite (see Figure 22.2). Asexual

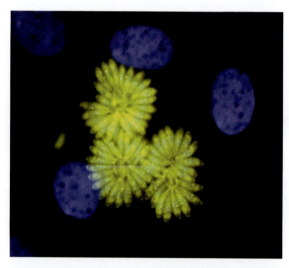

Figure 22.2 Fluorescence microscopy of a mature schizont of *S. neurona* growing in cultured bovine turbinate host cells. The yellow fluorescent protein-expressing schizont consists of multiple merozoites that will escape the infected host cell and reinvade new cells. Host cell nuclei are labeled with 4′,6-diamidino-2-phenylindole (blue). (Photo courtesy of Dr. Sriveny Dangoudoubiyam.)

reproduction of *S. neurona* occurs by endopolygeny, which is distinct from *T. gondii* and *N. hughesi* endodyogeny and allows for effective discrimination between these parasite species. The normal intermediate hosts for *S. neurona* are various small mammals including skunks [75], raccoons [76], armadillos [77], and cats [78]. Like other members of the genus *Sarcocystis*, *S. neurona* forms latent sarcocysts in muscle tissues of their intermediate hosts, which serve as the source of infection for the opossum-definitive host through scavenging and carnivorism. Opossums are opportunistic omnivores that rely heavily on carrion for their diet, so it is easy to appreciate the efficiency of the *S. neurona* life cycle. Indeed, the presence of *S. neurona* sporocysts has been observed previously in approximately 20–25% of opossums sampled [79–81], so it is apparent that these animals are commonly infected.

Horses become infected with *S. neurona* by ingesting food or water that has been contaminated with the infective sporocysts shed by the opossum into the environment. Unlike the normal small mammal intermediate hosts, however, mature sarcocysts are not readily found in equids. Consequently, the horse is considered a dead-end host that does not support completion of the *S. neurona* life cycle. This position has been challenged, however, with the demonstration of *S. neurona* sarcocysts in a 4-month-old foal with clinical signs of EPM [82]. Further work is required to assess the capacity of *S. neurona* to form sarcocysts in equids, but this finding suggests that long-term latent infection may occur in horses.

Interestingly, opossums can serve as the definitive host for several species of *Sarcocystis* [83, 84], and it was believed at one time that *S. neurona* was synonymous with *Sarcocystis falcatula*, thus implicating birds as an intermediate host for *S. neurona* [85]. However, it is now apparent that *S. neurona* and *S. falcatula* are distinct species with biological and molecular differences [86–89]. Although one report described *S. neurona* sarcocysts in muscle tissues of brown-headed cowbirds [90], it remains uncertain whether birds play a major role in the natural life cycle of *S. neurona*.

The life cycle of *N. hughesi* is unknown, so the major route of transmission to horses is unclear. The closely related parasite *Neospora caninum* utilizes canids as definitive hosts [91–93], but it has not been demonstrated that dogs are also a definitive host for *N. hughesi*. Vertical transmission from infected dam to developing fetus is known to be an efficient mode of *N. caninum* transmission in cattle (reviewed extensively in Ref. [94]), and there is now evidence that transplacental passage of *N. hughesi* can occur in horses [95, 96].

Epidemiology

Consistent with the geographic range of the opossum definitive hosts, EPM caused by *S. neurona* is a disease of North, Central, and South America. Most horses with a diagnosis of EPM outside this region appear to have spent some time in the endemic area. However, neurologic

horses with consistent clinical signs, positive *S. neurona* Western blot (WB) test results, and no history of travel in the American continent have been reported [97]. The nature of the infection in these horses is unclear, and may be due to cross-reaction in WB analysis, as observed for horses in Europe [98]. Horses in the United States have a variable but generally high prevalence of antibodies to S. *neurona*. Studies in various regions of the United States have shown seroprevalence against *S. neurona* ranging from approximately 15% in wild horses in Wyoming to 89% in horses in Oklahoma [99–106]. Seroprevalence studies in Central (Costa Rica) and South America (Brazil and Argentina) have similarly shown that horses in these regions are commonly exposed to *S. neurona* [107–110].

The prevalence of antibodies to *N. hughesi* in horses is generally lower than *S. neurona* seroprevalence and has varied substantially depending on geography and the assay used to detect antibodies. While seroprevalence over 10% [34, 111–113], and greater than 30% in some regions [102, 106], has been reported, other studies have detected antibodies against *N. hughesi* in much lower proportions of horses examined (i.e., <3%) [106–110, 114, 115]. Geographic differences certainly may account for some of the variation that has been observed. However, studies that have used WB analysis to confirm results suggest that seroprevalence to *N. hughesi* may be commonly overestimated [106, 109, 115]. While the annual incidence of *N. hughesi* infection may be uncertain, it is quite apparent that the range of *N. hughesi* extends beyond the Americas, with seropositive horses reported in Europe [111, 112], Asia [114], and New Zealand [106].

All horses are believed to be susceptible to the development of EPM, but epidemiological surveys have suggested that the average age of affected horses is approximately 3.5–4.5 years [116, 117]. The age range of reported cases is from 2 months [118] to 24 years [119]. Standardbred and Thoroughbred horses have been overrepresented in some studies [117, 120], but this finding is inconsistent and may reflect selection bias. Horses of all breeds appear to be affected and there is no gender bias. Most cases appear to be individual cases and "outbreaks" of EPM do not appear to occur.

Despite the often high rate of exposure to *S. neurona*, only a small percentage (an estimated 0.1–0.2%) of horses develop clinical EPM annually [121]. It is not well understood what factors are responsible for the progression from asymptomatic infection to full-blown clinical disease, but this is a major hindrance to EPM diagnosis and disease control. The number of *S. neurona* sporocysts ingested may contribute to the occurrence of natural cases of EPM, as suggested by experimental challenge of horses [29]. Differences in the virulence of parasite strains may also be involved. Although the population biology of *S. neurona* is characterized by fairly modest genetic diversity [122–126], antigenic differences between isolates of *S. neurona* have been documented [126–128]. As such, it is conceivable that other phenotypic differences, such as virulence, may exist between parasite strains. However, this has not been examined critically, so it remains unclear whether some *S. neurona* strains have greater capacity to cause EPM. Other potential factors that may increase susceptibility to EPM include physiologic stress associated with transport, training, showing, and pregnancy [129]. Indeed, one model used to induce EPM incorporated long-range transport to cause stress in horses immediately prior to oral challenge with *S. neurona* sporocysts [130]. It is assumed that stress leads to some degree of immune suppression, which is commonly implicated in exacerbating protozoan parasite infections. Paradoxically, inclusion of a second transport did not result in more severe neurologic signs [131]. Additionally, treatment of horses with immunosuppressive doses of steroids did not result in significantly worse histopathologic changes in the CNS, although clinical signs were slightly more severe in the immunosuppressed horses than in non-immunosuppressed horses [28]. While it seems likely that stress can play a role in the development of EPM, it is apparent that the interaction is complex and not fully understood at this time.

Pathophysiology

Gross lesions in the CNS of EPM horses are sometimes inapparent. When present, lesions are random and multifocal and are more commonly seen in the spinal cord but can occur in the brain or brainstem [132]. Gross lesions typically consist of areas of hemorrhage or brownish-red discoloration, sometimes with mild swelling and edema. Microscopically, lesions contain infiltrates of lymphocytes and macrophages that form prominent perivascular cuffs. Eosinophils and multinucleated giant cells are commonly present. Inflammation can extend into the adjacent neuropil with associated degeneration of tissue. Schizonts and/or merozoites of *S. neurona* are associated with the areas of inflammation but may be difficult to identify using standard staining procedures (e.g., hematoxylin and eosin) and are more readily observed after immunohistochemical labeling (see Figure 22.3). Parasites can be numerous and easily detected in some cases. Paradoxically, however, it is common that few organisms will be present even when lesions are substantial, thus suggesting that disease pathogenesis is at least partly immune based. While it is apparent that considerable deficiencies remain in our understanding of the pathophysiology of this disease, significant advances have been made in recent years to investigate *S. neurona* infection and EPM by utilizing

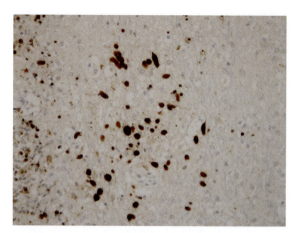

Figure 22.3 Extensively infected CNS tissue from a horse with EPM. Immunohistochemical labeling with anti-*S. neurona* rabbit serum showing numerous parasites (brown). (Photo courtesy of Breanna Gaubatz.)

genetically modified strains of mice, newly developed infection models, and molecular techniques.

The development of *S. neurona* has been carefully examined in immunodeficient mouse strains, in which there is a gut phase, with sporozoites found in the small intestinal villi as well as the Peyer's patches within hours of inoculation [133]. By 1 day after inoculation, organisms could be found in the mesenteric lymph nodes and pancreas. Parasitemia was observed on days 1–8 after infection, and organisms were found in numerous tissues by 1 week after infection. Parasites were found in brain by day 5 after infection [133]. Thus, in immunodeficient mice, it appears that there is a hematogenous distribution of parasites occurring rapidly and with widespread seeding of tissues.

In a similar challenge study performed in immunocompetent ponies, organisms were recovered from the mesenteric lymph nodes from day 1 to 7 postinfection, from the liver between day 2 and 7 postinfection, and from the lung between day 5 and 9 postinfection [134]. In addition, histologic changes consistent with *S. neurona* infection were found in the CNS of one pony on postinfection day 9. These findings suggest lymphatic dissemination and an early and transient parasitemia with hematogenous dissemination. Parasitemia in horses is rarely noted, but it has been observed in immunodeficient horses [135] and in one immunocompetent horse following challenge with *S. neurona* [31]. Generally, however, infection is not seen in extra-neural tissues of naturally infected horses.

The mechanism by which parasites enter the CNS is unknown; however, one attractive hypothesis is that the organism infects lymphocytes, which then carry the organism to the CNS during tissue surveillance, referred to as a "Trojan Horse" mechanism [31]. This method of CNS infection is supported by the observation that leukocytes can be infected with *S. neurona* [136] and clinical signs have been observed in immunocompetent horses following the intravenous injection of *S. neurona*-infected autologous lymphocytes [31]. Alternatively, or perhaps also, the organism may enter the CNS directly through the cytoplasm of infected endothelial cells after hematogenous dissemination [133].

Resistance to *S. neurona* is presumed to be due to the combined effects of humoral and cellular immunity. Following infection, there is a relatively rapid production of antibodies. In horses challenged with live *S. neurona* organisms orally, all horses seroconverted within 32 days [28], while in another study, horses challenged with a larger number of organisms seroconverted by day 13 after infection (if stressed by transport) and by day 30 if not stressed [130]. In immunocompetent mice, a vigorous humoral response is also noted, with seroconversion and increased B cell numbers and proportions associated with the development of germinal centers in lymphoid tissue [137].

It has been demonstrated that antibody to various apicomplexan parasites, including *S. neurona*, can be protective. For example, treatment of immunocompromised patients using plasma hyperimmunized against *Cryptosporidium parvum* can eliminate clinical signs [138]. This has been shown to be a direct result of the presence of antibodies to specific cell surface proteins [139]. Antibodies against SAGs of *T. gondii* and *N. caninum* have been found to inhibit infection of host cells [140–144], thus implicating a functional role for the SAG proteins in host cell attachment and invasion by these parasites. Using a serum neutralization assay, it has been similarly demonstrated that antibodies to the *S. neurona* surface protein Sn16 (now designated SnSAG2 [61]) block cellular infection, while antibodies directed against Sn30 (believed to comprise SnSAG1 and SnSAG4 [61]) had no inhibitory effect [145]. This is in contrast to a more recent study in which infectivity and clinical signs of EPM were reduced in horses vaccinated with recombinant SnSAG1 protein [146]. However, this study utilized a very small sample size (five infected control horses) and all animals (control and vaccinated) developed neurologic abnormalities. The possible protective role of antibodies against SnSAG surface proteins is further complicated by the antigenic diversity that exists amongst *S. neurona* isolates. In particular, the major surface antigen SnSAG1 has been shown to be absent from some *S. neurona* isolates, including strains isolated from EPM-affected horses [12, 128], which instead express alternative major SAGs [126, 127]. These findings are consistent with another study demonstrating that only 18 of 26 EPM-affected horses (as determined by postmortem) had measurable

antibody to the SnSAG1 surface protein [147]. Clearly, further work is needed to elucidate the roles of the *S. neurona* cell surface proteins in infectivity and pathogenicity and the potential immune protection provided by antibodies against these surface proteins.

While the effects of circulating antibody are likely to be very important, cell-mediated immunity is necessary for the elimination of most intracellular pathogens. In immunocompetent mice, there is a significant increase in both total CD8+ splenocytes and in the percentage of CD8+ peripheral blood lymphocytes following infection with *S. neurona* [137]. One study in horses found that peripheral blood CD4+ lymphocytes were slightly decreased in seropositive horses that were demonstrating clinical signs, when compared to asymptomatic, seropositive horses. In this group, there was no change in the CD8+ subset [148]. A small study of naturally infected horses found that there was no difference in peripheral blood or cerebrospinal fluid (CSF) lymphocyte subsets in EPM-affected horses, although the total T-cell number (CD5+) in CSF was higher in EPM-affected horses (93.2 vs. 73.2%; $p = 0.07$) [149]. Another study of 17 horses with EPM demonstrated that there was an increased number of infiltrating T cells in the CNS compared to normal horses [150].

Mouse studies have confirmed the importance of CD8+ T cells in protection against *S. neurona* encephalopathy in that species. Endothelitis and meningoencephalitis developed in CD8 knock out (KO) mice following challenge with *S. neurona*, highlighting the importance of this cell subset in protection against *S. neurona* [151]. The CD8+ T cells (aka cytotoxic T cells) are one important source of interferon gamma (IFN-γ), which is widely recognized as being important in the elimination of the related parasite *T. gondii* [152].

IFN-γ has also been found to be critical for protection against *S. neurona*-induced neurologic disease in mice. Infection of IFN-γ KO mice leads to fulminant neurologic disease [87]. Following infection with *S. neurona*, severe combined immunodeficiency (SCID) mice do not develop neurologic disease, yet maintain a persistent low level parasitemia following infection with *S. neurona* [135]. SCID mice are unable to mount adaptive immune responses, yet have natural killer (NK) cells that have the ability to secrete IFN-γ. When SCID mice were treated with neutralizing anti-IFN-γ antibody, neurologic disease resulted [135]. These findings support the critical importance of IFN-γ in protection against *S. neurona*.

These data also suggest an important role of the NK cell, which has been found to be critically important in the protection of other species from protozoan parasites [153]. However, when NK cells were depleted in mice that were then infected with *S. neurona*, neurologic disease did not result [135]. This could be due to a failure to eliminate all NK cells with some residual IFN-γ production or the production of IFN-γ by non-NK cells. IFN-γ secreted by sensitized T cells activates macrophages, enabling them to kill intracellular organisms by promoting phagosome–lysosome fusion. One important mechanism by which activated macrophages kill parasite-infected target cells is via the production of nitric oxide (NO).

Nitric oxide is a multifunction molecule that acts as a neurotransmitter, vasodilator, and immune mediator. It occurs as three isoforms (inducible nitric oxide synthase (NOS), endothelial NOS, and neuronal NOS), and all three have been reported in mammalian CSF [154]. Increased quantities of NO have been found in association with infections of various parasitic protozoa, including *Babesia bovis* [155], *Trypanosoma cruzi* [156], *T. brucei*, and *Plasmodium falciparum*, underscoring the importance of this protective mechanism in parasitic infections [157].

In horses with EPM induced using the transport stress model, as well as in naturally occurring EPM, a decreased concentration of NO in the CSF was found to be associated with the severity of clinical signs [158]. A clear interpretation of these results is not immediately obvious; however it was suggested that the decrease could be simply a result of infection and NO was not protective. This is supported by work in iNOS and eNOS KO mice, in which it was found that these mice were resistant to the development of CNS illness when infected with *S. neurona* [159]. It is important to recognize, however, that the iNOS KO mice had IFN-γ present in low concentrations, suggesting that only very low concentrations of IFN-γ are necessary for protection, and further highlighting the central role of IFN-γ in protection against *S. neurona*.

Epidemiologic studies have suggested that stress has at least a permissive effect upon the development of EPM. However, there is also evidence that the presence of the organism may itself be immunosuppressive. Cell-mediated immune responses to mitogens have been shown to be reduced in horses with EPM [148], but it is unclear if this was a cause or effect of infection. In other studies, lymphocytes from EPM positive horses had suppressed blastogenic responses when co-incubated with SnSAG1 protein that was not observed in lymphocytes from EPM negative horses, nor when either cell type was stimulated with Con A [160]. This represents an antigen-specific immunosuppression of cellular response. Furthermore, IFN-γ messenger RNA production was diminished in lymphocytes from EPM positive horses [160]. These were *in vitro* studies, which may not directly represent the *in vivo* situation, but even local immunosuppression in the microenvironment of the parasite is perhaps significant in an infected animal. In an *in vivo* challenge model, it has been demonstrated that EPM-affected horses had a diminished proliferative response to mitogens as soon as 2 days after infection

[161]. Hence, although it appears that the parasite itself induces some immunosuppressive effects, the unique environment of the CNS may also have a role in the pathophysiology of the infection.

Infection of the CNS is somewhat unique in that the CNS is considered an "immune-privileged site." This refers to the observation that the immune response in this tissue, while fully competent, differs from that of other tissues. Specifically, the immune system of the CNS appears to function to clear any infecting organism while minimizing inflammation [162]. This is perceived to have some survival benefit for the horse, for it may be that the inflammatory response in the CNS is more damaging than the initial insult that provokes it [162]. Modifications within the CNS to mediate the inflammatory response include a lack of conventional lymphatics, the presence of a blood–brain barrier (BBB) which minimizes but does not totally prohibit cellular surveillance of the CNS, and the presence of immunosuppressive cytokines that down-regulate the vigor of the immune response [163, 164]. A primary cytokine involved in immune privileged tissues is transforming growth factor-β (TGF-β). This cytokine has numerous immune functions, depending upon its concentration and other cytokines present. TGF-β has been found in the CSF of many mammalian species and is considered one of the primary immunosuppressive cytokines in this tissue [165]. Mice infected with *T. cruzi* develop greater parasite burdens and die sooner when treated with TGF-β than untreated controls [166]. Even more dramatically, the *T. cruzi*-resistant mouse strain (C57BL/6×DBA/2F1) had a 50% mortality when treated with TGF-β compared to 0% mortality in untreated mice [166]. In addition, TGF-β blocks the production of IFN-γ [167], which may be the mechanism responsible for decreased parasite clearance in the presence of TGF-β. In mice, IFN-γ production was decreased when cells were coincubated with CSF, an effect that was reversed when TGF-β was blocked with specific monoclonal antibodies, thus confirming its role [164].

TGF-β has been documented to be present in the CSF of the horse and its concentration was found to be less in the CSF of horses with EPM [168]. Contrary to findings in mice, treatment of equine lymphocytes with CSF enhanced IFN-γ production, an effect which was not significantly affected by the application of TGF-β monoclonal antibodies [168]. These findings suggest that TGF-β is immunomodulatory in equine CSF; however, there appears to be other immunomodulatory proteins present as well.

Clinical signs

Once the organism has infected the nervous system, it leads to localized inflammation with clinical neurologic abnormalities that are dependent upon the anatomic

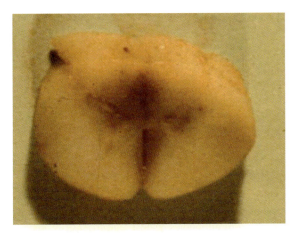

Figure 22.4 Gross view of a cross-section of a spinal cord with an EPM lesion, observed as brown discoloration around the dorsal fissure.

site of the infection in the CNS (Figure 22.4). In general, *S. neurona*-induced neurologic disease results in clinical signs of muscle atrophy and ataxia, with asymmetry (i.e., the three "*A's*" of EPM) (Figures 22.5 and 22.6). Symmetrical illness can be seen, however, and its presence should not lead one to exclude a diagnosis of EPM. Spinal cord symptoms predominate, leading to early signs of ataxia, stumbling, or weakness. Atrophy of the gluteal muscles is the most commonly affected muscle (54%), but any muscle can be involved, including the tongue [117]. In one series of cases, the progression of illness was most commonly chronic (47%) but was considered to be acute in 42% and per-acute in 11% of cases [117]. Cranial nerve signs have been reported in up to 12% of reported cases [117]. These signs include muscle wasting of the temporalis and masseter muscles, head tilt, or dysphagia. Cerebral signs can also be seen, although rarely, and these include blindness, seizure activity, and altered mentation.

Diagnosis

Due to the variable and sometimes subtle presentation of clinical signs and the inherent complexities of the diagnostic tests, clinical diagnosis of EPM remains a challenging task for veterinarians. However, an accurate diagnosis can now be achieved by careful interpretation of clinical and ancillary diagnostic laboratory testing. Diagnosis is dependent upon the following:

1 Confirming the presence of clinical signs that are consistent with EPM
2 Ruling out other potential causes of the observed clinical signs by appropriate means (CSF evaluation, cervical radiography, serology, etc.)

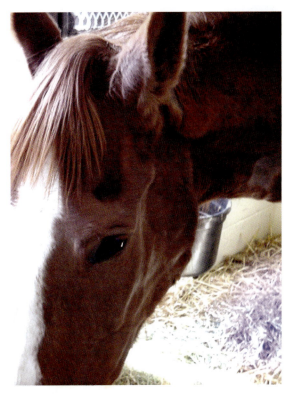

Figure 22.5 Masseter muscle atrophy in a horse with EPM.

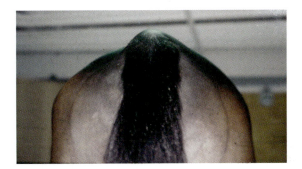

Figure 22.6 Left-sided gluteal muscle atrophy in a horse with EPM.

3 Using immunodiagnostic testing to demonstrate the presence of antibodies against *S. neurona* or *N. hughesi*, in CSF to assess intrathecal production.

Clinical examination

A thorough physical and neurological examination remains the keystone of the EPM diagnosis [169]. Conclusive evidence of CNS disease must be present for a diagnosis of EPM to be considered. Musculoskeletal disease should be ruled out, if possible, by appropriate means. This may involve flexion tests and local nerve or joint blocks. Concurrent disease is possible and must be considered. The classic clinical signs of EPM have been well described and include gait abnormalities, and/or signs of cranial nerve, brainstem, or cerebral disease [170]. Asymmetry of clinical signs is a hallmark of the disease, although symmetrical deficits can be seen.

Once a physical examination is completed, ancillary testing is important to gather further information. The nature and extent of ancillary testing will be determined by the results of the neurologic exam; however, most commonly this will include radiographs of the cervical spine along with serum and CSF collection and evaluation.

Eliminate other potential causes

In the evaluation of a horse with potential EPM, it is important to consider a list of potential rule-outs in addition to EPM to help direct a full diagnostic evaluation. This will commonly include disorders such as cervical compressive myelopathy, trauma, or viral or bacterial neurologic disease, for example. Other causes include equine degenerative encephalomyelopathy, lower motor neuron disease, or developmental abnormalities. Survey radiographs, serology, and CSF collection and analysis are all important components of a full evaluation. A full clinical examination to document the presence or absence of other clinical abnormalities, historical information, and routine clinicopathologic testing (CBC, serum chemistry profile) are usually warranted. A lameness examination is very important and should be carefully done to eliminate disease of the musculoskeletal system, as it is much more commonly affected than the CNS. If all such testing is negative, the probability of EPM increases, particularly if immunodiagnostic testing supports the diagnosis.

Cervical radiographs are indicated for the evaluation of any horses that have neuroanatomic localization of the clinical signs to the cervical region. While EPM does not cause radiographic changes, it is important to rule out other causes of spinal ataxia, such as cervical compression, fracture, or cervical process joint arthritis, which may be present. If evidence of cervical compression is found, then myelography should be pursued.

CSF collection and evaluation is also recommended for full evaluation of the horse with CNS disease. CSF should be evaluated for red blood and nucleated cell count, total protein, and glucose concentrations, as well as a cytologic examination. A full evaluation of the CSF is important in identifying horses with viral or bacterial meningoencephalitis, tumors, or trauma. The CSF is usually normal in horses with EPM.

CSF concentration of the enzyme creatine kinase (CK) has been reported to have value in the differentiation of horses with EPM from those with cervical compressive myelopathy [171]. However, other research has questioned the validity of this approach, indicating that the CSF CK can become increased from traumatic puncture of the dura [172]. As in testing of any biochemical constituent of the CSF, the quality of the spinal fluid collection is important, and a traumatic tap or one in which multiple penetrations were necessary to obtain fluid should lead to careful consideration of the validity of any constituent. This does not, in itself, automatically invalidate the use of the CSF CK concentrations as a diagnostic aid. Hence, in the authors' opinion, the use of CSF CK assay continues to have value on a properly collected sample (i.e., atraumatically).

Immunodiagnostic testing

Detection of antibodies against *S. neurona* or *N. hughesi* has been commonly used to aid antemortem diagnosis of EPM (Table 22.1). However, it is quite apparent that horses can be infected by these parasites without any clinical consequences. Therefore, the simple presence of antibodies in the blood has little diagnostic value. Detection of parasite-specific antibodies in CSF was logically proposed as an indicator of intrathecal antibody production and CNS infection. However, blood contamination of the CSF sample during collection as well as normal passive transfer of circulating antibody (i.e., within plasma) across an intact and healthy BBB [173] will lead to the detection of antibodies within the CSF of clinically normal horses. Given these challenges, it is not surprising that veterinary practitioners were often frustrated by the results obtained with the early EPM tests. Thankfully, the tools and methodologies for EPM immunodiagnosis have improved substantially since the initial test offerings. As discussed in greater detail later, the development of semi-quantitative assays now permit demonstration of intrathecal antibody production against the parasite, which accurately identifies horses suffering from EPM.

Serologic tests

The WB test (a.k.a. immunoblot) was the first assay developed for the detection of *S. neurona*-specific antibodies and represented a great step forward in understanding and diagnosing EPM [174]. This assay has been used for EPM diagnosis for nearly two decades and continues to be offered by several diagnostic testing laboratories.

In the time since it was developed, the conventional WB (cWB) test has been modified in attempts to improve the accuracy and/or to make the assay semi-quantitative. One permutation of the cWB uses bovine serum against *Sarcocystis cruzi* to "block" cross-reacting antigen [175]. This modified Western blot (mWB) was reported to have sensitivity and specificity approaching 100%. However, the study was performed on only a small number (a total of 6) of EPM-positive horses, and

Table 22.1 Summary of commercially available serologic tests for EPM diagnosis.

Test type and source	Test principle	Comments
SnSAG2, SnSAG4/3, NhSAG1 ELISAs, Equine Diagnostic Solutions, LLC	Detects antibodies to parasite surface antigens (*S. neurona* or *N. hughesi*)	Semi-quantitative, end-point titer provided
Immunofluorescence Antibody Test (IFAT), University of CA, Davis	Detects antibodies to whole parasites (*S. neurona* or *N. hughesi*)	Semi-quantitative, end-point titer provided
Western Blot, Equine Diagnostic Solutions, LLC	Detects antibodies to unknown *S. neurona* antigens	Non-quantitative
Western blot (modified), Michigan State University	Detects antibodies to immunodominant antigens after blocking with *S. cruzi* antibodies	Non-quantitative
Western blot, Neogen, Inc.	Detects antibodies to immunodominant *S. neurona* antigens	Quasi-quantitative, RQ report provided
SnSAG1 ELISA, Antech, Inc.	Detects antibodies to single *S. neurona* surface antigen	Semi-quantitative, end-point titer provided. Lower sensitivity
SnSAG1,5,6 stall-side test, Prota, LLC	Detects antibodies to *S. neurona* surface antigens	Non-quantitative. No description of assay validation

subsequent evaluation of the mWB by other investigators found a lower sensitivity/specificity of 89 and 69%, respectively [176]. An alternative interpretation of the cWB used by a commercial testing laboratory (Neogen, Inc) involves measuring the intensity of the primary low molecular weight (~17 kDa) band to yield a unitless number referred to as the "relative quotient" (RQ). The use of the RQ has not been found to improve diagnostic efficiency, although in one study the RQ did decrease slightly during treatment [177] (Table 22.1).

While development of the WB test was a tremendous boost to EPM diagnosis, the WB technique is primarily a research tool. Consequently, multiple "second generation" serologic assays have been developed to provide greater throughput and be more informative. Two assays developed using whole *S. neurona* merozoites as antigen were the *S. neurona* direct (serum) agglutination test (SAT) [8] and the indirect fluorescent antibody test (IFAT) [176, 178]. Both the SAT and the IFAT can be used to obtain an end-point antibody titer, which is a large improvement over the nonquantitative result provided by the WB test. The SAT is advantageous since it can be used for detection of antibodies in multiple different animal species, and the assay has been employed in a variety of research studies [179–183]. However, the SAT has not been routinely employed for EPM diagnosis and is not presently offered as a commercial test. The IFAT was optimized and validated at the University of California-Davis [176, 178], and testing is currently available from the University of California Veterinary Diagnostic Laboratory. Although specialized instrumentation is needed (i.e., a fluorescence microscope), interpretation of parasite fluorescence requires expertise, and concerns have been raised about cross-reactivity with the nonpathogenic species

S. fayeri, serologic results from the IFAT should be generally accurate when the assay is performed by individuals with proper training [184].

Enzyme-linked immunosorbent assays (ELISAs) are easy to perform, are generally less expensive and laborious, and provide a more objective interpretation of results relative to the other existing assays, particularly the WB. Several ELISAs have been developed using *S. neurona* antigens that have been expressed in *E. coli* as recombinant proteins [147, 185, 186]. These ELISAs are all based on the family of related surface antigens (SnSAGs), which are expressed by *S. neurona* merozoites [60, 61]. The SnSAGs are good serologic targets since they are abundant and immunogenic, and their incorporation into the ELISA format allows for relatively high-throughput testing that gives an objective, quantitative result. However, all of the SnSAGs are not equally appropriate for use in serologic assays since immunologic and molecular analyses have shown that there is antigenic diversity between different strains of *S. neurona* [12, 126–128, 187].

ELISAs based on recombinant forms of the SnSAG2, SnSAG3, and SnSAG4 surface antigens have been shown to be very accurate for detecting and quantifying antibodies against *S. neurona* in equine serum and CSF samples [147, 186]. Although all three antigens performed well, the best serologic accuracy was achieved with the recombinant SnSAG2 (rSnSAG2) antigen, which had a sensitivity and specificity of 95.5 and 92.9%, respectively, when used to test a set of characterized equine serum samples. To improve the ELISAs, a polyvalent antigen was created by fusing portions of both SnSAG3 and SnSAG4 into a single chimeric protein (rSnSAG4/3) [186]. Use of rSnSAG4/3 in ELISA yielded sensitivity and specificity of 95.2 and 100%, respectively, for detecting antibodies against *S. neurona*. The rSnSAG2 ELISA and the rSnSAG4/3 ELISA are presently run concurrently (designated SnSAG2, 4/3; Equine Diagnostic Solutions, LLC), thereby reducing the negative impact of antigenic diversity in the *S. neurona* population and the varied immune responses that occur in different horses. Homologues of the SnSAG2, SnSAG3, and SnSAG4 antigens can be identified in the related parasite *S. falcatula*. However, this does not hinder the specificity of the SnSAG2, 4/3 ELISA results since *S. falcatula* is incapable of infecting and causing seroconversion in horses [86]. Furthermore, extensive validation studies have shown that the SnSAG ELISAs are specific and do not cross-react with serum from horses infected with other species of *Sarcocystis* [98, 147]. Hence, these surface proteins are valuable immunologic markers of infection with *S. neurona*.

An ELISA based on the SnSAG1 surface antigen has been described for EPM diagnosis [185] and is currently offered by Antech, Inc. This test provides an end-point titer and values greater than 1:100 in serum are reported to indicate active infection. This test and cutoff point has not been rigorously evaluated, however, and the cutoff values used for a positive diagnosis appear to be arbitrary. More critically, the SnSAG1 protein has been shown to be absent from multiple *S. neurona* isolates [12, 128, 187], which explains the relatively poor accuracy achieved with this antigen in independent studies examining antibody detection [147] and EPM diagnosis [188]. An assay that combines SnSAG1 with the two alternative major SnSAGs, SnSAG5 [127] and SnSAG6 [126], is presently offered as a stall-side test (Prota LLC). However, there are no published reports describing validation of this assay, so it is unclear whether the test can provide an accurate detection of antibodies to *S. neurona*.

Two serologic assays are currently offered for detecting antibodies against *N. hughesi* in equine samples. An ELISA based on the major parasite surface antigen NhSAG1 [115] was available from Equine Diagnostic Solutions, LLC, while an IFAT using whole *N. hughesi* tachyzoites was offered by the University of California Veterinary Diagnostic Laboratory. The NhSAG1 ELISA exhibited high accuracy for antibody detection (94% sensitivity and 95% specificity) when compared to *N. hughesi* WB results for 1006 equine samples [115]. The *N. hughesi* IFAT sensitivity and specificity for detecting antibodies against *N. hughesi* was reported to be 100 and 71.4%, respectively, at a cutoff of 1:320 [189]. However, these results were based on a very small sample set (three naturally infected, seven experimentally infected, and seven naïve horses), so it is likely that the *N. hughesi* IFAT actually provides lower sensitivity but higher specificity than this reported value.

Serodiagnosis of CNS infection

As emphasized earlier, the simple presence of *S. neurona*- or *N. hughesi*-specific antibodies in the serum indicates only exposure of the horse to the parasite, but not necessarily infection of the CNS and active disease. Moreover, it is now apparent that the simple presence of parasite-specific antibodies in CSF is not a definitive indicator of CNS infection and EPM since blood contamination of the CSF sample during collection or the normal movement of circulating (plasma) antibody across an intact and healthy BBB [173] can both yield a false positive result. However, testing has been improved greatly by the development of semi-quantitative assays that give information about the amount of antibody present in the sample (i.e., IFAT and ELISAs), since this allows for diagnostic methods that can accurately reveal active infection in the CNS.

Intrathecal antibody production is a key feature of CNS infection that results in greater amounts of pathogen-specific antibodies in the CSF than would be present due to normal passive transfer across the BBB. The Goldmann-Witmer coefficient (*C* value) and the antigen-specific antibody index (AI) are tests of proportionality that compare the amount of antigen-specific antibody in the serum versus the CSF to assess whether intrathecal production has occurred. These methods have been used in human medicine to diagnose CNS infections caused by a variety of pathogens [190–192], including the apicomplexan *T. gondii* [193, 194]. The value of these indices for diagnosing EPM caused by *S. neurona* has been demonstrated by applying the *C* value and the AI to SnSAG2 ELISA results from 29 clinical cases (15 CVM and 14 EPM) [195]. The *C* value performed best in this study, achieving 86% sensitivity and 100% specificity for diagnosis. The study also reaffirmed the prior finding [196] that blood contamination of CSF has no adverse affect on assay results until more than 10 000 RBCs/µl are present in the sample. Therefore, minor iatrogenic contamination during CSF collection is not a concern and can be ignored.

Many EPM cases exhibit CSF titers that greatly exceed what will occur due to normal passive transfer of antibodies across the BBB. Consequently, calculation of a simple ratio of serum:CSF titers can serve as a proxy for the specific CSF indices (i.e., *C* value or AI), thereby reducing expense as measurement of albumin or IgG concentrations in the serum and CSF is not required. In studies using SnSAG2, 4/3 ELISAs to examine a large collection of horses with neurologic disease, the serum:CSF titer ratio was sufficient in many cases to reveal intrathecal antibody production and an accurate diagnosis of EPM [197, 198]. These studies found that the optimal serum:CSF titer ratio cutoff is 100 when using SnSAG2, 4/3 ELISAs; the ratio of 100:1 approximates the normal partitioning of proteins (e.g., albumin or IgG) between the blood and CSF of horses [195, 199]. At this cutoff, the serum:CSF ratio provided diagnostic accuracy of approximately 93% sensitivity and 83% specificity for the collection of 128 cases examined [198]. Moreover, 33 of the 44 EPM cases exhibited serum:CSF ratios of 25 or less, with nine horses having profound CSF antibody titers that approached or exceeded their serum titers (i.e., ratio of 1.6 or lower). Although not as accurate as the serum:CSF ratio, high CSF titers alone were also good evidence of intrathecal antibody production and active CNS infection, providing 93% sensitivity and 75% specificity at a SnSAG2, 4/3 titer cutoff of 1:10 [198]. Collectively, these findings suggest that use of the more thorough and laborious C value or AI can be limited to cases when the ELISA titer result is not compelling (e.g., the serum:CSF ratio equals the cutoff of 100) or when a condition that compromises the BBB is suspected.

Statistical modeling of IFAT results for a sample set of naturally and experimentally infected horses suggested CSF testing was minimally informative and that EPM diagnosis could be achieved from serum titers alone [200]. However, subsequent studies have shown that serum antibody titers are not a good indicator of EPM, and much greater diagnostic information is obtained from antibody titers in the CSF [197, 198]. The discrepant appraisals of serum results for EPM diagnosis likely arise from differences in the authenticity of the sample sets used for these studies. Specifically, the sample set used in the study by Duarte *et al.* [200] had a high proportion of seronegative horses in the non-EPM population (i.e., 85 of 97 naturally infected horses) [178], which is not consistent with the seroprevalence of *S. neurona* in many parts of the United States [99–106] as well as Central and South America [107–110]. A sampling from most geographic regions where *S. neurona* is endemic will reveal numerous seropositive horses exhibiting signs of neurologic disease not due to EPM, and some of these horses will exhibit serum titers that are relatively high. As shown in subsequent studies examining sample sets that better represent the equine population in the Americas [197, 198], serum antibody titers against *S. neurona* are only weakly correlated with EPM and are not a good criterion for diagnosis.

In conclusion, accurate antemortem diagnosis of EPM can be achieved by careful neurologic examination to confirm CNS abnormalities, elimination of other neurologic diseases by radiography and CSF evaluation, and measurement of parasite-specific antibodies in serum and CSF to reveal intrathecal antibody production. The utility of the serum:CSF ratio, C-value, and antigen-specific AI was established using the SnSAG2, 4/3 ELISAs, but similar analyses will likely be valid with other serologic tests that can reliably quantify parasite-specific antibodies (including *N. hughesi*), such as the

IFAT [178]. However, titer results from different assays are not directly comparable, so the optimal ratio cutoff for each serologic test will need to be determined empirically.

Treatment

The use of antiprotozoal compounds is the cornerstone of treatment for EPM. Recognition of the etiologic role of protozoa in EPM led to the use of trimethoprim and sulfonamide compounds to treat horses [201]. The clinical results from many investigators were favorable and this class of drug was widely used in the treatment of EPM for many years. Various new compounds have been developed subsequently and are licensed for treatment of EPM in the United States. In addition to ponazuril, which was the first FDA-approved EPM medication, diclazuril and a sulfadiazine/pyrimethamine combination drug (ReBalance®) are currently approved for treatment of EPM.

A widely used and recommended drug for the treatment of EPM is ponazuril (Marquis®, Bayer Animal Health), dosed at 5 mg/kg per day for a minimum of 28 days. Ponazuril is a benzeneacetonitrile compound that is related to the herbicide atrazine and may act by inhibiting apicoplast and/or mitochondrial function in the parasite [202, 203]. Ponazuril is technically considered to be a coccidiostat based upon *in vitro* analysis [204]. The significance of this finding *in vivo*, however, is totally unknown, and is probably unimportant as efficacy studies between coccidiocidal and coccidiostatic drugs provide similar outcomes.

Ponazuril is well absorbed orally and achieves a steady state concentration of 0.16±0.06 mg/l in the CSF of horses treated with 5 mg/kg body weight [205]. *In vitro* studies have documented that concentrations of 0.1 μg/ml resulted in a 94.4% reduction in *S. neurona* production [206]. The time to reach steady state concentrations of ponazuril in the CSF of horses is approximately 1 week. For this reason, it has become commonplace to give an initial loading dose in an effort to achieve therapeutic concentrations more quickly. While the clinical value of this approach has not yet been demonstrated, maximum CSF concentrations of ponazuril were achieved within 28 h when horses were given a loading dose of 15 mg/kg body weight (3× the normal dosage) [207]. Additionally, feeding 2 ounces of corn oil immediately before administering ponazuril results in blood concentrations that are 25% higher than if no corn oil is given [208]. The author (MF) routinely recommends this approach.

A field efficacy study of 101 horses demonstrated approximately 60% efficacy, with 8% relapse within 90 days following the termination of treatment [177].

Animals typically responded within 10 days and often continued to improve even after treatment stopped at 28 days. The baseline neurologic score did not influence outcome in that study. However, success was defined as improvement by one clinical grade, which may be considered unacceptable in severe cases [177]. In clinical cases, the author routinely reevaluates the animal at the end of the treatment period and then makes a determination if further treatment is needed. In general, if there has been a clinical response, yet the horse remains abnormal, a second month of ponazuril is recommended. Extended dosing may reduce the occurrence of relapse, but this has not been empirically evaluated. If finances are limited, treatment can be stopped after 28 days, but the horse should be reexamined in one month to ensure that there is no deterioration.

Toxicity studies have found ponazuril to be very safe, with no systemic toxicity, even at high doses (30 mg/kg body weight) for up to 56 days [209]. Uterine edema was noted in mares given 30 mg/kg body weight each day for 30 days, however [209]. Treatment of breeding stallions with 10 mg/kg body weight did not affect androgenic hormone production nor spermatogenesis [210]. Ponazuril has been used without obvious problems in pregnant mares, but the use of ponazuril in pregnant animals is off-label and owners should be made aware of this fact (Table 22.2).

Diclazuril (Protazil®, Merck Animal Health) is chemically very similar to ponazuril. Diclazuril is administered at 1 mg/kg body weight as alfalfa-based pellets that are top dressed in the daily grain ration. In a study of 49 horses, diclazuril had a success rate of 58%, when success was defined as improvement by a minimum of one clinical grade [204]. Recent investigation of diclazuril pharmacokinetics has shown that a dose of 0.5 mg/kg body weight (50% of the recommended dose) is sufficient to attain concentrations in plasma and CSF that will inhibit *S. neurona* growth in culture (Dr. N. Pusterla, pers. commun.). Further study is needed, but these findings suggest that effective treatment of EPM may be possible with lower doses of diclazuril.

Historically, a combination of sulfonamide and pyrimethamine (S/P) has been used to treat EPM. This was based upon the effectiveness of this class of compounds against malaria and other protozoan infections [201]. This combination has been compounded, but recently a premixed version of this combination has achieved FDA approval and can be purchased (ReBalance, PRN Pharmacal). The sulfonamide component of this compound competes with para-aminobenzoic acid to inhibit dihydropteroate synthetase activity, while pyrimethamine targets dihydrofolate reductase, which collectively inhibits folate metabolism. The synergistic effects of these compounds block synthesis of nucleic acids and amino acids, ultimately leading to parasite death. A field efficacy study reported a success rate of 57% after several months of treatment [204]. Weaknesses of S/P suspension in the treatment of EPM include the prolonged duration of treatment required to affect a positive response and the toxicity of the compound. Toxicity includes anemia, fetal loss, and fetal abnormalities. A benefit of S/P combination is the lower cost, yet this may be offset by the extended dosing interval required.

Pyrimethamine has historically been given in combination with sulfa drugs in the treatment of EPM. There is, however, some evidence to suggest a synergistic effect of pyrimethamine when used with the triazine-group antiprotozoals. While not empirically evaluated in horses with EPM, it may be beneficial to add this drug to the treatment regimen in refractory cases, but the effectiveness of this approach is not known at this time.

The broad-spectrum antimicrobial nitazoxanide (NTZ) was approved for the treatment of EPM and marketed as Navigator® (Idexx Pharmaceuticals, Inc.). Although treatment with NTZ was effective against EPM, there were prominent concerns about adverse side effects (e.g., colic, diarrhea, and laminitis). Subsequently, NTZ has been removed from the market and is no longer available. Decoquinate is an anti-protozoal drug that has

Table 22.2 Comparative summary of clinical efficacy for various approved drugs for the treatment of EPM.

Drug	N1	N2	Duration (d)	Dose (mg/kg)	Days follow-up	Success %
Ponaz	53	47	28	5	90	60
Ponaz	60	55	28	10	90	58
S/P	48	26	90–270	20/1	various	61
DCZ	72	49	28	1	20	58

DCZ, diclazuril; N1, number enrolled; N2, number completed; Ponaz, ponazuril; S/P, sulfadiazine pyrimethamine combination.

been used to treat coccidiosis in poultry, cattle, sheep, and goats. Decoquinate in combination with the immunomodulator levamisole is currently being investigated for treatment of EPM; however, results are not available at the present time.

The duration of treatment for EPM is difficult to determine, and when to terminate treatment in any one particular horse remains problematic. Duration of treatment appears to be more important than peak concentrations (as long as they exceed minimum inhibitory concentrations). Hence, the author's approach is to evaluate horses after 1 month of treatment with ponazuril or diclazuril. If improvement has been noted, but clinical signs remain, then a further month of treatment is recommended. If finances are limiting, or the horse appears clinically normal, then treatment can be discontinued, but the horse should be examined 1 month after treatment is completed to ensure that there has been no relapse. Alternatively, a 1–2 month course of S/P can be given to help minimize the chance of recrudescence.

Treatment until the CSF WB becomes negative has been advocated by some clinicians in the past [211]. Experience has dictated that this is an unachievable goal for most cases. Antibodies can have a lengthy half-life, so horses will exhibit positive titers for long periods. Therefore, antibody-negative CSF is not recommended as a treatment goal.

Ancillary treatments may include various anti-inflammatory drugs such as phenylbutazone, flunixen meglumine, DMSO (IV or oral), or steroids. Corticosteroids can be used to help stabilize horses with serious neurologic abnormalities during the early period of treatment. Long-term steroids should be avoided due to their unknown effects upon immune clearance of the organism, however. It has been observed that some horses initially worsen slightly and transiently with treatment, and hence prophylactic use of NSAIDs to ameliorate this "treatment crisis" is sometimes advised. In the author's experience, this is rarely a problem, particularly in minimally affected horses. In seriously affected horses, prophylactic anti-inflammatory treatment is probably advisable for the first week. Additional ancillary treatments, such as vitamin E and homeopathic medications, have not been demonstrated to have any value, and use of these compounds or approaches is not recommended.

Immunostimulants have been recommended by some on the presumption that immunosuppression is a component of the pathophysiology of EPM. Levamisole (1 mg/kg PO daily), EqStim™ (5 ml IM on day 1, 3 and 7, then monthly), or Equimune IV™, (1.5 ml IV weekly for 3 weeks) have all been advocated; however, there is no specific information to suggest that these have any positive effect. One potential beneficial immune modulator, however, is parapox ovis virus immunomodulator (Zylexis™, Pfizer Animal Health). While licensed as an aid in the treatment of horses with EHV-1 and EHV-4, parapox ovis immunomodulator has been demonstrated to increase IFN-γ secretion in treated horses. As IFN-γ is considered a key cytokine in the treatment of EPM, this compound might have use in select animals.

Prognosis

Based upon clinical experience and reported efficacy studies, it appears that 60% of affected horses will improve by at least one neurologic grade after treatment. Up to 20% may recover completely, that is, return to neurologic normalcy. Prompt treatment of suspect and less severe cases are more likely to have the best outcome, and a success rate of up to 80% has been suggested for such cases [204].

Prevention

The prevention of EPM remains a poorly investigated area. Simple measures such as removing spilled grain, fallen fruit, and animal or bird feed which might attract the opossum definitive host to the horse's environment are probably useful. Grain stores should be secured such that opossums cannot gain access and contaminate feed. Removal of opossums in an effort to reduce pasture contamination is probably futile.

The use of pharmaceutical agents to prevent EPM has been demonstrated by continuous pretreatment with ponazuril in horses [212]. At 5 mg/kg body weight once daily, the incidence of clinical EPM was dramatically reduced following challenge with infective sporocysts. This treatment did not completely eliminate clinical disease, however. While effective, it is not likely to be cost-effective to maintain a horse on the drug continuously, but may be useful in particular situations in which the risk of contracting EPM is increased, such as associated with stressful events, showing, or shipping. Intermittent (weekly) dosing with ponazuril at 20 mg/kg body weight reduced CSF antibody development in challenged horses and may be a more cost-effective option than continuous treatment. Other pharmaceutical approaches, such as the use of pyrantel pamoate, have not proven effective and are not advised.

Protective immunization would be an ideal preventative against EPM. However, an effective EPM vaccine will likely prove difficult to achieve. There have been successes in developing effective vaccines against apicomplexan parasites; most notable perhaps are vaccines against *Eimeria* spp. that can reduce coccidiosis in poultry and other domestic animals. However, the etiology and pathogenesis of coccidiosis is comparatively simple relative to EPM. Moreover, the interplay between the equine immune system and *S. neurona* is highly complex and remains generally enigmatic. Therefore, continued basic research on the parasite and equine immunity is needed to devise logical approaches to developing a safe and effective EPM vaccine.

An EPM vaccine consisting of killed *S. neurona* merozoites combined with an adjuvant was previously given a conditional license for commercial use. However, this product has been withdrawn from the market due to the inability to demonstrate efficacy.

References

[1] Rooney, J.R., Prickett, M.E., Delaney, F.M. *et al.* (1969) Focal myelitis-encephalitis in horses. *Cornell Vet*, 60, 494–501.

[2] Beech, J. and Dodd, D.C. (1974) *Toxoplasma*-like encephalomyelitis in the horse. *Vet Pathol*, 11, 87–96.

[3] Dubey, J.P. (1976) A review of *Sarcocystis* of domestic animals and of other coccidia of cats and dogs. *J Am Vet Med Assoc*, 169, 1061–1078.

[4] Dubey, J.P., Davis, S.W., Speer, C.A. *et al.* (1991) *Sarcocystis neurona* n. sp. (Protozoa: Apicomplexa), the etiologic agent of equine protozoal myeloencephalitis. *J Parasitol*, 77, 212–218.

[5] Davis, S.W., Speer, C.A. and Dubey, J.P. (1991) In vitro cultivation of *Sarcocystis neurona* from the spinal cord of a horse with equine protozoal myelitis. *J Parasitol*, 77, 789–792.

[6] Davis, S.W., Daft, B.N. and Dubey, J.P. (1991) *Sarcocystis neurona* cultured in vitro from a horse with equine protozoal myelitis. *Equine Vet J*, 23, 315–317.

[7] Dubey, J.P., Mattson, D.E., Speer, C.A. *et al.* (1999) Characterization of a *Sarcocystis neurona* isolate (SN6) from a naturally infected horse from Oregon. *J Eukaryot Microbiol*, 46, 500–506.

[8] Dubey, J.P., Mattson, D.E., Speer, C.A. *et al.* (2001) Characteristics of a recent isolate of *Sarcocystis neurona* (SN7) from a horse and loss of pathogenicity of isolates SN6 and SN7 by passages in cell culture. *Vet Parasitol*, 95, 155–166.

[9] Granstrom, D.E., Alvarez, O., Jr, Dubey, J.P. *et al.* (1992) Equine protozoal myelitis in Panamanian horses and isolation of *Sarcocystis neurona*. *J Parasitol*, 78, 909–912.

[10] Granstrom, D.E., MacPherson, J.M., Gajadhar, A.A. *et al.* (1994) Differentiation of *Sarcocystis neurona* from eight related coccidia by random amplified polymorphic DNA assay. *Mol Cell Probes*, 8, 353–356.

[11] Mansfield, L.S., Schott, H.C., Murphy, A.J. *et al.* (2001) Comparison of *Sarcocystis neurona* isolates derived from horse neural tissue. *Vet Parasitol*, 95, 167–178.

[12] Marsh, A.E., Johnson, P.J., Ramos-Vara, J. *et al.* (2001) Characterization of a *Sarcocystis neurona* isolate from a Missouri horse with equine protozoal myeloencephalitis. *Vet Parasitol*, 95, 143–154.

[13] Marsh, A.E., Denver, M., Hill, F.I. *et al.* (2000) Detection of *Sarcocystis neurona* in the brain of a Grant's zebra (*Equus burchelli bohmi*). *J Zoo Wildl Med*, 31, 82–86.

[14] Dubey, J.P., Benson, J. and Larson, M.A. (2003) Clinical *Sarcocystis neurona* encephalomyelitis in a domestic cat following routine surgery. *Vet Parasitol*, 112, 261–267.

[15] Forest, T.W., Abou-Madi, N., Summers, B.A. *et al.* (2000) *Sarcocystis neurona*-like encephalitis in a Canada lynx (*Felis lynx canadensis*). *J Zoo Wildl Med*, 31, 383–387.

[16] Cooley, A.J., Barr, B. and Rejmanek, D. (2007) *Sarcocystis neurona* encephalitis in a dog. *Vet Pathol*, 44, 956–961.

[17] Dubey, J.P., Chapman, J.L., Rosenthal, B.M. *et al.* (2006) Clinical *Sarcocystis neurona*, *Sarcocystis canis*, *Toxoplasma gondii*, and *Neospora caninum* infections in dogs. *Vet Parasitol*, 137, 36–49.

[18] Vashisht, K., Lichtensteiger, C.A., Miller, L.A. *et al.* (2005) Naturally occurring *Sarcocystis neurona*-like infection in a dog with myositis. *Vet Parasitol*, 133, 19–25.

[19] Lindsay, D.S., Thomas, N.J. and Dubey, J.P. (2000) Biological characterisation of *Sarcocystis neurona* isolated from a Southern sea otter (*Enhydra lutris nereis*). *Int J Parasitol*, 30, 617–624.

[20] Dubey, J.R., Rosypal, A.C., Rosenthal, B.M. *et al.* (2001) *Sarcocystis neurona* infections in sea otter (*Enhydra lutris*): evidence for natural infections with sarcocysts and transmission of infection to opossums (*Didelphis virginiana*). *J Parasitol*, 87, 1387–1393.

[21] Mylniczenko, N.D., Kearns, K.S. and Melli, A.C. (2008) Diagnosis and treatment of *Sarcocystis neurona* in a captive harbor seal (*Phoca vitulina*). *J Zoo Wildl Med*, 39, 228–235.

[22] Dubey, J.R., Johnson, G.C., Bermudez, A. *et al.* (2001) Neural sarcocystosis in a straw-necked ibis (*Carphibis spinicollis*) associated with a *Sarcocystis neurona*-like organism and description of muscular sarcocysts of an unidentified *Sarcocystis* species. *J Parasitol*, 87, 1317–1322.

[23] Dubey, J.P., Hamir, A.N., Niezgoda, M. *et al.* (1996) A *Sarcocystis neurona*-like organism associated with encephalitis in a striped skunk (*Mephitis mephitis*). *J Parasitol*, 82, 172–174.

[24] Dubey, J.P. and Hedstrom, O.R. (1993) Meningoencephalitis in mink associated with a *Sarcocystis neurona*-like organism. *J Vet Diagn Invest*, 5, 467–471.

[25] Dubey, J.P. and Hamir, A.N. (2000) Immunohistochemical confirmation of *Sarcocystis neurona* infections in raccoons, mink, cat, skunk, and pony. *J Parasitol*, 86, 1150–1152.

[26] Gerhold, R.W., Howerth, E.W. and Lindsay, D.S. (2005) *Sarcocystis neurona*-associated meningoencephalitis and description of intramuscular sarcocysts in a fisher (*Martes pennanti*). *J Wildl Dis*, 41, 224–230.

[27] Britton, A.P., Dubey, J.P. and Rosenthal, B.M. (2010) Rhinitis and disseminated disease in a ferret (*Mustela putorius furo*) naturally infected with *Sarcocystis neurona*. *Vet Parasitol*, 169, 226–231.

[28] Cutler, T.J., MacKay, R.J., Ginn, P.E. *et al.* (2001) Immunoconversion against *Sarcocystis neurona* in normal and dexamethasone-treated horses challenged with *S. neurona* sporocysts. *Vet Parasitol,* 95, 197–210.

[29] Sofaly, C.D., Reed, S.M., Gordon, J.C. *et al.* (2002) Experimental induction of equine protozoan myeloencephalitis (EPM) in the horse: effect of *Sarcocystis neurona* sporocyst inoculation dose on the development of clinical neurologic disease. *J Parasitol,* 88, 1164–1170.

[30] Fenger, C.K., Granstrom, D.E., Gajadhar, A.A. *et al.* (1997) Experimental induction of equine protozoal myeloencephalitis in horses using *Sarcocystis* sp. sporocysts from the opossum (*Didelphis virginiana*). *Vet Parasitol,* 68, 199–213.

[31] Ellison, S.B., Greiner, E., Brown, K.K. *et al.* (2004) Experimental infection of horses with culture-derived *Sarcocystis neurona* merozoites as a model for equine protozoal myeloencephalitis. *Int J Appl Res Vet Med,* 2, 79–89.

[32] Marsh, A.E., Barr, B.C., Madigan, J. *et al.* (1996) Neosporosis as a cause of equine protozoal myeloencephalitis. *J Am Vet Med Assoc,* 209, 1907–1913.

[33] Hamir, A.N., Tornquist, S.J., Gerros, T.C. *et al.* (1998) *Neospora caninum*-associated equine protozoal myeloencephalitis. *Vet Parasitol,* 79, 269–274.

[34] Cheadle, M.A., Lindsay, D.S., Rowe, S. *et al.* (1999) Prevalence of antibodies to *Neospora* sp. in horses from Alabama and characterisation of an isolate recovered from a naturally infected horse. *Int J Parasitol,* 29, 1537–1543.

[35] Dubey, J.P., Liddell, S., Mattson, D. *et al.* (2001) Characterization of the Oregon isolate of *Neospora hughesi* from a horse. *J Parasitol,* 87, 345–353.

[36] Cusick, P.K., Sells, D.M., Hamilton, D.P. *et al.* (1974) Toxoplasmosis in two horses. *J Am Vet Med Assoc,* 164, 77–80.

[37] Dubey, J.P., Lindsay, D.S., Saville, W.J.A. *et al.* (2001) A review of *Sarcocystis neurona* and equine protozoal myeloencephalitis (EPM). *Vet Parasitol,* 95, 89–131.

[38] Simpson, C.F. and Mayhew, I.G. (1980) Evidence for *Sarcocystis* as the etiologic agent of equine protozoal myeloencephalitis. *J Protozool,* 27, 288–292.

[39] Levine, N.D. (1970) Taxonomy of the Sporozoa. *J Parasitol,* 56 (Suppl), 208–209.

[40] Levine, N.D. (1988) *The Protozoan Phylum Apicomplexa,* CRC Press, Boca Raton, FL.

[41] Blackman, M.J. and Bannister, L.H. (2001) Apical organelles of Apicomplexa: biology and isolation by subcellular fractionation. *Mol Biochem Parasitol,* 117, 11–25.

[42] Sam-Yellowe, T.Y. (1996) Rhoptry organelles of the apicomplexa: their role in host cell invasion and intracellular survival. *Parasitol Today,* 12, 308–316.

[43] Soldati, D., Dubremetz, J.F. and Lebrun, M. (2001) Microneme proteins: structural and functional requirements to promote adhesion and invasion by the apicomplexan parasite *Toxoplasma gondii*. *Int J Parasitol,* 31, 1293–1302.

[44] Tomley, F.M. and Soldati, D.S. (2001) Mix and match modules: structure and function of microneme proteins in apicomplexan parasites. *Trends Parasitol,* 17, 81–88.

[45] Morrissette, N.S. and Sibley, L.D. (2002) Cytoskeleton of apicomplexan parasites. *Microbiol Mol Biol Rev,* 66, 21–38 table of contents.

[46] Cesbron-Delauw, M.F. (1994) Dense granule organelles of *Toxoplasma gondii*: their role in the host–parasite relationship. *Parasitol Today,* 10, 293–296.

[47] Dobrowolski, J. and Sibley, L.D. (1997) The role of the cytoskeleton in host cell invasion by *Toxoplasma gondii*. *Behring Inst Mitt,* 99, 90–96.

[48] Dobrowolski, J.M., Carruthers, V.B. and Sibley, L.D. (1997) Participation of myosin in gliding motility and host cell invasion by *Toxoplasma gondii*. *Mol Microbiol,* 26, 163–173.

[49] Dobrowolski, J.M. and Sibley, L.D. (1996) *Toxoplasma* invasion of mammalian cells is powered by the actin cytoskeleton of the parasite. *Cell,* 84, 933–939.

[50] Meissner, M., Schluter, D. and Soldati, D. (2002) Role of *Toxoplasma gondii* myosin A in powering parasite gliding and host cell invasion. *Science,* 298, 837–840.

[51] Carruthers, V.B. (2002) Host cell invasion by the opportunistic pathogen *Toxoplasma gondii*. *Acta Trop,* 81, 111–122.

[52] Dubremetz, J.F., Garcia-Reguet, N., Conseil, V. *et al.* (1998) Apical organelles and host-cell invasion by Apicomplexa. *Int J Parasitol,* 28, 1007–1013.

[53] Dubremetz, J.F. and Schwartzman, J.D. (1993) Subcellular organelles of *Toxoplasma gondii* and host cell invasion. *Res Immunol,* 144, 31–33.

[54] Zhou, X.W., Kafsack, B.F., Cole, R.N. *et al.* (2005) The opportunistic pathogen *Toxoplasma gondii* deploys a diverse legion of invasion and survival proteins. *J Biol Chem,* 280, 34233–34244.

[55] Lekutis, C., Ferguson, D.J., Grigg, M.E. *et al.* (2001) Surface antigens of *Toxoplasma gondii*: variations on a theme. *Int J Parasitol,* 31, 1285–1292.

[56] Howe, D.K. and Sibley, L.D. (1999) Comparison of the major antigens of *Neospora caninum* and *Toxoplasma gondii*. *Int J Parasitol,* 29, 1489–1496.

[57] Marsh, A.E., Howe, D.K., Wang, G. *et al.* (1999) Differentiation of *Neospora hughesi* from *Neospora caninum* based on their immunodominant surface antigen, SAG1 and SRS2. *Int J Parasitol,* 29, 1575–1582.

[58] Cesbron-Delauw, M.F. (1995) The SAG2 antigen of *Toxoplasma gondii* and the 31-kDa surface antigen of *Sarcocystis muris* share similar sequence features. *Parasitol Res,* 81, 444–445.

[59] Eschenbacher, K.H., Sommer, I., Meyer, H.E. *et al.* (1992) Cloning and expression in *Escherichia coli* of cDNAs encoding a 31-kilodalton surface antigen of *Sarcocystis muris*. *Mol Biochem Parasitol,* 53, 159–167.

[60] Ellison, S.P., Omara-Opyene, A.L., Yowell, C.A. *et al.* (2002) Molecular characterisation of a major 29 kDa surface antigen of *Sarcocystis neurona*. *Int J Parasitol,* 32, 217–225.

[61] Howe, D.K., Gaji, R.Y., Mroz-Barrett, M. *et al.* (2005) *Sarcocystis neurona* merozoites express a family of immunogenic surface antigens that are orthologues of the *Toxoplasma gondii* surface antigens (SAGs) and SAG-related sequences. *Infect Immun*, 73, 1023–1033.

[62] Zhu, G., Marchewka, M.J. and Keithly, J.S. (2000) *Cryptosporidium parvum* appears to lack a plastid genome. *Microbiology*, 146 (Pt 2), 315–321.

[63] McFadden, G.I., Reith, M.E., Munholland, J. *et al.* (1996) Plastid in human parasites. *Nature*, 381, 482.

[64] Kohler, S., Delwiche, C.F., Denny, P.W. *et al.* (1997) A plastid of probable green algal origin in Apicomplexan parasites. *Science*, 275, 1485–1489.

[65] Lang-Unnasch, N., Reith, M.E., Munholland, J. *et al.* (1998) Plastids are widespread and ancient in parasites of the phylum Apicomplexa. *J Parasitol*, 28, 1743–1754.

[66] Fast, N.M., Kissinger, J.C., Roos, D.S. *et al.* (2001) Nuclear-encoded, plastid-targeted genes suggest a single common origin for apicomplexan and dinoflagellate plastids. *Mol Biol Evol*, 18, 418–426.

[67] Fichera, M.E. and Roos, D.S. (1997) A plastid organelle as a drug target in apicomplexan parasites. *Nature*, 390, 407–409.

[68] Vollmer, M., Thomsen, N., Wiek, S. *et al.* (2001) Apicomplexan parasites possess distinct nuclear-encoded, but apicoplast- localized, plant-type ferredoxin-NADP+ reductase and ferredoxin. *J Biol Chem*, 276, 5483–5490.

[69] Ralph, S.A., van Dooren, G.G., Waller, R.F. *et al.* (2004) Tropical infectious diseases: metabolic maps and functions of the *Plasmodium falciparum* apicoplast. *Nat Rev Microbiol*, 2, 203–216.

[70] Gornicki, P. (2003) Apicoplast fatty acid biosynthesis as a target for medical intervention in apicomplexan parasites. *Int J Parasitol*, 33, 885–896.

[71] Fenger, C.K., Granstrom, D.E., Langemeier, J.L. *et al.* (1995) Identification of opossums (*Didelphis virginiana*) as the putative definitive host of *Sarcocystis neurona*. *J Parasitol*, 81, 916–919.

[72] Dubey, J.P., Lindsay, D.S., Kerber, C.E. *et al.* (2001) First isolation of *Sarcocystis neurona* from the South American opossum, *Didelphis albiventris*, from Brazil. *Vet Parasitol*, 95, 295–304.

[73] Hammond, D.M. and Long, P.L. (1973) *The Coccidia – Eimeria, Isospora, Toxoplasma, and Related Genera*, University Park Press, Baltimore, MD.

[74] Levine, N.D. (1985) *Veterinary Protozoology*, Iowa State University Press, Ames, IA.

[75] Cheadle, M.A., Yowell, C.A., Sellon, D.C. *et al.* (2001) The striped skunk (*Mephitis mephitis*) is an intermediate host for *Sarcocystis neurona*. *Int J Parasitol*, 31, 843–849.

[76] Dubey, J.P., Saville, W.J., Stanek, J.F. *et al.* (2001) *Sarcocystis neurona* infections in raccoons (*Procyon lotor*): evidence for natural infection with sarcocysts, transmission of infection to opossums (*Didelphis virginiana*), and experimental induction of neurologic disease in raccoons. *Vet Parasitol*, 100, 117–129.

[77] Cheadle, M.A., Tanhauser, S.M., Dame, J.B. *et al.* (2001) The nine-banded armadillo (*Dasypus novemcinctus*) is an intermediate host for *Sarcocystis neurona*. *Int J Parasitol*, 31, 330–335.

[78] Dubey, J.P., Saville, W.J., Lindsay, D.S. *et al.* (2000) Completion of the life cycle of *Sarcocystis neurona*. *J Parasitol*, 86, 1276–1280.

[79] Dubey, J.P. (2000) Prevalence of *Sarcocystis* species sporocysts in wild-caught opossums (*Didelphis virginiana*). *J Parasitol*, 86, 705–710.

[80] Dubey, J.P., Black, S.S., Rickard, L.G. *et al.* (2001) Prevalence of *Sarcocystis neurona* sporocysts in opossums (*Didelphis virginiana*) from rural Mississippi. *Vet Parasitol*, 95, 283–293.

[81] Elsheikha, H.M., Murphy, A.J. and Mansfield, L.S. (2004) Prevalence of *Sarcocystis* species sporocysts in Northern Virginia opossums (*Didelphis virginiana*). *Parasitol Res*, 93, 427–431.

[82] Mullaney, T., Murphy, A.J., Kiupel, M. *et al.* (2005) Evidence to support horses as natural intermediate hosts for *Sarcocystis neurona*. *Vet Parasitol*, 133, 27–36.

[83] Dubey, J.P. and Lindsay, D.S. (1999) *Sarcocystis speeri* N. sp. (Protozoa: Sarcocystidae) from the opossum (*Didelphis virginiana*). *J Parasitol*, 85, 903–909.

[84] Dubey, J.P., Rosenthal, B.M. and Speer, C.A. (2001) *Sarcocystis lindsayi* n. sp. (Protozoa: Sarcocystidae) from the South American opossum, *Didelphis albiventris* from Brazil. *J Eukaryot Microbiol*, 48, 595–603.

[85] Dame, J.B., MacKay, R.J., Yowell, C.A. *et al.* (1995) *Sarcocystis falcatula* from passerine and psittacine birds: synonymy with *Sarcocystis neurona*, agent of equine protozoal myeloencephalitis. *J Parasitol*, 81, 930–935.

[86] Cutler, T.J., MacKay, R.J., Ginn, P.E. *et al.* (1999) Are *Sarcocystis neurona* and *Sarcocystis falcatula* synonymous? A horse infection challenge. *J Parasitol*, 85, 301–305.

[87] Dubey, J.P. and Lindsay, D.S. (1998) Isolation in immunodeficient mice of *Sarcocystis neurona* from opossum (*Didelphis virginiana*) faeces, and its differentiation from *Sarcocystis falcatula*. *Int J Parasitol*, 28, 1823–1828.

[88] Marsh, A.E., Barr, B.C., Tell, L. *et al.* (1999) Comparison of the internal transcribed spacer, ITS-1, from *Sarcocystis falcatula* isolates and *Sarcocystis neurona*. *J Parasitol*, 85, 750–757.

[89] Tanhauser, S.M., Yowell, C.A., Cutler, T.J. *et al.* (1999) Multiple DNA markers differentiate *Sarcocystis neurona* and *Sarcocystis falcatula*. *J Parasitol*, 85, 221–228.

[90] Mansfield, L.S., Mehler, S., Nelson, K. *et al.* (2008) Brown-headed cowbirds (*Molothrus ater*) harbor *Sarcocystis neurona* and act as intermediate hosts. *Vet Parasitol*, 153, 24–43.

[91] Dubey, J.P., Jenkins, M.C., Rajendran, C. *et al.* (2011) Gray wolf (*Canis lupus*) is a natural definitive host for *Neospora caninum*. *Vet Parasitol*, 181, 382–387.

[92] Gondim, L.F., McAllister, M.M., Pitt, W.C. *et al.* (2004) Coyotes (*Canis latrans*) are definitive hosts of *Neospora caninum*. *Int J Parasitol*, 34, 159–161.

[93] McAllister, M.M., Dubey, J.P., Lindsay, D.S. *et al.* (1998) Dogs are definitive hosts of *Neospora caninum*. *Int J Parasitol*, 28, 1473–1478.

[94] Dubey, J.P., Schares, G. and Ortega-Mora, L.M. (2007) Epidemiology and control of neosporosis and *Neospora caninum*. *Clin Microbiol Rev*, 20, 323–367.

[95] Antonello, A.M., Pivoto, F.L., Camillo, G. *et al.* (2012) The importance of vertical transmission of *Neospora* sp. in naturally infected horses. *Vet Parasitol*, 187, 367–370.

[96] Pusterla, N., Conrad, P.A., Packham, A.E. *et al.* (2011) Endogenous transplacental transmission of *Neospora hughesi* in naturally infected horses. *J Parasitol*, 97, 281–285.

[97] Pitel, P.H., Pronost, S., Gargala, G. *et al.* (2002) Detection of *Sarcocystis neurona* antibodies in French horses with neurological signs. *Int J Parasitol*, 32, 481–485.

[98] Arias, M., Yeargan, M., Francisco, I. *et al.* (2012) Exposure to *Sarcocystis* spp. in horses from Spain determined by western blot analysis using *Sarcocystis neurona* merozoites as heterologous antigen. *Vet Parasitol*, 185, 301–304.

[99] Bentz, B.G., Granstrom, D.E. and Stamper, S. (1997) Seroprevalence of antibodies to *Sarcocystis neurona* in horses residing in a county of southeastern Pennsylvania. *J Am Vet Med Assoc*, 210, 517–518.

[100] Bentz, B.G., Ealey, K.A., Morrow, J. *et al.* (2003) Seroprevalence of antibodies to *Sarcocystis neurona* in equids residing in Oklahoma. *J Vet Diagn Invest*, 15, 597–600.

[101] Blythe, L.L., Granstrom, D.E., Hansen, D.E. *et al.* (1997) Seroprevalence of antibodies to *Sarcocystis neurona* in horses residing in Oregon. *J Am Vet Med Assoc*, 210, 525–527.

[102] Dubey, J.P., Mitchell, S.M., Morrow, J.K. *et al.* (2003) Prevalence of antibodies to *Neospora caninum*, *Sarcocystis neurona*, and *Toxoplasma gondii* in wild horses from central Wyoming. *J Parasitol*, 89, 716–720.

[103] Rossano, M.G., Kaneene, J.B., Marteniuk, J.V. *et al.* (2001) The seroprevalence of antibodies to *Sarcocystis neurona* in Michigan equids. *Prev Vet Med*, 48, 113–128.

[104] Saville, W.J., Reed, S.M., Granstrom, D.E. *et al.* (1997) Seroprevalence of antibodies to *Sarcocystis neurona* in horses residing in Ohio. *J Am Vet Med Assoc*, 210, 519–524.

[105] Tillotson, K., McCue, P.M., Granstrom, D.E. *et al.* (1999) Seroprevalence of antibodies to *Sarcocystis neurona* in horses residing in northern Colorado. *J Equine Vet Sci*, 19, 122–126.

[106] Vardeleon, D., Marsh, A.E., Thorne, J.G. *et al.* (2001) Prevalence of *Neospora hughesi* and *Sarcocystis neurona* antibodies in horses from various geographical locations. *Vet Parasitol*, 95, 273–282.

[107] Dubey, J.P., Kerber, C.E. and Granstrom, D.E. (1999) Serologic prevalence of *Sarcocystis neurona*, *Toxoplasma gondii*, and *Neospora caninum* in horses in Brazil. *J Am Vet Med Assoc*, 215, 970–972.

[108] Hoane, J.S., Gennari, S.M., Dubey, J.P. *et al.* (2006) Prevalence of *Sarcocystis neurona* and *Neospora* spp. infection in horses from Brazil based on presence of serum antibodies to parasite surface antigen. *Vet Parasitol*, 136, 155–159.

[109] Dangoudoubiyam, S., Oliveira, J.B., Viquez, C. *et al.* (2011) Detection of antibodies against *Sarcocystis neurona*, *Neospora* spp., and *Toxoplasma gondii* in horses from Costa Rica. *J Parasitol*, 97, 522–524.

[110] Dubey, J.P., Venturini, M.C., Venturini, L. *et al.* (1999) Prevalence of antibodies to *Sarcocystis neurona*, *Toxoplasma gondii* and *Neospora caninum* in horses from Argentina. *Vet Parasitol*, 86, 59–62.

[111] Bartova, E., Sedlak, K., Syrova, M. *et al.* (2010) *Neospora* spp. and *Toxoplasma gondii* antibodies in horses in the Czech Republic. *Parasitol Res*, 107, 783–785.

[112] Pitel, P.H., Pronost, S., Romand, S. *et al.* (2001) Prevalence of antibodies to *Neospora caninum* in horses in France. *Equine Vet J*, 33, 205–207.

[113] Villalobos, E.M., Furman, K.E., Lara Mdo, C. *et al.* (2012) Detection of *Neospora* sp. antibodies in cart horses from urban areas of Curitiba, Southern Brazil. *Brazilian J Vet Parasitol*, 21, 68–70.

[114] Gupta, G.D., Lakritz, J., Kim, J.H. *et al.* (2002) Seroprevalence of *Neospora*, *Toxoplasma gondii* and *Sarcocystis neurona* antibodies in horses from Jeju island, South Korea. *Vet Parasitol*, 106, 193–201.

[115] Hoane, J.S., Yeargan, M.R., Stamper, S. *et al.* (2005) Recombinant NhSAG1 ELISA: a sensitive and specific assay for detecting antibodies against *Neospora hughesi* in equine serum. *J Parasitol*, 91, 446–452.

[116] Boy, M.G., Galligan, D.T. and Divers, T.J. (1990) Protozoal encephalomyelitis in horses: 82 cases (1972–1986). *J Am Vet Med Assoc*, 196, 632–634.

[117] Mayhew, I.G., De Lahunta, A., Whitlock, R.H. *et al.* (1977) Equine protozoal myeloencephalitis. *Proc Ann Conven Amer Assoc Equine Pract*, 22, 107–114.

[118] Gray, L.C., Magdesian, K.G., Sturges, B.K. *et al.* (2001) Suspected protozoal myeloencephalitis in a two-month-old colt. *Vet Rec*, 149, 269–273.

[119] MacKay, R.J., Davis, S.W. and Dubey, J.P. (1992) Equine protozoal myeloencephalitis. *Comp Cont Ed Pract Vet*, 14, 1359–1367.

[120] Fayer, R., Mayhew, I.G., Baird, J.D. *et al.* (1990) Epidemiology of equine protozoal myeloencephalitis in North America based on histologically confirmed cases. *J Vet Intern Med*, 4, 54–57.

[121] NAHMS. *Equine Protozoal Myeloencephalitis (EPM) in the U.S.* In: USDA:APHIS:VS, ed. Fort Collins, CO: Centers for Epidemiology and Animal Health; 2001.

[122] Asmundsson, I.M., Dubey, J.P. and Rosenthal, B.M. (2006) A genetically diverse but distinct North American population of *Sarcocystis neurona* includes an overrepresented clone described by 12 microsatellite alleles. *Infect Genet Evol*, 6, 352–360.

[123] Elsheikha, H.M., Schott, H.C., 2nd and Mansfield, L.S. (2006) Genetic variation among isolates of *Sarcocystis neurona*, the agent of protozoal myeloencephalitis, as revealed by amplified fragment length polymorphism markers. *Infect Immun*, 74, 3448–3454.

[124] Rejmanek, D., Miller, M.A., Grigg, M.E. *et al.* (2010) Molecular characterization of *Sarcocystis neurona* strains from opossums (*Didelphis virginiana*) and intermediate hosts from Central California. *Vet Parasitol*, 170, 20–29.

[125] Sundar, N., Asmundsson, I.M., Thomas, N.J. *et al.* (2008) Modest genetic differentiation among North American populations of *Sarcocystis neurona* may reflect expansion in its geographic range. *Vet Parasitol*, 152, 8–15.

[126] Wendte, J.M., Miller, M.A., Nandra, A.K. *et al.* (2010) Limited genetic diversity among *Sarcocystis neurona* strains infecting southern sea otters precludes distinction between marine and terrestrial isolates. *Vet Parasitol*, 169, 37–44.

[127] Crowdus, C.A., Marsh, A.E., Saville, W.J. *et al.* (2008) SnSAG5 is an alternative surface antigen of *Sarcocystis neurona* strains that is mutually exclusive to SnSAG1. *Vet Parasitol*, 158, 36–43.

[128] Howe, D.K., Gaji, R.Y., Marsh, A.E. *et al.* (2008) Strains of *Sarcocystis neurona* exhibit differences in their surface antigens, including the absence of the major surface antigen SnSAG1. *Int J Parasitol*, 38, 623–631.

[129] Saville, W.J., Morley, P.S., Reed, S.M. *et al.* (2000) Evaluation of risk factors associated with clinical improvement and survival of horses with equine protozoal myeloencephalitis. *J Am Vet Med Assoc*, 217, 1181–1185.

[130] Saville, W.J., Stich, R.W., Reed, S.M. *et al.* (2001) Utilization of stress in the development of an equine model for equine protozoal myeloencephalitis. *Vet Parasitol*, 95, 211–222.

[131] Saville, W.J., Sofaly, C.D., Reed, S.M. *et al.* (2004) An equine protozoal myeloencephalitis challenge model testing a second transport after inoculation with *Sarcocystis neurona* sporocysts. *J Parasitol*, 90, 1406–1410.

[132] Mayhew, I.G. and Delahunta, A. (1978) Neuropathology. *Cornell Vet*, 68, 106–147.

[133] Dubey, J.P. (2001) Migration and development of *Sarcocystis neurona* in tissues of interferon gamma knockout mice fed sporocysts from a naturally infected opossum. *Vet Parasitol*, 95, 341–351.

[134] Elitsur, E., Marsh, A.E., Reed, S.M. *et al.* (2007) Early migration of *Sarcocystis neurona* in ponies fed sporocysts. *J Parasitol*, 93, 1222–1225.

[135] Sellon, D.C., Knowles, D.P., Greiner, E.C. *et al.* (2004) Depletion of natural killer cells does not result in neurologic disease due to *Sarcocystis neurona* in mice with severe combined immunodeficiency. *J Parasitol*, 90, 782–788.

[136] Lindsay, D.S., Mitchell, S.M., Yang, J. *et al.* (2006) Penetration of equine leukocytes by merozoites of *Sarcocystis neurona*. *Vet Parasitol*, 138, 371–376.

[137] Witonsky, S.G., Gogal, R.M., Jr, Duncan, R.B. *et al.* (2003) Protective immune response to experimental infection with *Sarcocystis neurona* in 57BL/6 mice. *J Parasitol*, 89, 924–931.

[138] Tzipori, S., Robertson, D., Cooper, D. *et al.* (1987) Chronic cryptosporidiosis and hyperimmune bovine colostrum. *Lancet*, ii, 344–345.

[139] Doyle, P.S., Crabb, J. and Peterson, C. (1993) Anti-*Cryptosporidium parvum* antibodies inhibit infectivity in vitro and in vivo. *Infect Immun*, 61, 4079–4084.

[140] Grimwood, J. and Smith, J.E. (1992) *Toxoplasma gondii*: the role of a 30-kDa surface protein in host cell invasion. *Exp Parasitol*, 74, 106–111.

[141] Grimwood, J. and Smith, J.E. (1996) *Toxoplasma gondii*: the role of parasite surface and secreted proteins in host cell invasion. *Int J Parasitol*, 26, 169–173.

[142] Hemphill, A. (1996) Subcellular localization and functional characterization of Nc-p43, a major *Neospora caninum* tachyzoite surface protein. *Infect Immun*, 64, 4279–4287.

[143] Mineo, J.R., McLeod, R., Mack, D. *et al.* (1993) Antibodies to *Toxoplasma gondii* major surface protein (SAG-1, P30) inhibit infection of host cells and are produced in murine intestine after peroral infection. *J Immunol*, 150, 3951–3964.

[144] Mineo, J.R. and Kasper, L.H. (1994) Attachment of *Toxoplasma gondii* to host cells involves major surface protein SAG-1 (P30). *Exp Parasitol*, 79, 11–20.

[145] Liang, F.T., Granstrom, D.E., Zhao, X.M. *et al.* (1998) Evidence that surface proteins Sn14 and Sn16 of *Sarcocystis neurona* merozoites are involved in infection and immunity. *Infect Immun*, 66, 1834–1838.

[146] Ellison, S. and Witonsky, S. (2009) Evidence that antibodies against recombinant SnSAG1 of *Sarcocystis neurona* merozoites are involved in infection and immunity in equine protozoal myeloencephalitis. *Can J Vet Res*, 73, 176–183.

[147] Hoane, J.S., Morrow, J., Saville, W.J. *et al.* (2005) Enzyme-linked immunosorbent assays for detection of equine antibodies specific to *Sarcocystis neurona* surface antigens. *Clin Diagn Lab Immunol*, 12, 1050–1056.

[148] Tornquist, S.J., Boeder, L.J., Mattson, D.E. *et al.* (2001) Lymphocyte responses and immunophenotypes in horses with *Sarcocystis neurona* infection. *Equine Vet J*, 33, 726–729.

[149] Furr, M., Pontzer, C. and Gasper, P. (2001) Lymphocyte phenotype subsets in the cerebrospinal fluid of normal horses and horses with equine protozoal myeloencephalitis. *Vet Ther*, 2, 317–324.

[150] Scott, P.R., Witonsky, S., Robertson, J. *et al.* (2005) Increased presence of T lymphocytes in central nervous system of EPM affected horses. *J Parasitol*, 91, 1499–1502.

[151] Witonsky, S.G., Gogal, R.M., Jr, Duncan, R.B., Jr *et al.* (2005) Prevention of meningo/encephalomyelitis due to *Sarcocystis neurona* infection in mice is mediated by CD8 cells. *Int J Parasitol*, 35, 113–123.

[152] Suzuki, Y., Orrelman, M., Schreiber, R. *et al.* (1988) Interferon-gamma: the major mediator of resistance against *Toxoplasma gondii*. *Science*, 240, 516–518.

[153] Denkers, E.Y., Gazzinelli, R.T., Martin, D. *et al.* (1993) Emergence of NK1.1+ cells as effectors of IFN-gamma dependent immunity to *Toxoplasma gondii* in MHC class I-deficient mice. *J Exp Med*, 178, 1465–1472.

[154] Dawson, V.L. and Dawson, T.M. (1996) Nitric oxide actions in neurochemistry. *Neurochem Int*, 29, 97–110.

[155] Stich, R.W., Shoda, L., Dreewes, M. *et al.* (1998) Stimulation of nitric oxide production in macrophages by *Babesia bovis*. *Infect Immun*, 66, 4130–4136.

[156] Metz, G., Carlier, Y. and Vray, B. (1993) *Trypanosoma cruzi* upregulates nitric oxide release by IFN-gamma-preactived macrophages, limiting cell infection independently of the respiratory burst. *Parasite Immunol*, 15, 693–699.

[157] Shoda, L., Kegerreis, K., Suarez, E. *et al.* (2001) DNA from protozoan parasites *Babesia bovis*, *Trypanosoma cruzi*, and *T. Brucei* is mitogenic for B lymphocytes and stimulates macrophage expression of interleukin-12, tumor necrosis factor alpha, and nitric oxide. *Infect Immun*, 69, 2162–2171.

[158] Njoku, C.J., Saville, W.J., Reed, S.M. *et al.* (2002) Reduced levels of nitric oxide metabolites in cerebrospinal fluid are associated with equine protozoal myeloencephalitis. *Clin Diagn Lab Immunol*, 9, 605–610.

[159] Rosypal, A.C., Lindsay, D.S., Duncan, R., Jr *et al.* (2002) Mice lacking the gene for inducible or endothelial nitric oxide are resistant to sporocyst induced *Sarcocystis neurona* infections. *Vet Parasitol*, 103, 315–321.

[160] Spencer, J.A., Ellison, S.E., Guarino, A.J. *et al.* (2004) Cell-mediated immune responses in horses with equine protozoal myeloencephalitis. *J Parasitol*, 90, 428–430.

[161] Witonsky, S., Ellison, S., Yang, J. *et al.* (2008) Horses experimentally infected with *Sarcocystis neurona* develop altered immune responses in vitro. *J Parasitol*, 94, 1047–1054.

[162] Cserr, H.F. and Knopf, P.M. (1992) Cervical lymphatics, the blood-brain barrier and the immunoreactivity of the brain: a new view. *Immunol Today*, 13, 507–512.

[163] Taylor, A. and Streilein, J. (1996) Inhibition of antigen stimulated effector T cells by human cerebrospinal fluid. *Neuroimmunomodulation*, 3, 112–118.

[164] Taylor, A.W. (1996) Neuroimmunomodulation in immune privilege: role of neuropeptides in ocular immunosuppression. *Neuroimmunomodulation*, 3, 195–204.

[165] Wilbanks, G. and Streilein, J. (1992) Fluids from immune privileged sites endow macrophages with the capacity to induce antigen-specific immune deviation via a mechanism involving transforming growth factor-b. *Eur J Immunol*, 22, 1031–1036.

[166] Silva, J.C., Twardzik, D. and Reed, S. (1991) Regulation of *Trypanosoma cruzi* infection *in vitro* and *in vivo* by transforming growth factor b (TGF-b). *J Exp Med*, 174, 539–545.

[167] Letterio, J. and Roberts, A. (1997) TGF-b; a critical modulator of immune cell function. *Clin Immunol Immunopathol*, 84, 244–250.

[168] Furr, M. and Pontzer, C. (2001) Transforming growth factor beta concentrations and interferon gamma responses in cerebrospinal fluid of horses with equine protozoal myeloencephalitis. *Equine Vet J*, 33, 721–725.

[169] Furr, M., MacKay, R., Granstrom, D. *et al.* (2002) Clinical diagnosis of equine protozoal myeloencephalitis (EPM). *J Vet Intern Med*, 16, 618–621.

[170] Lindsay, D.S., Thomas, N.J., Rosypal, A.C. *et al.* (2001) Dual *Sarcocystis neurona* and *Toxoplasma gondii* infection in a Northern sea otter from Washington state, USA. *Vet Parasitol*, 97, 319–327.

[171] Furr, M.O. and Tyler, R.D. (1990) Cerebrospinal fluid creatine kinase activity in horses with central nervous system disease: 69 cases (1984–1989). *J Am Vet Med Assoc*, 197, 245–248.

[172] Jackson, C., DeLahunta, A., Divers, T.J. *et al.* (1996) The diagnostic utility of cerebrospinal fluid creatine kinase activity in the horse. *J Vet Intern Med*, 10, 246–251.

[173] Furr, M. (2002) Antigen-specific antibodies in cerebrospinal fluid after intramuscular injection of ovalbumin in horses. *J Vet Intern Med*, 16, 588–592.

[174] Granstrom, D.E., Dubey, J.P., Davis, S.W. *et al.* (1993) Equine protozoal myeloencephalitis: antigen analysis of cultured *Sarcocystis neurona* merozoites. *J Vet Diagn Invest*, 5, 88–90.

[175] Rossano, M.G., Mansfield, L.S., Kaneene, J.B. *et al.* (2000) Improvement of western blot test specificity for detecting equine serum antibodies to *Sarcocystis neurona*. *J Vet Diagn Invest*, 12, 28–32.

[176] Duarte, P.C., Daft, B.M., Conrad, P.A. *et al.* (2003) Comparison of a serum indirect fluorescent antibody test with two Western blot tests for the diagnosis of equine protozoal myeloencephalitis. *J Vet Diagn Invest*, 15, 8–13.

[177] Furr, M., Kennedy, T., MacKay, R. *et al.* (2001) Efficacy of ponazuril 15% oral paste as a treatment for equine protozoal myeloencephalitis. *Vet Ther*, 2, 215–222.

[178] Duarte, P.C., Daft, B.M., Conrad, P.A. *et al.* (2004) Evaluation and comparison of an indirect fluorescent antibody test for detection of antibodies to *Sarcocystis neurona*, using serum and cerebrospinal fluid of naturally and experimentally infected, and vaccinated horses. *J Parasitol*, 90, 379–386.

[179] Jordan, C.N., Kaur, T., Koenen, K. *et al.* (2005) Prevalence of agglutinating antibodies to *Toxoplasma gondii* and *Sarcocystis neurona* in beavers (*Castor canadensis*) from Massachusetts. *J Parasitol*, 91, 1228–1229.

[180] Lindsay, D.S., Rosypal, A.C., Spencer, J.A. *et al.* (2001) Prevalence of agglutinating antibodies to *Sarcocystis neurona* in raccoons, *Procyon lotor*, from the United States. *Vet Parasitol*, 100, 131–134.

[181] Mitchell, S.M., Richardson, D.J., Cheadle, M.A. *et al.* (2002) Prevalence of agglutinating antibodies to

Sarcocystis neurona in skunks (*Mephitis Mephitis*), raccoons (*Procyon lotor*), and opossums (*Didelphis Virginiana*) from Connecticut. *J Parasitol*, 88, 1027–1029.

[182] Stanek, J.F., Stich, R.W., Dubey, J.P. *et al.* (2003) Epidemiology of *Sarcocystis neurona* infections in domestic cats (*Felis domesticus*) and its association with equine protozoal myeloencephalitis (EPM) case farms and feral cats from a mobile spay and neuter clinic. *Vet Parasitol*, 117, 239–249.

[183] Yabsley, M.J., Jordan, C.N., Mitchell, S.M. *et al.* (2007) Seroprevalence of *Toxoplasma gondii*, *Sarcocystis neurona*, and *Encephalitozoon cuniculi* in three species of lemurs from St. Catherines Island, GA, USA. *Vet Parasitol*, 144, 28–32.

[184] Saville, W.J., Dubey, J.P., Oglesbee, M.J. *et al.* (2004) Experimental infection of ponies with *Sarcocystis fayeri* and differentiation from *Sarcocystis neurona* infections in horses. *J Parasitol*, 90, 1487–1491.

[185] Ellison, S.P., Kennedy, T. and Brown, K.K. (2003) Development of an ELISA to detect antibodies to rSAG1 in the horse. *J Appl Res Vet Med*, 1, 318–327.

[186] Yeargan, M.R. and Howe, D.K. (2011) Improved detection of equine antibodies against *Sarcocystis neurona* using polyvalent ELISAs based on the parasite SnSAG surface antigens. *Vet Parasitol*, 176, 16–22.

[187] Hyun, C., Gupta, G.D. and Marsh, A.E. (2003) Sequence comparison of *Sarcocystis neurona* surface antigen from multiple isolates. *Vet Parasitol*, 112, 11–20.

[188] Johnson, A.L., Burton, A.J. and Sweeney, R.W. (2010) Utility of 2 immunological tests for antemortem diagnosis of equine protozoal myeloencephalitis (*Sarcocystis neurona* infection) in naturally occurring cases. *J Vet Intern Med*, 24, 1184–1189.

[189] Packham, A.E., Conrad, P.A., Wilson, W.D. *et al.* (2002) Qualitative evaluation of selective tests for detection of *Neospora hughesi* antibodies in serum and cerebrospinal fluid of experimentally infected horses. *J Parasitol*, 88, 1239–1246.

[190] Tumani, H., Nolker, G. and Reiber, H. (1995) Relevance of cerebrospinal fluid variables for early diagnosis of neuroborreliosis. *Neurology*, 45, 1663–1670.

[191] Dorta-Contreras, A.J. and Reiber, H. (1998) Intrathecal synthesis of immunoglobulins in eosinophilic meningoencephalitis due to *Angiostrongylus cantonensis*. *Clin Diagn Lab Immunol*, 5, 452–455.

[192] Lejon, V., Reiber, H., Legros, D. *et al.* (2003) Intrathecal immune response pattern for improved diagnosis of central nervous system involvement in trypanosomiasis. *J Inf Dis*, 187, 1475–1483.

[193] Contini, C., Fainardi, E., Cultrera, R. *et al.* (1998) Advanced laboratory techniques for diagnosing *Toxoplasma gondii* encephalitis in AIDS patients: significance of intrathecal production and comparison with PCR and ECL-western blotting. *J Neuroimmunol*, 92, 29–37.

[194] Potasman, I., Resnick, L., Luft, B.J. *et al.* (1988) Intrathecal production of antibodies against *Toxoplasma gondii* in patients with toxoplasmic encephalitis and the acquired immunodeficiency syndrome (AIDS). *Ann Intern Med*, 108, 49–51.

[195] Furr, M., Howe, D., Reed, S. *et al.* (2011) Antibody coefficients for the diagnosis of equine protozoal myeloencephalitis. *J Vet Intern Med*, 25, 138–142.

[196] Finno, C.J., Packham, A.E., David Wilson, W. *et al.* (2007) Effects of blood contamination of cerebrospinal fluid on results of indirect fluorescent antibody tests for detection of antibodies against *Sarcocystis neurona* and *Neospora hughesi*. *J Vet Diagn Invest*, 19, 286–289.

[197] Johnson, A.L., Morrow, J.K. and Sweeney, R.W. (2013) Indirect fluorescent antibody test and surface antigen ELISAs for antemortem diagnosis of equine protozoal myeloencephalitis. *J Vet Intern Med*, 27, 596–599.

[198] Reed, S.M., Howe, D.K., Morrow, J.K. *et al.* (2013) Accurate antemortem diagnosis of equine protozoal myeloencephalitis (EPM) based on detecting intrathecal antibodies against *Sarcocystis neurona* using the SnSAG2 and SnSAG4/3 ELISAs. *J Vet Intern Med*, 27, 1193–1200.

[199] Andrews, F.M., Geiser, D.R., Sommardahl, C.S. *et al.* (1994) Albumin quotient, IgG concentration, and IgG index determinations in cerebrospinal fluid of neonatal foals. *Am J Vet Res*, 55, 741–745.

[200] Duarte, P.C., Ebel, E.D., Traub-Dargatz, J. *et al.* (2006) Indirect fluorescent antibody testing of cerebrospinal fluid for diagnosis of equine protozoal myeloencephalitis. *Am J Vet Res*, 67, 869–876.

[201] Beech, J. (1974) Equine protozoal myeloencephalitis. *Vet Med Small Anim Clin*, 69, 1562–1566.

[202] Harder, A. and Haberkorn, A. (1989) Possible mode of action of toltrazuril: studies on two *Eimeria* species and mammalian and *Ascarus suum* enzymes. *Parasitol Res*, 76, 8–12.

[203] Mitchell, S.M., Zajac, A.M., Davis, W.L. *et al.* (2005) The effects of ponazuril on development of apicomplexans in vitro. *J Eukaryot Microbiol*, 52, 231–235.

[204] MacKay, R.J. (2006) Equine protozoal myeloencephalitis: treatment, prognosis and prevention. *Clin Tech Equine Pract*, 5, 9–16.

[205] Furr, M. and Kennedy, T. (2001) Cerebrospinal fluid and serum concentrations of ponazuril in horses. *Vet Ther*, 2, 232–237.

[206] Lindsay, D.S., Dubey, J.P. and Kennedy, T.J. (2000) Determination of the activity of ponazuril against *Sarcocystis neurona* in cell cultures. *Vet Parasitol*, 92, 165–169.

[207] Reed SM, Wendel M, King S, et al. Pharmacokinetics of ponazuril in horses. Proceedings of the Annual Convention of American Association of Equine Practitioners, December 1–5, 2012, Anaheim, CA; 2012: p. 572.

[208] Furr M.Unpublished observation.

[209] Kennedy, T., Campbell, J. and Selzer, V. (2001) Safety of ponazuril 15% oral paste in horses. *Vet Ther*, 2, 223–231.

[210] Welsh, T.H., Bryan, T.M., Johnson, L. *et al.* (2002) Characterization of sperm and androgen production by testes from control and ponazuril-treated stallions. *Theriogenology*, 58, 389–392.

[211] Fenger, C.K. (1998) Treatment of equine protozoal myelo-encephalitis. *Comp Cont Ed Pract Vet*, 20, 1154–1157.

[212] Furr, M., McKenzie, H., Saville, W.J.A. *et al.* (2006) Prophylactic administration of ponazuril reduces clinical signs and delays seroconversion in horses challenged with *Sarcocystis neurona*. *J Parasitol*, 92, 637–643.

23 Parasitic Infections of the Central Nervous System

Martin Furr

Marion duPont Scott Equine Medical Center, Virginia-Maryland Regional College of Veterinary Medicine, Leesburg, USA

Parasitic infections of the equine central nervous system (CNS) are relatively uncommon; they lead to very severe disease when present, however. Several different parasitic organisms have been documented to infect the CNS of the horse (Table 23.1). One author has suggested that *Strongylus vulgaris* is the most commonly involved parasite, but based upon the number of reports in the clinical literature, *Halicephalobus gingivalis* appears to be the most common. This may reflect nothing more than a reporting bias, however, and the true prevalence of different parasites causing equine meningoencephalitis is unknown.

The general features of parasitic infections of the CNS are an acute onset of asymmetric deficits that are progressive. Clinical signs are quite variable and there are no pathognomonic clinical features to distinguish verminous myeloencephalitis from myeloencephalitis arising from other causes. Few successfully treated cases have been reported, as diagnosis is most commonly made by postmortem examination (Table 23.2).

Organisms and clinical syndromes

Halicephalobus (Micronema) gingivalis

Halicephalobus gingivalis is a free-living saprophytic nematode (Order Rhabditata and Family Rhabditidae) that is normally found in soil, manure, and decaying humus [1]. Some confusion regarding the classification of this parasite has occurred, and it was originally named as a species of *Micronema*. It was subsequently found that *Micronema* was already in use for a fish genus, and it was recommended that the parasite be moved to the genus *Halicephalobus* [2]. More recently, the parasite has been cultured from a mandibular lesion in a horse and studied in more detail, and the authors established *H. gingivalis* as a valid species, with *H. deletrix* considered a synonym [3].

The parasite was first described in the nasal tumor of a horse [4] and has subsequently been reported to cause a variety of neurologic and non-neurologic infections of horses. Infections of bone [5, 6], testicles [7], eye [7], kidney [7, 8], mammary gland [9], granulomatous skin lesions [10], and CNS [5–8, 11–14] have all been reported. Meningoencephalitis of humans has also been reported [15, 16]. The parasite appears to have a wide geographic distribution as infections have been reported in the United States, Canada, Scotland, United Kingdom, and Italy, among others.

Clinical signs of CNS infection with *H. gingivalis* are variable and depend upon the location of the parasite within the CNS. In most cases, ataxia is present and may be associated with encephalitic signs, although more focal lesions have been reported. These include a classic case of cauda equina syndrome [12] as well as ocular parasitism, which progressed to encephalitis [17]. In many cases, there were non-neurologic signs that were coincident with or preceded the neurologic signs; these included renal disease, granulomatous masses of the head, nasal discharge and sinusitis, and uveitis. The large number of reports in which there is an association with masses/swellings on the head would suggest that this is a normal route of infection (i.e., infection of skin lesions, with subsequent migration); however, there may also be hematogenous dissemination. Infections have been seen without any signs of swellings or masses, and these cases may represent direct invasion up to the nasopharynx and through the cribiform plate.

Strongylus vulgaris

Due to the extensive tissue migration associated with *S. vulgaris* infection, it is perhaps not surprising that occasional migration through the CNS occurs. When aberrant infection of the CNS occurs, a wide variety of clinical signs can occur which reflect the location of the parasite within the CNS. Two general syndromes have been reported, however—a chronic ataxia and an acute, progressive encephalitis [18]. Clinical signs in the

Equine Neurology, Second Edition. Martin Furr and Stephen Reed.
© 2015 John Wiley & Sons, Inc. Published 2015 by John Wiley & Sons, Inc.
Companion website: www.wiley.com/go/furr/neurology

Table 23.1 List of parasites that have been documented to cause myeloencephalitis in horses.

Organisms

Halicephalobus gingivalis
Strongylus vulgaris
Angiostrongylus cantonensis
Hypoderma (bovis and lineatum)
Draschia megastoma
Parelaphostrongylus tenuis
Trypanosoma evansi
Trypanosoma equiperdum
Setaria digitata
Setaria labiatopapillosa

Table 23.2 Clinical signs reported to be caused by parasites in the horse.

Clinical signs

Ataxia
Alterations in consciousness
Seizures
Cauda equina syndrome
Blindness
Dementia
Circling
Dysphagia
Laryngeal paralysis
Hyperesthesia
Muscular weakness
Recumbency
Dog-sitting

Specific details and references given in text.

encephalitic form include blindness, dementia, circling, and dysphagia [19].

In one well-investigated case of verminous myelitis in a donkey, there was an asymmetric hind limb weakness and ataxia localized to the thoracolumbar spinal cord. The clinical signs progressed to involve more anterior regions of the spinal cord over a period of several days, and the donkey was killed. A postmortem examination found long tortuous lesions extending over several vertebral segments, corresponding to the cranial progression of the parasite in the spinal cord [20].

Experimental induction of verminous myeloencephalitis via intracarotid injection of fourth- and fifth-stage larvae of *S. vulgaris* resulted in variable neurologic signs in five of eight ponies [21]. Two ponies died acutely. Blindness was frequently observed, as well as hyperesthesia, gait deficits, convulsions, and laryngeal paralysis.

Peripheral white blood cell counts did not change following infection [21]. It appears from postmortem examinations that damage from migration of *S. vulgaris* can occur and then heal, as evidenced by healed tortuous tracts within the CNS of horses with relatively mild clinical illness [18]. In these reports, however, clinical signs may not have been carefully recorded and it is unlikely that the result of such infection is benign.

In clinical cases, the pathophysiology is believed to involve an embolic shower of larvae from parasite-induced granulomas in the heart or ascending aorta. All six horses in one report had verminous thrombotic masses, supporting this view. Alternatively, individual larvae have been found to enter the spinal cord and migrate [20].

Hypoderma bovis and *Hypoderma lineatum*

Intracranial myiasis has been reported to be fairly common in the 19th century in Europe; however, it has been very uncommonly reported in more recent times [19, 22]. Presumably, the widespread and frequent use of anthelmintics and the decreasing practice of housing horses with cattle have diminished the frequency of the condition. Larvae of both *Hypoderma lineatum* and *Hypoderma bovis* have been described in the CNS of horses [22, 23]. The larvae apparently enter the CNS via large foramina such as the foramen magnum, intervertebral foramina, or optic foramina. Once within the CNS, the migration of the larvae through CNS parenchyma results in inflammation, hemorrhage, and tissue destruction.

Reported clinical histories include a relatively abrupt onset of clinical signs that are usually asymmetric and progressive. Ataxia and muscular weakness, circling, blindness, and seizures have been seen, with a clinical course of from 1 to 15 days [22, 23]. There is an apparent predisposition for the brain, as Olander reported the larvae to be in the brain in 15 of 16 cases [22].

Setaria

Infection of the CNS with *Setaria* spp. (Nematoda:Filarioidea) appears to be a fairly common illness in Central and Southeast Asia, resulting in a condition referred to colloquially as "Kumri," which means "weak back" in Hindustani [24]. The illness has been described in India and China by British veterinarians beginning in the late 1800s and is due to CNS infestation with *Setaria digitata* [25]. A closely related species, *Setaria labiatopapillosa*, has been described in a single horse in the United States [26]. There are apparently regional differences in incidence in which disease is more common in low-lying areas with high seasonal rainfall [24].

Clinical signs observed from either parasite appear to be similar, and spinal ataxia with posterior weakness predominates. Signs of involvement of the cauda equina were reported in one horse [26], and cerebral lesions were noted in two horses in Japan [27]. Fever or other systemic signs of illness are not apparent, and clinical signs from infection of non-nervous tissue are limited to the wonderfully descriptive "worm-in-the-eye" as quoted by Innes, 1952, from "Hippopathology, Vol III, (1843)" [25]. That this illness could indeed be due to *Setaria* spp. is supported by a report of a *Setaria* spp. surgically recovered from the eye of a horse with uveitis [28]. Neurologic signs appear in most cases to be abrupt in onset and progressive, although historical accounts describe variability in the severity and rapidity of progression [25].

Few detailed reports of pathologic changes can be found; however, single or multifocal areas of inflammation with hemorrhage and necrosis have been described [25–27]. One report described tract-like lesions as well as individual random foci of necrosis [26]. Parasite cross-sections may be seen histologically.

Draschia megastoma

Larval *D. megastoma* are deposited on moist surfaces of the horse by feeding flies. Ingested larvae reach the stomach where they mature and survive in granulomatous masses, but larvae deposited at other sites may migrate widely, occasionally finding their way to the brain. A single case of nervous system disease resulting from infection with *D. megastoma* has been reported [29]. In this case, an acute onset of asymmetric brainstem disease was described, followed by a 5 week course of improvement and then worsening leading to euthanasia.

Angiostrongylus cantonensis

Normally, *A. cantonensis* is a lungworm of rats in which the third- and fourth-stage larvae migrate through the CNS. It is possible to acquire infective larvae by direct ingestion of larvae on the intermediate host (snails, slugs, or freshwater prawns) or by invasion of traumatized skin.

A. cantonesis has been described in two foals in Australia [30]. Clinical signs included a "dog-sitting" posture and inability to stand in one, and ataxia followed by recumbency in the other. Treatment of one foal with ivermectin was attempted, yet progression of clinical signs was rapid and both foals were humanely destroyed due to the severity of their clinical condition. Postmortem examination found meningitis and larval parasite within the CNS with variable degrees of inflammation. Eosinophilic inflammation was a prominent component in one foal. *A. cantonensis* myeloencephalitis has been described in a horse in the United States, which demonstrated weakness and severe ataxia, decreased nociception, and cauda equina syndrome. Cerebrospinal fluid (CSF) analysis found a normal total protein but increased nucleated cell count (0.9×10^9 cells/l) composed primarily of mononuclear cells (80%) and 10% eosinophils [31]. Treatment of this horse

was unsuccessful, and the parasite was recovered and cultured postmortem. The route of infection in these horses was not determined.

Parelaphostrongylus tenuis

Adult *P. tenuis* ("meningeal worm") live in the cranial subarachnoid space and surrounding cranial venous sinuses, primarily of cervidae. Eggs are deposited into the venous circulation and are embolized to the lungs, forming granulomas. The eggs hatch and release first-stage larvae that escape from the granulomas, penetrate the airways and are carried up the mucociliary escalator, swallowed, and passed in host feces. The L1 infect terrestrial mollusks, grow to L3 (infective stage), and are ingested along with vegetation during grazing. The L3 penetrate the abdomen and migrate to the spinal cord by 10 days after infection. The larvae develop in the spinal cord and subsequently migrate to the cranial subarachnoid space where they mature and lay eggs [32, 33]. *P. tenuis* is usually silent in whitetail deer but causes neurologic disease in other North American cervids and other ungulates such as sheep, goats, llamas, and antelopes. Cattle appear to be highly resistant to infection, and horses have been exceedingly rarely reported to be infected.

A parasite proposed to be *P. tenuis* has been found in one horse associated with a syndrome of acquired dorsal grey matter myelitis and cervical scoliosis [34]. It was proposed that the parasite migrated up spinal nerves into the dorsal grey columns, inducing a unilateral degeneration that results in the clinical signs. Although the dorsal grey column has been identified as a preferred site for the development of *P. tenuis*, the parasite of the report was not conclusively identified and was not found in the other five horses of the study with cervical scoliosis. Hence, it is premature to suppose that all cases of adult cervical scoliosis are due to parasitic migration.

P. tenuis has been conclusively demonstrated to cause myeloencephalitis in another horse, however. A 6-month-old Arabian foal was found to have acute onset of marked spastic tetraparesis and ataxia, as well as an abnormal head position [32]. CSF harvested from this foal antemortem demonstrated a mildly increased total protein (116 mg/dl; upper limit of normal 100 mg/dl) and 1200 cells/μl of which 40% were neutrophils, 58% lymphocytes, and only a few eosinophils were seen. On pathologic examination, there was a diffuse multifocal to coalescing eosinophilic granulomatous inflammation, with sections of both mature and immature worms and eggs seen. Morphologic features suggested that this was *P. tenuis*, and this was later conclusively confirmed by PCR techniques [35]. Intraocular *P. tenuis* has also been reported in a horse with no other clinical signs. This was successfully treated by surgical removal with no visual impairment [36].

Diagnosis

Antemortem diagnosis of verminous myeloencephalitis is difficult. There is little about the anamnesis or clinical signs that are unique in such cases. Horses with *Halicephalobus*-induced myeloencephalitis may have signs of kidney disease or granulomatous swellings of the skin or head; those with *Hypoderma* infections may have skin warbles. Most horses have a history of abrupt onset of asymmetric CNS disease which is usually progressive. If seizures or abnormal behavior are present, then leukoencephalomalacia should be considered.

Routine serum chemistry analysis and CBC are unlikely to be altered in cases of verminous myeloencephalitis. Nonspecific changes in the serum biochemistry analysis, such as dehydration or increased muscle enzyme activity, may exist secondary to recumbency or an inability to drink and maintain hydration. A stress leukogram may be seen in animals that are anxious and distressed.

The most rewarding diagnostic test is probably the CSF evaluation. The nature of the changes in the CSF is likely to be dependent upon the number and size of organisms, as well as the duration of clinical disease and collection site. Nonspecific signs of inflammation are often present and an eosinophilic pleocytosis is expected; surprisingly, it is not commonly reported and the absence of eosinophilia in the CSF should not exclude parasites as the cause of a neurologic illness.

In one reported study of eight ponies, larval *S. vulgaris* (2–11 larvae/horse) were inoculated via intracarotid injection, and CSF parameters after injection were reported [21]. Unfortunately, collection of CSF occurred at variable times after infection and in only four ponies. In those cases, CSF white blood cell counts varied from 0 to 1080 cells/μl and total protein ranged from 31.5 to 175 mg/dl [21]. Neutrophils and lymphocytes predominated and eosinophils (1%) were only reported in one pony [21]. These findings differ somewhat from another model in which 250 000 L2 larvae of *Ascaris suum* were given via

intracarotid injection to five ponies followed by sequential neurologic examination and CSF collection and analysis [37]. In these ponies, a WBC pleocytosis (mean 156.2 total nucleated cells/μl) was found to peak at 1 week postinjection and to be composed of primarily eosinophils (117.2 cells/μl). This abated fairly quickly, however, and by 3 weeks postinjection, the eosinophil count was down to a mean of 13.4 cells/μl [36] (Tables 23.3 and 23.4). These two studies vary considerably in their design; however, they demonstrate wide range of clinicopathologic findings in the CSF of horses with verminous myeloencephalitis. This is also reflected by examination of findings from clinical cases in which such data is reported.

In a horse with severe CNS disease from *D. megastoma*, the lumbosacral CSF was described as "normal" [29], while in a horse with *S. labiatopapillosa*, the CSF was originally described as normal, then was found upon repeat analysis a few days later to be mildly xanthochromic and to have an increased nucleated cell count and total protein [26]. Changes in the CSF of two horses with *H. gingivalis* infection included a mild xanthochromia and normal to mildly increased total protein (69 and 81 mg/dl) [13]. A mild pleocytosis (25 and 81 nucleated cells/μl) was observed in both horses, but eosinophils were only observed in one case (1 eosinophil/l) and lymphocytes predominated in both cases [13]. In another case, there was a marked CSF pleocytosis (2030 cells/μl) of which "only a few" were eosinophils [6].

It would appear from these results that mild to moderate increase of total protein and cell count, along with evidence of hemorrhage (as xanthochromia) are consistent with verminous myeloencephalitis. Neutrophilia is common, and eosinophilia is only inconsistently seen, with the notable exception of the high eosinophil count in one *A. cantonensis* case. Clearly, many parasites cause severe inflammation and local tissue necrosis with subsequent cellular infiltration. The changes in CSF with verminous encephalitis may vary depending upon the parasite or number of organisms, time since initial infection, and timing of the CSF collection.

Table 23.3 Selected cerebrospinal fluid variables in ponies following inoculation with larvae of *Ascaris suum*.

Week PI	Total RBC (cells/μl)	Total WBC (cells/μl)	Lymphocytes (cells/μl)	Eosinophils (cells/μl)	Total protein (mg/dl)
0	2.2	2.2	1.6	0	38.0
1	63.0	156.2	33.0	117.2	69.6
2	4.8	67.2	19.6	43.8	65.8
3	149.0	61.4	40.2	13.4	58.5

Adapted from Ref. [37].
PI, postinfection.

Table 23.4 Cerebrospinal fluid results in various cases of verminous myeloencephalitis.

Xanthochromia	Nucleated cell count	Neutrophil	Macrophage	Lymphocyte	Eosinophil	Total protein	Organism
Negative	2.03×10^9/l	Mostly			Few	0.89 g/dl	*Halicephalobus* [6]
	0.9×10^9/l	10%	80%		10%		*A. cantonensis* [31]
	1200 cells/ml	40%		58%	2%	116 mg/dl	*P. tenuis* [32]
	60 cells/µl					710 mg/dl	*Halicephalobus* [12]
2+	81 cells/µl	~8 µl	40/µl	~33 µl	0	114 mg/dl	*Halicephalobus* [26]
	25 cells/µl	~4 µl	6/µl	~14 µl	~1 µl	69 mg/dl	*Halicephalobus* [26]
Mild	9988 cells/µl	~7191 µl	1199/µl	1398/µl	~200 µl	550 mg/dl	*S. vulgaris* [20]
Mild	Increased					Increased	*Setaria* [34]
	1563×10^6/l	18×10^6/l	219×10^6/l	120×10^6/l	1206×10^6/l		*Angiostrongylus* [30]
Not reported	35 cells/µl	~9 µl	~20 µl		~6 µl	100 mg/dl	*Halicephalobus* [28]

Normal values are 0.005×10^9/l or <5 cells/µl (cell count), and 0.7 g/dl or <90 mg/dl (total protein).

In some cases, larvae may be seen in CSF [19]. When present, these provide a high degree of confidence in the diagnosis. This appears most likely to occur in cases of *Halicephalobus* and is unlikely in cases of *S. vulgaris* or larval myiasis, due to the size of the parasite.

Just as it is hard to confirm verminous encephalitis antemortem, it is equally difficult to rule it out; hence, it may be prudent to assume that it is present, and treat for it, if CSF findings are consistent and no other etiology is determined.

Treatment

Treatment of verminous myeloencephalitis has not been documented in the literature as successful; however, as it is so difficult to confirm verminous myeloencephalitis antemortem, the true incidence of successful treatment is unknown. In one parasite challenge study, lesions were noted upon postmortem in horses that had not demonstrated obvious clinical signs; hence, it appears possible that recovery can occur [21]. One recent report has described a compelling cases of verminous encephalitis that was successfully treated with a high dose of fenbendazole (50 mg/kg PO q24h for 3 days), as well as anti-inflammatory drugs and supportive care [38]. Most modern anthelmintics have efficacy against the parasites reported to cause verminous encephalitis; however, their ability to achieve effective concentration in the CNS and CSF is unknown. There are no studies reporting the efficacy of any of the drugs for the treatment of verminous myeloencephalitis, and recommendations are anecdotal at best. The amount of tissue necrosis and inflammation produced by most large parasites is such that local (CSF and CNS)

Table 23.5 Anthelmintics of potential use in cases of verminous myeloencephalitis.

Drugs	Doses
Fenbendazole	60 mg/kg once
Fenbendazole	50 mg/kg once per day for 2–3 days
Thiabendazole	440 mg/kg once
Diethyl carbamazine (DEC)	50–100 mg/kg repeated in 3 days
Trichlorfon	40 mg/kg

Adapted from Refs. [19, 29].

concentrations in the area of the infection are probably high. It is probably best to use antiparasitic agents that provide a rapid kill to minimize the progression of damage. Combinations of fenbendazole and ivermectin or moxidectin are reasonable, and ivermectin should probably not be used alone, due to its "slow-kill" action and questionable penetration of the BBB. It has been suggested that treatment may result in an acute worsening of the clinical signs due to inflammation associated with parasite death; however, there is no objective information available to support this position. Clearly, if parasite is present within the CNS, anthelmintic treatment is required and control of associated inflammation is important (Table 23.5).

The use of anti-inflammatory drugs for CNS disease is discussed in detail in Chapter 4; however, a general course of treatment would involve the use of intravenous DMSO, nonsteroidal anti-inflammatory drugs, and corticosteroids.

Other neuroinvasive parasites

Trypanosoma infections

The hemoflagellate protozoa of the genus *Trypanosoma* are pathogenic to several mammalian species, including horses, resulting in a variety of clinical disorders, including meningoencephalitis. Both *Trypanosoma evansi* and *Trypanosoma equiperdum* are important pathogens worldwide, although eradicated in North America.

The hind limb ataxia arising from the CNS form of *T. evansi* infection is referred to as *mal das cadeiras* in Brazil or *mal de caderas* in the Spanish-speaking South American countries; in Asian countries, it is referred to as "Surra." *T. evansi* is an important disease affecting horses, mules, and camels in North Africa, the Middle East, Asia, Indonesia, and the Philippines, and Central and South America [39]. In South America, a number of animals can serve as reservoirs, including capybaras, coatis, small marsupials, and armadillos [40]. The organism is transmitted host to host, mechanically from the mouth parts of the biting flies of the genus *Tabanus* and *Stomoxys*; transmission is enhanced by high-density housing of horses and during periods of high insect population (i.e., during the wet season) [39]. An incubation period of 1–2 weeks follows, after which time there are large numbers of parasites present in the blood, but only transiently. Parasitemia is associated with fever and progressive anemia, ventral edema, weight loss, and the development of CNS abnormalities [39, 41]. Neurologic signs appear to be variable, with generalized weakness and progressive hindlimb paralysis, as well as restlessness and circling [39–42]. In one report of an outbreak in Brazil affecting up to 100 horses, 23 horses infected with *T. evansi* were clinically examined, and of these, nine horses had CNS disease [40]. Neurologic signs included marked ataxia, blindness, circling, hyperexcitability, depression, and head tilt. Eight of the nine horses also had chronic wasting. The duration of neurologic signs was from 2 to 20 days and most of the horses died. Detailed pathologic examination found cerebral edema with gelatinous yellowing and malacia, primarily of the white matter of the brain. Microscopically there was severe perivascular lymphoplasmacytic meningoencephalitis, necrosis, edema and hemorrhage [40]. These findings are similar to that described in another report of the pathology of *T. evansi* [41].

Diagnosis of *T. evansi* infection is suggested by observation of the clinical syndrome (chronic wasting, anemia, weakness, and perhaps neurologic abnormalities) in a known endemic area. Diagnostic aids include direct observation of trypanosomes in blood or tissue fluids; however, parasitemia may be transitory. Mouse inoculation tests may also be performed [41] and an indirect ELISA test has been described [40, 42]. The mouse inoculation test is considered the most sensitive technique41, while the ELISA test had a low sensitivity but was considered useful for screening [42].

Pathologic findings in horses with Surra demonstrated nonspecific changes including emaciation, subcutaneous and ventral edema, and enlarged lymph nodes. Histologically, there is a generalized nonsuppurative meningoencephalitis affecting both white and grey matter of the brain. Extensive lymphocytic/plasmacytic perivascular cuffing was seen, and neuronal necrosis was not considered a prominent feature [41].

Treatment of Surra is commonly attempted with suramin at a dose of 10 mg/kg BW IV, and then repeated in 1 week [39]. Other drugs that can be used include isometamidium chloride (Samorin, Rhone Merieux) at 0.25–2 mg/kg BW IM. Phenylarsonate (Cymelarsen, Rhone Merieux) is effective against resistant strains of *T. evansi*, but it has not been evaluated in horses [39]. Dimenazine at 3.5 mg/kg BW has been used; however, resistance may be widespread and it was ineffective, and associated with toxicity, in a group of horses and mules in Thailand [42].

Dourine, caused by *T. equiperdum*, has a very extensive geographic range; however, it is not restricted by climate and due to the movement of breeding animals internationally could be seen worldwide. Dourine is a venereal disease that results primarily in local infection of the genitalia, with swelling, edema, and discharge. Skin ulcerations may also occur and fever is sporadic [37]. Neurologic signs may occur later in the infection, and horses demonstrate ataxia and stumbling, with muscle spasms of the hindquarters and facial paralysis [39]. Nervous system involvement is described as invariably fatal [39].

The neurologic signs are reported to occur coincident with the presence of trypanosomes in the CSF, and hence observation of organism from CSF would be confirmatory.

References

[1] Bowman, D.D. (ed.) (1999) Helminths, in *Georgis' Parasitology for Veterinarians*, 7th edn, W.B. Saunders Co, Philadelphia, PA, pp. 109–234.

[2] Andrassy, L. (1973) Uber vier homonyme nematodengathungen. *Nemathologia*, 19, 403–404.

[3] Anderson, R.C., Linder, K.E. and Peregrine, A.S. (1998) *Halicephalobus gingivalis* (Stefanski, 1954) from a fatal infection in a horse in Ontario, Canada with comments on the validity of *H. deletrix* and a review of the genus. *Parasitology*, 5, 255–261.

[4] Anderson, R.V. and Bemrick, W.J. (1965) *Micronema deletrix* n. sp. a saprophagus nematode inhabiting a nasal tumour of the horse. *Proc Helminthol Soc Wash*, 32, 74–75.

[5] Keg, P.R., Mirck, M.H., Dik, K.J. *et al.* (1984) *Micronema deletrix* infection in a Shetland pony stallion. *Equine Vet J*, 16, 471–475.

[6] Brojer, J.T., Parsons, D.A., Linder, K.E. *et al.* (2000) *Halicephalobus gingivalis* encephalomyelitis in a horse. *Can Vet J*, 41, 559–561.

[7] Kinde, H., Mathews, M., Ash, L. *et al.* (2000) *Halicephalobus gingivalis (H. deletrix)* infection in two horses in southern California. *J Vet Diagn Invest*, 12, 162–165.

[8] Blunden, A.S., Khalil, L.F. and Webbon, P.M. (1987) *Halicephalobus deletrix* infection in a horse. *Equine Vet J*, 19, 255–260.

[9] Greiner, E.C., Calderwood-Mays, M.B. and Smart, G.C. (1991) Verminous mastitis in a mare caused by a free living nematode. *J Parasitol*, 77, 320–322.

[10] Johnson, K.H. and Johnson, D.W. (1966) Granulomas associated with *Micronema deletrix* in the maxillae of a horse. *J Am Vet Med Assoc*, 149, 155–159.

[11] Stone, W.M., Stewart, T.B. and Peckham, J.C. (1970) *Micronema Deletrix* Anderson and Bemrick, 1965 in the central nervous system of a pony. *J Parasitol*, 56, 986–987.

[12] Johnson, J.S., Hibler, C.P., Tillotson, K.M. *et al.* (2001) Radiculomeningomyelitis due to Halicephalobus gingivalis in a horse. *Vet Pathol*, 38, 559–561.

[13] Darian, B.J., Belknap, J. and Nietfeld, J. (1988) Cerebrospinal fluid changes in two horses with central nervous system nematodiasis (*Micronema deletrix*). *J Vet Intern Med*, 2, 201–205.

[14] Cantile, C., Rossi, G., Braca, G. *et al.* (1997) A horse with *Halicepholobus deletrix* encephalitis in Italy. *Eur J Vet Pathol*, 3, 29–33.

[15] Hoogstraten, J. and Young, W.G. (1975) Meningo-encephali-myelitis due to the saprophagus nematode, *Micronema deletrix*. *J Can Sci Neurol*, 2, 121–126.

[16] Shadduck, J.A., Kebelacker, D.J. and van Telford, Q. (1979) *Micronema deletrix* meningo-encephalitis in an adult man. *Am J Clin Pathol*, 72, 640–643.

[17] Rames, D.S., Miller, D.K., Barthel, R. *et al.* (1995) Ocular *Halicepholobus* (syn. *Micronema*) *deletrix* in a horse. *Vet Pathol*, 32, 540–542.

[18] Little, P.B. (1972) Cerebrospinal nematodiasis of equidae. *J Am Vet Med Assoc*, 160, 1407–1413.

[19] Lester, G.D. (1992) Parasitic encephalomyelitis in horses. *Comp Cont Ed Pract Vet*, 14, 1624–1630.

[20] Mayhew, I.G., Brewer, B.D., Reinhard, M.K. *et al.* (1984) Verminous (*Strongylus vulgaris*) myelitis in a donkey. *Cornell Vet*, 74, 30–37.

[21] Little, P.B., Lwin, U.S. and Fretz, P.B. (1974) Verminous encephalitis of horses: experimental induction with *Strongylus vulgaris* larvae. *Am J Vet Res*, 35, 1501–1510.

[22] Olander, H.J. (1967) The migration of *Hypoderma lineatum* in the brain of a horse. *Vet Pathol*, 4, 477–483.

[23] Hadlow, W.J., Ward, J.K. and Krinsky, W.L. (1977) Intracranial myiasis by *Hypoderma bovis* (Linneus) in a horse. *Cornell Vet*, 67, 272–281.

[24] Innes, J.R.M. and Pillai, C.P. (1955) Kumri-so-called lumbar paralysis-of horses in Ceylon (India and Burma), and its identification with cerebrospinal nematodiasis. *Br Vet J*, 3, 223–235.

[25] Innes, J.R.M. (1952) Cerebrospinal nematodiasis: a nervous disease of animals caused by immature nematodes (*Setaria digitata*) and its relationship to Kumri of horses in India. *Indian Vet J*, 29, 81–86.

[26] Frauenfelder, H.C., Kazacos, K.R. and Lichtenfels, J.R. (1980) Cerebrospinal nematodiasis caused by a filariid in a horse. *J Am Vet Med Assoc*, 177, 359–362.

[27] Yoshihara, T., Oikawa, M., Kanemaru, T. *et al.* (1987) Two cases of cerebrospinal setariosis in the racehorses. *Bull Equine Res Inst*, 24, 14–22.

[28] Jemelka, E.D. (1976) Removal of *Setaria digitata* from the anterior chamber of the equine eye. *Vet Med Small Anim Clin*, 71, 673–675.

[29] Mayhew, I.G., Lichtenfels, J.R., Greiner, E.C. *et al.* (1982) Migration of a spiruroid nematode through the brain of a horse. *J Am Vet Med Assoc*, 180, 1306–1311.

[30] Wright, J.D., Kelly, W.R., Wadell, A.H. *et al.* (1990) Equine neural angiostrongylosis. *Aust Vet J*, 68, 58–60.

[31] Costa, L.R.R., McClure, J.J., Snider, T.G. and Stewart, T.B. (2000) Verminous meningoencephalomyelitis by *Angiostrongylus (=Parastrongylus)cantonensis* in an American miniature horse. *Equine Vet Ed*, 12, 2–6.

[32] Tanabe, M., Kelly, R., de La Hunta, A. *et al.* (2007) Verminous encephalitis in a horse produced by nematodes in the family protostrongylidae. *Vet Pathol*, 44, 119–122.

[33] Kontrimavichus, V.L., Delyamure, S.L. and Boev, S.N. (1985) Metastrongyloids of domestic and wild animals, in *Fundamentals of Nematology*, vol. 26 (ed. V.S. Kothekar), Oxonian Press, New Delhi, pp. 94–156.

[34] van Biervliet, J., De Lahunta, A., Ennulat, D. *et al.* (2003) Acquired cervical scoliosis in six horses associated with dorsal grey column chronic myelitis. *Equine Vet J*, 35, 86–92.

[35] Tanabe, M., Gerhold, R.W., Beckstead, R.B. *et al.* (2010) Molecular confirmation of *Parelaphostronglus tenuis* infection in a horse with verminous encephalitis. *Vet Pathol*, 47, 759.

[36] Reinstein, S.L., Lucio-Forster, A., Bowman, D.D. *et al.* (2010) Surgical extraction of an intraocular infection of Parelaphostronguylus tenuis in a horse. *J Am Vet Med Assoc*, 237, 196–199.

[37] Honor, D. Cerebrospinal fluid analysis in normal ponies and in ponies with experimentally induced central nervous system disease. PhD Dissertation. Purdue University, West Lafayette University. 1987;Thesis 36006.

[38] Wilford, S., Weller, R. and Dunkel, B. (2013) Successful treatment of a horse with presumed parasitic encephalitis. *Equine Vet Ed*, 25, 601–604.

[39] Luckins, A.G. (1994) Equine trypanosomiasis. *Equine Vet Ed*, 6, 259–262.

[40] Rodrigues, A., Fighera, R.A., Souza, T.M. *et al.* (2009) Neuropathology of naturally occurring *Trypanosoma evansi* infection of horses. *Vet Pathol*, 46, 251–258.

[41] Seiler, R.J., Omar, S. and Jackson, A.R.B. (1981) Meningoencephalitis in naturally occurring *Trypanosoma evansi* infection (Surra) of horses. *Vet Pathol*, 18, 120–122.

[42] Tuntasuvan, D., Jarabrum, W., Viseshakul, N. *et al.* (2003) Chemotherapy of surra in horses and mules with diminazene aceturate. *Vet Parasitol*, 110, 227–233.

24 Miscellaneous Infections of the Central Nervous System

Martin Furr

Marion duPont Scott Equine Medical Center, Virginia-Maryland Regional College of Veterinary Medicine, Leesburg, USA

Cryptococcus

The encapsulated yeast-like fungus *Cryptococcus* is an opportunistic pathogen of debilitated or immunologically compromised individuals. The organism is commonly found in pigeon feces and associated contaminated soil and infections are acquired primarily via aerosolation [1]. The organism can survive for long periods in soil. It is not contagious and cases occur sporadically. *Cryptococcus neoformans* [1–7] is most commonly implicated, although infections with *C. albidus* and *C. laurentii* have been seen [8].

Cryptococcus is spherical (2–10 micrometers in diameter) and is surrounded by a thick mucoid capsule that does not stain with hematoxylin and eosin (H&E). The capsule can be stained by mucicarmine, as well as periodic acid–Schiff and Gomori's methenamine silver [9]. It reproduces by narrow-based budding, which distinguishes it from *Blastomyces*.

Virulence factors for *Cryptococcus* include the presence of a capsule, the production of melanin, and thermotolerance [10]. The ability to grow and replicate at body temperature is key and is controlled by multiple genes; mutated temperature-sensitive strains are recognized and are avirulent. Virulent *Cryptococcus* organisms elaborate melanin that impairs antibody formation, depresses lymphoproliferation, and downregulates TNF-α production, as well as impairing phagocytosis of the organism. Blocking of phagocytosis is also an important consequence of the thick capsule [10].

Infection with *Cryptococcus* results in chronic granulomatous infections, typically of the respiratory tract leading to rhinitis [11, 12], sinusitis [5] or pneumonia [8], and occasionally meningitis and encephalitis [1–6, 13, 14]. There appears to be a predilection of the organism for the central nervous system (CNS), the meninges in particular, as one author reported that 10 of 40 reported cases had CNS involvement [10]. The reason that the CNS and meninges appear to be so commonly involved is not known at the present time. Organisms may reach the CNS by direct encroachment from a granulomatous mass in the head (sinus or postorbital mass in one case [5]) or perhaps by hematogenous dissemination from pulmonary or other infections. In humans, immunocompromised individuals are at greater risk, and this is also likely to be true in horses, as was demonstrated in one case [6]. Several reports are noted from Australia, where an association with the Eucalyptus plant (*Eucalyptus camaldulensis*) has been suggested [8].

Clinical signs

Clinical signs can vary depending upon the location of the infection within the CNS; however, diffuse signs of encephalitis seem to predominate. Asymmetric signs were reported in one horse [14]. Depression and anorexia are often noted, as is gait stiffness, hyperesthesia, and ataxia. Sudden death was reported in one horse [4]. Variable types and degrees of cranial nerve deficits may also be seen, including blindness, nystagmus, and fixed and dilated pupils [1, 6, 7]. Hind limb paralysis, rectal and bladder paralysis, penile paralysis, and gluteal muscle wasting have all been reported [3, 14]. In many cases, the cardinal signs are normal, although mild fever and anorexia may be seen. Blindness was noted in a horse with a postorbital mass, leading to pressure necrosis of the optic nerve as the granulomatous mass bulged into the cranial cavity displacing the left cerebral hemisphere [5], while blindness associated with optic neuritis was reported in another horse [6] (Table 24.1).

Equine Neurology, Second Edition. Martin Furr and Stephen Reed.
© 2015 John Wiley & Sons, Inc. Published 2015 by John Wiley & Sons, Inc.
Companion website: www.wiley.com/go/furr/neurology

Table 24.1 Clinical signs reported in horses with cryptococcal meningitis.

Nervous system signs
Depression
Anorexia
Stiff gait
Hyperesthesia
Head tilt
Ataxia
Blindness
Nystagmus
Dilated pupils
Hind limb paralysis
Penile paralysis
Bladder paralysis
Gluteal wasting

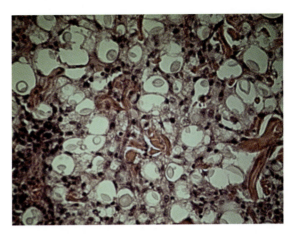

Figure 24.1 Postmortem brain sample from a horse with *Cryptococcus*, stained with H&E. Note clear zone around organism resulting in "soap-bubble appearance."

Diagnosis

The antemortem diagnosis of cryptococcal meningitis is challenging, as the clinical signs are nonspecific. Peripheral white blood cell counts are variable in reported cases, and serum biochemistry results highlight only nonspecific changes resulting from dehydration and recumbency. The diagnosis is primarily dependent on the analysis of cerebrospinal fluid (CSF). CSF results are very poorly reported from previous studies; however, discolored, turbid fluid with an increased total protein and white blood cell count is expected; variable degrees of hemorrhage may also be seen. A mixed inflammatory reaction with roughly equal numbers of neutrophils and macrophages was observed in one case [13], while in another horse, a total nucleated cell count of 1315 cells/l with a total protein of 616.5 mg/dl was reported [6]. Upon microscopic examination, budding yeasts surrounded by a thick, nonstaining capsule may be seen, but non- or poorly encapsulated form may also be observed in the CSF [6]. The presence of the capsule can be demonstrated by performing an India ink counterstain, which reveals a clear "halo" around a central organism. The organism is readily cultured on standard fungal media, and the sediment from 15 to 20 ml of CSF should be inoculated to enhance recovery [10]. Serum and CSF titers can be determined using commercially available antigens for *C. neoformans* capsular antigens, which were strongly positive in the CSF in one horse [6].

Postmortem examination reveals the surface of the brain/spinal cord to be covered with small nodules. Meninges may be thick and discolored yellow, with a gelatinous exudate on the surface [4]. Wet mount of a surface impression may reveal thick-walled capsular organisms. Histologic analysis finds a granulomatous inflammatory reaction, with few deep organisms surrounded by minimal local inflammation [1]. In H&E-stained tissues, there is a clear, unstained "halo" around the organism; multiple organisms clustered together results in a "soap bubble" appearance. Mucicarmine stains the capsule rose-red and the cell pink and is considered the preferred stain as it differentiates *Cryptococcus* from *Coccidioides* or *Blastomyces*, which do not stain with mucicarmine (Figure 24.1).

Treatment

Treatment of horses with cryptococcal meningitis is not well reported and recommendations for treatment must be extrapolated from human medicine. In humans, a two-phase treatment protocol is advised by some authors [15]. In a group of non-HIV-infected humans with cerebral cryptococcosis, best results were obtained using a treatment protocol of amphotericin B intravenously and intrathecally (phase 1), followed by oral fluconazole (phase 2). During phase 1, intrathecal treatment was administered two to three times per week until the CSF culture was negative. Amphotericin B should be diluted (1 mg/ml) in sterile water for injection and mixed with autologous CSF. Due to the irritant properties of amphotericin B, corticosteroids can be given either intrathecally or systemically. Phase 2 of the combination protocol employs long-term oral fluconazole or itraconazole until the CSF is culture negative three times, 1 week apart. Treatment duration in a human study ranged up to 16 months in one case, with an average of about 7 months [15]. Overall success using the two-phase approach was 97.5%, while monotherapy with fluconazole, itraconazole, or amphotericin B had a much lower success rate and more recurrences [15]. Another study reported that amphotericin B combined with flucytosine improved survival in human patients with cryptococcal meningitis, while combining fluconazole to amphotericin B had no additive effect [16]. The effectiveness of these approaches has not been investigated in horses, although successful treatment of one horse with pulmonary cryptococcosis was reported using 0.35–0.5 mg/kg amphotericin B diluted in 1 l of D5W, once per day for 31 days, given slowly IV. Muscle tremors, pyrexia, and tachycardia were observed and were controlled with flunixen [17].

Fluconazole dosed at 14 mg/kg BW loading and 5 mg/kg SID results in a concentration of drug in the CSF of horses that is considered adequate for the treatment of many fungi [18]. Fluconazole has been used to successfully treat nasal granulomas caused by *Cryptococcus*, as well as one horse with cryptococcal meningitis [6]. Fluconazole (5 mg/kg BW SID) following an initial loading dose was administered for 197 days after which time it was discontinued. Treatment was monitored by serial CSF titers using a latex agglutination assay and CSF analyses. Although total nucleated cell counts and total protein of CSF were normal by day 157 of treatment, it was reported that rare capsular fragments of the organism persisted. In this horse, blindness resolved, although mild ataxia persisted after treatment was discontinued [6].

Treatment of another horse with cryptococcal meningitis was attempted using amphotericin B, to which it responded transiently, and then worsened prompting euthanasia [13]. Amphotericin B (100 mg, then increased to 150 mg) was diluted in 4000 ml of 5% dextrose and administered IV over 4 h. This was given every other day for a total of 12 treatments. Intrathecal treatment with 50 mg amphotericin B was also performed. A deteriorating condition and seizures the day following the intrathecal treatment prompted euthanasia, and the authors suggested that a lower dose of intrathecal amphotericin B (15 mg) would have been advisable [13].

Obviously, treatment of cryptococcal meningitis is challenging, and a poor prognosis must be given for equine cases due to the expense and complexities associated with long-term management of a neurologic horse. Appropriate supportive care as well as long-term anti-inflammatory and anti-fungal medications is required. The experience of the cases reported earlier, however, suggests that successful treatment is possible using fluconazole. Inadequate information exists to determine if the two-phase protocol of intravenous and intrathecal amphotericin B, followed by oral fluconazole as sometimes used in humans, would be advisable in horses. The seizures noted following intrathecal administration of amphotericin B suggests caution and the use of a conservative dose.

Amebic meningoencephalitis

Free-living amebas of the genera *Acanthamoeba* and *Balamuthia* are distributed worldwide in fresh and brackish water. It is believed that the organisms gain entry via the ethmoturbinates, respiratory tract, or skin wounds, or ascend via the optic or olfactory nerves.

Amebic encephalitis is rarely reported in horses; however, the few reported cases did not survive. In one case of meningoencephalitis caused by the amebic organism *Balamuthia mandrillaris* (previously referred to as "leptomyxid ameba"), a horse showed acute signs of salivation and stumbling, which progressed to recumbency over a 2 day period prompting euthanasia [19]. No aspects of clinical pathology or CSF analysis were reported. Postmortem examination found numerous small (3 micrometers), irregularly shaped pale tan lesions in the midbrain and cervical spinal cord. Upon microscopic examination, these were associated with extensive necrosis with perivascular inflammatory cell infiltrates. Both trophozoites and cyst forms of a parasite were observed and immunohistochemical staining confirmed them to be *B. mandrillaris*.

In another report, four horses were found to have amebic infections, with three of the four demonstrating neurologic signs; amebas were observed histologically and recovered from the brain. These were confirmed to be either *B. mandrillaris* or species of *Acanthamoeba* [20]. Clinical signs included ataxia, recumbency, and depression; evidence of pulmonary disease was observed in several of the horses. It was speculated that hematogenous dissemination from the lung was the source of the CNS infection [20].

Antemortem diagnosis of amebic infections is challenging, even in humans, and is based upon demonstration of a mononuclear pleocytosis and increased total protein of the CSF. Magnetic resonance imaging studies may demonstrate multiple, diffuse hypodense lesions in the brain, and brain biopsy may reveal organisms. These modalities are not readily available nor employed for equine cases, and antemortem diagnosis in horses is unlikely.

Treatment is symptomatic (anti-inflammatory drugs and supportive care), along with anti-amebic compounds. Fluconazole, amphotericin B, and miconazole demonstrate some activity against the parasite, but there is a high mortality in human patients and a grave prognosis must be given if diagnosed antemortem [21].

Mycotic encephalitis

Fungal infections other than *Cryptococcus* have also been incriminated in equine neurologic disease, albeit rarely [22–25]. Reported cases appear to have most commonly occurred secondary to guttural pouch mycosis, although in one horse it was believed to be secondary to fungal sinusitis [25]. Clinical signs reflect brainstem and cerebral disease, with dysphagia, head shaking, ataxia, blindness, and seizures occurring variably. In one case, CSF taken from the atlantooccipital space found a CSF pleocytosis (79 cells/mm [3]), composed predominately of mononuclear cells but also demonstrating 19% neutrophils [23]. A strong positive Pandy test was present and fungal elements were not seen.

Histopathologic examination finds numerous areas of inflammation and necrosis, characterized by infiltration with neutrophils and mononuclear cells, thrombosis of vessels, and fungal elements. The fungus may obtain access to the brain by direct migration up a cranial nerve; however, hematogenous dissemination was considered most likely in one case, due to the degree of thrombosis and lack of obvious cranial nerve involvement [22].

Prognosis for such cases is very poor, but if treatment is attempted, the use of antifungal medications (as above) and anti-inflammatory drugs would be indicated.

Neuroborreliosis

Infection with *Borrelia burgdorferi* is widely distributed in the Northern Hemisphere [26, 27] and results in a syndrome of dermatitis, myalgia, arthritis and aseptic meningitis in humans [28]. Similar clinical signs have been ascribed to the horse; however, there is very little evidence confirming CNS disease in the vast majority of these cases. A compelling diagnosis for neuroborreliosis was made in one horse demonstrating clinical signs of abnormal mentation, head tilt, flaccid paralysis of the tail, and dysphagia [29]. The diagnosis in this case was based upon a high *B. burgdorferi* titer and the presence of spirochetes in the brain on postmortem examination [29]. Neuroborreliosis was also diagnosed in a horse with myalgia and neck stiffness, ataxia, and head tilt. CSF from this horse had inflammatory changes characterized by increased total protein (175 mg/dl) and total nucleated cell count (69 cells/l) with 82% neutrophils. Polymerase chain reaction (PCR) testing was positive for *B. burgdorferi* DNA [30]. Treatment with oxytetracycline was initially successful, and then the horse relapsed and was euthanized due to the severity of its neurologic abnormalities. Postmortem examination found congestion and hyperemia of the meninges, with lymphohistiocytic leptomeningitis and peripheral radiculoneuritis. Unfortunately, postmortem PCR testing, culture, and special staining for *B. burgdorferi* were all negative [30]. It is of interest that this horse also demonstrated laboratory evidence of common variable immunodeficiency; the role that this condition may have had in its illness is unknown.

Neuroborreliosis was also confirmed as the cause of neurologic abnormalities in two horses using PCR techniques. Both horses demonstrated a long history of waxing and waning neurologic problems including muscle and back soreness and hyperesthesia, ataxia, muscle wasting, and facial paralysis in one and gluteal muscle atrophy in the other [31]. Postmortem examination found thickened meninges with fibrous adhesions to the dura, with mild hemorrhage and purulent tan subdural deposits. Histopathologic findings included non-suppurative meningitis and radiculoneuritis, with occasional lymphoplasmacytic perivascular encephalitis. Spirochetes were observed in the dura mater of the brain and spinal cord of both horses, and quantitative PCR found high copy numbers for the *ospC* and *flaB* genes in one horse. *B. burgdorferi* DNA was recovered from the spinal cord of one horse and the identity was consistent with *ospA* and *ospC* genes [31]. These pathologic findings were similar to those seen in a horse reported from the UK [32].

From these reports, it appears that the clinical signs associated with Lyme neuroborreliosis can be varied. Nonspecific and nonlocalizing muscle soreness and gait abnormalities progressing to ataxia have been reported and may be associated with focal muscle wasting, mentation changes, or hyperesthesia. These signs may progress over a period of months before becoming overtly recognizable. An association with a history of lameness, joint swelling, or uveitis is also sometimes observed and suggestive. Methods for clinical diagnosis of equine neuroborreliosis are not validated, but elimination of other more likely pathogens, presence of a high titer, and residence in an endemic area would be supportive. A high serum titer alone, however, is not conclusive because it is not possible to differentiate exposure from active infection. Determining CSF anti-*B. burgdorferi* titers and calculating specific CSF antibody index (as described in Chapter 3) are likely to provide a more robust diagnosis and can be performed using either the conventional ELISA or the latex bead assay. This technique has been described in the diagnosis of a horse with a clinical diagnosis of neuroborelliosis [33]. Treatment recommended for non-nervous system Lymes disease is a prolonged antibiotic course using either oxytetracycline, doxycycline, or minocycline. Minocycline (4 mg/kg PO BID) may be preferable as it achieves higher concentrations in the CSF and aqueous fluids than doxycycline [27]. The value of these treatments in CNS infections is not yet proved at this time.

References

[1] Welsh, R.D. and Stair, E.L. (1995) Cryptococcal meningitis in a horse. *J Equine Vet Sci*, 15, 80–82.

[2] Cho, D.Y., Pace, L.W. and Beadle, R.E. (1986) Cerebral cryptococcosis in a horse. *Vet Pathol*, 23, 207–209.

[3] Barton, M.D. and Knight, I. (1972) Cryptococcal meningitis of a horse. *Aust Vet J*, 48, 534.

[4] Irwin, C.F.P. and Rac, R. (1957) Cryptococcus infection in a horse. *Aust Vet J*, 33, 97–98.

[5] Scott, E.A., Duncan, J.R. and McCormack, J.E. (1974) Cryptococcosis involving the postorbital area and frontal sinus in a horse. *J Am Vet Med Assoc*, 165, 626–627.

[6] Hart, K.A., Flaminio, M., LeRoy, B.E. *et al.* (2008) Successful resolution of cryptococcal meningitis and optic neuritis in an adult horse with oral fluconazole. *J Vet Intern Med*, 22, 1436–1440.

[7] Teuscher, E., Vrins, A. and Lemaire, T. (1984) A vestibular syndrome associated with *Cryptococcus neoformans* in a horse. *Zentralbl Veterinärmed A*, 31, 132–139.

[8] Riley, C.B., Bolton, J.R., Mills, J.N. *et al.* (1992) Cryptococcosis in seven horses. *Aust Vet J*, 69, 135–139.

[9] Zachary, J.F. (2007) Nervous system: fungi and algae, in *Pathologic Basis of Veterinary Disease* (eds M.D. McGavin and J.F. Zachary), Mosby, St. Louis, MO, pp. 890–893.

[10] Kohn, C. (2007) Miscellaneous fungal diseases, in *Equine Infectious Diseases*, 1st edn (eds D. Sellon and M. Long), W.B. Saunders, St Louis, MO, pp. 431–445.

[11] Corrier, D.E., Wilson, S.R. and Scrutchfield, W.L. (1984) Equine cryptococcal rhinitis. *Comp Contin Ed Pract Vet* , 6, S556–S558.

[12] Phillips, M.T. (1969) Equine cryptococcus. *Southwestern Vet*, 22, 147–148.

[13] Steckel, R.R., Adams, S.B., Long, G.G. *et al.* (1982) Antemortem diagnosis and treatment of cryptococcal meningitis in a horse. *J Am Vet Med Assoc*, 180, 1085–1089.

[14] Barclay, W.P. and de Lahunta, A. (1979) Cryptococcal meningitis in a horse. *J Am Vet Med Assoc*, 174, 1236–1238.

[15] Yao, Z., Liao, W. and Chen, R. (2005) Management of cryptococcosis in non-HIV-related patients. *Med Mycol*, 43, 245–251.

[16] Day, J.N., Chau, T.T., Wolbers, M. *et al.* (2013) Combination antifungal therapy for cryptococcal meningitis. *N Engl J Med*, 368, 1291–1302.

[17] Begg, L.M., Hughes, K.J., Kessell, A. *et al.* (2004) Successful treatment of cryptococcal pneumonia in a pony mare. *Aust Vet J*, 82, 686–689.

[18] Latimer, F.G., Carmen, M.H., Campbell, N.B. and Papich, M.G. (2001) Pharmacokinetics of fluconazole following intravenous and oral administration and body fluid concentrations of fluconazole following repeated oral dosing in horses. *Am J Vet Res*, 62, 1606–1611.

[19] Kinde, J., Visvesvara, G.S., Barr, B.C. *et al.* (1998) Amebic meningoencephalitis caused by *Balamuthia mandrillaris* (leptomyxid ameba) in a horse. *J Vet Diagn Invest*, 10, 378–381.

[20] Kinde, H., Read, D., Daft, B. *et al.* (2007) Infections caused by pathogenic free-living amebas (*Balamuthia mandrillaris* and *Acanthomoeba* sp.) in horses. *J Vet Diagn Invest*, 19, 317–322.

[21] Intalapaporn, P., Suankratay, C., Shuangshoti, S. *et al.* (2004) *Balamuthia mandrillaris* meningoencephalitis: the first case in southeast Asia. *Am J Trop Med Hyg*, 70, 666–669.

[22] McLaughlin, B.G. and O'Brien, J.L. (1986) Guttural pouch mycosis and mycotic encephalitis in a horse. *Can Vet J*, 27, 109–111.

[23] Wagner, P.C., Miller, R.A., Gallina, A.M. *et al.* (1978) Mycotic encephalitis associated with a guttural pouch mycosis. *J Equine Med Surg*, 2, 355–359.

[24] Hatziolos, B.C., Sass, B., Albert, T.F. *et al.* (1975) Blindness in a horse probably caused by gutturomycosis. *Zentralbl Veterinarmed B*, 22, 362–371.

[25] Hunter, B. and Nation, P.N. (2011) Mycotic encephalitis, sinus osteomyelitis, and guttural pouch mycosis in a 3 year old Arabian colt. *Can Vet J*, 52, 1339–1341.

[26] Madigan, J.E. (1993) Lyme disease (Lyme borreliosis) in horses. *Vet Clin North Am Equine Pract*, 9, 429–434.

[27] Divers, T.J. (2013) Equine Lymes disease. *J Equine Vet Sci*, 33, 488–492.

[28] Shapiro, E.D. and Gerber, M.A. (2000) Lyme disease. *Clin Infect Dis*, 31, 533–542.

[29] Burgess, E.C. and Mattison, M. (1987) Encephalitis associated with *Borrelia burgdorferi* infection in a horse. *J Am Vet Med Assoc*, 191, 1457–1458.

[30] James, F.M., Engiles, J.B. and Beech, J. (2010) Meningitis, cranial neuritis, and radiculoneuritis associated with *Borrelia burgdorferi* infection in a horse. *J Am Vet Med Assoc*, 237, 1180–1185.

[31] Imai, D.M., Barr, B.C., Daft, B. *et al.* (2011) Lyme neuroborreliosis in 2 horses. *Vet Pathol*, 48, 1151–1157.

[32] Hahn, C.N., Mayhew, I.G., Whitwell, K.E. *et al.* (1996) A possible case of Lyme borreliosis in a horse in the UK. *Equine Vet J*, 28, 84–88.

[33] Wagner B, Glaser A, Bartol J, et al. A New Sensitive Lyme Multiplex Assay to Confirm Neuroborreliosis in Horses: A Case Report. Proceedings of the 57th Annual Convention of American Association of Equine Practitioners (AAEP), Baltimore, MD, July 21, 2011:70–75.

25 Disorders Associated with Clostridial Neurotoxins: Botulism and Tetanus

Martin Furr

Marion duPont Scott Equine Medical Center, Virginia-Maryland Regional College of Veterinary Medicine, Leesburg, USA

Neurologic disease resulting from infection with clostridial organisms is not common, but results in severe disease when they occur. The clostridial neurotoxins are some of the most potent biological toxins known, leading to the clinical conditions of botulism (a flaccid paralysis) and tetanus (a tetanic paralysis). Both toxins exert their effects by inhibiting neurotransmitter release, but the anatomic localization of the inhibition results in the markedly different clinical signs. For the clostridial neurotoxins to alter neurotransmitter release, they must bind to and be internalized into the nerve terminal. The toxins first bind to large negatively charged molecules (polysialogangliosides) on the nerve terminal. After this, the ganglioside/toxin complex binds to a second specific protein receptor on the nerve terminus surface. The specific nature of this receptor is believed to determine the subsequent internalization and differential localization of the toxins within the nerve. After internalization into the nerve terminal, tetanus toxin migrates retrograde along the motor neuron to the spinal cord and brainstem. Botulism toxin remains at the nerve terminus of the neuromuscular junction (NMJ).

Once the cell body is reached, tetanus toxin is moved by transsynaptic exchange into the terminus of inhibitory motor neurons of the spinal cord. Tetanus toxin cleaves vesicle-associated membrane protein (VAMP) (synaptobrevin), a "docking protein" required for exocytosis of neurotransmitter, which in the spinal inhibitory interneuron is glycine and gamma aminobutyric acid (GABA) [1–3]. In contrast, botulinum toxin remains within the nerve terminus of the NMJ and blocks acetylcholine release by attacking proteins responsible for neurotransmitter exocytosis at the NMJ. Specifically, botulism toxin types A and E cleave SNAP-25, serotypes B, D, F and G inactivate VAMP (synaptobrevin), and serotype C inactivates syntaxin [3] (Table 25.1 and Figure 25.1).

Tetanus

Tetanus is a neurologic disease resulting from the toxin of *Clostridium tetani*. *C. tetani* is a gram-positive, obligate anaerobic bacillus. Occasionally it forms long filaments in culture [4]. The organism exists primarily in spore form and is common in the gastrointestinal (GI) tract of animals, and subsequently is a common soil organism. Spores are highly resistant to environmental extremes and antimicrobials but can be destroyed by heating to 239°F (115°C) for 20 min [4]. *C. tetani* produces three toxins: (i) tetanospasmin (neurotoxin), (ii) hemolysin, and (iii) a peripherally acting non-spasmogenic toxin. Tetanospasmin is responsible for the characteristic clinical features of tetanus, and antibodies to this toxin are protective [4].

Neurologic disease is seen following infection of wounds with *C. tetani* spores. Clostridial growth occurs in conditions of a low O_2 tension, and hence deep penetrating wounds are common sources of infection. Wounds with a large amount of tissue necrosis or impaired blood supply can also provide a favorable environment for the growth of the organism. Tetanus has been observed following castration, metritis, retained placenta, and injection abscesses in adult horses [5]. In a case series of 20 horses with tetanus, puncture wounds to the distal limbs were the most common wound history, with lacerations and sole abscesses being very common, and wounds to the head were also reported but infrequently [6]. The umbilicus has been implicated as a site of infection in neonates [5]. The time from wound occurrence until development of neurologic signs can vary greatly, with the average reported in one cases series to be 9 days, with a range of 2–21 days [6]. Other authors have stated that clinical signs may occur months after the injury, due to prolonged viability of spores in tissues [5].

Equine Neurology, Second Edition. Martin Furr and Stephen Reed.
© 2015 John Wiley & Sons, Inc. Published 2015 by John Wiley & Sons, Inc.
Companion website: www.wiley.com/go/furr/neurology

Table 25.1 Clostridial neurotoxins and their target proteins.

Toxin	Target
Tetanus toxin	VAMP (synaptobrevin)
Botulinum toxin	
A	SNAP-25
B	VAMP (synaptobrevin)
C	SNAP-25 and syntaxin
D	VAMP (synaptobrevin)
E	SNAP-25
F	VAMP (synaptobrevin)
G	VAMP (synaptobrevin)

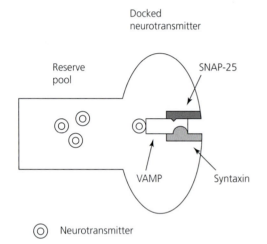

Figure 25.1 Schematic demonstrating the relationship of botulinum toxins at the motor end plate.

Clinical signs

The clinical signs of tetanus observed in horses are due to the effects of the neurotoxin on striated and smooth muscles. Examination reveals a diffuse, symmetrical hypertonicity and hyperresponsiveness of all muscle groups. The severity and rate of progression of clinical signs vary depending upon the dose of neurotoxin and the size, age, and immune status of the infected animal. Initial signs observed may reflect the location of the injury, but in almost all cases progress rapidly to a diffuse, symmetrical tetanic spasm of muscles. The most common clinical signs are hyperesthesia and prolapse of the third eyelid, both of which were seen in 85% of cases [6].

Early signs include reluctance or inability to feed off the ground due to spasm of the neck muscles, a mildly stiff gait, or hyperresponsiveness to external stimuli such as sound or unexpected motion (exaggerated "startle" response). Contraction of the facial muscles results in an "anxious" expression with retracted lips, flared nostrils, and erect ears (*risus sardonicus*). Prolapse of the nictitating membrane is seen due to retraction of the globe. Prolapse of the nictitating membrane can be accentuated ("flick of the haw") by tapping on the forehead or making a sudden noise. Progressive tetany of skeletal muscles results in a stiff gait, with rigid extension of the neck and limbs, resulting in the classic "sawhorse" stance. Spasms of muscles may result in a ventral or lateral arching of the neck or back. Dysphagia may occur due to involvement of the muscles of mastication and swallowing, and retention of feces and urine can occur. Spasm of the muscles of mastication (trismus) and elevation of the tail head are also commonly seen.

The tetanus toxin also affects the autonomic system, and in humans labile hypertension and tachycardia are commonly seen [7, 8]. Tachycardia is commonly seen in horses with tetanus; however, it is difficult to conclusively state if this is due to the direct action of the toxin on the autonomic nervous system, or rather a response to the discomfort, anxiety, and struggling that the horse may experience when afflicted with tetanus.

As the severity of the tetany progresses, horses usually become recumbent. Efforts to stand result in clonic/tonic spasms, which may be confused with convulsions. In this case, however, the horse remains conscious of its surroundings and responds to external stimuli—this is not observed in horses with seizures. Prolonged and uninhibited muscle contraction can result in fracture of long bones, and self-induced trauma during this activity can be severe.

Death usually occurs due to paralysis of respiratory muscles and is seen within 5–7 days of the initial clinical signs. Bloating associated with GI stasis may result in colic and/or respiratory embarrassment. Complications such as aspiration pneumonia, rhabdomyolysis, and subsequent renal disease can be seen and may be severe and fatal. The reported mortality rate is high (up to 75%) and is highly dependent on prior immunization status [6]. Those horses that had been vaccinated within 1 year of the intoxication had a significantly higher survival rate.

Treatment

Treatment of tetanus in the adult horse is a considerable challenge and the general principles of treatment are (i) destruction of *C. tetani* organism, (ii) neutralization of unbound toxin, and (iii) control of muscle spasms. In addition, good nursing care is of particular importance in overall response.

Destruction of the organism is achieved most commonly with the use of appropriate antibiotics, combined with wound debridement if possible. Historically, penicillin has been recommended in the veterinary literature at various dosages up to 50 000 IU/kg for the first

2 days of treatment [5]. The chemical structure of peni-cillin is similar to GABA, an important inhibitory neuro-transmitter, and penicillin may act as a competitive antagonist [7]. High doses of penicillin may therefore synergize with tetanus toxin to block GABA activity and worsen clinical signs. Recent comparative studies in human tetanus have demonstrated metronidazole to be superior to penicillin and is the preferred antimicrobial [7]. Other antibiotics of value include erythromycin, doxycycline, and chloramphenicol. If the wound cannot be adequately debrided, then increasing the antimicro-bial dosage is a reasonable course of action. Antimicrobial treatment should be continued for at least 10 days, the ultimate goal being to ensure death of the spore form of the bacteria in tissues. The value of hyperbaric oxygen therapy in horses with tetanus (to aid clearance of the organism) is unknown, but may be considered.

Neutralization of toxin is achieved by treatment with tetanus antitoxin (TAT), in most cases given either IV or IM. TAT will neutralize only circulating toxin, however, and has no effect upon toxin that has entered the ner-vous system or is within neurons. Recommended dos-ages of TAT vary widely and the optimum dose is not known. Doses of TAT as high as 2.5 million IU (once) or 220 IU/kg q12 h have been suggested by some authors. Others have suggested that a dose of 5–10 000 IU is probably adequate, as the amount of circulating toxin is usually very low. One study suggests that daily treatment with TAT (2500 IU subcutaneously for 3 days) following an initial dose had better outcomes [6]. In those horses in which adequate wound debridement cannot be obtained, or in which clinical signs have been present for more than 1 day, higher dosages of TAT are justified. It is important that TAT be given before aggressive wound debridement occurs, as a release of toxin may occur during or following this procedure.

An alternative means of neutralizing tetanus toxin is via intrathecal (subarachnoid) administration of TAT. This means of delivery bypasses the blood–CSF barrier and allows at least some unbound toxin to be neutral-ized. In one study, this mode of treatment was consid-ered to result in a rapid halt of the progression of the clinical signs, with a survival of 77%, as compared to a survival of 50% in historical controls [9]. In another report, 16 horses with a field diagnosis of tetanus were treated with 30 000 IU TAT intrathecally, and of these 10 horses (62.5%) recovered; 77% of horses that were not recumbent at the time of treatment recovered [10]. No seizures were noted among the horses of this study, which was reported in another case series using intra-thecal administration of TAT [9]. Using intrathecal therapy with TAT, the progression of signs was halted, but not reversed, and hence this therapy is obviously most beneficial early in the course of illness. In another study, five horses treated with intrathecal TAT did not survive; however, treated horses in this study were very severely affected prior to administering the TAT [6]. If clinical signs are allowed to progress, and intrathecal TAT is considered a treatment of last resort, then results are likely to be poor. In addition, this treatment is not without potential complications as seizures were reported in one of the five horses following intrathecal TAT [6]. The risks of anesthesia must be considered if the atlantooccipital (AO) site is used.

Intrathecal administration of TAT can be performed at either the AO or lumbosacral site, and there is no clear benefit of one site over the other. AO administration requires general anesthesia; however, the bulk flow of cerebrospinal fluid (CSF) from a cranial to caudal direction may ensure the most opportunity for toxin–antitoxin interaction. A total of 5–30 000 IU of TAT is slowly admin-istered after removal of an equal volume of CSF. The con-comitant use of 20–100 mg prednisolone sodium succinate has been advocated to minimize meningeal inflammation but is an unproven adjunctive therapy.

In addition to TAT, it is important to provide active immunization using tetanus toxoid at the earliest oppor-tunity. This should be administered at standard dosages and at a site distant from the injection site from the TAT to minimize interaction. Naturally occurring infection does not appear to result in protection against future disease.

Control of muscle spasms is often difficult in horses with tetanus but is important in the overall success of management. The ideal drug or drug combination has not been determined, but a number of options exist. Centrally acting muscle relaxants, such as methocarba-mol and glycerol guaiacolate, are probably the best choice as they block polysynaptic reflex activity in the brainstem and spinal cord. Methocarbamol (10–20 mg/kg q8 h) is relatively inexpensive and efficacious in mild cases. Glycerol guaiacolate has a very short duration of action, and horses with tetanus given this drug often go down, but it has been suggested that it can be used by slow continuous infusion, titrated to effect. Diazepam reduces anxiety and muscle spasms by potentiating the release of GABA and has been proven beneficial in humans with severe tetanus [11, 12]. It is quite useful in horses with tetanus, particularly when combined with alpha-2 agonists such as xylazine [6]. Chlorpromazine or acepromazine are probably the most commonly employed, and are useful in mild cases, but are often ineffective in more severe cases.

On an interesting historical note, one of the earliest reported drugs for the treatment of tetanus in the horse was curare, which was reported to be used in two horses with tetanus in 1835, as reported by McIntyre [13]. Several other historical attempts were described by Smithcors, and though the initial beneficial clinical effects of the curare were apparently quiet remarkable, all the horses died within a few hours [13].

Overall management of horses with tetanus is very important in the outcome of the case. Horse that cannot eat or drink should be appropriately supported using an indwelling nasogastric tube, or intravenously. Repeated passage of a nasogastric tube should be minimized due to the risk of aspiration pneumonia in a dysphagic horse, and intravenous fluids may be optimal. Manual evacuation of the bladder and rectum may be necessary. Horses can be aided to remain standing by use of a sling if they will tolerate it, and they should be maintained in a quiet, darkened stall with minimal stimulation. Horses that are recumbent have a very poor prognosis, and early euthanasia should be considered.

Diagnosis

There is no specific antemortem test for the diagnosis of tetanus in the horse. Clinical signs are quite characteristic; however, given the very low prevalence of this disease in most horse-rearing areas, it is often "forgotten" as a possibility. Clinical signs of diffuse, symmetrical muscle tetany, prolapsed nictitating membranes, and history of recent wound or trauma provide strong evidence for tetanus. The clinical signs could be confused with azoturia/exertional rhabdomyolysis; however, the clinical history would in most cases be revealing. Hypomagnesemia can result in muscle fasciculations, tetany, and *risus sardonicus*. This can be ruled out with an assay of serum magnesium. Poisoning with strychnine will also result in very similar clinical signs. As noted earlier, in horses that are recumbent, tetanic paddling can resemble seizure activity, and this possibility should be ruled out by careful neurologic examination.

Clinical chemistry evaluation is often unremarkable in horses with tetanus or may reflect nonspecific changes of infection, dehydration, or increased muscle activity from muscle spasms and recumbency. Electromyography will reflect prolonged insertional activity, and nerve conduction velocities are normal. CSF evaluation is unremarkable. Serum antibody titers for *C. tetani* may be performed but are unlikely to add significant diagnostic value during the clinical phase of the disease.

Postmortem examination reveals no findings specific for tetanus. Signs of recumbency may be seen, as well as evidence of a penetrating, infected wound. Culture of infected tracts and confirmation of the presence of *C. tetani* by appropriate microbiological methods would support the final diagnosis. Smears made from infected wounds will demonstrate the characteristic "badminton racket" or "drumstick" appearance. Presence of toxin can be confirmed by homogenizing tissue and treating with 50% ethanol for 1 h. The homogenate is then centrifuged and the 0.2 ml of supernate injected into the muscle of naïve and antitoxin-treated mice. Clinical signs of tetanus, or death, will be observed in the unprotected mice within 3 days [4].

Prophylaxis

The control of tetanus is readily achieved by active immunization with any number of commercially available vaccines. Most require an initial vaccine series, followed by annual revaccination. Vaccinated horses with injuries and deep wounds, or those undergoing elective surgical procedures should be given a booster. Vaccine titers probably last up to at least 4 years following a booster [14]. In a review of 20 cases, however, horses that had been vaccinated within 1 year of the illness had a better prognosis than those that had not been vaccinated within 1 year of the wound [6]. This suggests that antibody titers had declined to suboptimal concentrations.

Unvaccinated horses, or those in which the vaccination history is unknown, should receive 1500 IU of TAT following injury, or before emergency surgery. Tetanus toxoid should be administered at the same time, at a separate site from the TAT, and then boostered if the horse is unvaccinated. There is an association of acute hepatic necrosis (Theiler's disease) following TAT administration; however, this should not be an argument against the use of TAT in those circumstances.

Pregnant mares that were vaccinated in the last month of pregnancy generally provide adequate passive immunity to tetanus in colostrum, which may last up to 3 months of age. Hence, it is reasonable to begin tetanus prophylaxis at 3 months of age. In addition, TAT (1500 IU, IM) can be given to foals at birth if there is any question regarding the mare's vaccination status or the foal's consumption of colostrum. It has been recommended that foals should be given toxoid at 3, 4, and 6 months of age and then annually thereafter [6].

Botulism

Botulism is caused by intoxication with the exotoxin of *Clostridium botulinum* (*botulinum neurotoxin*). The organism was recovered from the soil in 18.5% of soil samples tested in the United States. *C. botulinum* produces several different subtypes of toxin, which are identified as type A, B, C_1, C_2, D, E, F, and G [15]. The distribution of the different toxin subtypes varies, however, with type A found in west of the US Rocky Mountains and type C found most commonly in Europe. Some cases of equine botulism from type C, however, have been reported from Florida, California, New England, Arizona, and Canada, and hence may not be as uncommon in the United States as was once thought [16–20]. Type-C botulism has also been reported in Australia [21]. Type-B toxin is most commonly found in the Mid-Atlantic region of the United States, and Kentucky, and historically is the most commonly reported cause of botulism in the United States (>85%)

[22]. More recent reports of type-A mediated disease may suggest that it is more common than previously supposed, however. Type-A intoxication has been documented to arise from contamination of forage (hay) and grass clippings [23, 24]. Type-B botulism seems to be most commonly associated with silage, while type C appears to be more commonly seen when forage is contaminated with carcasses, and in one outbreak of type-C botulism, fur and tissue of an unidentified mammal were found in the hay cubes that caused botulism in 38 horses [19]. Type-D botulism is rare in horses but was suspected in one outbreak of botulism in horses in California [25]. The use of large and round bale hay has also been incriminated as a risk factor for botulism in horses, and storing the bales in plastic bags appears to increase the risk [26, 27]. Apparently, the common practice of storing such hay outdoors, where it can become wet, leads to proper conditions for the growth of *C. botulinum*. Any form of wet hay however, even small square bales, can be a source of botulism toxin [28]. While individual cases on a premise can be seen, outbreaks involving large numbers of horses can be seen due to feed contamination [19, 20, 24]. This is an important observation as all horses on a premise should be evaluated once a single case is observed.

Like other organism of the genus *Clostridium*, *C. botulinum* forms spores which withstand extremes of temperature and humidity and which vegetate and grow under anaerobic conditions and an alkaline or neutral pH (pH > 4.5). Once the organism begins to grow, the toxin is elaborated. Sporulation, replication, and toxin elaboration cannot occur in an acidic environment (pH < 6), and hence poorly made silage has been a source of intoxication [29, 30]. The increased incidence of botulism in Europe has been proposed to be associated with the increased use of grass silage, in many cases associated with type-B botulism [31, 32].

Pathophysiology

There are three major mechanisms by which intoxication occurs in equine botulism. Ingestion of preformed toxin ("forage poisoning") from the environment is probably the most common source of intoxication in adult horses. A second source is elaboration of toxin from *C. botulinum* infection in wounds (wound botulism), such as castration sites [33]. One case of wound botulism was associated with an injection site abscess [34] and infection of umbilical remnants of foals is also considered wound botulism. A final mechanism is the ingestion of *C. botulinum* spores, which then vegetate and produce toxin within the GI tract (toxicoinfectious botulism) [35, 36]. This is usually attributed to type-B toxin, although this mechanism was also assumed in several reported outbreaks of type-A botulism [22, 24]. It has been proposed that inflammatory sites within the

GI tract, such as gastric ulcers, may be sites for toxin production, yet this hypothesis remains unproven [36].

Clinical signs

The clinical signs of botulism are fundamentally derived from a consideration of the pathophysiology of the disorder. The botulism toxin results in a diffuse, flaccid paralysis and loss of muscle strength. Clinical abnormalities are symmetrical, which is an important observation in evaluating such cases, and all aspects of the clinical examination findings reflect this fact. The clinical signs are the same regardless of the mechanism of infection and recent reports suggest that the clinical signs associated with different toxin types are similar, although there may be differences in toxin potency, with type A seemingly more toxic than types B or C [24].

Clinical signs can be seen at any time from 12 h to 10 days following ingestion of the toxin [22]. Initial signs often include subtle signs of dysphagia or muscular weakness or horses may be found dead. The severity of clinical signs and the rapidity of progression depend upon the amount of toxin ingested. Early clinical signs that may be seen include generalized muscle weakness leading to a lowered head carriage, slow eating, and a shuffling gait with toe dragging. Colic has been the initial presenting complaint in some reports [18, 22].

Constitutional signs are usually normal, although mild dehydration may be seen as the condition progresses and horses are unable to drink. Tachycardia may be seen in horses that struggle to stand, but heart rate is normal early in the course of the disease. Constipation, urine dribbling, or bladder distention may be seen. In more severe cases, an exaggerated respiratory effort, associated with a normal or reduced respiratory rate may be seen; aspiration pneumonia may be present.

A thorough neurologic examination will reveal mydriasis and ptosis generally early in the clinical course of the illness. A slow pupillary light reflex may be seen, but this is often difficult to assess and equivocal. Tail tone is often diminished in clinical cases; however, it has been reported to be variable in experimental induction of the disease [37]. Muscle trembling and fasciculations of large muscle groups is common in standing horses. Tongue tone is diminished and delayed retraction of the tongue when pulled from the horse's mouth is commonly seen. Horses normally retract the tongue very quickly; horses with botulism will withdraw the tongue slowly and with difficulty and may be unable to do so. Dysphagia is commonly observed, and this can be tested by the horse's ability to swallow a stomach tube. In addition, prolonged time to consume a standard amount of grain has been used in experimental cases and was considered a good means to evaluate dysphagia ("grain test"). Normal horses were found to consume a 250 ml cup of grain in less than 2 min, while horses with experimentally induced botulism ate much more slowly and with greater difficulty [37]. The value of this test in clinical cases is not clearly established. Adult horses can be seen to immerse their entire muzzle under water to drink, and nursing foals will spill milk when nursing. These signs may be seen in other causes of dysphagia and are not specific to botulism.

Horses are weak but are not ataxic. Proprioceptive deficits are not present, but horses may be too weak to properly position the limb; careful observation is required to differentiate between the two. Stumbling and tripping are often seen, as horses do not pick their feet up when walking. This leads to a shuffling, slow gait. The head is typically held lower than normal and in severe cases may lead to head edema and respiratory stridor.

In foals, the clinical signs above can also be seen, but more commonly foals present with a history of excessive recumbency and muscle fasciculations ("shaker foal syndrome"). Foals are typically bright and alert when down—usually in a normal, sternal position. They may stand and appear to be normal for several minutes, then are observed to demonstrate diffuse fine muscle fasciculations that progress to coarse muscle trembling, and then stumbling followed by recumbency. When lying down, the muscle fasciculations cease and the foal looks normal once again. This cycle may be repeated several times or may progress rapidly to complete recumbency rapidly, depending upon the dose of toxin acquired and the time since intoxication.

Diagnosis

A presumptive diagnosis of botulism is based upon history and physical examination findings. An abrupt onset of diffuse, symmetrical weakness in a horse with normal mentation and the absence of central nervous system abnormalities support the diagnosis. Ancillary diagnostic testing includes complete blood cell count, serum biochemistry analysis, and CSF evaluation.

Clinical pathology results are within normal limits in most cases, although results may reflect dehydration or muscle damage from recumbency. In cases of wound botulism, the CBC may reflect signs of infection. CSF evaluation is normal in horses with botulism and helps to rule out many infectious and traumatic illnesses.

The clinical signs of botulism are fairly characteristic in the more advanced stages but can be confusing early in the course of the disease. The absence of abnormal constitutional signs and clinical pathology results help to eliminate many infectious and toxic conditions. The "grain test" can be used as a screening procedure; however, it is important to rule out other causes of slow eating (e.g., depression, dental disease, fractured jaw, and oral foreign body). Principal diagnostic rule-outs for diffuse weakness and muscle fasciculations include

white muscle disease, hyperkalemic period paralysis (HYPP), electrolyte abnormality (hypocalcemia, hypomagnesemia) and ionophore, white snake root, lead, and organophosphate toxicity. Rabies and yellow star thistle toxicity can result in dysphagia, but rabies will result in hyperexcitability and diffuse CNS inflammation. HYPP can be confused with botulism, but signs are episodic and is associated with an increase in potassium concentrations, of which neither is seen with botulism. Dysphagia can be caused by guttural pouch mycosis and this can be confirmed or ruled out by endoscopic examination (Table 25.2).

A diagnosis is further supported by (i) finding preformed toxin in the feed, GI contents, or wounds of an affected horse, (ii) demonstration of *C. botulism* spores in the GI contents or feed, or (iii) detection of an antibody response in a convalescent patient [22]. Definitive diagnosis requires confirmation of toxin in serum, plasma, GI contents or wounds.

A mouse bioassay (MBA) is the most sensitive test for the detection of botulinum toxin. Serum from a suspect horse is injected into ICR Swiss Webster mice and they are observed for signs of botulism. Additional mice are pretreated with polyvalent antiserum, and if protected, the presence of botulism toxin is confirmed. If necessary, further testing can be conducted using specific monovalent antiserum to determine specific toxin type. The MBA is rarely positive in clinical cases, however, because the horse is so susceptible to the toxin that it may demonstrate clinical signs when concentrations of toxin are so low that it does not produce clinical signs in the mice. Only a few cases have been reported in which the presence of circulating toxin was confirmed.

An ELISA test has been developed for the assay of fluids for the presence of type C and D botulinum toxin. This test is not considered as specific as the MBA, due to cross reactivity with *C. novyi*. This test is not available commercially at the present time. A PCR test for the type-B neurotoxin gene has also been developed and validated for equine samples [38]. A sensitivity or 96% and specificity of 95% has been reported for this test,

Table 25.2 Differential considerations for botulism and tetanus.

Tetanus	Botulism
Exertional rhabdomyolysis	White muscle disease
	HYPP
Hypomagnesemia	Hypocalcemia
Strychnine toxicity	White snakeroot toxicity
Laminitis	Ionophore toxicity
	Lead intoxication
	Organophosphate toxicity

which is available by submission to the Botulism Laboratory of New Bolton Center, Kennett Square, PA.

Given the difficulty and rarity of detecting circulating toxin, botulism is most commonly supported by finding *C. botulinum* spores in feed or GI content. Spores are rarely reported in the feces of normal horses but are found in up to 70% of shaker foals [22]. In one study, 3.2% of normal horses were found to have *C. botulinum* spores in feces [22].

Detection of antibody in serum of affected (but non-vaccinated) horses has been reported and may prove to be a useful means of confirming infection [22].

Electromyography has been described as a means to diagnose botulism in horses. Repetitive nerve stimulation produces a decremental response in evoked muscle. This is rarely described in the horse and one author has reported it to be of minimal value in the diagnosis of botulism in horses [22, 39].

Treatment

The fundamental principle of treating botulism in horses is the neutralization of circulating toxin. This is readily achieved by the administration of botulism antitoxin. The disease is highly fatal if horses are not treated with antitoxin, although mildly affected horses may survive. At the present time, there are two commercial sources for botulism antiserum: a trivalent (types A, B, and C) antitoxin (Lake Immunogenics, Ontario, NY) or a monovalent antitoxin (type B) (Plasvacc, Templetone, CA). In the authors' experience, one treatment is usually adequate. Clinical signs may progress for a period of 12–24 h after antitoxin treatment, as antitoxin has no effect after the toxin has been internalized into the neuron. Early treatment is critical and will minimize the severity of the clinical signs.

Elimination of the organism may be necessary in cases of wound or toxicoinfectious botulism. In wound botulism, tissue debridement and disruption of the anaerobic environment are the most effective and may be aided by the use of antibiotics. Aminoglycosides, tetracyclines, and procaine penicillin are known to potentiate neuromuscular weakness and should be avoided. Potassium penicillin is preferred. Antibiotic treatment probably does not clear organism in the intestine and their use in such cases may not be justified.

A variety of compounds have been proposed to counter the physiologic effects of botulinum toxin. Neostigmine and 4-aminopyridine will increase acetylcholine release in the NMJ and result in increased muscular strength in horses with botulism. The increased strength, however, is very temporary and overall mortality is higher in horses treated with these compounds, as they exhaust the acetylcholine (ACH) that is present. Therefore, they should not be used.

Nursing care of horses with botulism is critical to overall success. Affected horses should be maintained in a quiet environment such that they can conserve energy and do not have to compete with other animals. Horses frequently develop ileus and withholding food is often necessary. Treatment with mineral oil to soften stool may aid passage, and manual evacuation of the rectum and bladder is sometimes necessary. If horses are able to remain standing, they often develop dependent edema of the head, as it remains in a dependant position. The head can be tied up and nasotracheal tubes can be passed to maintain a patent airway and block muzzle swelling. Hydration status can be maintained with oral fluids, or if ileus is present, using intravenous fluids. Horses may aspirate food material and can develop aspiration pneumonia, and hence they may need to be withheld from eating. Nutritional support is necessary and can be achieved by feeding a slurry through a feeding tube, or more effectively, using intravenous nutrition. Antibiotic treatment is necessary in horses with aspiration pneumonia. Ocular lubricants are useful as some horses develop dry-eye.

Horses with botulism should not be maintained in a sling, as this tends to exhaust them and leads to increased mortality. Severely affected animals develop respiratory distress due to hypoventilation, which is the ultimate cause of death. Use of a sling compresses the chest and further compromises respiration. Mechanical ventilation is required in severe cases, and is highly rewarding in foal cases, but is probably not possible in horses that weigh more than 400 lbs. Horses that are recumbent usually remain so for about 7–10 days, so treatment of such animals should not begin unless the owner is committed to a lengthy hospitalization. Horses that are recumbent can be maintained on a king-size human water bed. These beds are particularly comfortable (apparently) as the water can be warmed, and it distributes the horse's weight; the bed should be filled only enough to "lift" the hip bones off the ground. Horses maintained in this manner seem to rest comfortably and not struggle as they do on other types of padding. In addition, there is little to no skin excoriation from small movements that are often seen with recumbent horses on some types of padding. Muscular recovery takes up to 10 days which is the time required for regeneration of docking proteins in the NMJ—to return to full strength may take up to 1 month [22]. Improvement in muscle strength may be noted prior to this but will not be complete and will be dependent on the initial degree of weakness present. The more severe the weakness, the longer the recovery takes (Figure 25.2).

Prognosis

The outcome is dependent on the amount of toxin present, and perhaps also the toxin type, as well as the horse's age. It is difficult to compare survival between

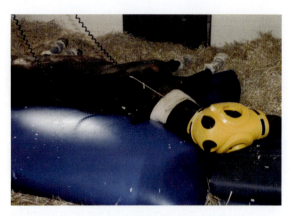

Figure 25.2 An adult horse with botulism being cared for on a human king-size waterbed. These are very useful for managing recumbent horses.

different toxin types due to differences in reporting and treatment; however, the case fatality rate in several type-A outbreaks described by Johnson et al. [24] found a mean case mortality of approximately 90%, with a median case mortality of 100%, while a large outbreak of type C had an 80% case fatality rate [19], and a mean, combined case fatality rate of about 70% was seen in several outbreaks involving type-B toxin [28, 29, 33].

As it is not generally possible to know the toxin type or amount consumed at the time of initial examination, prognosis is difficult. In general, horses that are able to stand at the time that definitive treatment (e.g., appropriate antitoxin) is administered usually do well, while those that are recumbent at the time of antitoxin treatment have a much lower chance of survival (perhaps no better than 20%). In one report of horses treated with the appropriate antitoxin, only one of three horses recumbent at the time of treatment survived, while six of seven horses that were standing at the time of treatment survived [19]. Success of treatment of adults is often determined by the complications of recumbency, with pneumonia and decubital ulceration being the most common complications. Foals are much easier to maintain overall and have a higher survival rate than adults. Johnson reported a survival rate of 96% in foals treated at a hospital [40].

Prophylaxis

In North America, a vaccine against type-B botulism is currently available. An initial vaccination is followed by a booster in 3 weeks, with annual revaccination recommended. The vaccine appears to be highly effective, but infection with other serotypes is possible as there is no cross-protection between different toxin types. Horses that reside in an endemic area should be vaccinated, as well as horses that are feed round bale hay or silage.

Pregnant mares in endemic areas should be vaccinated and given a booster 4–6 weeks before anticipated foaling. Foals from unvaccinated mares can be transiently and passively protected using the antitoxin, or vaccinated with the toxoid, although it is not labeled for foals.

References

[1] Coleman, E.S. (1998) Clostridial neurotoxins: tetanus and botulism. *Comp Cont Ed Pract Vet*, 20, 1089–1096.

[2] Bleck, T. (1986) Pharmacology of tetanus. *Clin Neuropharmacol*, 9, 103–120.

[3] Montecucco, C. and Shiavo, G. (1994) Mechanism of action of tetanus and botulinum neurotoxins. *Mol Microbiol*, 13, 1–8.

[4] Timoney, J.F., Gillespie, J.H., Scott, F.W. *et al.* (1988) The genus Clostridium, In: *Hagan and Bruner's Microbiology and Infectious Diseases of Domestic Animals* (eds J.F. Timoney, J.H. Gillespie, F.W. Scott and J.E. Barlough), Comstock Publishing Associates, Ithaca, NY, pp. 214–222.

[5] Hahn, C.N., Mayhew, I.G. and MacKay, R.J. (1999) Diseases of the brainstem and cranial nerves, In: *Equine Medicine and Surgery*, 5th edn (eds P.T. Colahan, A.M. Merritt, J.N. Moore and I.G. Mayhew), Mosby, St. Louis, MO, pp. 931–944.

[6] Green, S.L., Little, C.B., Baird, J.D. *et al.* (1994) Tetanus in the horse: a review of 20 cases (1970–1990). *J Vet Intern Med*, 8, 128–132.

[7] Goonetilleke, A. and Harris, J.B. (2004) Clostridial neurotoxins. *J Neurol Neurosurg Psychiatry*, 74 (s3), 35–39.

[8] Wright, D.K., Lalloo, U.G. and Nayiager, S. (1989) Autonomic nervous system dysfunction in severe tetanus: current perspectives. *Crit Care Med*, 17, 371–375.

[9] Muylle, E., Oyaert, W., Ooms, L. *et al.* (1975) Treatment of tetanus in the horse by injections of tetanus antitoxin into the subarachnoid space. *J Am Vet Med Assoc*, 167, 47–48.

[10] Fisher, R.J. (2005) The treatment of tetanus in horses using intrathecal injection of tetanus antitoxin. *UK Vet*, 10, 1–3.

[11] Odusote, K.A., George, B.O. and Femi-Pearse, D. (1976) Favorable prognosis of prolonged coma associated with large doses of diazepam in severe tetanus. *Trop Geogr Med*, 28, 194–198.

[12] Weinstein, L. (1973) Current concepts: tetanus. *N Engl J Med*, 289, 1293–1296.

[13] Smithcors, J.F. (1956) The treatment of tetanus with curare – a little known chapter in veterinary history. *J Am Vet Med Assoc*, 129, 303–305.

[14] Jansen, B.C. and Knoetze, P.C. (1979) The immune response of horses to tetanus toxoid. *Onderstepoort J Vet Res*, 46, 211–216.

[15] Horowitz, B.Z. (2005) Botulinum toxin. *Crit Care Clin*, 21, 825–839.

[16] MacKay, R.J. and Berkhoff, G.A. (1982) Type C toxicoinfectious botulism in a foal. *J Am Vet Med Assoc*, 180, 163–164.

[17] Semrad, S. and Peek, S. (2002) Equine botulism. *Comp Cont Ed Pract Vet*, 24, 169–172.

[18] Heath, S.E., Bell, R.J. and Harland, R.J. (1988) Botulinum type C intoxication in a mare. *Can Vet J*, 29, 530–531.

[19] Kinde, H., Betty, R.L. and Ardans, A. (1991) Clostridium botulinum type-C intoxication associated with consumption of processed hay cubes in horses. *J Am Vet Med Assoc*, 199, 742–746.

[20] Schoenbaum, M.A., Hall, S.M., Glock, R.D. *et al.* (2000) An outbreak of type C botulism in 12 horses and a mule. *J Am Vet Med Assoc*, 217, 365–368.

[21] Hutchins, R. (1994) Preliminary report on an outbreak of botulism. *Aust Equine Vet*, 12, 54–55.

[22] Whitlock, R.H. and Buckley, C. (1997) Botulism. *Vet Clin N Am Equine Pract*, 13, 107–128.

[23] Ostrowski, S.R., Kubiski, S.V., Palmero, J. *et al.* (2012) An outbreak of equine botulism type A associated with feeding grass clippings. *J Vet Diagn Invest*, 24, 601–603.

[24] Johnson, A.L., McAdams, S.C., Whitlock, R.H. *et al.* (2010) Type A botulism in the United States: a review of the past ten years (1998–2008). *J Vet Diagn Invest*, 22, 165–173.

[25] Switzer, J.W., Jensen, M. and Reimann, H.P. (1984) An outbreak of suspected type D botulism in horses in California. *Calif Vet*, 7, 14–17.

[26] Hunter, J.M., Rohrbach, B.W., Andrews, F. *et al.* (2002) Round bale grass hay: a risk factor for botulism in horses. *Comp Cont Ed Pract Vet*, 24, 169–172.

[27] Broughton, J. and Parsons, L. (1985) Botulism in horses fed big bale silage. *Vet Rec*, 117, 674.

[28] Wichtel, J.J. and Whitlock, R.H. (1991) Botulism associated with feeding alfalfa hay to horses. *J Am Vet Med Assoc*, 199, 471–474.

[29] Ricketts, S.W., Greet, T.C.R., Glyn, P.J. *et al.* (1984) Thirteen cases of botulism in horses fed big bale silage. *Equine Vet J*, 16, 515–518.

[30] Divers, T.J., Bartholomew, R.C., Messick, J.B. *et al.* (1986) Clostridium botulinum type B toxicosis in a herd of cattle and a group of mules. *J Am Vet Med Assoc*, 188, 382–386.

[31] Goehring, L.S., van Maanen, C. and van Oldruitenborgh-Oosterbaan, S. (2005) Neurologic syndromes among horses in The Netherlands. A 5 year retrospective survey (1999–2004). *Vet Q*, 27, 11–20.

[32] Haagsma, J., Haesebrouck, F., Devriese, L. *et al.* (1990) An outbreak of botulism type B in horses. *Vet Rec*, 127, 206.

[33] Bernard, W., Divers, T.J., Whitlock, R.H. *et al.* (1987) Botulism as a sequel to open castration in a horse. *J Am Vet Med Assoc*, 191, 73–74.

[34] Mitten, L.A., Hinchcliff, K.W., Holcombe, S.J. *et al.* (1994) Mechanical ventilation and management of botulism secondary to an injection abscess in an adult horse. *Equine Vet J*, 26, 420–423.

[35] Swerczek, T.W. (1980) Experimentally induced toxicoinfectious botulism in horses and foals. *Am J Vet Res*, 41, 348–350.

[36] Swerczek, T.W. (1980) Toxicoinfectious botulism in foals and adult horses. *J Am Vet Med Assoc*, 176, 217–220.

[37] Whitlock, R.H. (1995) Botulism type C experimental and field cases in the horse. *Proc Ann Meet Am Coll Vet Int Med*, 13, 720–723.

[38] Johnson, A.L., Sweeney, R.W., McAdams, S.C. *et al.* (2012) Quantitative real-time PCR for detection of the neurotoxin gene of *Clostridium botulinum* type B in equine and bovine samples. *Vet J*, 194, 118–120.

[39] Divers, T.J., Bartholemew, R.C., Messick, J.B. *et al.* (1992) Equine motor neuron disease: a new cause of weakness, trembling, and weight loss. *Comp Cont Ed Equine Pract*, 14, 1223–1226.

[40] Johnson, A.L. (2013) Advances in the diagnosis and treatment of botulism. *Proc Ann Meet Am Coll Vet Int Med*, 31, 209–212.

26 Neurodegenerative Disorders

Robert J. MacKay

College of Veterinary Medicine, University of Florida, Gainesville, USA

Equine degenerative myeloencephalopathy

History and epidemiology

Since the original description in 1976 [1], equine degenerative myeloencephalopathy (EDM) and the related condition neuroaxonal dystrophy (NAD) [2] have been reported throughout the world in horses and ponies of many different breeds and in other equids including donkeys, Przewalski's horses, and zebras [3, 4]. The clinical signs of EDM and NAD are identical and the associated central nervous system (CNS) lesions are thought to be on a continuum with EDM lesions more widely distributed than are those of NAD [3, 4]. For the rest of this section, both conditions will be referred to as EDM.

Clinical signs usually begin within the first year of life and, with only a few reported exceptions, all have begun by 3 years of age [5]. A hereditary basis for the condition has been strongly suggested by the results of breeding studies or pedigree analyses in Morgan, Appaloosa, and Lusitano horses [4, 6, 7]. The mode of inheritance was suspected to be polygenic or dominant with variable expression [4, 6]. A familial basis also has been suspected because of clustering of cases among the progeny of particular Standardbreds, Paso Finos, Norwegian Fjord horses, Arabians, Welsh ponies, Haflingers, and Quarter Horses [8].

Overcrowding, lack of access to fresh green forage, pelleted feed, and poor quality hay were thought to be risk factors on two affected premises [9]. In another study, significant risk factors were exposure to insecticides/repellents, exposure to wood preservatives such as creosote, and time spent on dirt lots [5]. Time spent on green pasture was a protective factor. By contrast, several clusters of cases in Oregon and California occurred in horses on pasture [7, 8]. In the California series, the pasture was growing on volcanic soil that was deficient in selenium and vitamin E [8].

With rare exceptions [5, 10], there has been a consistent association reported between EDM and marginal or low serum/plasma vitamin E concentration. Published normal ranges for α tocopherol vary with age, location, season, diet, and use; however, a commonly accepted scheme classifies results >2.0 μg/ml as normal, 1.5–2.0 μg/ml as marginal, and <1.5 μg/ml as deficient [9, 11]. Healthy horses sharing feedstuffs and environment with affected horses usually also have low vitamin E although foals in an Appaloosa family with hereditary EDM had significantly lower plasma vitamin E than did age-matched normal pasture mates [12]. This difference was maintained continuously from 6 weeks to 10 months of age. During the approximately 15 years after it was first recognized, EDM was one of the most prevalent causes of spinal cord disease in horses presented to teaching hospitals in the United States [5]. Although no surveillance data have been published in recent years, it is widely believed that prevalence of EDM in the United States may have declined over the last 20 years.

Cause and pathogenesis

EDM most closely resembles vitamin E deficiency of humans and other animals [4, 8, 11]. The neuroprotective effects of vitamin E relate to inhibition of oxidation of CNS membrane lipids and facilitation of axonal transport of macromolecules [11]. Consistent with the notion of vulnerability of the CNS to oxidant damage in horses with low vitamin E, markers of oxidative injury were identified in CNS neurons of two horses with EDM [13]. Although familial isolated vitamin E deficiency of humans is caused by mutations in the α-tocopherol transfer protein (α-TTP) gene, expression of α-TTP mRNA was similar in four unaffected horses and four horses with EDM from a group of related Quarter Horse weanlings and yearlings [8]. Also, on the basis of an association analysis performed using single-nucleotide polymorphisms (SNPs) in the region and direct sequencing of the α-TTP gene, it is

Equine Neurology, Second Edition. Martin Furr and Stephen Reed.
© 2015 John Wiley & Sons, Inc. Published 2015 by John Wiley & Sons, Inc.
Companion website: www.wiley.com/go/furr/neurology

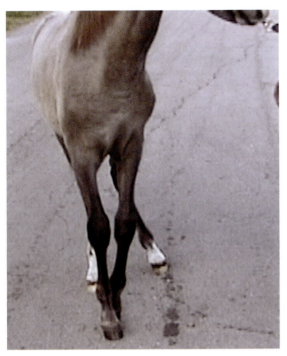

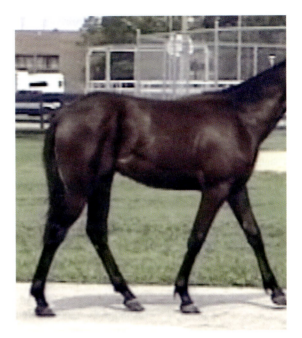

Figure 26.2 Two-beat "pacing" gait at walking speed in a yearling American Paso Fino filly. Limb ataxia was first noticed at approximately 1 month of age. The sire of this filly produced at least 15 other progeny that developed EDM.

Figure 26.1 Interference between thoracic limbs (left) and collapse of and picoting around the pelvic limbs in a 4-month-old Andalusian filly. This filly had shown clinical signs of limb ataxia and weakness since approximately 1 week of age. A full sibling born a year earlier also developed signs of EDM shortly after birth.

unlikely that genetic mutations in the gene are responsible for EDM [14]. Low serum vitamin E in horses with EDM is not explained by impaired intestinal absorption: oral vitamin E tolerance tests were normal in affected horses [12]. It is reasonable to speculate that there is a defect in at least one of the more than 30 known proteins involved in vitamin E absorption, transport, and metabolism [14]. For example, mutation-associated defects have been described in a lipoprotein carrier, an hepatic transfer protein, and a vitamin E receptor site [11, 12].

Clinical signs

EDM has an acute to occasionally insidious onset of symmetric ataxia and paresis of the trunk and limbs (Figure 26.1). The onset of clinical signs typically is between 1 and 12 months of age but has been seen in neonates and in mature horses [3, 4]. Posture and gait are wide-based. There is notable hypometria (spasticity) in affected limbs. Signs typically are considerably more severe in the pelvic limbs and the thoracic limbs may be clinically normal. In two recent reports, it was noted that limb weakness was only seen in horses with moderate or severe ataxia and was not recognized in many horses that were mildly ataxic [4, 8]. Some horses

with EDM adopt a two-beat lateral ("pacing") gait at walking speed (Figure 26.2). Long spinal reflexes such as the cervicofacial, laryngeal adductor (slap), and cutaneous trunci may be reduced or absent, especially in longstanding cases. Neurogenic muscle atrophy is not seen in horses with EDM and recently reported cases occurred in horses with body condition scores of five to six out of nine [4, 8]. Signs of brain dysfunction were not reported until recently. Among a group of Quarter Horses with EDM (NAD) 77/88 were described as dull or obtunded and minimally responsive to light flashes, sudden movement, or loud noises [8]. An electroencephalogram performed on one affected horse revealed dominant states of drowsiness to slow-wave sleep. Reduced or absent menace responses were noted in 33/88 Quarter Horses and 4/6 Lusitanos with EDM [4, 8]. Vision, pupillary light reflexes, ophthalmologic examinations, and electroretinograms were normal.

Signs may not worsen after initial onset; others progress for days to months before stabilizing. Only rarely does the condition progress to recumbency.

Laboratory findings

There is no antemortem diagnostic test for EDM. Plasma/serum vitamin E concentrations of EDM horses and pasture mates are often marginal or low. Because vitamin E concentrations within individual horses vary considerably over time (especially if they are low), it is recommended that three blood samples be taken over the course of 24 h [11, 12]. Samples must not be visibly hemolyzed and should be stored so that the blood is not in contact with the rubber stopper. Plasma creatine kinase (CK) and aspartate aminotransferase (AST) activities may be slightly to moderately high because of increased recumbency [7].

Diagnosis

Diagnosis antemortem is presumptive only and is made primarily by suggestive signalment and clinical signs with exclusion of competing diagnoses. EDM should be suspected in horses with symmetric limb ataxia that began within the first year of life and for which results of standard neurologic workups (cervical vertebral radiographs, cerebrospinal fluid (CSF) analysis, immunoassay for *S. neurona* antibody) have not implicated another diagnosis. Low or marginal serum/plasma vitamin E concentration (≤2.0 µg/ml) is supportive of the diagnosis.

Differential diagnoses include conditions associated with spinal cord compression, particularly cervical vertebral stenotic myelopathy, occipitoatlantoaxial malformation and vertebral trauma, inflammatory spinal cord diseases including equine protozoal myeloencephalitis (EPM) and West Nile virus myeloencephalitis, or spinal cord ischemia associated with equine herpesvirus 1 myeloencephalopathy or fibrocartilaginous myelopathy.

Necropsy findings

There are no abnormal gross necropsy findings. Histologic changes develop in the spinal cord and brain stem [11, 4, 7, 8]. In horses with NAD there are lesions in the lateral and medial cuneate, gracilis, and thoracic nuclei characterized by spheroid formation with vacuolation, loss of somata, astrogliosis, and lipofuscin pigment accumulation. Additionally, in horses with EDM, axonal necrosis and demyelination involve the dorsal and ventral spinocerebellar tracts and ventromedial funiculi of the cervicothoracic spinal cord. No histologic lesions were found to explain observations of dull mentation [15] and abnormal menace responses [4, 8] in recently reported case series.

Treatment and prevention

It is unlikely that EDM can be cured even if treated early. Slight to no improvement was seen in affected horses supplemented with 2000–8000 IU of vitamin E daily [7, 9, 15]. The type of vitamin E and the method of supplementation have important effects on its bioavailability. Natural water-soluble vitamin E (RRR-α-tocopherol) is up to twofold more active than synthetic vitamin E (D,L-α-tocopherol or all-rac-α-tocopherol). Absorption requires fat so bioavailability of vitamin E is negligible or low unless given with feed or vegetable oil.

Consistent with the notion that EDM is associated with some interaction between metabolic defect and

vitamin E deficiency, vitamin E supplementation appears to be at least partially effective prophylaxis and is recommended in circumstances in which there is familial predisposition, processed feed, lack of access to pasture, and exposure to insecticides or wood preservatives. In one study, the incidence of EDM was reduced from 36% over 3 years to 9% in the following year by supplementation of foals with 1500 IU vitamin E daily [9]. Similar results were seen in three other outbreaks [8, 9, 16]. Obviously, sensible genetic, nutritional, and other management practices alone could greatly reduce or eliminate the risk of EDM.

Equine motor neuron disease

Equine motor neuron disease (EMND) is an acquired degenerative disorder of the somatic lower motor neurons of the spinal cord and brainstem.

History and epidemiology

EMND was first reported in 1990 in 11 horses from 4 northeastern states [17]. Hundreds more cases occurred in the northeastern region of the United States over the subsequent 20 years and other cases were scattered elsewhere across the country [18, 19]. Additional solitary cases or outbreaks of EMND were reported in Great Britain, Canada, Ireland, Switzerland, Belgium, Japan, Brazil, and the Netherlands [18–20]. Annual incidence of EMND cases in the United States peaked in about 1997 and has now declined to low levels with less than one new admission annually to Cornell University College of Veterinary Medicine's Equine Animal Hospital [21].

The disease usually occurs sporadically, with only one case on a given premise at any time; however, one or more additional cases have occurred on the same premise within 2 years of the original diagnosis [18]. An unusual cluster of more than 80 cases was seen among horses in a city police cavalry in Brazil during the 1990s [18]. The age range of reported cases is 2–27 years [19, 22] with a mean of 9 years and estimated maximal risk at 16 years of age [23, 24].

In the United States, age and Quarter Horse breed [23] and age, breed, duration of residence, lack of recent rabies vaccination, exercising in a dirt paddock, a history of cribbing or coprophagia, use of pelleted feed (alone or with sweet feed), and use of vitamin/mineral supplements lacking vitamin E/selenium were significant nutritional risk factors in multivariate logistic regression models [24]. Most important, after controlling for other significant risk factors, a strong negative association was demonstrated between serum vitamin E concentration and EMND risk [25]. Interestingly, 13/32 cases in Europe had part- or full-time exposure to pasture, yet all had low plasma vitamin E, suggesting that bioavailability of ingested vitamin E was low in these pastured horses [22]. A horse in Finland developed EMND despite supplementation with 300 mg α-tocopherol daily for the previous 10 years [26]. In that case, daily supplementation with excessive amounts of iron was suggested as a possible cause. In the United States, horses with EMND that had normal access to pasture had enteric or hepatic disease, presumably resulting in malabsorption of vitamin E [19, 27].

Cause and pathogenesis

EMND is a spontaneous, progressive, sporadic, even solitary, condition that closely resembles progressive spinal muscular atrophy, a variant of amyotrophic lateral sclerosis (ALS; Lou Gehrig's disease) of humans [23]. Between 5 and 10% of ALS cases are considered familial and most of these are associated with mutations in the Cu/Zn superoxide dismutase (SOD1) gene. Sequencing of SOD1 mRNA (as cDNA) from horses with EMND did not reveal any known mutations [28]. Although sporadic ALS is likely multifactorial, it is widely believed that oxidative stress is involved in the final common pathways of neuronal injury. Evidence of systemic oxidant stress in horses with EMND includes the dominant involvement of oxidatively active type 1 myofibers in atrophied skeletal muscles and the abundant deposits of ceroid lipofuscin found in the retinal pigmented epithelium and in the endothelium of spinal cord capillaries [19, 29]. Such deposits are thought to be the end products of peroxidation of membrane polyunsaturated fatty acids [30]. Pathologic protein aggregates are found in neurons and glial cells of humans with ALS or other neurodegenerative diseases and these prion-like aggregations may be the final common pathway for a variety of destructive processes, including oxidative injury [31]. One of the most abundant and well-studied components of ALS protein aggregates is TAR DNA-binding protein 43 (TDP-43), aggregates of which may impair regulation of RNA granules and functioning of protein degradation pathways [31]. A possible role for aggregation in the pathogenesis of EMND is suggested by the finding of TDP-43 immunoreactivity in the nuclei of neurons from EMND cases but not in those from normal horses [32].

In addition to the epidemiologic evidence for an association between hypovitaminosis E and EMND, the disease has been reproduced experimentally by prolonged feeding of vitamin E–deficient diets. After 21–28 months on a diet deficient in vitamin E but high in the pro-oxidant transition elements Fe and Cu, four of eight horses developed clinical signs of EMND that were confirmed histologically [33]. In a separate experiment, four of ten horses on the vitamin E–deficient diet but with normal Fe and Cu developed clinical signs of EMND after 18–37 months and the remaining horses had histologic evidence of the disease in peripheral nerve biopsies and/or at necropsy [34]. Taken together, the results of these experiments and epidemiologic studies confirm that a diet low in vitamin E is a strong risk factor for EMND. Left unresolved is whether or not vitamin E intake is the *only* responsible nutritional or management factor influencing the development of EMND in these experimental horses and in other affected horses around the world.

Clinical signs

The clinical signs of EMND reflect motor denervation of skeletal muscles. Signs of muscle weakness and atrophy dominate the clinical presentation [18–20, 27, 33]. It is estimated that clinical signs of weakness occur when 30% of motor neurons become diseased or dysfunctional [34]. At the onset of weakness, there is usually noticeable muscle wasting, although signs occasionally occur in normally muscled horses. In four horses that developed EMND when fed a vitamin E–deficient diet, there was mean weight loss of 92 kg at the time signs of limb weakness first occurred [18]. In rare cases, the atrophy may advance insidiously without sudden weakness. Typically, however, there is acute onset of trembling in antigravity muscles, generalized sweating, and frequent episodes of recumbency. When standing in one place, horses with EMND adopt a characteristic "horse-on-a-ball" stance with the limbs gathered close together under the body (Figure 26.3) [35]. Affected horses lack the strength necessary to engage the stay apparatus of the pelvic limbs when standing still; thus, they constantly shift weight between the pelvic limbs and have great difficulty standing in a confined area such as a stocks. Acutely affected horses are more comfortable walking than

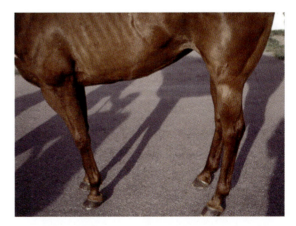

Figure 26.3 Characteristic gathering of feet under the body ("horse on a ball") in a horse with acutely presenting EMND. This 13-year-old Quarter Horse mare had been kept on a sand lot and fed bleached grass hay and sweet feed for the previous 10 years. There was sudden-onset muscle trembling and recumbency 2 days before this photograph was taken.

standing still although even brief walking exercise may cause signs of distress such as sweating, tachypnea, and nasal flaring. Typically, at the walk, protraction phases appear somewhat short and hypometric. Horses with EMND do not have signs of ataxia such as interference between limbs or circumduction of the pelvic limbs.

In most horses with acute EMND, the head is carried below the shoulders, usually reflecting obvious wasting of the neck muscles (Figure 26.4) [18]. The tail head is

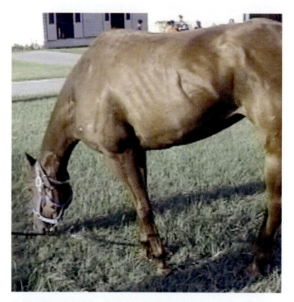

Figure 26.4 Because of weakness of the neck muscles, the horse shown in Figure 26.4 spends most of its time either recumbent or with the head held below the withers.

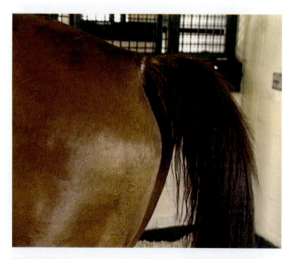

Figure 26.5 Elevation of the tailhead in the horse shown in Figure 26.4.

elevated in many cases because of atrophy and contracture of the dorsal coccygeal muscles [18] (Figure 26.5). If not present at the onset of neurologic signs, widespread muscle atrophy develops quickly (days to weeks) and is most obvious in the quadriceps, triceps, and gluteal muscles.

Despite the frequent occurrence of pathologic changes in the motor nuclei of cranial nerves V, VII, XII and the nucleus ambiguus, noticeable atrophy of the masseters and tongue has not been reported. The only clinical signs possibly ascribable to cranial nerve involvement are weak palpebral tone, dilated pupils, and sluggish pupillary light reflexes reported in a horse examined in the United Kingdom [36] and lip flaccidity and head tilt in an affected horse in Japan [37].

In some 40% of cases, fundoscopic examination reveals a horizontal band of pigment above the optic disc at the tapetal–nontapetal junction [18, 30]. The pigment may be brown-black to yellow-brown and has a reticulated or mosaic appearance. Surprisingly, problems with vision have not been reported even in EMND horses with severe pigment retinopathy [30].

The frequency distribution of the most important clinical signs of EMND in three published case series is shown in Figure 26.6.

Laboratory findings

Available data for clinicopathologic testing of clinical and experimental cases of EMND are shown in Table 26.1. Typical cases have below-range plasma/serum vitamin E concentration. However, as a stand-alone test, vitamin E is quite nonspecific: [35] normal pasture-mates of experimentally induced [33] or naturally occurring [27] EMND horses often also have low vitamin E. In healthy pasture-fed horses, vitamin E concentrations are variable during the day and often drop transiently below the normal range [12]. For this reason, it is recommended that plasma (or serum) from serial blood collections throughout the day be combined for the purpose of vitamin E assay [12]. It has recently been reported that horses with *vitamin E–responsive muscle atrophy and weakness*, a syndrome related to EMND, may have normal serum but low muscle concentration of vitamin E, presumably because of impaired transfer of vitamin E into tissues [38]. Vitamin E concentration can be measured in snap-frozen muscle biopsies of at least 250 mg.

Mild to moderately high plasma or serum CK and AST activities are found during the initial rapid progression of clinical signs but muscle enzyme activities may be normal in chronic stable cases (Table 26.1).

Changes in cytology of CSF are not seen in EMND; however, there may be increased total protein concentration and CK activity (Table 26.1) [18, 19]. IgG index is high in many cases, suggesting the presence of intrathecally produced IgG.

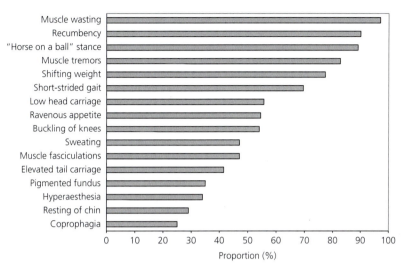

Figure 26.6 Aggregate frequency distribution of clinical signs in horses from three published case series.

Table 26.1 Clinicopathologic parameters of value in the evaluation of horses with equine motor neuron disease.

Source/analyte	EMND	Normal[a] (range/control)	References
Plasma/serum			
Vitamin E (μg/ml)	0.255±0.159	2.0–4.0 (R)	18
	0.4–1.5	2.0–4.4 (R)	22
	0.76±0.70	2.15±1.66 (C)	25
	0–1.22	0.108–2.56 (C)	27
CK (U/l)	301±365	<200 (R)	40
	875–3820		29
	149–3508		27
	482–9303	143–531 (R)	19
AST (U/l)	367±169	<275 (R)	40
	538–974		29
LDH (U/l)	1160±787	<420 (R)	40
CSF			
TP (mg/dl)	17–166	0–90 (R)	27
	34–145	0–70 (R)	17
Serum/CSF			
IgG index	0.1–9.7	<0.272 (R)	27

[a] Normal ranges (R) or controls (C) used in cited reference.
AST, aspartate aminotransferase; CK, creatine kinase; CSF, cerebrospinal fluid; LDH, lactate dehydrogenase; TP, total protein.

Ancillary tests
Needle electromyography
Needle electromyography (EMG) can be performed in the standing or recumbent, anesthetized horse. Horses with EMND often have abnormal EMG findings including prolonged insertional activity and pathologic spontaneous activity such as fibrillation potentials and trains of positive sharp waves [35]. Signs of denervation are found in facial muscles as well as appendicular and epaxial muscles [19]. Standing EMG is preferred in order to avoid anesthesia in weak compromised animals; however, interpretation of these studies is difficult because of movement artifacts associated with reluctance of affected horses to stand in one place. The use of sedation and caudal epidural anesthesia (lidocaine, 0.2 mg/kg) was reported to facilitate the procedure in a horse with EMND [36]. Techniques for quantitative analysis of motor action potentials have been published and results are abnormal in horses with EMND [39, 40]. Regardless of the EMG technique used, abnormal results are nonspecific as to cause, suggesting only denervation or myopathy [35].

Glucose absorption/metabolism
Oral glucose tolerance tests in horses with EMND were intermediate or abnormal in approximately 50% of reported cases whereas results of oral xylose absorption tests were normal or slightly low [18, 27, 40]. It appears that increased glucose metabolism, possibly associated with increased glucose sensitivity, rather than reduced intestinal absorption, is the cause of abnormal oral glucose tolerance in horses with EMND. Euglycemic clamp results from one horse showed a 5.4-fold increase in insulin sensitivity compared with control horses [41].

Nerve biopsy
Biopsy of the ventral branch of the spinal accessory nerve allows reliable antemortem diagnosis of EMND, at least in subacute and chronic cases [19, 42]. A 5-cm section of

the nerve is excised as it courses over and into the medial belly of the sternocephalicus muscle. The procedure can be performed either in the standing or recumbent, anesthetized patient and does not induce visible muscle atrophy at the surgical site. A positive histologic result is evidence of mild to severe Wallerian degeneration of axons and Schwann cell proliferation. Chronic cases are marked by loss of myelinated fibers, presence of compact Büngner's bands, and increased endoneurial collagen. Positive predictive value of nerve histology for EMND was 77.4% and negative predictive value was 90% [42]. False negative results appeared to be most likely in acute cases (<2 weeks). Nerve biopsy has largely been supplanted as an initial test by evaluation of sacrocaudalis dorsalis medialis (SCDM) muscle biopsies (see next section).

Muscle biopsy

The initial invasive procedure of choice is biopsy of the SCDM tailhead muscle [19, 43]. This muscle is rich in type I myofibers, a fiber type that is highly sensitive to the effects of denervation. The muscle sample is obtained under local anesthesia, placed on a tongue depressor, and sent chilled or in 10% formalin for histologic examination (Figure 26.7). In stained histologic sections, there is neurogenic atrophy characterized by variable numbers of angular atrophied myofibers, defined as fiber cross-sections with at least two concave sides that meet to form at least one point around the cellular margin [38]. Atrophied muscle fibers are of both types, but type I fibers predominate. The use of muscle biopsy has high sensitivity for EMND (>90%) but relatively low specificity [19]. In chronic EMND cases, histology of nerve biopsies may have higher sensitivity for diagnosis than does muscle histology [19]. A recently described syndrome of EMND-like clinical signs and low serum vitamin E without evidence of neurogenic atrophy, known as vitamin E–responsive muscle atrophy and weakness [38], may represent a variant form or early stage of EMND. Biopsies of SDCM from eight affected horses lacked the angular atrophied myofibers expected in denervated muscle but instead had evidence of myogenic atrophy, with anguloid muscle fibers (two or less slightly concave sides per cell), and an abnormal, "moth-eaten" appearance of the mitochondria of myofibers revealed by stains for any of several different mitochondrial enzymes. The authors suggested that these cases of vitamin E–responsive muscle atrophy and weakness may account for the <10% of false negatives reported when using SCDM biopsy results for diagnosis of EMND [19].

Diagnosis

Antemortem diagnosis of EMND usually is not difficult. It is based on typical clinical signs, age of 2 years or older, and diet low in green forage and high in carbohydrate. Needle EMG findings of denervation, especially in the deep limb muscles, are difficult technically because of movement artifact in weak horses, but are supportive of the diagnosis as are the findings of mild to moderately high plasma CK and AST activities and low plasma vitamin E concentration. Finally, evidence of denervation in muscle or nerve biopsies in the context of the preceding clinical and laboratory findings is tantamount to a definitive diagnosis of EMND. Occasionally, in cases of insidiously progressive EMND, especially in nonendemic areas, diagnosis is only made postmortem.

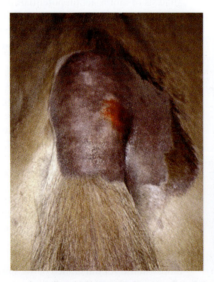 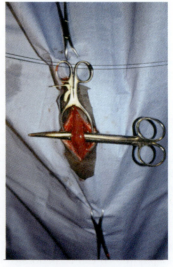

Figure 26.7 Location over the tailhead of biopsy site (rectangle in left image) and isolation, elevation, and removal of a section of the right sacrocaudalis dorsalis muscle (right).

Differential diagnoses include diseases with presentations that resemble some component of EMND. These may include laminitis, colic, EPM, myopathies, grass sickness, and botulism.

Necropsy findings

Although there is obvious weight loss in horses with EMND, fat deposits noted postmortem are usually within normal limits [17, 20, 43]. In acute cases, there is widespread degeneration and loss of somatic motor neurons in the ventral horns of the spinal cord accompanied by degenerative axonal changes in the ventral roots and peripheral nerves. All brainstem cranial nerve somatic motor nuclei, except those of cranial nerves III, IV, and VI, are variably involved. Most affected neurons are swollen, markedly chromatolytic and diffusely argyrophilic while severely affected neurons are shrunken or vacuolated. In chronic "burn out" cases, there are glial scars consisting of astrocytes and lipofuscin-laden microglia. Additional deposits of ceroid lipofuscin are found in the retinal epithelium and occasionally in the liver and intestine. Relatively minor neurodegenerative changes may be found in dorsal root ganglia. By contrast with grass sickness, there are minimal or no lesions in the autonomic nervous system. In skeletal muscles, there is angular atrophy of all myofiber types with some selectivity for type I fibers. Atrophied fibers are intermingled among normal fibers and fascicles. Involvement of the deeper muscles of the limbs may be grossly evident as pale discoloration. As described earlier in the Muscle Biopsy section, muscle from horses with vitamin E–responsive muscle atrophy and weakness syndrome lack histologic evidence of neurogenic atrophy but rather show anguloid myofiber atrophy and distinctive mitochondrial morphology in sections stained for mitochondrial enzymes [38].

Treatment

The only treatment recommended for horses with EMND is vitamin E supplementation. This can be supplied in good quality grass and alfalfa hay or by vitamin E supplementation (at least 10 IU/kg). Natural vitamin E (RRR-α-tocopherol) has higher bioavailability and potency than synthetic vitamin E (*all-rac*-α-tocopherol acetate or D,L-α-tocopherol) [11]. While vitamin E treatment appears logical, there has been no clinical trial that has evaluated the efficacy of treatment. In one recent report, mean ± SD serum vitamin E of six long-term resident horses improved from 0.52 ± 0.37 to $1.49 \pm 0.64\,\mu g/ml$ 9 weeks after moving to a new location even though feeding was unchanged and there was no pasture access at either location. The authors speculated that the relatively rural location of the second site may have reduced the oxidant stress associated with the densely populated, industrial environment of the original location.

The frequent clinical observation that many EMND horses have increased [35] appetite may be explained by an estimate that daily caloric requirement of horses could be twice that of normal horses [15]. Thus, as part of the convalescent program of surviving horses, high quantity and quality of pasture, hay, and concentrate is recommended.

Clinical course

Within 6 weeks after onset of signs, approximately 40% of horses progressively deteriorate and are euthanized while a similar number undergo marked improvement in clinical signs (usually following relocation to another premise and/or administration of antioxidants) [18]. These "recovered" horses look normal but may recrudesce under the pressure of intensive training or competition [17]. Horses with vitamin E–responsive muscle atrophy and weakness [38] presumably fall into this class. In the remaining 20%, the disease appears to "burn out" and such horses survive with permanent and obvious muscle wasting and emaciation.

Equine grass sickness

History and epidemiology

Grass sickness is a debilitating, often fatal, dysautonomia of equids associated with full-time access to pasture [44]. Because lesions are also found in somatic lower motor neurons, it has been suggested that it is more accurate to describe grass sickness as a polyneuropathy rather than a dysautonomia. A comparable fatal polyneuropathy has also long been recognized in the Patagonia region of South America where it is known as "mal seco." [45] Equine grass sickness (EGS) is endemic in Scotland, England, and Wales and has also been reported from western Europe, Cyprus, Hungary, the Falkland islands, and Colombia with isolated cases in Australia, Ethiopia, and the United States [44, 46–49]. The single case reported in the United States involved a 6-year-old female mule in Kansas with signs of colic [47]. Between 2000 and 2009, an annual average of 141 cases of EGS were reported to the UK-wide national surveillance scheme [50].

Epidemiological studies conducted since the early 1970s have identified high horse density, full-time grazing, a recent change in pasture or premises, previous occurrence of the disease on the premises, lack of hay in the diet, pasture disturbance, mechanical removal of horse manure from pastures, sandy or loamy soils, recent deworming with ivermectin, and good bodily condition as risk factors [44, 50–57]. Cases occur throughout the year with peak numbers in the spring and a smaller peak in the autumn. The risk of disease was highest in horses aged 2–7 years (peak 5–6 years) although cases have been reported in horses from

2 months to 27 years of age. Horses of all breeds, ponies, donkeys, Przewalski's horses, and zebras are affected. Males and females are equally represented in recent surveillance data [50]. Protective factors included contact with previous cases, daily feeding of hay or hay-lage, chalky soil, manual removal of feces from pastures, pasture grass mowing, and co-grazing with ruminants.

Cause and pathogenesis

Theories as to the cause of EGS have included mineral or vitamin deficiencies or exposure to toxic plants, secondary metabolites and trace minerals in pasture grass, insects, mycotoxins, viruses, or bacterial toxins [56, 58, 59]. Although the clinical syndrome of EGS has not been reproduced experimentally, the characteristic neuropathology has been induced by administration of serum from acute cases into the peritoneal cavity or parotid salivary gland [60, 61]. The activity was found in a >30-kDa fraction of serum and has been further characterized recently in an effort, not yet realized, to develop a diagnostic serum test and to determine the mechanism of toxic effect [62].

Over the last 20 years, an hypothesis originally developed in the 1920s [63] has been resurrected, namely, that EGS is a toxicoinfectious form of botulism involving a type C strain commonly carried by birds [64]. Strong support for this hypothesis has been (i) the demonstrated association between EGS and the presence in ileal contents of *C. botulinum* type C, type C1 neurotoxin (BoNT/C) [64], and anti-BoNT/C IgA [65]; (ii) the observation that horses with EGS have significantly lower serum antibodies to *C. botulinum* and BoNT/C than do pasture-mate controls [66, 67], and; (iii) presence of rising titers of specific IgG antitoxin in chronic EGS cases. *Clostridium botulinum* type C is unique among clostridial organisms in that its major toxin, BoNT/C, possesses potent and nonspecific neurotoxicity *in vitro*, probably via action on cellular syntaxin [64]. It has been hypothesized that toxin production and absorption occur in the ileum due to overgrowth from normal intestinal flora and/or to spore germination in association with nutritional or environmental triggers involving factors such as changes in feed, pasture, and weather conditions and parasite status [44, 46]. An EGS pilot study in 100 horses involving use of a formaldehyde-inactivated *C. botulinum* type C toxoid vaccine (Febrivac BOT) marketed for use in mink was begun in 2012 and a trial of at least 1000 horses is scheduled to begin in 2014 that is powered to detect a vaccine-associated fourfold reduction in EGS incidence.

Clinical signs

The major clinical signs of grass sickness reflect dysfunction of the autonomic nervous system, particularly of the gastrointestinal (GI) tract [44, 68]. There is

dysphagia, gastric and small intestinal dilation, nasogastric reflux, colonic impaction, and colic. Clinical presentations are classified as acute (course of <48 h), subacute (2–7 days) and chronic (>7 days) [69]. Since 2000, 66% of reported cases have been acute or subacute, with 34% classified as chronic [44]. Acutely affected horses may be found dead or in abdominal crisis with signs of colic, tachycardia, generalized sweating, nasogastric reflux including spontaneous nasal regurgitation of stomach contents, absence of intestinal borborygmi, and abdominal distension. Rectal palpation and transabdominal ultrasonography reveal distended loops of small intestine and gas-filled large bowel. Affected horses are unable to swallow food or water and thick ropy saliva may drool from the mouth. Fine muscle fasciculations similar to those seen with EMND may affect the triceps and quadriceps. Horses with subacute EGS survive long enough to develop colonic impactions and secondary large intestinal tympany. Chronic EGS may develop insidiously and only a minority of these cases show mild, intermittent colic. There is patchy sweating and/or pilo-erection on the neck, flanks and behind the shoulders (Figure 26.8). Typically, the appetite is reduced and there are varying degrees of difficulty in chewing and swallowing; however, salivation, accumulation of fluid in the stomach and impaction are not usual features. There is often bilateral ptosis with ventral deviation of the eye-lashes secondary to loss of sympathetic eyelid tone. Because of suppression of normal nasal secretions there is a characteristic dry crusty nasal exudate (rhinitis sicca). Fecal production is reduced and feces are unusually firm and small. There is rapid and severe weight loss.

Acute and subacute cases are invariably fatal. Death occurs from gastric rupture, circulatory compromise, cardiopulmonary failure or, most commonly, from

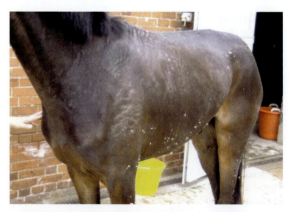

Figure 26.8 Horse with chronic EGS showing patchy sweating around the neck and residues of salt elsewhere on the body reflecting previous sweating. (Image courtesy of Dr. IG Mayhew.)

euthanasia. Before the 1980s, it was thought that chronic EGS also was usually fatal or associated with hopeless emaciation. EGS is very unlikely to recur in recovered horses [57].

Diagnosis
Definitive diagnosis requires histopathologic examination of autonomic neurons for chromatolytic changes [44, 70]. Antemortem, the sample of choice is an ileal biopsy which typically is obtained during exploratory celiotomy or laparoscopy of horses presenting with signs of colic [71]. The diagnostic accuracy of this test may be improved by use of a decision tree based solely on neuronal density and intensity of immunohistochemical staining of synaptophysin, an abundant integral membrane protein of synaptic vesicles [72]. Nasal and rectal biopsies have been investigated for diagnostic accuracy, but currently are regarded as unreliable for diagnosis in the live horse [71].

There is no confirmatory blood test for EGS. Nonspecific abnormalities are consistent with severe dehydration, hypovolemia, stress, loss of GI secretions, and anorexia [73]. Peritoneal fluid protein concentration may be high although nucleated and red cell counts usually are normal. Serum concentrations of numerous acute phase proteins, including α2 macroglobulin, serum amyloid A, ceruloplasmin, haptoglobin, and orosomucoid are high but such changes are not specific to EGS [71, 74].

In EGS cases with ptosis, topical application of 0.5 ml 0.5% phenylephrine eyedrops results in normalization of the eyelash angle within 30 min and is supportive of the diagnosis (Figure 26.9) [75].

Treatment and prevention
All cases of acute and subacute EGS are considered incurable and therefore require euthanasia on humane grounds as soon as possible after diagnosis. Treatment of selected chronic cases involves excellent nursing care and provision of palatable, easily swallowed food and high energy concentrates. Clinical recovery occurs in about 50% of selected treated cases [44].

Current efforts at prevention involve minimization of known risk factors and introduction of suspected protective practices. Thus, in endemic areas, horse owners are advised to avoid exposure to pastures where previous cases have occurred, minimize disturbance of pasture or soil, prevent overgrazing of pasture, and avoid the "overuse" of ivermectin dewormers. On the other hand, owners are encouraged to co-graze horses with ruminants, mow pastures regularly, remove feces by hand, and supplement pasture feeding with hay or haylage. These practices are particularly important during seasonal and climatic risk periods, and for young horses in good bodily condition, especially those recently imported.

Necropsy findings
Gross necropsy findings in horses with EGS include esophageal ulceration, fluid distension of the stomach and small intestines, impaction of the large colon and/or cecum and the presence of inspissated mucus within the small colon and rectum. Subacute and chronic cases do not have gastric and small intestinal distension but do have variable degrees of large intestinal impaction and often rhinitis sicca [68]. Histologic lesions of neuronal degeneration are most evident in the autonomic ganglia, gut wall nerve plexuses, brain and spinal cord [69, 76]. There is chromatolysis, nuclear eccentricity, nuclear degenerative changes, cell death and neuronophagia, cytoplasmic vacuolation and spheroid formation.

Cerebellar degeneration

The most commonly reported cerebellar neurodegenerative conditions of horses are inherited abiotrophies. A distinct apparently inherited cerebellar condition of Oldenburg foals is characterized by multifocal cerebellar degeneration and an invariably fatal outcome [77]. A syndrome of progressive ataxia associated with cerebellar degeneration was identified in one American Miniature Horse foal and anecdotal evidence for an additional two cases was cited [78]. An unusual case of NAD with cerebellar signs was reported in a Pony of the Americas foal [79]. Cerebellar degeneration and lipofuscin accumulation associated with presumed toxicosis has been described in Gomen disease of horses in New Caledonia [80]. Induced mannosidosis with neurovisceral degeneration involving the cerebellum has been reported for poisoning by swainsonine-containing plants in the United States, Australia, and Brazil [81–83].

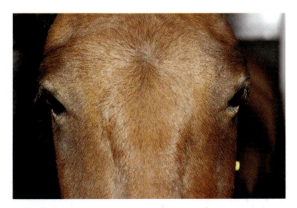

Figure 26.9 Phenylephrine test in horse with EGS; 0.5 ml of 0.5% phenylephrine has been applied to the right eye. Note the elevation of the eyelid in the treated eye. (Image courtesy of Dr. IG Mayhew.)

Cerebellar abiotrophy

History and epidemiology

The term abiotrophy refers to spontaneous premature degeneration resulting from an inborn error of development [84]. Syndromes of cerebellar abiotrophy (CA) have been described for Arabian [85], Gotland Pony [86, 87], and Eriskay Pony foals [88]. The Gotland breed developed in isolation on Gotland island off the coast of Sweden but stallions of other breeds were introduced in the late nineteenth century in an attempt to improve the breed and this practice was continued through a period of precipitous population decline in the early twentieth century and up until the studbook was closed in 1971 [87]. Two such stallions are now found in the pedigrees of most Gotland ponies with CA (a condition known locally as *slinger*). Because both highly represented stallions and the many Welsh Pony stallions introduced subsequently are likely part Arabian, it has been argued that the genetic defect responsible for slinger may be the Arabian CA mutation and may have arrived via outcrossing [87]. Genetic testing is expected to resolve this issue in the near future. The modern Eriskay pony is claimed by its breed society to be one of the few pure pony breeds left in the western islands of Scotland, with origins dating back to Norse and Celtic invasions [89]. Because the population declined to about 20 animals in the early 1970s, the surviving population certainly is the product of intense inbreeding.

Cause and pathogenesis

In Arabians with CA, degeneration only begins after formation of the cerebellum and is characterized by apoptosis of Purkinje cells [90]. The likely genetic basis for CA in Arabians was recently identified as a SNP on horse chromosome 2 in the *TOE1* gene and is designated *TOE1*:g.2171G>A SNP [91]. Thus, the *TOE1*:g.2171G>A SNP genotype A/A is associated with CA, horses with A/G genotypes are clinically normal heterozygotic carriers of the mutation, and G/G is the wild-type genotype. The *TOE1* mutation is thought to exert its effect by downregulation of expression of the 3′-located *MUTYH* gene. *MUTYH* encodes a DNA glycosylase involved in repair of oxidative damage to genomic DNA during organogenesis and mitochondrial DNA during postnatal life. This gene is abundantly expressed in the cerebellums of normal horses; expression is significantly lower in CA foals [91]. The mode of inheritance is single Mendelian autosomal recessive [85, 91, 92]. The CA-SNP allele A was found in 19.7% of approximately 4200 Arabian horses and is well represented in Egyptian, Spanish, and Polish lineages [91, 92]. Among tested horses, 1.4% were homozygous (A/A). Nine of the homozygotes were clinically normal which, taken together with the observed range of ages of onset, is evidence for variable expression of the CA trait.

The allele was also present at low frequency in the Bashkir Curly Horse, a breed that used Arabians as foundation stock, and in Welsh Ponies and Trakehners, breeds that allow outcrossing with Arabians [93].

Clinical signs

Signs of CA typically begin in foals between 6 weeks and 4 months of age; however, foals may be affected at or shortly after birth. Among 18 confirmed or suspected cases, signs were present at birth in 4 (22%), began at ≤3 months of age in 10 (56%), 3–6 months in 2 (11%), and >6 months in 2 (11%) [77, 94–96]. The first signs noticed are incoordination, base-wide posturing in the thoracic limbs, and head tremors. The head tremor usually is a coarse bobbing in either the horizontal or vertical plane. When the head is extended toward the dam's udder or toward offered food, the head tremor becomes more pronounced. Because the menace response pathway involves the cerebellar cortex ipsilateral to the tested eye, CA foals can see normally, but lack a menace response (i.e., a CA foal will not blink in response to a hand gesture toward the eye although it may move its head away). Affected foals walk with a swaying, lurching gait and may even wobble side-to-side or back and forth while standing still. Thoracic limbs may appear stiff or there may be exaggerated flexion ("paddling") during the protraction phase. Gait abnormalities are most obvious when movement is initiated and during turns. Normal strength is preserved even in severely ataxic foals and blindfolding does not exacerbate clinical signs. All clinical signs are exaggerated by stimulation of affected foals. Such hyperresponsiveness means CA foals are difficult to halter-train and lead; even normal handling often causes an affected foal to pull away or even flip over backwards. Severely affected foals that fall often panic and struggle for some time before standing.

Diagnosis

The diagnosis in an Arabian foal with compatible clinical signs is strongly supported by demonstration of homozygosity for the CA allele. This test requires submission of 20–30 hairs with roots and is submitted to the Veterinary Genetics Laboratory at the University of California, Davis (http://www.vgl.ucdavis.edu/services/horse.php). Hematologic and serum chemistry findings are usually normal. Some foals have high CSF protein concentration and CK activity, consistent with active neurodegeneration at the time of CSF collection [95]. Magnetic resonance (MR), and possibly computed tomography imaging of affected foals may reveal atrophy of the cerebellum and relatively abundant CSF surrounding the cerebellum in foals with CA [97]. Morphometric quantification of the areas of the cerebellum, cerebellar CSF, and brain in median T2-weighted

MR images of the heads of 5 CA horses and 15 normal horses demonstrated significant reduction of the median cerebellum: brain ratio in CA horses (17.6% vs. 20.3%) and a corresponding significant increase in the cerebellar CSF: brain ratio (16.3% vs. 9.4%) (Figure 26.10)

[98]. Using a cutoff value of 11% for the latter variable, its sensitivity in identifying CA-affected horses was 100% and specificity was 93.3%.

Signs may be stable after onset or get worse for up to several months. It is rare, however, for CA foals to become persistently recumbent. Modest improvement has been noted in some mildly affected horses once they become adults [77]. Foals with CA seldom succumb to direct effects of the condition, but most are euthanized because of severe clinical signs and poor prognosis.

Necropsy findings

Gross appearance of the affected brain is usually described as normal; however, the ratio of cerebellar to whole brain weight is usually <8%, while normal ratios are ≥8%. The characteristic histologic lesion is thinning of the cerebellar cortex affecting both granular and molecular layers [77, 85, 94–96]. There is marked reduction in the number of Purkinje cells in the granular layer, and some of those remaining show degenerative changes (swelling, shrinkage, and hyperchromasia of the perikaryon). There is relative sparing of the Purkinje cells of the nodulus and flocculi [95]. Vacuolation may be noted in the olivary nuclei [94]. Mineralized neuronal cell bodies may be found in the thalamus adjacent to the third ventricle (Figure 26.11).

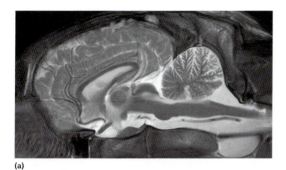

(a)

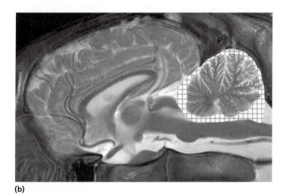

(b)

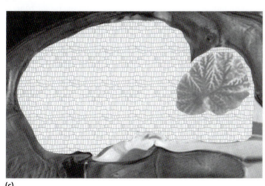

(c)

Figure 26.10 Outline of MRI morphometric calculations on mid representative median T2-weighted MRI of horse with cerebellar abiotrophy (a). The cerebellum, its surrounding CSF space, and the whole brain were outlined manually, and the ratio of the area of the cerebellum and the area of the cerebellum plus its surrounding CSF space (checkered pattern) was calculated (b). To obtain the relative cerebellar size, the area of the cerebellum was put into a ratio with the area of the whole brain (irregular pattern) (c). (Reproduced with permission from Ref. [98].)

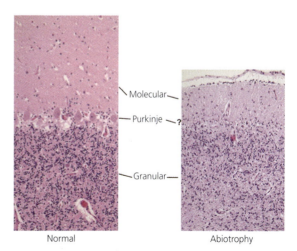

Normal   Abiotrophy

Figure 26.11 Cross-section of the cerebellar cortex from normal foal and foal with cerebellar abiotrophy. Note the thinning of the molecular layer, absence of Purkinje cells, and decreased cellularity of the granular layer of the CA specimen.

References

[1] Mayhew IG, Delahunta A, Whitlock RH, et al. Equine degenerative myeloencephalopathy. *J Am Vet Med Assoc* 1977;170:195–201.

[2] Beech J. Neuroaxonal dystrophy of the accessory cuneate nucleus in horses. *Vet Pathol* 1984;21:384–393.

[3] Miller MM, Collatos C. Equine degenerative myeloencephalopathy. *Vet Clin North Am Equine Pract* 1997;13:43–52.

[4] Finno CJ, Higgins RJ, Aleman M, et al. Equine degenerative myeloencephalopathy in Lusitano horses. *J Vet Intern Med* 2011;25:1439–1446.

[5] Dill SG, Correa MT, Erb HN, et al. Factors associated with the development of equine degenerative myeloencephalopathy. *Am J Vet Res* 1990;51:1300–1305.

[6] Beech J, Haskins M. Genetic studies of neuraxonal dystrophy in the Morgan. *Am J Vet Res* 1987;48:109–113.

[7] Blythe LL, Hultgren BD, Craig AM, et al. Clinical, viral, and genetic evaluation of equine degenerative myeloencephalopathy in a family of Appaloosas. *J Am Vet Med Assoc* 1991;198:1005–1013.

[8] Aleman M, Finno CJ, Higgins RJ, et al. Evaluation of epidemiological, clinical, and pathological features of neuroaxonal dystrophy in Quarter Horses. *J Am Vet Med Assoc* 2011;239:823–833.

[9] Mayhew IG, Brown CM, Stowe HD, et al. Equine degenerative myeloencephalopathy: a vitamin E deficiency that may be familial. *J Vet Intern Med* 1987;1:45–50.

[10] Gandini G, Fatzer R, Mariscoli M, et al. Equine degenerative myeloencephalopathy in five Quarter Horses: clinical and neuropathological findings. *Equine Vet J* 2004;36:83–85.

[11] Finno CJ, Valberg SJ. A comparative review of vitamin E and associated equine disorders. *J Vet Intern Med* 2012;26:1251–1266.

[12] Blythe LL, Craig AM, Lassen ED, et al. Serially determined plasma alpha-tocopherol concentrations and results of the oral vitamin E absorption test in clinically normal horses and in horses with degenerative myeloencephalopathy. *Am J Vet Res* 1991;52:908–911.

[13] Wong DM, Ghosh A, Fales-Williams AJ, et al. Evidence of oxidative injury of the spinal cord in 2 horses with equine degenerative myeloencephalopathy. *Vet Pathol* 2012;49:1049–1053.

[14] Finno CJ, Famula T, Aleman M, et al. Pedigree analysis and exclusion of alpha-tocopherol transfer protein (ttpa) as a candidate gene for neuroaxonal dystrophy in the American Quarter Horse. *J Vet Intern Med* 2013;27:177–185.

[15] Finno CJ, Aleman M, Ofri R, et al. Electrophysiological studies in American Quarter horses with neuroaxonal dystrophy. *Vet Ophthalmol* 2012;15:3–7.

[16] Liguori V, Vichi G, De Iuliis P. Ten cases of *EDM* in an Italian Saddle horse breeding farm. *Ippologia* 2010;21:19–22.

[17] Cummings JF, Delahunta A, George C, et al. Equine motor neuron disease – a preliminary-report. *Cornell Vet* 1990;80:357–379.

[18] Divers TJ, Mohammed HO, Hintz HF, et al. Equine motor neuron disease: a review of clinical and experimental studies. *Clin Tech Equine Pract* 2006;5:24–29.

[19] Divers TJ, Mohammed HO, Cummings JF. Equine motor neuron disease. *Vet Clin North Am Equine Pract* 1997;13:97–105.

[20] Divers TJ, De Lahunta A, Hintz HF, et al. Equine motor neuron disease. *Equine Vet Ed* 2001;13:63–67.

[21] Devilbiss BA, Mohammed HO, Divers TJ. Perception of equine practitioners regarding the occurrence of selected equine neurologic diseases in the northeast over a 10-year period. *J Equine Vet Sci* 2009;29:237–246.

[22] Mcgorum BC, Mayhew IG, Amory H, et al. Horses on pasture may be affected by equine motor neuron disease. *Equine Vet J* 2006;38:47–51.

[23] Mohammed HO, Cummings JF, Divers TJ, et al. Risk factors associated with equine motor-neuron disease – a possible model for human MND. *Neurology* 1993;43:966–971.

[24] de la Rúa-Domènech R, Mohammed HO, Cummings JF, et al. Intrinsic, management, and nutritional factors associated with equine motor neuron disease. *J Am Vet Med Assoc* 1997;211:1261–1267.

[25] de la Rúa-Domènech R, Mohammed HO, Cummings JF, et al. Association between plasma vitamin E concentration and the risk of equine motor neuron disease. *Vet J* 1997;154:203–213.

[26] Syrja P, Cizinauskas S, Sankari SM, et al. Equine motor neuron disease (EMND) in a horse without vitamin E deficiency: a sequela of iron excess? *Equine Vet Ed* 2006;18:122–126.

[27] Divers TJ, Mohammed HO, Cummings JF, et al. Equine motor neuron disease – findings in 28 horses and proposal of a pathophysiological mechanism for the disease. *Equine Vet J* 1994;26:409–415.

[28] de la Rúa-Domènech R, Wiedmann M, Mohammed HO, et al. Equine motor neuron disease is not linked to Cu/Zn superoxide dismutase mutations: sequence analysis of the equine Cu/Zn superoxide dismutase cDNA. *Gene* 1996;178:83–88.

[29] Palencia P, Quiroz-Rothe E, Rivero JLL. New insights into the skeletal muscle phenotype of equine motor neuron disease: a quantitative approach. *Acta Neuropathol (Berl)* 2005;109:272–284.

[30] Riis RC, Jackson C, Rebhun W, et al. Ocular manifestations of equine motor neuron disease. *Equine Vet J* 1999;31:99–110.

[31] Blokhuis AM, Groen EJN, Koppers M, et al. Protein aggregation in amyotrophic lateral sclerosis. *Acta Neuropathol (Berl)* 2013;125:777–794.

[32] El-Assaad I, Di Bari JA, Yasuda K, et al. Differential expression of tar DNA-binding protein (tdp-43) in the

central nervous system of horses afflicted with equine motor neuron disease (EMND): a preliminary study of a potential pathologic marker. *Vet Res Commun* 2012;36: 221–226.

[33] Divers TJ, Cummings JE, De Lahunta A, et al. Evaluation of the risk of motor neuron disease in horses fed a diet low in vitamin E and high in copper and iron. *Am J Vet Res* 2006;67:120–126.

[34] Mohammed HO, Divers TJ, Summers BA, et al. Vitamin E deficiency and risk of equine motor neuron disease. *Acta Vet Scand* 2007;49:17.

[35] Wijnberg ID. Equine motor neuron disease. *Equine Vet Ed* 2006;18:126–129.

[36] Kyles KWJ, Mcgorum BC, Fintl C, et al. Electromyography under caudal epidural anaesthesia as an aid to the diagnosis of equine motor neuron disease. *Vet Rec* 2001;148: 536–538.

[37] Sasaki N, Yamada M, Morita Y, et al. A case of equine motor neuron disease (EMND). *J Vet Med Sci* 2006;68: 1367–1369.

[38] Bedford HE, Valberg SJ, Firshman AM, et al. Histopathologic findings in the sacrocaudalis dorsalis medialis muscle of horses with vitamin E-responsive muscle atrophy and weakness. *J Am Vet Med Assoc* 2013;242:1127–1137.

[39] Wijnberg ID, Back W, De Jong M, et al. The role of electromyography in clinical diagnosis of neuromuscular locomotor problems in the horse. *Equine Vet J* 2004;36: 718–722.

[40] Benders NA, Dyer J, Wijnberg ID, et al. Evaluation of glucose tolerance and intestinal luminal membrane glucose transporter function in horses with equine motor neuron disease. *Am J Vet Res* 2005;66:93–99.

[41] Van Der Kolk JH, Rijnen K, Rey F, et al. Evaluation of glucose metabolism in three horses with lower motor neuron degeneration. *Am J Vet Res* 2005;66:271–276.

[42] Jackson CA, Delahunta A, Cummings JF, et al. Spinal accessory nerve biopsy as an ante mortem diagnostic test for equine motor neuron disease. *Equine Vet J* 1996;28: 215–219.

[43] Valentine BA, Delahunta A, George C, et al. Acquired equine motor-neuron disease. *Vet Pathol* 1994;31: 130–138.

[44] Wylie CE, Proudman CJ. Equine grass sickness: epidemiology, diagnosis, and global distribution. *Vet Clin North Am Equine Pract* 2009;25:381–399.

[45] Uzal FA, Robles CA. Mal seco, a grass sickness-like syndrome of horses in Argentina. *Vet Res Commun* 1993;17: 449–457.

[46] Hedderson EJ, Newton JR. Prospects for vaccination against equine grass sickness. *Equine Vet J* 2004;36: 186–191.

[47] Wright A, Beard L, Bawa B, et al. Dysautonomia in a six-year-old mule in the United States. *Equine Vet J* 2010;42: 170–173.

[48] Protopapas KF, Spanoudes KAM, Diakakis NE, et al. Equine grass sickness in Cyprus: a case report. *Turk J Vet Anim Sci* 2012;36:85–87.

[49] Schwarz B, Brunthaler R, Hahn C, et al. Outbreaks of equine grass sickness in Hungary. *Vet Rec* 2012; 170:75.

[50] Wylie CE, Proudman CJ, Mcgorum BC, et al. A nation-wide surveillance scheme for equine grass sickness in Great Britain: results for the period 2000–2009. *Equine Vet J* 2011;43:571–579.

[51] Gilmour JS, Jolly GM. Some aspects of the epidemiology of equine grass sickness. *Vet Rec* 1974;95:77–81.

[52] Doxey DL, Gilmour JS, Milne EM. The relationship between meteorological features and equine grass sickness (dysautonomia). *Equine Vet J* 1991;23:370–373.

[53] Mccarthy HE, Proudman CJ, French NP. Epidemiology of equine grass sickness: a literature review (1909–1999). *Vet Rec* 2001;149:293–300.

[54] Wood JL, Milne EM, Doxey DL. A case-control study of grass sickness (equine dysautonomia) in the United Kingdom. *Vet J* 1998;156:7–14.

[55] French NP, Mccarthy HE, Diggle PJ, et al. Clustering of equine grass sickness cases in the United Kingdom: a study considering the effect of position-dependent reporting on the space-time K-function. *Epidemiol Infect* 2005;133:343–348.

[56] Newton JR, Wylie CE, Proudman CJ, et al. Equine grass sickness: are we any nearer to answers on cause and prevention after a century of research? *Equine Vet J* 2010;42:477–481.

[57] Newton JR, Hedderson EJ, Adams VJ, et al. An epidemiological study of risk factors associated with the recurrence of equine grass sickness (dysautonomia) on previously affected premises. *Equine Vet J* 2004;36:105–112.

[58] Mcgorum BC, Pirie RS, Fry SC. Quantification of cyanogenic glycosides in white clover (*Trifolium repens* L.) from horse pastures in relation to equine grass sickness. *Grass Forage Sci* 2012;67:274–279.

[59] Michl J, Modarai M, Edwards S, et al. Metabolomic analysis of *Ranunculus* spp. as potential agents involved in the etiology of equine grass sickness. *J Agric Food Chem* 2011;59:10388–10393.

[60] Gilmour JS, Mould DL. Experimental studies of neurotoxic activity in blood fractions from acute cases of grass sickness. *Res Vet Sci* 1977;22:1–4.

[61] Gilmour JS. Experimental reproduction of the neurological lesions associated with grass sickness. *Vet Rec* 1973;92: 565–566.

[62] Malekinejad H, Bull S, Rahmani F, et al. Cytotoxic effects of serum from equine grass sickness cases on Neuro-2a and PC12 Tet-Off cell lines: implication for using in vitro methods as antemortem diagnostic tools. *J Equine Vet Sci* 2012;32:53–59.

[63] Tocher JF, Brown W, Tocher JW, et al. "Grass sickness" investigation report. *Vet Rec* 1923;3:37–45, 75–89.

[64] Hunter LC, Miller JK, Poxton IR. The association of *Clostridium botulinum* type C with equine grass sickness: a toxicoinfection? *Equine Vet J* 1999;31:492–499.

[65] Nunn FG, Pirie RS, Mcgorum B, et al. Preliminary study of mucosal IgA in the equine small intestine: specific IgA in cases of acute grass sickness and controls. *Equine Vet J* 2007;39:457–460.

[66] Hunter LC, Poxton IR. Systemic antibodies to *Clostridium botulinum* type C: do they protect horses from grass sickness (dysautonomia)? *Equine Vet J* 2001;33: 547–553.

[67] Mccarthy HE, French NP, Edwards GB, et al. Equine grass sickness is associated with low antibody levels to *Clostridium botulinum*: a matched case-control study. *Equine Vet J* 2004;36:123–129.

[68] Cottrell DF, Mcgorum BC, Pearson GT. The neurology and enterology of equine grass sickness: a review of basic mechanisms. *Neurogastroenterol Motil* 1999;11:79–92.

[69] Hahn CN, Mayhew IG, De Lahunta A. Central neuropathology of equine grass sickness. *Acta Neuropathol* 2001;102:153–159.

[70] Milne EM, Pirie RS, Mcgorum BC, et al. Evaluation of formalin-fixed ileum as the optimum method to diagnose equine dysautonomia (grass sickness) in simulated intestinal biopsies. *J Vet Diagn Invest* 2010;22:248–252.

[71] Ireland JL, Newton JR. Improving antemortem diagnosis of equine grass sickness. *Vet Rec* 2011;168:261–262.

[72] Waggett BE, Mcgorum BC, Shaw DJ, et al. Evaluation of synaptophysin as an immunohistochemical marker for equine grass sickness. *J Comp Pathol* 2010;142:284–290.

[73] Johnson P, Dawson AM, Mould DL. Serum protein changes in grass sickness. *Res Vet Sci* 1983;35:165–170.

[74] Doxey DL, Milne EM, Gilmour JS, et al. Clinical and biochemical features of grass sickness (equine dysautonomia). *Equine Vet J* 1991;23:360–364.

[75] Hahn CN, Mayhew IG. Phenylephrine eyedrops as a diagnostic test in equine grass sickness. *Vet Rec* 2000;147:603–606.

[76] Doxey DL, Pogson DM, Milne EM, et al. Clinical equine dysautonomia and autonomic neuron damage. *Res Vet Sci* 1992;53:106–109.

[77] Palmer AC, Blakemore WF, Cook WR, et al. Cerebellar hypoplasia and degeneration in the young Arab horse: clinical and neuropathological features. *Vet Rec* 1973;93: 62–66.

[78] Fox J, Duncan R, Friday P, et al. Cerebello-olivary and lateral (accessory) cuneate degeneration in a juvenile American miniature horse. *Vet Pathol* 2000;37:271–274.

[79] Brosnahan MM, Holbrook TC, Ritchey JW. Neuroaxonal dystrophy associated with cerebellar dysfunction in a 5-month-old Pony of the Americas colt. *J Vet Intern Med* 2009;23:1303–1306.

[80] Legonidec G, Kuberski T, Daynes P, et al. A neurologic disease of horses in New Caledonia. *Aust Vet J* 1981;57: 194–195.

[81] Kirkpatrick JG, Burrows GE. Locoism in horses. *Vet Hum Toxicol* 1990;32:168–169.

[82] Huxtable CR, Dorling PR. Poisoning of livestock by *Swainsona* spp – current status. *Aust Vet J* 1982;59:50–53.

[83] Loretti AP, Colodel EM, Gimeno EJ, et al. Lysosomal storage disease in Sida carpinifolia toxicosis: an induced mannosidosis in horses. *Equine Vet J* 2003;35:434–438.

[84] Delahunta A. Abiotrophy in domestic animals – a review. *Can J Vet Res* 1990;54:65–76.

[85] Debowes RM, Leipold HW, Turnerbeatty M. Cerebellar abiotrophy. *Vet Clin North Am Equine Pract* 1987;3:345–352.

[86] Bjorck G, Everz KE, Hansen HJ, et al. Congenital cerebellar ataxia in the Gotland Pony breed. *Zentralbl Veterinarmed A* 1973;20:341–354.

[87] Brostrom L. Slinger and cerebellar abiotrophy in horses – a literature review. Master's Thesis. Uppsala, Swedish University of Agricultural Sciences, Department of Animal Breeding and Genetics, 2011.

[88] Mayhew IG, ed. Congenital, genetic, and familial disorders. *Large Animal Neurology*, 2 ed. Oxford: Wiley-Blackwell; 2008:183–224.

[89] The eriskay pony society. http://www.eriskaypony.com/theeriskaypony.htm. Accessed November 29, 2014.

[90] Blanco A, Moyano R, Vivo J, et al. Purkinje cell apoptosis in Arabian horses with cerebellar abiotrophy. *J Vet Med A Physiol Pathol Clin Med* 2006;53:286–287.

[91] Brault LS, Cooper CA, Famula TR, et al. Mapping of equine cerebellar abiotrophy to ECA2 and identification of a potential causative mutation affecting expression of MUTYH. *Genomics* 2011;97:121–129.

[92] Brault LS, Famula TR, Penedo MCT. Inheritance of cerebellar abiotrophy in Arabians. *Am J Vet Res* 2011;72: 940–944.

[93] Brault LS, Penedo MCT. The frequency of the equine cerebellar abiotrophy mutation in non-Arabian horse breeds. *Equine Vet J* 2011;43:727–731.

[94] Baird JD, Mackenzi. CD. Cerebellar hypoplasia and degeneration in part Arab horses. *Aust Vet J* 1974;50:25–28.

[95] Turner Beatty M, Leipold HW, Cash W, et al. Cerebellar disease in the horse. *Proc Ann Meet Amer Assoc Equine Pract* 1985;21:241–255.

[96] Dungworth DL, Fowler ME. Cerebellar hypoplasia and degeneration in a foal. *Cornell Vet* 1966;56:17–24.

[97] Pongratz MC, Kircher P, Lang J, et al. Diagnostic evaluation of a foal with cerebellar abiotrophy using magnetic resonance imaging (MRI). *Pferdeheilkunde* 2010;26:559–562.

[98] Cavalleri JMV, Metzger J, Hellige M, et al. Morphometric magnetic resonance imaging and genetic testing in cerebellar abiotrophy in Arabian horses. *BMC Vet Res* 2013;9:105.

27 Equine Hepatic Encephalopathy

Tom Divers

College of Veterinary Medicine, Cornell University, Ithaca, USA

Hepatic encephalopathy (HE) is a neurologic disorder associated with liver failure. HE is common in horses with either acute or chronic liver failure and may also occur in foals with portosystemic shunts. There are also two primary hyperammonemia syndromes in horses that have similar clinical and laboratory findings (increased ammonia) similar to HE; these two syndromes are primary enteric hyperammonemia syndrome seen mostly in adult horses and a presumed inherited ammonia metabolism deficit in young Morgan horses.

Pathophysiology

The pathophysiology of HE is complex and likely involves several gut-derived neurotoxins, cerebral and systemic inflammation, cerebral vascular dysfunction, and neuroendocrine abnormalities. High concentrations of blood and cerebrospinal fluid (CSF) ammonia have been most commonly incriminated as causing the pathophysiologic events of HE. Ammonia (NH_3) is believed to pass the blood–brain barrier (BBB) by diffusion, while the less toxic or nontoxic ionized ammonia (NH_4^+) is limited to the transcellular route for translocation. Ammonia is believed to play a key role in the development of HE, with glutamate, NMDA (*N*-methyl-D-aspartate) receptor activity and increased glutamine all playing a central role in ammonia metabolism and HE [1]. Increased NH_3 in the brain results in increased metabolism of ammonia by astrocytes and the resulting accumulation of glutamine which is known to disrupt water balance in the brain leading to cytotoxic edema [2]. Inflammation and ammonia-induced free radical production in the brain may also cause vasogenic edema [3]. Increased ammonia concentrations in the brain may have direct effects on pH, membrane potential and neurotransmission, in addition to cellular metabolism and cerebral water balance [4]. Although undoubtedly the most important single neurotoxin involved in HE, ammonia should not be considered as the sole cause. In fact, a moderate number of horses with HE do not have blood ammonia values above the reported normal range. Other neurotransmitters are frequently discussed as playing role in HE, but their association has not been well documented. These neurotransmitters include endogenous benzodiazepine-like compounds, mercaptans, monoamine, and aromatic aminoacids [5].

Increased BBB permeability for ammonia may also play an integral role in HE. The BBB is the physical and metabolic barrier separating the peripheral circulation from the central nervous system (CNS) and regulates exchanges between the two [6]. Changes in BBB permeability may be due to both structural alterations in tight junctions and inflammatory vascular effects and functional changes. Increases in blood ammonia, metalloproteinase activity, and endotoxin may increase permeability of the BBB in liver failure permitting transport of other neurotoxins to the brain [7].

Systemic inflammation and sepsis from endotoxemia or bacterial translocation are often part of the syndrome of HE. Breakdown products of injured hepatocytes in addition to systemic inflammatory cytokine production increases free radical and metalloproteinase concentrations, which can have severe systemic effects in addition to increasing permeability of the BBB [8]. The toxic effect of these events on the brain with HE is believed to result in both cytotoxic (intracellular swelling without increased permeability of BBB) and vasogenic (increased permeability of BBB levels to net gain of fluid) brain edema.

Equine Neurology, Second Edition. Martin Furr and Stephen Reed.
© 2015 John Wiley & Sons, Inc. Published 2015 by John Wiley & Sons, Inc.
Companion website: www.wiley.com/go/furr/neurology

Causes

The causes of HE include any disorder that results in diffuse hepatocellular dysfunction. Predominantly biliary diseases, such as cholangiohepatitis, are much less likely to result in HE than are diseases that cause more fulminant hepatocyte dysfunction (e.g., Theiler's disease). The diseases that are most likely to cause HE include Theiler's disease, pyrrolizidine alkaloid toxicosis, any cause of chronic fibrosis, *Cassia occidentalis* seed ingestion, phosphide/phosphine poisoning, hepatic lipidosis, iron toxicosis, panicum hay, alsike clover, and less commonly neoplasia and bacterial cholangiohepatitis [9–19]. Portosystemic shunt in foals and hyperammonemia in Morgan foals and primary hyperammonemia in horses will also have signs identical to HE because of the marked elevation in ammonia in those cases [20–22] (Table 27.1).

Clinical signs

The clinical signs of HE in horses may be mild with only depression, anorexia, and frequent yawning. In other cases, the signs can be fulminant and include head pressing, blindness, circling, and coma [23, 24] (Figures 27.1 and 27.2). Ataxia can be noticeable in some cases while absent in others. Rarely, ataxia may precede HE signs or icterus in acute liver failure (e.g., Theiler's disease). Clinical examination may reveal decreased muscle tone of the lower lips, delayed or absent response to touching the inner nares and cortical blindness often accompanied by mydriasis. These signs are all a result of the cortical disease that occurs with HE. A scoring system has been devised to describe the severity of clinical signs, and it may prove useful in monitoring (Table 27.2).

Other clinical signs associated with liver failure and not attributable to HE include jaundiced membranes, discolored plasma and urine, colic, photosensitization, and weight loss in more chronic cases [23, 24].

Laryngeal paralysis or dysphagia (presumably due to HE and functional disturbance in the nucleus ambiguous)

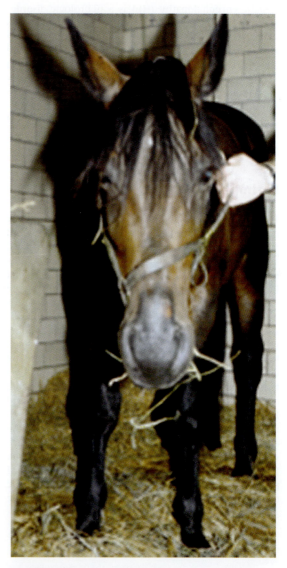

Figure 27.1 A 13-year-old Standardbred mare with Theiler's disease and hepatic encephalopathy. The mare had an acute onset of head pressing, biting the wall and hay without purposefully eating. Ataxia was also present and marked jaundice was noted upon examination of mucus membranes.

Table 27.1 Differential diagnoses for the encephalopathic horse.

Head trauma
Viral encephalitis (including WNV, EEE, WEE, VEE, and Rabies virus)
Equine protozoal myeloencephalitis (EPM)
Intracranial abscess (including *Streptococcus*, *Rhodococcus*, and *Listeria*)
Leukoencephalomalacia (moldy corn toxicosis)
Verminous encephalitis (e.g., *Halicephalobus* spp.)
Organophosphate toxicity
Nigropallidal encephalomalacia (yellow star-thistle toxicosis)
Hepatic encephalopathy
Hyperammonemia
Hyponatremia
Heavy metal toxicosis (arsenic, lead)
Intracranial neoplasia (cholesterol granuloma, etc.)
Adverse drug reactions (e.g., fluphenazine)
Meningitis

Additional considerations discussed in previous sections.
EEE, eastern equine encephalitis; VEE, Venezuelan equine encephalitis; WEE, western equine encephalitis; WNV, west Nile virus.

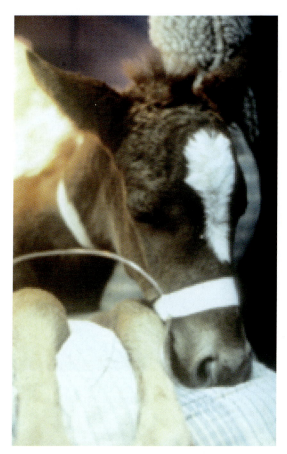

Figure 27.2 A 5-week-old foal with hepatic encephalopathy caused by Tyzzer's disease. The foal had severe hypoglycemia and metabolic acidosis in addition to marked elevations in serum bilirubin, bile acids, ammonia, and hepatic-derived enzymes.

Table 27.2 Clinical staging of HE according to neurologic observations.[a]

Stage	Clinical observations
1	Subtle forebrain disturbances often dismissed as unusual behavior for the animal. Often missed.
2	Episodic drowsiness, irritability, disorientation, constant pacing, and/or circling. Head pressing may also be observed.
3	Inappropriate responses to stimuli, stupor, aggression, fear, somnolence, depression, yawning, and ptyalism.
4	Recumbency, loss of motor control, periodic unconsciousness, and coma. Seizures are infrequently observed.

Adapted from Barton (2004).
[a] Ref. [25].

and gastric impaction/rupture (presumably due to autonomic nerve dysfunction) are additional findings with HE in horses [26, 27].

Laboratory findings

Almost all cases of HE have laboratory evidence of hepatic disease (elevated liver derived enzymes in the serum) and dysfunction (increased serum direct and indirect bilirubin and serum bile acid concentration) [23]. On very rare occasions with severe chronic fibrosis and HE, liver-derived serum enzymes may be unremarkable. This is presumably due to marked fibrosis and loss of most functional hepatocytes [24]. Other common laboratory findings supportive of hepatic failure include prolonged prothrombin and partial thromboplastin time, increased blood lactates (both D- and L isomers), increased globulins, decreased albumin, and decreased blood urea nitrogen (most common with prolonged hepatic fibrosis). Two other laboratory findings that are believed to be directly related to HE are hyperammonemia and hypoglycemia. Increased blood ammonia is common, but certainly not always above normal range in horses with HE. Hypoglycemia is rather uncommon in adult horses with HE but common in young foals with HE.

The normal range of blood ammonia varies between laboratories, but it is generally less than 90 μmol/l. Many cases of HE have concentrations in the 100–200 range; a few cases are greater than 200 and many cases are at the upper normal range, 70–90. Horses with HE as a result of liver failure generally do not have ammonia concentrations as high as those seen with primary enteric hyperammonemia, (Figure 27.3) portosystemic shunts, or Morgan foal hyperammonemia syndrome that often have blood ammonia concentrations of greater than 300 μmol/l [20–22]. Metabolic acidosis, mostly due to lactic acidosis, is common in horses with HE. Although primary respiratory alkalosis resulting from hyperventilation is a common finding in humans with HE, this is rare in horses and most horses with HE have a metabolic acidosis. A unique finding with liver failure in the horse is polycythemia in many cases.

Pathologic findings

Pathologic findings in the CNS of horses with HE consist of reactive astrocytosis in gray matter, Alzheimer type II cells, and cerebral edema [28]. Alzheimer type II cells (enlarged astrocytes with basophilic nucleoli which appear to be metabolically hyperactive) are closely associated with increased blood and CSF ammonia; these cells are also routinely found in the brain of horses dying from primary intestinal hyperammonemia [29] (Figure 27.4).

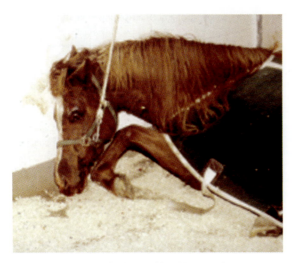

Figure 27.3 A 7-year-old thoroughbred horse with primary enteric hyperammonemia. The horse presented with colic and encephalopathic signs (blind with normal pupillary light response, head pressing, circling). Alzheimer type II cells were found in the brain on necropsy. All liver enzymes and function test were normal except for ammonia being greater than 366 μmol/l. The horse was hyperglycemic and had a metabolic acidosis.

Treatment

Treatments for HE revolve around decreasing enteric-derived neurotoxins (primarily ammonia); decreasing cerebral edema; correcting glucose, electrolyte, and acid–base abnormalities; and maintaining perfusion and oxygenation to the brain and other vital organs. Providing specific treatment for the liver disease *per se* (i.e., hepatic lipidosis or bacterial cholangiohepatitis) is imperative; but in many cases of liver failure, there are no specific treatments for the hepatic disease and only supportive care, as outlined later, can be provided. Additionally, general supportive treatments that inhibit both systemic and neuroinflammation, reduce oxidative stress and prevent multiple organ dysfunction are recommended.

Horses with HE can have propulsive (compulsive forward movement) cortical signs, which may require sedation in order to properly attend the horse and prevent injury to the horse or humans. A low dose of detomidine (5–10 μg/kg IV) may suffice. It is important to not overly sedate a horse with HE as that might cause excessive lowering of the head in the standing horse and promote cerebral edema in addition to the potential negative effects on the brain, liver, and other organ perfusion. If additional seizure or propulsive behavior control are required, phenobarbital administration could be used short term. Although phenobarbital is metabolized in the liver, as are many drugs, it may have a protective and prolonged effect

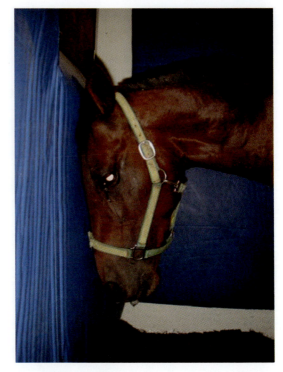

Figure 27.4 Head pressing behavior in an encephalopathic Quarterhorse. (Photo courtesy of The Ohio State University Veterinary Teaching Hospital.)

on the brain during metabolic or oxidative stress. If phenobarbital is used, respiration and blood oxygenation should be monitored and appropriate treatment (e.g., intranasal oxygen) provided, if necessary, and therapeutic drug monitoring performed. Diazepam should not be used in horses with HE as it will induce astrocyte swelling and worsen HE. Ideally, sedatives should be avoided in HE [3] (Table 27.3). Pregabalin (4 mg/kg PO, Q 8-12 H) can be used.

The next stepwise treatment for HE would be to correct intravascular fluid, electrolyte, and glucose abnormalities. A normal or slightly high-sodium-content fluid with additional potassium chloride (20 mEq/l) added is an acceptable initial crystalloid therapy for HE. Supplemental potassium is generally recommended since horses with HE are anorexic and would most likely be deficient in total body potassium (TBP) and hypokalemia is known to increase proximal tubular ammoniogenesis with the increased ammonia being returned to circulation and worsening the symptoms of HE [30]. Hypokalemia can also have adverse effects of other organ systems (e.g., cardiovascular).

One of the most important goals in the treatment of HE is to promote reduction of blood and CSF ammonia concentration [31]. The primary means for reduction of

Table 27.3 Suggested drug dosages for HE therapeutics.

Drug	Dose
Metronidazole	10–15 mg/kg PO TID
Neomycin	10–50 mg/kg PO BID-QID for 2 days
Sodium ampicillin	10 mg/kg IV/IM QID
Potassium penicillin	22,000 IU/kg IV QID
Gentamicin sulfate	6.6 mg/kg IV SID
Lactulose	0.3–0.5 ml/kg PO QID
Omeprazole	4 mg/kg PO SID
Minocycline	4 mg/kg PO BID
Sarmazenil	0.04 mg/kg IV Q 4-6 H
L-carnitine	25–50 mg/kg PO SID
Mineral oil	10–16 ml/kg PO SID
Sodium sulfate	1 g/kg PO SID for 3 days

blood/CSF ammonia is to reduce the production or absorption of ammonia from the gut. Therapeutic options include neomycin (10 mg/kg PO q8h) or another poorly absorbed antibiotic. Metronidazole has equal effect on decreasing intestinal ammonia production, but it is well absorbed, metabolized by the liver and may have neurotoxic effects. It may be preferred to combine neomycin with lactulose. Neomycin decreases ammonia production via its effect upon the gastrointestinal microbial population by decreasing ammonia-producing bacteria. Lactulose, a poorly absorbed carbohydrate, decreases ammonia when its metabolism in the large bowel results in increased H^+ production and conversion of some ammonia ions (NH_3) to poorly absorbed NH_4^+ (ammonium) salts. Orally administered antibiotics should not be prolonged beyond 1–3 days to lower the risk of antibiotic-associated diarrhea. It would be ideal if the treatments softened the stool (a cathartic effect) without causing diarrhea.

Other oral treatments that have been used to lower enteric ammonia production include probiotics and in humans the antimicrobial rifaximin. Probiotics, prebiotics, and symbiotics (probiotic with lactulose) may all have some efficacy in treating HE by modulating the gut flora [32]. They may decrease ammonia production and endotoxin absorption, but they are not proven to be beneficial in HE studies.

Treatments to decrease neuroinflammation and disruption of the BBB are mostly unproven but include N-acetylcysteine, minocycline, neurosteroids such as progesterone, or allopregnanolone and hypothermia [2, 6, 7]. Treatments to support energy metabolism and antioxidant activity to the brain include B vitamins, vitamin C and DMSO although all are unproven. Treatment of cerebral edema with mannitol or hypertonic saline may have some temporary effect in decreasing cerebral edema [33].

Controlled clinical trials showed that flumazenil had a transient beneficial effect in only a subpopulation of HE patients. Their presumed positive effect in those cases was from inhibition of benzodiazepine receptor ligands, which may play a role in the pathogenesis of HE by increasing GABAergic tone [34].

Another commonly recommended treatment for HE is oral supplementation of the branched chain amino acids (BCAAs) valine, leucine, and isoleucine. Their role in treating HE is controversial with some reports demonstrating beneficial effects possibly via improved glucose metabolism, decrease protein and muscle catabolism, and as an alternative pathway (in muscle) for ammonia detoxification [35]. They may, therefore, be of particular benefit in the treatment of HE caused by hepatic lipidosis, but other reports point out concerns of BCCA administration increasing glutamine synthesis and worsening of HE [36].

There are no highly effective, safe, and specific treatments for decreasing ammonia that is present in the blood and CSF of patients with HE. Glycerol phenylbutyrate has been used in human clinical studies, sometimes combined with BCAA, to lower ammonia by providing an alternative to ammonia to urea pathway with excretion of phenylacetylglutamine in the urine [36, 37].

Prognosis

In one retrospective study evaluating a large number of horses with liver disease, the most useful noninvasive prognostic indicator was the severity of clinical signs including stage of hepatic encephalopathy. In a study of 116 horses with hepatic disease, 13.8% demonstrated signs of HE, and those with HE were greater than five times more likely to die within 6 months compared to horses with liver disease that did not show signs of HE [25]. Increased plasma fibrinogen concentrations and subnormal serum creatinine concentrations had a direct association with nonsurvival [25]. Prognosis can depend on the underlying hepatic disease. For instance, pyrrolizidine alkaloid toxicity carries a poor to guarded long-term prognosis, but horses may survive many years after a diagnosis is confirmed. Regardless of the cause, the prognosis is considered poor for horses with hepatic disease and neurologic dysfunction. Some authors have reported up to 40% of horses with HE survive beyond 6 months, a finding that certainly justifies attempted therapy on a short-term basis.

References

[1] Sørensen M. Update on cerebral uptake of blood ammonia. *Metab Brain Dis* 2013;28:155–159.
[2] Desjardins P, Du T, Jiang W, et al. Pathogenesis of hepatic encephalopathy and brain edema in acute liver failure: role of glutamine redefined. *Neurochem Int* 2012;60:690–696.

[3] Lachmann V, Görg B, Bidmon HJ, et al. Precipitants of hepatic encephalopathy induce rapid astrocyte swelling in an oxidative stress dependent manner. *Arch Biochem Biophys* 2013;536:143–151.

[4] Rose CF. Ammonia-lowering strategies for the treatment of hepatic encephalopathy. *Clin Pharmacol Ther* 2012;92:321–331.

[5] Palomero-Gallagher N, Zilles K. Neurotransmitter receptor alterations in hepatic encephalopathy: a review. *Arch Biochem Biophys* 2013;536:109–121.

[6] Cui W, Sun CM, Liu P. Alterations of blood-brain barrier and associated factors in acute liver failure. *Gastroenterol Res Pract* 2013;2013:841707.

[7] Jayakumar AR, Ruiz-Cordero R, Tong XY, et al. Brain edema in acute liver failure: role of neurosteroids. *Arch Biochem Biophys* 2013;536:171–175

[8] Coltart I, Tranah TH, Shawcross DL. Inflammation and hepatic encephalopathy. *Arch Biochem Biophys* 2013;536:189–196.

[9] Aleman M, Nieto JE, Carr EA, et al. Serum hepatitis associated with commercial plasma transfusion in horses. *J Vet Intern Med* 2005;19:120–122.

[10] Peek SF, Divers TJ. Medical treatment of cholangiohepatitis and cholelithiasis in mature horses: 9 cases (1991–1998). *Equine Vet J* 2000;32:301–306.

[11] de Lanux-Van GV. Tansy ragwort poisoning in a horse in southern Ontario. *Can Vet J* 2000;41:409–410.

[12] Pearson EG. Liver failure attributable to pyrrolizidine alkaloid toxicosis and associated with inspiratory dyspnea in ponies: three cases (1982–1988). *J Am Vet Med Assoc* 1991;198:1651–1654.

[13] Nation PN. Alsike clover poisoning: a review. *Can Vet J* 1989;30:410–415.

[14] Divers TJ, Warner A, Vaala WE, et al. Toxic hepatic failure in newborn foals. *J Am Vet Med Assoc* 1983;183:1407–1413.

[15] Ossedryver SM, Baldwin GI, Stone BM, et al. *Indigofera spicata* (creeping indigo) poisoning of three ponies. *Aust Vet J* 2013;9:143–149.

[16] Easterwood L, Chaffin MK, Marsh PS, et al. Phosphine intoxication following oral exposure of horses to aluminum phosphide-treated feed. *J Am Vet Med Assoc* 2010;236:446–450.

[17] Johnson AL, Divers TJ, Freckleton ML, et al. Fall Panicum (*Panicum dichotomiflorum*) hepatotoxicosis in horses and sheep. *J Vet Intern Med* 2006;20:1414–1421.

[18] Mogg TD, Palmer JE. Hyperlipidemia, hyperlipemia, and hepatic lipidosis in American miniature horses: 23 cases (1990–1994). *J Am Vet Med Assoc* 1995;207:604–607.

[19] Polkes AC, Giguère S, Lester GD, et al. Factors associated with outcome in foals with neonatal isoerythrolysis (72 cases, 1988–2003). *J Vet Intern Med* 2008;22:1216–1222.

[20] McConnico RS, Duckett WM, Wood PA. Persistent hyperammonemia in two related Morgan weanlings. *J Vet Intern Med* 1997;11:264–266.

[21] Peek SF, Divers TJ, Jackson CJ. Hyperammonaemia associated with encephalopathy and abdominal pain without evidence of liver disease in four mature horses. *Equine Vet J* 1997;29:70–74.

[22] Fortier LA, Fubini SL, Flanders JA, et al. The diagnosis and surgical correction of congenital portosystemic vascular anomalies in two calves and two foals. *Vet Surg* 1996;25:154–160.

[23] Bergero D, Nery J. Hepatic diseases in horses. *J Anim Physiol Anim Nutr (Berl)* 2008;92:345–355.

[24] McGorum BC, Murphy D, Love S, et al. Clinicopathological features of equine primary hepatic diseases: a review of 50 cases. *Vet Rec* 1999;145:134–139.

[25] Hurcombe S. Equine Hepatic Encephalopathy. In: Furr M, Reed S, eds. *Equine Neurology*. Ames:Wiley;2008:257–268.

[26] Hughes KJ, McGorum BC, Love S, et al. Bilateral laryngeal paralysis associated with hepatic dysfunction and hepatic encephalopathy in six ponies and four horses. *Vet Rec* 2009;164:142–147.

[27] Milne EM, Pogson DM, Doxey DL. Secondary gastric impaction associated with ragwort poisoning in three ponies. *Vet Rec* 1990;126:502–504.

[28] Thumburu KK, Taneja S, Vasishta RK, et al. Neuropathology of acute liver failure. *Neurochem Int* 2012;60:672–675.

[29] Johns IC, Del Piero F, Wilkins PA. Hepatic encephalopathy in a pregnant mare: identification of histopathological changes in the brain of a mare and fetus. *Aust Vet J* 2007;85:337–340.

[30] Weiner ID, Wino CS. Hypokalemia – consequences, causes, and corrections. *J Am Soc Nephrol* 1997;8:1179–1188.

[31] Poh Z, Chang PE. A current review of the diagnostic and treatment strategies of hepatic encephalopathy. *Int J Hepatol* 2012;2012:480309.

[32] Sekhar MS, Unnikrishnan MK, Rodrigues GS, et al. Synbiotic formulation of probiotic and lactulose combination for hepatic encephalopathy treatment: a realistic hope? *Med Hypotheses* 2013;81:167–168.

[33] Mohsenin V. Assessment and management of cerebral edema and intracranial hypertension in acute liver failure. *J Crit Care* 2013;28:783–791.

[34] Als-Nielsen B, Gluud LL, Gluud C. Benzodiazepine receptor antagonists for hepatic encephalopathy. *Cochrane Database Syst Rev* 2004;2:CD002798.

[35] Dam G, Ott P, Aagaard NK, et al. Branched-chain amino acids and muscle ammonia detoxification in cirrhosis. *Metab Brain Dis* 2013;28:217-220.

[36] Holecek M. Branched-chain amino acids and ammonia metabolism in liver disease: therapeutic implications. *Nutrition* 2013;29:1186–1191.

[37] Rockey DC, Vierling JM, Mantry P, et al. Randomized, double-blind, controlled study of glycerol phenylbutyrate in hepatic encephalopathy. *Hepatology* 2014;59:1073–1083.

28   Cervical Vertebral Stenotic Myelopathy

Amy L. Johnson[1] and Stephen Reed[2]

[1] New Bolton Center, University of Pennsylvania School of Veterinary Medicine, Kennett Square, USA
[2] Rood and Riddle Equine Hospital, Lexington, USA

Introduction

Cervical vertebral stenotic myelopathy (CVSM) is a common cause of ataxia in horses and other animals. Early manuscripts describing this problem indicate genetic predisposition as a known risk factor [1]. Further studies have shown the problem is a developmental abnormality which might have genetic predisposition and environmental influences. CVSM is characterized by ataxia and weakness, caused by narrowing of the cervical vertebral canal and compression of the spinal cord often in combination with malalignment and malformation of the cervical vertebrae. Stenosis of the vertebral canal, anywhere from the first cervical vertebral body (C1) to the first thoracic vertebral body (T1), is the most important abnormality in CVSM.

Neurologic gait deficits in horses have been recognized since at least 1860 [2] and the term "Wobblers syndrome" was introduced in 1938 to describe several clinically observed abnormalities [3]. CVSM is the main cause of "Wobblers syndrome" and older synonyms for CVSM include equine sensory ataxia, equine incoordination, and spinal ataxia [4]. As malformation, malarticulation, or malalignment of one or more cervical vertebrae generally leads to CVSM, the disease has also been referred to as cervical vertebral malformation (CVM) or cervical vertebral instability (CVI). At the present time either cervical vertebral compressive myelopathy (CVCM) or CVSM seem to be the most commonly used and appropriate terms.

Types of CVSM

Rooney distinguished three types of CVSM [5]. In type I, the vertebral column is fixed in flexed position at the site of malarticulation/malformation, which generally occurs at C2–C3, but has been observed at other sites as well. Type I CVSM is uncommon and often present at birth. In type II CVSM, symmetrical overgrowth of the articular processes causes spinal cord compression during flexion of the neck. Type II lesions occur most often in sucklings and weanlings and are generally found in the mid-cervical region. Type III CVSM is characterized by asymmetrical overgrowth of one articular process that leads to compression of the spinal cord either directly by bony proliferation, or indirectly by associated soft tissue hypertrophy. Type III is most often seen in mature horses but can begin as early as 1–3 years of age. This lesion most often affects C5–C6 and C6–C7 [6].

More recent publications divide CVSM into two broad categories or classes of horses; one affecting young horses (Type I, which correlates with Rooney's Type II) and one affecting older horses (Type II, which correlates with Rooney's Type III) [7, 8]. In both types of CVSM, morphological changes of the cervical vertebrae cause stenosis of the vertebral canal and spinal cord compression. Type I CVSM, the condition of young horses, is observed most often in Thoroughbreds and is a multifactorial disease including such factors as gender, inheritance, diet, trauma, and rate of growth [9, 10]. These factors cause developmental abnormalities of the cervical vertebral column including malformation of the vertebral canal, enlargement of the physes, extension of the dorsal aspect of the vertebral arch, angulation sometimes with fixation between adjacent vertebrae, and malformation of the articular processes as a result of osteochondrosis [11]. Type II CVSM, the condition of older horses, affects all breeds and involves osteoarthritic changes of the articular processes. These changes often include malformation with degenerative joint disease of the articular processes, wedging of the vertebral canal, periarticular proliferation with or without a synovial or epidural cyst, and overt fractures of the articular processes [11, 12]. It is important to note that many older horses will have bony abnormalities of the cervical

Equine Neurology, Second Edition. Martin Furr and Stephen Reed.
© 2015 John Wiley & Sons, Inc. Published 2015 by John Wiley & Sons, Inc.
Companion website: www.wiley.com/go/furr/neurology

vertebral column; however, only a small percentage of horses develop clinical signs as a result of spinal cord compression [13].

Epidemiology

CVSM is the leading cause of noninfectious spinal ataxia in the horse [9, 14–17] and is estimated to affect 1.3–2% of Thoroughbred horses [5] but has also been identified in many other breeds including Arabians, Morgans, and Appaloosas [9, 16, 18, 19]. Breeds described as predisposed to CVCM include Thoroughbred, Quarter Horse, Warmblood, and Tennessee Walking Horse [11, 12, 16]. A large case-control study showed that Thoroughbreds, Tennessee Walking Horses, and Warmbloods were overrepresented compared to Quarter Horses, whereas Arabians and Standardbreds were underrepresented [20].

Male horses are more likely to be affected than female horses [6, 8, 9, 12, 14–16, 20, 21]. Age is significantly associated with a diagnosis of CVSM; horses less than 7 years of age are more likely to be diagnosed with CVCM than horses 10 years or older [20]. Horses with type 1 CVSM are generally younger at time of diagnosis than horses with type 2 CVSM [8]. Although the horse is often 1–2 years of age at presentation to a veterinarian, the onset of the condition was likely much earlier. The onset of clinical signs is dependent upon the degree of compression or repeated trauma to the spinal cord.

Clinical examination

History
Young horses often have a history of a recent period of rapid growth or weight gain, and foals might have high milk-producing dams or be larger than similarly aged unaffected foals. Although a common historical finding is acute onset of ataxia or gait abnormalities following trauma, that is, a fall or halter-breaking accident, in many cases the horse will have been mildly ataxic prior to the observed trauma. In fact, the mild neurologic deficits might have caused the traumatic incident that resulted in exacerbation of the neurologic signs. In other cases, the onset is more insidious and weeks or months pass before neurologic deficits are recognized. Older horses (with type II CVSM) more commonly have a more chronic history of performance problems, inability to progress in training, possible lameness, reluctance to bend, neck stiffness, tripping, or even behavior issues.

Physical examination
Physical examination might reveal abrasions around the heels or medial aspect of the thoracic limbs due to interference, and short, squared hooves due to excessive toe-dragging. Although the physical examination is often unremarkable, many young horses affected with CVSM have signs of developmental orthopedic disease such as physitis or physeal enlargement of the long bones, joint effusion secondary to osteochondrosis, and flexural limb deformities. Stewart et al. demonstrated the increased incidence of osteochondrosis in horses with CVSM [22]. Evidence of damage to nerve roots or spinal nerves such as cervical pain, atrophy of cervical musculature, and cutaneous hypalgesia adjacent to affected cervical vertebrae is rare in young horses. These signs are more common in older horses with arthropathies of the caudal cervical vertebrae; these horses might demonstrate focal muscle wasting, focal sweating, or palpable bony abnormalities of the vertebral articular processes. Reluctance to raise or lower the head or bend the neck laterally is more commonly observed in older horses.

Neurologic examination
Complete neurologic examination is described elsewhere in this text; but in general, horses with CVSM should have a normal attitude/mental status, normal cranial nerve function, and normal spinal reflexes. The thoracolaryngeal reflex, which is the adductory movement of the arytenoid cartilages of the larynx in response to a slap on the thorax (slap test), might be diminished in horses with cervical spinal cord disease. A negative result for this test does not exclude the possibility of cervical spinal cord disease, however [23].

Gait examination will reveal upper motor neuron paresis and general proprioceptive ataxia compatible with compression and damage of the cervical spinal cord white matter. Ataxia and spasticity followed by weakness are usually observed in the pelvic limbs first and then progress to the thoracic limbs [16, 24]. Signs tend to remain more severe in the pelvic than thoracic limbs and are often relatively symmetric, although many horses with CVSM show some asymmetry. Asymmetric signs are more common in horses with significant degenerative joint disease of the articular processes and lateral compression of the spinal cord [17]. In a standing horse, general proprioceptive deficits might be present such as an abnormally wide-based stance, abnormal limb placement, and delayed limb positioning. Ataxia and paresis are more easily observed at a walk than at faster gaits and horses often demonstrate truncal sway, irregular and unpredictable stride length and foot placement with a tendency to have a longer stride, an over-reaching or "floating" thoracic limb gait, circumduction of the outside limb, pivoting on the inside limb, toe-dragging or scuffing, delayed protraction, and stumbling. The horse may exhibit an exaggerated, stiff-legged or spastic movement. These signs will be exacerbated when the horse is circled, led up and down a hill or over obstacles, and when the horse's head is elevated during the neurologic examination. In young horses, clinical signs of ataxia often progress and then stabilize. This cycle of progression followed by stabilization can occur several times prior to final confirmation of the diagnosis.

Neuropathophysiology

The characteristic signs of CVSM are the result of lesions in the white matter of the cervical spinal cord, specifically damage to the ascending general proprioception pathways (causing ataxia) and to the descending upper motor neuron pathways (causing paresis) [4]. Progression of disease is due to prolonged compression or repeated trauma to the spinal cord, with initial damage to superficial white matter followed by gradual spread to deeper areas. The lateral funiculi are especially susceptible to degeneration by pressure or compression. Controversy exists regarding the presence of altered blood supply to the spinal cord, and its potential role in the pathogenesis of CVSM [16].

A cervical spinal cord compressive lesion produces more severe pelvic limb than thoracic limb ataxia in part because of the more superficial anatomic location of the proprioceptive tracts from the pelvic limbs, the dorsal and ventral spinocerebellar tracts, compared with those of the thoracic limbs, the cuneocerebellar and cranial (rostral) spinocerebellar tracts [4, 25]. Disparity in signs between the pelvic and thoracic limbs might also be explained by the greater distance of the pelvic limbs from the center of gravity of the horse and the greater percentage of upper motor neuron synapses in the gray matter of the cervical intumescence [4]. Obvious signs of disturbance of the ascending general somatic afferent pathway, characterized by decreased nociception, occur rarely.

Differential diagnoses for spinal ataxia

Important differential diagnoses for spinal ataxia in a young horse include CVSM, equine protozoal myeloencephalitis (EPM), trauma, equine degenerative myeloencephalopathy (EDM), and equine herpesvirus 1 myeloencephalopathy (EHV-1). Less common causes of spinal ataxia and weakness include rabies, viral encephalitides (Eastern, Western, Venezuelan, and West Nile), brain abscesses, neoplasia, and hepatoencephalopathy. Congenital anomalies and malformations of the vertebral column which could cause compression of the cervical spinal cord are reported infrequently, including occipitoatlantoaxial malformation (OAAM), butterfly vertebrae, hemivertebrae, block vertebrae, atlantoaxial

subluxation, and atlantoaxial instability [19]. Spinal cord compression can also result from traumatic injury [26], vertebral fracture [27–29], vertebral neoplasia [30], discospondylitis [31, 32], diskospondylosis [33], intervertebral disk protrusion [31, 34], arachnoid diverticulum [35], unusual parasite migration [36], and spinal hematomas [37]. A more complete discussion of the differential diagnosis of horses with spinal ataxia is found in Chapter 8.

Diagnostic techniques

The diagnosis of CVSM is generally based on a detailed history, the signalment, recognition of spinal ataxia on neurologic examination, imaging findings consistent with vertebral canal stenosis, and elimination of other possible causes of spinal ataxia. The "gold standard" for confirmation of the diagnosis remains a postmortem examination [6, 9].

Blood and cerebrospinal fluid analysis
Hematologic and serum biochemical parameters are generally unremarkable in horses with CVSM. Cerebrospinal fluid (CSF) analysis is normal in the majority of cases, but CSF analysis remains an important ancillary diagnostic tool in the evaluation of equine neurologic disorders [38]. Xanthochromia, subtle elevation of the white blood cell count, and a rare increase in aspartate transaminase activity have occasionally been demonstrated in CSF from horses with CVSM [16]. Examination of CSF CK activity was once thought to be a useful diagnostic test for horses with CVSM; however, horses with confirmed disease usually did not have increased activity, presumably because the rate of release of CK is too slow to allow accumulation of the enzyme [39]. Cerebrospinal fluid electrophoresis has been described as an aid to diagnose cervical compression. Furr et al. demonstrated that CSF high-resolution electrophoresis revealed a less prominent β_2-globulin fraction and more frequent post-β peaks in horses with compressive disease when compared to horses without neurologic disease [40]. Cytokine gene expression in CSF has also been evaluated and might be helpful in differentiating horses with CVSM from horses with other neurologic diseases and clinically healthy horses [41]. However, in the authors' opinion the true value of CSF analysis in horses suspected of having CVSM is immunologic testing to rule out differential diagnoses such as EPM.

Plain radiography
Lateral radiographs of the cervical vertebrae, obtained in the standing horse, can be subjected to subjective, semiquantitative, and objective analyses. Most horses with CVSM have bony malformations of the cervical vertebrae,

although exceptions exist. The five characteristic bony malformations of the cervical vertebrae in horses with CVSM are "flare" of the caudal vertebral epiphysis of the vertebral body, abnormal ossification of the articular processes, malalignment between adjacent vertebrae, extension of the dorsal laminae, and degenerative joint disease of the articular processes [9, 14–16, 19] (Figure 28.1). Degenerative joint disease characterized by osteochondrosis and/or osteoarthrosis of the articular processes is a common lesion identified on cervical vertebral radiographs in horses affected with both type I and type II CVSM, and is a defining feature of type II CVSM [9, 12] (Figure 28.2a, b).

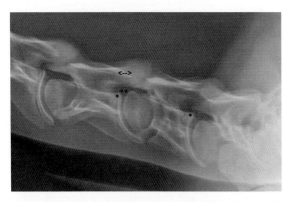

Figure 28.1 Survey radiograph of the caudal cervical vertebral column (C5–C7) of an abnormal 6 month-old Thoroughbred colt. Several characteristic bony malformations of CVSM are present, including flare of the caudal epiphysis of the vertebral body (*), malalignment between adjacent vertebrae (++), and extension of the dorsal lamina (< -- >).

Several caveats exist to subjective interpretation of equine cervical radiographs. Most importantly, subjective assessment of cervical radiographs does not adequately discriminate between horses with and without CVSM [15]. Compressive lesions can develop at vertebral sites that are not affected by bony malformation, and sites with malformation do not always cause compression [16, 22]. Evaluation of degenerative joint disease is particularly challenging, both in terms of radiographic technique and interpretation. Articular process disease is most common in the caudal cervical region, where overlying muscle is thickest and dorsoventral views difficult to obtain. There is limited visualization of the articular process joints in laterolateral radiographs, and oblique views are difficult to interpret unless ideal technique is used [42]. Even when degenerative joint disease is radiographically obvious, the significance of such change is often unclear. Age of the horse appears to contribute to the presence of degenerative joint disease, but disease has not been shown to correlate with clinical signs of neurologic disease [43].

Many investigators have attempted to improve radiographic interpretation by obtaining more objective values. Minimum sagittal diameter (MSD) values were published for horses under anesthesia [16]; however, magnification made these values impossible to interpret and unreliable in cervical vertebral radiographs obtained in standing horses. Subsequently, a noninvasive, semi-quantitative, radiographic CVSM scoring system was developed for foals in which multiple radiographic characteristics were considered, one of which was stenosis of the vertebral canal. The presence of stenosis was assessed by the corrected MSD (ratio of MSD: vertebral body length) in which the MSD was measured either

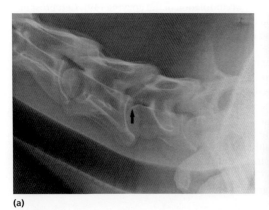

(a)

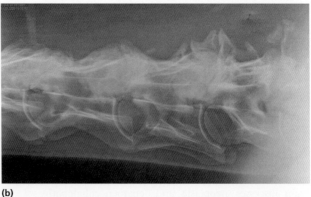

(b)

Figure 28.2 (a) Survey radiograph of the caudal cervical vertebral column of an abnormal 3-year-old National Show Horse gelding. Note the degenerative joint disease of the articular processes between C6–C7 with ventral bony proliferation that obscures the intervertebral foramina (arrow). (b) Survey radiograph of the caudal cervical vertebral column of an abnormal teenage Thoroughbred mare. Severe degenerative joint disease of the articular processes is present at all articulations, with extensive osteophytes.

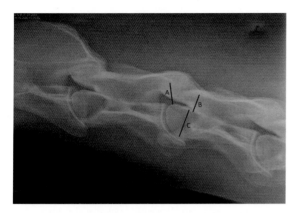

Figure 28.3 Survey radiograph of the third and fourth cervical vertebrae of a normal adult horse. The intervertebral sagittal ratio (A:C) is determined by A (minimum sagittal diameter between two adjacent vertebrae) and C (sagittal height of the maximum dimension of the cranial aspect of the caudal vertebral body). The intravertebral sagittal ratio (B:C) is determined by B (minimum sagittal diameter within a vertebra) and C (sagittal height of the maximum dimension of the cranial aspect of the same vertebral body).

intravertebral or intervertebral [11]. Using this scoring system, foals with signs of CVSM were successfully distinguished from normal foals [11].

An intravertebral ratio method of canal diameter assessment was developed for use in adult horses based on an a similar method that improved accuracy of diagnosis of cervical spinal stenosis in people [12]. This method is still frequently used and requires direct lateral radiographs. The sagittal ratio is the ratio of the MSD:sagittal height of the maximum dimension of the cranial aspect of the vertebral body (Figures 28.3 and 28.4). Assessment of this ratio is therefore independent of radiographic magnification. A ratio of less than 50% at C4, C5, or C6 or a ratio of less than 52% at C7 is associated with a high likelihood (likelihood ratio: 26.1–41.5) of having cervical stenotic myelopathy (Table 28.1). The sensitivity and specificity of this ratio method is greater than 89% at each vertebral site using suggested cut-offs of less than 52% for C4, C5, and C6 and less than 56% for C7 [12]. Although this method is relatively accurate in detecting CVSM, it does not accurately identify the site(s) of compression for any individual horse [7].

More recently, inclusion of intervertebral MSD measurements for assessing canal height has been proposed as a way to increase the accuracy of using standing survey radiographs to diagnose CVSM in horses and assist in identifying sites of compression [33, 44, 45] (Figures 28.3 and 28.4). When intra- and intervertebral MSD ratios were applied to a small group of horses, including 8 horses with necropsy-confirmed CVSM and

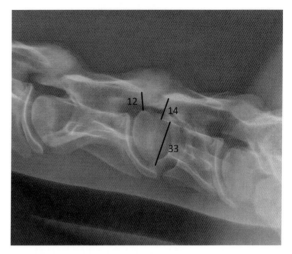

Figure 28.4 Survey radiograph of the fifth and sixth cervical vertebrae of the same colt as in Figure 28.1. The intervertebral sagittal ratio (12:33) was calculated to be 36% and the intravertebral sagittal ratio (14:33) was calculated to be 42%.

Table 28.1 Cervical vertebral sagittal ratio measurements given with the proportion horses affected with CVSM and the likelihood ratios.[a]

	C4	C5	C6	C7
Sagittal ratio (%)	<50	<50	<50	<52
Proportion affected[b] (%)	86 (30/35)	78 (29/37)	83 (34/41)	82 (27/33)
Likelihood ratio	28.6	26.1	41.5	39.0

[a] Data from Rush Moore et al. [12].
[b] Percentage of horses affected with CVSM that had sagittal ratios less than 50–52% at the site of compression.

18 horses without CVSM, all horses with CVSM had at least one MSD ratio less than or equal to 0.485, and the smallest intervertebral ratio always indicated a site of compression [45]. One reason that intervertebral MSD ratios were more accurate at determining site of compression could be that most (11/14) sites of compression were intervertebral rather than intravertebral. However, when this method was used to compare ratios of compressed sites to noncompressed sites in both CVSM and non-CVSM cases, there was significant overlap between values [7].

Overall, MSD ratios are relatively accurate at predicting a diagnosis of CVSM, with inter-vertebral MSD ratios slightly superior to intravertebral MSD ratios, but neither should be used to predict the site of compression in a CVSM case due to unacceptable sensitivity and specificity [7, 12, 24]. Furthermore, an observer agreement study using two examiners revealed that cervical vertebral ratios varied by 5–10% within and between examiners, suggesting that clinicians should be cautious when applying these ratios in practice to avoid misdiagnosis [46]. Therefore, myelography remains the diagnostic tool of choice for antemortem diagnosis of CVSM and location of specific sites of compression.

Myelography

Myelography is required to confirm a diagnosis of focal spinal cord compression and to identify the location and number of lesions, particularly if surgical treatment is to be considered or pursued [6, 12, 14, 47]. The technique for performing a myelogram has been described using a nonionic, water-soluble contrast agent (iopamidol, iohexol) administered through the atlanto-occipital space into the subarachnoid space after withdrawal of an equal volume of CSF [38, 47]. Radiographs are taken in neutral, flexed, and extended positions of the neck. A technique for standing myelography via lumbosacral puncture has also been described [48] but does not always result in adequate cervical images and is rarely utilized due to concerns about adverse reactions and patient comfort.

Myelography allows detection of static and dynamic compression. Static compression is defined by narrowing of the vertebral canal with subsequent compression of the spinal cord regardless of neck position, whereas dynamic compression is only evident in certain neck positions. By definition static stenosis is noticeable in neutral views, but extension of the neck may exacerbate this compression suggesting a degree of coexisting dynamic compression. The most common sites for static stenosis are at C5–C6 and C6–C7 [6, 9, 49] (Figure 28.5). Dynamic compression is most commonly seen in flexed views at more cranial sites,

including C3–C4 and C4–C5 (Figure 28.6a, b). However, narrowing of the vertebral canal can occur at any site within the cervical vertebral column, and stenosis at more than one site is not uncommon [9, 12, 14, 16].

Several criteria for evaluating equine myelograms have been proposed but continue to be the source of some debate. These criteria include a reduction of thickness of the contrast columns to less than 2 mm [47] and attenuation of both the dorsal and ventral contrast columns by greater than 50% at diametrically opposed sites [15]. Currently, complete attenuation of the ventral contrast column with 50% attenuation of the dorsal contrast column compared to the maximal height of the dorsal contrast column within the cranial vertebral body is most commonly used as myelographic evidence of compression [50]. The accuracy of this criterion has recently been questioned, and the use of the minimal sagittal dural diameter (MSDD), which is the sagittal diameter of the dural space measured intervertebrally, has been advocated to more precisely define the sites of spinal cord compression [24, 44, 51] (Figure 28.7, Table 28.2). MSDD greater than 20% smaller than the largest dural diameter measured within the cranial vertebra has been suggested as a potentially more accurate criterion [52]. However, when these various myelographic criteria for compression are critically evaluated, it becomes clear that none yields high sensitivity and specificity at all cervical articulations [7, 52].

It is important to recognize that standard myelographic views, performed in lateral recumbency, are best at identifying dorsoventral compression and not ideal for identifying lateral or dorsolateral compression. Signs that can indicate lateral compression of the spinal cord on laterolateral myelogram images include blanching of the overall contrast column, widening of the sagittal shadow of the spinal cord, and the appearance of two dorsal borders to the contrast column if asymmetric dorsolateral compression is present [53].

As can be seen, although myelography is currently considered one of the most accurate antemortem tests, it has several limitations. As described, no consensus for diagnosis of compression exists. Most myelographic studies only include laterolateral images of the vertebral column despite the fact that horses often have dorsolateral spinal cord compression, which would be best viewed with ventrodorsal or oblique radiographic images [52, 54]. Finally, although myelography is considered more likely to accurately identify the site of compression, it may not be superior to plain radiography in differentiating horses with CVSM from horses without CVSM. In one study, direct comparison of myelography to radiography in the diagnosis of CVSM was performed using 108 postmortem-confirmed cases (77 with CVSM, 31 without) [55]. Using MSD measurements from plain radiographs resulted in higher sensitivity (87%) and specificity (94%) than myelography

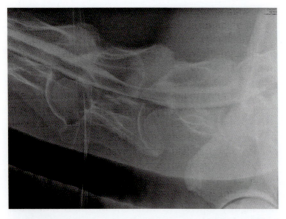

Figure 28.5 Cervical myelogram of an 8-year-old Thoroughbred gelding demonstrating static compression of the cervical spinal cord at C6–C7.

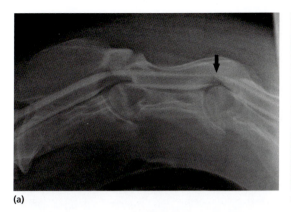

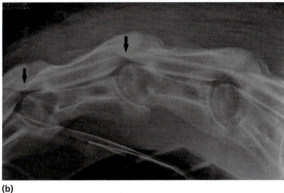

(a)   (b)

Figure 28.6 (a, b). Cervical myelogram of the same gelding as in Figure 28.2a. Dynamic compression is present at C3–C4 and C4–C5 (arrows).

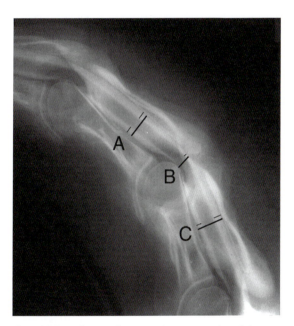

Figure 28.7 Myelogram demonstrating compression of the cervical spinal cord at C4–C5. Measurements of the dorsal contrast column, the ventral contrast column, and the sagittal dural diameter are given (Table 28.2). The dorsal contrast column reduction is 67% and the sagittal dural diameter reduction is 45%.

Table 28.2 Measurements of the dorsal contrast column, the ventral contrast column, and the sagittal dural diameter for the myelogram shown in Figure 28.2.

Line	Dorsal CC (mm)	Ventral CC (mm)	SDD (mm)
A	7	5	22
B (intervertebral)	3	0	12
C	7	5	22

CC, contrast column; SDD, sagittal dural diameter.

been evaluated in the horse [17]. In a postmortem study involving six horses with CVSM, CECT images could be obtained from C1–T1. CVSM lesions were accurately detected and significant additional information was obtained regarding location and severity of the lesions [17]. The main indications for CECT are presurgical evaluation of the cervical vertebral column and spinal cord at sites that are suspected to have dynamic compressive lesions and evaluation of lateral compressive lesions in horses strongly suspected to have CVSM without myelographic evidence. Depending on the patient aperture and table size, evaluation of C1–C7 is possible with CECT.

Magnetic resonance

Magnetic resonance (MR) imaging is the imaging modality of choice for people and dogs with compressive myelopathy and has been evaluated for horses [56]. A postmortem study was performed on 39 ataxic and 20 neurologically normal horses using a 1.5 Tesla magnet after removal of the head and neck from the body at T1 or T2. Although subjective evaluation of MR images allowed differentiation of horses with cervical vertebral disease from horses with other causes of ataxia and normal horses, MR imaging did not allow

(56% sensitivity and 83% specificity), although correct identification of the site(s) of compression was not evaluated.

Computed tomography

Contrast-enhanced computed tomography (CECT) is considered more useful than myelography to diagnose and characterize vertebral stenosis in humans, and has accurate identification of the site of compression, as an MR diagnosis of spinal cord compression had only poor to slight agreement with histology. This finding is somewhat surprising when compared to results in people and dogs. Additional studies are warranted to evaluate the accuracy of MR in the diagnosis of CVSM in horses as compared to plain radiography and myelography.

Endoscopy

A technique for epiduroscopy and myeloscopy has been developed using an open approach to the epidural and subarachnoid spaces [57]. Cervical vertebral canal endoscopy potentially allows identification of compressive lesions as well as spinal cord lesions that could only be identified by direct visualization. Successful completion of the procedure has been described in six healthy horses and one neurologic horse [58, 59]. Complications included an increase in mean arterial pressure during epiduroscopy, minor hemorrhage at the insertion site and introduction of air into the subarachnoid space during myeloscopy, transient ataxia in one horse after recovery, and transient subclinical meningitis [58]. Although the sensitivity and specificity of this technique are unknown, myeloscopy correctly identified the site of compression, which was misdiagnosed by myelography, in the single clinical case evaluated [59].

A technique for arthroscopic evaluation of cervical articular process joints has been described recently [60]. Good visualization of the cartilage surfaces was achieved and complications were minimal, although only three clinical cases were reported.

To summarize the current state of diagnostic testing, no single modality is sufficient for accurate diagnosis [61]. The most accurate diagnosis for any individual horse is achieved through careful consideration of all available information, including history, signalment, neurologic examination findings, imaging studies, and other ancillary tests to eliminate other possible differential diagnoses. Of all the widely available imaging modalities, MSD ratios best predict a diagnosis of CVSM, but do not reliably identify sites of compression. Myelography is necessary for surgical planning but does not have well-established criteria for compression; experience of the observer likely contributes to diagnostic accuracy. As for many neurologic diseases, histopathology remains the gold-standard diagnostic test.

Postmortem examination and histopathology

On gross examination of the vertebral column, bony abnormalities and malformations such as those detected by radiography might be present. Narrowing

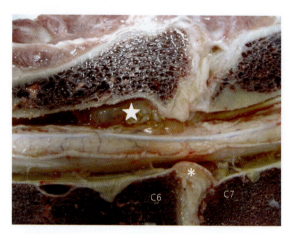

Figure 28.8 Postmortem image of a sagittal section of the C6–C7 articulation of the same horse as in Figure 28.5. Cranial is to the left and dorsal is to the top of the image. Narrowing of the vertebral canal is evident dorsal to the intervertebral disc (*) and an epidural cyst is present within the dorsal vertebral canal of C6 (star).

of the vertebral canal frequently occurs through soft tissue swelling and proliferation, or through thickening of the ligaments between the vertebral bodies, and particularly of the lateral ligamentum flavum [21, 62, 63]. The presence of cysts and bony proliferations also leads to compression of the spinal cord. (Figure 28.8) Changes in the ligament and the development of cysts are often associated with degenerative changes in the articular processes of the vertebral bodies [63]. Abnormal biomechanical forces or instability of articulations result in stretching and tearing of the ligamentum flavum and joint capsule with subsequent fibrovascular and fibrocartilaginous proliferation, osteosclerosis of the dorsal lamina, and osteophyte formation on the articular processes [9]. Horses with CVSM have decreased differentiation of cartilage and osteopetrosis, sometimes associated with osteonecrosis and osteoclasia in the cervical vertebrae. Similar lesions can be present in the costochondral junctions and seem to be associated with osteochondrosis dissecans [16] (Figure 28.9).

On gross evaluation of the spinal cord, lesions might [64] or might not [65] be detected. The characteristic finding is a focal pressure-induced lesion in the cervical spinal cord, affecting especially the white matter when examined microscopically [16]. A pressure-induced lesion can be identified by recognizing flattening of the fixed spinal cord in a transverse section, when compared to adjacent segments, or a decrease in height of the spinal cord.

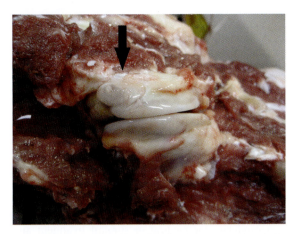

Figure 28.9 Postmortem dissection showing an osteochondral fragment associated with a cervical articular process.

At the level of compression, prominent features of the focal lesion include neuronal fiber swelling and degeneration, occasional spheroids, astrocytic gliosis, increased macrophage activity, and increased perivascular collagen. Myelin degeneration or loss was reported to be greatest in the ventral and lateral funiculi [64]. Vessels at the site of a primary lesion may also be surrounded by increased collagen indicating a process of fibrosis [16]. In more severe cases vacuolated spongy degeneration of the white matter may be seen [65]. Proximal and distal segments and stumps of injured axons swell and may resemble spheroids that are characteristically seen in EDM. However, the spheroids in EDM are found primarily in the gray matter, whereas the spheroids in CVSM are more commonly found in the white matter [16].

Wallerian or Wallerian-like neuronal fiber degeneration can be observed related to but distant from the focal lesion. The secondary neuronal fiber degeneration is characterized by a loss of myelin and axons. In areas of marked fiber degeneration perivascular fibrosis in the white matter is often evident. Astrocytic gliosis is a prominent and persistent finding in areas of neuronal degeneration in horses with chronic CVSM [64]. The characteristic pattern of fiber degeneration and developing gliosis can be used to map the site of an undetected primary lesion and allow further sections to be examined until the primary lesion is detected. Cranial to the compressive lesion the degeneration occurs in ascending white matter tracts, predominantly in the dorsal funiculi and the spinocerebellar tracts on the surface of the lateral funiculi. Caudal to the lesion the degeneration occurs in descending tracts deep in the lateral funiculi and in the ventral funiculi, adjacent to the median sulcus and below the pia [66].

The relative roles of direct injury to nervous tissue and alterations in spinal cord blood supply are not clearly defined in CVSM. Return of function following a partial focal compressive myelopathy has not been shown to be dependent on remyelination of those axons that remain intact and may be due to adaptation of remaining nervous tissue.

Treatment

Medical treatment

Choice of medical treatment for CVSM depends in part on type of lesion, severity and chronicity of clinical signs, and age of the horse. In the immediate period following an acute onset of ataxia and paresis, medical therapy is aimed at reducing cell swelling and edema formation, thereby reducing compression on the spinal cord. Anti-inflammatory drugs such as corticosteroids, nonsteroidal anti-inflammatory drugs, and dimethyl sulfoxide are the most commonly used treatments.

For horses less than 1 year of age, changes in management may influence the development of CVSM. These changes include restricted exercise and diet, along with alterations in the concentrations of trace nutrients such as copper and zinc in the diet. The "paced growth" program, for which efficacy has been suggested in young horses with early clinical or radiographic signs of CVSM [67], includes stall rest and a diet that restricts protein and carbohydrate intake. Proponents of this diet suggest that bone growth should be retarded, bone metabolism should be enhanced, and the vertebral canal diameter should enlarge and relieve spinal cord compression. However, controlled studies demonstrating efficacy are lacking, and it is unclear whether the strict diet provides any additional benefit to time alone. It is important that the selected diet meet minimum requirements of essential nutrients, and during the period of growth retardation the patient should be under careful nutritional supervision [68]. In young horses supplementation with vitamin E/selenium is recommended as EDM is an important differential diagnosis which might improve following vitamin E administration [69]. General recommendations for a paced diet include restricting protein and carbohydrates to 65–75% National Research Council (NRC) recommendations, maintaining balanced vitamin and mineral intake (minimum 100% NRC requirements), supplementing vitamins A and E at three times NRC recommendations, and supplementing selenium to 0.3 ppm.

In adult horses with compressive lesions of the spinal cord, the options for medical therapy are restricted to stabilizing a horse with acute neurologic deterioration and injecting the articular joints with corticosteroids, chemical mucopolysaccharides such as hyaluronate sodium, or both in an attempt to reduce soft tissue swelling and stabilize or prevent bony proliferation [70, 71]. Injecting articular joints is most beneficial in horses that demonstrate zero or only minimal neurologic deficits (grade 0–2), and that have moderate to significant degenerative joint changes evident on radiographs of the cervical vertebral column. Horses that fit into this last category are generally older horses (>5 years) that are in training and have developed osteoarthritic changes, usually in the caudal cervical vertebral joints.

Surgical treatment
General considerations
The aim of surgical treatment is to stop repetitive trauma to the spinal cord, which is caused by narrowing of the vertebral canal, and thereby to allow the inflammation in and around the spinal cord to resolve. Restoration or maintenance of adequate blood supply to the spinal cord is vital to reduction of edema and removal of inflammatory mediators from the affected site. Surgical management of horses that have been diagnosed with spinal cord compression involves the use of a ventral stabilization procedure. The surgical technique was initially described in 1979 [72] and in the hands of some surgeons is now considered a routine procedure. However, several factors must be considered carefully and discussed with the patient's owners and caregivers prior to recommending surgical treatment for any individual horse. These include whether or not the horse is a good surgical candidate, expectations for improvement and return to use, cost of surgical treatment and rehabilitation, insurance issues, and safety and liability concerns.

The best surgical candidates are young horses with only one or two myelographic lesions, a short duration of mild to moderate clinical signs, and no evidence of concurrent disease such as EPM. However, surgical success has been reported in less than ideal candidates, including horses undergoing tri-level interbody fusion [73, 74]. Horses that might have EPM based on antibody titers in CSF should undergo antiprotozoal therapy prior to considering cervical surgery.

It is important for the owner to have realistic expectations and to be aware that the final determination of the results might not be known until the end of the recovery period, which usually takes 6 months–1 year. Following interbody fusion surgery an improvement of 1–2 out of 5 grades is expected. There is a low probability that a horse will improve more than 3 out of 5 grades, so severely affected horses (grade 4 or 5) are highly unlikely to return to normal neurologic function. Although normal neurologic function is not always required for breeding stock, the potential heritability of vertebral canal stenosis must be considered.

Discussion of cost with the owner must include estimates of initial diagnostic testing, transportation costs for the horse to ship to a surgical facility or for an experienced surgeon to travel to a local facility, surgical expenses, postoperative care, and rehabilitation, as well as general maintenance costs of the horse for the duration of the recovery period. A structured rehabilitation program is essential to success, and the owner must commit to spending time with the horse daily or paying for this service.

Horses with CVSM and insurance policies present an additional set of issues for the owner and the veterinarian. In the authors' opinion, there are several important insurance aspects for consideration. The most common questions encountered are whether the horse is a candidate for medical or surgical treatment and when the horse becomes a candidate for humane destruction. The response to the first question is impacted by several factors including the severity of clinical signs, the number of sites affected, the owners' commitment to the horse, and the economic value of the horse combined with the cost for performing surgery. Whether a horse is a candidate for humane destruction is governed by guidelines established by the American Association of Equine Practitioners (AAEP) Insurance committee on behalf of the AAEP. Important criteria for euthanasia include inhumane suffering, chronic and incurable pain necessitating pain-relieving medication, a chronic and incurable condition, and an animal that is a danger to itself, other animals, or its handlers. Some insurance underwriters have established a "wobbler clause" which in general says that for a horse with CVSM to be a candidate for humane destruction it must have severe clinical signs (at least grade 3/5) as well as myelographic confirmation of a surgical lesion. This statement is a generality and in no way do the authors intend to interpret the policy guidelines of any insurance underwriter or company. Depending on the policies issued, mortality claims may or may not be granted. It is uncommon but not unprecedented for insurance agencies to take over ownership of the affected horse and salvage it for athletic or breeding purposes. Severely affected animals and affected animals for which treatment is not an option or not effective are generally humanely destroyed.

Safety is of utmost importance both before after surgical treatment of CVSM. In the authors' opinion, it is essential for everyone involved with the patient, including all potential handlers and caregivers, to be aware of what signs a horse with neurological disease might show. In most cases, a horse with neurological gait deficits less than a grade 4 can be managed in a fashion similar to other horses. A horse with grade 4 neurologic gait deficits may fall with normal movements, and therefore needs to be handled in a very careful fashion.

Opposition to surgical treatment of CVSM has generally been focused on postoperative safety concerns during performance, although 30 years of experience with this procedure has allayed some of these fears. Concerns regarding safety of the horse following surgery are based on the assumption that neurons do not regenerate completely following vertebral body stabilization, and thus even if the compression is alleviated, irreversible neuronal damage could make a horse unsuitable for performance activities. There is clear evidence in people, dogs, and horses with cervical compressive myelopathies that surgical intervention results in improvement in neurologic signs in the majority of patients [10, 75–77]. Without pre- and postoperative histopathology (an impossibility!), one cannot know whether improvement is due to healing of damaged neurons or compensatory mechanisms in remaining neurons. Regardless, determination of safety for the horse's intended use should be evaluated on a case-by-case basis by performance of thorough neurologic examinations.

In response to the question of liability, it is the authors' opinion that the owner has ultimate responsibility for the horse and therefore assumes the "lion's share" of liability. However, in more than 35 years of managing horses with neurological disease of varying severity, we are unaware of any instance in which an owner or handler has been injured as the result of managing an affected horse. Notwithstanding this fact, it is very important that owners be aware of their responsibility to inform all potential handlers and/or riders of the horse's diagnosis as well the impact it might have on the horse's ability to be exercised.

Surgical technique

There have been a number of technical changes since an adaptation of the Cloward technique (anterior interbody fusion) was first described as a treatment for cervical vertebral malformation [72]. The Cloward technique utilized the principle of dynamic compression that results from having a circular bone dowel hammered into a slightly smaller diameter hole drilled between adjacent vertebra that need to be stabilized. The next significant modification was the use of a stainless steel circular implant that had numerous holes to allow for the cancellous bone from the drilling procedure to be used as an autologous graft resulting in an osseous fusion [78]. This technique was used for over two decades with great success although there was occasional implant migration and an increased incidence of postoperative vertebral fractures from forcing the oversized implant into pathological bone.

The use of the threaded BAK implant for the stabilization of lumbar vertebrae in people led to the development of the Seattle Slew implant in 2000. This implant, a partially or fully threaded cylinder, is screwed into a previously drilled and threaded site. The implant site is prepared using a Kerf cleaning instrument so that a peninsula of bone is left to accelerate fusion.

This procedure should be performed in an appropriate surgical facility where the patient can be placed on a table in dorsal recumbency with the neck in a cervical brace. Good lighting, reliable aspiration, positive-pressure anesthesia with blood pressure and cardiac monitoring, and intraoperative imaging (C-arm or digital radiography) are all necessary for performing this procedure. The use of the Seattle Slew implant requires a number of specifically designed instruments that are commercially available. In addition, a general instrument pack for standard opening and closing, large curved osteotome, orthopedic hammer, depth gauge, Deaver and Inge retractors, aspiration tips and hoses, orthopedic reamers with nitrogen hoses and tank and regulators, and large roungers are all necessary. The use of a Hall drill to prepare and remove excessive intervertebral disc is also recommended.

Prior to performing the surgical procedure, an endoscopic examination is performed to evaluate recurrent laryngeal nerve function. If laryngeal paralysis is present, the approach to the vertebral column should be on the dysfunctional side of the trachea (i.e., left side if a left-sided paralysis) to prevent damage to the normal nerve during retraction. Failure to do so might result in bilateral laryngeal paralysis that could seriously compromise the horse's airway and recovery from anesthesia. Other routine preoperative evaluations such as screening clinicopathologic tests are also recommended.

Preoperative antibiotics and tetanus toxoid are administered as standard for the surgical facility. Nonsteroidal anti-inflammatory drugs are also administered preoperatively unless anesthesia dictates they be withheld until after completion of the procedure. Corticosteroids are usually only administered to the very ataxic patients (>3.5/5 grade). Clipping and preliminary cleaning of the ventral cervical area before anesthesia will assist in reducing anesthesia time. After induction and intubation, the patient is placed in dorsal recumbency on a well-padded surgical table. The neck is placed in a cervical brace that is designed to hold a radiology plate intraoperatively. After standard clipping, shaving, and skin preparation, the cervical vertebrae that are to be fused are located by obtaining a radiographic image after 14 gauge needles have been placed subcutaneously over the vertebral bodies. In mature horses, the vertebral bodies are approximately a hands' width apart. Care should be taken to have the needles on the cassette side of the cervical area to reduce any parallax problem. The second cervical vertebra needs to be included so the characteristic formation of C2 can be used as a reference. Standard toweling and draping technique is utilized as for any sterile procedure. Small towel clamps are used to mark the position of the needles to prevent any confusion that palpation of needles through the towels and drapes could cause, which could result in selection of the wrong site.

A 20 cm skin incision is made on ventral midline centered over the intervertebral area that is to be fused. The ventral cervical subcutaneous muscle is also incised down to the sternothyrohyoideus muscles. The thickness of these muscles is quite variable depending on the patient's age and degree of neurological deficits. The fascia is separated from the side of the trachea with blunt finger and scissor dissection deeper to the carotid sheath. The recurrent laryngeal nerve and vagosympathetic trunk are identified so they can be protected from excessive trauma during retraction. Using large hand-held retractors, the trachea and sternocephalicus muscles are separated to expose the ventral aspect of the vertebral bodies. The longus colli muscle overlies the vertebral bodies, but usually the ventral spine of the cranial body can be palpated through the muscle (except for C6, which has a ventral spine so small that palpation is not possible.) A 4 cm incision is made over the ventral spine parallel with the muscle fibers down to the spine. The muscle insertion on the spine is elevated with a large blunt elevator (a sharp osteotome can be used, but the possibility of injury to the esophagus is increased). The spine is isolated using two pairs of Inge retractors. The spine is removed using a large curved osteotome and orthopedic hammer down to the level of the intervertebral disc appearing on the anterior aspect of the posterior vertebra. At this time, a small exploratory hole is drilled with a 16 mm drill through a matching drill guide that has been placed with the posterior edge of the drill guide on the epiphyseal scar of the anterior vertebra (a distinct white undulating line in young and middle age patients). The test hole is drilled to a depth of 8–10 mm and bone removed. The very white intervertebral disc should now be visible. Two to three marker pins are then placed through a marker pin guide to assist in drilling the implant hole with the disc in the center of the hole. An intraoperative image is obtained and the marker pin with the most ideal location is selected. If there is no ideal placement, then repeating this procedure is recommended. After the correct pin placement site has been determined, then the pin guide and other pins are removed. This pin will then be placed into the center hole of the guide bar to assist in placing the large drill guide in the correct location. The drill guide is secured in place by the use of an orthopedic hammer and impacter. The implant site is then prepared by using a series of thin core saw, thick core saw, large pointed drill, and large flat drill. The depth of each should be set to 20 mm by premeasuring the set rings on the drill guide. Then, the #1 Kerf cleaner is placed into

the drill guide and the Kerf is started. The drill guide is removed and the tap is used to countersink the leading aspect of the implant site to allow the use of the 1 mm larger #2 Kerf cleaner. The Kerf cleaner is then drilled by hand to a depth of 25–30 mm (there are guide lines on the Kerf cleaner set at 10 mm increments) and an intraoperative image is obtained with the #2 Kerf cleaner in place to determine the correct depth. Ideally, the depth should not be any closer than 10 mm from the spinal canal to reduce the risk of fractures during recovery. After the depth has been determined, the site is tapped and the threaded implant is twisted into place with an inserter until it is very secure. A partially threaded implant is used; but if it does not become secure, a fully threaded implant is used to provide a more secure implant. Care must be exercised when using a fully threaded implant as the design allows for it to be self-tapping, and it could be possible to twist it all the way to the spinal canal.

After the implant placement has been confirmed with another image, the harvested bone graft (obtained by saving the drilling debris on a sterile sponge that has been soaked with blood) is firmly placed into and over the implant. The longus colli muscle is reapposed by using a two-layer closure with zero PDS. The surgery site is then examined for any foreign debris and thoroughly flushed. The ventral cervical muscles are reapposed in a two layer closure with zero PDS in a simple continuous pattern. Skin staples are used on the skin. Recovery from anesthesia can usually follow routine procedures although a determination about the likelihood of the horse requiring special assistance can be made by the way it recovered following its myelogram.

The modifications of the procedures have resulted in reduction in surgery time, better bony fusion, less pain, and improved outcome for the horse (Figure 28.10). Since the inception of the modern procedure, more than 2000 horses have benefited from use of these procedures and long-term survival appears to be greater than 80%, although this has never been critically reviewed and published.

In some of the early literature describing the surgical techniques for CVSM, a subtotal dorsal decompressive laminectomy was described. In this procedure, the caudal aspect of the vertebral arch of the cranial vertebrae and the cranial aspect of the vertebral arch of the caudal vertebrae are removed [71, 79]. The surgical technique is challenging and requires specific positioning with a sternal brace; the horse is place in lateral recumbency with the neck in maximal flexion and the body tilted such that the feet are lower than the neck and the neck is higher than the rest of the body. A dorsal midline skin incision is centered over the affected intervertebral space and extended through nuchal fat and

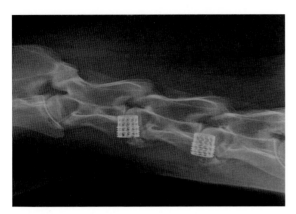

Figure 28.10 Lateral survey postoperative radiograph of the same gelding as in Figures 28.2a and 28.6 demonstrating bilevel placement of partially threaded implants. Adequate fusion and clinical improvement were observed and the gelding returned to expected level of use.

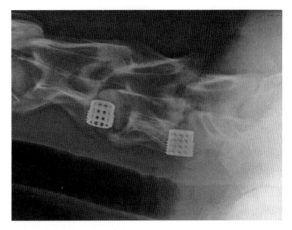

Figure 28.11 Lateral survey postoperative radiograph of a 4-year-old Warmblood gelding that sustained complications during recovery from anesthesia, resulting in fracture of the caudal C6 vertebral body and severe narrowing of the vertebral canal. The gelding's neurologic status showed no improvement at 12 months postoperatively.

then through the funicular and lamellar ligamentum nuchae. After retraction of the lamellar ligamentum nuchae and dorsal muscles, sharp dissection is used to remove the tendinous insertions of the multifidus muscles and the ligamentum nuchae at their attachments to the spinous processes of the vertebrae. The interspinous ligament and ligamentum flavum (interarcuate ligament) are removed with scissors and then a high-speed air drill is used to remove the dorsal laminae from the cranial then caudal vertebrae in a subtotal manner. Rounding the corners of the bone removal site is believed to help reduce the development of stress risers and reduce postoperative fracture. Once the impinging bone is removed, an autogenous fat graft is placed over the exposed dura prior to closure. This surgery offers almost immediate decompression of the spinal cord; however, the technique is technically demanding and carries a high risk of serious complications.

Locking compression plate fixation has been proposed as an alternative to Kerf cut cylinder (KCC) fixation. This method has been reported in a 3-month-old foal; revision surgery was required 11 days postoperatively due to screws backing out, but the foal's neurologic signs eventually improved by 2.5 grades [80]. *In vitro* studies were conducted to compare the strength of the locking compression plate fixation to traditional KCC fixation [81, 82]. The mechanical properties of the LCP constructs were considered superior to the KCC in this model, although it did not assess the effect of repetitive loading nor could it predict in vivo behavior, as bony ingrowth occurs through the holes of the KCC and increases stability. Anecdotally, this procedure has been used in adult horses with success but results are not yet published.

Reported nonfatal complications associated with surgical intervention include transient worsening of ataxia, seroma formation, implant failure or migration, vertebral fracture, (Figure 28.11) right laryngeal hemiplegia, and colitis [10, 80]. Fatal complications included vertebral body fracture, spinal cord edema, and implant failure [10].

Postoperative care

Recommendations for aftercare vary according to surgeon preference as well as case specifics. In general, at least 1 month of strict stall rest is recommended. A second month of stall rest with hand-walking follows; the horse is initially walked for 5–10 min twice daily and gradually increased to 30 min 2–3 times daily. If the horse is comfortable and healing is progressing well, small paddock turnout is introduced during the third month. Neurologic reevaluation by a veterinarian is recommended prior to beginning turnout. Cervical radiographs are often repeated 3–6 months postoperatively to assess the position of the implant(s) and healing prior to turnout in a large pasture or return to forced exercise.

Usually, a month or more of unlimited turnout is provided prior to return to forced exercise (long-lining, lunging, or riding) at 4–6 months postoperatively. During this turnout period, ground work in hand should be performed as a form of physical therapy to improve proprioception and balance. This ground work should be performed without restriction of the horse's head and neck movements, so that the horse is free to assume a comfortable head and neck position. Exercises include walking patterns (circles, serpentines, figure eights) on both flat surfaces and inclines, as well as walking over cavaletti poles or other 4–6″ obstacles. Initially, only one obstacle should be used; and as the horse masters this task, additional obstacles can be added in more complex patterns. Also, the poles can be raised slowly up to 12″ at one end so that the limbs on one side of the horse's body must be raised higher to clear the obstacle. Additionally, standing exercises such as "carrot stretches" to improve the horse's cervical range of motion can be added during this time period; again, the horse should be encouraged but not forced to move its head and neck in any given direction.

Exercise under saddle most commonly begins about 6 months postoperatively, but less severely ataxic horses with good recoveries sometimes can be ridden 4 months postoperatively, and more severely ataxic horses might not regain enough function to be ridden until 9–12 months. Full neurologic examination by a veterinarian is strongly recommended prior to beginning work under saddle. A slow return to previous level of exercise is recommended, with 2–4 weeks of walking prior to the addition of trot work, and a slow increase in the amount of trot work (from 5 to 20 or 30 min/session) over the course of a month prior to the addition of any canter work. Owners should anticipate a full year of recovery time prior to the horse being in "normal" work although obviously some horses require less or more time than this.

Prognosis

Regardless of treatment selected, the response and the prognosis depend largely on the age of the horse, the severity of neurologic deficits, the duration of neurologic signs, and the expected level of performance. Generally, a horse with CVSM will be able to survive but performance might be impaired. Without treatment, the prognosis in all types of CVSM is usually poor to guarded, as there is continued damage to the cervical spinal cord with an increasing chance of severe cord destruction following trauma.

The initial response to medical therapy with anti-inflammatory drugs in cases of acute spinal cord damage is generally good, however, if bony malformations or soft tissue proliferations exist, neurologic deficits will remain. Young horses treated medically with a low-protein, low-energy "paced" diet and stall confinement showed good results; in a study population of 18 young horses (<1 year of age) with a presumptive diagnosis of CVSM, 83% improved and had at least one racing start [11]. These cases were not confirmed by myelography or histology, and it is unclear whether diet, exercise restriction, or time led to the perceived improvement, if there was any

change at all. When medical treatment was evaluated in a population of Thoroughbreds containing slightly older horses (mainly 1–2 years of age), only 21/70 (30%) had at least one racing start [83]. For older horses with significant arthropathies, articular joint injections with corticosteroids often result in reduced soft tissue swelling [70, 71]. However, these injections generally need to be repeated at variable intervals. Again, the prognosis depends on the severity of neurologic deficits and the severity of the degenerative joint changes.

The clinical response to ventral stabilization depends on the ability to detect all compressed sites and the accuracy of the diagnosis. Optimal outcomes are achieved if surgical intervention is pursued shortly after the first clinical signs develop. Overall, if return to use is considered, a success rate of 45–60% is estimated based on review of the literature [73]. An early study [10] evaluating 73 horses with CVSM that had surgical intervention (cervical vertebral interbody fusion ($n=63$) or dorsal laminectomy ($n=10$)) indicated that neurologic function improved in 77% of horses, and 46% achieved athletic function. Only 4/10 horses undergoing dorsal laminectomy improved. A shorter duration of clinical signs prior to intervention was positively associated with neurologic improvement and return to function, whereas age and number of compressive lesions did not affect outcome. Based on the experiences of the authors, owners and veterinarians can expect clinical improvement in approximately 80% of horses undergoing surgery (Reed, S. Unpublished observation). Although clinical improvement can be somewhat variable, approximately 63% of the horses return to athletic function and another 15% are suitable for breeding. About 10% have poor response to treatment but can be turned out and live a relatively normal life at pasture, while the final 12% fail to improve sufficiently (Reed, S. Unpublished observation).

Pathogenesis

The pathogenesis of CVSM is not fully understood but appears to be multifactorial, potentially involving genetic predisposition, trauma, exercise, and nutrition. Early on a genetic predisposition to CVSM in horses was suspected based on the frequency of CVSM in certain families of Thoroughbreds; [3, 84]; however, lack of many close relationships in a group of 47 horses with CVSM gave rise to thoughts on other etiologic factors [1]. Although some investigators have failed to demonstrate genetic determination of CVSM [85, 86], others believe that genetic factors that determine the length of the neck, cervical vertebral biomechanics, and body size play a significant role in the development of CVSM [5, 87, 88]. In the most recent investigation of the heritability of CVSM, Reed reported a suspicion that affected horses inherited a predisposition for increased sensitivity to environmental factors influencing cartilage growth [89].

Cartilage growth and osteochondrosis dissecans are likely linked to the development of CVSM because osteochondrotic type lesions are frequently seen in vertebrae involved in myelocompressive lesions [88]. Osteochondrosis of the articular processes might result in instability and malalignment of adjacent vertebrae, secondary osteoarthritis of the articular processes, and hypertrophy of soft tissue structures. All of these changes might contribute to spinal cord compression [9, 21, 22, 62, 63]. Multiple investigators have shown that horses with CVSM have an increased incidence and severity of degenerative joint changes in the axial skeleton [1, 16, 22, 62] and Wagner et al. demonstrated that although offspring from horses with CVSM did not develop myelocompressive lesions themselves, this group did have a high incidence (45%) of osteochondrotic lesions in both the axial and appendicular skeleton [86].

Despite the high incidence of osteochondrosis, the importance of degenerative joint disease to the pathogenesis of CVSM in young horses remains unclear. Rooney proposed that malformation of the articular processes is the predisposing lesion and essential in the pathogenesis of CVSM [5]. Binkhorst, however, found only 8% correlation between lesions of the articular processes and histologic changes in the spinal cord; [62] similarly, Stewart et al. reported that the site of the most severe osteochondrotic lesions did not always correlate with the site of vertebral stenosis [22]. This finding suggests that osteochondrosis of the articular processes is not the direct cause of CVSM, and that the primary factor in the pathogenesis of CVSM in young horses is insufficient diameter of the cervical vertebral canal. This is why Hurtig and Pool suggest CVSM is a manifestation of developmental orthopedic disease, but does not belong in the osteochondrosis syndrome [90]. However, the positive correlation between osteochondrosis and CVSM could indicate that the pathogenesis of both conditions is similar [22, 89].

In contrast to young horses in which the role of degenerative joint disease in the pathogenesis of CVSM appears controversial, in older horses (>4 years) CVSM is generally associated with significant arthropathies of the caudal cervical articular processes. In these horses, the compression of the spinal cord can be attributed to the bony and soft tissue proliferation at the affected articular processes. This finding is supported by the improvement many of these horses show when medical and surgical treatment leads to reduction of the bony proliferation as evidenced radiographically. The genesis of the degenerative joint disease in older horses

with CVSM is speculative, but external trauma is thought to be important [33], and exercise might have a role.

Dietary factors might also contribute to the development of osteochondrosis and CVSM [67, 91]. An accelerated rate of gain, but not of growth has been related to osteochondrosis and CVSM in horses; however, controlled investigations have failed to confirm this relationship [92]. Nutritional factors that have been associated with the incidence of developmental orthopedic disease are an imbalance in the calcium/phosphorus ratio, copper deficiency, excessive zinc, excessive protein, and excessive carbohydrate. The three most important nutritional factors appear to be excessive digestible energy, excessive phosphorus, and copper deficiency [91].

Carbohydrate excess in the diet is thought to contribute to developmental orthopedic disease through an endocrine imbalance involving elevation of serum insulin concentrations and decreased serum thyroxin concentrations, resulting in a lack of cartilage maturation [93, 94]. This theory prompted the previously described recommendation for a "paced growth" program to prevent and treat CVSM [67]. Savage et al. demonstrated that diets high in digestible energy consisting of both carbohydrate and corn oil components caused osteochondrotic lesions in foals, and that this result was not solely due to an excessive average daily weight gain [95]. Feeding high-digestible energy diets might result in endocrinologic alterations that affect local cartilaginous factors and selectively activate genes that cause a specific alteration in matrix phenotype [91].

A dietary calcium/phosphorus imbalance has been implicated in CVSM [62] and particularly excessive phosphorus (388% of the requirement) appears to be correlated with an increased incidence and severity of osteochondrotic lesions in foals [95].

Copper deficiency leads to defective lysyl oxidase, which is a copper-dependent enzyme required for proper maturation of connective tissues. A low copper diet (15 ppm) produced three times as many osteochondrotic lesions of the appendicular and seven times as many osteochondrotic lesions of the axial skeleton, as compared to the number of lesions in foals fed a high copper (55 ppm) diet [92]. However, copper supplementation did not eliminate developmental orthopedic disease, supporting the presence of other etiologic factors. Similar results were obtained when foals fed 7 ppm of copper had a much higher incidence of macroscopic osteochondrosis than foals fed 30 ppm of copper [96]. Zinc has an antagonistic effect to copper and potentially diets with excessive zinc could cause secondary copper deficiency [97], but this has not been proven in the horse.

Conclusion

CVSM is the most common noninfectious cause of spinal ataxia in the horse. Stenosis of the cervical vertebral canal and subsequent myelocompression is the cause of this neurologic disease. Although the etiology of CVSM is not fully understood, diagnostic and therapeutic options for affected horses have continued to improve. The specificity and sensitivity of predicting CVSM from survey radiographs using the sagittal ratio method are high; however, myelography remains necessary for localization of compressive lesions. Further research is required in the field of antemortem diagnostic testing to define criteria to evaluate myelograms and evaluate the use of advanced imaging techniques such as MR and CT. Ventral interbody fusion has proven to be an effective surgical procedure; however, complete recovery does not occur in all horses, and risks associated with postoperative performance must be carefully considered by the owners.

References

[1] Dimock, W.W. and Errington, B.J. (1939) Incoordination of equidae: Wobblers. *J Am Vet Med Assoc*, 95, 261–267.

[2] Mayhew, E. (1860) *The Illustrated Horse Doctor*, W. H. Allen and Co., London.

[3] Errington, B.J. (1938) Causes of "Wobblers". *Vet Bull Supp Army Med Bull*, 32, 153–155.

[4] De Lahunta, A. (1983) *Veterinary Neuroanatomy and Clinical Neurology*, W.B. Saunders Co, Philadelphia.

[5] Rooney, J.R. (ed.) (1969) Disorders of the nervous system, in *Biomechanics in Lameness*, Williams and Wilkins, Baltimore, pp. 219–233.

[6] Wagner, P.C., Grant, B.D. and Reed, S.M. (1987) Cervical vertebral malformation. *Vet Clin North Am Equine Pract*, 3, 385–396.

[7] Van Biervliet, J. (2007) An evidence-based approach to clinical questions in the practice of equine neurology. *Vet Clin North Am Equine Pract*, 23, 317–328.

[8] Oswald, J., Love, S., Parkin, T.D. *et al.* (2010) Prevalence of cervical vertebral stenotic myelopathy in a population of Thoroughbred horses. *Vet Rec*, 166, 82–83.

[9] Powers, B.E., Stashak, T.S., Nixon, A.J. *et al.* (1986) Pathology of the vertebral column of horses with cervical static stenosis. *Vet Pathol*, 23, 392–399.

[10] Rush Moore, B., Reed, S.M. and Robertson, J.T. (1993) Surgical treatment of cervical stenotic myelopathy in horses: 73 cases (1983–1992). *J Am Vet Med Assoc*, 203, 108–112.

[11] Mayhew, I.G., Donawick, W.J., Green, S.L. *et al.* (1993) Diagnosis and prediction of cervical vertebral malformation in thoroughbred foals based on semi-quantitative radiographic indicators. *Equine Vet J*, 25, 435–440.

[12] Rush Moore, B., Reed, S.M., Biller, D.S. *et al.* (1994) Assessment of vertebral canal diameter and bony malformations of the cervical part of the spine in horses with cervical stenotic myelopathy. *Am J Vet Res*, 55, 5–13.

[13] Van Biervliet, J., Mayhew, J. and de LaHunta, A. (2006) Cervical vertebral compressive myelopathy. *Clin Tech Equine Pract*, 5, 54–59.

[14] Nixon, A.J., Stashak, T.S. and Ingram, J. (1982) Diagnosis of cervical vertebral malformation in the horse. *Proc Am Assoc Equine Pract*, 28, 253–266.

[15] Papageorges, M., Gavin, P.R., Sande, R.D. *et al.* (1987) Radiographic and myelographic examination of the cervical vertebral column in 306 ataxic horses. *Vet Radiol*, 28, 53–59.

[16] Mayhew, I.G., De Lahunta, A., Whitlock, R.H. *et al.* (1978) Spinal cord disease in the horse. *Cornell Vet*, 68 (Suppl 6), 1–207.

[17] Rush Moore, B., Holbrook, T.C., Stefanacci, J.D. *et al.* (1992) Contrast-enhanced computed tomography and myelography in six horses with cervical stenotic myelopathy. *Equine Vet J*, 24, 197–202.

[18] Wilson, W.D., Hughes, S.J., Ghoshal, N.G. *et al.* (1985) Occipitoatlantoaxial malformation in two non-Arabian horses. *J Am Vet Med Assoc*, 187, 36.

[19] Reed, S.M. and Rush, B.R. (1999) Developmental vertebral anomalies, in *Equine Surgery* (eds J.A. Auer and J.A. Stick), W.B. Saunders, Philadephia, pp. 423–428.

[20] Levine, J.M., Ngheim, P.P., Levine, G.J. *et al.* (2008) Associations of sex, breed, and age with cervical vertebral compressive myelopathy in horses: 811 cases (1974–2007). *J Am Vet Med Assoc*, 233, 1453–1458.

[21] Gerber, H., Ueltschi, G., Diehl, M. *et al.* (1989) Untersuchungen an der Halswirbelsäule des Pferdes—eine klinisch-radiologische Studie. *Schweiz Arch Tierheilkd*, 131, 311–321.

[22] Stewart, R.H., Reed, S.M. and Weisbrode, S.E. (1991) Frequency and severity of osteochondrosis in horses with cervical stenotic myelopathy. *Am J Vet Res*, 52, 873–879.

[23] Newton-Clarke, M.J., Divers, T.J., De Lahunta, A. *et al.* (1994) Evaluation of the thoraco-laryngeal reflex ("slap test") as an aid to the diagnosis of cervical spinal cord and brainstem disease in horses. *Equine Vet J*, 26, 358–361.

[24] Tomizawa, N., Nishimura, R., Sasaki, N. *et al.* (1994) Efficacy of the new radiographic measurement method for cervical vertebral instability in wobbling foals. *J Vet Med Sci*, 56, 1119–1122.

[25] Andrews, F.M. and Adair, H.S., III (1999) Anatomy and physiology of the nervous system, in *Equine Surgery* (eds J.A. Auer and J.A. Stick), W.B. Saunders, Philadelphia, pp. 405–412.

[26] Mayhew, I.G. (1996) Equine neurology and nutrition. *Proc AEVA Bain-Fallon Mem Lect*, 18, 1–73.

[27] Chiapetta, J.R., Baker, J.R. and Feeney, D.A. (1985) Vertebral fracture, extensor hypertonia of thoracic limbs, and paralysis of the pelvic limbs (Schiff-Sherrington syndrome) in an Arabian foal. *J Am Vet Med Assoc*, 186, 387.

[28] Rashmir-Raven, A., DeBowes, R.M., Hudson, L. *et al.* (1991) Vertebral fracture and paraplegia in a foal. *Prog Vet Neurol*, 2, 197–202.

[29] Pinchbeck, G. and Murphy, D. (2001) Cervical vertebral fracture in three foals. *Equine Vet Educ*, 1, 24–28.

[30] Schott, H.C., II, Major, M.D., Grant, B.D. *et al.* (1990) Melanoma as a cause of spinal cord compression in two horses. *J Am Vet Med Assoc*, 196, 1820–1822.

[31] Furr, M.O., Anver, M. and Wise, M. (1991) Intervertebral disk prolapse and diskospondylitis in a horse. *J Am Vet Med Assoc*, 198, 2095–2096.

[32] Colbourne, C.M., Raidal, S.L., Yovich, J.V. *et al.* (1997) Cervical discospondylitis in two horses. *Aust Vet J*, 75, 477–479.

[33] Mayhew, I.G.J. (1999) The diseased spinal cord. *Proc Am Assoc Equine Pract*, 45, 66–84.

[34] Yovich, J.V., Powers, B.E. and Stashak, T.S. (1985) Morphologic features of the cervical intervertebral disks and adjacent vertebral bodies of horses. *Am J Vet Res*, 46, 2372–2377.

[35] Allison, N. and Moeller, R.B., Jr (2000) Spinal ataxia in a horse caused by an arachnoid diverticulum (cyst). *J Vet Diagn Invest*, 12, 279–281.

[36] Hestvik, G., Ekman, S. and Lindberg, R. (2006) Onchocercosis of an intervertebral joint capsule causing cervical vertebral stenotic myelopathy in a horse. *J Vet Diagn Invest*, 18, 307–310.

[37] Gold, J.R., Divers, T.J., Miller, A.J. *et al.* (2008) Cervical vertebral spinal hematomas in 4 horses. *J Vet Intern Med*, 22, 481–485.

[38] Andrews, F.M., Matthews, H.K. and Reed, S.M. (1990) The ancillary techniques and tests for diagnosing equine neurologic disease. *Vet Med*, December, 1325–1330.

[39] Furr, M.O. and Tyler, R.D. (1990) Cerebrospinal fluid creatine kinase activity in horses with central nervous system disease: 69 cases (1984–1989). *J Am Vet Med Assoc*, 197, 245–248.

[40] Furr, M., Chickering, W.R. and Robertson, J. (1997) High resolution protein electrophoresis of equine cerebrospinal fluid. *Am J Vet Res*, 58, 939–941.

[41] Pusterla, N., Wilson, W.D., Conrad, P.A. *et al.* (2006) Comparative analysis of cytokine gene expression in cerebrospinal fluid of horses without neurologic signs or with selected neurologic disorders. *Am J Vet Res*, 67, 1433–1437.

[42] Withers, J.M., Voûte, L.C., Hammond, G. *et al.* (2009) Radiographic anatomy of the articular process joints of the caudal cervical vertebrae in the horse on lateral and oblique projections. *Equine Vet J*, 41, 895–902.

[43] Down, S.S. and Henson, F.M. (2009) Radiographic retrospective study of the caudal cervical articular process joints in the horse. *Equine Vet J*, 41, 518–524.

[44] Mayhew, I.G. and Green, S.L. (2002) Radiographic diagnosis of equine cervical vertebral malformation. *Proc Annu Meet Am Coll Vet Intern Med*, 20, 382–383.

[45] Hahn, C.N., Handel, I., Green, S.L. *et al.* (2008) Assessment of the utility of using intra- and intervertebral minimum sagittal diameter ratios in the diagnosis of cervical vertebral malformation in horses. *Vet Radiol Ultrasound*, 49, 1–6.

[46] Scrivani, P.V., Levine, J.M., Holmes, N.L. *et al.* (2011) Observer agreement study of cervical-vertebral ratios in horses. *Equine Vet J*, 43, 399–403.

[47] Neuwirth, L. (1992) Equine myelography. *Compend Contin Educ Pract Vet*, 14, 72–78.

[48] Rose, P.L., Abutarbush, S.M. and Duckett, W. (2007) Standing myelography in the horse using a nonionic contrast agent. *Vet Radiol Ultrasound*, 48, 535–538.

[49] Reed, S.M., Newberry, J., Norton, K. *et al.* (1985) Pathogenesis of cervical vertebral malformation. *Proc Am Assoc Equine Pract*, 31, 37–42.

[50] Nyland, T.G., Blythe, L.L., Pool, R.R. *et al.* (1980) Metrizamide myelography in the horse: clinical, radiographic, and pathologic changes. *Am J Vet Res*, 41, 204–211.

[51] Van Biervliet, J., Scrivani, P.V., Divers, T.J. *et al.* (2002) Evaluation of a diagnostic criterion for spinal cord compression during cervical myelography. *Proc Annu Meet Coll Vet Intern Med*, 20, 769.

[52] van Biervliet, J., Scrivani, P.V., Divers, T.J. *et al.* (2004) Evaluation of decision criteria for detection of spinal cord compression based on cervical myelography in horses: 38 cases (1981–2001). *Equine Vet J*, 36, 14–20.

[53] Mayhew, I.G. (ed.) (1989) Tetraparesis, paraparesis and ataxia of the limbs, and episodic weakness, in *Large Animal Neurology: A Handbook for Veterinary Clinicians*, 1st edn, Lea and Febiger, Philadelphia, pp. 246–258.

[54] Schmidburg, I., Pagger, H., Zsoldos, R.R. *et al.* (2012) Movement associated reduction of spatial capacity of the equine cervical vertebral canal. *Vet J*, 192, 525–528.

[55] Mayhew, I.G. and Green, S.L. (2000) Accuracy of diagnosing CVM from radiographs. *Proc Br Equine Vet Assoc Annu Congr, Equine Vet J Ltd, Newmarket*, 39, 74–75.

[56] Mitchell, C.W., Nykamp, S.G., Foster, R. *et al.* (2012) The use of magnetic resonance imaging in evaluating horses with spinal ataxia. *Vet Radiol Ultrasound*, 53, 613–620.

[57] Prange, T., Derksen, F.J., Stick, J.A. *et al.* (2011) Endoscopic anatomy of the cervical vertebral canal in the horse: a cadaver study. *Equine Vet J*, 43, 317–323.

[58] Prange, T., Derksen, F.J., Stick, J.A. *et al.* (2011) Cervical vertebral canal endoscopy in the horse: intra- and post operative observations. *Equine Vet J*, 43, 404–411.

[59] Prange, T., Carr, E.A., Stick, J.A. *et al.* (2012) Cervical vertebral canal endoscopy in a horse with cervical vertebral stenotic myelopathy. *Equine Vet J*, 44, 116–119.

[60] Pepe, M., Angelone, M., Gialletti, R. *et al.* (2014) Arthroscopic anatomy of the equine cervical articular process joints. *Equine Vet J*, 46, 345–351.

[61] Hudson, N.P.H. and Mayhew, I.G. (2005) Radiographic and myelographic assessment of the equine cervical vertebral column and spinal cord. *Equine Vet Educ*, 17, 34–38.

[62] Binkhorst, G.J., (1986). Het ataxie syndroom bij jonge paarden. Inaugural Dissertation, Utrecht University, Utrecht, the Netherlands.

[63] Gruys, E., Beynen, A.C., Binkhorst, G.J. *et al.* (1994) Neurodegeneratieve aandoeningen van het centrale zenuwstelsel bij het paard. *Tijdschr Diergeneeskd*, 119, 561–567.

[64] Yovich, J.V., Gould, D.H. and LeCouteur, R.A. (1991) Chronic cervical compressive myelopathy in horses: patterns of astrocytosis in the spinal cord. *Aust Vet J*, 68, 334–337.

[65] Tomizawa, N., Nishimura, R., Sasaki, N. *et al.* (1994) Relationships between radiography of cervical vertebrae and histopathology of the cervical cord in wobbling 19 foals. *J Vet Med Sci*, 56, 227–233.

[66] Summers, B.A., Cummings, J.F. and de Lahunta, A. (1995) *Veterinary Neuropathology*, Mosby, St. Louis.

[67] Donawick, W.J., Mayhew, I.G., Galligan, D.T. *et al.* (1989) Early diagnosis of cervical vertebral malformation in young Thoroughbred horses and successful treatment with restricted, paced diet and confinement. *Proc Am Assoc Equine Pract*, 35, 525–528.

[68] Kronfeld, D.S., Meacham, T.N. and Donoghue, S. (1990) Dietary aspects of developmental orthopedic disease in young horses. *Vet Clin North Am Equine Pract*, 6, 451–465.

[69] Mayhew, I.G., Brown, C.M., Stowe, H.D. *et al.* (1987) Equine degenerative myeloencephalopathy: a vitamin E deficiency that may be familial. *J Vet Intern Med*, 1, 45–50.

[70] Grisel, G.B., Grant, B.D. and Rantanen, N.W. (1996) Arthrocentesis of the equine cervical facets. *Proc Am Assoc Equine Pract*, 42, 197–198.

[71] Grant, B.D. (1999) Surgical treatment of developmental disorders of the spinal column, in *Equine Surgery*, 1st edn (eds J.A. Auer and J.A. Stick), W. B. Saunders, Philadelphia, pp. 429–435.

[72] Wagner, P.C., Bagby, G.W., Grant, B.D. *et al.* (1979) Surgical stabilization of the equine cervical spine. *Vet Surg*, 8, 7–12.

[73] Walmsley, J.P. (2005) Surgical treatment of cervical spinal cord compression in horses: a European experience. *Equine Vet Educ*, 17, 39–43.

[74] Huggons, N. (2007) Tri-level surgical treatment of cervical spinal cord compression in a Thoroughbred yearling. *Can Vet J*, 48, 635–638.

[75] Kumar, V.G., Rea, G.L., Mervis, L.J. *et al.* (1999) Cervical spondylotic myelopathy: functional and radiographic long-term outcome after laminectomy and posterior fusion. *Neurosurgery*, 44, 771–777 discussion 777–778.

[76] Hacker, R.J. (2002) Threaded cages for degenerative cervical disease. *Clin Orthop Relat Res*, 394, 39–46.

[77] Rusbridge, C., Wheeler, S.J., Torrington, A.M. *et al.* (1998) Comparison of two surgical techniques for the management of cervical spondylomyelopathy in Dobermans. *J Small Anim Pract*, 39, 425–431.

[78] DeBowes, R.M., Grant, B.D., Bagby, G.W. *et al.* (1984) Cervical vertebral interbody fusion in the horse: a comparative study of bovine xenografts and autografts supported by stainless steel baskets. *Am J Vet Res*, 45, 191–199.

[79] Nixon, A.J. and Stashak, T.S. (1983) Dorsal laminectomy in the horse. I. Review of the literature and description of a new procedure. *Vet Surg*, 12, 172–176.

[80] Reardon, R., Kummer, M. and Lischer, C. (2009) Ventral locking compression plate for treatment of cervical stenotic myelopathy in a 3-month-old warmblood foal. *Vet Surg*, 38, 537–542.

[81] Reardon, R., Bailey, R., Walmsley, J. *et al.* (2009) A pilot in vitro biomechanical comparison of locking compression plate fixation and kerf-cut cylinder fixation for ventral fusion of fourth and fifth equine cervical vertebrae. *Vet Comp Orthop Traumatol*, 22, 371–379.

[82] Reardon, R.J., Bailey, R., Walmsley, J.P. *et al.* (2010) An in vitro biomechanical comparison of a locking compression plate fixation and kerf cut cylinder fixation for ventral arthrodesis of the fourth and the fifth equine cervical vertebrae. *Vet Surg*, 39, 980–990.

[83] Hoffman, C.J. and Clark, C.K. (2013) Prognosis for racing with conservative management of cervical vertebral malformation in Thoroughbreds: 103 cases (2002–2010). *J Vet Intern Med*, 27, 317–323.

[84] Dimock, W.W. (1950) "Wobblers" – an hereditary disease in horses. *J Hered*, 41, 319–323.

[85] Falco, M.J., Whitwell, K. and Palmer, A.C. (1976) An investigation into the genetics of "Wobbler disease" in Thoroughbred horses in Britain. *Equine Vet J*, 8, 165–169.

[86] Wagner, P.C., Grant, B.D., Watrous, B.J. *et al.* (1985) A study of the heritability of cervical vertebral malformation in horses. *Proc Am Assoc Equine Pract*, 31, 43–50.

[87] Rooney, J.R. (1972) Etiology of the Wobbler syndrome. *Mod Vet Pract*, 53, 42.

[88] Stashak, T.S., Nixon, A.J. and Powers, B.E. Pathology associated with cervical vertebral malformation (CVM) in the horse. Proceedings of the Veterinary Orthopedic Society, Salt Lake City, Vol. 12; 1985, p. 41.

[89] Reed, S.M. Cervical vertebral stenotic myelopathy: pathogenesis. Proceedings of the International Equine Neurology Conference, July 11–13, 1997. Cornell University, New York, Vol. 1; 1997, pp. 45–49.

[90] Hurtig, M.B. and Pool, R.R. (1996) Pathogenesis of equine osteochondrosis, in *Joint Disease in the Horse* (eds C.W. McIllwraith and G.W. Trotter), W.B. Saunders, Philadelphia, pp. 335–338.

[91] Savage, C.J. (1998) Etiopathogenesis of osteochondrosis, in *Current Techniques in Equine Surgery and Lameness* (eds N.A. White II and J.N. Moore), W.B. Saunders, Philadelphia, pp. 318–322.

[92] Knight, D., Weisbrode, S.E., Schmall, L.M. *et al.* (1990) The effects of copper supplementation on the prevalence of cartilage lesions in foals. *Equine Vet J*, 22, 426–432.

[93] Glade, M.J. and Belling, T.H., Jr (1984) Growth plate cartilage metabolism, morphology and biochemical composition in over- and underfed horses. *Growth*, 48, 473–482.

[94] Glade, M.J. and Luba, N.K. (1987) Serum triiodothyronine and thyroxine concentrations in weanling horses fed carbohydrate by direct gastric infusion. *Am J Vet Res*, 48, 578–582.

[95] Savage, C.J., McCarthy, R. and Jeffcott, L. (1993) Effects of dietary energy and protein on induction of dyschondroplasia in foals. *Equine Vet J*, (Suppl 16), 74–79.

[96] Hurtig, M.B., Green, S.L. and Dobson, H. (1993) Correlative study of defective cartilage and bone growth in foals fed a low-copper diet. *Equine Vet J*, (Suppl 16), 66–73.

[97] Knight, D.A., Gabel, A.A., Reed, S.M. *et al.* (1985) Correlation of dietary mineral to incidence and severity of metabolic bone disease in Ohio and Kentucky. *Proc Am Assoc Equine Pract*, 31, 445–461.

29 Electrolyte Abnormalities and Neurologic Dysfunction in Horses

Ramiro E. Toribio

College of Veterinary Medicine, The Ohio State University, Columbus, USA

Maintaining intra- and extracellular electrolyte values within narrow limits is essential to the function of excitable cells (neurons, muscle fibers, cardiac conduction system). In nervous tissue, changes in transmembrane ion gradients (membrane potential) could disrupt glial cell and neuron activity, which will clinically manifest as deficiency (depression, paralysis, coma) or release (excitability, spasticity, seizures). Similarly, substances that influence or mimic electrolytes, could alter brain cell biology. Most of the information in this chapter is derived from human or comparative studies; however, equine-specific information will be provided when available.

While many ions are essential for the function excitable tissue, sodium (Na^+), potassium (K^+), chloride (Cl^-), calcium (Ca^{2+}), magnesium (Mg^{2+}), bicarbonate (HCO_3^-), and phosphate (P_i) are the most important. Concentrations of Na^+, Cl^-, Ca^{2+}, and HCO_3^- are higher in the extracellular fluid (ECF), while K^+, Mg^{2+}, and P_i concentrations are higher in the cell. Their shifts across the cell membrane occur by simple diffusion (channels) and facilitated diffusion (carrier proteins, energy-dependent processes). Organic osmolytes (e.g., myo-inositol) and nonpermeable anionic particles such as proteins (Donnan effect) also influence ionic dynamics across the cell membrane. Ions move in a downward (passive transport) or an upward gradient (active transport). The movement of water across the cell membrane (osmosis) is as important as that of ions in neuron and glial cell physiology and pathophysiology. Ligands, hormones, toxins, endogenous by-products, drugs, energy depletion, and hypoxia can disturb ion and water dynamics, with detrimental effects to nervous tissue.

The cell membrane potential

The *membrane potential* is defined as the electrical difference between the inner and outer side the cell membrane. At resting state, the membrane potential is negative and values depend on cell type, ranging from −40 to −80 mV (*resting potential*). The membrane potential is the result of changes in permeability to Na^+, K^+, Ca^{2+}, and Cl^-; however, Na^+, K^+, and Cl^- are the main determinants (Goldman voltage equation). Ionized magnesium modulates cation channels and processes that require energy. The role of P_i in the action potential (AP) is indirect, as the source of energy (ATP). The movement of these ions is determined by intra- and extracellular concentrations, channels (Na^+ channels, Ca^{2+} channels, NMDA receptor (NMDAR), α-amino-3-hydroxy-5-methyl-4-isoxazolepropionic acid (AMPA) receptor (AMPAR), $GABA_A$ receptor ($GABA_A$R)), transporters (plasma membrane calcium ATPase (PMCA)), co-transporters (K^+/Cl^- co-transporter, $Na^+/K^+/2Cl^-$ co-transporter (NKCC)), and exchangers (Na^+/K^+ ATPase, Na^+/Ca^{2+} exchanger (NCX)).

The AP is a phenomenon by which the cell membrane potential increases (depolarization) and decreases (repolarization) at high speeds. The AP is essential for excitable cells to sense and communicate (stimulation, suppression) at short and long distances, and for endocrine and neuroendocrine cells to release endocrine and paracrine factors.

Ultimately, disturbances in membrane potentials (resting and APs) explain many of the signs of pathological processes afflicting the central (CNS) and peripheral (PNS) nervous systems.

Sodium

Sodium is the most abundant ion in the ECF. It controls extracellular volume, blood volume, cell volume, blood pressure, tissue perfusion, osmolality, and influences the pH. Due to its osmotic properties, it also determines the movement of water across compartments. Sodium distributes rapidly between plasma and the interstitial fluid (ICF), reaching equilibrium in 15–20 min.

Equine Neurology, Second Edition. Martin Furr and Stephen Reed.
© 2015 John Wiley & Sons, Inc. Published 2015 by John Wiley & Sons, Inc.
Companion website: www.wiley.com/go/furr/neurology

Extracellular Na⁺ concentrations are regulated by gastrointestinal (GI) absorption, renal excretion, and various homeostatic systems (natriuretic peptides, renin–angiotensin–aldosterone system, vasopressin) that control water and Na⁺ balance. Thus, GI and renal disorders, as well as endocrine dysfunction (e.g., adrenal insufficiency) could indirectly alter brain function via their actions on Na⁺ concentration.

In the case of the CNS, the movement of Na⁺ across cell membranes is determined by its extracellular concentrations, other ions (e.g., Ca^{2+}, Mg^{2+}, and K^+), neurotransmitters (e.g., glutamate, acetylcholine), hormones (e.g., insulin), energy (e.g., ATP), oxygen and osmolytes (e.g., glutamine, myo-inositol), and water.

Disturbances in plasma Na⁺ concentrations are a common clinical problem in human patients admitted to ICU's [1]. For example, one large-scale study found that many cases of dysnatremia were acquired after patients were admitted and Na⁺ abnormalities were associated with a poor prognosis [1]. Dysnatremias are also frequent in hospitalized horses and foals [2]; however, large-scale studies on the prevalence of Na⁺ disorders and their association with severity of disease are lacking in the equine literature.

Hyponatremia

Hyponatremia is defined as a serum Na⁺ concentration below 134 mEq/l (134 mmol/l) [2–4]. It can be hypovolemic (Na⁺ depletion), euvolemic (increased body water, normal Na⁺), or hypervolemic (increase in Na⁺ with greater increase in water). Hypervolemic and hypovolemic hyponatremic states are documented in all species. Hyponatremia could also be divided into hypotonic, isotonic, or hypertonic; however, only hypotonic hyponatremia has clinical relevance to disorders of the CNS. Pseudohyponatremia is characterized by normal plasma osmolality, low Na⁺ concentrations, no clinical signs related to Na⁺ imbalance, and occurs with displacement of water by hyperproteinemia, hyperlipidemia, or hyperglycemia.

Causes of hyponatremia

In general terms, a decrease in Na⁺ intake, increase in water consumption or retention, or Na⁺ waste could lead to hyponatremia. These include conditions that result in water retention (renal failure, congestive heart failure, hypervasopressinemia), excessive water administration (iatrogenic), behavior (polydipsia, water intoxication), Na⁺ loss (renal failure, sweating, GI disease), solute redistribution (uroabdomen), endocrinopathies (adrenal insufficiency, vasopressin), and drugs (diuretics). Water intoxication can be a consequence of psychogenic polydipsia or administration of hypotonic solutions.

Hyponatremia is a hallmark of uroperitoneum in foals. Due to their milk-based diet (low in Na⁺, high in K⁺) [5, 6] and the fact that equine renal excretion is low

for Na⁺ and Cl⁻, but high for K⁺, when the urinary bladder ruptures, a large volume of a hyponatremic, hypochloremic, and hyperkalemic solution accumulates in the abdomen. Solute equilibration between the abdominal fluid and the ECF leads to hyponatremia, hypochloremia, hyperkalemia, and azotemia.

Unlike other species, there is limited data on drugs causing hyponatremia in horses. In one case report, a 9-year-old Quarterhorse gelding developed iatrogenic hypoadrenocorticism with multiple electrolyte abnormalities following chronic administration of stanozolol [7]. Diuretics, in particular the thiazides, may cause hyponatremia [8]. The syndrome of inappropriate antidiuretic hormone secretion (SIADH) characterized by excessive secretion of vasopressin is a frequent cause of hyponatremia in people [3, 9–11]. This syndrome occurs with nonosmotic release of vasopressin, and includes meningitis, head injury, some malignancies, and drugs (citalopram, carbamazepine, clofibrate, morphine) [3, 9–11]. At present, there are no reports of SIADH in horses. The use of carbamazepine may have implications in equine medicine as this drug has been recommended for the treatment of idiopathic head-shaking in horses [12]. The administration of desmopressin for the treatment of hemostatic disorders or diabetes insipidus in people has been shown to cause dilutional hyponatremia [3, 13, 14].

Pathophysiology of hyponatremia and the central nervous system

Hyponatremic encephalopathy is a major cause of human mortality. A factor leading to a negative outcome in people with this condition is the inability of the brain to adapt to hyponatremia and regulate its volume, resulting in swelling and neurological damage [15]. This is further complicated by the expansion of nervous tissue in a rigid cranial vault, with the consequent increase in intracranial pressure (ICP), reduced cerebral perfusion pressure (CPP), ischemia, cell injury, permanent damage, and even death [16].

Hyponatremia creates a gradient for water to move into the CNS, leading to cerebral edema and neuronal injury. This is particularly true in patients with prolonged hyponatremia that have made intracellular adaptations to a hypoosmolar state through organic osmolytes (idiogenic osmoles) and in which a rapid correction in extracellular Na⁺ concentrations triggers excessive water influx into glial cells and neurons, cellular swelling, cytotoxicity, axon demyelination, cerebral edema, and death [15].

Cell volume and glial cells

To better understand the process of hyponatremic neuropathy, it is necessary to briefly examine the structure of the blood–brain barrier (BBB). The BBB represents a complex homeostatic system that regulates electrolytes and water in the extracellular compartment of the CNS [15]. It separates the brain from the systemic circulation, including substances that could be harmful to neurons and glial cells (e.g., glutamate). Water moves across the BBB by a number of mechanisms, including osmosis and water transport systems. Most of the BBB consists of endothelial cells and astrocytes. Aquaporin water channels, in particular aquaporin 1 (AQP1) and aquaporin 4 (AQP4) in glial cells are crucial for cerebral water regulation. There is evidence that AQP4 participates in the pathogenesis of brain edema from hyponatremia [17]. In fact, the astrocyte is essential for water balance as they contain most of the intracellular water in the brain, are rich in AQP4, and will swell in the early stages of hyponatremia or brain edema to protect neurons from water influx [15]. Through energy-dependent mechanisms (e.g., Na^+/K^+ ATPase) Na^+ ions will be extruded, water will follow, cell volume will be restored, and brain edema reduced.

Hypoxemia is a complicating factor during hyponatremia as the mechanisms that regulate Na^+ transport and neuronal adaptation to hyponatremia are energy- and oxygen-dependent. Hypoxia impairs astrocyte volume regulation and by itself can cause cerebral edema. A depletion in energy (ATP, phosphocreatine) initiates cellular accumulation of L-lactate and other by-products that will further lower the cellular pH and the ability to adapt to the hypoosmolar environment [15, 18]. Intracellular Na^+ and extracellular K^+ concentrations will increase, in part due to Na^+/K^+ ATPase failure. Water and Cl^- will follow Na^+ and astrocytes will swell. As a compensatory mechanism to correct extracellular K^+, the $Na^+/K^+/2Cl^-$ co-transporter (NKCC) will be activated by K^+, ischemia, and glutamate, and the increased cellular uptake of K^+ will worsen cellular swelling and excitotoxicity [19]. This understanding of NKCC could have therapeutic implications to equine cerebral edema, as bumetanide and furosemide inhibit NKCC, and could potentially reduce edema by dual actions (diuresis, astrocyte effect). While outside the focus of this chapter, there is evidence that Na^+/K^+ ATPase inhibition and NKCC activation contribute to glial and neuronal volume expansion in brain and spinal cord trauma [19]. The function of other energy-dependent cell membrane proteins that maintain the ionic balance (NCX, PMCA) can also be disrupted.

Vasopressin can have detrimental effects on water handling by the brain during hyponatremia [20]. It reduces cerebral blood flow, impairs oxygen delivery to astrocytes, lowers ATP synthesis, decreases intracellular pH, induces vasogenic brain edema, and increases cellular water influx [15, 20–23].

During cerebral injury (trauma, ischemia, hypoxia, edema, hyponatremia) Ca^{2+} influx is a major determinant of cytotoxity as it activates phospholipases, endonucleases, caspases, and proteases (calpains). Calcium enters brain cells through glutamate receptor channels (NMDAR, AMPAR, mGluR), voltage-gated Ca^{2+} channels, NCX, and transient receptor potential vanilloid channels (TRPVs). PMCA and NCX are the main keepers of intracellular Ca^{2+} at very low concentrations, and therefore protect the cell against Ca^{2+} build up. In severe neuronal injury, caspases and calpains disrupt or even reverse the function of NCX and PMCA [24, 25], altering their ability to restore intracellular Ca^{2+}. In addition, Ca^{2+} may leak from intracellular organelles to further cellular damage.

Glutamate/glutamine cycle and hyponatremia

Most glutamate, GABA, and glutamine in the brain result from recycling rather than transport from systemic circulation because they can be cytotoxic in high concentrations and are blocked by the BBB from getting into the CNS [26]. The synthesis of these amino compounds is controlled by the glutamate–GABA-glutamine cycle [26]. Glutamate and GABA released by neurons are taken by astrocytes to be converted to glutamine. Astrocytes have higher glutamine synthetase activity than neurons, and are the main source of glutamine in the brain. Subsequently, glutamine is taken by neurons as a precursor for glutamate or GABA. This information is a great example of how glial cell dysfunction could influence neuronal activity.

Hypoosmotic conditions stimulate the release of glutamate by astrocytes and reduce the conversion of glutamate to glutamine [26]. This decreased conversion is a consequence of activation of volume-regulated anion channels that impair glutamine synthetase function [26]. Taken together, increased glutamate and decreased glutamine release from swollen astrocytes in part explains the hyperexcitable state of humans and animals with hyponatremia.

Osmolytes (idiogenic osmoles, idiosmoles)

Cerebral edema occurs with acute hyponatremia but rarely in chronic hyponatremia. This difference is the result of a series of adaptive and compensatory processes. In the sequence of events to correct the effects of cerebral hyponatremia, osmolytes and water will be moved from neurons and glial cells to the interstitial space, then to the CSF, and subsequently to systemic circulation. The efflux of inorganic osmolytes (Na^+, K^+, Cl^-) occurs rapidly (hours) to reduce cellular swelling while organic osmolytes (idiosmoles; creatine, betaine, glycine, taurine, urea, myo-inositol, sorbitol, N-acetylaspartate (NAA), glutamine, and choline-containing compounds) are extruded slowly (days) to regulate cell volume [27]. This will persist as long as the ECF remains hypoosmolar. During correction of hyponatremia, intracellular osmolytes will be slowly restored. However, in individuals with chronic or severe hyponatremia who have made intracellular adaptations to the prevailing hypotonicity, rapid correction may overwhelm compensatory processes and brain damage may ensue. Brain myo-inositol, creatine, NAA, and choline-containing compounds were associated with serum Na^+ concentrations in human patients with hypo- and normonatremia [27, 28].

Osmotic demyelination syndromes (central myelinolysis)

Central pontine myelinolysis (CPM) is a specific form (pons, brainstem) of hyponatremic encephalopathy [3, 10, 11]. It occurs as a consequence of rapid correction of Na^+ concentrations in patients with chronic and severe hyponatremia that have adjusted to the hypotonic environment. High cerebral ionic concentrations without adequate levels of organic osmolytes contribute to the development of CPM [28]. This is well documented in people, dogs, and laboratory animals [3, 10, 11, 27–30]. Extrapontine myelinolysis is another osmotic demyelination syndrome affecting other areas of the brain [11].

Hypovolemic hyponatremic encephalopathy was reported in a foal with diarrhea [31]. Water consumption resulted in rapid hyponatremia and hypotonicity. The foal developed blindness, loss of menace response, and seizures. Signs resolved after treatment with hypertonic saline solution (7.2%). To prevent the development of pontine and extrapontine myelinolysis, at least in people, it is recommended to correct hyponatremia at a rate of no more than 8–12 mEq/l/day (see section "Treatment of Hyponatremia") [32]. Similar recommendations may apply to domestic animals.

Clinical signs

Clinical signs of hyponatremia reported in horses include depression, blindness, reduced menace response, and seizures [31, 33]. The serum Na^+ concentration necessary to initiate clinical signs is variable and depends on the magnitude and the speed at which hyponatremia developed. Concurrent problems such as hypoxia, hypoglycemia, or liver disease may exacerbate the signs of hyponatremia. In experimental studies in rabbits, animals that develop hyponatremia (119 ± 1 mEq/l) acutely (2–3 h) showed grand mal seizure activity and 86% died. All rabbits had moderate to marked cerebral edema with greater than 17% increase in brain water content compared to normonatremic controls. Rabbits with a slower development of hyponatremia (3.5 days) and a serum Na^+ of 122 ± 2 mEq/l were asymptomatic despite a 7% increase in brain water content. Rabbits with 16 days of hyponatremia with a serum Na^+ 99 ± 3 mEq/l were weak, anorectic, lethargic, and unable to walk.

These subjects had a 7% increase in brain water content and low brain osmolality (218 ± 12 mOsm/kg) [34]. These findings support that in hyponatremic patients, clinical signs are correlated with the magnitude and duration of hyponatremia, increased in cerebral water, and concurrent losses of brain osmolytes [34].

One foal with seizures had a serum Na^+ concentration of 99 mEq/l [35]. The foal remained lethargic and depressed, with an absent menace when serum Na^+ was 113 mEq/l. In another foal with diarrhea, seizures were observed associated with a serum Na^+ of 117 mEq/l [33]. Hyponatremia was also observed in two foals with rhabdomyolysis, with serum Na^+ values of 117–119 mEq/l, with no obvious neurologic abnormalities [36]. Hence, it seems that the presence of neurologic signs is variable when the serum Na^+ is 115–120 mEq/l, and clinical signs are likely to develop when values are less than 115 mEq/l.

Treatment of hyponatremia

Factors to consider in the treatment of hyponatremia include onset of hyponatremia (acute <48 h; chronic >48 h), severity of hyponatremia, presence of neurological signs, and volemia [3, 10, 11, 37]. The next step would be the selection of the replacement solution as well as the rate of Na^+ administration. Recent review articles in human intensive care medicine have been critical to the traditional therapeutic approach to hyponatremia [37, 38]. Because free water excess (FWE) is the main cause of hyponatremia in people, ideally FWE should be calculated [10]. FWE is calculated as:

$$FWE = body\ weight \times (140 - serum\ Na^+)/140\ [10].$$

Once this is calculated, the rate of correction should be determined. One would want to remove about one third of the FWE in 24 h to avoid overcorrection of serum Na^+. Depending on urine production, concurrent disease, and whether neurological signs are present, isotonic or hypertonic (3–7.2%) NaCl solutions are recommended. A gradual increase in blood Na^+ concentration is indicated rather than bolus dosing to prevent overcorrection and possible CPM. If hyponatremia developed rapidly, correction can be rapid, but in severe or chronic hyponatremia the maximum accepted rate of correction is 8–12 mEq/l in 24 h [3, 10, 11, 37–39]. However, specific recommendations for horses have not been established. One method is to calculate the Na^+ deficit and correct serum sodium concentration to 120 mEq/l using hypertonic saline by bolus infusion, followed by slow correction (over 24 h) of the remaining deficit. Sodium deficit is calculated as follows:

$$Na^+\ deficit = 0.6 \times BW\ (kg) \times (desired\ Na^+ - measured\ Na^+)\ [31]$$

This formula differs from the used for calculating Na^+ deficit in the ECF, which uses the term 0.3 instead of 0.6 for

Table 29.1 Sodium content of various solutions used for the treatment of hyponatremia.

Sodium concentration (%)	Sodium concentration (mEq/l)
0.45	77
0.9 (isotonic)	154
3	513
5	855
7.2	1232

water content. Treatment in horses can be achieved with hypertonic, isotonic, or hypotonic saline solutions. An empirical dose of 2 ml/kg of a 7.2% hypertonic saline solution has been used successfully in equids, in addition to restricting the ingestion of free water [31]. A more conservative approach is to use isotonic NaCl with the goal of correcting Na$^+$ by 10 mEq/l in 24 h. The sodium concentrations of various solutions are presented in Table 29.1.

Osmotic demyelinating syndromes (e.g., CPM) may occur after rapid restoration of normonatremia [3, 10, 16, 39], and can have permanent consequences. Risk factors identified for the development of CPM in people include chronic hyponatremia with rapid Na$^+$ restoration, concurrent hypokalemia, liver disease, poor nutrition, and cutaneous burns [3, 10, 16, 39]. There are no published cases of CPM in the horse; however, it should be considered when treating horses or foals with hyponatremia. Seizures have been observed in foals immediately following rapid correction of hyponatremia with hypertonic (M. Furr, pers. commun.) and isotonic solutions (R. Toribio, pers. obs.).

Frequent monitoring of serum Na$^+$ concentration is recommended after bolus treatment, then every 6–8 h during Na$^+$ repletion. In cases of iatrogenic hyponatremia or psychogenic polydipsia, fluid restriction with careful monitoring of serum electrolytes is indicated, providing there are no ongoing losses of total body fluid (i.e., diarrhea, renal failure, and third spacing). If hyponatremia is associated with excessive fluid loss (e.g., diarrhea), water restriction is contraindicated [21].

Furosemide may be considered in animals with water retention, to limit the expansion of the ECF, and to lower the risk of CPM [2, 19, 40, 41]. By inhibiting NKCC in glial cells and the choroid plexus, furosemide reduces brain cell swelling, ICP, and CSF production [2, 19, 40, 41]. Furosemide decreased CSF production, brain edema, and ICP in experimental cats [40, 41]. Furosemide also has been advocated as a supplementary drug to reduce the rate of saline administration [42]. Doses of furosemide in horses are 0.5–1 mg/kg IV q8–24 h. It can also be given as a continuous rate infusion (CRI) with a loading dose of 0.12 mg/kg followed by a rate of 0.12 mg/kg/h (3 mg/kg/q24 h) [43].

For people with chronic hyponatremia or hyponatremia secondary to water retention (e.g., SIADH), the development of drugs that block vasopressin actions (vaptans) is shifting the therapeutic approach to hyponatremia [3, 9–11, 37, 38, 44]. Aquaretics block vasopressin V1/V2 (conivaptan) or V2 (tolvaptan) receptors [9, 10, 44, 45]. Vaptans have not been evaluated in horses; however, they should be considered in animals that fail to respond to water restriction and Na$^+$-containing solutions, or that have evidence of euvolemic (e.g., SIADH) or hypervolemic (e.g., congestive heart failure) hyponatremia [3, 11, 38, 44]. Vaptans are contraindicated in hypovolemic hyponatremia (e.g., diarrhea) [44].

Desmopressin may be indicated to correct overcorrection or to re-lower Na$^+$ when neurological signs develop after treatment [3, 32, 39]. In fact, the concurrent combination of 3% saline solution with desmopressin is being promoted as a simple strategy for safe correction of severe hyponatremia [32].

For most cases of hyponatremia, if the primary problem is resolved, the long-term prognosis is good.

Hypernatremia

Hypernatremia, defined as a serum Na$^+$ concentration over 144 mEq/l (144 mmol/l) [2, 35, 46, 47], is a hyperosmolar condition from decreased total body water in relation to the solute content. Some considered hypernatremia to be a problem of water balance rather than a disturbance in Na$^+$ homeostasis. Hypernatremia occurs secondary to excessive Na$^+$ ingestion/administration or from excessive loss of body water, and may result from dehydration, diabetes insipidus, from water restriction, diuretics, and excessive Na$^+$ intake or administration.

Many of the neurological signs of hypernatremia do not result from increased Na$^+$ concentrations but rather from inappropriate osmotherapy. Brain shrinkage caused by hypernatremia can result in vascular rupture, cerebral bleeding, subarachnoid hemorrhage, and permanent neurologic damage or death. Neurologic signs of hypernatremia are poorly documented in horses. Pigs with severe hypernatremia or salt poisoning may develop cerebral edema and eosinophilic meningoencephalitis [48, 49]. Clinically, there is blindness, disorientation, seizures, even death. Cattle also show neurological signs with salt intoxication, but do not develop cerebral eosinophilic infiltration.

To counteract the effects of hypernatremia, solutes (Na$^+$, K$^+$) move in and water out of the cells. As an adaptive response, shrunken brain cells gain additional organic solutes (osmolytes) and tissue restitution occurs when water moves back after therapy. This leads to normalization of brain volume. The same principles discussed in the hyponatremia section in regard to idiogenic osmoles apply to hypernatremia but in the opposite direction.

Slow correction of a hypertonic state reestablishes brain volume and osmolality usually without inducing cerebral edema. The risk of rapid correction is that excessive water moves into the hypertonic cerebral interstitium resulting in edema [46, 47].

Fatal hypernatremia was described in a 2-year-old Standardbred gelding secondary to an ependymoma of the neurohypophysis which was suspected of causing impingement on the hypothalamic thirst center [50]. Many diseases that cause a loss of total body water such as severe dehydration due to illness or water deprivation can result in hypernatremia in horses. In foals, hypernatremia is the result of reduced milk intake, renal disease, or iatrogenic (drugs, Na$^+$-containing solutions). Of interest, it is not unusual for sick newborn foals to develop "idiopathic hypernatremia," which can be refractory to treatment for days. We speculate this could be the result of increased aldosterone secretion and/or renal vasopressin resistance [51]. It is also possible that many critically ill foals cannot handle large Na$^+$ loads. We have also observed hypernatremia in sick full term and premature foals receiving commercial milk replacers (R. Toribio, pers. obs.).

Clinical signs of hypernatremia

Signs reflect CNS dysfunction and are prominent when the rise in serum Na$^+$ concentration is rapid (hours) or large. General signs in people include hyperpnea, muscle weakness, restlessness, insomnia, lethargy, and intense thirst. Orthostatic hypertension and tachycardia are observed secondary to hypovolemia. Reported neurologic signs in the horse are prolapsed nictitating membrane, myoclonus, altered consciousness that is directly proportional to the severity of hypernatremia, persistent tail swishing, and coma [22].

Treatment of hypernatremia

The key concepts in treating hypernatremia are correction of hypertonicity and management of the underlying cause [2]. Like hyponatremia, demyelinating syndromes are observed in chronically affected hypernatremic patients following the rapid restoration of normonatremia [52, 53]. During correction, frequent monitoring of serum electrolyte concentrations is indicated. Treatment goals and methods for correcting hypernatremia are listed in Table 29.2.

The rate of fluid administration should be calculated using the following formula, where the change in serum Na$^+$ represents the change in serum Na$^+$ after administering the selected fluid: [46]

$$\frac{\text{Change in serum Na}^+}{\text{(mEq/l)}} = \frac{\text{Infusate [Na}^+] - \text{serum [Na}^+]}{\text{Total body water (TBW)} + 1}$$

where TBW = BW (kg) × 0.6 for horses; BW(kg) × 0.7 for foals.

For example, in a 60 kg foal with a serum [Na$^+$] of 160 mmol/l, treatment with 0.45% NaCl (i.e., 77 mmol/l

Table 29.2 Treatment goals and methods for correction of hypernatremia.

	Acute	Chronic
Goal	Lower serum [Na$^+$] to 140–145 mEq/l	Lower serum [Na$^+$] to 140–145 mEq/l
Preferred route	Enteral	Enteral
Fluid types	Water (oral)	Water (oral)
	0.25% NaCl	0.25% NaCl
	0.45% NaCl	0.45% NaCl
	5% dextrose	5% dextrose
	0.45 NaCl/2.5% dextrose	0.45 NaCl/2.5% dextrose
Correction rate	Reduce serum [Na$^+$] by 1 mEq/l/h	Reduce serum [Na$^+$] by 0.5 mEq/l/h

Na$^+$) and 5% dextrose would result in a decrease of 2.0 mmol/l in the serum [Na$^+$] for each liter administered. In animals with central diabetes insipidus, replacement therapy with vasopressin analogs such as desmopressin is indicated. Vasopressin may of value if the goal of treatment is to reduce water excretion. This treatment will not work with nephrogenic diabetes insipidus.

Potassium

Potassium is the major intracellular cation. Approximately 98% of the total K$^+$ in the body is intracellular. The remaining 2% is extracellular, of which roughly 0.4% is measurable [54]. As mentioned earlier, the ratio between intra- and extracellular K$^+$ concentrations is critical to maintain the membrane potentials in excitable tissue. A number of membrane proteins (pumps, channels) are important for this charge difference. Serum K$^+$ concentrations mainly depend on the dietary intake and the equine diet is rich in K$^+$ [55]. Potassium disorders (mostly hypokalemia) are common in hospitalized human patients [54], and from clinical experience, this also seems to be the case in horses.

Potassium disturbances can be attributed to (i) abnormal K$^+$ intake (too little or too much), (ii) abnormal K$^+$ distribution between the intra- and extracellular spaces, or between compartments, or (iii) abnormalities of K$^+$ excretion.

Unlike disorders of Na$^+$, neurological signs from K$^+$ disturbances are rare.

Hypokalemia

Hypokalemia is defined as a serum K$^+$ concentration below 3.5 mEq/l (3.5 mmol/l) [3–5]. Hypokalemia is often observed in critically ill patients, but clinical manifestations are rarely documented or go unnoticed in horses.

A potential explanation for this is that intracellular K^+ concentrations are likely normal or signs occur concurrent with other electrolyte abnormalities (hypochloremia, hypomagnesemia, hypophosphatemia). A low serum K^+ does not imply depletion of intracellular K^+. Pseudo-hypokalemia, similar to pseudohyponatremia, can be caused by hyperlipemia and hyperproteinemia.

Low extracellular K^+ concentrations hyperpolarize the cell membrane, leading to prolongation of the AP and refractory period. Signs of hypokalemia are mainly muscular. Clinically, this manifests as muscle weakness, fasciculations, paralysis, and cardiac dysrhythmias. Horses subjected to forced anorexia over a 7 day period had a reduction in skeletal muscle K^+ concentration from 91.1 mEq/l (day 0) to 73.6 mEq/l (day 7), with a change in resting membrane potential favoring hyper-polarization from −105.84 mV (day 0) to −100.93 mV (day 7) [56]. This highlights the importance of maintaining a steady dietary intake of K^+ in horses. Hypokalemic myopathy can occur in any species including horses. Affected animals may show ventroflexion of the neck, muscular weakness, exercise intolerance, stiff gait, pain on palpation of affected muscles, and dysrhythmias [56].

Causes of hypokalemia

Extracellular K^+ concentrations decrease secondary to reduced GI absorption (disease, anorexia, lack of food, or low dietary content of K^+), increased renal excretion (renal disease, endocrinopathies, hypomagnesemia, drugs), excessive sweating, or redistribution between compartments (hormones, drugs, alkalosis). A number of GI disorders could directly or indirectly result in hypokalemia, including proximal enteritis, nasogastric reflux (hypochloremia, alkalosis), and enterocolitis. Hypochloremia activates the renin–angiotensin–aldosterone system (RAAS), and aldosterone increases the urinary excretion of K^+.

Renal diseases rarely cause hypokalemia in horses. Excessive mineralocorticoid activity or use of drugs with aldosterone activity (e.g., isoflupredone) can increase the urinary excretion of K^+ [57]. Redistribution between intra- and extracellular compartments occurs with numerous conditions (hyperlipemia, hyperglycemia, hypomagnesemia, hyperinsulinemia, enteritis, pH status) or treatments (e.g., insulin, β-adrenergic agonists).

Hypomagnesemia is often associated with hypokalemia and could worsen its clinical presentation. In fact, hypokalemia can remain refractory to treatment unless a normal magnesium concentration is restored. Ionized magnesium is a cofactor in processes that regulate K^+ and require ATP (e.g., Na^+/K^+ ATPase). In this case, a low Mg^{2+} concentration contributes to intracellular K^+ depletion due to a cellular inability to maintain K^+ inside. Ionized magnesium is also an inhibitor of the renal outer medullary potassium channel (ROMK), a K^+ inwardly rectifying channel that is required for K^+ recycling and

Table 29.3 Clinical signs of hypokalemia in the horse.

Severity	Clinical signs
Mild	Tiredness, lethargy, and mild muscle weakness
Moderate	Muscle weakness, fasciculations, and dysrhythmias
Severe	Muscle weakness, rhabdomyolysis, myoglobinuria, paralysis, respiratory arrest, and fatal dysrhythmias

secretion. A decrease in Mg^{2+} concentration increases ROMK activity and kaliuresis [58, 59].

Insulin (and glucose indirectly) increases the activity of the Na^+/K^+ ATPase, which will translate as hypokalemia, but intracellular K^+ concentrations would be normal or elevated. These horses may not show clinical signs. On the other hand, insulin resistance could, in the long term, result in hypokalemia due to urinary wasting of K^+ and inability to maintain K^+ intracellularly (depletion). Clinical signs of hypokalemia in horses are listed in Table 29.3.

Diagnosis

Diagnosis of hypokalemia is based on clinical signs, evidence of preexisting disease, history of anorexia, renal and GI diseases, and measurement of serum K^+ concentrations. However, plasma K^+ concentrations are poorly correlated with intracellular K^+ concentrations. Measuring intracellular K^+ concentration is clearly impractical; however in animals with prolonged disease and hypokalemia, one should assume some degree of intracellular K^+ depletion.

Assessment of renal function may be prudent, especially in cases where dietary intake is reduced, no other systemic clinical signs are evident, and inappropriate excretion of K^+ is suspected. Measuring the fractional excretion may reveal excessive K^+ excretion.

Electrocardiographic (ECG) changes associated with hypokalemia include increased P wave amplitude, prolongation of the P-R interval, Q-T interval prolongation, reduced T wave amplitude, and T wave inversion [23]. These changes can arise in any number of clinical situations leading to hypokalemia.

Treatment of hypokalemia

Oral and intravenous preparations of K^+ salts (usually potassium chloride) are available. Potassium phosphate is a good option in animals with concurrent hypophosphatemia. In the treatment, is important to consider current deficit, on-going losses, maintenance, and sequestration. The following formula can be used to calculate the ECF K^+ deficit:

$$K^+ \text{ deficit} = 0.3 \times BW \text{ (kg)} \times (4.0 - \text{measured serum } K^+)$$

where 0.3 is the ECF volume and 4.0 is the desired K^+ concentration.

It is important that the intravenous K^+ administration rate does not exceed 0.5 mEq/kg/h. Furthermore, intravenous fluids containing glucose and bicarbonate or bicarbonate precursors (lactated Ringer's solution) may exacerbate hypokalemia by promoting intracellular K^+ shift.

Hyperkalemia

Hyperkalemia is a serious and life-threatening electrolyte abnormality. It is defined as a serum K^+ concentration greater than 4.5 mEq/l (4.5 mmol/l) [2, 53, 60]. Increased serum K^+ concentration reduces the activity of excitable membranes, especially in cardiac muscle, but also skeletal muscle and neurons. Excessive extracellular K^+ causes cardiac flaccidity and decreases the conduction of APs through the atrioventricular node [54]. Heart rate and cardiac output subsequently decrease.

Causes of hyperkalemia

Hyperkalemia from excessive ingestion of K^+ is rare in horses, especially if they have normal renal function. Horses have a high urinary excretion of K^+ and renal injury often results in hyperkalemia [61]. More commonly, hyperkalemia is linked to excessive K^+ administration (iatrogenic; drugs containing K^+), transcellular shift (acidosis), redistribution between compartments (uroperitoneum), cell lysis (hemolysis, rhabdomyolysis, tumor lysis, blood transfusions), metabolic acidosis, adrenal insufficiency, and hyperkalemic periodic paralysis (HYPP). Hyperkalemia can also be spurious arising from laboratory error or improper blood sample handling. Hyperkalemia is a consistent finding in foals with a ruptured urinary bladder and subsequent uroperitoneum (see discussion in section "Hyponatremia").

Clinical signs are muscular, cardiac, and neurological; however, muscular and cardiac signs predominate. They are usually not apparent until serum K^+ exceeds 7.0 mEq/l, although early ECG changes may be present at concentrations greater than 6.0 mEq/l [54]. Muscular signs include muscle fasciculations, weakness, and flaccid paralysis. Cardiac signs include conduction disturbances with risk of sudden death. The ECG findings in horses with hyperkalemia include flattening to absent P waves, prolongation of the P-R interval, widening QRS complexes with a bizarre "sine wave" appearance, and finally ending in ventricular asystole or fibrillation at serum levels around 8–10 mEq/l [2, 54, 56]. Neurological signs may include depression, weakness, and paralysis.

Hyperkalemic periodic paralysis

HYPP is the clinical presentation of a genetic disorder affecting Quarterhorses, Paint horses, Appaloosas, and any horses carrying bloodlines traceable to the sire Impressive (AQHA #0767246). It is unknown if the mutation in this stallion was inherited or spontaneously occurred. The typical phenotype of affected horses is a heavy musculature. Hyperkalemic periodic paralysis is homologous to human *adynamia episodica hereditaria* or *Gamstorp episodic adynamy*, first reported in 1950 [62].

Pathophysiology

Hyperkalemic periodic paralysis has an autosomal dominant mode of inheritance, of variable penetrance [63]. Due to its association with a heavily muscular phenotype, this genetic disorder is more common in halter horses. Episodes are characterized by intermittent attacks of weakness, muscle fasciculations, and/or paralysis. Precipitating factors include high K^+ diets, K^+ containing drugs, fasting, anesthesia, cold weather, stress, strenuous exercise, rest after exercise, and concurrent diseases [64, 65].

Affected horses have a missense mutation in the α–subunit gene (*SCN4A*) of the Na^+ channel (chromosome 17q) resulting in an amino acid substitution from phenylalanine to leucine (F1419L) [66, 67]. The consequence of this defect is an impairment of Na^+ channel inactivation. Muscle fibers in affected horses are "leaky" to Na^+ and closer to the depolarization threshold (–55 mV in affected vs. –70 mV control) [68]. The excessive movement of Na^+ across the membrane and failure of muscle fibers to repolarize due to persistent channel activity results in continuous muscle depolarization, fasciculations, weakness, and paralysis [64–68]. The increase in extracellular K^+ concentrations further increases Na^+ conductance, depolarization and efflux of K^+. A concurrent hyperkalemia may be present during episodes; however, normal horses undergoing intensive exercise may have serum K^+ concentrations comparable to those of affected horses, suggesting that K^+ concentrations *per se* are not responsible for the clinical signs [68]. In fact, many HYPP horses have serum K^+ concentrations in the normal range during episodes.

As the cell membrane depolarizes and approaches the threshold potential, it becomes hyperexcitable, which is manifested as myotonic activity. With subsequent depolarizations the muscle cell membrane becomes refractory and paralysis occurs [68].

Gene nomenclature classifies homozygous normal horses as N/N, heterozygotes as N/H and homozygous affected as H/H. One genetic survey found the mutant frequency (H) in the Quarterhorse population was 4.4% [69].

Clinical signs of HYPP

Hyperkalemic periodic paralysis is classified as a myotonic disorder (characterized my muscular irritability, contractility, and delayed relaxation). Other myotonic disorders of horses include *myotonia congenita* and *myotonia dystrophica*.

Both H/H and N/H genotypes can show episodes; however, signs are more frequent and severe in H/H [65]. In general, clinical signs begin by 3 years of age and are recurrent in nature [65, 70]. In H/H animals, signs may occur as early as few days of age [65]. Upper airway obstruction occurs more often in H/H horses and young foals [71]. Foals may have upper airway obstruction or dysphagia from laryngeal paralysis and pharyngeal collapse. Rarely N/H foals will show signs at early age. In one report, a 7-month-old Quarterhorse filly developed myotonia, fasciculations, and sweating with a concurrent hyperkalemia 150 min after the induction of general anesthesia with halothane [70]. This filly was heterozygous (N/H) [70].

Horses are typically conscious and alert to visual, audible, and tactile stimuli. Episodes typically last for 30–60 min (range 20–240 min). Interestingly, the resting membrane potential tends to become more negative with increasing age, so the number of clinical episodes appears to decrease with age.

Diagnosis of HYPP

Genetic testing using DNA from equine hair bulbs or whole blood is performed. Tests are reported as N/N (normal), N/H (heterozygous or carrier), or H/H (affected). If a suspect animal dies suddenly, collection of hair sample and genetic testing is recommended, especially if that animal has progeny with unknown status. Increased K^+ concentration in aqueous humor may support hyperkalemia at the time of death. Provocative K^+ challenge testing can be done, but is not recommended.

The American Quarter Horse Association (AQHA) recognizes HYPP as an undesirable trait. From AQHA (www.aqha.com): "Foals born in 1998 and later and descendants of Impressive will have a statement placed on their Certificates of Registration that recommends testing for the condition unless test results indicating the foal is negative (N/N) are on file with AQHA." Under AQHA rule 205, Impressive foals born 2007 or later are required to be tested for HYPP, and any H/H animal will not be eligible for registration. Heterozygote (N/H) and unaffected animals (N/N) will be labeled as such in the certificate. Only tests performed by a licensed laboratory will be accepted by AQHA. These include the Veterinary Genetics Laboratory at The University of California, Davis (www.vgl.ucdavis.edu).

The same pathophysiological information described for Quarter horses applies to American Paint horses and Appaloosas. Genetic testing for HYPP is not required by the American Paint Horse Association. The American Appaloosa Association requires DNA testing of any horse descendant of Impressive and carriers will not be registered. The Appaloosa Horse Club requires foals born after 2007 from an Impressive parent to be tested and results noted in the certificate.

Serum K^+ concentrations can be normal but are often elevated, usually around 5.0–11.7 mEq/l [72]. Recovery is related to normalization of serum K^+ concentrations. Serum CK and AST activities tend to be normal or mildly elevated [68]. Microscopically, there are no abnormalities in muscle fiber architecture. This contrasts with paramyotonia syndromes in humans that have fiber destruction, vacuolar myopathy, sarcoplasmic reticulum dilation, and fusion of T-tubules.

Electromyography (EMG) abnormalities can be present at rest and during an episode. Complex repetitive discharges, myotonic potentials, fibrillation wave, and positive sharp waves can be seen [65, 68]. Insertional and resting activity (myopotentials) can be observed in clinically normal or affected animals. Prolonged insertional activity is pronounced as well as spontaneous myotonic discharges in doublets or triplets [65, 68, 73].

Treatment of HYPP

Treatment for HYPP depends in some degree on the severity of the attack. Recommended treatments are intended to induce an intracellular shift of K^+. In severe cases, intracellular dextrose and sodium bicarbonate should be given; intravenous calcium gluconate can also be administered but should not be mixed with calcium-containing solutions as it may result in precipitation. Insulin is not a practical treatment in horses, and epinephrine can be used as a last resort or in those animals in which other treatments are not available. In very severe cases, tracheostomy may be required if there is upper airway obstruction. In mildly affected horses, oral supplementation with soluble carbohydrates (i.e., Karo syrup) are helpful; molasses should be avoided due to its high K^+ content. Acetazolamide (2–3.0 mg/kg PO, q8–12 h) may be useful [65, 68, 71].

Prevention of future attacks may be achieved using daily administration of acetazolamide at 2.0–3.0 mg/kg PO q8–12 h. Acetazolamide is a carbonic anhydrase inhibitor and a K^+ wasting diuretic. The benefits of acetazolamide in preventing or attenuating HYPP episodes are unclear, but acetazolamide can activate skeletal muscle Ca^{2+}-activated K^+ channels [74]. In addition, acetazolamide has been shown to stabilize blood glucose and K^+ by stimulating insulin secretion [74, 75]. Avoid feeding alfalfa hay, molasses containing feed, K^+-containing salt blocks, and provide regular exercise. Take precautions when using drugs with K^+ (e.g., K^+ penicillin). Establish a set feeding and exercise regime, and avoid sudden changes. Pasture turnout may be beneficial.

Prognosis is good to guarded. Because episodes are unpredictable only people with knowledge of the clinical signs should ride affected horses. Treatment recommendations for horses with acute clinical signs of HYPP are listed in Table 29.4.

Table 29.4 Treatment recommendations for horses with acute onset of HYPP.

Acute, severe	Mild to moderate
Dextrose IV (0.2–0.5 mg/kg)	Oral soluble carbohydrate (e.g. Karo syrup)
Sodium bicarbonate (1–2 mEq/kg)	Acetozolamide (2.0–3.0 mg/kg PO, q8–12 h)
Calcium gluconate (23% solution; 0.2–0.4 ml/kg IV)	Consider acute treatments if no correction
Epinephrine (3–6 ml of 1:1000, IM)	
Tracheostomy	

Table 29.5 Conditions associated with hypocalcemia.

Enterocolitis	Furosemide administration
Sepsis	Excessive administration of $NaHCO_3$
Endotoxemia	Oxalate ingestion
Colic	Hypoparathyroidism
Endurance exercise	Hypomagnesemia
Pregnancy	Cantharidin toxicosis
Lactation (lactation tetany)	Liver disease
Transportation (transit tetany)	Dystocia
Acute renal failure	Malignant hyperthermia
Rhabdomyolysis	Magnesium toxicity
Pleuropneumonia	Retained placenta
Heat stroke	Postoperative myopathy
Pancreatitis	

Calcium

Calcium is a regulatory ion that participates in multiple cellular processes. It is required for neuromuscular excitability, muscle contraction, enzymatic activation, hormone secretion, cell division, cell membrane stability, and blood coagulation [76]. Most calcium in the body (99%) is in the skeleton, providing support against gravity, protecting internal organs, hosting blood-forming elements, and serving as a reservoir for calcium. The remaining calcium (1%) is in the cell membrane, mitochondria, endoplasmic reticulum (0.9%), and in the extracellular fluid (0.1%). In equine blood, total calcium (tCa) is found in a free or ionized form (Ca^{2+}; 50–58%), bound to proteins (40–45%) and complexed to anions such as citrate, bicarbonate, phosphate, and lactate (5–10%) [76, 77]. It is the ionized fraction (Ca^{2+}) that modulates neuromuscular activity. Therefore, Ca^{2+} deviations from its narrow limits can result in neurological signs.

Hypocalcemia

Hypocalcemia is defined as a serum tCa concentration below 11 mg/dl (2.75 mmol/l) or a Ca^{2+} concentration below 6 mg/dl (1.5 mmol/l) [76, 77]. Many pathological conditions associated with hypocalcemia have been documented in the horse (Table 29.5).

Causes of hypocalcemia

Hypocalcemia can be the result of parathyroid gland dysfunction (hypoparathyroidism), systemic illness (sepsis, endotoxemia), GI disease, acute renal failure, tissue sequestration, and hypomagnesemia [76, 78–80]. Horses may develop hypocalcemia secondary to the ingestion of oxalates. If the ingestion is excessive signs of hypocalcemia may develop. Detailed information on the pathogenesis of hypocalcemia in horses is described elsewhere [77, 78].

Clinical signs of hypocalcemia

The signs of hypocalcemia are the result of increased neuromuscular excitability and decreased smooth muscle contractility, and their severity relates to the magnitude of hypocalcemia. These include hyperexcitability, synchronous diaphragmatic flutter (SDF, thumps), ileus, tetany, ataxia, stupor, muscle fasciculations, seizures, recumbency, and death [76, 77]. Rarely horses with Ca^{2+} greater than 5 mg/dl will show clinical signs, or signs may be mild enough to be noticed.

Extracellular Ca^{2+} binds to Na^+ fast channels, decreasing their permeability to Na^+ influx, thus raising the depolarization threshold. In hypocalcemia, the threshold is decreased, making nervous and muscular tissue "more excitable." This manifests as tetany, ataxia, seizures, peripheral neuropathies, weakness and muscle fasciculations [76, 77]. Seizures were observed in four neonatal foals with hypocalcemia [81]. Critically ill foals often develop hypocalcemia, which can lead to other clinical signs (e.g., ileus, seizures) [81]. In adult horses, the prognosis for refractory hypocalcemic seizures is guarded [76, 82].

Synchronous diaphragmatic flutter develops when depolarization of the right atrium stimulates APs in the phrenic nerve as it crosses over the heart. Clinically, there is a rhythmic movement on the flank from diaphragmatic contractions that are synchronous with the heartbeat [76].

Horses with hypochloremic metabolic alkalosis from Cl^- losses (duodenitis/jejunitis, excessive sweating) can develop ionized hypocalcemia due to increased Ca^{2+} binding to plasma proteins (mainly albumin); this also applies to Mg^{2+} [83]. Hyperventilation and respiratory alkalosis can also induce ionized hypocalcemia (and hypomagnesemia) [76].

Lactation tetany (eclampsia) occurs in mares from the end of gestation up to weaning. This is more common in draft breeds; however, any mare producing large volumes of milk, eating low-calcium diets or lush pastures, or performing physical activity is at higher risk to develop hypocalcemia. Signs in these mares include hypersalivation, dysphagia, hyperhidrosis, anxiety, muscle fasciculations, tremors, tachypnea, and ataxia [76, 77].

Diagnosis of hypocalcemia

The diagnosis of hypocalcemia is based on clinical signs, preexisting or ongoing disease, and measurement of serum PTH, tCa, Ca^{2+}, and Mg^{2+} concentrations. Urinary fractional excretion of calcium may help in determining the cause of hypocalcemia. Compared to other species, horses have a high fractional excretion of calcium (up to 10%) [76–78]. Horses with hypoparathyroidism have hypocalcemia, hyperphosphatemia, low or normal PTH concentrations, and increased urinary excretion of calcium [76–78]. Abnormal EMG activity (fibrillation potentials, polyphasic motor unit APs) during hypocalcemia indicates neuromuscular hyperirritability [83].

Treatment of hypocalcemia

The goal of treatment is to prevent or reduce the severity of clinical signs from hypocalcemia. During treatment, it is important to consider calcium deficit, maintenance, losses, and sequestration (third spacing). Serum Ca^{2+} gives a better estimate of the calcium status than tCa; however, it is not necessarily routine to measure Ca^{2+} and most treatment decisions can be based on tCa concentrations. Parenteral calcium therapy is crucial in horses showing signs of hypocalcemia. One comparative advantage of horses is that they can handle large amounts of parenteral calcium, in particular if renal function is normal. Empirically, adding 50 ml of 23% calcium gluconate per 5 l of lactated Ringer's solution (twice maintenance rate) is sufficient to restore normocalcemia in horses with mild hypocalcemia. Higher doses (100–200 ml) may be required in animals with severe hypocalcemia and clinical signs. In animals with chronic or refractory hypocalcemia, oral supplementation with calcium carbonate (limestone; 100–300 g/horse/day) or dicalcium phosphate (100–200 g/horse/day) is indicated. Without knowing the cause of hypocalcemia the use of vitamin D is questionable; however, some horses with hypoparathyroidism may benefit from active vitamin D (calcitriol; $1,25(OH)_2D_3$) (R. Toribio, pers. obs.). Often, horses with neuromuscular signs of hypocalcemia also have hypomagnesemia, and signs may not resolve until they receive magnesium supplementation [76, 77, 84]. Therefore, it is recommended to measure Mg^{2+} in any horse with hypocalcemia, in particular those with clinical signs as combined therapy may be required [76, 77, 84].

The ionized calcium deficit can be calculated with the following formula [77]:

$$Ca^{2+} \text{ deficit} = \frac{(6.5 - \text{measured } [Ca^{2+}])(10)(0.3)(BW)}{Ca^{2+} \text{ ratio}}$$

where 6.5 is the desired Ca^{2+} in mg/dl, 10 is a multiplication factor from mg/dl to mg/l (or kg), 0.3 is the ECF, and the Ca^{2+} ratio is $[Ca^{2+}]$ divided by tCa concentration.

For lactation tetany, 23% calcium gluconate (150–300 ml/500 kg BW) can be given slowly IV, over 10–30 min. It is important to monitor heart rate and rhythm during treatment. Do not administer calcium solutions in the same IV line as bicarbonate solutions, as this may cause precipitation.

Hypercalcemia

Hypercalcemia in horses is linked to hyperparathyroidism, hypercalcemia of malignancy, vitamin D intoxication, and chronic renal failure [76]. Clinical signs of hypercalcemia in horses in general are subtle unless it is severe (tCa > 18 mg/dl). Due to the Na^+ channel blocking properties of Ca^{2+}, hypercalcemia hyperpolarizes the cell membrane, which clinically translates as hypoexcitability, depression, disorientation, ataxia, hyporreflexia, muscle weakness, and cardiac arrhythmias. Other signs that may develop include polyuria/polydipsia, dehydration, and hypercoagulability [61, 76, 83]. Horses with secondary hyperparathyroidism develop skeletal problems, but rarely neurological signs are present.

Chronic hypercalcemia in general carries a guarded to poor prognosis. If clinical signs are present, loop diuretics (furosemide, 1–2 mg/kg, IV, BID) may be indicated. This is a palliative treatment until the primary cause is identified and treated.

Magnesium

Magnesium (Mg) is the fourth most abundant cation in the body and the second most abundant intracellular cation after K^+ [85]. The distribution of Mg resembles that of K^+. The body contains 0.05% magnesium per body weight of which 60% is in the skeleton (0.5–1% bone ash), 38% in soft tissue (intracellular), and 1–2% in the extracellular fluid. Serum Mg concentrations are not a reliable indicator of the body status of magnesium [86]. Cells with higher metabolic activity have higher Mg content. Most equine diets supply adequate amounts of Mg.

In circulation, total magnesium (tMg) can be free or ionized (Mg^{2+}), bound to proteins, or chelated to organic anions (carbonate, lactate, citrate). Ionized Mg is the active electrolyte for most biological functions. In the horse, 60% of the serum tMg is Mg^{2+}, 30% is protein-bound, and 10% is complexed to anions [61, 86–88].

The same principles that apply to calcium in regard to ionization apply to magnesium. Serum tMg concentrations depend on protein concentrations (albumin), whereas Mg^{2+} concentrations depend on the acid–base status. Alkalosis decreases Mg^{2+} and the opposite occurs with acidosis. Conditions leading to alkalosis (nasogastric reflux, duodenitis/jejunitis, exercise-associated alkalosis) can cause ionized hypomagnesemia.

Intestinal absorption and renal excretion control serum Mg^{2+} concentrations. In horses, most Mg^{2+} absorption occurs in the small intestine with approximately 25% being absorbed in the proximal small intestine, 30–35% in the distal small intestine, and 5–10% in the large colon [89–91]. The kidneys play a major role in regulating serum Mg concentrations by controlling tubular reabsorption, mainly in the thick ascending limb of the loop of Henle [84]. Renal excretion of Mg is matched to GI absorption; Mg absorbed in excess is excreted by the kidneys. Renal tubular reabsorption rate is regulated by dietary availability of Mg, serum Ca^{2+} and Mg^{2+} concentrations, and hormones [84].

Magnesium and the central nervous system

Magnesium is directly or indirectly (via ATP) required in neurological processes involving ion traffic and neurotransmitter release. Intracellular Mg^{2+} binds to negatively charged molecules (ATP, DNA, RNA), enzymes, and other proteins. All reactions that utilize ATP require Mg^{2+} since the intracellular substrate is the complex $Mg^{2+} \cdot ATP$. By interacting with cellular proteins Mg^{2+} affects the cell cycle and stabilizes the cell membrane. Relevant to CNS physiology, Mg^{2+} interacts with Ca^{2+} in the intra- and extracellular compartments. These interactions can be additive, synergistic, or antagonistic. For example, hypocalcemia can alter neuronal function and the magnesium status can worsen the severity of clinical signs.

Magnesium is required for the activity of the Na^+/K^+ ATPase, Ca^{2+}/K^+ ATPase, Na^+/Ca^{2+} exchanger (NCX), PMCA, NMDAR, and other proteins involved in neuronal function. The neuroprotective actions of Mg^{2+} are mainly due to its ability to compete with Ca^{2+} in a number of proteins (e.g., NCX and NMDAR) that increase intracellular Ca^{2+} concentrations. As previously mentioned, NCX can be reversed during brain injury and Mg^{2+} can block intracellular accumulation of Ca^{2+} [24, 92]. Ionized Mg may also protect brain cells against free radical injury and neurotoxicity [93].

The NMDAR is a cation-selective (Ca^{2+}, Na^+) channel that mediates neuronal excitability. Its activation by glutamate allows Ca^{2+} influx, which can trigger excitotoxic death. This process is blocked by cations such as Zn^{2+} and Mg^{2+} [94, 95]. The protective effects of Mg^{2+} may be relevant in reducing NMDAR activity in acute brain injury. This is important in the neonatal brain where the

NMDAR is a predominant mediator of excitotoxicity [94]. In the developing brain, susceptibility to hypoxia is determined by the lipid composition, the rate of lipid peroxidation, antioxidant status, modulation of the NMDAR, and intracellular Ca^{2+} influx [94]. Ionized Mg influences these mechanisms and may be useful in preventing irreversible damage.

In the CNS, Mg^{2+} is a modulator of the response to pain. Similar to ketamine, Mg^{2+} controls Ca^{2+} entry into neurons by antagonizing the NMDAR, which is translated as reduced excitability or nociception. This information has been useful in the management of acute and chronic pain as excessive nociception increases pain hypersensitivity (wind-up syndrome). Of the multiple receptors involved with calcium fluxes and pain, the NMDAR is essential in central sensitization to pain [96].

Hypomagnesemic conditions are well described in the literature, whereas hypermagnesemic conditions are rarely encountered. Normal serum tMg in the horse is 0.6–0.9 mmol/l (1.4–2.2 mg/dl) and Mg^{2+} is 0.45–0.66 mmol/l (0.9–1.5 mg/dl) [35, 61, 78, 88].

Hypomagnesemia

Hypomagnesemia is well described in large animals including horses [84, 97], and it is a common finding in critically ill horses and foals [78, 84, 91, 98]. Hypomagnesemia was identified as the most common electrolyte abnormality in critically ill canine and feline patients [99]. Chronic hypomagnesemia is often associated with inadequate dietary Mg^{2+} intake, while acute hypomagnesemia is the result of multiple pathologies. While clinical hypomagnesemia is more common in ruminants, it has been documented in horses [84, 100–103]. Primary hypomagnesemia is typically observed in animals feeding exclusively on fresh rapidly growing pastures that are low in magnesium content [84, 97, 100–103]. Hypomagnesemia can result in neuromuscular disturbances; however, these are rare in horses.

Causes of hypomagnesemia

Magnesium disorders may occur with GI and renal diseases, sepsis, endotoxemia, endocrine disorders, alterations of the acid–base status, and cell lysis [84]. Stress hormones such as catecholamine and insulin can worsen the clinical signs of hypomagnesemia by stimulating intracellular Mg^{2+} shifts [97]. The severity of hypomagnesemia is the result of reduced dietary intake, excessive mobilization of endogenous stores, increased urinary excretion, tissue redistribution, or a combination of them [84].

Clinical signs of hypomagnesemia

Numerous clinical signs of hypomagnesemia result from Mg depletion at the synaptic terminals and neuromuscular junctions. Ionized Mg blocks signal transmission via inhibition of Ca^{2+}-dependent, presynaptic excitation–secretion coupling [84, 97, 104]. Ionized Mg depletion contributes to tetany by increasing the release of acetylcholine at the neuromuscular junctions and delaying its degradation by acetylcholinesterase [84, 97]. Early clinical signs include restlessness, extreme alertness, muscular weakness, muscle fasciculations, and SDF. Some animals may become ataxic, excitable, aggressive, vocalizing, and develop tetanic episodes. Animals with severe hypomagnesemia may become recumbent, show opisthotonus and paddling movements. Seizure activity, ventricular fibrillation, coma, and sudden death can also occur [84].

Cardiac rhythm disturbances can occur and include ventricular dysrhythmias, supraventricular tachycardia, and atrial fibrillation. Electrocardiographic (ECG) findings characteristic of hypomagnesemia include prolongation of the P-R interval, ST segment depression, peaked T waves, and widening of the QRS complex. [84]

Hypomagnesemia and concurrent hypokalemia are frequent findings in foals and horses, in particular those with sepsis and GI disease [78, 84, 91, 98]. As previously discussed, Mg^{2+} is a co-factor for the Na^+/K^+ ATPase and pump failure leads to intracellular K^+ depletion and intracellular accumulation of Na^+ [59]. This lowers the resting membrane potential facilitating spontaneous depolarization activity and impairment of AP propagation. This phenomenon has been demonstrated in studies on Purkinje fiber function, where increased excitability can lead to the development of dysrhythmias [105, 106].

Foals fed a magnesium-deficient diet (7–8 mg mg/kg) developed nervousness, tetany in response to loud noises, muscular tremors, and ataxia [102]. In these foals, serum tMg concentrations decreased from 0.78 mmol/l (day 0) to 0.53 mmol/l (day 7) after being placed on this diet. Some of these foals became comatose, exhibited hyperhydrosis, seizure activity, and death. Necropsy evaluation revealed severe aortic and pulmonary artery mineralization around 30–35 days after foals were placed in this diet. The total serum magnesium concentrations at which these severe neurologic signs occurred was 0.7 ± 0.4 mg/dl [102].

Transportation and lactation were identified as precipitating causes of tetany in two Thoroughbred broodmares that developed hypocalcemia and hypomagnesemia [107]. Both animals responded well to intravenous calcium borogluconate and magnesium chloride therapy [107].

Adult horses with a neurological signs such as aberrant behavior, hyperexcitability with or without ataxia, stringhalt and SDF associated with hypomagnesemia have been observed (R. Toribio, pers. obs. and M. Furr, pers. commun.). In most cases, clinical signs resolve quickly with magnesium treatment. Assessing serum Mg^{2+} and Ca^{2+} concentrations is warranted in horses with unexplained neurological signs or hypocalcemia.

Diagnosis

The diagnosis of hypomagnesemia is based on clinical signs, concurrent diseases, and determination of serum tMg and Mg^{2+} [84]. Serum Mg^{2+} gives a more accurate assessment of the Mg status than tMg. However, as long as hypomagnesemia is not the result of alkalosis, tMg concentrations give a good estimate of the Mg status. Ideally, serum Ca^{2+} concentrations should be measured as well because hypocalcemia is a frequent finding in these horse, while prolonged hypercalcemia can indirectly induced Mg depletion [61, 76, 83].

Changes in the electromyogram (EMG) have been in subclinical hypomagnesemic horse and are identical to the changes observed in subclinical hypocalcemia. These changes represent nerve hyperirritability [83].

Treatment of hypomagnesemia

The recommended dose rate for magnesium sulfate ($MgSO_4$) in horses ranges from 25 to 150 mg/kg/day IV in 0.9% NaCl or other polyionic balanced electrolyte solutions. For adult horses with neurological signs, 10–25 g of $MgSO_4$ can be given IV in crystalloid fluids over 10–20 min (20–50 mg/kg). Subsequently, it can be supplemented with crystalloid fluids or as a CRI (50–200 mg/kg/day). Most commercial crystalloid solutions lack magnesium salts, and will need supplemental Mg added. Magnesium for oral administration is available as $MgSO_4$, MgO, $MgCO_3$, and magnesium gluconate. Epson salt ($MgSO_4$) is the cheapest oral alternative to parenteral $MgSO_4$ (up to 200 mg/kg/day PO), but high doses can be laxative and induce somnolence [108]. Frequent monitoring of serum Ca^{2+} and Mg^{2+} concentrations is important to adjust dosing and reduce side effects. Some horses may require daily oral supplementation of Mg. A similar $MgSO_4$ dosing regimen (25–200 mg/kg/day) can be used in foals. $MgSO_4$ can be given as a bolus (40–50 mg/kg, IV) over a few minutes, in replacement fluids, or via CRI. For foals with ischemic encephalopathy and seizures a loading dose of 25–50 mg/kg in crystalloid solution over 10 min followed by 25–50 mg/kg, every 6 h, or a CRI of 50–200 mg/kg/day have been suggested, although safety and efficacy studies are lacking.

Hypermagnesemia

Because Mg^{2+} regulates membrane ion transport, blocks Ca^{2+} channels, inhibits excitatory channels (NMDAR), and hyperpolarizes the cell membrane; signs of hypermagnesemia include depression, somnolence, ataxia, hypotension, muscle weakness, and paralysis. Few reports of hypermagnesemia are found in horses, with no well-described syndromes of primary hypermagnesemia. Most cases of hypermagnesemia in people and animals are iatrogenic. Conditions associated with cell lysis (rhabdomyolysis, tumor lysis, hemolysis) may cause secondary hypermagnesemia, and horses with chronic renal failure may develop hypermagnesemia [84]. Improper sample handling can lead to spurious hypermagnesemia.

One case report describes hypermagnesemia in two horses treated for large colon impaction using $MgSO_4$ and dioctyl sodium succinate (DSS) [108]. Both horses received a lower than the recommended dose of $MgSO_4$ and their serum tMg concentrations were several folds higher than normal. Clinical signs included weakness, sweating, muscle tremors, flaccid paralysis, tachycardia, tachypnea, and recumbency. Horses recovered after treatment with calcium gluconate and intravenous fluids [108]. It was speculated that the combination of cathartics with DSS may have enhanced intestinal absorption of Mg^{2+}. Treatment for acute hypermagnesemia includes 0.9% NaCl, furosemide, and parenteral administration of calcium salts.

Magnesium as a therapeutic agent in brain injury

Magnesium salts have been recommended for human and animal patients with brain injury and hypoxia [83, 103, 109–112]. Although Mg^{2+} infusions are used in humans with brain and spinal injury, the benefits remain unclear [83, 109–112]. The rationale is that Mg^{2+} decreases free radical injury, modulates NMDAR, and antagonizes the cytotoxic effects of intracellular Ca^{2+} [83, 93–95, 104, 109–112]. Activation of NMDAR by glutamate allows intracellular Ca^{2+} influx that results in neuronal excitability, protease activation, and death. This process is blocked by cations such as Zn^{2+} and Mg^{2+} [94, 95, 112]. In addition, by blocking Ca^{2+} channels in vascular smooth muscle, Mg^{2+} prevents Ca^{2+} entry, resulting in cerebral vasodilation [54]. Under this premise, Mg^{2+} has been used to treat foals with hypoxic ischemic encephalopathy and horses with brain injury [103, 113, 114]. However, controlled studies on the efficacy of Mg^{2+} therapy to equine adults or neonates with acute CNS dysfunction are lacking.

Most clinical studies have failed to demonstrate a positive effect of $MgSO_4$ on outcome [109, 111, 112, 115], which differs from observations in experimental conditions of brain injury where $MgSO_4$ has shown to be beneficial [115, 116]. This discrepancy could arise because in experimental conditions $MgSO_4$ was given before ischemia was induced, which does not mimic clinical events. In support of using $MgSO_4$, a recent study found that $MgSO_4$ infusion immediately after hypoxic ischemia was induced to preterm lambs was protective [117]. Even though there is not clear clinical

evidence that parenteral Mg^{2+} salts are protective in horses with acute brain injury, the potential benefits may outweigh the risks.

Phosphate

Phosphorus (P) has regulatory and structural functions. It represents 1% of the body weight with most (85%) located in the bone matrix as hydroxyapatite. Around 15% is in blood and soft tissues with less than 0.1% in the extracellular fluid [118]. Phosphate is the main intracellular anion, existing in organic and inorganic (P_i) forms. Intracellular concentrations of P_i are 20–40 folds higher than in the extracellular fluid.

Blood P_i concentrations are influenced by age, physiological status, activity, dietary phosphate content, diurnal variations, disease, glycemia, hormones, acid–base status, and quality of sample (pH, hemolysis, hyperlipemia, hyperproteinemia, and gammopathies). Serum P_i concentrations are controlled by intestinal absorption and renal reabsorption, by vitamin D, PTH, and phosphatonins [76]. The kidney is the major regulator of P_i concentrations [76]. In adult horses, serum P_i ranges from 3.0–5.0 mg/dl (0.96–1.6 mmol/l) while in healthy foals concentrations are greater (5.0–9.0 mg/dl; 1.6–2.6 mmol/l). Similar to K^+ and Mg^{2+}, serum P_i is an unreliable indicator of body stores.

Phosphate is essential for muscle contraction, neurological function, cell proliferation and differentiation, cell membrane integrity, enzyme activity, electrolyte transport, oxygen transport, gene transcription, and in the intermediary metabolism of proteins, carbohydrates and fats [76, 119]. The functions of P_i are closely linked to other ions (Mg^{2+}, K^+, Ca^{2+}, Na^+). Proteins and enzymes involved in the trans-membrane movement of ions (PMCA, NCX, Na^+/K^+ ATPase) indirectly require P_i as these are ATP-dependent processes. It is not unusual for horses with hypophosphatemia to have concurrent hypokalemia and hypomagnesemia [84]. Unfortunately, these abnormalities often go unnoticed in equine patients.

There is limited information on the association between serum P_i concentrations and equine neurological diseases. In general, signs of hypophosphatemia in horses manifest when serum P_i concentrations are below 1.0 mg/dl (0.32 mmol/l). These include neuromuscular irritability, muscle weakness, muscle fasciculations, arrhythmias, decreased gastrointestinal motility, and cell lysis (hemolysis, rhabdomyolysis) [77]. Of these, muscle fasciculations seem to be the most common, in particular in ponies and miniature horses (R. Toribio, pers. obs.) Hypophosphatemia can result in hypoxia due to reduced erythrocyte levels of 2,3-bisphosphoglycerate, shifting the hemoglobin dissociation curve to the left, and impairing oxygen release.

Hypophosphatemia has also been associated with pontine myelinolysis in people [120]. The extracellular P_i deficit can be calculated with the following formula:

$$P_i \text{ deficit} = BW \times (\text{desired } P_i - \text{measured } P_i) \times 10$$
$$(\text{conversion from dl to l}) \times 0.3 \text{ ECF}$$

Treatment of hypophosphatemia is based on the use of injectable and oral phosphate salts. Potassium phosphate is the parenteral solution of choice for acute hypophosphatemia as it also provides K^+. Sodium phosphate is a good alternative for animals with normo- or hyperkalemia. Sick horses can be supplemented via nasogastric intubation with chemical grade potassium or sodium phosphate salts. A number of products formulated for cattle that contain calcium, magnesium and potassium can be used in horses. Phosphate enemas containing monobasic and dibasic sodium phosphate are used intravenously in ruminants to treat hypophosphatemia, and can be used enterally in horses. It is important to monitor serum P_i and Ca^{2+} concentrations during aggressive treatment as high phosphate doses can cause hyperphosphatemia and hypocalcemia.

Hyperphosphatemia in horses is less frequent, often associated with cell lysis; and if neurological signs develop, likely result from hypocalcemia.

References

[1] Lee JW. Fluid and electrolyte disturbances in critically ill patients. *Electrolyte Blood Press* 2010;8:72–81.

[2] Johnson PJ. Electrolyte and acid-base disturbances in the horse. *Vet Clin North Am Equine Pract* 1995;11:491–514.

[3] Sterns RH, Hix JK, Silver S. Treatment of hyponatremia. *Curr Opin Nephrol Hypertens* 2010;19:493–498.

[4] Palmer BF. Hyponatremia in the intensive care unit. *Semin Nephrol* 2009;29:257–270.

[5] Ullrey DE, Struthers RD, Hendricks DG, Brent BE. Composition of mare's milk. *J Anim Sci* 1966;25:217–222.

[6] Schryver HF, Oftedal OT, Williams J, Soderholm LV, Hintz HF. Lactation in the horse: the mineral composition of mare milk. *J Nutr* 1986;116:2142–2147.

[7] Dowling PM, Williams MA, Clark TP. Adrenal insufficiency associated with long-term anabolic steroid administration in a horse. *J Am Vet Med Assoc* 1993;203:1166–1169.

[8] Nelson JM, Robinson MV. Hyponatremia in older adults presenting to the emergency department. *Int Emerg Nurs* 2012;20:251–254.

[9] Decaux G. The syndrome of inappropriate secretion of antidiuretic hormone (SIADH). *Semin Nephrol* 2009;29: 239–256.

[10] Lien YH, Shapiro JI. Hyponatremia: clinical diagnosis and management. *Am J Med* 2007;120:653–658.

[11] Sterns RH, Nigwekar SU, Hix JK. The treatment of hyponatremia. *Semin Nephrol* 2009;29:282–299.

[12] Newton SA, Knottenbelt DC, Eldridge PR. Headshaking in horses: possible aetiopathogenesis suggested by the results of diagnostic tests and several treatment regimes used in 20 cases. *Equine Vet J* 2000;32:208–216.

[13] Das P, Carcao M, Hitzler J. DDAVP-induced hyponatremia in young children. *J Pediatr Hematol Oncol* 2005;27: 330–332.

[14] Olowokure O, Fishman M, Cromwell C, Aledort L. DDAVP for von Willebrand menorrhagia—severe hyponatraemia, haemolysis, seizure, coma.!! Caution. *Haemophilia* 2009;15:837.

[15] Ayus JC, Achinger SG, Arieff A. Brain cell volume regulation in hyponatremia: role of sex, age, vasopressin, and hypoxia. *Am J Physiol Renal Physiol* 2008;295:F619–F624.

[16] Soupart A, Decaux G. Therapeutic recommendations for management of severe hyponatremia: current concepts on pathogenesis and prevention of neurologic complications. *Clin Nephrol* 1996;46:149–169.

[17] Papadopoulos MC, Verkman AS. Aquaporin-4 and brain edema. *Pediatr Nephrol* 2007;22:778–784.

[18] Videen JS, Michaelis T, Pinto P, Ross BD. Human cerebral osmolytes during chronic hyponatremia. A proton magnetic resonance spectroscopy study. *J Clin Invest* 1995; 95:788–793.

[19] Pasantes-Morales H, Vazquez-Juarez E. Transporters and channels in cytotoxic astrocyte swelling. *Neurochem Res* 2012;37:2379–2387.

[20] Rosenberg GA, Estrada E, Kyner WT. Vasopressin-induced brain edema is mediated by the V1 receptor. *Adv Neurol* 1990;52:149–154.

[21] Dickinson LD, Betz AL. Attenuated development of ischemic brain edema in vasopressin-deficient rats. *J Cereb Blood Flow Metab* 1992;12:681–690.

[22] Hertz L, Chen Y, Spatz M. Effects of arginine vasopressin on water space in astrocytes and in whole brain. *Am J Physiol Endocrinol Metab* 2000;278:E1175–E1176.

[23] Sarfaraz D, Fraser CL. Effects of arginine vasopressin on cell volume regulation in brain astrocyte in culture. *Am J Physiol* 1999;276:E596–E601.

[24] Cross JL, Meloni BP, Bakker AJ, et al. Modes of neuronal calcium entry and homeostasis following cerebral ischemia. *Stroke Res Treat* 2010;2010:316862.

[25] Bano D, Nicotera P. Ca2+ signals and neuronal death in brain ischemia. *Stroke* 2007;38:674–676.

[26] Hyzinski-Garcia MC, Vincent MY, Haskew-Layton RE, et al. Hypo-osmotic swelling modifies glutamate-glutamine cycle in the cerebral cortex and in astrocyte cultures. *J Neurochem* 2011;118:140–152.

[27] Restuccia T, Gomez-Anson B, Guevara M, et al. Effects of dilutional hyponatremia on brain organic osmolytes and water content in patients with cirrhosis. *Hepatology* 2004;39:1613–1622.

[28] Lien YH, Shapiro JI, Chan L. Study of brain electrolytes and organic osmolytes during correction of chronic

hyponatremia. Implications for the pathogenesis of central pontine myelinolysis. *J Clin Invest* 1991;88:303–309.

[29] Churcher RK, Watson AD, Eaton A. Suspected myelinolysis following rapid correction of hyponatremia in a dog. *J Am Anim Hosp Assoc* 1999;35:493–497.

[30] O'Brien DP, Kroll RA, Johnson GC, et al. Myelinolysis after correction of hyponatremia in two dogs. *J Vet Intern Med* 1994;8:40–48.

[31] Lakritz J, Madigan J, Carlson GP. Hypovolemic hyponatremia and signs of neurologic disease associated with diarrhea in a foal. *J Am Vet Med Assoc* 1992;200:1114–1116.

[32] Sood L, Sterns RH, Hix JK, et al. Hypertonic saline and desmopressin: a simple strategy for safe correction of severe hyponatremia. *Am J Kidney Dis* 2013;61:571–578.

[33] Kortz GD, Madigan JE, Lakritz J, Goetzman BW. Cerebral oedema and cerebellar herniation in four equine neonates. *Equine Vet J* 1992;24:63–66.

[34] Arieff AI, Llach F, Massry SG. Neurological manifestations and morbidity of hyponatremia: correlation with brain water and electrolytes. *Med (Baltim)* 1976;55:121–129.

[35] Navarro M, Monreal L, Segura D, et al. A comparison of traditional and quantitative analysis of acid-base and electrolyte imbalances in horses with gastrointestinal disorders. *J Vet Intern Med* 2005;19:871–877.

[36] Perkins G, Valberg SJ, Madigan JM, et al. Electrolyte disturbances in foals with severe rhabdomyolysis. *J Vet Intern Med* 1998;12:173–177.

[37] Patel GP, Balk RA. Recognition and treatment of hyponatremia in acutely ill hospitalized patients. *Clin Ther* 2007;29:211–229.

[38] Qiu Y, Qiu M. Is hyponatremia mistreated? Challenging the current paradigm. *Med Hypotheses* 2013;80:810–812.

[39] Sterns RH, Hix JK, Silver SM. Management of hyponatremia in the ICU. *Chest* 2013;144:672–679.

[40] Reulen HJ. Vasogenic brain oedema. New aspects in its formation, resolution and therapy. *Br J Anaesth* 1976;48:741–752.

[41] Melby JM, Miner LC, Reed DJ. Effect of acetazolamide and furosemide on the production and composition of cerebrospinal fluid from the cat choroid plexus. *Can J Physiol Pharmacol* 1982;60:405–409.

[42] Cluitmans FH, Meinders AE. Management of severe hyponatremia: rapid or slow correction? *Am J Med* 1990;88:161–166.

[43] Johansson AM, Gardner SY, Levine JF, et al. Furosemide continuous rate infusion in the horse: evaluation of enhanced efficacy and reduced side effects. *J Vet Intern Med* 2003;17:887–895.

[44] Lehrich RW, Ortiz-Melo DI, Patel MB, Greenberg A. Role of vaptans in the management of hyponatremia. *Am J Kidney Dis* 2013;62:364–376.

[45] Palm C, Pistrosch F, Herbrig K, Gross P. Vasopressin antagonists as aquaretic agents for the treatment of hyponatremia. *Am J Med* 2006;119:S87–S92.

[46] Adrogue HJ, Madias NE. Hypernatremia. *N Engl J Med* 2000;342:1493–1499.

[47] Lindner G, Funk GC. Hypernatremia in critically ill patients. *J Crit Care* 2013;28:216–220.

[48] Zachary JF. Nervous system. In: Zachary JF, McGavin MD, eds. *Pathologic Basis of Veterinary Diseases*. St. Louis:Elsevier Mosby;2012:771–872.

[49] Smith DL. Poisoning by sodium salt: a cause of eosinophilic meningoencephalitis in swine. *Am J Vet Res* 1957;18:825–850.

[50] Heath SE, Peter AT, Janovitz EB, et al. Ependymoma of the neurohypophysis and hypernatremia in a horse. *J Am Vet Med Assoc* 1995;207:738–741.

[51] Dembek KA, Onasch K, Hurcombe SD, et al. Renin–angiotensin–aldosterone system and hypothalamic-pituitary-adrenal axis in hospitalized newborn foals. *J Vet Intern Med* 2013;27:331–338.

[52] Mastrangelo S, Arlotta A, Cefalo MG, et al. Central pontine and extrapontine myelinolysis in a pediatric patient following rapid correction of hypernatremia. *Neuropediatrics* 2009;40:144–147.

[53] Levin J, Hogen T, Patzig M, et al. Pontine and extrapontine myolinolysis associated with hypernatraemia. *Clin Neurol Neurosurg* 2012;114:1290–1291.

[54] Schaefer TJ, Wolford RW. Disorders of potassium. *Emerg Med Clin North Am* 2005;23:723–727.

[55] National Research Council (U.S.), Committee on Nutrient Requirements of Horses. In: *Nutrient Requirements of Horses*, 6th rev. ed. Washington, DC:National Academies Press; 2007.

[56] Johnson PJ, Goetz TE, Foreman JH, et al. Effect of whole-body potassium depletion on plasma, erythrocyte, and middle gluteal muscle potassium concentration of healthy, adult horses. *Am J Vet Res* 1991;52:1676–1683.

[57] Picandet V, Leguillette R, Lavoie JP. Comparison of efficacy and tolerability of isoflupredone and dexamethasone in the treatment of horses affected with recurrent airway obstruction ("heaves"). *Equine Vet J* 2003;35:419–424.

[58] Yang L, Frindt G, Palmer LG. Magnesium modulates ROMK channel-mediated potassium secretion. *J Am Soc Nephrol* 2010;21:2109–2116.

[59] Huang CL, Kuo E. Mechanism of hypokalemia in magnesium deficiency. *J Am Soc Nephrol* 2007;18:2649–2652.

[60] Constable PD, Hinchcliff KW, Muir WW, III. Comparison of anion gap and strong ion gap as predictors of unmeasured strong ion concentration in plasma and serum from horses. *Am J Vet Res* 1998;59:881–887.

[61] Toribio RE, Kohn CW, Rourke KM, et al. Effects of hypercalcemia on serum concentrations of magnesium, potassium, and phosphate and urinary excretion of electrolytes in horses. *Am J Vet Res* 2007;68:543–554.

[62] Cox J. An episodic weakness in four horses associated serum hyperkalemia and the similarity of the disease to

hyperkalemic paralysis in man. *Proc Am Assoc Equine Pract* 1985;31:383.

[63] Naylor JM, Robinson JA, Crichlow EC, Steiss JE. Inheritance of myotonic discharges in American quarter horses and the relationship to hyperkalemic periodic paralysis. *Can J Vet Res* 1992;56:62–66.

[64] Aleman M. A review of equine muscle disorders. *Neuromuscul Disord* 2008;18:277–287.

[65] Finno CJ, Spier SJ, Valberg SJ. Equine diseases caused by known genetic mutations. *Vet J* 2009;179:336–347.

[66] Rudolph JA, Spier SJ, Byrns G, et al. Periodic paralysis in quarter horses: a sodium channel mutation disseminated by selective breeding. *Nat Genet* 1992;2:144–147.

[67] Cannon SC, Hayward LJ, Beech J, Brown RH, Jr. Sodium channel inactivation is impaired in equine hyperkalemic periodic paralysis. *J Neurophysiol* 1995;73:1892–1899.

[68] MacLeay JM. Channelopathies: aberrations of ion and electrolyte flux. In: Reed SM, Bayly WM, Sellon DC, eds. *Equine Internal Medicine*. St. Louis:Saunders/Elsevier; 2010:506–508.

[69] Bowling AT, Byrns G, Spier S. Evidence for a single pedigree source of the hyperkalemic periodic paralysis susceptibility gene in quarter horses. *Anim Genet* 1996;27: 279–281.

[70] Bailey JE, Pablo L, Hubbell JA. Hyperkalemic periodic paralysis episode during halothane anesthesia in a horse. *J Am Vet Med Assoc* 1996;208:1859–1865.

[71] Carr EA, Spier SJ, Kortz GD, Hoffman EP. Laryngeal and pharyngeal dysfunction in horses homozygous for hyperkalemic periodic paralysis. *J Am Vet Med Assoc* 1996;209: 798–803.

[72] Spier S, Valberg S, Carr E. Update on hyperkalemic periodic paralysis. *Proc Am Assoc Equine Pract* 1995;31: 231–233.

[73] Robinson JA, Naylor JM, Crichlow EC. Use of electromyography for the diagnosis of equine hyperkalemic periodic paresis. *Can J Vet Res* 1990;54:495–500.

[74] Tricarico D, Barbieri M, Mele A, et al. Carbonic anhydrase inhibitors are specific openers of skeletal muscle BK channel of K+-deficient rats. *FASEB J* 2004;18:760–761.

[75] Alberts MK, Clarke CR, MacAllister CG, Homer LM. Pharmacokinetics of acetazolamide after intravenous and oral administration in horses. *Am J Vet Res* 2000;61: 965–968.

[76] Toribio RE. Disorders of calcium and phosphate metabolism in horses. *Vet Clin North Am Equine Pract* 2011;27: 129–147.

[77] Toribio RE. Disorders of calcium and phosphorus. In: Reed SM, Bayly WM, Sellon DC, eds. *Equine Internal Medicine*. St. Louis:Saunders/Elsevier;2010:1277–1291.

[78] Toribio RE, Kohn CW, Chew DJ, et al. Comparison of serum parathyroid hormone and ionized calcium and magnesium concentrations and fractional urinary clearance of calcium and phosphorus in healthy horses and horses with enterocolitis. *Am J Vet Res* 2001;62: 938–947.

[79] Hudson NP, Church DB, Trevena J, et al. Primary hypoparathyroidism in two horses. *Aust Vet J* 1999;77: 504–508.

[80] Aguilera-Tejero E, Estepa JC, Lopez I, et al. Polycystic kidneys as a cause of chronic renal failure and secondary hypoparathyroidism in a horse. *Equine Vet J* 2000;32: 167–169.

[81] Beyer MJ, Freestone JF, Reimer JM, et al. Idiopathic hypocalcemia in foals. *J Vet Intern Med* 1997;11:356–360.

[82] Richardson JD, Harrison LJ, Edwards GB. Two horses with hypocalcaemia. *Vet Rec* 1991;129:98.

[83] Wijnberg ID, van der Kolk JH, Franssen H, Breukink HJ. Electromyographic changes of motor unit activity in horses with induced hypocalcemia and hypomagnesemia. *Am J Vet Res* 2002;63:849–856.

[84] Toribio RE. Magnesium and disease. In: Reed SM, Bayly WM, Sellon DC, eds. *Equine Internal Medicine*. St. Louis:Saunders/Elsevier;2010:1291–1296.

[85] Altura BM, Altura BT. Role of magnesium in pathophysiological processes and the clinical utility of magnesium ion selective electrodes. *Scand J Clin Lab Invest Suppl* 1996;224:S211–S234.

[86] Stewart AJ, Hardy J, Kohn CW, et al. Validation of diagnostic tests for determination of magnesium status in horses with reduced magnesium intake. *Am J Vet Res* 2004;65:422–430.

[87] Lopez I, Estepa JC, Mendoza FJ, et al. Fractionation of calcium and magnesium in equine serum. *Am J Vet Res* 2006;67:463–466.

[88] Toribio RE, Kohn CW, Hardy J, Rosol TJ. Alterations in serum parathyroid hormone and electrolyte concentrations and urinary excretion of electrolytes in horses with induced endotoxemia. *J Vet Intern Med* 2005;19:223–231.

[89] Hintz HF, Schryver HF. Magnesium metabolism in the horse. *J Anim Sci* 1972;35:755–759.

[90] Hintz HF, Schryver HF. Magnesium, calcium and phosphorus metabolism in ponies fed varying levels of magnesium. *J Anim Sci* 1973;37:927–930.

[91] Stewart AJ. Magnesium disorders in horses. *Vet Clin North Am Equine Pract* 2011;27:149–163.

[92] Levitsky DO, Takahashi M. Interplay of Ca(2+) and Mg(2+) in sodium-calcium exchanger and in other Ca(2+)-binding proteins: magnesium, watchdog that blocks each turn if able. *Adv Exp Med Biol* 2013;961:65–78.

[93] Weglicki WB. Hypomagnesemia and inflammation: clinical and basic aspects. *Annu Rev Nutr* 2012;32:55–71.

[94] Mishra OP, Fritz KI, Ivoria-Papadopoulos M. NMDA receptor and neonatal hypoxic brain injury. *Ment Retard Dev Disabil Res Rev* 2001;7:249–253.

[95] Levenson CW. Regulation of the NMDA receptor: implications for neuropsychological development. *Nutr Rev* 2006;64:428–432.

[96] Latremoliere A, Woolf CJ. Central sensitization: a generator of pain hypersensitivity by central neural plasticity. *J Pain* 2009;10:895–926.

[97] Martens H, Schweigel M. Pathophysiology of grass tetany and other hypomagnesemias. Implications for clinical management. *Vet Clin North Am Food Anim Pract* 2000;16:339–368.

[98] Hurcombe SD, Toribio RE, Slovis NM, et al. Calcium regulating hormones and serum calcium and magnesium concentrations in septic and critically ill foals and their association with survival. *J Vet Intern Med* 2009;23:335–343.

[99] Dhupa N, Proulx J. Hypocalcemia and hypomagnesemia. *Vet Clin North Am Small Anim Pract* 1998;28:587–608.

[100] Rook JA, Storry JE. Magnesium in the nutrition of farm animals. *Nutr Abstr Rev* 1962;32:1055–1077.

[101] Johansson AM, Gardner SY, Jones SL, Levine JY. Hypomagnesemia in hospitalized horses. *J Vet Intern Med* 2003;17:860–867.

[102] Harrington DD. Pathologic features of magnesium deficiency in young horses fed purified rations. *Am J Vet Res* 1974;35:503–513.

[103] Wong DM, Wilkins PA, Bain FT, Brockus CW. Neonatal encephalopathy in foals. *Comp Cont Educ Vet* 2011;33:E1–E10.

[104] Rosol TJ, Capen CC. Pathophysiology of calcium, phosphorus, and magnesium metabolism in animals. *Vet Clin North Am Small Anim Pract* 1996;26:1155–1184.

[105] Roden DM, Iansmith DH. Effects of low potassium or magnesium concentrations on isolated cardiac tissue. *Am J Med* 1987;82:18–23.

[106] Whang R. Magnesium and potassium interrelationships in cardiac arrhythmias. *Magnesium* 1986;5:127–133.

[107] Meijer P. Two cases of tetany in the horse (author's transl). *Tijdschr Diergeneeskd* 1982;107:329–332.

[108] Henninger RW, Horst J. Magnesium toxicosis in two horses. *J Am Vet Med Assoc* 1997;211:82–85.

[109] Temkin NR, Anderson GD, Winn HR, et al. Magnesium sulfate for neuroprotection after traumatic brain injury: a randomised controlled trial. *Lancet Neurol* 2007;6: 29–38.

[110] van den HC, Vink R. The role of magnesium in traumatic brain injury. *Clin Calcium* 2004;14:9–14.

[111] Sen AP, Gulati A. Use of magnesium in traumatic brain injury. *Neurotherapeutics* 2010;7:91–99.

[112] Arango MF, Bainbridge D. Magnesium for acute traumatic brain injury. *Cochrane Database Syst Rev* 2008;CD005400.

[113] MacKay RJ. Brain injury after head trauma: pathophysiology, diagnosis, and treatment. *Vet Clin North Am Equine Pract* 2004;20:199–216.

[114] Wilkins PA. Magnesium infusion in hypoxic ischemic encephalopathy. *Proc Annual Meet Amer Coll Vet Intern Med* 2001;19:242–244.

[115] Siemkowicz E. Magnesium sulfate solution dramatically improves immediate recovery of rats from hypoxia. *Resuscitation* 1997;35:53–59.

[116] Hallak M, Hotra JW, Kupsky WJ. Magnesium sulfate protection of fetal rat brain from severe maternal hypoxia. *Obstet Gynecol* 2000;96:124–128.

[117] Goni-de-Cerio F, Alvarez A, Lara-Celador I, et al. Magnesium sulfate treatment decreases the initial brain damage alterations produced after perinatal asphyxia in fetal lambs. *J Neurosci Res* 2012;90:1932–1940.

[118] Tenenhouse HS. Regulation of phosphorus homeostasis by the type iia na/phosphate cotransporter. *Annu Rev Nutr* 2005;25:197–214.

[119] Endres DB, Rude RK. Mineral and bone metabolism. In: Burtis CA, Ashwood ER, Bruns DE, eds. *Tietz Textbook of Clinical Chemistry and Molecular Diagnostics*. St. Louis: Saunders/Elsevier;2006:1891–1963.

[120] Geerse DA, Bindels AJ, Kuiper MA, et al. Treatment of hypophosphatemia in the intensive care unit: a review. *Crit Care* 2010;14:R147.

30 Cervical Articular Process Disease, Fractures, and Other Axial Skeletal Disorders

Richard Hepburn

B & W Equine Hospital, Gloucestershire, UK

Cervical spinal cord compression has traditionally been thought to refer solely to intravertebral canal narrowing due to vertebral malformation; however, this assumption underestimates the relevance of disease within the vertebral articular process joints (APJs) and the contiguous ligamentum flavum (LF) [1]. Osteoarthritis and osteochondrosis share many pathophysiologic similarities and commonly occur within the APJs, which are in close proximity to the dorsolateral white matter of the spinal cord [2–5]. There is increasing pathological, diagnostic imaging and clinical evidence of the importance of dorsolateral compression not just in combination with vertebral canal malformation, but as a separate entity in both young and old horses. This observation could influence the way cervical spinal cord compression, particularly in younger horses, is diagnosed and treated. As well as developmental or nutritional disease, the axial skeleton is also subject to trauma. The cervical spine is more mobile and less protected than the thoracolumbar spine; hence, thoracolumbar disease is less likely to cause neurologic disease, but it is often more severe when it does occur. Diseases of the vertebral body and the intercentral joints are rare, are most commonly of a traumatic, infectious or neoplastic etiology, and can have a variable neurologic presentation. An understanding of the vertebral anatomy and how it relates to the spinal cord it encloses, and what pathological changes can occur, is vital to identifying APJ/LF disease and treating it effectively.

Anatomy of the articular process joints

The seven vertebrae within the equine neck articulate with one another by both an intercentral articulation and via paired zygapophyseal synovial joints known as articular process joints (APJs) or more colloquially as "facets" [6]. They are located dorsolaterally on each vertebra and are dorsal to the intervertebral foramen. Within each joint, the caudal articular process of the cranial vertebra sits axially to the cranial articular process of the caudal vertebra [7]. The intervertebral foramen represents the space between the articular process of the cranial vertebra and the vertebral body of the caudal vertebra. In the dorsoventral plane, the APJs are oval in shape, with margins that are wedge-shaped cranioventrally and rounded dorsocaudally [8]. Multiple outpouches extend from the basic oval shape (Figure 30.1): lateral outpouch (from the lateral gap between cranial and caudal articular processes, it extends laterally and dorsolaterally); medial outpouch (positioned dorsolaterally within the vertebral canal, it extends ventromedially from the medial gap between articular processes); cranial outpouch (wedge shaped, positioned along the lateral curve of the cranial vertebra); and caudal outpouch (extends caudally from the tip of the cranial articular process along the dorsal surface of the body of the caudal vertebra).

Spanning the dorsal half of the vertebral canal as thin elastic sheets contiguous with the APJ capsule, and connecting the adjacent vertebral arches, is the ligamentum flavum (LF) (Figure 30.2) or interarcuate ligament [9, 10]. The cervical APJs have the largest joint capsules in the axial skeleton [6, 11]. Their articular surfaces are located progressively more laterally from C2 to C7 [12]. The lateral separation of the synovial surfaces also gets progressively wider from C2 to C7, then moves closer to the midline from T1 caudally [13]. The angle of the APJ articular surface relative to the floor of the vertebral canal becomes gradually steeper from C2 to C7 [8]. A significant increase in cervical APJ volume also occurs caudally from C2 to C7 [8], as does intervertebral

Equine Neurology, Second Edition. Martin Furr and Stephen Reed.
Companion website: www.wiley.com/go/furr/neurology

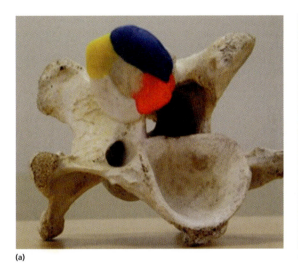

(a)

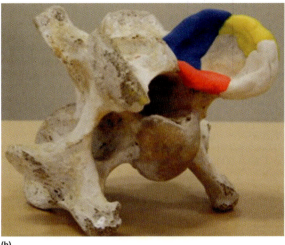

(b)

Figure 30.1 Representation of the positions of the outpouches of the right articular process joint between C5 and C6 (a) oblique caudocranial view of C5 (b) oblique craniocaudal view of C6 (red, medial outpouch; yellow, lateral outpouch; blue, caudal outpouch; and white, cranial outpouch).

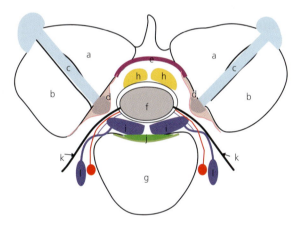

Figure 30.2 Cross-sectional drawing depicting the relationship between the APJ/LF and contents of the vertebral canal, at the level of an intervertebral foramen (a, caudal articular process of the cranial vertebra; b, cranial articular process of the caudal vertebra; c, APJ space; d, APJ medial joint capsule; e, ligamentum flavum; f, spinal cord within dura mater; g, intervertebral disc; h, epidural fat; i, ventral longitudinal venous plexus; j, dorsal longitudinal ligament; k, cervical segmental nerve; and l, vertebral vein and artery).

foramina length and height [14]. The result is an increasingly laterally positioned, upright, medial orientation and wider joint space in the caudal articulations. Individual right and left APJs have variable joint margins, but are significantly related in shape, volume, and medial outpouch into the vertebral canal [8].

Articular cartilage covers the osseous ends of diarthrodial joints; it is an avascular and aneural load-bearing connective tissue that absorbs impact and shearing forces, whilst allowing frictionless motion of the joint [15]. The synovial surfaces of the cervical APJs are almost flat [13]. Variously sized intra-articular synovial folds, which contain synovial membrane, synoviocytes and adipose, are commonly found in the equine cervical spine [11], and in man have been described throughout the vertebral column [16]. They are thought to function as passive space fillers, ensuring the articular cartilage is covered with synovial fluid during all ranges of motion. It contains innervated adipose tissue that may be important in proprioceptive feedback [17]. Multiple epaxial muscles attach to the vertebral bodies, articular processes, and their articular margins.

The shape of the atlanto-occipital (AO) and atlantoaxial (AA) joints allows movement in all three directions [12]. The AO joint is a hinge-like ginglymus joint; C1–C2 is a trochoid pivot joint [13]. Within the remaining cervical articulations, the greatest lateral movement occurs at C6 [18]. The greatest range of flexion–extension motion occurs at C3–C4 and the smallest at C5–C6 [12]. This could indicate that C5–C6 is a "low motion, high pressure" joint, predisposing it to osteoarthritic change. The general shape of the cervical APJs *in vitro* is not affected by neck flexion [8], however extension results in a significant reduction in intervertebral foramina dimensions from C4 to T1 [14]. Vertebral canal dimensions are also affected by motion, with size reduction occurring dorsolaterally and ventrolaterally, rather than dorsoventrally, reflecting the noncircular nature of the vertebral canal [19]. The normal vertebral formula is cervical 7, thoracic 18, lumbar 6, sacral 5, and caudal (coccygeal) 15–21 [20]. Variation in the L6/S5 formula appears common in many breeds. The thoracic vertebrae have dorsal spinous processes that change in height, with T5/T6 typically forming the highest point at the withers. The spinous processes then reduce in height and have a caudal inclination to T14; T15 has an upright dorsal process, and the remaining thoracic and lumbar vertebrae have a cranial inclination. The articular surface of the thoracolumbar APJs is horizontally to tangentially oriented, whereas in the lumbar surfaces are vertically oriented [21]. The lumbar APJs are wider than those found in the thoracic spine [22]. *In vitro*, the stiffness of the thoracolumbar spine is 2–7 times greater than the cervical stiffness [23]. Lateral flexion is greatest in the cranial thoracic vertebrae (T6), then reduces through to L5/6 [18]. Flexion–extension is greatest at the lumbosacral joint, as it has the largest APJ and intercentral joint size [21].

Pathological changes within APJs

As with any other diathrodial joint, APJ disease can be broadly split into developmental (osteochondrosis, OC) and degenerative (osteoarthritis, OA) etiologies. Interestingly, it has been observed that many of the general morphological characteristics of OA closely resemble the deranged endochondral differentiation processes seen in OC, leading to similar clinical outcomes [2]. Postmortem studies in horses of varying ages with spinal ataxia have shown dorsolateral spinal cord compression associated with APJ/LF pathology [3–5, 24]. The contiguous anatomy of the APJ and LF is seen pathologically, with degeneration occurring simultaneously in both structures as part of both OA and OC. Within OA moderate fraying and fibrillation of articular cartilage, villous proliferation of the synovial membrane, joint capsule hypertrophy, and production of new bone at the articular margins occurs [3, 4]. In younger horses (<6 years old), OC lesions are more varied with profound malformation and instability of the APJs, osteochondritis dissecans (OCD) lesions, subchondral bone cysts and extradural synovial cysts described. Paracrine release of growth factors and pro-inflammatory cytokines from adipose within the synovial folds of the APJs may contribute to development of OA [16]. The LF becomes increasingly rigid due to hypertrophy, fibrovascular proliferation and thickening of the confluent dorsomedial aspect of the joint capsule. Hemorrhage within the ligament and necrosis of marginal fat have also been found. The fibrocartilagenous attachment of the LF to vertebral dorsal lamina becomes enlarged and osteosclerotic. Extradural synovial cysts can cause spinal compression either alone, or as part of the APJ/LF process [3, 4, 25]. In man, these are termed "degenerative intraspinal cysts"

and arise from within degenerated APJs, but also from within the ligamentum flavum, leading to either myelopathy or compression of spinal outflow [26].

Within the thoracolumbar spine APJ OA is uncommon. Pathological changes typical for OA are reported including subchondral sclerosis, osteophytosis, and narrowing of the joint space [27]. Progression to the point of ankylosis can occur, and articular process fractures appear common; yet, thoracolumbar APJ disease is rarely associated with spinal compression or neurologic signs [28, 29].

The most likely etiology for the degenerative changes within the APJ/LF is abnormal articulation stress placed upon the vertebrae, particularly repeated loading strain (flexion–extension, and torsion) [30]. This is a logical part of OA in older horses; however, repeated strain may also be a component of OC, causing production of excessive fibrocartilage that after endochondral ossification resembles osteophytosis [2]. This retention of cartilage matrix at the insertion site of the LF occurs in young horses with spinal ataxia, but not in controls [3].

Neuropathophysiology

At the level of a cervical intervertebral foramen, working from dorsal to ventral within the vertebral canal (Figures 30.2 and 30.3), the joint capsule of the APJ and LF form the outer margin of the epidural space, which

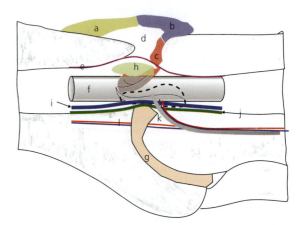

Figure 30.3 Sagittal section drawing depicting the relationship between the APJ/LF and contents of the vertebral canal at an intervertebral articulation (a, lateral outpouch of the APJ; b, caudal outpouch of the APJ; c, medial outpouch of the APJ; d, caudal articular process of the cranial vertebra; e, ligamentum flavum; f, spinal cord within dura mater; g, intervertebral disc; h, epidural fat; i, ventral longitudinal venous plexus; j, dorsal longitudinal ligament; k, cervical segmental nerve; and l, vertebral vein and artery, dotted line represents the intervertebral foramen).

itself encircles the spinal cord and contains semifluid fat, alveolar connective tissue, ventral longitudinal spinous venous sinuses, lateral intervertebral venous plexus (located at 5 and 7 o'clock); and through which the ventral and dorsal root nerves pass [9, 31]. Next are the fibrous dura mater, subdural space, arachnoid mater, subarachnoid space, pia mater, and then the spinal cord itself. Spinal branches of the vertebral artery and intervertebral vein enter and exit through the intervertebral space [32].

The spinal cord of each of the eight cervical segments is relatively long—longer than the corresponding segment in small animals [33]. The cross-sectional area of the equine spinal cord increases in the caudal cervical segments from C5. The APJ/LF oppose the dorsal and lateral funiculi of the white matter of the spinal cord, which contain the ascending proprioceptive tracts of the fasciculus gracilis and cuneatus, and spinocerebellar and spinocuneocerebellar tracts respectively; and the descending upper motor neuron tracts [9, 34]. Sensory (pinprick, temperature, and some touch) fibers also ascend within the spinothalamic tracts within the lateral funiculus.

The neck has eight cervical nerves; the first emerges from the lateral foramen of the atlas and the second between the atlas and the axis. The third to seventh cervical nerves emerge from the intervertebral foramina between adjacent cervical vertebrae, whilst the eighth is between C7 and T1. The sixth to eighth cervical nerves contribute to the brachial plexus. The cervical nerves contain dorsal and ventral root nerves; the dorsal branch contains sensory afferent nerves of the general somatic and general proprioceptive systems [35]; the ventral root contains general somatic efferent and general visceral efferent lower motor neurons. Branches of the vertebral sympathetic nerve, which runs adjacent to the vertebral artery within the paravertebral foramina, join with the spinal root nerves and provide local autonomic innervation [33]. The cutaneous trunci reflex, the cervical (cutaneous coli) and cervicofacial reflexes have segmental sensory input via the dorsal root nerves. The motor pathways of the cervical cutaneous coli reflex are not fully understood, but likely include ventral spinal nerves. Motor input to the cutaneous trunci is via the lateral thoracic nerve, which itself originates from ventral spinal nerves from spinal segments C8–T1 [35].

Compression can lead to both functional and physical neuronal alteration [5]. Functional alteration represents clinically relevant changes in neuronal activity without histologic damage, and could occur where compression is intermittent or is yet to reach the threshold at which rapid physical neuronal degeneration occurs [36]. Histologic evidence of compression is seen as axonal swelling or degeneration, spheroidosis, myelin degeneration or loss, astrocytic gliosis, increased macrophage

activity, and/or perivascular fibrosis [5]. These changes are greatest at the site of compression and most prominent in the lateral and ventral funiculi, as well as the gracile fascicle. Cranial to the site of compression Wallerian degeneration is found in superficial portions of the lateral funiculi and in the middle of the dorsal funiculi [36]. Caudally, it is present in the ventral funiculi adjacent to the ventral median fissure and in the middle of the lateral funiculi.

Clinical presentation of cervical APJ disease

It is important to appreciate that whilst horses with a developmentally narrowed vertebral canal would be predisposed to compression from APJ/LF pathology; compression can occur *without* evidence of vertebral canal malformation [1, 4]; that is, it is possible for spinal compression in younger horses to be solely due to APJ/LF pathology, leading to a clinical presentation similar to the compressive myelopathy seen in older horses with APJ/LF OA [5]. In this author's experience, this appreciation is vital to interpretation of orthogonal cervical radiographs, as alteration in mean sagittal ratios will not occur with APJ/LF compression alone.

Historically, the name given to cervical spinal cord compression was based on the neck position in which compression occurred rather than the origin of the compression itself; cervical vertebral instability was characterized by narrowing of the sagittal diameter of the vertebral canal during neck flexion, and cervical static stenosis referred to compression irrespective of neck position [3]. This terminology has made appreciation of the role of APJ/LF pathology difficult. The recent definition of two broad types of cervical vertebral compressive myelopathy (CVCM) is based more upon etiology but is still potentially misleading [37, 38]. Type 1 CVCM describes a developmental disease in which a caudally extended vertebral arch and a dorsoventrally narrowed vertebral canal (vertebral malformation) is the primary compressing lesion. Secondary soft tissue compression from OC changes within the APJ/LF can be present. This condition is similar to developmental orthopedic disease in the appendicular skeleton; indeed the frequency and severity of appendicular OC lesions can be greater in CVCM horses compared to normal controls [39]. Type 2 CVCM describes a similar clinical presentation in older horses (8–25 years old at onset) due to APJ/LF OA; this presentation has also been termed caudal cervical arthropathy [40, 41]. Exactly, where younger horses with compression solely due to APJ/LF OC fit into this classification is unclear; previously young horses (4 years old) with APJ/LF changes described as OA have been included in type 2 [40]. Instead this author recommends considering spinal cord compression due to APJ/LF disease in three, rather than two scenarios, although their neurologic presentation is very similar:

Type 1 CVCM. Young horses (<4 years) with APJ/LF disease and concurrent vertebral canal malformation

Type 2 CVCM. Young horses (<4 years) with APJ/LF disease as the sole cause of spinal compression

Type 3 CVCM. Older horses with APJ/LF disease as the sole cause of spinal compression

Any age delineator for these types is likely to be arbitrary given the individual variation in the timing of vertebral physeal closure. Radiographic closure of the cranial physis starts ventrally and is usually complete by 2 years of age, whereas the caudal physis starts closing dorsally and is usually complete by 4–5 years of age [42]. Morphological closure occurs much later, with the cranial physes of C3–7 closed by 3 years, whereas the caudal physes are present and discontinuous at 6–9 years but absent at 12 years [33]. How this relates to the potential for osteochondritis-like APJ disease to occur is unclear. It is this author's experience that young horses with spinal cord compression due to APJ/LF alone are typically older than those with APJ/LF pathology in addition to vertebral canal malformation. In all cases, neurologic examination describes deficits that neuro-anatomically localize to the cervical spine. A multicenter study of CVCM found a median thoracic limb ataxia grade of 2/5, and a pelvic limb grade of 3/5 [43]. Over 40% of the cases were described as having asymmetric neurologic deficits; however, this was not associated with any specific pathologic asymmetry. In most cases, the asymmetry was not pronounced, while horses with primary APJ/LF disease demonstrate a greater degree of asymmetry—these are subjective assessments, however and will vary greatly between individual cases. Cervical hyperesthesia was associated with the presence of APJ osteophytosis, but not with any other type of gross CVCM lesion. The median duration of clinical signs prior to diagnosis was 28 days (range 1–730). This author's experience of APJ/LF cases would reflect this, with a typical presentation being grade 2–3 thoracic and pelvic limb ataxia and dysmetria, and grade 2–3 pelvic limb upper motor neuron paresis. Clinically, this is seen as forelimb hypermetria and hindlimb spasticity that is exaggerated during backing up and hill walking; forelimb pivoting and hindlimb circumduction during tight circling; and weakness and uncontrolled distal limb pronation during tail pulling whilst walking. Gait deficits can be symmetric or asymmetric. Muscle atrophy is typically minimal and when present localized to the dorsal midline and rump. Horses may present with a history of being neurologically normal in the preceding 12 months or they may have a more prolonged (5–200 day) but nonprogressive history of neurologic dysfunction including tripping and stumbling, particularly downhill

and altered performance (unbalanced, refusing to jump, weak behind, "clumsy") [40, 44]. In some cases, a single bout of shoulder/neck trauma that may have occurred days to years previously is reported. Often, a thorough orthopedic examination has failed to define a problem. Cervical hyperesthesia is seen as an exaggerated skin prick responses over the neck compared to the trunk; and is variably present in CVCM cases [43]. Hyperesthesia is significantly associated with APJ osteophytosis, but it is also found more commonly in horses with acute onset neurological signs [40]. In this author's experience, the differences between young horses with sole APJ/LF pathology from those with concurrent vertebral canal malformation are sole APJ/LF disease tends to occur in older animals (3–6 years); it causes neurological gait deficits that are less severe and more similar in grade and presentation to those seen in horses with type 2 CVCM; muscle atrophy is less obvious; and the onset of disease is more insidious and less progressive compared to those with concurrent canal malformation.

Mechanical neck pain should be considered distinctly from hyperesthesia, and describes an inability to display a normal range of neck motion. The basic mechanisms causing pain in diseased joints are incompletely understood [45] and even less is known on the origin of primary APJ neck pain in the horse. Unfortunately, the clinical presentation is variable and nonspecific. In more severe cases, the horse may be unable to lower the neck to graze, necessitating a "giraffe-like" stance. Often, the rider notes neck stiffness, poor bending when working in a circle, or even violent throwing of the head into the air; however, all these signs are not specific to neck pain, occurring with orthopedic problems such as lameness or back pain [10]. Neck flexibility should be assessed from side to side and up and down. Many normal horses resist forced manipulation, and many ignore feed incentives, or merely move to get to them, making interpretation difficult. Positioning the opposite side of the trunk against a wall can help, with the incentive positioned initially at the elbow, then the mid thorax and then the stifle [18]. The clinician needs to distinguish between the horse properly flexing the neck, and inappropriate twisting of the head on the neck, however this is very subjective. As neck pain is often positional, observing for an altered neck carriage or stiffness whilst the horse moves in hand, on the lunge and when ridden can be helpful. The incidence of mechanical neck pain in ataxic horses with APJ/LF disease is unknown; but in this author's experience, it is uncommon and inconsistent.

A syndrome of episodic, transient, marked neck pain, stiffness, and lowered head carriage is reported that can resolve with careful manipulation of the neck base [10]. In this author's experience, a history of running away or bucking the rider off, and cutaneous hyperreflexia may also be present. In between episodes, these horses are often completely normal, although mild (grade 1/5) gait deficits may be present. No definitive cause has been established, although marked radiographic enlargement of the caudal APJs is typically found, which raises the possibility of cervical radiculopathy being present [46]. In this author's experience, these cases can respond to corticosteroid medication of the affected APJ; however, this may need to be repeated frequently (2–3 times per year).

Diagnosis of APJ/LF cervical spinal cord compression

When considering the two scenarios of cervical spinal cord compression solely due to APJ/LF pathology (young horses due to OC, older horses due to OA), this author applies the same decision criteria and analyzes all results in series and in parallel. There should be suitable neurological deficits that localize to the cervical spinal cord, with or without signs of spinal segment nerve compression; significant changes in the appearance of individual APJs on lateral plain radiographs; an absence of significant APJ asymmetry on oblique lateral plain radiography; and an absence of vertebral canal malformation shown either by normal mean sagittal ratios, or if these are abnormal then an absence of dorsoventral myelographic compression at that site. In regions where equine protozoal myeloencephalopathy (EPM) is prevalent, an appropriate negative test result could be added to these criteria.

Cervical radiography

The majority of the data assessing the utility of plain radiography and its derived measurements (mean sagittal diameter, mean sagittal ratio) in CVCM has focused on dorsoventral compression [47], whereas APJ/LF compression occurs in a dorsolateral plane. There is minimal data comparing radiographic changes of the APJ/LF alone, with either myelography or the gold standard of neurohistopathology, making objective diagnosis difficult [1]. This diagnostic problem is compounded in areas where noncompressive disease such as EPM is common.

Cervical radiography is performed with the horse standing and standard techniques for lateral-lateral and lateral oblique projections have been thoroughly described [7, 48] (Figures 30.4 and 30.5).

Careful positioning of the neck is important to minimize rotation, which will artifactually reduce intervertebral foramina size and increase APJ size. Lateral images that show rotation should be repeated, and a complete set of images from the occiput to T1 should be obtained. Normal variation of the radiographic anatomy of the APJs exists; in particular, C7 can have a small dorsal spinous process which on lateral projection can be

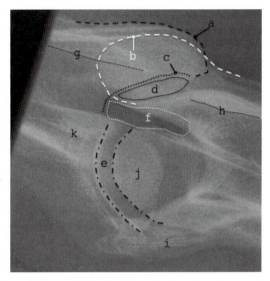

Figure 30.4 Lateral–lateral radiograph of C4–C5, with normal APJs, cranial is to the left (a, abaxial margin of caudal articular process of C4; b, abaxial margin of cranial articular process of C5; c, dorsal contour of d, crescent shaped radiolucent area caused by a groove on the axial border of the caudal articular process; e, intercentral joint space; f, intervertebral foramen; g, dorsal lamina of C4; h, dorsal lamina of C5; I, cranial tubercle of transverse process of C5; j, cranial epiphysis of C5; and k, caudal epiphysis of C4).

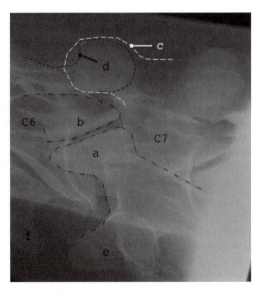

Figure 30.5 Left 50° ventral to right-dorsal oblique view of C6–C7, tangential to the right C6–C7 APJ space, cranial is to the left (a, Left cranial articular process of C7; b, left caudal articular process of C6; c, right cranial articular process of C7; d, right caudal articular process of C6; e, cranial tubercle of left transverse process of C7; and f, caudal tubercle left transverse process of C6).

superimposed over the APJs of C6–7 giving a false appearance of dorsal osteophytosis.

Several pathologic changes can be recognized on cervical lateral radiographs [47]:

1 Epiphyseal enlargement and dorsal extension of the caudal epiphysis of the vertebral body
2 Caudal extension of the dorsal aspect of the vertebral arch over the cranial epiphysis of the adjacent vertebra
3 Osteochodrotic change, including incomplete ossification of the articular processes
4 Abnormal dorsal angulation/malarticulation/mild subluxation of adjacent vertebrae
5 Osteophytosis of the APJ

The author recommends a greater focus on more critical and detailed description of the change in radiographic appearance of the cervical APJs by applying a novel grading scheme [41] (Table 30.1):

Arthropathy and irregular radiographic enlargement of the margins of the C6–C7 APJs has been anecdotally described as a normal variation in mature horses [10]; however, an age effect on worsening APJ grade was only found at C5–C6 [41]. No significant association between clinical disease and radiographic grade was reported; however, the numbers of horses with ataxia was small. Preliminary analysis of a larger population of horses with spinal ataxia that fulfill the authors decision criteria, in a region free of EPM, has shown an increased proportion of horses to have grades 3b and 4b at C5–C6 and C6–C7, and grade 4b at C6–C7 (R. Hepburn and J. Butler, unpublished observation) suggesting that ventral osteophytosis could be a more useful radiographic predictor of neurologically significant APJ/LF disease. In this population, C6–C7 was the most commonly implicated articulation (Figure 30.6).

Oblique lateral views of the caudal cervical articulations (C5–T1) should be routinely taken, and are particularly important in cases where there is asymmetry of the neurological deficits, or where possible spinal outflow compression is suspected. The primary beam is positioned tangential to the joint space of the APJ furthest from the X-ray machine, allowing assessment of its width and regularity; the axial margin of the closer APJ and the intervertebral foramen can also be identified [7]. Marked facet asymmetry can be found on oblique lateral projection that was not apparent on the lateral view. In this author's experience, marked asymmetry has a negative effect on prognosis; however, empirical support for this position is currently not found (Figure 30.7).

Table 30.1 Proposed scoring system for horses with articular process joint arthritis.

Grade	Radiographic findings
1	No enlargement of the APJ either dorsally or ventrally.
2	The dorsal margin of the APJ is enlarged by osteophytosis, but there is none on the ventral margin; the intervertebral foramen is readily visible.
3a	The intervertebral foramen is reduced in size by osteophytosis on the ventral margin of the APJ, the reduction is not sufficient to obscure the foramen (the ventral aspect of the APJ does not overly the dorsocaudal epihpysis). There is no osteophytosis dorsally.
3b	The ventral enlargement of the APJ by periarticular new bone is sufficient to obscure the foramen (the ventral aspect of the APJ overlies the dorsocaudal epihpysis). There is no osteophytosis dorsally.
4a	Osteophytosis is present on the dorsal and ventral margins of the APJ in approximately equal amounts. The increased overall size of the APJ seen dorsal to the vertebral canal is <1.5× the size of the vertebral canal immediately below. The intervertebral foramen is reduced in size by osteophytosis on the ventral margin of the APJ; the reduction is not sufficient to obscure the foramen (the ventral aspect of the APJ does not overly the dorsocaudal epihpysis).
4b	Osteophytosis is present on the dorsal and ventral margins of the APJ, with the ventral osteophytosis most prominent. The increased overall size of the APJ seen dorsal to the vertebral canal is <1.5× the size of the vertebral canal immediately below. The ventral enlargement of the APJ by periarticular new bone is sufficient to obscure the foramen (the ventral aspect of the APJ overlies the dorsocaudal epihpysis).
5a	Osteophytosis is present on the dorsal and ventral margins of the APJ, with the dorsal osteophytosis most prominent. The increased overall size of the APJ seen dorsal to the vertebral canal is >1.5× the size of the vertebral canal immediately below. The intervertebral foramen is reduced in size by osteophytosis on the ventral margin of the APJ, the reduction is not sufficient to obscure the foramen (the ventral aspect of the APJ does not overly the dorsocaudal epihpysis).
5b	Severe osteophytosis is present on the dorsal and ventral margins of the APJ in approximately equal amounts. The increased overall size of the APJ seen dorsal to the vertebral canal is >1.5× the size of the vertebral canal immediately below. The ventral enlargement of the APJ by periarticular new bone is sufficient to obscure the foramen (the ventral aspect of the APJ overlies the dorsocaudal epihpysis).

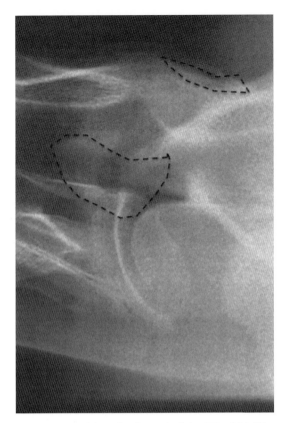

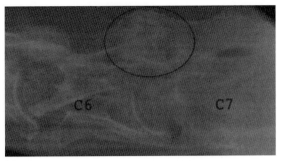

(a)

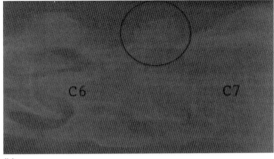

(b)

Figure 30.7 (a) Left 50° ventral to right-dorsal oblique and (b) right 50° ventral to left-dorsal oblique views of the C6–C7 articulation in a 12-year-old Warmblood mare with CVCM, asymmetric cutaneous colli reflexes and reduced neck lateral flexion. Marked, irregular enlargement of the left APJ, and reduced size of the right APJ are seen.

Figure 30.6 Lateral–lateral radiograph of the APJs of C6–C7, cranial is left, showing grade 4b dorsal and ventral osteophytosis (dotted lines delineate).

In order to exclude the possibility of vertebral canal malformation this author calculates intravertebral mean sagittal ratios (MSRs) at all articulations, using a cut off value of >0.52 for C3–C4 to C5–C6, and >0.56 for C6–C7, although the low sensitivity in some individual cases must be acknowledged [38]. Cervical myelography under general anesthesia is a relatively straightforward procedure that has traditionally been used to define the site of spinal cord compression when the intention is surgery; however given the increased appreciation of the significance of APJ/LF pathology, this author routinely uses myelography to exclude vertebral canal malformation. For instance, if an individual articulation has significant APJ/LF changes, and a separate one has an abnormal MSR or signs of malarticulation, cervical myelography can be used to assign significance to each site. APJ/LF disease most commonly affects the caudal cervical articulations, where myelography is more sensitive and specific on neutral views rather than flexed [49]. In addition to these, the use of anatomically realistic extended views is recommended as reduced vertebral canal dimensions occur during *in vivo* extension, and extension of the caudal articulations occurs during exercise [14, 50, 51]. The degree of extension should mimic the head/neck positions that occur when ridden: where the neck is raised and the bridge of the nose is vertical; and where is neck is raised and extended, and the bridge of the nose is in front of the vertical [50]. Specific decision criteria should be used to identify compression during extension and flexion at individual articulations [49]. Unfortunately, this information is not available for anatomically realistic extended views; instead, the author applies the same criteria as in interpreting neutral views, but only assigns significance when any criteria is at least 1.5× that found at adjacent articulations. When concurrent APJ changes and a narrow MSR are found at a single articulation, it may be possible, though technically challenging, to assign relative significance to dorsoventral compression (from vertebral canal malformation) versus dorsolateral compression (from APJ pathology), by attempting oblique lateral projections. As no decision criteria exist for these views, critical comparison with adjacent articulations is required.

Radiographic examination of the thoracolumbar spine is more challenging due to the presence of ribs, whose articulations are close to the APJs, and the increased depth of tissue. Standardized lateral and oblique techniques are described [48].

Nuclear scintigraphy

Clinically, normal horses have increased radiopharmaceutical uptake (IRU) in the APJs of C5–C7, reflecting the increased mobility of these joints; and in the dens of the axis, making scintigraphy relatively insensitive and nonspecific [52]. Timed images should be obtained from each side, looking for asymmetry in IRU and shape. Fractures often do not have prominent IRU, so the shape of the articular process and vertebral body should be carefully assessed, as it may be the only indication [10].

Ultrasonography

A large variation in the outline of APJs, caused by the irregularity of the insertions of the epaxial muscles, is found on transcutaneous ultrasonography, making identification of osteophytosis or APJ enlargement difficult [11]. Ultrasonography is only useful for assessment of epaxial swellings and for ultrasound guided APJ injections.

Computed tomography and magnetic resonance imaging

Unfortunately computed tomography (CT) and magnetic resonance (MR) imaging are of little value due to size limitations and the inability to alter neck position, but both have been used post mortem and have greatly increased our knowledge of APJ/LF spinal cord compression [5, 8, 14].

Neurophysiologic testing

Electromyography has not been studied in cervical ataxia; however, transcranial magnetic stimulation has shown significantly different evoked motor responses in cases of CVCM when compared to normal horses [53]. This could be a useful ancillary test to differentiate between mild ataxia and lameness.

Treatment of cervical APJ/LF disease

The response of ataxic horses with APJ osteoarthritis to nonsteroidal anti-inflammatory drugs (NSAIDs) and reduced exercise or rest is poor [10]. Instead intra-articular administration of corticosteroid under ultrasound guidance is recommended, although there is little published evidence of its efficacy. A study of 33 sport horses with spinal ataxia attributable to CVCM, in addition to 26 with other cervical disease (neck pain, obscure lameness), reported that overall 32% returned to full function and 39% improved [54]. The overall

effect was of variable duration (<1 month to 5 years); however in 55%, it was less than 6 months. It is difficult to draw conclusions from this study as the number with ataxia was small and not analyzed separately, the diagnostic criteria were poorly defined, the response was owner assessed, and the treatment was variable in dose and drug used. Preliminary analysis of a larger population of horses aged over 8 years with spinal ataxia, that fulfill this authors APJ/LF disease inclusion criteria has shown a >80% positive response rate (defined as all limbs neurological gait grade ≤1) (R. Hepburn, unpublished observation). All horses received either triamcinolone acetonide when treating 2 APJs (8 mg/joint, 16 mg max dose) or methylprednisolone acetate when treating 4 APJs (40 mg/joint, 160 mg max dose); with follow up neurological examination performed at 1, 4, and 12 months. Neurological resolution occurred over 1–4 months, and lasted 1–5 years; with repetition of the treatment yielding a similar response. Serial radiography of affected APJs did not show significant progression in the grade of the OA change.

Application of the same approach to a smaller population of horses aged 4–8 years, but with the inclusion of myelography if a MSR is abnormal to exclude vertebral canal malformation, has shown a >60% positive response rate, with a duration of response lasting between 2 and 8 years (R. Hepburn, unpublished observation). The reduced response rate in younger horses with sole APJ/LF compression reflects the variety and increased severity of pathological changes that occurs in OC.

Cervical APJ injection technique

The horse should be sedated (0.01 mg/kg detomidine HCl) and a 10 cm^2 area dorsal to the transverse process of the affected vertebra clipped and prepared aseptically. A micro-convex or phased array probe (6–10 MHz, 4–10 cm depth), is ideal as the small footprint facilitates easy needle placement, the probe itself should be placed inside a sterile glove or probe cover that has been filled with a small amount of acoustic gel. A standardized ultrasound image aids orientation—the author always positions the probe reference dorsal, with the screen reference to the right, and holds the probe in a transverse orientation. The probe is placed 6–8 cm dorsal to the palpable transverse process, angled 10–20° downward and slightly cranially, and then moved ventrally until the APJ margins are imaged. If the vertebral body is imaged the probe should be moved cranially or caudally to image the articular process and then joint. The APJ margins are seen as two crescent-shaped hyperechoic contours that cast acoustic shadows, separated by the anechoic joint space. With the joint space in the middle of the screen, the depth of the joint should be noted (typically about 4–5 cm). The probe is then held in a

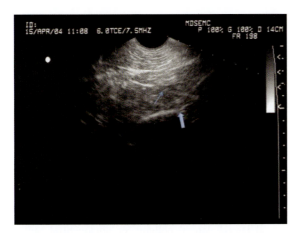

Figure 30.8 Ultrasound image acquired for direct injection of the articular process joint. The small arrow indicates the advancing needle, while the large arrow indicates the joint space between two adjacent articular processes.

fixed position, and a 12.5 cm 18G spinal needle is inserted ~1 cm dorsal to the probe, with its long axis parallel to the long axis of the probe, at a downward angle so that the needle crosses the center of the ultrasound image at the depth of the joint. The needle is then advanced toward and into the joint. If repositioning is required, it can be confusing. The skin acts as a pivot: to move the tip of the needle dorsally, the hub should be moved ventrally and vice versa. This approach is accurate, with 89% injections being either intraarticular or intracapsular, with a further 9% within 1 mm of the APJ capsule [55]. Injection should be directly visualized as hyperechoic sparkling within the joint space. An alternative technique exists, where the ventral margin of the facet is injected, with the needle positioned ventral to the probe, with the joint space appearing as a step like structure [56]. The author does not recommend this technique given the proximity to the intervertebral foramen and risk of dural injection (Figures 30.8 and 30.9).

Other axial skeletal disorders

Discospondylitis
Intercentral joint anatomy
The cervical intervertebral disks entirely comprise fibrocartilage, and are widest immediately beneath the dorsal longitudinal ligament [10]. The discs are thickest in the cervical and lumbar regions, and thinnest in the middle thoracic region. Fibrocartilage joins the vertebral bodies and is continuous with the dorsal longitudinal ligament that forms the ventral floor of the vertebral canal.

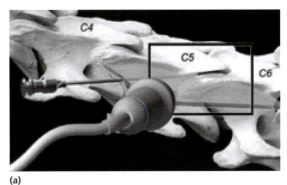

(a)

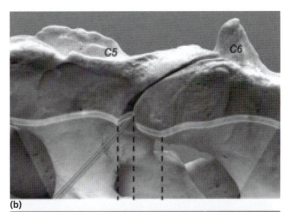

(b)

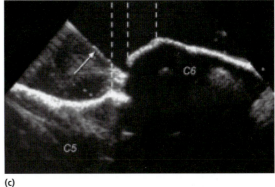

(c)

Figure 30.9 (a) The ultrasound transducer and sector ultrasound beam are depicted on C5–6. The spinal needle is properly positioned within the ultrasound beam and the tip of the needle is in the C5–6 joint. The black box outlines the location of (b). (b) Closeup view of C5–6 showing the ultrasound beam and spinal needle. The spinal needle is within the ultrasound beam. The image corresponds to the ultrasound image. Bony landmarks on the vertebrae are "connected" to the ultrasound image by dotted lines. The spinal needle (arrow) is hyperechoic. Note the reverberation artifacts on the left margin of the image, distal to the spinal needle. C5, fifth cervical vertebra; C6, sixth cervical vertebra. Reprinted with permission from Ref. [56].

Clinical findings

Discospondylitis is a rare primary cause of neurological disease, but could predispose to APJ/LF disease as a result of dorsal bulging of the dorsal longitudinal ligament reducing the overall vertebral canal size, or by increasing intervertebral mobility [10]. Commonly reported sites for discospondylitis include C3–C4, C6–C7, C7–T1, and T11–T13 [57]. Clinically, it is more likely to present as severe mechanical neck pain, reduced neck mobility, intermittent forelimb lameness, or severe back pain. When spinal compression does occur, the clinical signs are determined anatomically. Compression in the thoracolumbar region (T3–L3) would present as normal thoracic limbs, pelvic limb spasticity and paresis, cutaneous trunci hypalgesia caudal to the lesion, possibly associated with focal sweating, urinary incontinence with normal tail and anal tone [35]. Compression in the lumbosacral region (L4 caudally) cord segments presents as normal thoracic limbs, marked pelvic limb paresis and ataxia, with shortened strides; hypalgesia of the tail, anus and pelvic limbs from the level of the lesion; urinary incontinence; and obstipation. Diagnosis is typically made radiographically, where a loss of normal opacity of the cranial and caudal vertebral endplates, and alteration of the intercentral joint space is seen (Figure 30.10).

Vertebral fractures

Cervical vertebral fractures are usually traumatic: rotational or headlong falls at speed, falling sideways onto the neck base or pulling back whilst tied up. In adults,

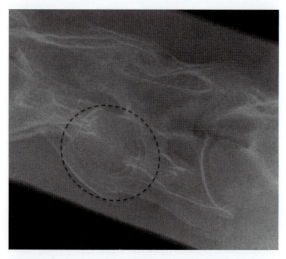

Figure 30.10 Lateral–lateral radiograph of C5–C7 showing complete ankylosis of the C5–C6 intercentral joint (dotted circle) due to chronic discospondylitis. Moderate changes within the APJs of C5–C6 and C6–C7 are also seen. This 12-year-old Thoroughbred mare had a history of chronic neck stiffness and low-grade neck pain.

the vertebral body or arch of C3–C6, and the articular processes or APJs of C5–C7 are most commonly affected [24]. Vertebral body fractures may also involve the adjacent intervertebral disc and dorsal longitudinal ligament [10]. In foals, atlas and axis fractures are also common, typically through the separate ossification center of the dens (odontoid peg). This can also fracture in adults [58]. In all cases, clinical signs are immediate and include focal guarding pain, neck stiffness or abnormal neck position/inability to move the neck, muscle contracture, and focal sweating; soft tissue swelling is not always present. Spinal ataxia is often not present, but when it is can be of variable severity and duration. Thoracic limb lameness may also be present, as can persistent pawing. Diagnosis is confirmed with lateral–lateral, lateral oblique, or dorsoventral radiographs. In young horses, it is important not to confuse physes and separate ossification centers with fragments. Acute treatment involves strict stall confinement, and cross tying is not recommended due to the risk of pulling back. Food and water should be offered from an elevated position, and hay should be loose to limit excessive neck movement. Foals with mid-cervical fractures can be stabilized in a neck cast or with a neck cradle; this is contraindicated with fractures of C1–C2 or C6–C7 as it will encourage fracture movement. This author advocates the use of corticosteroids in the acute stage in ataxic horses (dexamethasone 0.05–0.1 mg/kg IV). It is difficult to give an accurate prognosis, but many non-displaced vertebral body and articular process fractures will heal within 6–9 months, with a good prognosis for return to athletic function. Repeat neurological examination and radiography every 6 weeks is recommended. If ataxia persists, or significant focal muscle atrophy develops then the prognosis is poor, as this is often associated with callus formation and resultant spinal cord and nerve root compression. Horses with severe ataxia or displaced fractures have a very poor prognosis (Figure 30.11).

Thoracolumbar fractures appear to occur more commonly and unless they cause interruption of the vertebral canal or intervertebral foramina are typically neurologically silent; they are more likely to cause hindlimb lameness or back pain [28]. When neurological disease is present, it can range from transient focal sweating and prolonged cutaneous hypalgesia, to complete hemiparesis/hemiplegia with urinary and fecal retention that warrants euthanasia.

Cervical vertebral epidural hematomas

Cervical vertebral epidural hematomas are most commonly associated with trauma or coagulopathy, originating from the ventral internal plexus, spinal branch of the vertebral artery, or the intervetebral vein [32]. The hematoma typically occurs asymmetrically in the caudal

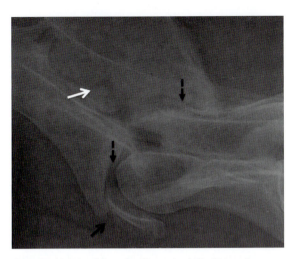

Figure 30.11 Lateral–lateral radiograph of C2–C3 in a 6-year-old Warmblood gelding with a history of recent neck trauma. A displaced fracture of the caudal epiphysis of C2 (black arrow), involving the intercentral joint, extending to an irregular, lucent fracture line within the vertebral arch (white arrow) is found. The APJs and intercentral joint of C2–C3 are ventrally subluxated (dotted arrows). This horse was euthanatized due to severe guarding neck pain and abnormal neck position; only mild signs of spinal ataxia were present.

cervical region and is confined within the vertebral canal between the dura mater and the ventral aspect of the articular process. Ataxia and paresis affecting all four limbs, and neck pain occur. Diagnosis is difficult as survey radiographs are usually normal, as is lumbosacral CSF analysis. Myelography or CT (in suitably sized horses) can demonstrate the site of compression, but not its cause. Presumptive diagnosis is by exclusion and relies on history, clinical signs and negative radiography. Treatment involves supportive care, recovery is typically prompt and complete unless callus formation occurs with concurrent periosteal damage.

Vertebral subluxation

Subluxation of C5–C6 or C6–C7 is an unusual cause of mild-to-moderate hindlimb ataxia, dysmetria and paresis in adults; in younger horses, C3–C4 is the most common articulation [10, 48]. Lateral radiographs typically show dorsal displacement of the head of C6 or C7 and subluxation of the associated intercentral joint; APJ enlargement and asymmetry is often also found. Occasionally, the subluxation occurs in a ventral direction. This condition carries a poor prognosis, although if the origin of the lesion is APJ OA, intra-articular corticosteroid medication could be beneficial, however the effect is often transient. Thoracolumbar subluxation is rare and typically traumatic in origin, presenting very similarly to a vertebral fracture [28].

Vertebral neoplasia

Vertebral lymphoma, melanoma, fibrosarcoma, myeloma, and hemangiosarcoma have all been described at the level of the vertebral canal to cause spinal cord compression [59]. Cases are usually advanced when diagnosed, with neurological signs dependent on location and degree of compression or vertebral weakness/instability. Associated soft tissue swelling or pain, or evidence of spinal outflow compression may also be present. Depending on the origin of the mass osteolysis of the vertebral body, or an irregular radiolucency may be found radiographically, this is easier with cervical than thoracolumbar masses. Cervical myelography can identify extra-dural compression, provided the lesion is compressing in a dorsoventral plane; CT may be able to identify lesions located cranial to C4 or beyond in smaller animals. Chemotherapy is rarely available or affordable; and would likely require some measure of inter-vertebral stabilisation.

Vertebral osteomyelitis

Vertebral osteomyelitis rarely occurs, but it is more common in younger animals secondary to hematogenous spread to physeal growth plates, which are predisposed by their slow rate of blood flow [60]. Bacterial infection results in destruction, remodeling and instability of the vertebra, and may extend to abscessation within the paravertebral tissues. Various pathogens have been isolated: *Aspergillus* spp., *Mycobacterium bovis* in adults; *Rhodococcus equi*, *Klebsiella* spp., *Streptococcus* spp., *Escherichia coli*, and *Actinobacillus* spp. in foals. Fever, pain and stiffness over the affected vertebrae often precede development of neurological deficits typical of spinal compression at that level. Radiographic signs include osteoproliferative change, osteolysis, sclerosis and associated soft tissue swelling; however, osteomyelitis may not be radiographically evident until 2–8 week after onset of clinical signs when up to 50% of the vertebra has undergone demineralization. Nuclear scintigraphy or CT (in the cranial neck) should be used to identify early cases. Aggressive long-term broad spectrum antimicrobial therapy is required. In adults, the combination of penicillin G and enrofloxacin, or chloramphenicol is recommended; in foals, a macrolide or chloramphenicol is recommended. Surgical debridement is advisable, though not often possible. As the diagnosis is rarely made until the infective process has extended peridurally, the condition carries a grave prognosis.

Intervertebral disk prolapse

Intervertebral disk prolapse is rarely reported in the horse; however, several cases have been described [61–64]. In one case, the prolapse was associated with discospondylitis [61], while in the majority of the other cases, no evidence of discospondylitis was observed and the etiology was considered to be trauma [62–64]. Described cases demonstrate a fairly abrupt onset of moderate-to-severe ataxia, consistent with spinal cord disease as all reported cases are associated with cervical vertebrae; neck pain is consistently reported. Constitutional signs and routine clinicopathologic evaluation are usually unremarkable, and the cerebrospinal fluid is typically normal, although increased CSF_{CK} was reported in one horse [61]. Standard radiographs demonstrate a collapse of the intervertebral space, with accompanying sclerosis of vertebral endplates, or an irregular roughened appearance to the vertebral endplate; in some cases abnormalities could not be detected. Myelography demonstrates extradural compression of the dye column. Treatment options are limited; surgical decompression via a ventral slot has been unsuccessfully attempted in one horse. Euthanasia is usually recommended if the horse demonstrates significant ataxia and associated pain.

References

[1] Hahn, C.N., Handel, I., Green, S.L. *et al.* (2008) Assessment of the utility of using intra- and intervertebral minimum sagittal diameter ratios in the diagnosis of cervical vertebral malformation in horses. *Vet Radiol Ultrasound*, 49, 1–6.

[2] Dreier, R. (2010) Hypertrophic differentiation of chondrocytes in osteoarthritis: the developmental aspect of degenerative joint disorders. *Arthritis Res Ther*, 12, 216–227.

[3] Powers, B.E., Stashak, T.S., Nixon, A.J. *et al.* (1986) Pathology of the vertebral column of horses with cervical static stenosis. *Vet Pathol*, 23, 392–399.

[4] Trostle, S.S., Dubielzig, R.R. and Beck, K. (1993) Examination of frozen cross sections of cervical spinal intersegments in nine horses with cervical vertebral malformation: lesions associated with spinal cord compression. *J Vet Diagn Invest*, 5, 423–431.

[5] Mitchell, C.W., Nykamp, S.G., Foster, R. *et al.* (2012) The use of magnetic resonance imaging in evaluating horses with spinal ataxia. *Vet Radiol Ultrasound*, 53, 613–620.

[6] Dyson, S.J. (2003) The cervical spine and soft tissues of the neck, in *Diagnosis and Management of Lameness in the Horse* (eds M.W. Ross and S.J. Dyson), W.B. Saunders, St. Louis, pp. 522–531.

[7] Withers, J., Voute, L., Hammond, G. and Lischer, C. (2009) Radiographic anatomy of the articular process joints of the caudal cervical vertebrae in the horse on lateral and oblique projections. *Equine Vet J*, 41, 895–902.

[8] Claridge, H., Piercy, R., Parry, A. and Weller, R. (2010) The 3D anatomy of the cervical articular process joints in the horse and their topographical relationship to the spinal cord. *Equine Vet J*, 42, 726–731.

[9] King, A.S. (1993) *Physiological and Clinical Anatomy of the Domestic Mammals. Volume 1: Central Nervous System*, 2nd edn, Oxford University Press, Oxford.

[10] Dyson, S.J. (2011) Lesions of the equine neck resulting in lameness or poor performance. *Vet Clin North Am Equine Pract*, 27, 417–437.

[11] Berg, L.C., Nielsen, J.V., Thoefner, M.B. and Thomsen, P.D. (2003) Ultrasonography of the equine cervical region: a descriptive study in eight horses. *Equine Vet J*, 35, 647–655.

[12] Zsoldos, R.R., Groesel, M., Kotschwar, A. *et al.* (2010) A preliminary modelling study on the equine cervical spine with inverse kinematics at walk. *Equine Vet J Suppl*, 42 (38), 516–522.

[13] Clayton, H.M. and Townsend, H.G.G. (1989) Kinematics of the cervical spine of the adult horse. *Equine Vet J*, 21, 189–192.

[14] Sleutjens, J., Voorhout, G., Van Der Kolk, J.H. *et al.* (2010) The effect of ex vivo flexion and extension on intervertebral foramina dimensions in the equine cervical spine. *Equine Vet J Suppl*, 42 (38), 425–430.

[15] Martel-pelletier, J. and Pelletier, J. (2010) Is osteoarthritis a disease involving only cartilage or other articular tissues? *Joint Dis Rel Surg*, 21, 2–14.

[16] Webb, A.L., Collins, P., Rassoulian, H. and Mitchell, B.S. (2011) Synovial folds—a pain in the neck? *Man Ther*, 16, 118–124.

[17] Benjamin, M., Redman, S., Milz, S. *et al.* (2004) Adipose tissue at entheses: the rheumatological implications of its distribution. A potential site of pain and stress dissipation? *Ann Rheum Dis*, 63, 1549–1555.

[18] Clayton, H., Kaiser, L., Lavagnino, M. and Stubbs, N. (2012) Evaluation of intersegmental vertebral motion during performance of dynamic mobilization exercises in cervical lateral bending in horses. *Am J Vet Res*, 73, 1153–1159.

[19] Schmidburg, I., Pagger, H., Zsoldos, R.R. *et al.* (2012) Movement associated reduction of spatial capacity of the equine cervical vertebral canal. *Vet J*, 192, 525–528.

[20] Stubbs, N.C., Hodges, P.W., Cowin, G. *et al.* (2006) Functional anatomy of the caudal thoracolumbar and lumbosacral spine in the horse. *Equine Vet J Suppl*, 38 (36), 393–399.

[21] Johnston, C., Holm, K., Faber, M. *et al.* (2010) Effect of conformational aspects on the movement of the equine back. *Equine Vet J Suppl*, 42 (34), 314–318.

[22] Cousty, M., Firidolfi, C., Geffroy, O. and David, F. (2011) Comparison of medial and lateral ultrasound-guided approaches for periarticular injection of the thoracolumbar intervertebral facet joints in horses. *Vet Surg*, 40, 494–499.

[23] Pagger, H., Schmidburg, I., Peham, C. and Licka, T. (2010) Determination of the stiffness of the equine cervical spine. *Vet J*, 186, 338–341.

[24] Nixon, A.J. (1996) Fractures of the vertebrae, in *Equine Fracture Repair* (ed. A. Nixon), W.B. Saunders, Philadelphia, pp. 299–312.

[25] Fisher, L.F., Bowman, K.F. and Macharg, M.A. (1981) Spinal ataxia in a horse caused by a synovial cyst. *Vet Pathol*, 18, 407–410.

[26] Machino, M., Yukawa, Y., Ito, K. and Kato, F. (2012) Cervical degenerative intraspinal cyst: a case report and literature review involving 132 cases. *BMJ Case Reports*, epub (Nov 28), 1–5.

[27] Girodroux, M., Dyson, S. and Murray, R. (2009) Osteoarthritis of the thoracolumbar synovial intervertebral articulations: clinical and radiographic features in 77 horses with poor performance and back pain. *Equine Vet J*, 41, 130–138.

[28] Stubbs, N.C., Riggs, C.M., Hodges, P.W. *et al.* (2010) Osseous spinal pathology and epaxial muscle ultrasonography in Thoroughbred racehorses. *Equine Vet J Suppl*, 42 (38), 654–661.

[29] Johnson, P.J., Johnson, G.C. and Pace, L.W. (1997) Thoracic vertebral malformation in two horses. *Equine Vet J*, 29, 493–496.

[30] Laynon, L. and Rubin, C.T. (1984) Static vs dynamic loads as an influence on bone remodelling. *J Biomech*, 17, 897–905.

[31] Prange, T., Derksen, F.J., Stick, J. and Garcia-Pereira, F.L. (2011) Endoscopic anatomy of the cervical vertebral canal in the horse: a cadaver study. *Equine Vet J*, 43, 317–323.

[32] Gold, J.R., Divers, T.J., Miller, A.J. *et al.* (2008) Cervical vertebral spinal hematomas in 4 horses. *J Vet Intern Med*, 22, 481–485.

[33] Mayhew, I.G. The equine spinal cord in health and disease 1: The healthy spinal cord. Proceedings of the Annual Meeting, American Association of Equine Practitioners. 1999;67–84.

[34] Mackay, R.J. (2012) Anatomy and physiology of the nervous system, in *Equine Surgery*, 4th edn (eds J. Auer and J. Stick), Elsevier Saunders, St. Louis, pp. 665–675.

[35] De Lahunta, A. and Glass, E.N. (2009) Large animal spinal cord disease, in *Veterinary Neuroanatomy and Clinical Neurology*, 3rd edn (eds A. de LaHunta and E. Glass), Saunders Elsevier, St. Louis, pp. 285–318.

[36] Yovich, J.V., LeCouteur, R., Gould, D.H. and Coutel, R.A.L. (1991) Chronic cervical compressive myelopathy in horses: clinical correlations with spinal cord alterations. *Aust Vet J*, 68, 326–334.

[37] Mayhew, I.G. The equine spinal cord in health and disease 2: The diseased spinal cord. Proceedings of the Annual Meeting, American Association of Equine Practitioners. 1999;67–84.

[38] Van Biervliet, J., Mayhew, J. and De Lahunta, A. (2006) Cervical vertebral compressive myelopathy: diagnosis. *Clin Tech Equine Pract*, 5, 54–59.

[39] Stewart, R., Reed, S.M. and Weisbrode, S.E. (1991) Frequency and severity of osteochondrosis in horses with cervical stenotic myelopathy. *Am J Vet Res*, 52, 873–879.

[40] Levine, J.M., Adam, E., MacKay, R.J. *et al.* (2007) Confirmed and presumptive cervical vertebral compressive myelopathy in older horses: a retrospective study (1992–2004). *J Vet Intern Med*, 21, 812–819.

[41] Down, S.S. and Henson, F.M.D. (2009) Radiographic retrospective study of the caudal cervical articular process joints in the horse. *Equine Vet J*, 41, 518–524.

[42] Whitwell, K.E. and Dyson, S. (1987) Interpreting radiographs 8: equine cervical vertebrae. *Equine Vet J*, 19, 8–14.

[43] Levine, J., Scrivani, P., Divers, T. *et al.* (2010) Multicenter case-control study of signalment, diagnostic features, and outcome associated with cervical vertebral malformation-malarticulation in horses. *J Am Vet Med Assoc*, 237, 812–822.

[44] Maher, O., Aleman, M., Puchalski, S. and Snyder, J.R. Sport horses with neurologic deficits and cervical vertebral osteoarthrosis presenting within one year of prepurchase examination: 18 cases (2000–2007). Proceedings of XIV Congress of the Italian Society of Equine Practitioners (SIVE) and Veterinary European Equine Meeting (FEEVA). Venice, Italy;2008.

[45] McDougall, J.J. (2006) Arthritis and pain. Neurogenic origin of joint pain. *Arthritis Res Ther*, 8, 220.

[46] Rubinstein, S. and Pool, J. (2007) A systematic review of the diagnostic accuracy of provocative tests of the neck for diagnosing cervical radiculopathy. *Eur Spine J*, 307–319.

[47] Van Biervliet, J. (2007) An evidence-based approach to clinical questions in the practice of equine neurology. *Vet Clin North Am Equine Pract*, 23, 317–28.

[48] Butler, J.B., Colles, C., Dyson, S. *et al.* (2012) The spine, in *Clinical Radiology of the Horse*, 3rd edn (eds J.A. Butler, C.M. Colles, S.M. Dyson, K.E. Kold and P.W. Poulos), Wiley-Blackwell, Chichester, pp. 505–572.

[49] Van Biervliet, J., Scrivani, P.V., Divers, T.J. *et al.* (2004) Evaluation of decision criteria for detection of spinal cord compression based on cervical myelography in horses: 38 cases (1981–2001). *Equine Vet J*, 36, 14–20.

[50] Elgersma, A.E., Wijnberg, I.D., Sleutjens, J. *et al.* (2010) A pilot study on objective quantification and anatomical modelling of in vivo head and neck positions commonly applied in training and competition of sport horses. *Equine Vet J Suppl*, 42 (38), 436–443.

[51] Wijnberg, I.D., Sleutjens, J., Van Der Kolk, J.H. and Back, W. (2010 Nov) Effect of head and neck position on outcome of quantitative neuromuscular diagnostic techniques in Warmblood riding horses directly following moderate exercise. *Equine Vet J Suppl*, 42, 261–267.

[52] Didierlaurent, D., Contremoulins, V., Denoix, J.-M. and Audigie, F. (2009) Scintigraphic pattern of uptake of 99mTechnetium by the cervical vertebrae of sound horses. *Vet Rec*, 164, 809–813.

[53] Nollet, H., Van Ham, L., Dewulf, J. *et al.* (2003) Standardization of transcranial magnetic stimulation in the horse. *Vet J*, 166, 244–250.

[54] Birmingham, S.S.W., Reed, S.M., Mattoon, J.S. and Saville, W.J. (2010) Qualitative assessment of corticosteroid cervical articular facet injection in symptomatic horses. *Equine Vet Ed*, 22, 77–82.

[55] Nielsen, J.V., Berg, L.C., Thoefnert, M.B. and Thomsen, P.D. (2003) Accuracy of ultrasound-guided intra-articular

injection of cervical facet joints in horses: a cadaveric study. *Equine Vet J*, 35, 657–661.

[56] Mattoon, J.S., Drost, W.T., Gruric, M.R. *et al.* (2004) Technique for equine cervical articular process joint injection. *Vet Radiol Ultrasound*, 45, 238–240.

[57] Meehan, L., Dyson, S. and Murray, R. (2009) Radiographic and scintigraphic evaluation of spondylosis in the equine thoracolumbar spine: a retrospective study. *Equine Vet J*, 41, 800–807.

[58] Vos, N.J., Pollock, P.J., Harty, M. *et al.* (2008) Fractures of the cervical vertebral odontoid in four horses and one pony. *Vet Rec*, 162, 116–119.

[59] Raes, E.V., Durie, I., Wegge, B. *et al.* (2014) Imaging findings of a haemangiosarcoma in a cervical vertebra of a horse. *Equine Vet Ed*, 26, 548–551.

[60] Giguere, S. and Lavoie, J.P. (1994) *Rhodococcus equi* vertebral osteomyelitis in 3 quarter horse colts. *Equine Vet J*, 26, 74–77.

[61] Furr, M.O., Anver, M. and Wise, M. (1991) Intervertebral disk prolapse and diskospondylitis in a horse. *J Am Vet Med Assoc*, 198, 2095–2096.

[62] Foss, R.R., Genetzky, R.M., Riedesel, E.A. and Graham, C. (1983) Cervical intervertebral disk protrusion in two horses. *Can Vet J*, 24, 188–191.

[63] Stadler, P., Van Den Berg, S.S. and Tustin, R.C. (1988) Servikale Intervertebrale Diskus Prolaps in 'N Perd. *J S Afr Vet Assoc*, 5, 31–32.

[64] Nixon, A.J., Stashak, T.S., Ingram, J.T. *et al.* (1984) Cervical intervertebral disk protrusion in a horse. *Vet Surg*, 11, 154–158.

31 Congenital Malformation of the Nervous System

Martin Furr

Marion duPont Scott Equine Medical Center, Virginia-Maryland Regional College of Veterinary Medicine, Leesburg, USA

Malformations of the central nervous system (CNS) are reported to be common [1], yet few reports exist in the equine literature and congenital CNS malformations appear to be rare in the horse. Laugier and colleagues reported an incidence of 2.4% among 543 horses with neurologic disease examined by postmortem; this total excluded cases of cervical vertebral instability [2]. Similar results were observed in another study that found congenital defects of the thoracolumbar spine in 2.9% of 443 horses [3]. In another survey of 773 equine fetuses or foals less than 5 days of age, a single case of nervous system abnormality was found—a foal with cerebral agenesis [4]. In a study comprising 608 foals with congenital defects that resulted in death, hydrocephalus was found in 3%, and cleft cranium with meningoencephalocele was observed in 1.6% [5]. Exposure to infectious agents, teratogenic chemicals, and plant teratogens has been described, although the cause in most cases remain undetermined. Cerebellar and cerebral hypoplasia and hydrocephalus were observed in two aborted equine fetuses secondary to hydrops allantois [6]; however, the "cause" in most cases is unknown. Clinically recognized syndromes related to malformation of the CNS in horses remain few, however (Table 31.1).

Brain

Numerous disorders of brain development are described in veterinary species, each of which may result in variable degrees of cranial nerve disorders. Cerebral hypoplasia with an associated meningoencephalocele was observed in a Belgian foal that was born dead, and cerebral agenesis was described in another foal that was born dead [1, 4]. Agenesis of the corpus collosum with cerebellar hypoplasia and dilation of the fourth ventricle represent a syndrome termed the "Dandy–Walker syndrome." This has been described in two foals that displayed severe ataxia, truncal sway, seizures, an erratic breathing pattern and a wide, dome-shaped forehead [16, 17]. Diagnosis was confirmed by CT scanning and postmortem. One foal survived, but had persistent ataxia, nystagmus, occasional intention tremors, and became aggressive, eventually prompting euthanasia.

Congenital encephalomyelopathy was observed in a Quarter Horse foal [14]. The foal was affected at birth and was unable to stand, and had coarse rhythmic rear limb tremors that were exaggerated when the foal was assisted into a standing position. Vital parameters and mentation were normal. Forelimb reflexes were normal however rear limb reflexes (patellar reflex) were exaggerated bilaterally. Blood and cerebrospinal fluid (CSF) evaluation was unremarkable. Postmortem examination found no gross abnormalities, but histologic examination found enlarged axons in all white matter tracts, with myelin degeneration; astrocytosis and gliosis were seen as well [14]. The cause of the disorder was not determined, but a genetic disorder was suspected, as the dam had produced two other foals with similar clinical signs.

Hydrocephalus

Hydrocephalus is defined as an increase in the volume of CSF, which can be classified as either compensatory or obstructive (internal). Obstructive hydrocephalus can be observed following aqueductal stenosis, or may be seen secondary to suppurative bacterial meningitis or cholesterol granulomas in older animals. In compensatory hydrocephalus, the CSF increases in volume to replace parenchyma that has been destroyed or failed to develop [1]. Congenital hydrocephalus has been recognized in neonatal foals [7–11].

Congenital hydrocephalus in foals appears to be rare, and is of variable severity. Many foals are aborted or born dead [8]. The condition is often associated with dystocia due to the grossly enlarged head (Figure 31.1).

Equine Neurology, Second Edition. Martin Furr and Stephen Reed.

Table 31.1 Listing of reported congenital abnormalities of the central nervous system of horses.

Condition	References
Brain	
Cerebellar hypoplasia	6
Cerebral hypoplasia/agenesis	4
Hydrocephalus	7–11
Meningoencephalocele	5
Meningomyelocele	12
Meningocele	13
Congenital encephalomyelopathy	14
Syringomyelia	15
Dandy–Walker syndrome	16, 17
Spine and spinal cord	
Cervical vertebral instability	See Chapter 28
Occipitoatlantoaxial malformation	18, 19
Lordosis	
Kyphosis	20, 21
Scoliosis/torticollis	22, 23
Block vertebrae	
Hemivertebrae	21
Spina bifida	13
Anomolous cervical vertebrae	24
Oldenburg ataxia	25
Spinal dysraphism	25
Agenesis of the dens	26
Transitional vertebrae	27
Cleft vertebral centrum	28

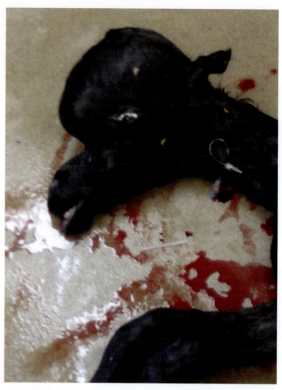

Figure 31.1 Hydrocephalus in a foal. (Photo courtesy of Dr. Stephen Reed.)

Hydrocephalus may be inherited, as one Standardbred stallion produced seven hydrocephalic foals out of a foal crop of 239 [8]. Inadequate numbers of foals were available for a full evaluation; however, the authors concluded that it was unlikely to be an X-linked or single autosomal-recessive defect.

Clinical signs resulting from hydrocephalus are variable. Foals may be born dead or they may be initially normal and develop clinical signs later (hours to days). Clinical signs reflect cerebral disease and include dullness, blindness, strabismus, and nystagmus; seizures may be seen as well.

Diagnosis is by observation and is aided in less obvious cases by radiography. An amorphous *ground glass* appearance may be seen, along with very thin cranial bones and the presence of open fontanels. Palpation of the skull may reveal open fontanels or areas of bone defect in the cranium. Ultrasonography can be used for confirmation [7]; however, CT or MRI is the optimal diagnostic imaging method. Some breeds, Arabians, in particular, typically have a very "domed" head at birth, and confirmation should be achieved before a diagnosis of hydrocephalus is made in these breeds.

Treatment of internal hydrocephalus has been attempted in one reported case, using a ventricular stent tunneled to the thoracic cavity to drain excess CSF. Although drainage of the excess CSF was achieved, the thoracic drain could not be placed, and the foal was euthanized on the first post-operative day due to complications and a grave prognosis [7] (Figure 31.1).

The spine and spinal cord

Reports regarding developmental defects of the equine vertebral column and spinal cord are sparse. Abnormalities of the vertebral column can include dorso-ventral deviations (kyphosis or lordosis) or lateral/rotational deviations (scoliosis), the direction of the deviation depending upon the specific shape of the developing vertebrae. Lordosis (ventral convexity) is usually seen in the thoracic area or extending over the thoracolumbar region, while kyphosis (dorsal convexity) is more commonly seen in the lumbar spine. Additional developmental abnormalities of the vertebrae include hemivertebrae.

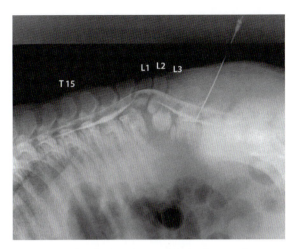

Figure 31.2 Left-right lateral view of the lumbar vertebrae. Lumbar myelography has been performed. Here, the needle is positioned at the L4–5 site with the needle tip placed in the ventral vertebral canal. In live horses, the optimal site for needle insertion during myelography is the lumbosacral site. Kyphosis of the lumbar vertebrae due to malformation of several lumbar vertebrae is visible. Dorsal deviation of the spinal cord and suspected compression of the spinal cord at L1 is noticeable. (Reprinted from Ref. [20].)

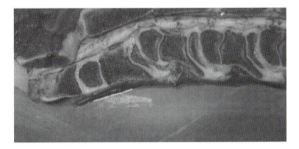

Figure 31.3 Sagittal section of the cervical spine of a foal. Note the wedge-shaped malformed cervical vertebra resulting in spinal compression.

Development of the vertebrae is complex, including three primary centers of ossification—one in the body and one for each side of the arch. Secondary ossification centers appear later at the top of the spinous process, the transverse processes, and the cranial and caudal epiphyses of the body. Improper timing or degree of ossification of these centers result in the abnormal shape of the vertebrae. If the central portion of the vertebrae does not form, then there are two unconnected hemivertebrae, which are termed "butterfly vertebrae." The so-called block vertebrae result from incomplete separation of the vertebral bodies or arches—these are usually stable and do not result in clinical signs.

Neurologic abnormalities may or may not result from these developmental abnormalities depending on their severity. Ataxia associated with severe kyphosis causing spinal cord compression has been described, and was demonstrated with a caudal myelogram [20]. Given their close proximity and intercalation, abnormalities of the ribs have also been seen in some cases [21], occasional impinging the brachial plexus or peripheral nerve roots with subsequent pain or dysfunction. Summers et al. report a foal with myelodysplasia and vertebral scoliosis [1]. The foal was reported to have no observable gait abnormality (Figures 31.2 and 31.3).

The meninges

Myelocele, meningomyelocele, and meningocele are rare congenital abnormalities of the spinal cord and meninges. A meningomyelocele is a protrusion of the meninges accompanied by portions of the spinal cord and associated nerve roots, while a myelocele involves prolapse of the dura mater. These defects are most commonly associated with spina bifida. A meningocele presents as a fluctuant mass that communicates with the spinal canal. A thoracic meningocele that was visible under the skin of the dorsal thorax that was successfully repaired has been reported in a foal [29]. This foal did not have obvious neurologic deficits. Meningomyelocele has also been described in the ventral cervical region of a foal that did not have spina bifida, but that did result in neurologic abnormalities [12].

Cervical spina bifida associated with a meningocele has been reported in an Appaloosa foal [13]. Other forms of myelodysplasia of the equine spinal cord have been reported including syringomyelia in a thoroughbred foal [15]. A prominent bunny-hopping gait with spasticity was observed in this foal.

Occipitoatalantoaxial malformation

The most commonly recognized and described syndrome associated with congenital vertebral abnormalities, with the exception of cervical vertebral instability, is occipitoatlantoaxial malformation (OAAM).

OAAM describes the syndrome of congenital disorders of the occiput, atlas, and axis. Although there are a number of variations, the basic abnormality involves fusion of the atlas and occiput, and hypoplasia of the atlas and dens [18, 19, 30]. Subluxation and scoliosis are variably seen. In addition, a foal with congenital luxation of the atlantoaxial joint has been described secondary to absence of the dens, and in which the occipitoatlantal joint appeared to be normal [26] (Figure 31.4).

The following are the four basic subtypes of the anomaly that are observed:

(i) Occipitalization (occipital bone-like modification) of the atlas and atlantization (atlas bone-like modification) of the axis (familial in Arabian horses),

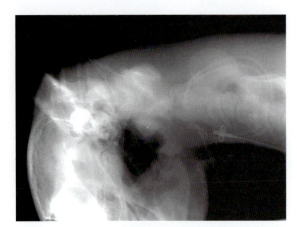

Figure 31.4 Radiograph of a foal which demonstrates occipitoatalantoaxial malformation. The dens is malformed and appears subluxated, and the atlas is malformed. (Photo courtesy of Dr. Robert MacKay.)

(ii) asymmetric malformations, (iii) Asymmetric atlantoaxial fusion, and (iv) OAAM with two atlases. A fifth type has been described which is comprised of changes similar to the familial Arabian form, but in non-Arabian horses [19].

Clinical neurologic signs in affected individuals can vary in onset and severity. Some affected horses may have only scoliosis without neurologic gait deficits [18]. Foals may be born dead due to compression of the medulla oblongata and spinal cord by unstable osseous structures, or the development of clinical signs may be delayed considerably. In the familial form, horses are usually noted to be affected at birth, but signs may not appear until later in life [18]. Clinical signs of pelvic limb ataxia did not develop until 3 years of age in one horse. A 3-year-old Quarterhorse had been ridden and shown successfully prior to demonstrating signs of incoordination and weakness [18].

Typically, neurologic abnormalities involve various degrees of ataxia and tetraparesis. Cutaneous hypalgesia of the cranial cervical area may be present, and scoliosis is variably present. In most cases, the horses have an abnormal head and neck carriage, with the neck extended. The atlas is usually palpably abnormal, and there may be visible swellings. An audible clicking sound is often heard when the horses' head is moved, associated with recurrent subluxation.

Diagnostic rule-outs include cervical trauma, other congenital malformations of the spinal cord, and cerebellar hypoplasia. Cervical compressive myelopathy should be considered, but usually it does not become apparent until later in life. Cerebellar hypoplasia can be differentiated by presence of intention tremors and dysmetria which is absent in horses with OAAM. The diagnosis is confirmed by radiography of the head and cranial cervical spine. Successful treatment has not been reported, and those cases with severe neurologic signs should be destroyed. Although not confirmed, it is considered that the defect in Arabian horses is hereditary; hence, affected horses should not be used for breeding.

References

[1] Summers BA. Malformations of the central nervous system. In: Summers BA, Cummings JF, de Lahunta A, eds. *Veterinary Neuropathology*, St. Louis:Mosby;1995:68–94.

[2] Laugier C, Tapprest J, Foucher N, et al. A necropsy survey of neurologic diseases in 4,319 horses examined in Normandy (France) from 1986 to 2006. *J Equine Vet Sci* 2009;29:561–568.

[3] Jeffcoat LB. Disorders of the thoracolumbar spine of the horse—a survey of 443 cases. *Equine Vet J* 1980;12:197–210.

[4] Collobert-Laugier C, Tariel G. Congenital abnormalities in foals. *Pratique Vétérinaire Equine* 1993;25:105–110.

[5] Crowe MW, Swerczek TW. Equine congenital defects. *Am J Vet Res* 1985;46:353–358.

[6] Waelchli RO, Ehrensperger F. Two related cases of cerebellar abnormality in equine fetuses associated with hydrops of fetal membranes. *Vet Rec* 1988;123:513–514.

[7] Foreman JH, Reed SM, Rantanen NW. Congenital internal hydrocephalus in a Quarter Horse foal. *J Equine Vet Sci* 1983;3:154–164.

[8] Ojala M, Ala-Huikku J. Inheritance of hydrocephalus in horses. *Equine Vet J* 1992;24:140–143.

[9] Carberry JT. A case of equine hydrocephalus. *N Z Vet J* 1979;27:158.

[10] Bester RC, Cimprich RE, Evans LH. Hydrocephalus in an 18-month-old-colt. *J Am Vet Med Assoc* 1976;168:1041–1042.

[11] Bowman RW. Congenital hydrocephalus in 2 foals. *Mod Vet Pract* 1980;61:862–864.

[12] Harmelin A, Egozi O, Nysaka A, et al. Ventral meningomyelocoele in a filly. *J Comp Pathol* 1993;109:93–97.

[13] Leathers CW, Wagner PC, Milleson BD. Cervical spina bifida with meningocele in an Appaloosa foal. *J Vet Orthop* 1979;1:55–58.

[14] Seahorn TL, Fuentealba IC, Illanes OG, et al. Congenital encephalomyelopathy in a Quarter Horse. *Equine Vet J* 1991;23:394–396.

[15] Cho DY, Leipold HW. Syringomyelia in a thoroughbred foal. *Equine Vet J* 1977;9:195–197.

[16] Cudd TA, Mayhew IG, Cottrill CM. Agenesis of the corpus collosum with cerebellar vermian hypoplasia in a foal resembling the Dandy-Walker syndrome: pre-mortem diagnosis by clinical evaluation and CT scanning. *Equine Vet J* 1989;21:378–381.

[17] Wong D, Winter M, Haynes J, et al. Dandy-Walker-like syndrome in a Quarter Horse colt. *J Vet Intern Med* 2007;21:1130–1134.

[18] Mayhew IG, Watson AG, Heissan JA. Congenital occipitoatlantoaxial malformations in the horse. *Equine Vet J* 1978;10:103–113.

[19] Wilson WD, Hughes SJ, Ghoshal NG, et al. Occipitoatlantoaxial malformation in two non-Arabian horses. *J Am Vet Med Assoc* 1985;187:36–40.

[20] de Heer N, Nout YS. Congenital kyphosis secondary to lumbar vertebral hypoplasia causing paraparesis in a Friesian foal. *Equine Vet Ed* 2011;23:231–234.

[21] Wong DM, Scarratt WK, Rohleder J. Hindlimb paresis associated with kyphosis, hemivertebrae and multiple thoracic vertebral malformations in a Quarter Horse gelding. *Equine Vet Ed* 2005;17:187–194.

[22] Boyd JS. Congenital deformities in two clydesdale foals. *Equine Vet J* 1976;8:161–164.

[23] Proctor PT. Foetal monstrosity in a thoroughbred mare resembling shistosomus reflexus. *Equine Vet J* 1982;14:340.

[24] Crochik SS, Barton MH, Eggleston RB, et al. Cervical vertebral anomaly and ventricular septal defect in an Arabian foal. *Equine Vet Ed* 2009;21:207–211.

[25] Huston R, Saperstein GT, Leipold HW. Congenital defects in foals. *J Equine Med Surg* 1977;1:46–61.

[26] Witte S, Alexander K, Bucellato M, et al. Congenital atlantoaxial luxation associated with malformation of the dens axis in a Quarter Horse foal. *Equine Vet Ed* 2005;17:175–178.

[27] Haussler KK, Stover SM, Willits NH. Developmental variation in lumbosacralpelvic anatomy of thoroughbred racehorses. *Am J Vet Res* 1997;58:1083–1091.

[28] Doige CE. Congenital cleft vertebral centrum and intra- and extraspinal cyst in a foal. *Vet Pathol* 1996;33:87–89.

[29] Van Hoogmoed L, Yarbrough TB, Lecouteur RA, et al. Surgical repair of a thoracic meningocele in a foal. *Vet Surg* 1999;28:496–500.

[30] Gonda C, Crisman M, Moon M. Occipitoatlantoaxial malformation in a Quarter Horse foal. *Equine Vet Ed* 2001;13:289–291.

32 Central Nervous System Trauma

Yvette S. Nout-Lomas

College of Veterinary Medicine, Colorado State University, Fort Collins, USA

Trauma to the central nervous system (CNS) is a significant cause of neurologic disease in horses; however, very few studies provide data on prevalence of traumatic CNS injury. The most recent report is an international multicenter study on causes of sudden death among racing Thoroughbreds, which shows CNS trauma to account for 18 out of 143 (13%) cases of sudden death in racing Thoroughbred horses [1]. In that study, spinal cord injury (SCI) was more commonly seen (60% of cases) than traumatic brain injury (TBI) [1]. An older study from Europe reported CNS trauma to account for 22% of neurologic disorders [2], which is similar to an Australia report in which CNS trauma accounted for 24% of neurological case [3]. Similar to other studies, trauma to the spinal cord was shown to be more prevalent than brain injury. Feige et al. reported a diagnosis of TBI in 5 out of 22 (23%) horses that were presented for traumatic neurologic disease, whereas 17 of the 22 (77%) were diagnosed with SCI [2]. Tyler et al. reported 47 cases of TBI and cranial nerve disease in 107 (44%) horses examined, whereas 60 horses in this group had SCI (56%) [3].

Although mechanisms of CNS cell damage, to a certain degree, are similar after TBI and SCI, there are a few processes with regards to etiology, pathophysiology, and treatment that are different for TBI and SCI. Clinical syndromes as a result of traumatic injury to the CNS can vary tremendously, but the most common are abnormal level of consciousness, abnormal behavior, cranial nerve deficits, vestibular disease, tetra- and paraparesis or paraplegia, and cauda equina syndrome. Treatment regimens for CNS injury are directed toward reducing inflammation and swelling, halting secondary injury mechanisms, and promoting regenerative and plasticity mechanisms to improve functional recovery. Prognosis depends primarily on severity of primary injury and on the neuroanatomic location and extent of CNS damage. Recovery of function in the short term can be helpful in determination of long-term prognosis.

Etiology

Traumatic brain injury

A review of 34 cases of TBI in horses found that in 44% of cases injury was sustained to the poll subsequent to rearing and falling over backward during halter training or restraint [4]. Other causes of head injury included struggling from entrapment in a fence or subsequent to becoming prone in a stall, recovery from anesthesia, collision with a tree, and kicks by another horse. The cause of trauma was unknown for 12 (35%) horses. Nine of the 15 horses in this report were less than 1 year of age [4].

Although traumatic injury to the head is reported to be common in horses, subsequent CNS injury was present in only half of the horses presented for head trauma had evidence of TBI [5]. The remaining horses typically present for fractures of the orbit; periorbital rim; and zygomatic, mandibular, or maxillary bones [5, 6]. Impact to the head causes bony deformation, which may be transient, or may result in fracture or separation of the bones of the calvarium. Fractures may be linear, stellate, compound, comminuted, or depressed and TBI may occur with or without fracture of the calvarium. Within the closed calvarium, the sum of the intracranial volumes of the brain, blood, and cerebrospinal fluid (CSF) is constant, and volume or pressure changes within one of these compartments will affect the volume or pressure of the other compartments (Monroe-Kellie Doctrine). For example, the presence of hematomas or brain swelling after trauma will rapidly lead to increased intracranial pressure (ICP) with subsequent reduction of cerebral perfusion pressure (CPP) and cerebral blood flow (CBF), with potential for further damage or herniation of brain matter.

Feary et al. reported fractures of the calvarium in 65% of TBI cases [4]. Impact sustained to the poll in horses that flip over backward can result in fracture of the bones on the side and base of the calvarium such as

Equine Neurology, Second Edition. Martin Furr and Stephen Reed.

© 2015 John Wiley & Sons, Inc. Published 2015 by John Wiley & Sons, Inc.

Companion website: www.wiley.com/go/furr/neurology

the petrous temporal, squamous temporal, and parietal bones. However, more commonly these bones remain intact and more serious injury occurs to the basilar bones as a result of strong traction forces from the rectus capitis ventralis muscles [7–9]. Fractures of the basilar (basisphenoid and basioccipital) and temporal bones associated with poll impact have been identified in 44% of TBI cases [4]. The ventral aspect of the basi-occipital and basisphenoid bones is the insertion site of the paired rectus capitis ventralis muscles, which are the main flexors of the head. They originate at the cervical vertebrae and sudden extension of the head stretches these muscles, which commonly results in fracture of the bony tubercles from the basilar bones. Additionally, adjacent large vessels are lacerated and hemorrhage into the retropharyngeal spaces or gut-tural pouches can occur [10]. In severe cases, transverse fracture of the basilar bones at the level of the basioc-cipital-basisphenoidal suture can occur. Young horses appear more susceptible to poll injury, likely due to a combination of behavioral responses and because the suture between the basilar bones remains open until 2–5 years of age. In most cases, the fracture site is stable and minimal displacement occurs. Despite this, serious damage of associated soft tissue such as subdural or subarachnoid bleeding around the brain stem and cranial nerve damage may occur. The cere-bellum is seldom severely damaged after poll impact [9], while the cerebral parenchyma is more commonly injured after being subjected to rapid acceleration–deceleration forces. Moreover, optic nerves and other attachments may be torn from the cerebral hemi-spheres [11].

Impact to the dorsal surface of the head may result in damage to the frontal or parietal bones with subsequent cerebral cortical injury or, more commonly, damage to the cervical vertebrae with subsequent SCI [9]. Also, cranial nerve XII may be injured as it exits the hypoglossal foramen. Furthermore, occipital cortical injury may occur and with frontal injuries the optic nerves may be stretched as described for poll impact injuries.

Another type of head injury that may lead to CNS damage is fracture of the petrous temporal bone associ-ated with temporohyoid osteoarthropathy. The cause of this disorder remains unknown [12, 13]. Temporohyoid osteoarthropathy is a chronic condition in which fusion of the temporal and stylohyoid bones, stricture of the external ear canal, and obliteration of the lumen of the tympanic bullae occur [12, 14, 15]. Forces applied to this immobilized joint can cause fractures of the skull of which a common sequela is damage to the vestibular apparatus or cranial nerve VII. Another sequela is extension of infection in the middle/inner ear to the brain stem, additional cranial nerves, or hindbrain.

Table 32.1 Classification of traumatic brain injury.

Mechanism	Blunt	Most common in horses
	Penetrating (e.g., gunshot)	Can occur with high or low velocity
	Blast	
Severity	Mild	Neurologic examination
	Moderate	
	Severe	
Morphology	Skull fracture	Vault
		Basilar—most common in horses
	Intracranial	Focal
		Diffuse (concussion, diffuse axonal injury)

TBI can be classified according to mechanism of injury, injury severity, and anatomical structures involved in the damage. This is shown in Table 32.1.

Spinal cord injury

Trauma to the vertebral column is typically caused by incidents such as collision with an immovable object or falling. A recent study demonstrated vertebral fractures to account for 10% of fatal musculoskeletal injuries in Quarter Horse racehorses [16]. Injury to the vertebral column can occur at all sites, but predilection sites for vertebral trauma in adult horses are the occipital-atlanto-axial region, the caudal cervical region (C5–T1), and the caudal thoracic region [17, 18]. Although trauma to or fractures of the cervical vertebrae are the most common [2, 3, 16–18], reports of injury at other sites along the vertebral column exist [16, 19–22]. Foals appear to be more susceptible to vertebral trauma than adults and frequently suffer injury to the cranial cervical (C1–3), and caudal thoracic (T15–18) regions [17]. Fractures elsewhere along the vertebral column occur as well; three foals with vertebral fractures between C3–6 have been described as well as SCI in a foal with a T10 vertebral fracture secondary to osteomyelitis [23, 24].

Hyperextension, hyperflexion, dislocation, and compression of the vertebral column can result in varying severities of osseous damage and/or SCI. When a horse nosedives with the head under the body, neck hyperflexion can lead to damage in the occipital-atlanto-axial and caudal cervical regions. Spinal cord injury, however, may or may not be associated with fracture of the vertebrae, and injury at the level of the occipital-atlanto-axial site is frequently not associated with fracture [18]. Tearing or avulsion of the ligaments of the dens can result in severe compression of the spinal cord at the level of the occipital-atlanto-axial region. Injury to the caudal cervical spinal cord can occur in the absence of a fracture, subsequent to local hemorrhage following a primary insult. Fractures of the mid-thoracic to cranial lumbar region are often associated with tremendous forces sustained when a horse lands on its back. These fractures are often unstable; however in horses, muscle spasms can temporarily stabilize these lesions [18].

Typically, the more severe the insult, the more the damage to the vertebral column, and the more severe the clinical signs due to soft tissue damage and osseous fragments compressing the spinal cord. With very severe injury, soft tissue structures supporting the vertebral column may be disrupted, resulting in dislocation of vertebrae. Both subluxation and luxation of vertebrae have been reported in horses [25, 26]. There is an increased incidence of luxations, subluxations, and epiphyseal separations in young horses which are likely due to the fact that cervical vertebral growth plate closure does not occur until 4–5 years of age [17]. Compression injuries are associated with shortening of the vertebral body and result from a head-on collision with an immovable object.

Pathophysiology

Traumatic brain injury

After trauma, forces are transmitted to the intracranial soft tissues, and the brain is consequently shaken within the uneven bony interior of the skull and/or directly damaged by osseous fragments or foreign bodies. Most severe damage generally takes place at the place of impact (coup), and/or opposite to the side of impact (contrecoup). Additionally, the brain is subjected to other forces after trauma, such as rotational and shock wave forces. The principal mechanisms of TBI are classified as focal brain damage due to contact injury resulting in contusion, laceration, and intracranial hemorrhage or diffuse brain damage due to acceleration–deceleration injury resulting in widespread axonal injury or brain swelling. Outcome from head injury is determined by two substantially different mechanisms/stages, the first being the primary insult (primary damage, mechanical damage) occurring at the moment of impact. In treatment terms, this type of injury is exclusively sensitive to preventive but not therapeutic measures. The second is the secondary insult (secondary damage, delayed nonmechanical damage) which represents consecutive pathological processes initiated at the moment of injury with delayed clinical presentation. In TBI, most secondary damage is caused by brain swelling, with an increase in ICP and a subsequent decrease in cerebral perfusion leading to ischemia. These types of injury are sensitive to therapeutic interventions.

Primary damage is a result of the biomechanical effects of the injury and is characterized by immediate and often irreversible damage to neuronal cell bodies, dendritic arborizations, axons, glial cells, and brain vasculature. This initial brain injury may be focal, multifocal, or diffuse. By contrast, secondary injury is a complex cascade of molecular, cellular, and biochemical events that can occur for days to months following the initial insult, resulting in delayed tissue damage. In addition, systemic alterations further contribute to the tissue damage. Hypoxia, ischemia, brain swelling, alterations in ICP, hydrocephalus, infection, breakdown of blood–brain barrier (BBB), impaired energy metabolism, altered ionic homeostasis, changes in gene expression, inflammation, and activation/release of autodestructive molecules occur and exacerbate the initial injury. Components of both primary and secondary CNS injury are shown in Table 32.2.

In humans, diffuse axonal injury is widely considered the most important pathology in severe TBI and accounts for a high percentage of mortality due to brain trauma [27–29]. More recently, there is evidence to suggest diffuse axonal injury also plays an important role in the pathophysiology of mild TBI in humans [30]. Diffuse axonal injury results from forces that rapidly rotate and deform the brain and, pathologically, encompasses a spectrum of abnormalities from primary mechanical breaking of the axonal cytoskeleton, to transport interruption, swelling, and proteolysis, through secondary physiological changes [31].

The cascade of secondary injury that results in necrotic and apoptotic cell death is reviewed in the literature on a regular basis [32–35]. Hemorrhage, ischemia, and the primary tissue damage lead to sequestration of vasoactive and inflammatory mediators at the injury site. Inflammation and endothelial damage causes derangements in normal cerebrovascular reactivity and contribute to a mismatch of oxygen delivery to tissue demand, resulting in local or diffuse ischemia. Uncontrolled glutamate release and failure of energy systems in neuronal and supporting tissues lead to elevated intracellular calcium concentrations and subsequent cell death.

A major consequence of ischemia is reduced delivery of oxygen and glucose. Blood flow interruption is responsible for disruption in ion homeostasis (especially calcium, sodium, and potassium), and a switch to anaerobic glycolysis resulting in lactic acid production and acidosis. Cell membrane lipid peroxidation with subsequent prostaglandin and thromboxane synthesis, formation of reactive oxygen species, NO, and energy failure also ensue. Because of the high metabolic rate and oxygen demand of the brain, disruption of blood flow rapidly compromises the energy-supplying processes and leads to impaired nerve cell function and

Table 32.2 Characteristics of primary injury and factors that play a role in the multidimensional cascade of secondary injury after CNS trauma.

Primary injury	Secondary injury	
	CNS	Systemic
1. Mechanical injury	1. Vascular:	1. Hypoxia
	(a) impaired regulation of local and systemic blood pressure	2. Hypotension
	(b) impaired cerebrovascular and spinal cord blood flow autoregulation	3. Hyperglycemia
2. Hemorrhage	(c) blood flow mismatch	4. Fever
	(d) breakdown of blood-brain and blood-spinal cord barrier	5. Seizures
3. Diffuse axonal injury	(e) vasospasm	
	2. Edema formation	
	3. Impaired oxygenation	
	4. Metabolic dysfunction	
	5. Ionic concentration alterations	
	6. Inflammatory tissue response	
	7. Excitotoxicity and neurotransmitter accumulation	
	8. Oxidative stress:	
	(a) reactive oxygen species	
	(b) lipid peroxidation	
	9. Influx of serum proteins, calpain proteases, and metalloproteinases	
	10. Cell death:	
	(a)necrosis	
	(b)apoptosis	

even cell death. Impaired mitochondrial function with subsequent energy depletion leads to a loss in maintenance of membrane potentials resulting in depolarization of neurons and glia. Cytotoxic edema develops through the failure of the sodium–potassium ATPase-dependent pump in the presence of hypoxia, and the subsequent influx of water that passively follows sodium and chloride. This type of edema occurs in gray and white matter and decreases the extracellular fluid volume [36]. If capillary endothelial cells are edematous, the capillary lumen size will diminish, creating an increased resistance to arterial flow. Capillary permeability is usually not directly affected in cytotoxic edema. Major decreases in cerebral function occur with cytotoxic edema, with stupor and coma being common signs [36]. In addition to cytotoxic edema, vasogenic edema develops as a result of disruption of the BBB, which includes damage of endothelial cells, degeneration of pericytes, and loss of astrocytes. Extravasation of blood components and water occurs resulting in increased extracellular fluid accumulation. Cerebral white matter is especially vulnerable to vasogenic edema, possibly owing to its low capillary density and blood flow. Vasogenic edema displaces cerebral tissue and increases ICP.

The principles of increased ICP are described by the Monro–Kellie doctrine which states that three nearly incompressible volumes (i.e., blood, CSF, and brain parenchyma) exist within the rigid cranial vault [37]. Consequently, an increase in volume of one of those compartments must increase ICP unless it is compensated by an equivalent decrease within other compartment volumes. Blood flow to the brain is controlled by changes in diameter of resistance blood vessels and CBF is controlled by autoregulation whereby the CPP (mean arterial blood pressure minus ICP) is maintained within a range of approximately 50–150 mmHg. Beyond these limits, CBF decreases at pressures below the lower limit and increases at pressures above the higher limit. Although there are no reports of these parameters in horses after TBI, Brosnan et al. have shown that in anesthetized healthy horses, horses are able to autoregulate CBF to some extent; however, a significant reduction in perfusion was seen when mean arterial blood pressure was lowered to 60 mmHg and when horses are tilted into the head-down position ICP increases and CBF decreases [38, 39].

Cerebral perfusion pressure is the stimulus to which the autoregulatory response of the vasculature responds. Cerebral autoregulation is altered unpredictably after

TBI, and it appears that the minimum acceptable CPP is higher than normal after trauma [40]. Increased ICP leads to a decreased CPP and subsequently reduces CBF. Reduced CBF results in areas of ischemia and subsequent restriction of delivery of substrates such as oxygen and glucose to the brain. Intracranial hypertension and cerebral hypoperfusion are associated with poor outcomes in humans with TBI, and presumably horses as well. The development of cerebral ischemia within the brainstem initiates a reflex during which systemic arterial pressure increases to preserve CPP and CBF. This systemic pressor response to intracranial hypertension is termed the "Cushing response." Persistently increased ICP and reduction of CBF result in increased sympathetic discharge (catecholamines) with subsequent myocardial ischemia and development of cardiac arrhythmias, which is referred to as the "brain–heart syndrome."

Vascular damage that occurs after head injury can occur intraaxial (intraparenchymal and intraventricular) or extraaxial (within the skull but outside the brain tissue). Extraaxial hemorrhage encompasses epidural (between dura mater and the skull), subdural (between the dura mater and arachnoid mater), and subarachnoid hemorrhage (between arachnoid mater and pia mater). In dogs, recent evidence suggests extraaxial hemorrhage to occur in 10% of animals with mild and over 80% of animals with severe head injury [34]. Evidence of hemorrhage into the CSF (increased red blood cells and erythrocytophagia) occurs commonly in horses with CNS trauma [6, 41]. Hematoma formation is of special concern because of the potential for devastating expansion within the rigid calvarium, as can occur with edema. These processes displace brain tissue, with possible sequelae being herniation, pressure necrosis, and brainstem compression. Additionally, hemorrhage around the interventricular foramen or mesencephalic aqueduct may obstruct CSF outflow and lead to hydrocephalus. Furthermore, elevation of ICP after TBI due to hemorrhage and development of edema is of particular concern.

Traumatic brain injury combines mechanical stress to brain tissue with an imbalance between CBF and metabolism, excitotoxicity, edema formation, and inflammatory and apoptotic processes. Understanding the multidimensional cascade of injury offers therapeutic options including the management of CPP, mechanical (hyper-)ventilation, therapy to improve oxygenation and to reduce ICP, and pharmacological intervention to reduce excitotoxicity and ICP.

Spinal cord injury

Spinal cord injury secondary to trauma is a dynamic process of which the severity is related to the velocity, degree, and duration of the impact and subsequent compression of nervous tissue. Blunt injuries to the spinal cord occur under a variety of loading conditions, including flexion, extension, axial load, rotation, and distraction. Forces that produce the primary mechanical insult to the spinal cord in their mildest form result in cord concussion with brief transient neurologic deficits, and in their most severe form result in complete and permanent paralysis. Cord concussion with transient neurologic deficits is a result of local axonal depolarization and transient dysfunction, whereas permanent paralysis is a result of primary tissue injury followed by spreading of secondary damage that expands from the injury epicenter.

Primary injury is the initial mechanical damage to the components of the spinal cord that follows acute insult. Blood vessels are broken, axons are disrupted, and neuron and glial cell membranes are damaged. Consequences of primary injury are predominantly visible in the central gray matter. Immediately after injury, the gray matter at the region of impact contains disrupted cells and blood; however, the surrounding white matter and the gray matter cranial and caudal to the impact region can appear remarkably intact. The reason for this is not entirely clear, but is most likely related to the rich blood supply and increased metabolic requirements for oxygen and glucose of the nerve cell bodies in the gray matter, and the biomechanical properties of the myelin ensheathed axons in the surrounding white matter. Ensuing pathophysiological processes involving ischemia, release of chemicals from injured cells, and electrolyte shifts alter the metabolic milieu at the level of the lesion and trigger a secondary injury cascade that substantially compounds initial mechanical damage (see Figure 32.1 and Table 32.2). These secondary injury processes do not necessarily coincide with the clinical picture, as pathologic changes may progress in severity for weeks to months, even in the face of clinical improvement.

Secondary injury is responsible for both expansion of the injury site and limiting restorative processes. Although mechanisms involved in this are not fully understood, some aspects of these processes are well described (Figure 32.1) and reviewed [43–46]. The phase of secondary injury is widely studied since this process progresses from minutes to months after injury and is, thus, considered to be a target for therapeutic interventions. Minimizing secondary injury through protection of neural elements that initially survived the mechanical injury would increase the quantity of spared tissue and could lead to improved recovery of function.

Acute injury results in immediate hemorrhage and cell destruction within the central gray matter. This early, often progressive, hemorrhage is one of the hallmarks of acute SCI. Loss of microcirculation involving predominantly capillaries and venules subsequently spreads over considerable distance cranial

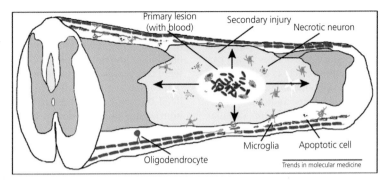

Figure 32.1 Secondary spinal cord injury. Initial trauma to the cord is directed to the central gray matter, where frank destruction occurs. The initial injury is followed by a cascade of biochemical events (secondary injury) that is thought to enlarge the area of cell death through necrosis and apoptosis. Neurons and glial cells at the margins of the expanding lesion represent a target for neuroprotection. When axons in the white matter are damaged, Wallerian degeneration can induce microglial activation and apoptotic cell death of oligodendrocytes long after the initial injury. This later microglial activation represents another potential target for treatments that reduce microglial activation and/or oligodendrocyte apoptosis. (Used with permission from Ref. [42], © Elsevier.)

and caudal to the site of injury. Furthermore, the cord swells within minutes of injury mainly due to hemorrhage and development of edema. The initial hemorrhage, edema, and hypoperfusion of the gray matter extends centripetally within minutes to hours of injury and results in central necrosis, white matter edema, and eventually, demyelination of axons through secondary injury processes. Spinal cord ischemia develops over several hours after injury and is considered one of the most important contributors to secondary injury. The mechanical disruption of the microvasculature causes petechial hemorrhage and intravascular thrombosis, which in combination with vasospasm of intact vessels and edema can lead to profound local hypoperfusion and ischemia. Cord swelling (e.g., tissue pressure) that exceeds venous blood pressure results in secondary ischemia, and loss of autoregulation makes the cord vulnerable to systemic hypotension. Spinal cord injury can therefore be markedly worsened under ischemic and hypoxic conditions, highlighting the importance of maintaining normotension after SCI.

During the ischemic/hypoxic state, cell metabolism is altered such that a shift occurs from aerobic to anaerobic metabolism, which is a less efficient method of energy production. Anaerobic metabolism results in lactic acid accumulation, causing acidosis in nervous tissue, thus decreasing glucose and oxygen consumption. Furthermore, lactic acid stimulates prostaglandin production, adenosine diphosphate release, platelet aggregation, thromboxane A2 release, vasospasm, vasoconstriction, and the inhibition of neurotransmitter release. In addition, in hypoxic states, the sodium–potassium ATPase-dependent cell pump is inhibited or damaged, resulting in the cell's inability to maintain its electrical polarity. Damage to this pump allows for

accumulation of potassium extracellularly and sodium intracellularly, which contributes to the development of edema.

Free radicals can cause progressive oxidation of fatty acids in cellular membranes (lipid peroxidation) through reactions with their unpaired electrons. Furthermore, oxidative stress can disable key mitochondrial respiratory chain enzymes, alter DNA/RNA and their associated proteins, and inhibit sodium–potassium ATPase. These changes can induce metabolic collapse and necrotic or apoptotic cell death and are considered important during the initial period of hypoperfusion, and perhaps even more important during the period of reperfusion. In addition to oxidative stress and membrane damage, NO production and excitatory amino-acid-induced calcium entry are considered important mediators of necrotic and apoptotic cell death [42].

Excitotoxicity refers to the deleterious cellular effects of excess glutamate and aspartate stimulation of ionotropic and metabotropic receptors. Extracellular concentrations of both of these excitatory amino acids are increased after acute SCI, which occurs through release from damaged neurons, decreased uptake by damaged astrocytes, and through depolarization-induced release. Ionotropic receptors include the N-methyl-D-aspartate (NMDA) and alpha-amino-3-hydroxy-5-methyl-4-isoxazole propionic acid (AMPA)/kainite receptors through which extracellular calcium and sodium can pass down a massive concentration gradient into the cell, or when activated can result in release of calcium from intracellular stores. Metabotropic glutamate receptors are coupled to G proteins that act as secondary intracellular messengers to mediate a wide spectrum of cellular functions. Furthermore, elevation of intracellular calcium concentration can occur through direct membrane damage and voltage-gated calcium channels triggered by membrane depolarization. Increased intracellular calcium concentrations can trigger a multitude of calcium-dependent processes that can lethally alter cellular metabolism, such as activation of lytic enzymes (calpains, phospholipase A2, proteases, and lipoxygenase), generation of free radicals, impairment of mitochondrial function, spasm of vascular smooth muscle, and binding of phosphates with subsequent depletion of cell energy sources. Sodium dysregulation is thought to be important in the pathophysiology of damage to axonal and glial components in the white matter through similar mechanisms that lead to elevated intracellular calcium concentrations.

The role of inflammation, both local and systemic, in acute SCI has gained much interest over the past decade, particularly because the effects of inflammatory cells can be both protective and damaging. After SCI, the injury site is rapidly infiltrated by blood-borne neutrophils, which can secrete lytic enzymes and cytokines. Later, blood-borne macrophages and monocytes are recruited, as well as locally activated resident microglia, both of which subsequently invade to phagocytize the injured tissue. These and other reactive cells produce cytokines such as tumor necrosis factor alpha, interleukins, and interferons, that mediate the inflammatory response and can further damage local tissue and recruit other inflammatory cells. It has been suggested that the early inflammatory phases are deleterious in nature, whereas the later inflammatory events appear to be protective. Systemic immune suppression is now well documented to occur after stroke, TBI, and SCI [47]. This CNS injury-induced immune depression is characterized by apoptosis of splenocytes, impaired production of cytokines from leukocytes and leukopenia. This reduced immune capacity is accompanied by a prolonged stress response in which levels of catecholamines and cortisol are elevated in the tissue, the circulation or both after SCI.

Clinical signs and diagnostics

Traumatic brain injury
Clinical signs associated with head trauma in the horse range from inapparent to recumbency with unconsciousness or death. In the 34 cases reviewed by Feary et al., the most common neurological deficit reported was ataxia (65%) [4]. This was followed by nystagmus (56%), abnormal mentation (56%), abnormal pupil size, symmetry, or pupillary light response (47%), and head tilt (44%) [4]. Noteworthy is that many horses presented with multiple neurological deficits; 29% of cases presented with a triad of clinical signs, namely ataxia, nystagmus, and abnormal mentation. Other deficits identified in this group of horses included prolonged recumbency (duration > 4 h), epistaxis, facial nerve paralysis, strabismus, seizure, otorrhea, dysphagia, blindness, and unconsciousness. Most horses (~80%) were tachycardic on presentation [4].

A complete physical examination is very important in head trauma cases, as fractures and other concurrent injuries are not uncommon and require identification and treatment. Life-threatening injuries should be attended to first and then a complete neurologic examination should be performed. Horses may be recumbent and/or intractable following a traumatic incident and examination and management of these horses can be difficult and dangerous [48]. Sedation may be necessary for examination. Although alpha 2 agonists may transiently cause hypertension, which may potentiate intracranial hemorrhage [18], xylazine has been found to cause a minor decrease in CSF pressure in normal, conscious horses [49]. It is believed that xylazine is probably a safe sedative to use in horses with head trauma, if the horse's head is not allowed to drop to such a low position that postural effects could lead to physiological increases of intracranial pressure [5].

Hemorrhage from the nose is typically venous blood originating from a paranasal sinus, ethmoturbinate, or nasal cavity. Occasionally, arterial blood is seen which most likely originates from larger vessels in the guttural pouches [9, 10]. Respiratory distress can occur associated with significant throat swelling after profuse hemorrhage into the guttural pouches. Furthermore, neurogenic pulmonary edema has been reported to occur. The pathophysiology of the development of neurogenic pulmonary edema appears to be associated with a sudden increase in ICP which upregulates sympathetic signal transduction to ensure brain perfusion. Immediate consequences are an increased tonus of venous and arterial vessels and increased myocardial function. However, if systemic vascular resistance increases excessively, left ventricular failure and finally pulmonary edema may result. Additionally, the presence of protein-rich edema fluid suggests altered endothelial permeability within the pulmonary circuit, which may be caused by the acute pressure increase and neurohumoral mechanisms.

The complete neurologic examination should include an assessment of the horse's mentation, cranial nerve function, posture, and ability to coordinate movements as well as its ability to regulate rate and range of motion. Also, reflex and nociceptive testing should be performed to investigate any concurrent SCI. Figure 32.2 provides an outline for localizing the level of brain injury based on the neurologic findings. Serial neurologic examinations, particularly during the first hours, are important for diagnostic and prognostic purposes, as well as assessing response to therapy. Pupil size, symmetry, and

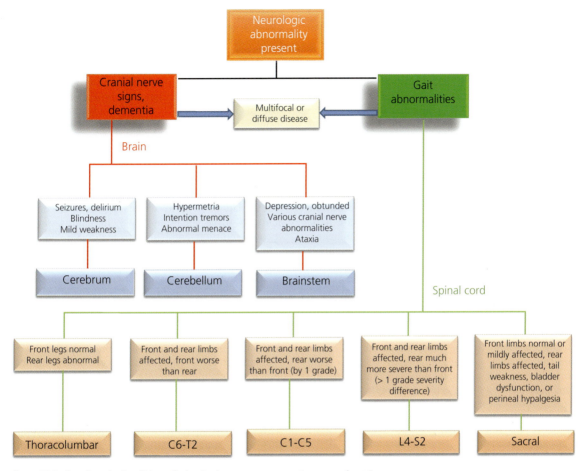

Figure 32.2 Flowchart for localizing a lesion in the nervous system in a recumbent horse.

response to light should be assessed in all horses, and followed carefully. A change from bilateral pupillary constriction to bilateral dilation with no response to light is a poor prognostic indicator [5].

The most common neurological syndromes following head trauma are a result of hemorrhage into the middle and inner ear cavities. Signs are those of central or peripheral vestibular disease and facial nerve damage and include recumbency, head tilt, neck turn, body lean, and circling, all toward the side of the lesion. The ipsilateral eye may be rotated ventrally and laterally, and there may be horizontal or rotary nystagmus with the fast phase away from the lesion [9, 18]. Facial paralysis on the same side as the lesion is seen with cranial nerve VII damage. Central vestibular disease is suspected when signs of brain stem disease of more cranial nerve deficits are present. Central vestibular lesions can result in a paradoxic vestibular syndrome, in which the lesion is located on the side opposite to that

which is expected from the clinical signs [9]. More serious trauma can lead to alterations of mentation and/or behavior.

The level of consciousness is affected by the degree of damage to the cerebrum and reticular activating system (RAS) in the brain stem. Immediately after cerebral injury, there is a period of concussion with unconsciousness for various periods of time; usually a horse recovers from this in minutes to hours. Comatose horses may have an irregular breathing pattern with periods of either Cheyne–Stokes breathing or hyperventilation. In some horses, seizures can occur after initial concussion; these are typically generalized seizures. Level of mentation and responsiveness to reflexes should be assessed and recorded. Injury to the occipital cortex can result in impairment of vision and menace response of the eye contralateral to the lesion; the pupillary light reflex should remain intact. Injury to the parietal cortex can result in decreased facial sensation on the contralateral side. Another sign of cerebral damage is dementia, or altered behavior, such as walking in circles (toward the side of the lesion), head pressing, hyperexcitability, or aggression [5, 9, 18].

Severe rostral brainstem injuries (mesencephalon) can be associated with coma and depression due to damage to the RAS. Strabismus, asymmetric pupil size, and loss of pupillary light response can be present due to damage to cranial nerve III. Apneustic or erratic breathing reflects a poor prognosis and bilaterally dilated and unresponsive pupils indicate an irreversible brainstem lesion. These lesions can occur immediately after injury, secondary to herniation of components of the cerebrum or cerebellum, or following hemorrhage. Severe brainstem injuries may result in a decorticate posture, characterized by rigid extension of neck, back, and limbs [9]. Injury to caudal parts of the brainstem (pons and medulla) results in dysfunction of multiple cranial nerves in addition to depression and limb ataxia and/or weakness. To make a distinction between a cranial cervical spinal cord and caudal brain stem lesion, careful assessment of the horse's mentation and function of cranial nerves X and XII is important [5, 9].

Signs of cerebellar injury occur infrequently and include intention tremor, broad-based stance, spastic limb movements, and absent menace response with normal vision. If multiple areas of the brain are damaged, this will be reflected in the different clinical signs. Multifocal damage or progression of disease through hemorrhage and/or secondary injury mechanisms is suggested when clinical signs are more widespread.

Diagnostic tools that are helpful in further defining cranial trauma in horses include radiography, computed tomography (CT), magnetic resonance imaging (MRI), endoscopy, nuclear scintigraphy (chronic cases), electrodiagnostics, and CSF analysis. Radiographs are used to determine the presence and severity of fractures, hemorrhage in cavities, or stylohyoid bone and/or bulla thickening. Subtle nondisplaced fractures and soft tissue damage, however, may not be easily detected radiographically and, in fact, fractures were identified radiographically in only 50% of cases with confirmed fractures [4]. The remainder were diagnosed using CT or via postmortem examination. CT is currently available in many equine hospitals, and it can be critical in the precise diagnosis of fractures in cases of head trauma and, in addition, provides information regarding soft tissue trauma, which may not be apparent on endoscopy and plain radiography [4, 50, 51]. Changes observed after TBI include changes in the size, shape, and position of the ventricles, deviation of the falx cerebri, and focal changes in brain opacity [9]. In humans, CT findings in TBI include cisternal compression, midline shift, epidural mass lesions, and

intraventricular blood or subarachnoid hemorrhage, to name a few. The Marshall and Rotterdam grading systems are used in combination with other diagnostics for prognostication purposes [52, 53], and there is good interobserver reproducibility between neuroradiologists and neurosurgeons in the interpretation of CT imaging features of TBI and calculation of those scores [54]. The cost of CT remains a major disadvantage of this technique; however, scanners have and will become more affordable and the ability to perform standing computer tomography significantly reduces the cost of the procedure. MRI offers a higher sensitivity for examination of soft tissue structures and has the ability to acquire images in all planes. In addition, it allows differentiation of gray/white matter, detection of abnormal tissue signals and mass effect shifts, swelling, edema, contusion, and hemorrhage [55, 56].

Substantial advancements are being made within the field of neuroimaging as a means of noninvasive evaluation of TBI patients. The current neuroimaging goals are no longer only for evaluation of gross anatomy, but also include evaluation of anatomical details such as tracts (white matter) and integrity of axons, blood flow, and function. In addition, many of these techniques are used to monitor patients and evaluate changes that occur over time. Multiple imaging modalities currently exist for this in humans, including (Doppler) ultrasound, CT, single photon emission CT (SPECT), positron emission tomography (PET), and MRI. These techniques continue to evolve with the development of advanced MRI techniques such as fractional anisotropy, fiber tractography, and diffusion tensor imaging [57, 58].

Additional ancillary diagnostics may include endoscopy, electrodiagnostics, and CSF analysis. Upper respiratory endoscopy is an important diagnostic for evaluation of cranial nerve function, stylohyoid bones, retropharyngeal area, and appearance of guttural pouches (Figure 32.3). Hemorrhage inside or within the wall of the guttural pouches may be indicative of injury to the longus capitis muscles as a result of poll trauma. Electrodiagnostics are typically not indicated immediately after TBI; however after stabilization or during recovery, these techniques may provide information about certain levels of (dys)function. For example, electroencephalograms are used for assessment of seizure activity, brainstem auditory evoked response is used for examination of vestibular function, and visual function is examined with visual evoked potential in combination with electroretinography. CSF analysis may not always be indicated after acute trauma, but may be useful for excluding other diseases. Cisternal CSF collection is contraindicated if increased ICP is suspected because of the possibility of brain herniation through the foramen magnum. Lumbosacral collection is a safer alternative

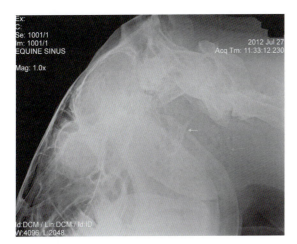

Figure 32.3 Lateral radiograph of a horses head with a basisphenoid fracture (noted at white arrow), which is displaced from the fracture bed by the pull of the longus colli muscles. At the double arrows, blood can be detected within the guttural pouch.

but can be normal despite a traumatic episode, especially in the acute phase. Increased red blood cell numbers and erythrocytophagia are suggestive of hemorrhage into the CSF following trauma. If the hemorrhage is recent or iatrogenic, the CSF usually clears with centrifugation; however if it persists, earlier hemorrhage should be suspected [59]. It has also been shown that CSF lactate concentrations are increased after trauma in horses [60].

Spinal cord injury

Clinical signs seen as a result of trauma reflect the extent and location of the injury. Neurologic signs are usually observed immediately after the accident, but may occur weeks to months after the initial insult because of delayed damage to the spinal cord caused by instability, arthritis, or bony callus formation at the site of impact. Clinical signs depend on the neuroanatomical location of injury and range from inapparent to severe incapacitating tetraparesis or tetraplegia (Figure 32.2). Lesions causing recumbency are mostly found in the caudal cervical or thoracic spinal cord, whereas lesions of non-recumbent horses are mostly found further cranial in the cervical spinal cord or in the lumbosacral cord [2]. Horses with vertebral fractures often display signs of pain in the acute phase, such as reduced willingness to move when asked to flex/extend/bend the neck or painful responses to palpation. Also pruritus affecting the dermatome associated with a C2 fracture has been reported in a pony [61].

Initial evaluation of the patient should be directed toward stabilization and correction of any life-threatening problems such as airway obstruction, hemorrhage, cardiovascular collapse, and pneumothorax. In addition, major long-bone fractures must be identified, as these may be the limiting factor for survival of the horse. Affected horses may be nervous or agitated as a result of pain and the inability to stand, and care should be taken when evaluating these horses. A systematic neurologic evaluation should then be performed in order to localize the site of injury (Figure 32.2). In recumbent horses, the use of a sling to assist standing may be a valuable diagnostic tool for localizing the site of injury and for assessing progression of disease and prognosis [48].

In animals, SCI usually occurs as a solitary lesion and the level of the lesion is typically diagnosed by neurologic examination. Depression or loss of a segmental spinal reflex implies damage to either the afferent, efferent, or connecting pathways of the reflex arc. However, after acute SCI, a phase of spinal shock can occur in which there is profound depression in segmental spinal reflexes caudal to the level of the lesion, even though reflex arcs are physically intact [62–64]. This "spinal shock" occurs in all species, however, appears to be of less clinical significance in veterinary species when compared to primates [64]. This is mostly due to spinal shock having a much shorter duration in dogs, cats, and rabbits when compared to humans. Anatomic differences (localization, significance, projection pattern) of the tracts for descending motor control and subsequent differences with respect to responses to injury (tracts damaged and regeneration/plasticity within the cord) in animals versus humans contributes to this more rapid recovery from spinal shock in nonprimates [64]. Another syndrome that occurs infrequently and is short-lived in the horse is the Schiff–Sherrington syndrome, in which extensor hypertonus is present in otherwise normal thoracic limbs in patients with a severe thoracic lesion [65, 66].

Cord injury typically results in damage that is worse in the large myelinated motor and proprioceptive fibers compared to the smaller or nonmyelinated nociceptive fibers. Therefore, ataxia and loss of proprioception and motor function will occur prior to the loss of deep pain [17]. Flaccid paralysis with hypo- or areflexia, muscular hypotonia, and neurogenic muscle atrophy are characteristic of a lower motor neuron lesion. Signs resulting from an upper motor neuron spinal cord lesion include loss of voluntary motor function, while muscle tone may be increased and spinal reflexes may be normal to hyperactive.

In horses, lesions in the C1 to T2 region are most common and result in various degrees of tetraparesis to recumbency (Figure 32.4). Thoracolumbar SCI can result in paraparesis to recumbency and horses may dog-sit. Sacral cord damage can result in fecal and urinary incontinence, loss of use of tail and anus, muscle

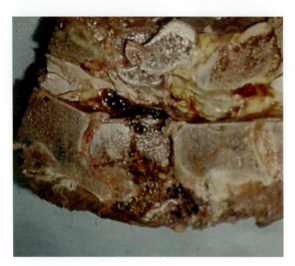

Figure 32.4 Postmortem photograph of a sagittal section of the vertebrae demonstrating a compression fracture of T1 vertebral body sustained after a horse fell with the neck in flexion underneath its body.

atrophy, and mild deficits of pelvic limb function. Sacrococcygeal cord injury can produce hypalgesia, hypotonia, and hyporeflexia of the perineum, tail, and anus, or total analgesia and paralysis of those structures. In addition to these clinical signs, loss of sensation can occur distal to the level of SCI. Furthermore, diffuse sweating can be seen as a result of loss of supraspinal input to the preganglionic cell bodies of the sympathetic system in the thoracolumbar intermediate gray. Patchy sweating can be seen with damage to specific preganglionic or postganglionic nerve fibers [17, 65].

Ancillary diagnostics that may aid in diagnosing or localizing SCI in horses include radiography, ultrasonography, myelography, CT, MRI, nuclear scintigraphy, CSF analysis, nerve conduction velocity studies, electromyography, and transcranial magnetic stimulation. Radiography remains the most commonly used imaging technique and is used to demonstrate fractures, luxations, subluxations, and vertebral compression. While plain, lateral radiographs of the cervical spine are very informative in itself, the addition of oblique images to the radiographic study will allow for better characterization of lateralized pathology [67]. Oblique radiographs result in separation of the paired anatomic structures (articular processes and transverse processes) and provide the opportunity to acquire orthogonal projections thereby enabling better evaluation of the individual joint for fracture, congenital abnormalities and degenerative changes. Oblique radiographs should be taken to better characterize abnormalities seen on the lateral radiographs or to image regions identified as abnormal on clinical examination. Ultrasound evaluation of the cervical spine provides complementary information in the assessment of facet or transverse process pathology [68]. Myelography may be required to confirm spinal cord compression and can be used at the level of the cervical, cranial thoracic, and sacral-coccygeal spinal cord, depending on the size of the horse. The main disadvantage of this technique is that it requires general anesthesia. CT and MRI techniques are in development, however, the size of the horse and equipment aperture size and costs limit its use to investigations of the cervical and cranial thoracic spinal cord [69]. Nuclear scintigraphy can be useful in diagnosing nondisplaced or occult fractures and soft tissue lesions. CSF analysis may be normal, especially in very acute or chronic cases, but common abnormalities following SCI include xanthochromia, mild-to-moderate increased red blood cell and total protein concentrations [17, 41]. Horses with SCI were found to have increased concentrations of the cytokines interleukin-6, interferon gamma, and transforming growth factor beta [41]. Nerve conduction velocity and electromyographic studies evaluate the lower motor neuron and aid in lesion localization. Electromyographic changes, however, may not develop until 4–5 days following nerve damage [70]. Transcranial magnetic stimulation allows detection of functional lesions in descending motor tracts through recording of magnetic motor-evoked potentials. This method has been validated and used to distinguish motor tract disorders from other causes of recumbency in clinical cases [71–73].

Neurocritical care: acute treatment and monitoring

Traumatic brain injury
Ischemia, hypoxia, and energy dysfunction are important determinants of secondary brain injury. The goal of acute treatment is to minimize cellular injury and salvage brain tissue that is undamaged or reversibly damaged. Initial treatment of TBI is, therefore, aimed at optimizing CBF, maintaining oxygenation and energy substrate delivery, and promoting ionic homeostasis. However, management of human patients with TBI remains mainly focused to ICP/CPP therapy, which alone appears not be enough to modify TBI prognosis [74]. This may be partly due to the complexity of TBI pathophysiology and the heterogeneity of TBI lesions, and there is now evidence that suggests that management of severe TBI patients is increasingly based on a more comprehensive approach that is not limited to ICP/CPP therapy, but also includes the individual optimization of CBF, oxygen, and energy substrate delivery guided by bedside brain multimodal monitoring [75, 76].

Parameters that are of interest during the care of the TBI patient include the following: (i) anatomy; (ii) function; (iii) brain, blood, and CSF pressures; (iv) CBF; and (v) oxygen and glucose metabolism [76]. Monitoring tools can be distinguished into radiography/tomography techniques that provide data at a specific time, and bedside monitors that are invasive or noninvasive, and continuous or noncontinuous. Anatomy is evaluated using neuroimaging techniques such as radiography, CT, and MRI. In addition perfusion studies can be performed using techniques such as CT and MR angiography, PET, and SPECT. Sequential clinical evaluation is central to physiological monitoring of the human and equine TBI patient. This is best done when the patient has normal oxygenation and arterial blood pressure and effects of pharmacological agents such as sedatives should be taken into account. In addition, electrophysiological measurements such as electroencephalography and evaluation of somatosensory evoked potentials may be of use in TBI, in particular to assist in determining prognosis.

Monitoring ICP and CPP is recommended in the Brain Trauma Foundation guidelines for the management of severe TBI [77], and should be considered in all patients with severe TBI. The significance of intracranial hypertension in predicting poor outcome from TBI has been well documented, and aside from its prognostic value, ICP monitoring also guides early diagnosis and management of intracranial hypertension. Several studies have now shown that ICP monitoring leads to reduced mortality and improved outcomes in humans with TBI [78, 79]. Noninvasive techniques that can be used in humans to screen for intracranial hypertension include transcranial Doppler ultrasonography derived pulsatility index and optic nerve ultrasonography; however, reliability of these techniques is questionable and ICP in humans is best monitored invasively, with a ventricular catheter or an intraparenchymal monitor [76]. CBF can be assessed noninvasively using transcranial Doppler ultrasonography, a technique based on movement of sound, or invasively using laser Doppler flowmetry or thermal diffusion flowmetry, techniques based on changes in light and temperature, respectively. Each of these techniques carries its advantages and disadvantages [76]. Methods to measure and monitor ICP and CPP have been described for use in foals and adult horses; however, these techniques have thus far not been evaluated in horses with neurological disease [38, 39, 80–82].

Monitoring of cerebral oxygenation after TBI can help guide therapy, as it allows one to calculate optimal ICP or CPP in individual patients, identify episodes of secondary brain injury before irreversible damage occurs, and inform prognosis. There are four broad methods to measure brain oxygenation: jugular venous bulb oximetry, direct brain tissue oxygen tension measurement, near-infrared spectroscopy, and oxygen-15 PET. The jugular bulb is the final common pathway for venous blood that drains the brain, and oxygen saturation at the jugular bulb indicates the balance between supply and oxygen consumption by the brain. Brain oxygen monitors were included in the treatment guidelines for human TBI in 2007 and utilize either electrochemical properties of metals or fluorescence techniques to indicate the balance between regional oxygen supply and cellular oxygen consumption. Near-infrared spectroscopy is a noninvasive technique that measures regional cerebral oxygen saturation. It has not yet been validated for use in TBI [76].

Brain metabolism can be assessed using cerebral microdialysis, which allows low-molecular-weight substances from the interstitial space (i.e., brain extracellular fluid) to be collected and sampled through a specialized catheter with a semipermeable dialysis membrane at its tip that is placed in the brain parenchyma. In TBI, the most commonly examined analytes are markers of cerebral energy metabolism (glucose, lactate, and pyruvate), neurotransmitters (glutamate), and cell damage (glycerol) [76].

Acute treatment of TBI should include emergency surgical treatment when there are open cranial fractures or if there is deterioration despite medical therapy. Once the patient is stabilized, repair of less life-threatening fractures can be considered. Initial stabilization requires normalization of mean arterial blood pressure and oxygenation. Shock should be prevented, rapidly diagnosed, and treated. A single episode of hypotension has been associated with increased morbidity and doubling of mortality in human TBI [32].

The underlying cause of hypotension in trauma patients is most commonly hemorrhage; therefore, intravascular fluid is intuitively the most effective way to restore blood pressure. Mean arterial blood pressure should be maintained within normal limits (in humans: >90 mmHg). Unlike the treatment of SCI where sympathetic outflow often is disrupted and pressor therapy is indicated, this is not commonly seen after TBI and the goal is to maintain normal mean arterial blood pressure and euvolemia by isotonic crystalloid fluid therapy. It is crucial to avoid overhydration as fluid loading may increase ICP and ventilation/perfusion complications related to pulmonary edema. Crystalloids are the fluid therapy of choice for maintenance of blood pressure, particularly in light of findings of the serum versus albumin fluid evaluation (SAFE) study [83], which determined no difference in outcomes between patients treated with albumin or normal saline, and in which subgroup analysis demonstrated an increased mortality in TBI patients that were treated with albumin. Recently a comparison of calculated osmolarity and measured *in vitro* osmolality suggested that human albumin solutions, Hartmann's solution, and, to a lesser extent, gelatin preparations are hypo-osmolar, and may, therefore, increase brain volume and ICP. The authors concluded that the osmolality of an infusion solution rather than the colloid osmotic pressure per se represents the key determinant in the pathogenesis of cerebral edema formation [84].

Trials have shown both higher systolic blood pressure and better survival in trauma patients resuscitated with hypertonic saline instead of isotonic crystalloids [32, 85], and meta-analysis found that patients who received hypertonic saline and dextran were about twice as likely to survive as those who received standard therapy [86]. Furthermore, hypertonic saline may decrease ICP in patients with intracranial hypertension. Hypertonic saline exerts its effect primarily by increasing serum sodium and osmolarity, thereby establishing an osmotic gradient. Water diffuses passively from cerebral intracellular and interstitial spaces into capillaries resulting in a reduction in ICP. Although mannitol works similarly, sodium chloride has a better reflection coefficient (1.0) than mannitol (0.9), making it a better osmotic agent. Hypertonic saline may also normalize resting membrane potential and cell volume by restoring normal intracellular electrolyte balance in injured cells. Furthermore, hypertonic saline has positive effects on CBF, oxygen consumption, and inflammatory response at a cellular level [87]. There is strong evidence that hypertonic saline is effective in reducing ICP and improving CPP [88]. Hypertonic saline was also shown to decrease mortality rates in severely injured human TBI patients compared with albumin infusions [89]. However, despite these data, more recent assessment of clinical trials of early administration to TBI patients has failed to show significant benefit of hypertonic saline on outcome [85, 90].

In humans, hypertonic saline is typically used as 3, 5, or 7.5% solutions, but a recent study showed beneficial effects using small-volume 23.4% hypertonic saline to reduce ICP [91]. In humans intravenous administration of a 4 ml/kg bolus of 3% hypertonic saline is given and then repeated until ICP is normalized or until a serum sodium concentration of 155 mmol/l is achieved. The serum sodium concentration is maintained at this concentration until ICP is stabilized and then gradually allowed to decrease. If ICP is still elevated after 3–4 days, furosemide is used in an effort to mobilize tissue sodium [92].

In horses, hypertonic saline can be administered intravenously as 5 or 7.5% NaCl solutions (4–6 ml/kg) over 15 min. A recent equine study showed that hypertonic saline administration (7.5%, 4 ml/kg) provided faster restoration of intravascular volume deficits than isotonic saline (0.9%, 4 ml/kg) in endurance horses receiving emergency medical treatment [93]. However,

more marked electrolyte changes should be expected with hypertonic saline administration and additional fluids after hypertonic saline administration likely are needed. Contraindications to the use of hypertonic saline include dehydration, ongoing intracerebral hemorrhage, hypernatremia, renal failure, hyperkalemic periodic paralysis, and hypothermia. Systemic side effects include potential for coagulopathy, excessive intravascular volume, and electrolyte abnormalities.

Blood transfusion may be indicated in situations of severe hemorrhage. Although hemoglobin deficiency adversely affects oxygen delivery to tissues and guidelines for traumatic injury traditionally have advocated aggressive treatment of anemia in TBI, a recent human study has demonstrated that similar to other critical care patients, blood transfusions negatively affected outcome in TBI patients [94]. The threshold for transfusion, thus, should be no different than in other critical care patients.

The use of carbohydrate-containing intravenous solutions should be avoided early in the treatment of head trauma patients. Glucose suppresses ketogenesis, and may increase lactic acid production by the traumatized brain, limiting the availability of nonglycolytic energy substrates [95]. Furthermore, carbon dioxide liberated from glucose metabolism could cause vasodilation and worsening of cerebral edema. It has been well established that maintaining blood glucose concentrations at 80–110 mg/dl through intensive insulin therapy reduces morbidity and mortality in human critical care patients [96]. However, neurointensivists have shown that intensive insulin therapy increases markers of cellular distress in the brain, and suggest that systemic glucose concentrations of 80–110 mg/dl are too low in TBI and may lead to cerebral hypoglycemia [97]. Moreover, two randomized controlled trials in humans identified increased episodes of hypoglycemia in the treatment groups [90]. Recommendations now are maintaining blood glucose concentrations at 120–140 mg/dl in TBI. Providing early nutritional support demonstrated beneficial treatment effect in two studies (zinc supplementation within 48 h and total parenteral nutrition within 72 h) [90].

In human medicine pharmacological and nonpharmacological measures to manage TBI are identified and have recently been reviewed [88, 90, 98]. Nonpharmacological measures used in the acute management of TBI include both noninvasive and invasive procedures. Noninvasive procedures include rapid intubation, adjusting head posture, body rotation, hyperventilation, hypothermia and hyperbaric oxygen, and are commonly used to help decrease ICP or improve cellular metabolism. Invasive procedures, such as CSF drainage and decompressive craniectomy, are generally used as a last resort when ICP is unresponsive to other treatments. Decompressive craniectomy has been used in normal dogs and was effective at reducing ICP [99]. Pharmacological strategies for the management of intracranial hypertension generally fall under one of three types: osmotic agents (diuretics), analgesics, or sedatives. Osmotic agents draw fluid from the cranial cavity, thereby reducing increased ICP. Analgesics and sedatives reduce the metabolic demands placed on injured or at risk neurons by limiting nociceptive stimulation and reducing overall brain activity.

When examining the evidence surrounding use of nonpharmacological interventions in the acute phase of TBI, beneficial effects were found for only five of the eight interventions (rapid intubation, decompressive craniectomy, CSF drainage, hypothermia, and hyperbaric oxygen) [88, 90]. Although nine of the investigated pharmacological interventions showed some benefit for treatment of TBI, these benefits rarely resulted in improved long-term patient outcomes [88, 90]. In these reviews, corticosteroids were found to be contraindicated. Tables 32.3 and 32.4 show a summary of these interventions and Figure 32.5 shows the most common methods that are currently used in sequence in human neurocritical care units to reduce elevated

ICP. Treatment to reduce ICP is commenced at pressures of 20–25 mmHg.

Mannitol has been the primary osmotherapeutic drug for the past four decades. However, current research is focused on the use of substitutes for mannitol, of which the most promising is hypertonic saline. Mannitol induces changes in blood rheology and increases cardiac output, leading to improved CPP and cerebral oxygenation. Improved cerebral oxygenation induces cerebral artery vasoconstriction and subsequent reduction in cerebral blood volume and ICP. There is strong evidence that mannitol reduces elevated ICP, but equally strong

Table 32.3 Nonpharmacological management techniques in human TBI [90, 100].

Nonpharmacological treatment modalities

---

1. **Rapid intubation** (prehospital): Improved neurological outcome compared to intubation in hospital.
2. **Head elevation**: Evidence suggests that 30° head elevation post TBI decreases elevated intracranial pressure and increases cerebral perfusion pressure.
3. **Body rotation**: No significant benefits.
4. **Hyperventilation**: High blood CO_2 levels cause cerebral vasodilation. However, no studies indicated that hyperventilation alone improved outcomes. Moreover, intense or prolonged hyperventilation may increase metabolic acidosis and has been associated with poorer outcomes.
5. **Hypothermia: Selective** brain cooling decreases elevated ICP and improves outcomes.
6. **Hyperbaric oxygen:** Hyperbaric oxygen may decrease mortality, but there is conflicting evidence about effect on functional recovery.
7. **CSF drainage:** There is strong evidence that CSF drainage effectively reduces intracranial pressure in the immediate phase; however, it does not address the underlying cause of elevated intracranial pressure.
8. **Decompressive craniectomy:** Reduces elevated intracranial pressure immediately after surgery. Conflicting data on long-term functional outcome.

In bold are those that have been proven most effective.

Table 32.4 Pharmacological management techniques in human TBI [99, 100].

Pharmacological

---

1. Propofol: In conjunction with morphine, reduces elevated ICP and the need for other ICP and sedative interventions.
2. Barbiturates: Believed to reduce increased ICP through the suppression of cerebral metabolism. There is conflicting data on its efficacy.
3. Opioids: Controversy persists regarding the effect of opioids on ICP and CPP. It has been reported that opioids can increase CBF, which may lead to an increase in ICP.
4. Midazolam: Does not affect ICP in TBI, and there is evidence to suggest it can cause hypotension and reduced CPP.
5. Mannitol: Reviewed in text.
6. **Hypertonic saline: Reviewed in text.**
7. **Corticosteroids: Reviewed in text.**
8. **Progesterone: Reviewed in text.**
9. Bradykinin anatonists: The kinin–kallikrein pathway is one of the components of the inflammatory cascade following TBI. There is some evidence that bradykinin antagonists prevent elevations of ICP following TBI.
10. **Dimethyl sulphoxide: Reviewed in text**
11. Cannabinoids: Synthetic, nonpsychotropic cannabinoids are thought to act as a noncompetitive NMDA antagonist to decrease glutamate excitotoxicity. However, there is strong evidence that they do not result in acute improvement in ICP or have benefits in long-term outcomes in people.
12. Calcium channel blockers: One study indicated beneficial effects on neurological outcome after nimodipine treatment.
13. Neuroprotection targeting glutamate excitotoxicity: None of the trials demonstrated beneficial effects.
14. **Methylphenidate: Reviewed in text**
15. Magnesium: No significant beneficial effects were seen; moreover, low-dose magnesium treatment was associated with worsening on neurological outcomes.

In bold are those that are of most interest to the equine practitioner. CBF, cerebral blood flow; CPP, cerebral perfusion pressure; ICP, intracranial pressure.

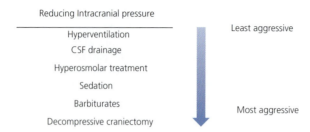

Figure 32.5 Common sequence of strategies used in treatment of human TBI to reduce intracranial pressure.

evidence that mannitol is less effective than hypertonic saline. With prolonged dosage, mannitol may diffuse through the BBB, potentially exacerbating any elevation in ICP. Mannitol has also been associated with significant diuresis, acute renal failure, hyperkalemia, hypotension, and rebound. For these reasons, it has been recommended that mannitol only be used when signs of elevated ICP or deteriorating neurological status suggest the benefits of mannitol may outweigh potential complications or adverse effects [88]. In horses, 20% mannitol can be administered at 0.25–2.0 mg/kg intravenously over 20 min. Horses receiving osmotic diuretics should be adequately hydrated.

Treatment with anti-inflammatories is likely the most commonly used treatment in equine TBI. Indications for use of anti-inflammatory treatment are to combat the inflammatory pathways of secondary injury mechanisms (cytokine release, free radicals), improve comfort level, and reduce fever. Fever occurs extremely commonly after TBI, and it has been well documented in animal models and in people to negatively affect outcome after TBI, through for example augmenting secondary injury mechanisms. It is proposed that a proactive approach should be taken toward reducing fever. In fact, hypothermia has been shown to be neuroprotective. Hypothermia results in decreased cellular metabolism and has been proven efficacious in treatment of TBI in experimental and clinical settings (Table 32.3). Neuroprotective effects include reduced release of excitotoxins, reduction of free radical and inflammatory mediator formation, and reduction of BBB disruption. Anti-inflammatory drugs that are common to equine practice include corticosteroids, nonsteroidal anti-inflammatories, dimethylsulfoxide (DMSO), and vitamin E.

Corticosteroids used in brain injury care have included dexamethasone, methylprednisolone, prednisolone, betamethasone, cortisone, hydrocortisone, prednisone, and triamcinolone. Research has noted focal lesions appear to respond well to corticosteroid therapy while diffuse intracerebral lesions and hematomas appear less responsive. The corticosteroid randomization after significant head injury (CRASH) trial is a large,

international, randomized placebo-controlled trial of the effect of early administration of 48 h infusion of methylprednisolone on risk of death and disability after head injury [101, 102]. The trial aimed to inform clinical decision-making in an area of increasing global health importance. Compared with placebo, the risk of death from all causes within 2 weeks was higher in the group allocated corticosteroids (21.1% vs. 17.9% deaths; relative risk 1.18 (95% CI 1.09–1.27); $P=0.0001$). The relative increase in deaths due to corticosteroids did not differ by injury severity or time since injury [101, 102]. This study shows that there is strong evidence that methylprednisolone increases mortality and should not be used in acute TBI management in humans. In addition, there is conflicting evidence regarding the effect of corticosteroids on ICP and evidence suggesting glucocorticoid administration may increase the risk of seizures [88]. What this means for the care of horses with head trauma is unclear. Although there are no studies that have evaluated corticosteroid use in horses with head trauma, there is anecdotal evidence to suggest treatment with dexamethasone may benefit horses with TBI in the acute phase and corticosteroid treatment is typically incorporated in suggested treatment strategies [103]. Reported dosages of dexamethasone for horses range from 0.1 to 0.25 mg/kg intravenously every 6–24 h for 24–48 h. A favorable response is expected within 4–8 h after administration.

Dimethylsulfoxide (DMSO) has been reported to result in strong diuresis, protect cells from mechanical damage, reduce edema in tissue by stabilizing cell membranes, and act as a free radical scavenger. It is also believed that DMSO increases tissue perfusion, thereby improving cell oxygenation, neutralizing metabolic acidosis, and decreasing intracellular fluid retention. In addition, there is evidence that DMSO transiently reduces increased ICP [88]. In horses, DMSO is administered at a dose of 0.9–1.0 g/kg intravenously.

Two more recently studied pharmaceuticals are progesterone and methylphenidate. Progesterone may modulate excitotoxicity, reconstitute the BBB, reduce cerebral edema, regulate inflammation, and decrease apoptosis. Two studies have shown that progesterone decreases mortality rates in TBI and one of those studies showed improve clinical outcome [104, 105]. Administration of progesterone was 1.0 mg/kg intramuscular injection followed once per 12 h for 5 consecutive days in one study [105] and 0.71 mg/kg at 14 ml/h for the first hour, followed by 0.5 mg/kg/h for the next 72 h in the other study [104]. Methylphenidate is a CNS stimulant with dopaminergic and slight noradrenergic activity. Neuroprotective effects have been attributed to methylphenidate like aspartate inhibitors. Treatment (0.3 mg/kg orally twice daily) was associated with shorter ICU and hospital stays [106].

Controlling seizure activity is very important after TBI, since seizure activity increases cerebral metabolic rate and is detrimental to secondary injury. It is not unusual for horses sustaining cranial trauma to develop seizures. Diazepam, midazolam, phenobarbital, or pentobarbital are drugs that can be used for to control seizures (see Chapter 7 for further discussion of control of seizures). Intractable seizures may necessitate general anesthesia. Agents useful for general anesthesia include guaifenesin, chloral hydrate, barbiturates, and gas anesthesia. Ketamine is not recommended as part of a balanced anesthesia regimen as it increases CBF and ICP. Barbiturates may also have a protective effect against ischemia following brain injury by lowering cerebral metabolism and by retarding peroxidation of lipids within brain cell membranes. In horses, phenobarbital at a dose of 5–10 mg/kg intravenously given to effect may be useful [103].

Antibiotic treatment is usually warranted in cases of head trauma, especially when fractures are involved. The presence of hemorrhage increases the possibility of septic meningitis. Antibiotic choice should be based on culture and sensitivity testing. Good empirical choices for broad-spectrum coverage include trimethoprim–sulfamethoxazole and penicillin in combination with gentamicin. Owing to disruption of the BBB, other antimicrobials probably penetrate into the CNS, and therefore their use may also be efficacious.

Nutritional support plays a role in the outcome following neurologic injury. In humans, it has been found that neurologic recovery from head injury occurs faster in patients receiving early adequate nutritional support [107]. If the horse is able to eat, and the gastrointestinal tract is functioning normally, water and good-quality hay should be available at all times. Horses with a poor appetite or those unable to swallow may have to be tube-fed using a gruel of alfalfa and complete feed pellets. Horses in which enteral feeding is not possible are candidates for total parenteral nutrition. Additionally, the use of thiamine may be of benefit in treating head injuries because thiamine aids in metabolism of lactic acid and is a necessary coenzyme in brain energy pathways.

Spinal cord injury

Treatment to reverse primary SCI does not currently exist and basic and clinical research treatment trials can be broadly classified into those directed at neuroprotection and those directed at neuroregeneration. Neuroprotective agents act to minimize the secondary injury after SCI and may, therefore, be considered acute. Neuroregenerative treatment modalities, on the other hand, are directed at promoting neuronal regeneration and reestablishing axonal pathways to restore neurological function in chronic SCI. This section describes some of the acute neuroprotective treatments.

Surgical intervention is warranted when there is need for stabilization, fracture repair, or evidence of a compressive lesion; it is not, however, routine practice. The use of medical treatment to stabilize the patient should always be instituted before surgery is performed. Acute SCI often results in impaired cardiopulmonary function such as impaired ventilation, bradycardia, and hypotension. This is particularly the case in severe lesions cranial to C5 (respiratory center affected) and cranial to T2 (origin of sympathetic outflow = thoracolumbar spinal cord). Systemic hypotension may exacerbate spinal cord hypoperfusion and ischemia, and maintaining systemic blood pressure has been shown to improve spinal cord perfusion. Volume resuscitation is clearly indicated in shock and for restitution of tissue perfusion. The current recommendation is to maintain euvolemic normotension, and because of sympathetic outflow disruption after cranial SCI, pressor therapy is commonly indicated in the treatment regimen. Maintaining normal mean arterial blood pressure is also important to consider during stabilization of the acutely injured horse, and is particularly important when horses undergo general anesthesia for various diagnostic/therapeutic procedures.

Similar to TBI, SCI has a complex multifactorial pathophysiology and likely requires a combinational treatment intervention for successful outcome. Many agents that could target different aspects of the secondary injury mechanisms have been investigated for use in SCI and are reviewed in the literature on a regular basis [43, 45, 46, 108, 109]. Table 32.5 lists acute neuroprotective and subacute to chronic neuroregenerative therapies, which have been employed in a clinical setting. Until now only methylprednisolone (MP) sodium succinate has been shown to be efficacious in both animal models and humans [42, 110–115]; however, MP has not demonstrated clinically significant effects, and when given in very high doses after SCI intravenously (35 mg/kg) in humans has been associated with significant side effects. MP is a synthetic glucocorticoid with four times more anti-inflammatory activity and 0.8 times less mineralocorticoid action compared with cortisol [116]. Beneficial effects of MP on neural tissue include inhibition of lipid

Table 32.5 Acute neuroprotective and subacute to chronic neuroregenerative therapies that have been employed in a clinical setting in human SCI [42].

Acute

1. **Methylprednisolone: Reviewed in text**
2. Nimodipine: A calcium channel blocker shown to improve blood flow to the spinal cord in laboratory settings, however, a randomized clinical study failed to show benefit.
3. Gacyclidine: An NMDA antagonist that blocks glutamate induced calcium influx. No significant benefits seen in trials.
4. Thyrotropin releasing hormone: Humans with incomplete injury had improved neurological recovery, however, patients with complete SCI demonstrated no benefit. Follow up study is necessary.

Subacute—chronic

1. GM1 ganglioside: No beneficial effect seen in human SCI.
2. Rho antagonist: In humans, Rho antagonists were applied during surgery within 7 days of injury extradurally and neurologic improvement was seen in a subset of patients. Further clinical trials to test efficacy in SCI patients are planned.
3. Anti-Nogo antibodies: Nogo-A is the most potent inhibitory molecule in myelin. Efficacy studies in humans are ongoing.
4. Acidic fibroblast growth factor: Beneficial effects seen in animals and humans with SCI. In humans, it was used in chronic SCI and applied directly to the cord.
5. Autologous activated macrophages: Activated macrophages have been injected into patient's spinal cord immediately caudal to the lesion within 14 days of injury. Improved functional outcomes were observed. Further clinical trials are underway.
6. Autologous mesenchymal stem cells: One study showed neurological improvement in one-third of patients with SCI. The time elapsed between injury and therapy and the number of cells injected correlated with improvement. Two other studies did not show improved recovery of function.
7. Olfactory mucosa autograft: Mixed results.

In bold are those that have been proven most effective.

peroxidation, eicosanoid formation, and lipid hydrolysis, including arachidonic acid release, maintenance of tissue blood flow and aerobic energy metabolism, improved elimination of intracellular calcium accumulation, reduced neurofilament degradation, and improved neuronal excitability and synaptic transmission. MP was selected for human clinical trials because the succinate radical has been shown to cross cell membranes more rapidly than other radicals [111]. It was subsequently evaluated in the National Acute Spinal Cord Injury Studies (NASCIS I, II, and III) and was shown to enhance neurological recovery [108, 111, 114, 117, 118]. Therapy was started within 8 h of injury using an initial bolus of 30 mg/kg intravenously for 15 min followed 45 min later by a continuous infusion of 5.4 mg/kg/h for 24 h. There

have been some reports on increased incidence of adverse effects after MP treatment in humans, such as hyperglycemia, pneumonia, longer hospital stay, and gastrointestinal complications [109], and in animals MP administration according to the doses recommended in the NASCIS II/III studies was associated with lymphocytopenia, intestinal necrosis, and eosinophilic pulmonary infiltrates [119]. Adapting the delivery of MP may provide safe and effective treatment and avoiding the effects of systemic steroids may be key to shifting the risk-benefit considerations. Recently remarkable protective, regenerative, and functional outcome after 1 week of the primary insult was demonstrated when MP was applied topically at the injury site encapsulated in poly-lactic-*co*-glycolic acid nanoparticle formulations [120]. Although MP is not a definitive treatment for SCI at this time, there may be a role for MP in treating SCI through improved indications and techniques.

The usefulness of high-dose MP treatment for spinal cord trauma in the horse remains to be investigated. In horses, corticosteroids, alone or in combination with other drugs, are likely the most commonly used drugs for acute CNS trauma. Reported dosages of dexamethasone for horses range from 0.1 to 0.25 mg/kg intravenously every 6–24 h for 24–48 h. A favorable response is expected within 4–8 h after administration. Horses on corticosteroid therapy should be monitored closely for the development of laminitis or Aspergillus pneumonia. If improvement in clinical signs is observed, the horse may be placed on oral prednisolone therapy (0.5–1.0 mg/kg tapered over 3–5 days) to decrease the chance of laminitis. The neuroprotective effect of corticosteroids is thought primarily to be mediated by free radical scavenging, but may include decreased catecholamines and glutamate, and decreased apoptosis-related cell death [121]. Other potential beneficial effects of corticosteroids include reduction in the spread of morphologic damage, prevention of the loss of axonal conduction and reflex activity, preservation of vascular membrane integrity, and stabilization of white matter neuronal cell membranes in the presence of central hemorrhagic lesions. Furthermore, their anti-inflammatory properties may be useful in reducing edema and fibrin deposition, as well as their ability to reverse sodium and potassium imbalance due to edema and necrosis. Another beneficial effect of corticosteroids is maintenance of normal blood glucose concentrations while maintaining electrolyte balance.

Estrogen and melatonin are two pharmaceuticals that show promise in animal models of SCI; however, neither of these has been used in (human) clinical practice yet. Other evaluated treatments are listed in Table 32.5.

The use of nonsteroidal anti-inflammatory drugs (NSAIDs) such as flunixin meglumine and phenylbutazone may decrease the inflammation associated with a traumatic episode, and may be beneficial in maintaining a normal rectal temperature. These compounds work by inhibiting cyclooxygenase, which converts arachidonic acid to inflammatory mediators (endoperoxides). In addition, the potential beneficial properties of DMSO, 1 g/kg intravenously as a 10–20% solution for three consecutive days followed by three treatments every other day, likely warrant inclusion of this drug in the treatment of SCI [5]. The exact mechanism of DMSO remains unknown and this treatment remains controversial as some researchers have found no positive effects on neurologic outcome from the use of DMSO. Although the free radical scavengers vitamin E and selenium have been shown to be beneficial in SCI, these antioxidants do not appear useful in the acute management because of the length of time required to achieve therapeutic concentrations in the CNS.

Similar to treatment for TBI, antibiotics are not always necessary for vertebral or spinal cord trauma; however, they are indicated for open fractures and secondary complications associated with a recumbent horse, such as pneumonia and decubital sores.

Repairing the CNS: regeneration and rehabilitation

Based on the pathophysiology of events that occur after TBI and SCI it is likely that single drug intervention would not be effective and evaluation of combinatorial treatment strategies is more common currently. Targeting multiple injury mechanisms that contribute to the secondary injury cascade may increase successful clinical trial outcomes.

This section describes aspects of chronic management of CNS trauma with emphasis on SCI. The CNS has an inadequate regenerative potential attributable to an unfavorable balance of abundant inhibitory signaling and inadequate intrinsic mitogenic capacity. Repair of the spinal cord requires knowledge of the mechanisms of the lesion itself, of axonal growth, of anatomical and functional organization of the spinal cord, as well as of other structures of the CNS. Studies on SCI have revealed an extensive potential for endogenous neuroplasticity (anatomical, neurochemical, and physiological) that could be manipulated by appropriate exogenous interventions (pharmacological, surgical, and rehabilitative). Neuroplasticity may occur via regeneration of damaged fibers or sprouting of undamaged fibers. Over recent years we have learned that (i) the CNS has the capacity to regrow axons after injury when some barriers are partially lifted, albeit incomplete; (ii) glial scar tissue at the site of the lesion can be manipulated so as to make it more permissive for axonal growth;

(iii) stem cells can participate in remyelinating fibers damaged but not cut by the lesions; and (iv) the spinal cord below the lesion possesses a repertoire of primarily autonomous sensorimotor functions that can potentially be rehabilitated [43].

During the secondary phase of injury, we see excessive release of neurotransmitters, inflammatory reactions, and apoptosis. During this period, the size of the astrocytes increases in a process termed "reactive gliosis," creating a glial scar at the site of injury. Inflammatory cells migrate toward the injury site and, although necessary for the body's response to injury, they can also have detrimental effects on CNS tissue. In the chronic phase of injury (days to years), apoptosis can continue and surviving cells can be further affected by impairments in channel and receptor functions. Finally, there can be significant scar formation along with demyelination of some fibers and Wallerian degeneration of axons that no longer have a target due to cell loss from the initial injury.

During all phases following SCI, the CNS undergoes substantial reorganization. These changes include synaptic plasticity, axonal sprouting, and cellular proliferation throughout the CNS. Some of the changes may involve the formation of new pathways to bypass the damaged regions, while other changes may involve reorganization in undamaged regions to take on new or modified functions. Of particular clinical importance are changes in electrophysiological properties and connectivity that result in hyperreflexia and spasticity [122].

One approach used to promote the regeneration and integration of injured axons across a spinal cord lesion is neural tissue transplantation, in which the intent is to provide a substrate that will support and guide axons toward a specified target. Much has been written about the sources of these tissues, with strong evidence of axonal growth into and through transplants of embryonic neural tissue, Schwann cells, segments of peripheral nerve, genetically modified fibroblasts, and stem cells. Other reports suggest that biomaterial scaffolds effectively maintain continuity between injured surfaces of the spinal cord to facilitate axon growth [123].

There are three parts to the general accepted model of locomotor control. The first part is the central pattern generator, or CPG, which is a spinal circuit generating a detailed locomotor rhythm of the limbs in which flexor and extensor muscles of one hindlimb are activated in opposite phases and in alternation with the other limb. The second part includes sensory afferents generating phasic signals to the CGP, allowing it to adapt to the environment. The third part involves descending pathways from the brain and brainstem that provide start/stop signals, steering, coordination, posture, and also neurochemical drive necessary for goal-oriented locomotion, interlimb coordination, and postural control [43].

Cyclic movements, such as locomotion, can elicit repetitive patterns of activation that may maximize the benefits to be derived from activity-dependent plasticity. By delivering an appropriately timed intervention that utilizes electrical stimulation to produce cyclic movements, it may be possible to maximize the therapeutic benefits by reversing the downregulation of receptors and other proteins, and directing plasticity to produce functional reorganization [123]. Repetitive motion exercises have been used in humans to accelerate or enhance recovery. These include passive exercise, active exercise, electrical stimulation, adaptive control of electrical stimulation, and neuromuscular electrical stimulation [122]. In addition, several studies have indicated that locomotor activity could significantly improve locomotor recovery. Mechanisms of improvements include increased corticospinal responses and cortical-dependent muscle unit coherence. There are also clinical observations suggesting that the spinal cord of humans also possesses some degree of autonomous intrinsic rhythmogenic potential. Therefore, it seems likely that, after a partial spinal lesion, neuroplastic changes occur at both the supraspinal and spinal levels and that rehabilitation approaches should aim at fostering locomotor training using techniques to reinforce both voluntary aspects of locomotion as well as to reinforce endogenous spinal mechanisms [43].

Prognosis

The prognosis for cranial trauma is dependent on severity of insult and early treatment, and is gauged by response to treatment. An early prognosis based on initial findings is important to establish for owners and thus can influence clinical decisions. However, in a study performed in human TBI patients, even with sophisticated clinical and radiological technologies, it was not possible to predict outcome on the first day after the accident with sufficient accuracy to guide early management [124]. Here again, it is important to highlight the value of repeated neurologic evaluations. In the horses with TBI reviewed by Feary et al., 62% survived to discharge from the hospital [4]. In the nonsurvivor group, mean packed cell volume was significantly higher (40%), compared to the survivor group (33%) [4]. Risk factors associated with nonsurvival included recumbency of more than 4h duration after initial evaluation (odds ratio, 18), and fracture of the basilar bone (odds ratio, 7.5). Time, good nursing care, and adequate nutritional support, especially in the recumbent horse, are vital for a positive outcome. Complications that may occur after TBI include development of meningitis, meningoencephalomyelitis, and pneumocephalus [125, 126]. In a recent review of 28 meningitis/meningoencephalomyelitis cases, 32% had a history of trauma and none of those horses survived. Pneumocephalus, or the presence of gas within any intracranial compartment (intraventricular, intraparenchymal, subarachnoid, subdural and epidural), was recently reported in five cases, four of which had a history of trauma [126]. Identification of gas within the cranial vault, indicative of a communication between extra- and intracranial spaces, warrants initiation of antimicrobial treatment to prevent establishment of a CNS infection.

Physical therapy is important in the rehabilitative process in spine-injured horses. Controlled exercise allows the unaffected parts of the nervous system to compensate for the affected parts by increasing strength and conscious proprioception. Exercise is especially helpful in improving weakness, ataxia, spasticity, and hypermetria. In recumbent horses, massage, therapeutic ultrasound, and hydrotherapy of affected muscle groups for 10–15 min at least twice a day is important. These measures help combat necrosis and muscle atrophy of the horse's dependent muscle groups. Passive flexion and extension of all limbs is helpful in maintaining full range of motion in recumbent horses.

Prognosis is based on response to therapy and is directly related to the time from injury to the institution of treatment. Horses that show rapid neurologic improvement have a fair-to-good prognosis. Recumbent horses or horses suffering from fractures or luxations have a guarded-to-poor prognosis. Horses that have lost deep pain sensation and have a functional or anatomical spinal cord transection have a grave prognosis. The longer the time from loss of deep pain to treatment, the poorer the prognosis. Partial or complete recovery of horses with spinal cord trauma may take weeks to months, so time and nursing care are required. It should be noted that in some cases with vertebral trauma fusion of an intervertebral articulation may result in so-called domino-effect compression of the spinal cord as a result of changes within the vertebral column cranial and/or caudal to the initial (semi) fused intervertebral joint. This process may take months to years to occur. This appears to occur more frequently with traumatically induced vertebral fusion than with successful surgical fusion undertaken for cervical vertebral stenotic myelopathy [26].

References

[1] Lyle, C.H., Uzal, F.A., McGorum, B.C. *et al.* (2011) Sudden death in racing Thoroughbred horses: an international multicentre study of post mortem findings. *Equine Vet J*, 43, 324–331.

[2] Feige, K., Fürst, A., Kaser-Hotz, B. and Ossent, P. (2000) Traumatic injury to the central nervous system in horses: occurrence, diagnosis and outcome. *Equine Vet Ed*, 12, 220–224.

[3] Tyler, C.M., Begg, A.P., Hutchins, D.R. and Hodgson, D.R. (1993) A survey of neurological diseases in horses. *Aust Vet J*, 70, 445–449.

[4] Feary, D.J., Magdesian, K.G., Aleman, M.A. and Rhodes, D.M. (2007) Traumatic brain injury in horses: 34 cases (1994–2004). *J Am Vet Med Assoc*, 231, 259–266.

[5] Reed, S.M. (1993) Management of head trauma in horses. *Comp Contin Ed Pract Vet*, 15, 270–273.

[6] Reed, S.M. (1987) Intracranial trauma, in *Current Therapy in Equine Medicine 3* (ed. N.E. Robinson), W.B. Saunders, Philadelphia, pp. 377–380.

[7] Stick, J.A., Wilson, J. and Kunze, D. (1980) Basilar skull fractures in three horses. *J Am Vet Med Assoc*, 176, 228.

[8] Ramirez, O., Jorgensen, J.S. and Thrall, D.E. (1998) Imaging basilar skull fractures in the horse: a review. *Vet Radiol Ultrasound*, 39, 391–395.

[9] MacKay, R.J. (2004) Brain injury after head trauma: pathophysiology, diagnosis, and treatment. *Vet Clin North Am Equine Pract*, 20, 199–216.

[10] Sweeney, C.R., Freeman, D.E., Sweeney, R.W. *et al.* (1993) Hemorrhage into the guttural pouch (auditory tube diverticulum) associated with rupture of the longus capitis muscle in three horses. *J Am Vet Med Assoc*, 202, 1129–1131.

[11] Martin, L., Kaswan, R. and Chapman, W. (1986) Four cases of traumatic optic nerve blindness in the horse. *Equine Vet J*, 18, 133–137.

[12] Walker, A.M., Sellon, D.C., Cornelisse, C.J. *et al.* (2002) Temporohyoid osteoarthropathy in 33 horses (1993–2000). *J Vet Intern Med*, 16, 697–703.

[13] Palus, V., Bladon, B., Brazil, T. *et al.* (2012) Retrospective study of neurological signs and management of seven English horses with temporohyoid osteoarthropathy. *Equine Vet Ed*, 24, 415–422.

[14] Blythe, L.L., Watrous, B.J., Schmitz, J.A. and Kaneps, A.J. (1984) Vestibular syndrome associated with temporohyoid joint fusion and temporal bone fracture in three horses. *J Am Vet Med Assoc*, 185, 775–781.

[15] Blythe, L.L. (1997) Otitis media and interna and temporohyoid osteoarthropathy. *Vet Clin North Am Equine Pract*, 13, 21–42.

[16] Sarrafian, T.L., Case, J.T., Kinde, H. *et al.* (2012) Fatal musculoskeletal injuries of Quarter Horse racehorses: 314 cases (1990–2007). *J Am Vet Med Assoc*, 241, 935–942.

[17] Reed, S.M. (1994) Medical and surgical emergencies of the nervous system of horses: diagnosis, treatment, and sequelae. *Vet Clin North Am Equine Pract*, 10, 703–715.

[18] Mayhew, IG. Equine neurology and nutrition. *Proceedings of the Eighteenth Bain-Fallon Memorial Lectures. 22–26th July, South Australia, Australia*; 1996: p. 18.

[19] Wagner, P.C., Long, G.G., Chatburn, C.C. and Grant, B.D. (1977) Traumatic injury of the cauda equina in the horse: a case report. *Equine Med Surg*, 1, 282–285.

[20] Collatos, C., Allen, D., Chambers, J. and Henry, M. (1991) Surgical treatment of sacral fracture in a horse. *J Am Vet Med Assoc*, 198, 877–879.

[21] Haussler, K.K. and Stover, S.M. (1998) Stress fractures of the vertebral lamina and pelvis in Thoroughbred racehorses. *Equine Vet J*, 30, 374–381.

[22] Tutko, J.M., Sellon, D.C., Burns, G.A. *et al.* (2002) Cranial coccygeal vertebral fractures in horses: 12 cases. *Equine Vet Ed*, 14, 250–254.

[23] Pinchbeck, G. and Murphy, D. (2001) Cervical vertebral fracture in three foals. *Equine Vet Ed*, 13, 24–28.

[24] Rashmir-Raven, A., DeBowes, R.M., Hudson, L. *et al.* (1991) Vertebral fracture and paraplegia in a foal. *Prog Vet Neurol*, 2, 197–202.

[25] Jeffcott, L.B. (1980) Disorders of the thoracolumbar spine of the horse: a survey of 443 cases. *Vet J*, 12, 197.

[26] Mayhew, I.G. (2009) Cervical vertebral fractures. *Equine Vet Ed*, 21, 536–539.

[27] Povlishock, J.T. (1992) Traumatically induced axonal injury: pathogenesis and pathobiological implications. *Brain Pathol*, 2, 1–12.

[28] Smith, D.H. and Meaney, D.F. (2000) Axonal damage in traumatic brain injury. *Neuroscientist*, 6, 483–495.

[29] Smith, D.H., Hicks, R. and Povlishock, J.T. (2013) Therapy development for diffuse axonal injury. *J Neurotrauma*, 30, 307–323.

[30] Browne, K.D., Chen, X.H., Meaney, D.F. and Smith, D.H. (2011) Mild traumatic brain injury and diffuse axonal injury in swine. *J Neurotrauma*, 28, 1747–1755.

[31] Johnson, V.E., Stewart, W. and Smith, D.H. (2013) Axonal pathology in traumatic brain injury. *Exp Neurol*, 246, 35–43.

[32] Ghajar, J. (2000) Traumatic brain injury. *Lancet*, 356, 923–929.

[33] Werner, C. and Engelhard, K. (2007) Pathophysiology of traumatic brain injury. *Br J Anaesth*, 99, 4–9.

[34] Sande, A. and West, C. (2010) Traumatic brain injury: a review of pathophysiology and management. *J Vet Emerg Crit Care*, 20, 177–190.

[35] Feala, J.D., Abdulhameed, M.D., Yu, C. *et al.* (2013) Systems biology approaches for discovering biomarkers for traumatic brain injury. *J Neurotrauma*, 30, 1101–1116.

[36] Fishman, R.A. (1975) Brain edema. *N Eng J Med*, 293, 706–711.

[37] Mokri, B. (2001) The Monro-Kellie hypothesis: applications in CSF volume depletion. *Neurology*, 56, 1746–1748.

[38] Brosnan, R.J., Esteller-Vico, A., Steffey, E.P. *et al.* (2008) Effects of head-down positioning on regional central nervous system perfusion in isoflurane-anesthetized horses. *Am J Vet Res*, 69, 737–743.

[39] Brosnan, R.J., Steffey, E.P., LeCouteur, R.A. *et al.* (2011) Effects of isoflurane anesthesia on cerebrovascular autoregulation in horses. *Am J Vet Res*, 72, 18–24.

[40] Bouma, G.J., Muizelaar, J.P., Bandoh, K. and Marmarou, A. (1992) Blood pressure and intracranial pressure-volume dynamics in severe head injury: relationship with cerebral blood flow. *J Neurosurg*, 77, 15–19.

[41] Pusterla, N., Wilson, W.D., Conrad, P.A. *et al.* (2006) Comparative analysis of cytokine gene expression in cerebrospinal fluid of horses without neurologic signs or with selected neurologic disorders. *Am J Vet Res*, 67, 1433–1437.

[42] Beattie, M.S. (2004) Inflammation and apoptosis: linked therapeutic targets in spinal cord injury. *Trends Mol Med*, 10, 580–583.

[43] Rossignol, S., Schwab, M., Schwartz, M. *et al.* (2007) Spinal cord injury: time to move? *J Neurosci*, 27, 11782–11792.

[44] Webb, A.A., Ngan, S. and Fowler, J.D. (2010) Spinal cord injury I: a synopsis of the basic science. *Can Vet J*, 51, 485–492.

[45] Cao, H.Q. and Dong, E.D. (2013) An update on spinal cord injury research. *Neurosci Bull*, 29, 94–102.

[46] Varma, A.K., Das, A., Wallace, G.T. *et al.* (2013) Spinal cord injury: a review of current therapy, future treatments, and basic science frontiers. *Neurochem Res*, 38, 895–905.

[47] Popovich, P. and McTigue, D. (2009) Damage control in the nervous system: beware the immune system in spinal cord injury. *Nat Med*, 15, 736–737.

[48] Nout, Y.S. and Reed, S.M. (2005) Management and treatment of the recumbent horse. *Equine Vet Ed*, 7, 416–432.

[49] Moore, R.M. and Trim, C. (1992) Effect of xylazine on cerebrospinal fluid pressure in conscious horses. *Am J Vet Res*, 53, 1558–1561.

[50] Lacombe, V.A., Sogaro-Robinson, C. and Reed, S.M. (2010) Diagnostic utility of computed tomography imaging in equine intracranial conditions. *Equine Vet J*, 42, 393–399.

[51] Avella, C.S. and Perkins, J.D. (2011) Computed tomography in the investigation of trauma to the ventral cranium. *Equine Vet Ed*, 23, 333–338.

[52] Marshall, L.F., Marshall, S.B., Klauber, M.R. *et al.* (1992) The diagnosis of head injury requires a classification based on computed axial tomography. *J Neurotrauma*, 9 (Suppl 1), S287–S292.

[53] Maas, A.I., Hukkelhoven, C.W., Marshall, L.F. and Steyerberg, E.W. (2005) Prediction of outcome in traumatic brain injury with computed tomographic characteristics: a comparison between the computed tomographic classification and combinations of computed tomographic predictors. *Neurosurgery*, 57, 1173–1182 discussion.

[54] Chun, K.A., Manley, G.T., Stiver, S.I. *et al.* (2010) Interobserver variability in the assessment of CT imaging features of traumatic brain injury. *J Neurotrauma*, 27, 325–330.

[55] Tucker, R.L. and Farrell, E. (2001) Computed tomography and magnetic resonance imaging of the equine head. *Vet Clin North Am Equine Pract*, 17, 131–144.

[56] De Zani, D., Zani, D.D., Binanti, D. *et al.* (2013) Magnetic resonance features of closed head trauma in 2 foals. *Equine Vet Ed*, 25(10), 493–498.

[57] Stroman, P.W., Bosma, R.L., Kornelsen, J. *et al.* (2012) Advanced MR imaging techniques and characterization of residual anatomy. *Clin Neurol Neurosurg*, 114, 460–470.

[58] Fox, W.C., Park, M.S., Belverud, S. *et al.* (2013) Contemporary imaging of mild TBI: the journey toward diffusion tensor imaging to assess neuronal damage. *Neurol Res*, 35, 223–232.

[59] Schwarz, B. and Piercy, R.J. (2006) Cerebrospinal fluid collection and its analysis in equine neurologic disease. *Equine Vet Ed*, 18, 313–320.

[60] Green, E.M. and Green, S. Cerebrospinal fluid lactic acid concentration: reference values and diagnostic implications of abnormal concentrations in adult horses. *Proceedings of the 8th Annual Meeting of American College Veterinary Internal Medicine. May 10, Washington, DC*; 1990: pp. 495–499.

[61] Scheffer, C.J., Dik, K.J. and Sloet van Oldruitenborgh-Oosterbaan, M.M. (2001) Ataxia and pruritus in a pony due to a cervical vertebral fracture. *Tijdschr Diergeneeskd*, 126, 419–422.

[62] Sherrington, C.S. (1898) Croonian lecture (1897): the mammalian spinal cord as an organ of reflex action. *Philos Trans*, 190B, 128–138.

[63] Ditunno, J.F., Little, J.W., Tessler, A. and Burns, A.S. (2004) Spinal shock revisited: a four-phase model. *Spinal Cord*, 42 (7), 383–395.

[64] Smith, P.M. and Jeffery, N.D. (2005) Spinal shock—comparative aspects and clinical relevance. *J Vet Intern Med*, 19, 788–793.

[65] DeLahunta, A. (ed.) (1983) Spinal cord disease, in *Veterinary Neuroanatomy and Clinical Neurology*, W.B. Saunders, Philadelphia, pp. 169–220.

[66] Chiapetta, J.R., Baker, J.R. and Feeney, D.A. (1985) Vertebral fracture, extensor hypertonia of thoracic limbs, and paralysis of the pelvic limbs (Schiff-Sherrington syndrome) in an Arabian foal. *J Am Vet Med Assoc*, 186, 387.

[67] Dimock, A.N. and Puchalski, S.M. (2010) Cervical radiology. *Equine Vet Ed*, 2, 83–87.

[68] Berg, L.C., Nielsen, J.V., Thoefner, M.B. and Thomsen, P.D. (2003) Ultrasonography of the equine cervical region: a descriptive study in eight horses. *Equine Vet J*, 35, 647–655.

[69] Mitchell, C.W., Nykamp, S.G., Foster, R. *et al.* (2012) The use of magnetic resonance imaging in evaluating horses with spinal ataxia. *Vet Radiol Ultrasound*, 53, 613–620.

[70] van Wessum, R., Sloet van Oldruitenborgh-Oosterbaan, M.M. and Clayton, H.M. (1999) Electromyography in the horse in veterinary medicine and in veterinary research—a review. *Vet Q*, 21, 3–7.

[71] Nollet, H., Deprez, P., van Ham, L. *et al.* (2004) Transcranial magnetic stimulation: normal values of magnetic motor evoked potentials in 84 normal horses and influence of height, weight, age and sex. *Equine Vet J*, 36, 51–57.

[72] Nollet, H., Van Ham, L., Deprez, P. and Vanderstraeten, G. (2003) Transcranial magnetic stimulation: review of the technique, basic principles and applications. *Vet J*, 166, 28–42.

[73] Nollet, H., Vanschandevijl, K., Van Ham, L. *et al.* (2005) Role of transcranial magnetic stimulation in differentiating motor nervous tract disorders from other causes of recumbency in four horses and one donkey. *Vet Rec*, 157, 656–658.

[74] Chesnut, R.M., Temkin, N., Carney, N. *et al.* (2012) A trial of intracranial-pressure monitoring in traumatic brain injury. *N Eng J Med*, 367, 2471–2481.

[75] Bouzat, P., Sala, N., Payen, J.F. and Oddo, M. (2013) Beyond intracranial pressure: optimization of cerebral blood flow, oxygen, and substrate delivery after traumatic brain injury. *Ann Intensive Care*, 3, 23.

[76] Le Roux, P. (2013) Physiological monitoring of the severe traumatic brain injury patient in the intensive care unit. *Curr Neurol Neurosci Rep*, 13, 331.

[77] Bratton, S.L., Chestnut, R.M., Ghajar, J. *et al.* (2007) Guidelines for the management of severe traumatic brain injury. II. Hyperosmolar therapy. *J Neurotrauma*, 24 (Suppl 1), S14–S20.

[78] Fakhry, S.M., Trask, A.L., Waller, M.A. and Watts, D.D. (2004) Management of brain-injured patients by an evidence-based medicine protocol improves outcomes and decreases hospital charges. *J Trauma*, 56, 492–499 discussion 499–500.

[79] Farahvar, A., Gerber, L.M., Chiu, Y.L. *et al.* (2012) Increased mortality in patients with severe traumatic brain injury treated without intracranial pressure monitoring. *J Neurosurg*, 117, 729–734.

[80] Kortz, G.D., Madigan, J.E., Goetzman, B.W. and Durando, M. (1995) Intracranial pressure and cerebral perfusion pressure in clinically normal equine neonates. *Am J Vet Res*, 56, 1351–1355.

[81] Brosnan, R.J., LeCouteur, R.A., Steffey, E.P. *et al.* (2002) Direct measurement of intracranial pressure in adult horses. *Am J Vet Res*, 63, 1252–1256.

[82] Brosnan, R.J., Steffey, E.P., LeCouteur, R.A. *et al.* (2002) Effects of body position on intracranial and cerebral perfusion pressures in isoflurane-anesthetized horses. *J Appl Physiol*, 92, 2542–2546.

[83] Finfer, S., Bellomo, R., Boyce, N. *et al.* (2004) A comparison of albumin and saline for fluid resuscitation in the intensive care unit. *N Eng J Med*, 350, 2247–2256.

[84] Van Aken, H.K., Kampmeier, T.G., Ertmer, C. and Westphal, M. (2012) Fluid resuscitation in patients with traumatic brain injury: what is a SAFE approach? *Curr Opin Anaesthesiol*, 25, 563–565.

[85] Bulger, E.M. and Hoyt, D.B. (2012) Hypertonic resuscitation after severe injury: is it of benefit? *Adv Surg*, 46, 73–85.

[86] Wade, C.E., Grady, J.J., Kramer, G.C. *et al.* (1997) Individual patient cohort analysis of the efficacy of hypertonic saline/dextran in patients with traumatic brain injury and hypotension. *J Trauma*, 42, S61–S65.

[87] Kempski, O. (2001) Cerebral edema. *Semin Nephrol*, 21, 303–307.

[88] Meyer, M.J., Megyesi, J., Meythaler, J. *et al.* (2010) Acute management of acquired brain injury. Part II: An evidence-based review of pharmacological interventions. *Brain Inj*, 24, 706–721.

[89] Myburgh, J., Cooper, D.J., Finfer, S. *et al.* (2007) Saline or albumin for fluid resuscitation in patients with traumatic brain injury. *N Engl J Med*, 357, 874–884.

[90] Lu, J., Gary, K.W., Neimeier, J.P. *et al.* (2012) Randomized controlled trials in adult traumatic brain injury. *Brain Inj*, 26, 1523–1548.

[91] Ware, M.L., Nemani, V.M., Meeker, M. *et al.* (2005) Effects of 23.4% sodium chloride solution in reducing intracranial pressure in patients with traumatic brain injury: a preliminary study. *Neurosurgery*, 57, 727–736 discussion 727–736.

[92] White, H., Cook, D. and Venkatesh, B. (2006) The use of hypertonic saline for treating intracranial hypertension after traumatic brain injury. *Anesth Analg*, 102, 1836–1846.

[93] Fielding, C.L. and Magdesian, K.G. (2011) 2011. A comparison of hypertonic (7.2%) and isotonic (0.9%) saline for fluid resuscitation in horses: a randomized, double-blinded, clinical trial. *J Vet Intern Med*, 25, 1138–1143.

[94] Carlson, A.P., Schermer, C.R. and Lu, S.W. (2006) Retrospective evaluation of anemia and transfusion in traumatic brain injury. *J Trauma*, 61, 567–571.

[95] Robertson, C.S., Goodman, J.C., Narayan, R.K. *et al.* (1991) The effect of glucose administration on carbohydrate metabolism after head injury. *J Neurosurg*, 74, 43–50.

[96] van den Berghe, G., Wouters, P., Weekers, F. *et al.* (2001) Intensive insulin therapy in the critically ill patients. *N Engl J Med*, 345, 1359–1367.

[97] Vespa, P., Boonyaputthikul, R., McArthur, D.L. *et al.* (2006) Intensive insulin therapy reduces microdialysis glucose values without altering glucose utilization or improving the lactate/pyruvate ratio after traumatic brain injury. *Crit Care Med*, 34, 850–856.

[98] Marklund, N., Bakshi, A., Castelbuono, D.J. *et al.* (2006) Evaluation of pharmacological treatment strategies in traumatic brain injury. *Curr Pharm Des*, 12, 1645–1680.

[99] Bagley, R.S., Harrington, M.L., Pluhar, G.E. *et al.* (1996) Effect of craniectomy/durotomy alone and in combination with hyperventilation, diuretics, and corticosteroids on intracranial pressure in clinically normal dogs. *Am J Vet Res*, 57, 116–119.

[100] Meyer, M.J., Megyesi, J., Meythaler, J. *et al.* (2010) Acute management of acquired brain injury. Part I: An evidence-based review of non-pharmacological interventions. *Brain Inj*, 24, 694–705.

[101] Roberts, I., Yates, D., Sandercock, P. *et al.* (2004) Effect of intravenous corticosteroids on death within 14 days in 10008 adults with clinically significant head injury (MRC CRASH trial): randomised placebo-controlled trial. *Lancet*, 364, 1321–1328.

[102] Edwards, P., Arango, M., Balica, L. *et al.* (2005) Final results of MRC CRASH, a randomised placebo-controlled trial of intravenous corticosteroid in adults with head injury-outcomes at 6 months. *Lancet*, 365, 1957–1959.

[103] Reed, S.M. (2007) Head trauma: a neurological emergency. *Equine Vet Ed*, 19, 365–367.

[104] Wright, D.W., Kellermann, A.L., Hertzberg, V.S. *et al.* (2007) ProTECT: a randomized clinical trial of progesterone for acute traumatic brain injury. *Ann Emerg Med*, 49, 391–402 402 e391–392.

[105] Xiao, G., Wei, J., Yan, W. *et al.* (2008) Improved outcomes from the administration of progesterone for patients with acute severe traumatic brain injury: a randomized controlled trial. *Crit Care*, 12, R61.

[106] Moein, H., Khalili, H.A. and Keramatian, K. (2006) Effect of methylphenidate on ICU and hospital length of stay in patients with severe and moderate traumatic brain injury. *Clin Neurol Neurosurg*, 108, 539–542.

[107] Young, B., Ott, L., Twyman, D. *et al.* (1987) The effect of nutritional support on outcome from severe head injury. *J Neurosurg*, 67, 668–676.

[108] Bracken, M.B. (2012) Steroids for acute spinal cord injury. *Cochrane Database Syst Rev*, 1, CD001046.

[109] Bydon, M., Lin, J., Macki, M. *et al.* (2013) The current role of steroids in acute spinal cord injury. *World Neurosurg*, 82(5), 848–854.

[110] Hall, E.D., Wolf, D.L. and Braughler, J.M. (1984) Effects of a single large dose of methylprednisolone sodium succinate on experimental posttraumatic spinal cord ischemia. Dose-response and time-action analysis. *J Neurosurg*, 61, 124–130.

[111] Bracken, M.B., Shepard, M.J., Collins, W.F., Jr *et al.* (1992) Methylprednisolone or naloxone treatment after acute spinal cord injury: 1-year follow-up data. Results of the second National Acute Spinal Cord Injury Study. *J Neurosurg*, 76, 23–31.

[112] Bracken, M.B. and Holford, T.R. (1993) Effects of timing of methylprednisolone or naloxone administration on recovery of segmental and long-tract neurological function in NASCIS 2. *J Neurosurg*, 79, 500–507.

[113] Bracken, M.B., Shepard, M.J., Holford, T.R. *et al.* (1997) Administration of methylprednisolone for 24 or 48 hours or tirilazad mesylate for 48 hours in the treatment of acute spinal cord injury. Results of the Third National Acute Spinal Cord Injury Randomized Controlled Trial. National Acute Spinal Cord Injury Study. *JAMA*, 277, 1597–1604.

[114] Bracken, M.B., Shepard, M.J., Holford, T.R. *et al.* (1998) Methylprednisolone or tirilazad mesylate administration after acute spinal cord injury: 1-year follow up. Results of the Third National Acute Spinal Cord Injury randomized controlled trial. *J Neurosurg*, 89, 699–706.

[115] Behrmann, D.L., Bresnahan, J.C. and Beattie, M.S. (1994) Modeling of acute spinal cord injury in the rat: neuroprotection and enhanced recovery with methylprednisolone, U-74006F and YM-14673. *Exp Neurol*, 126, 61–75.

[116] Hall, E.D. (1992) The neuroprotective pharmacology of methylprednisolone. *J Neurosurg*, 76, 13–22.

[117] Bracken, M.B., Shepard, M.J., Hellenbrand, K.G. *et al.* (1985) Methylprednisolone and neurological function 1 year after spinal cord injury. Results of the National Acute Spinal Cord Injury Study. *J Neurosurg*, 63, 704–713.

[118] Bracken, M.B., Shepard, M.J., Collins, W.F. *et al.* (1990) A randomized, controlled trial of methylprednisolone or naloxone in the treatment of acute spinal-cord injury. Results of the Second National Acute Spinal Cord Injury Study. *N Eng J Med*, 322, 1405–1411.

[119] Kubeck, J.P., Merola, A., Mathur, S. *et al.* (2006) End organ effects of high-dose human equivalent methylprednisolone in a spinal cord injury rat model. *Spine*, 31, 257–261.

[120] Chvatal, S.A., Kim, Y.T., Bratt-Leal, A.M. *et al.* (2008) Spatial distribution and acute anti-inflammatory effects of Methylprednisolone after sustained local delivery to the contused spinal cord. *Biomaterials*, 29, 1967–1975.

[121] Zurita, M., Vaquero, J., Oya, S. and Morales, C. (2002) Effects of dexamethasone on apoptosis-related cell death after spinal cord injury. *J Neurosurg*, 96, 83–89.

[122] Hillen, B.K., Abbas, J.J. and Jung, R. (2013) Accelerating locomotor recovery after incomplete spinal injury. *Ann N Y Acad Sci*, 1279, 164–174.

[123] Houle, J.D. and Cote, M.P. (2013) Axon regeneration and exercise-dependent plasticity after spinal cord injury. *Ann N Y Acad Sci*, 1279, 154–163.

[124] Kaufmann, M.A., Buchmann, B., Scheidegger, D. *et al.* (1992) Severe head injury: should expected outcome influence resuscitation and first-day decisions? *Resuscitation*, 23, 199–206.

[125] Toth, B., Aleman, M., Nogradi, N. and Madigan, J.E. (2012) Meningitis and meningoencephalomyelitis in horses: 28 cases (1985–2010). *J Am Vet Med Assoc*, 240, 580–587.

[126] Dunkel, B., Corley, K.T., Johnson, A.L. *et al.* (2013) Pneumocephalus in five horses. *Equine Vet J*, 45, 367–371.

33 Disorders of the Peripheral Nervous System

Martin Furr

Marion duPont Scott Equine Medical Center, Virginia-Maryland Regional College of Veterinary Medicine, Leesburg, USA

Trauma to peripheral nerves can be induced by various methods including pressure, stretch, or direct force (blows). These forces can arise from either internal (masses, fractures) or external sources. The range and degree of deficit that results from trauma are dependent on numerous issues, including the degree of force applied, the location, and the amount of soft tissue covering of the nerve. In addition, stretching of nerves can induce damage particularly of the brachial plexus, while transection of nerves can occur secondary to wounds or fractures.

Mechanical trauma induces changes that have been classified into one of the following three categories: neuropraxia, axonotmesis, or neurotmesis [1]. In clinical cases, a mixture of these types is expected. Neuropraxia results from mild compressive lesion primarily resulting in bruising and inflammation of the nerve; axonal integrity is maintained. This nerve injury is transient and usually resolves within 3–6 weeks. Axonotmesis is a more severe injury, resulting from a crushing of the nerve; the epineurium and perineurium remain intact. Neurotmesis is the most severe, and describes complete disruption of nervous and perineural tissues.

Mechanical injury to peripheral neurons results in a characteristic series of events to the nerve. In axonotmesis or neuronotmesis, a stereotypical response occurs in the neuron. Primary degeneration involves a separation of the distal segment from the nerve cell body, and there is complete disintegration of the myelin sheath and telodendria, termed "Wallerian degeneration." Schwann cells proliferate to remove cellular debris, and in doing so form *band fibers* (*protoplasmic bands*) along the length of the disintegrated segment. These band fibers help to guide the regenerating axon (neurites) to the nerve termination. The axons can regrow at a rate of about 1 mm/day [2]. Only axons that reach their proper endoneurial tubes will reinnervate the distal stump and its end organ.

Following a traumatic event, as swelling of the nerve or surrounding tissue progresses, a characteristic progression of dysfunction ensues. Large-diameter myelinated fibers are first compromised, resulting in loss of proprioceptive function in the affected region. Placement deficits and mild ataxia may be observed. Large myelinated motor fibers are next affected, resulting in paresis or paralysis of voluntary and reflex movement. Smaller sensory axons are next compromised, resulting in loss of sensation, and finally the smallest diameter fibers, responsible for the sensation of pain, become dysfunctional. Hence, the severity of the nerve injury can be assessed by clinical observation and the assessment of the various peripheral nerve functions [3]. Loss of deep pain perception implies a much more severe injury to the nerve than proprioceptive deficits.

It may be difficult to identify specific areas of cutaneous hypalgesia due to the widespread degree of overlapping of innervated zones. Loss of sensation over a wide area of the limb suggests multiple nerve damage. Autonomous zones, that is, areas that are innervated by only one specific sensory nerve, are limited in the horse, but their presence allows clinical evaluation of a specific nerve.

Following complete transaction, a muscle will lose approximately one-half its mass by 2 weeks post injury. This atrophy will continue to progress until the nerve heals and innervation of the muscle is reestablished. Scarring and fibrosis of the muscle may limit healing and failure to heal beyond 12 months is associated with a poor prognosis (Tables 33.1 and 33.2).

General treatment

In the acute phase, general treatments directed at minimizing inflammation are appropriate. Systemic administration of nonsteroidal anti-inflammatory agents is helpful

Equine Neurology, Second Edition. Martin Furr and Stephen Reed.

Table 33.1 Innervation and clinical signs associated with major nerves of the pectoral limb.

Nerve	Muscle	Spinal cord segment	Clinical signs
Suprascapular	Supraspinatus	C6,7	Lateral rotation and subluxation of shoulder
	Infraspinatus		Atrophy of supraspinatus and infraspinatus
Axillary	Deltoideus	C7,8	Atrophy of deltoid
Musculocutaneous	Biceps brachii	C7,8	Overextension of elbow
	Brachialis		Hypalgesia medial forearm
			Atrophy of brachialis and biceps brachii
Radial	Triceps	C8,T1	Non-weight-bearing
	Extensor carpi radialis		Inability to extend/lock elbow
	Common digital extensor		Dorsum of pastern on ground
	Lateral digital extensor		
	Ulnaris lateralis		
Median	Flexor carpi radialis	C8,T1,2	Goose-stepping gait
			Dragging of toe
			Hyperextension of carpus, fetlock, and pastern
Ulnar	Superficial digital flexor	T1,2	Goose-stepping gait
	Flexor carpi ulnaris		Dragging of toe
			Hyperextension of carpus, fetlock, and pastern
Brachial plexus	As above	C6, T2	Signs of radial and suprascapular nerve injury as above
			Atrophy of supra and infraspinatus, triceps, and extensor carpi

Table 33.2 Innervation and clinical signs associated with major nerves of the pelvic limb.

Nerve	Muscle innervated	Spinal cord segments	Clinical signs
Gluteal	Gluteals	L5,6, S1,2	Mild abduction
			Outward rotation of stifle
			Gluteal muscle atrophy
Femoral	Quadraceps	L4,5	Inability to bear weight; knuckling/buckling
			Lack of limb extension
			Absent patella reflex
			Loss of sensation (medial thigh)
			Quadriceps atrophy
Obturator	Adductor	L4,5,6	Abduction of rear limbs
	Gracilus		Lateral slipping
Sciatic	Semimembranosis	L6–S1	Poor limb flexion
	Semitendonosis		Extended stifle and hock/flexed fetlock
			Hypalgesia (stifle down)
Peroneal	Long and lateral digital extensors	L5,6,S1	Knuckling of fetlock
			Unable to flex hock and extend digits
			Hypalgesia (cranial portion of limb)

to minimize neuronal or perineuronal swelling which may further compromise the nerve. Topical nonsteroidal pastes may also be beneficial in this regard. Dimethyl sulfoxide (DMSO) is commonly employed for nerve and soft tissue inflammation and may be given systemically (0.5–1 gm/kg IV as a 20% solution) or topically. Corticosteroids (0.05–0.2 mg/kg IV) may also be beneficial in the acute phase. Cold water hosing (hydrotherapy)

or ice packs in the acute phases of the injury may help minimize the degree of inflammation. Stall confinement is prudent to minimize further injury, and wraps may be needed for support or protection from further injury.

After the acute phase has passed and local inflammation has resolved, limited exercise may be appropriate. This allows the horse to develop compensatory mechanisms and strength, but this may not be appropriate in all cases. Physical therapy in the form of hydrotherapy, muscle massages, therapeutic ultrasound, and passive flexion may help improve the horses comfort and maintain range of motion [4]. Specific treatments are further discussed below as appropriate.

Specific peripheral nerve syndromes

Facial nerve

Facial nerve injury occurs following traumatic compression of the nerve as is passes over the facial crest, or inflammation of the nerve as it passes through the middle ear or guttural pouch. Damage to the facial nucleus in the brainstem is possible, and maybe seen in cases of bacterial, viral or protozoal encephalitis, verminous encephalitis, or neoplasia. Damage is almost always unilateral, but bilateral disease may be seen in cases of encephalitis. Clinical signs of damage to the distal portion of the facial nerve include deviation of the muzzle away from the affected side, and collapse of the ipsilateral alar fold. This is most commonly seen following recumbency during anesthesia or a tight-fitting halter. Injury of the nerve proximal to branching or involvement of the facial nucleus results in muzzle deviation away from the side of injury, ptosis, and ear droop. Tear production may be impaired resulting in corneal damage. Involvement of the facial nucleus or medulla may also result in alterations in mentation and perhaps ataxia. Due to the proximity of the vestibular nerve, proximal injury may also be associated with signs of head tilt, nystagmus, or circling (Figure 33.1).

Treatment is nonspecific as described earlier for traumatic injury. If the paralysis is secondary to another condition (e.g., equine protozoal myeloencephalitis or EPM, bacterial meningitis, temporomandibular osteoarthropathy), then specific treatment for the inciting condition is also employed.

Radial nerve

Damage to the radial nerve most commonly occurs from external blows due to collision with stationary objects, motor vehicles, or following lateral recumbency in anesthesia. It is also commonly involved in lesions of the brachial plexus. The clinical signs associated with radial nerve injury are fairly typical, and include an inability to flex the shoulder, extend the limb, and fix the elbow. This results in an inability of the horse to bear weight on the limb [5, 6]. The elbow remains in a slightly flexed position, with the dorsum of the hoof resting on the ground (Figure 33.2).

Brachial plexus

Brachial plexus damage results from compression of the nerve roots comprising the brachial plexus, usually between the medial aspect of the scapula and the ribs [7].

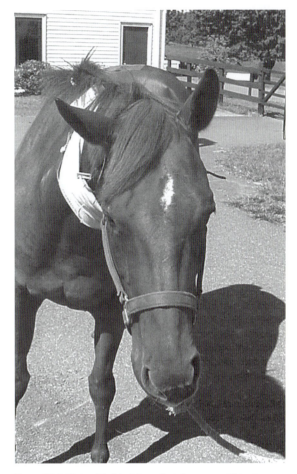

Figure 33.1 Right-sided facial paralysis in a mare. Note the dropped ear, muzzle deviation, and ptosis of the right eye. This suggests very proximal or central damage to the facial nerve. Profound mental depression was also present in this mare, and bacterial meningitis was diagnosed.

Stretching of the nerve roots may also lead to this injury. Clinical signs reflecting involvement of several different nerves may be seen in this condition, including a dropped elbow, inability to bear weight on the limb, and lateral deviation of the shoulder. Atrophy of the supraspinatus and infraspinatus muscles may be seen with this condition.

Musculocutaneous nerve

Injury to the musculocutaneous nerve is rare, and transaction does not result in obvious gait abnormalities [6]. Atrophy of the biceps and brachialis muscles, with hypalgesia of the medial aspect of the forearm, may be observed.

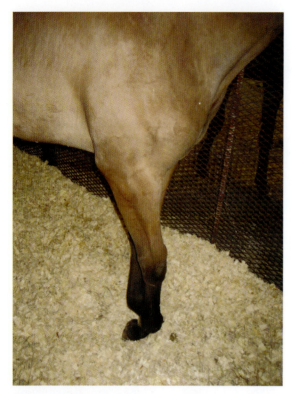

Figure 33.2 Radial nerve paralysis in a horse. Note dropped elbow and inability to extend distal limb. (Photo courtesy of Dr. Adriana Silva.)

Median and ulnar

Damage to the median and ulnar nerves may occur secondary to fracture of the humerus or following external trauma to the limb. Hyperextension of the carpus, fetlock, and pastern joints are seen, and the horse demonstrates a stiff, goose-stepping gait [6]. Hypalgesia of the medial distal aspect of the limb is seen with medial nerve damage, while the ulnar nerve innervates the lateral distal and caudal antebrachial aspect of the limb.

Suprascapular nerve damage ("sweeney")

Damage to the suprascapular nerve results in the clinical presentation known to horsemen for generations as "sweeney" (shoulder slip). The suprascapular nerve arises from the sixth and seventh cervical nerves and innervates the supraspinatus and infraspinatus muscles. The course of the nerve carries it across the cranial edge of the scapula. Although well protected by the brachiocephalicus, cutaneous colli and subclavian muscles, it is susceptible to trauma from collisions with other horses, fixed objects or kicks by nature of its adherence to the

scapula [2]. Classically, poorly fitted collars on draft animals were incriminated. Injury to the nerve from stretching can occur when horses stumble with the limb placed back. Hence, injury to the suprascapular nerve appears to be most frequent in horses that are worked over uneven ground [8]. In chronic cases, scar tissue can build up, further entrapping the nerve.

Clinical signs include atrophy of the supraspinatus and infraspinatus muscles, abduction of the limb during weightbearing, and an inability to advance the shoulder. These signs were also documented following selective anesthesia of the suprascapular nerve, indicating that damage to the suprascapular nerve alone is adequate to result in clinically relevant gait abnormalities [9]. Some horses will circumduct the affected leg. The lateral movement of the shoulder joint is best observed from the front, as the horse is walking toward the examiner. Diagnosis is made predominately by observation; however, electromyography (EMG) can be useful and will show denervation of involved muscles [10]. In cases resulting from direct trauma, some involvement of the brachial plexus is common. EMG will reveal denervation after about 1 week following induction. EMG evaluation should also include evaluation of muscles in the region other than the supraspinatus and infraspinatus. Denervation of other nerves suggests more widespread injury involving the brachial plexus and may influence prognosis (Figure 33.3).

Diagnosis is sometimes not straightforward in the acutely affected animal, in which localized swelling and pain may complicate the evaluation, and in which muscle atrophy is not present. Fractures of the shoulder should be considered, as well as localized infection or hematoma.

General treatment is as described earlier. Return of function can occur in several days of the damage is minimal, but several weeks may be necessary for reinnervation of the muscle. Based on anatomical studies and the anticipated regeneration rate for peripheral nerves (1 mm/day), function should return in about 70 days. Patients in which function has not returned in this period of time are suspected of having scar tissue entrapping the nerve [2]. Permanent fibrosis and contracture of affected muscles can occur with time, and it has been suggested that surgical decompression is recommended if there is no improvement after 90 days [2]. The procedure is described in detail in various textbooks of equine surgery, and the reader is referred to these for further discussion of the surgical technique.

Femoral nerve injury

The femoral nerve originates from the fourth and fifth lumbar spinal segments and innervates the quadriceps muscle. Injury has been observed following external trauma resulting in unilateral disease, or dystocia and

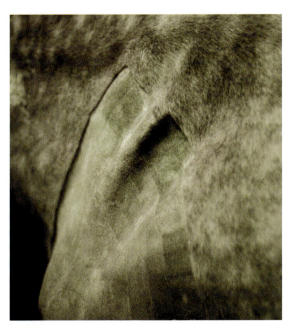

Figure 33.3 Supraspinatus and infraspinatus atrophy consistent with shoulder sweeney.

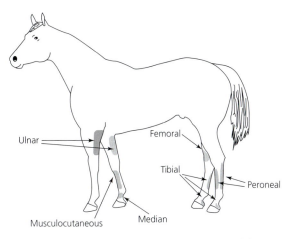

Figure 33.4 Autonomous zones of the major nerves of the front and rear limbs.

general anesthesia (bilateral disease) [11]. Femoral paralysis has been associated with abscesses, tumors, and aneurysms of the external iliac arteries, and fractures of the pelvis and femur [8].

Dysfunction of the femoral nerve leads to an inability to extend the stifle, and horses cannot support weight on the affected limb. Horses with bilateral disease may dog-sit. If able to stand, they adopt a characteristic crouching position with all joints flexed and standing on the toes, due to the action of the reciprocal apparatus. When walking, the limb is not advanced easily, and there is a decreased stride length. The patellar reflex is absent, and there may be hypalgesia or analgesia of the medial aspect of the rear limb above the hock. Atrophy of the quadriceps muscle will be noted within 1–2 weeks. Diagnosis is by observation, and is supported by history and EMG findings. Spinal cord disease at L4 and L5 can produce similar signs and should be considered, and severe muscle disease such as exertional rhabdomyolysis and recumbency myopathy can also produce similar clinical signs. Treatment is supportive and nonspecific, and the prognosis depends on the degree of compromise. Horses that remain standing or have only one affected leg may do well with time, although it is difficult to determine the extent of the damage for purposes of giving a prognosis.

Obturator nerve

The obturator nerve innervates the adductors of the thigh, and it may become damaged during difficult foaling. This appears to be far less common in mares than cows, but it has been reported to occur even without a history of dystocia [8]. Excessive traction during dystocia can lead to injury to this nerve be compressing the nerve between the fetus and the shaft of the ilium. Fractures of the sacrum or ilium could also lead to obturator paralysis. Clinical signs are the inability to adduct the rear limbs and horses will go "splay-legged," in some cases being unable to stand. Treatment is nonspecific control of inflammation, and good footing is imperative in managing such cases. Slings may be useful, but recovery of strength can take several weeks. The prognosis is guarded, and an approximate survival rate of 50% for postfoaling paralysis has been reported [8].

Sciatic nerve

The sciatic nerve supplies the extensor muscles of the hip and flexor muscles of the stifle, with the peroneal branch innervating the flexor muscles of the tarsus and extensors of the digit. The tibial branch innervates the digital flexor muscles. In the adult horse, the nerve is very deep and well protected; however in foals, it is more superficial and may be damaged by intramuscular injections. Pelvic fracture may damage the nerve, and inflammatory spinal cord disease, such as EPM, bacterial infection, or osteomyelitis can produce damage to the nerve. Sciatic nerve paralysis results in profound effects upon the gait; the limb hangs behind the horse with the stifle and hock extended. The foot cannot be advanced normally and must be dragged. If placed properly, the limb will bear weight, however. Hypalgesia extends over most of the thigh, with the exception of the medial aspect which is innervated by the femoral nerve.

The tibial branch of the sciatic nerve innervates the digital flexors. Paralysis is uncommon, but results in the fetlock resting in a flexed position. When moving, the limb is overflexed with the foot carried higher than normal, and the foot is placed on the ground with excessive force. Hence, the gait is very similar to that of stringhalt [8].

Flexors of the hock and extensors of the digits are innervated by the peroneal nerve. The nerve passes over the lateral condyle of the femur where it is susceptible to injury, typically from a kick from another horse. At rest, the horse holds the leg behind them, with the dorsum of the hoof resting on the ground. When moving, the foot cannot be advanced and is dragged forward, followed by an abrupt caudal movement during the weight bearing phase. If the foot is manually placed, the horse can bear weight on the limb. Prognosis is considered guarded, but many horses are reported to do well with time [8]. Treatment involves local anti-inflammatories and protection of the limb from injury during movement.

Polyneuritis equi

Polyneuritis equi (PNE) is an uncommon neurologic syndrome affecting horses of all ages and breeds. It has also been referred to as "cauda equina neuritis"; however, the observation that nerves outside of the cauda equina could be involved has suggested that the term "polyneuritis equi" is preferable. It was originally described by Drexler, in 1897 in a horse with tail and anal sphincter paralysis [12]. A case reported in 1833 bears similarities also, however [13]. The condition has been intermittently reported since that time in horses from North America and Europe [14–17]. There does not appear to be a breed, gender, or age predilection, with the youngest recorded case seen in a 17-month-old horse [18].

The etiology of the disorder is unknown; however, evidence suggests that it is an allergic-mediated polyneuropathy similar to Guillain–Barre syndrome of humans and experimental allergic neuritis (EAN) of laboratory rodents [19, 20]. Infections with equine herpesvirus-1 and camplylobacter, as well as immune-mediated reaction to Streptococcus species have been proposed, but there has not been confirmation [17]. Equine adenovirus-1 has been isolated from the spinal cord in two horses, suggesting a causal association; however, further work has not confirmed this report [21].

Research has demonstrated the presence of serum antibodies to the neuritogenic myelin protein P_2 in a number of animals with PNE [19, 22]. This is the same antigenic protein responsible for EAN, further supporting the putative pathophysiology of the disorder in horses. Lesions are characterized by a granulomatous inflammation of the roots of the affected nerves, with swelling and hemorrhage, and microscopic findings of hemorrhage, demyelination, axonal degeneration, granulomatous inflammation, and fibrosis. Inflammatory infiltrates in these lesions consist of lymphocytes, plasma cells, macrophages, eosinophils, and neturophils [21, 23, 24]. In addition, the cellular infiltrate is primarily composed of T-cells, with some B-cell infiltrates [25]. The antigenic specificity of the infiltrating cells was not investigated, but was assumed to be myelin.

Clinical signs

Clinical signs are typically a slowly progressive paralysis of the tail, anus, rectum, and bladder, with symmetrical hindlimb weakness and ataxia. Perineal hyperesthesia, followed by hypalgesia may be seen; in some cases, the area of hypalgesia is surrounded by a zone of hyperesthesia. Hence, perineal hyperesthesia may present as tail rubbing in the early stages. Penile prolapse with urine dribbling can be seen in males. Muscle atrophy is variably present. Cranial nerve dysfunction may also be seen coincident with or preceding the caudal signs. The cranial nerve signs are often asymmetric, in contrast to the caudal signs, although asymmetrical caudal signs have been reported [26]. Paralysis of masticatory and facial muscles, head tilt, nystagmus, tongue paralysis, and difficulty swallowing have all been reported. Impotence has been reported in stallions due to urospermia and erection failure [27] (Figure 33.5).

Diagnosis

Currently, no specific antemortem diagnostic test exists for the diagnosis of PNE. The diagnosis is primarily one of exclusion, supported by the presence of clinical signs of cauda equina syndrome and cranial nerve deficits. The presence of high serum concentrations of P_2 antibody is supportive; however, the test is not commercially available, and is not specific for PNE [19].

Routine clinicopathologic testing is indicated in the evaluation of horses with this presentation, and evidence of chronic inflammation is usually observed. Cerebrospinal fluid (CSF) is often abnormal. Xanthochromia, with a mildly increased cell count and total protein are common [14, 28]. Recently, the use of rectal ultrasound has been used to make an antemortem diagnosis based on enlargement and hypoechoic appearance of the extradural sacral nerve roots as they exited the ventral sacral foramina; iliac lymphadenopathy was also observed [29].

A number of rule outs should be considered prior to making a diagnosis of PNE. Equine herpesvirus-1 myeloencephalitis, rabies, sacral fracture, meningitis, sorghum cystitis, and verminous myelitis should all be considered. Evaluation as discussed in detail in Chapter 12 should be performed. A particularly

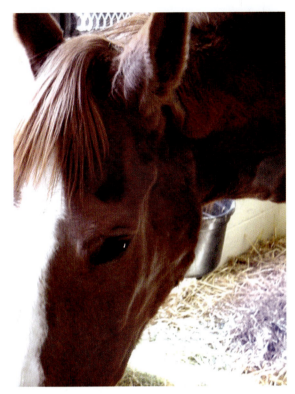

Figure 33.5 Masseter atrophy.

important consideration is EPM which can have a very similar clinical presentation. Horses with EPM do not usually have changes in the CSF, and definitive testing using serum/CSF antibody ratios will allow differentiation. See Chapter 22 for further discussion of EPM.

The definitive diagnosis is made on postmortem examination. Extradural and intradural nerve roots of the cauda equina are grossly thickened and have infiltration of inflammatory cells. Demyelination and axonal degeneration are present [23, 24, 30]. The changes are typically worse in the cauda equina, but changes of cranial nerves may also be observed.

Treatment

The primary treatment is palliative, including management of urinary and fecal incontinence, managing cystitis, and minimizing urine scalding. Horses that have difficulty eating may need tube feeding. Treatment with corticosteroids, preferably dexamethasone (0.05–0.1 mg/kg) has provided some palliative benefit, but most authors consider the effects short-lived. The condition is slowly progressive, but the overall outcome is generally poor.

References

[1] Seddon, H.J. (1943) Three types of nerve injury. *Brain*, 66, 237–288.

[2] Schneider, R.K. and Bramlage, L.R. (1990) Suprascapular nerve injury in horses. *Comp Contin Ed Pract Vet*, 12, 1783–1790.

[3] Blythe, L.L. (2003) Limb weakness, atrophy, and other signs of peripheral nerve disease, in *Current Therapy in Equine Medicine 5* (ed. N.E. Robinson), Saunders, St. Louis, pp. 735–740.

[4] Andrews, F.M., Mathews, H.K. and Reed, S.M. (1990) Medical, surgical and physical therapy for horses with neurologic disease. *Vet Med*, 85, 1229–1235.

[5] Rooney, J.R. (1963) Radial paralysis in the horse. *Cornell Vet*, 53, 328–331.

[6] Henry, R.W. Gait alterations in the equine pectoral limb produced by neurectomies. PhD Thesis. Ohio State University, Columbus, 1976.

[7] Mayhew, I.G. (1989) *Large Animal Neurology*, Lea and Febinger, Philadelphia.

[8] Han, C.N., Mayhew, I.G. and MacKay, R.J. (1999) Diseases of the peripheral (spinal) nerves, in *Equine Medicine and Surgery* (eds P.T. Colahan, A.M. Merritt, J.N. Moore and I.G. Mayhew), Mosby, St. Louis, pp. 975–980.

[9] Devine, D.V., Jann, H.W. and Payton, M.E. (2006) Gait abnormalities caused by selective anesthesia of the suprascapular nerve in horses. *Am J Vet Res*, 67, 834–836.

[10] Andrews, F.M. (1987) Electrodiagnostic aids in neurologic disease. *Vet Clin North Am Equine Pract*, 3, 293–322.

[11] Dyson, S., Taylor, P. and Whitwell, K. (1988) Femoral nerve paralysis after general anaesthesia. *Equine Vet J*, 20, 376–380.

[12] Drexler, H. (1897) Uber die combinierte chronische Schweiflahmungund Sphinkterenparalyse des Pferdes (Hammelschwanz). *Z Tiermed*, 279–299.

[13] Bainbridge, G. (1833) A case of palsy of the lips. *Veterinarian*, 16, 638.

[14] Rousseaux, C.G., Futcher, K.G., Clark, E.G. *et al.* (1984) Cauda equina neuritis: a chronic idiopathic polyneuritis in two horses. *Can Vet J*, 25, 214–218.

[15] Wright, J.A., Fordyce, P. and Edington, N. (1987) Neuritis of the cauda equina in the horse. *J Comp Pathol*, 97, 667–675.

[16] Greenwood, A.G., Barker, J. and McLeish, I. (1973) Neuritis of the cauda equine in a horse. *Equine Vet J*, 5, 111–115.

[17] Scarratt, K. and Jortner, B.S. (1985) Neuritis of the cauda equina in a yearling filly. *Comp Contin Ed Pract Vet*, 7, S197–S202.

[18] Vatistas, N.J., Mayhew, I.G., Whitwell, K.E. *et al.* (1991) Polyneuritis equi: a clinical review incorporating a case report of a horse displaying unconventional signs. *Prog Vet Neurol*, 2, 67–72.

[19] Kadlubowski, M. and Ingram, P.L. (1981) Circulating antibodies to the neuritogenic myelin protein, P2, in neuritis of the cauda equina of the horse. *Nature*, 293, 299–300.

[20] Hanhn, C.N. (2006) Miscellaneous disorders of the equine nervous system: Horners syndrome and polyneuritis equi. *Clin Tech Equine Pract*, 5, 43–48.

[21] Edington, N., Wright, J.A., Patel, J.R. *et al.* (1984) Equine adenovirus 1 isolated from cauda equina neuritis. *Res Vet Sci*, 37, 252–254.

[22] Fordyce, P.S., Edington, N., Bridges, G.C. *et al.* (1987) Use of an ELISA in the differential diagnosis of cauda equina neuritis and other equine neuropathies. *Equine Vet J*, 19, 55–59.

[23] Cummings, J.F., de Lahunta, A. and Timoney, J.F. (1979) Neuritis of the cauda equina, a chronic idiopathic polyradiculoneuritis in the horse. *Acta Neuropathol*, 46, 17–24.

[24] Yvorchuk-St Jean, K. (1987) Neuritis of the cauda equina. *Vet Clin North Am Equine Pract*, 3, 421–427.

[25] van Galen, G., Cassart, D., Sanderson, C. *et al.* (2008) The composition of the inflammatory infiltrate in three cases of polyneuritis equi. *Equine Vet J*, 40, 185–188.

[26] Bazargani, T.T., Rafia, S., Helan, J.A. and Moaddab, S.H. (2010) Occurrence of unilateral posterior polyneuritis in an 8-year-old crossbred mare. *J Equine Vet Sci*, 30, 711–714.

[27] Held, J.P., Vanhooser, S., Prater, P. *et al.* (1989) Impotence in a stallion with neuritis cauda equine: a case report. *J Equine Vet Sci*, 9, 67–68.

[28] White, P.L., Genetzky, R.M., Pohlenz, J.F. *et al.* (1984) Neuritis of the cauda equina in a horse. *Comp Contin Ed Pract Vet*, 6, S217–S223.

[29] Aleman, M., Katzman, S.A., Vaughan, B. *et al.* (2009) Antemortem diagnosis of polyneuritis equi. *J Vet Intern Med*, 23, 665–668.

[30] Summers, B. (1995) Diseases of the peripheral nervous system, in *Veterinary Neuropathology* (eds B. Summers, J.F. Cummings and A. de Lahunta), Mosby, St. Louis, pp. 402–501.

34 Equine Neurotoxic Agents and Conditions

Martin Furr

Marion duPont Scott Equine Medical Center, Virginia-Maryland Regional College of Veterinary Medicine, Leesburg, USA

Specific neurointoxications appear to be rare in the horse, yet there remain a substantial number of compounds which can result in neurologic illness, either as a primary or secondary illness. Any horse that is severely shocky or compromised might well demonstrate weakness and ataxia as a secondary sign, yet not have specific neurologic disease. This is often difficult to discriminate in the clinical setting. Compounds discussed in the following text demonstrate specific neurotoxic properties in the horse, or result in clinical signs in which neurologic deficits are a major presenting sign. The effects of many of the compounds are very poorly described in the equine species and literature, and are represented by very few cases.

Pharmaceutical toxicity

Fluphenazine

In veterinary medicine and equine practice in particular, the phenothiazine derivative tranquilizers have been an important contribution to the management of many conditions. The most commonly used compounds of this class, promazine and acetylpromazine, have a wide margin of safety, but a short duration of action. In conditions in which longer duration of activity is desired other phenothiazine formulations that are not approved for use in the horse have been used including fluphenazine, perphenazine, and pipothiazine. These extended duration phenothiazines are used in humans as an antipsychotic, and they act by blocking dopamine receptors in the limbic region of the brain; as a group, they are referred to as neuroleptics [1]. In addition, however, they also block dopamine receptors in the striatum, leading to a variety of side effects referred to as the "extrapyramidal syndrome" (EPS). This syndrome is characterized by involuntary muscle spasms, particularly of the head and neck and proximal extremities (dystonia), as well as a motor restlessness, which causes the patient to pace or rock uncontrollably (akathisia).

Although not approved for use in the horse, fluphenazine has been used as a long-term sedative for horses with behavioral problems. Conventional doses given to adult horses range from 25 to 50 mg intramuscularly, every 3–4 weeks. This dosage is not based on any known pharmacokinetic analysis, and the metabolism and clearance of the drug are totally unknown in the horse. Horses have demonstrated typical EPS-like signs following these doses; it has also been observed in horses in which it had been used previously with no observed complications.

In reported cases, the clinical signs have been noted to begin at 14–36 h after administration [2, 3]. Clinical signs include restlessness and agitation, accompanied by sweating and muscle tremors. Uncontrollable gross body movements may occur, with the horse crashing into walls and staggering. Characteristically, there are writhing movements of the head and neck associated with a repetitive striking movement of one or both front legs. Horses are commonly noted to refuse to move forward. The clinical presentation can be confused with a seizure, and can lead to self-induced injury to the horse, as well as put owners or handlers at risk of injury. Horses suffering from this condition are not typically aggressive toward people, but affected horses must be handled with caution.

Treatment is symptomatic and has involved the use of various sedatives and/or anticonvulsants for immediate control, in some cases coupled with the anticholinergics benztropine or diphenhydramine hydrochloride [1–3]. The severity of the condition will dictate treatment, and not all drugs appear to work in all cases. Xylazine or detomidine will provide transient relaxation in many cases, sometimes lasting only several minutes. Phenothiazine tranquilizers should be avoided, due to the potential to worsen the clinical signs. Combinations of intravenous pentobarbital (4.8 mg/kg loading dose and 1.2 mg/kg maintenance as needed) and phenobarbital (1 mg/kg) have been reported to control the clinical signs and allow the horse to stand quietly and eat [2]. In another report, a horse responded to intravenous administration of diphenhydramine hydrochloride (0.6 mg/kg). Clinical signs abated within minutes and remained absent for another 18 h, after which time a second dose given with equal effect. The authors experience with the use of diphenhydramine for the control of EPS is variable, with some horses not responding at all. Benztropine (0.035 mg/kg PO q12 h; 0.018 mg/kg IV, q12 h) has been used in horses with EPS resulting from fluphenazine toxicity with good results [3]. In most reported cases, as well as the author's clinical experience, most horses recover within 5–7 days with no long-term effects.

One case of EPS associated with administration of the neuroleptic pipothiazine palmitate (250 mg IM) has been described, with clinical signs identical to fluphenazine [4]. Clinical signs in this case occurred 5 days after injection, and the horse recovered over several days with empirical clinical management using diazepam (10 mg q4 h).

Ivermectin and moxidectin

Overdose with the anthelmintic ivermectin can result in neurologic disease. A 10× dose of ivermectin given to a zebra foal resulted in depression, ataxia and blindness which began approximately 12 h after administration [5]. The zebra recovered and was considered normal by 5 days after ingestion. Other reported cases were also foals, which were inadvertently given an entire syringe of product. Clinical signs were similar, and one foal died 18 h after ingestion associated with severe bradycardia [5]. This is similar to other reports in which a 10× overdose orally to adult horses resulted in blindness, ataxia, and depression, which persisted for 4 days [6]. With injectable ivermectin, doses of 15× resulted in mild neurologic signs (mydriasis) [6]. Lower doses of ivermectin (2×–3×) have been reported to cause toxic signs in foals that have had a previous neurologic disease.

Toxicity associated with ivermectin has also been observed in horses given an appropriate dosage, however. Three horses given a normal dosage of ivermectin demonstrated signs of toxicity; two horses recovered with conservative treatment. Reasons for why these three horses out of a group of five treated had signs of toxicity was not determined [7]. In addition, an outbreak of ivermectin toxicity was observed in six horses given a standard dosage of ivermectin but which had also consumed a large amount of *Solanum eleagnifolium* (Silverleaf nightshade) and *Solanum dimidiatum* (Western horse nettle). It was hypothesized that gastrointestinal irritation led to enhanced absorption of the ivermectin as serum concentrations of ivermectin were higher than pharmacokinetic studies would suggest [8]. However, the blood concentrations that resulted were inadequate to cause the clinical signs

seen, and it was further supposed that toxins from the Solanum plants might have either damaged the blood–brain barrier (BBB), leading to increased cerebrospinal fluid (CSF) concentrations of ivermectin, or there might have been interaction between the solanum toxins and ivermectin [8].

Clinical signs of ivermectin toxicity include mydriasis, ataxia, blindness, and recumbency. Muscle tremors are often present, and horses may also have signs of hyperesthesia and agitation. Tachycardia is commonly reported, and there is no fever. Facial nerve abnormalities are often reported, with paralysis of the lips; due to the degree of depression the head may be held low with secondary passive congestion. Excessive salivation may be seen. Defecation and urination are occasionally affected.

Ivermectin causes paralysis of nematodes and arthropods by potentiating the release of gamma aminobutyric acid (GABA) [9]. GABA is an inhibitory neurotransmitter found in the central nervous system (CNS) of vertebrates and peripheral nervous system of invertebrates and blocks postsynaptic transmission of nerve impulses by hyperpolarization of neuronal membranes [10, 11]. This is the basis for neurotoxicity; however, ivermectin does not readily cross the BBB, hence the potential for toxicity is minimized. Mutation in a multidrug resistance gene (*mdr*1) in Collie dogs results in a deletion of the P-glycoprotein of the BBB which is important in excluding ivermectin from the CNS [12]. Dogs with this genotype are very sensitive to the effects of ivermectin. No such genetic trait has been observed in horses; however, it is possible that there are similar conditions that might make some animals more sensitive to the drug than others.

Overdose with moxidectin has also resulted in neurologic signs in horses [13, 14]. Moxidectin is a macrolide anthelmintic which is structurally similar to the avermectins, but is in the chemical class of milbemycims. Overdose with moxidectin can result in signs of coma, dyspnea, depression, ataxia, trembling, seizures, and muscle weakness [14]. The approximate dose at which these signs were seen was from 1.0 to 5.0 mg/kg, which is 2.5–13 times the approved label dosage of 0.4 mg/kg. Clinical signs have been seen in young foals (<4 months of age) after a single dosage of 5× the label dose, or three consecutive daily doses of 3× the label dose [15].

Most reported cases are in foals, with adults seemingly less commonly affected. This has been proposed to be due to an increased sensitivity of foals to the toxic effects of the drug, but may simply be that foals are more likely than adults to be given an overdose due to the nature of the drug delivery system (i.e., an oral dose syringe). Failure of the syringe locking mechanisms or intentional administration of the entire tube has both been reported as causes of the overdose. The mechanism of toxicity is believed to be similar to that of ivermectin.

Clinical signs are noted from 6 to 18 h after administration and signs persisted for 36–168 h. In contrast to ivermectin overdosage, blindness has not been reported with moxidectin overdose.

Treatment of either ivermectin or moxidectin overdose is primarily supportive. If an overdose is quickly identified, oral activated charcoal can be given. Intravenous fluid support may be necessary for severely affected animals. Dimethylsulfoxide and/or corticosteroids can be given; however, their efficacy for the treatment of this condition is unknown. Control of seizures and self-induced injury may be required, and should be determined on a case-by-case basis.

Picrotoxin has been recommended as a reversal agent for ivermectin toxicosis in dogs, as it functions as a GABA-receptor antagonist [11]. It is reported to have a narrow margin of safety, and it has been used in the treatment of ivermectin toxicity of calves with no discernible effect [16]. Hence, the use of picrotoxin in horses, although it has not been empirically evaluated, is not recommended at this time. Sarmazenil (0.04 mg/kg IV q2 h) blocks chloride conductance and theoretically may be useful in ivermectin and moxidectin toxicity. It has been used in foals with ivermectin or moxidectin toxicity with mixed results; no effect in a foal with ivermectin overdose, and good effect in a foal with moxidectin toxicity [17, 18].

Intravenous administration of 20% lipid emulsion has been reported to be effective in one foal with ivermectin toxicity, presumably by acting as a "lipid sink" to remove the lipophilic ivermectin from the CNS into the peripheral circulation to be metabolized [17]. This was temporally associated with an improvement in clinical signs, and assay of blood ivermectin concentrations, although these results are not confirmatory that it was effective. Hence, treatment with lipid emulsion may represent a reasonable and cost effective adjunct to treatment of ivermectin toxicosis.

The majority of reported cases have recovered with supportive care; however, affected foals have died despite intensive supportive care, and adult horses have been euthanized due to the severity of the condition.

Tentative diagnosis can be determined by the clinical signs and history of exposure. No typical clinical chemistry abnormalities are expected with ivermectin or moxidectin overdose. Serum, plasma, liver, kidney, or adipose tissue can be assayed, but toxic levels in horses are not known [14].

Haloxon

Bilateral laryngeal paralysis has been reported following the use of haloxon as an anthelmintic in foals. At doses of 1 and 2 g, every 14 days several foals developed dyspnea after three doses of haloxon. A stiff gait was also described premortem, but this was not evaluated in detail. Biopsy of the recurrent laryngeal nerves found nerve cell death, Wallerian degeneration, and demyelination [19].

Levamasol

Levamasol is occasionally used in the horse as an anthelmintic and potential immunomodulator. The toxic dose is 20 mg/kg BW, and clinical signs (sometimes resulting in death) have been seen within 1 h of administration [20]. Hyperexcitability, muscle tremors, hyperactivity, excessive sweating, and lacrimation have been reported [21]. Treatment is supportive, and clinical signs generally resolve within 12 h in survivors.

Propylene glycol

Propylene glycol is commonly present in the veterinary environment and is used to treat bovine ketosis. Due to the similarity of appearance and storage, inadvertent administration of propylene glycol has occurred in horses [22–24]. Oral dosing of 3/4 gallon of propylene glycol in a clinical patient resulted in severe depression and ataxia, and doses of 1/2 to 1 gallon resulted in depression and ataxia, which was transient and resolved within 3 days with no specific treatment. Two gallons of propylene glycol administered to an adult horse resulted in recumbency, followed by severe diarrhea; the horse died after 3 days [23]. Treatment is supportive; administration of activated charcoal may be beneficial.

Ionophores

Ionophore compounds are polyether antibiotics that include the compounds monensin, lasalocid, salinomycin, narasin, and maduromycin. Although primarily a cardiotoxin, signs of neurologic disease can be seen with acute ionophore toxicity. Toxicity with monensin is the most commonly reported, presumably because it has been in commercial use for the longest time, although toxicity with salinomycin has also been reported [25–27]. Horses gain access to the ionophores due to mixing errors or accidental feeding with treated cattle feed.

The ionophores are a family of compounds that transport specific alkali metal cations across cell membranes [25]. Specifically, ionophores are selective in their influence on the movement of sodium and potassium ions between intracellular and extracellular spaces. A secondary influence on calcium is also recognized. In fact, the myocardial and skeletal muscle toxicity of ionophores is probably related to the increase in intracellular calcium, which initiates a series of events leading to cell death [28, 29].

Neurologic abnormalities associated with ionophore toxicity are depression and ataxia which are noted within 24–48 h of consumption of monensin. Horses demonstrate weakness of the rear limbs, reluctance to move and stumbling. They may lie down and then stand frequently, until such time that they remain recumbent [30, 31]. Profuse sweating is noted in horses with monensin, but not lasalocid intoxication [27]. Poisoning with salinomycin results in similar clinical signs, although some horses showed acute swelling of the masseter and eyelid regions [26]. It is unclear if the neurologic signs observed are simply a result of the combined effects of abdominal pain, myopathy and shock, or if a specific neuropathy is present, as the nervous system is such cases has not been carefully examined. Other conditions to consider in the list of differential diagnoses are exertional myopathy, intoxication with white snakeroot or coffee senna, blister beetle intoxication, nutritional myodegeneration, or primary myocardial disease.

Diagnosis of ionophore intoxication antemortem is challenging, and is greatly aided by a careful history suggesting a feed change or the possibility of consumption of intoxicated feeds. Clinical signs are not specific, but typically laboratory evaluation will demonstrate hemoconcentration, hypokalemia, and hypocalcemia [25, 27, 31].

Horses appear to be very sensitive to the effects of ionophores, and feed containing 279 ppm monensin is lethal to adult horses, while feed with 125 ppm monensin is toxic, although not fatal [30]. The LD50 of monensin for horses has been estimated to be 2–3 mg/kg body weight, while 20 mg/kg body weight is fatal [30]. The LD50 of lasalocid for horses has been estimated to be 21.5 mg/kg body weight [31].

Treatment for ionophore toxicity is primarily supportive, as there is no specific antidote. The use of Vitamin E and selenium is suggested in other species but is unproven in the horse [27].

Environmental toxins

Bromide
Methyl bromide has been used as a soil fumigant and ingestion of hay from fumigated fields has resulted in signs of ataxia in horses [32]. Clinical signs include ataxia, an "ambling" gait, and dragging of the feet. Hay from the fumigated field was found to have a bromide concentration of 6800 ppm, and serum from affected horses had a bromide concentration of 36.9 mEq/l [32]. In a test feeding, horses developed clinical signs after 7 days of consuming the affected hay. This resulted in a total consumption of 49 g of bromide ion per day. Prognosis for bromide intoxication is variable, and eliminating the source of bromide and supportive care has sometimes been successful.

Urea
Poisoning with urea is rare in the horse, but has been reported to occur occasionally [33]. Horses may become intoxicated by accidental feeding of ammonia or by gaining access to urea treated cattle feeds. Aimless wandering, incoordination, depression, head pressing, convulsions, and death have been observed in ponies feed 450 g of ammonia. Diagnosis is made by detection of increased blood and/or CSF ammonia concentrations in the absence of liver disease. Treatment is supportive and the prognosis is considered poor, although there are limited equine reports to confirm this position.

Organophosphates
Organophosphates are commonly used as animal insecticides and parasiticides, plant insecticides, herbicides, rodenticides, and insect repellants. There is a bewildering array of organophosphate formulations, each with subtle differences in its metabolism, toxic potential and clinical effects.

Organophosphates are readily absorbed from the gastrointestinal tract or through skin [20]. They exert their toxic action by irreversible inhibition of cholinesterase and pseudocholinesterase, resulting in the accumulation of acetylcholine at neuromuscular junctions, cholinergic synapses within the CNS, and parasympathetic postganglionic sites [20]. Clinical signs are a direct consequence of this overstimulation.

Profuse salivation, lacrimation, and nasal discharge are observed due to the stimulation of muscarinic cholinergic sites. Due to increased secretion and muscular contraction, abdominal pain and diarrhea may be seen. Bradycardia, miosis, sweating, and frequent urination are observed. Neurologic abnormalities include muscle stiffness and fasciculations, tremors, and a stiff, awkward gait. Anxiety, nervousness, and hyperactivity may be seen due to the diffuse CNS stimulation arising from overstimulation of the nicotinic cholinergic receptors.

The clinical syndrome of organophosphate toxicity is fairly characteristic, and coupled with a history of exposure should provide a presumptive diagnosis. Confirmation is best attempted antemortem by determining cholinesterase activity in blood or other body tissue. Blood cholinesterase activity of greater than 25% of normal are considered confirmatory [20]. Differential considerations include carbamate toxicity, blister beetle, botulism, colic, and pheochromocytoma.

Treatment of organophosphate intoxication is most readily attempted with atropine sulfate. A dose of 0.2 mg/kg BW has been recommended, with 1/4 given IV and the remainder subcutaneously or intramuscularly. This can be repeated as necessary at 3–6 h intervals, with the minimum amount possible used to minimize the risk of gut stasis and colic [20]. Muscle fasciculations may not be affected by atropine treatment.

Other treatment options include use of an oxime compound, 2-PAM (praladoxime chloride). This will free the organophosphate from the receptor. The recommended dose varies between 20 and 50 mg/kg BW IV, and it should be given after atropine to optimize its action. Phenothiazine tranquilizers, succinylcholine, and morphine should specifically be avoided in suspect organophosphate intoxication cases.

Carbamates

Intoxication with the carbamate pesticides results in clinical signs that are very similar to the organophosphates. As the carbamates are reversibly bound to the cholinesterase receptor they can be removed by spontaneous hydrolysis and consequently the clinical signs resulting from intoxication tend to be short-lived (36–48 h).

Diagnosis is as for the organophosphates, and chemical analysis of tissues or fluids are often unrewarding. Confirmation of the compound in stomach contents may be helpful in confirming exposure.

Recommended treatment is atropine sulfate (0.2 mg/kg BW, 1/4 IV and the remainder subcutaneously or intramuscularly). The oxime compounds should not be used in cases of suspected carbamate toxicity, as they are of no benefit and may in fact worsen the clinical signs in cases of carbaryl poisoning. Activated charcoal can be given, but mineral oil should be avoided as it may enhance absorption of the compound [20].

Nicotine

Nicotine sulfate has been used as a plant insecticide, premise spray, and historically as an ectoparaciticide. In addition, the shrub pituri (*Duboisia hopwoodii*) is widely distributed in Western Australia, and it contains nicotine; horses have been poisoned by grazing the plant [34]. The lethal dose of nicotine in the horse is reported to be 100–300 mg [20]. Nicotine is readily absorbed from the oral mucosa, gastrointestinal tract, respiratory tract, and intact skin.

Nicotine stimulates autonomic nervous system ganglia, neuromuscular junctions, and some synapses in the CNS by interaction with the nicotonic receptor and subsequent depolarization of the postsynaptic membrane. In larger concentrations, this initial depolarization is immediately followed by blockade of the receptor. Death is due to paralysis of respiratory muscles, owing to blockade of the neuromuscular junction.

Clinical signs of intoxication include signs of cholinergic stimulation (agitation, nervousness, salivation, tachypnea, diarrhea), shortly followed by depression, muscle weakness, ataxia, and an increased heart rate. In humans, low blood pressure, mental confusion, and weak pulse are prominent [35]. Seizures may occur, and progression to prostration and death due to respiratory paralysis can occur [20].

Diagnosis is established by the clinical signs of cholinergic stimulation followed by paralysis, accompanied by a history of potential exposure. There are no characteristic clinicopathological changes, and no observable abnormalities on postmortem. The odor of tobacco may be present in gut content if the toxin is ingested. There is no antidote, and treatment is supportive and empirical. Activated charcoal can be given, and the horse washed if the exposure was cutaneous. Atropine is not considered to be of value.

Mercury

Intoxication of horses with mercury has only rarely been reported, but chronic ingestion of grain treated with fungicidal mercury compounds can be a source of intoxication [36]. Clinical signs of ataxia, hypermetria, muscle trembling, and head bobbing were noted. Chronic ingestion of phenylmercuric acetate (0.672 mg/kg for 191 days) resulted in dermatitis, gingival swelling and necrosis, weight loss, and masseter muscle atrophy. Dullness, depression, and weakness were also seen. It is unclear if these signs were associated with primary neurologic disease, or were merely secondary signs [37]. Poisoning with mercuric chloride did not result in neurotoxicity [38]. One horse suffered intoxication from a mercuric blister applied to treat a leg injury, but the clinical signs included renal failure and dermatitis; no neurologic signs were noted [39]. In another horse treated with a mercury blister (mercury chloride in herb and alcohol base; 5.3% mercury) for a leg wound, mercury toxicity ensued and was expressed as renal failure, colic, and ventral edema [40]. No clinical neurologic signs were detected, but neuronal necrosis and edema of the brain was evident on postmortem examination [40].

Lead

Horses become exposed to lead via ingestion of forage contaminated by aerial fallout of lead surrounding smelting plants or highway rights of way, chewing on surfaces painted with lead-based paint, or from ingestion of lead-based orchard herbicidal sprays. These sources lead to the chronic form of lead toxicity ("plumbism"). Acute lead intoxication appears to be very uncommon in the horse due to their selective eating habits; however, it has been reported from ingestion of paint and motor oil [41, 42]. In developed countries, public health policies to decrease environmental contamination with lead has probably resulted in the seemingly less common presentation of this disorder in the horse in recent years.

A daily intake of 1.7 mg/kg for several months will result in classic signs of chronic lead toxicity [43]. This corresponds to the average daily consumption of forage with 80 ppm lead (dry weight). Limited data are available on acute toxicity of horses with lead, but one horse was given 1000 mg of lead/kg with only nonspecific clinical signs [44].

Lead disrupts nerve transmission, probably by interference with the availability of calcium [45]. Lead also interfered with the uptake of dopamine and the metabolism of GABA [45]. Motor nerves are more susceptible than sensory nerves. This is consistent with the clinical presentation.

Chronic ingestion of lead commonly leads to signs of peripheral neuropathy. The most commonly noted neurologic signs in horses include dysphagia and abnormal phonation (roaring) due to pharyngeal and laryngeal paralysis. Other clinical signs include facial paralysis, muscle weakness with ataxia, dysmetria of the tongue and lips, and anal sphincter paresis. Cerebral signs such as depression are rare in horses, but can be seen in severe intoxications. Inhalation pneumonia may develop secondary to the dysphagia. Colic and protein losing enteropathy with ventral edema have been reported occasionally. Joint swelling and lameness can be seen in young growing animals. A blue "lead line" around the base of the teeth has also been reported in the horse. In a summary of reported lead intoxications of the horse, roughened hair coat was the most common clinical signs (53% of cases) and weight loss was seen in 36% [41]. Neurologic signs, such as incoordination (20% of cases) or laryngeal dysfunction (44% of cases), were commonly seen as well.

Clinical chemistry analysis of horses with lead toxicity is usually normal, although nonspecific changes may be noted in horses with colic or pneumonia. Hypoproteinemia is occasionally seen, and mild dehydration may be seen in horses with colic or dysphagia. White blood cell counts are usually normal unless the illness is complicated by pneumonia or colic. Anemia was reported in 22% of reported cases [41], and is usually mild when seen [42]. Immature RBCs and basophilic stippling are sometimes seen.

Diagnosis is supported by clinical signs and history of exposure, accompanied by assays of blood or urine for lead. Concentration of blood lead greater than 0.35 ppm should be considered significant; however, lower values do not rule out lead toxicity due to sequestration of lead in bone [42]. In addition, there seems to be little correlation of blood lead concentrations and the severity of the clinical signs. An increase of urine lead concentration (>1 ppm) following chelation treatment is also supportive of lead poisoning. Anemia or dehydration can alter blood concentrations and interpretation of blood lead concentrations in such animals should be done with caution. In cases of chronic poisoning blood lead concentrations may be low, due to redistribution of lead to peripheral tissues. CSF evaluation is usually normal, and electromyography (EMG) findings in one horse with lead intoxication were normal [41]. Assay of liver or kidney can be used to confirm lead intoxication.

Other inferential assays for lead toxicity include increased urine delta aminolevulinic acid (>200 mg/dl), but alteration of this compound appears to be inconsistent in the horse. In addition, the presence of increased free erythrocytoporphyrin concentrations correlates directly with blood lead concentrations. These assays are rarely used in clinical practice [42, 46].

Recommended treatment is chelation with 6.6% calcium disodium EDTA (calcium versenate). This will mobilize lead from peripheral tissues and enhance clearance. The recommended dosage is 50–100 mg/kg of calcium versenate given intravenously once per day for 3 days, then repeated after a nontreatment interval of 4 days. Repeated blood and urine assays should reveal decreasing concentrations, and treatment can be discontinued when normal values are obtained. The duration of treatment necessary to obtain clearance is unknown, but in two reported cases, 10 days total of treatment was adequate [41]. In addition to chelation therapy, thiamine (1 mg/kg, once/day) can be given, and is reported to be beneficial. Ancillary treatments are dictated by the nature of the horses other clinical problems. Long-term prognosis is unknown, but mild clinical signs may persist.

Strychnine

Strychnine is used as a rodenticide and has only rarely been reported to cause toxicity in the horse [47]. Clinical signs appear rapidly following ingestion, and include apprehension, nervousness, and muscle stiffness, followed by violent tetanic seizures. The seizures may be interspersed between periods of relaxation.

Strychnine competitively antagonizes the inhibitory neurotransmitter glycine in the spinal cord, resulting in hyperexcitation of muscles. No specific antidote exists, and treatment is supportive and empirical. Control of seizures with pentobarbital or phenobarbital is recommended. Chloral hydrate has also been suggested as a sedative; however, availability may be an issue, and the author has seen little effect from the use of chloral hydrate in the horse. The centrally acting muscle relaxant methocarbamol (150 mg/kg BW) and guaifenesin (110 mg/kg IV) can be given as needed [20]. Activated charcoal can be given in an effort to neutralize the toxin.

Molluscicides

The molluscicides metaldehyde and methiocarb have been incriminated in the horse only very rarely. Horses become intoxicated by inadvertent consumption of the compounds placed around ornamental plants or crops [20]. Horses may be more susceptible than dogs to the effects of metaldehyde, and ingestion of a single dose of 60 mg/kg BW and 120 mg/kg BW resulted in the death of two horses [48, 49]. Methiocarb has been reported to result in toxicity at an estimated dosage of 100–125 g [50, 51].

Clinical signs observed with both compounds include nervousness and anxiety, sweating, and muscle fasciculations progressing to tremors and seizures. Death occurred rapidly (within a few hours) in horses intoxicated with metaldehyde, while one horse intoxicated with methiocarb lived and clinical signs resolved after 12 h [51].

Diagnosis is by observation of clinical signs and a history of exposure. Analysis of stomach content for acetaldehyde has been suggested, and a formaldehyde-like odor may be recognized in the stomach in cases with metaldehyde toxicity [20]. Treatment of intoxication is supportive, including administration of activated charcoal, intravenous fluid support, and control of seizure activity with phenobarbital and valium. Methocarbamol (150 mg/kg BW) may be beneficial to control muscle fasciculation.

The antidote for methiocarb is atropine sulfate, which can be given as needed. Supportive care as discussed earlier is also beneficial.

4-Aminopyridine

Intoxication with 4-aminopyridine (a bird repellant often mixed with grain) has been reported in one horse, which had signs of profuse sweating, behavioral abnormalities, fluttering of the eyelids, and convulsions [52]. The estimated lethal dose is 2–3 mg/kg BW. The mechanism of action is not known, but the overall effect is CNS stimulation. No specific antidote is known. Diagnosis has been confirmed by HPLC of stomach content [52].

Amitraz

There is one report of intoxication following topical application of the acaricide amitraz [53]. Topical application of a 0.025% solution resulted in clinical signs of colic and large colon impactions, tranquilization, depression, and ataxia. It appears that intoxication is due to chemical breakdown of the amitraz to the highly toxic chemical 3,5-dimethylphenyl N-methyl formamidine during storage prior to application [53]. Treatment is symptomatic, and affected horses recovered completely over a period of several days.

Plant- and forage-associated intoxications

White snakeroot and Rayless goldenrod

White snakeroot is a common plant in wooded areas of the eastern and central United States, extending as far north as Michigan [20]. Rayless goldenrod, or jimmyweed, is a shrub primarily found in the southwest United States. The toxic principle of both plants is tremetol, a fat-soluble alcohol. Ingestion of these plants

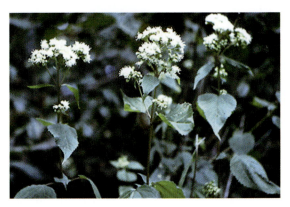

Figure 34.1 Typical appearance of white snakeroot. (Photo courtesy of Dr. Blair Meldrum.)

results in a clinical syndrome referred to as the "trembles," due to the characteristic muscle fasciculations that they produce. An interesting historical note is that tremetol in milk from cows consuming white snakeroot was responsible for the condition known as "milk sickness" in humans (Figure 34.1).

The mechanism of action of the toxin is unknown, but clinical signs will result from ingestion of 1–10% of body weight of the green plant and may be fatal [54]. The plant remains toxic after drying and in hay. Clinical signs of toxicity can appear up to 3 weeks after exposure to the plant. Predominant clinical signs are dilated pupils, depression, a stiff gait with muscle tremors, patchy sweating, and cardiac arythmias [54]. Dysphagia and hypersalivation have also been seen [55].

Increased muscle enzyme activity is typically noted, along with hemoglobinuria, hyperglycemia, and acidosis [20, 54]. Postmortem findings include colitis, renal tubular necrosis, pericarditis, myocarditis, and myositis [54]. Diagnosis is supported by the clinical observation of muscle tremors associated with myositis and cardiomyopathy, and the potential for exposure to the plant. Assay of body fluids for the toxic principle have not been successful [20]. There is no specific antidote, and treatment is symptomatic.

Solanaceae species

Several members of the Solanum family have been reported to cause toxicity in the horse. Plants within this family contain either the atropine-like or solanum alkaloids. *Datura* spp. (jimsonweed), *Atropa belladonna* (deadly nightshade), and *Dubosia* spp. (corkwoods) contain atropine alkaloids. These plants are generally unpalatable but can become included in hay, where they retain toxicity. Ingestion of an unknown quantity of jimsonweed resulted in the death of 11 out of 15 ponies with clinical signs of depression, excessive urination, diarrhea, mydriasis, muscle spasms, and convulsions [55]. Physostigmine can be used to effect in horses affected by the atropine containing plants. Black night-shade (*Solanum nigram*) contains the solanum alkaloid toxin and ingestion by horses results in colic, ataxia, weakness, tremors and convulsions.

Nigropallidal encephalomalacia

Ingestion of yellow star-thistle (*Centaurea solstitialis*), and Russian knapweed (*Acroptilon repens*, previously *Centaurea repens*) result in a syndrome referred to as nigropallidal encephalomalacia (NE) [56–59]. In addition, it has been suggested that the Malta star-thistle (*Centaurea melitensis*), native to Central Texas, may also cause the disease, but specific reports cannot confirm this [60].

These plants are abundant in nonimproved or nonirrigated fallow pastures in their native range, where they tend to persist in the summer and late fall. This corresponds to the prevalence of clinical illness; in one report a peak of cases was seen in midsummer (June and July) and another peak in the fall (October and November) [55]. The plant remains toxic in hay [61]. Cases due to yellow star-thistle have also been documented in Australia and Argentina [62].

Yellow star-thistle is most abundant in the United States in California, southern Oregon, and Idaho, and is spreading eastward, with sporadic distribution. Yellow star-thistle has a single erect woody stem, 1–6 ft in height, topped with a cluster of bright yellow flowers. Russian knapweed has a broader distribution in the mountain states and has been confirmed in Colorado, Utah, and Washington. The plant is a perennial, 1–3 ft in height, topped with solitary, cone-shaped pinkish to blue-white flowers (Figure 34.2).

The toxic principle is currently not identified, although a variety of possible compounds have been suggested. The sesqeuterpine lactone repin has been investigated. More recently, the compound dihydro-methylpyrane (DDMP) has been suggested to be the cause, as it has been shown to be cytotoxic to various regions of the brain [60]. Confirmation of this compound in intoxicated horses or the plants themselves is apparently lacking at the present time.

Clinical signs appear after the horses have had a continuous and protracted ingestion of the plant; occasional consumption does not result in observable clinical abnormalities. Feeding trials suggest that a horse must consume between 59 and 200% of their body weight (yellow star-thistle) or 59–63% of their body weight (Russian knapweed) for a period of 3–11 weeks before clinical signs occur [61]. It is considered that some horses will actively seek out the plant once exposed to it; it is not usually grazed if more suitable forage is present. The onset of clinical signs is abrupt and primarily affects the muscles of mastication and

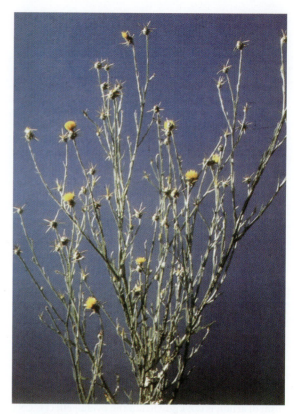

Figure 34.2 Yellow star thistle (*Centaurea solstitialis*). (Photo courtesy of Dr. Blair Meldrum.)

prehension. Hypertonicity of the facial muscles result in a "wooden" expression, and the mouth is held partially open with the lips retracted. The tongue may be moved, but often curls on the side to form a "trough." Horses have a good appetite, but cannot move food into the pharynx; hence, weight loss develops quickly. Horses may immerse their entire head, down to the eyes, in water troughs to drink, and some adopt unusual eating methods, such as "scooping" the feed into their mouths. Circling, depression, yawning, or "frenzied" behavior can be variably seen. Gait deficits appear to be minimal, although conscious proprioceptive deficits may be seen. Death is most commonly due to starvation or dehydration. Animals of all ages can be affected, but younger animals appear to be more susceptible, with a mean age of 2 years reported [63] (Figure 34.3).

Diagnosis is dependent on the characteristic clinical signs, combined with confirmation of access to the toxic plants. Clinicopathologic abnormalities are nonspecific and reflect anorexia and dehydration. Antemortem diagnosis with MRI has demonstrated cavitation of the substantia nigra, but this is not a widely available procedure [64]. Postmortem findings are characteristic, with sharply circumscribed areas of liquifactive necrosis of the substantia nigra or globus pallidus, usually bilaterally symmetrical (Figure 34.4).

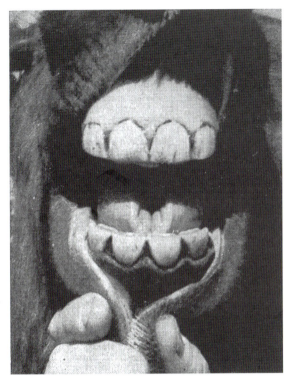

Figure 34.3 Typical lateral curling of the tongue in a horse with nigropallidal encephalomalacia.

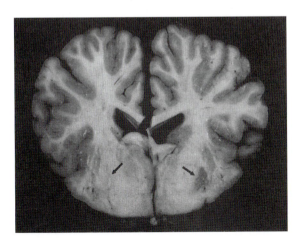

Figure 34.4 Gross postmortem photograph demonstrating the necrosis of the globus pallidus (arrows) in a horse with nigropallidal encephalomalacia.

There is no specific treatment other than removal from the source of toxin, and nursing care; recovery is unlikely.

Bracken fern

Bracken fern (*Pteridium aquilinum*) is widely distributed across North America, primarily in the northern and western regions. The condition is reported to be well known in the United Kingdom, and was first reported in Germany in 1897 [65]. The plant grows in forested areas and abandoned fields or roadways which are being re-forested. The entire plant is toxic in its natural state or when dried as in hay. Intoxications tend to occur in late summer or fall when forage is limited, but can occur at any time of the year. It has been reported that horses can acquire a fondness for the plant and seek it out [65]. Hay containing 20% bracken fern is considered hazardous [63, 65].

The toxic principle of bracken fern is thiaminase, and clinical signs result from the depletion of thiamine. Thiamine is an important cofactor in energy production, catalyzing the decarboxylation of pyruvate to acetyl CoA [20]. In a group of experimentally poisoned horses, blood thiamine concentration dropped from 8.5 to 1.5 µg/dl, and blood pyruvate concentrations increased from 2.2 to 6.2 mg/dl [55]. Neurologic dysfunction is presumed to arise from cellular energy failure.

The most prominent clinical abnormality associated with bracken fern intoxication is ataxia, which begins approximately 1 month after consumption begins, and progresses over several days. All four limbs are typically involved [65]. This may be associated or preceded by weight loss, and bradycardia and anorexia are usually present [63, 66]. If ingestion continues, muscle fasciculations and tremors progressing to terminal convulsions may be seen. Clinical signs and progression are similar to experimentally induced thiamine deficiency using amprolium; however, blindness was also seen in the horses of that report [63, 67]. A "tucked-up" appearance with an arched back are commonly reported and appear to be a consistent clinical observation.

Diagnosis is established by the observation of consistent clinical signs (i.e., ataxia of all four limbs, with bradycardia and muscle tremors), combined with the observation of bracken fern in the diet. It must be noted, however, that clinical signs can occur for a period of time after bracken is removed from the diet. There are no pathognomonic clinicopathologic changes on routine laboratory analysis. Decreased blood thiamine and RBC transketolase concentrations (a surrogate for thiamine assay) and increased blood lactate and pyruvate concentrations are expected.

Treatment is removal of bracken from the diet, and administration of thiamin intramuscularly (0.25–0.50 mg/kg BW once/day). A loading dose of 5–10 mg/kg of thiamine can be given on the first day of treatment, but this should be diluted in fluids and given slowly, due to the reported potential for adverse reactions [20]. Oral thiamin can also be given orally at 0.5–1 g twice/day [66]. Thiamine replacement therapy is reported to provide rapid resolution of clinical signs in naturally occurring disease, but slower return to normalcy (5–7 days) was seen in amprolium-induced thiamine deficiency [67]. Treatment is usually successful if treatment begins prior to the terminal phase of muscle tremors and convulsions. Necessary duration of treatment apparently depends upon the severity of the condition, but several doses may be needed before complete resolution is achieved.

A similar syndrome is observed following intoxication with *Equisetum arvense* (horse tail, scouring rush), which also produces a thiaminase [68]. This plant remains toxic in hay, but is generally considered unpalatable otherwise [63]. Diets containing 20% *E. arvense* fed for 2 weeks has been adequate to induce disease [68]. Treatment and management is as for bracken fern.

Hypochoeris

Stringhalt has been recognized in the horses for centuries and has been described as having one of two forms: the conventional or classic form of the disease, and Australian stringhalt. The classic form of the disease is considered to occur worldwide and is defined by its clinical signs with little other information available. Surgery is usually curative [69, 70]. Australian stringhalt (AS) was traditionally reported in Australia and New Zealand associated with ingestion of the weed *Hypochoeris radicata* (flatweed) [71]; however, this form of stringhalt has been reported in North America [70, 72].

The plant is an invader of disturbed soils, and is often seen in stressed pastures. While originally described in Australia and New Zealand, flatweed is widely distributed in North America, particularly the Pacific Northwest, California, and Northeastern United States [70, 73]. Flatweed is very similar in appearance to the common dandelion, the major difference being that flatweed has a solid stalk, and the stalk of the common dandelion is hollow [70].

Horses with stringhalt demonstrate a very characteristic gait, the severity of which is variable. The syndrome is characterized by exaggerated hock flexion varying from stiffness, which is only seen during periods of excitation, to a marked flexion in which the foot of the affected leg strikes the abdomen. With classic stringhalt, only one leg may be affected, and no other clinical signs are seen. With the Australian form, signs are usually bilateral. Horses sometimes are almost unable to move forward without "bunny-hopping." The rear limbs are most commonly affected, although front limb stiffness can be seen in the Australian (but not classic)

form. Recumbency may result in very severe cases. Excitement, turning sharply, going downhill, and prolonged exercise will all exacerbate the gait abnormalities. In addition to gait deficits, laryngeal hemiplegia was observed in 10 of 11 horses with AS [71]. The severity of clinical signs with AS is variable, and a grading scale has been described. Muscle atrophy of the long and lateral digital extensor muscles is most commonly observed, although generalized hind-limb muscle atrophy has been seen [71].

Most cases of AS have been associated with ingestion of *H. radicata* (flatweed, false dandelion), although other plants have been suggested including *Taraxicum officinal* and *Lathyrus species*. The toxic principle is not identified and may be a mycotoxin. *H. radicata* has a worldwide distribution, including North and South America, Europe, Australia, New Zealand, and Japan [69, 74]. Intoxication tends to occur in situations in which there are large amounts of the weed (>30% of available forage), which occurs in situations of severely overgrazed pastures, often in late summer or fall [72]. Outbreaks with a large number of affected individuals, or sporadic cases can be seen. The duration of time to the onset of signs is not clearly established, but it takes at least 2 weeks, and signs may progress once noted, particularly if consumption continues [71].

Australian stringhalt is a distal axonopathy, and affected horses demonstrate axonal degeneration and demyelination. This is responsible for the clinical signs seen of peripheral neuropathy (neurogenic muscle atrophy, laryngeal hemiplegia). The pathogenesis of the gait deficit is more complex, and probably involves disruption of the reflex arc responsible for motor tone, with damage leading to disinhibition of upper motor neurons.

Diagnosis is made by observation of the characteristic clinical signs, which are clear in the severe form. Neurologic deficits consistent with hypertonicity and hyperflexion, involving both rear limbs, associated with laryngeal hemiplegia and exposure to the plant are adequate to confirm the diagnosis. Electromyography will reveal spontaneous electrical activity of the affected muscles, positive sharp waves, and fibrillation potentials, suggesting denervation [72]. Nerve conduction studies find a marked reduction in nerve conduction, and a decremental response to repetitive nerve stimulation [71]. Clinicopathologic evaluation is normal, as are serum vitamin E and selenium concentrations. Pathologic examination will reveal peripheral nerve degeneration and muscle atrophy and spinal cord, brain, or brainstem pathology is not observed.

Treatment primarily involves removal of the horse from the source of toxin, and in cases of AS this appears to result in some resolution of clinical signs, although this usually takes many months and recovery is often incomplete [71]. A 1 week course of treatment with thiamine has been advocated, but results appear to be inconsistent and it is difficult to attribute clinical improvement to the treatment [71, 72]. In addition, phenytoin (15 mg/kg BW/os q24 h) for 3 weeks has been advocated, also with inconsistent results [72]. Better results were reported with a dosage of phenytoin of 15 mg/kg BW q12 h [75]; however, the effectiveness of this therapy remains unconfirmed [74]. Treatment with the centrally acting muscle relaxant mephenisin has been reported, but with equivocal results [76]. Some success has been reported with the use of the GABA inhibitor baclofen (1 mg/kg q8 h) [75] but it had no effect in another report [74].

Leukoencephalomalacia

Equine leukoencephalomalacia (ELEM) (moldy corn disease, cornstalk disease) has been recognized for many years. Reference to it can be found in literature of the nineteenth century. The association with moldy corn has been known since 1902, when a feeding trial of affected corn resulted in clinical signs consistent with the natural outbreak [77]. Outbreaks have been reported in which large numbers of horses died; up to 5000 horses died in Iowa during 1934–1935 [78]. Even though the cause has been recognized for more than a century, outbreaks still occur, with one fairly recent outbreak resulting in the death of 14 horses of a group of 66, and another resulting in the death of 6 out of 10 horses on another farm [79, 80]. The attack rate on any particular farm varied from 14 to 41% in one summary report, with a case fatality rate ranging from 26 to 100% [81].

The disease is most commonly reported in the eastern and Midwestern United States; however, it appears to have a worldwide distribution [82–84]. The toxin is elaborated primarily by *Fusarium moniliforme*, and *Fusarium proliferatum* [85–87]. The toxic principle is the mycotoxin fumonisin, of which fumonisin B1 is the most commonly reported, although fumonisin B2 and B3 have been shown to be present in contaminated corn and will cause the same clinical syndrome [80, 86]. Fumonisin B1 and B2 appear to have similar toxic potential, although fumonisin B3 is much less toxic [85]. Intoxication is almost exclusively associated with contamination of corn, and both white and yellow varieties appear to be affected. Environmental conditions that favor toxin production include a period of drought during the growing season, with cool moist conditions during pollination and kernel formation [85]. Infected corn may be fed directly, or can be part of a grain mix or pelleted feed [81]. There is poor correlation between the concentration of toxin in feed and the visual appearance of the grain [88].

The toxin acts by inhibiting the synthesis of sphingosine from sphinganine via inhibition of ceramide synthetase [85, 86, 89]. As a result, the ratio of sphinganine to sphinogosine rises several fold and may be useful in the early detection of intoxication. Clinical signs are presumed to result from this alteration of sphingolipid metabolism. In addition, fumonisin B1 has been shown to alter the permeability of porcine endothelial cells [89]. If a similar phenomenon occurs in equine endothelial cells, this could explain the protein exudation and edema which occurs in the CNS with fumonisin intoxication.

Horses appear to be the most sensitive to the effects of the fumonisin toxin, with concentrations as low as 8–10 ppm resulting in clinical disease [90]. Clinical signs of intoxication occur abruptly, usually after 7–10 days of high dose of the toxin, or prolonged ingestion of a low dose of the toxin [85]. Higher doses of toxin favor hepatotoxicity, while chronic ingestion of lower concentrations is more associated with neurologic disease [85].

Clinical signs of fumonisin neurotoxicosis include the abrupt onset of depression, blindness, and ataxia. Clinical signs rapidly progress to hyperexcitability, headpressing, and delirium. Fumonisin B1 demonstrates dose-dependent characteristics, and when given intravenously at 0.01 mg/kg body weight no clinical signs are seen. At a dose of 0.05 mg/kg body weight, however, horses developed recognizable neurologic signs 8–13 days after dosing began [91]. These signs included tongue weakness, ataxia, mentation changes, and proprioceptive abnormalities. Mentation changes progressed in some horses to intermittent dementia. More severe signs were seen at higher doses [91]. Sudden death can be observed without prior recognition of neurologic disease.

Clinical signs reflect severe forebrain disease that must be differentiated from viral encephalitis, meningitis or cerebral abscessation, parasitic encephalitis, botulism, hepatoencephalopathy, other intoxications, or trauma. The observation of pink to reddish-brown mold on corn provides presumptive information, although failure to observe this does not rule fumonisin intoxication out. Clinical chemistry analysis of blood may reveal alterations in liver enzymes, as well as other, nonspecific changes associated with recumbency, stress or dehydration. Direct fumonisin assay of body fluids does not appear to have value and is not routinely done in clinical cases.

CSF evaluation recovers fluid which is xanthochromic, with an elevated total protein count. A mean CSF total protein concentration of 197 mg/dl was found in 10 horses with neurologic signs after intravenous dosing with fumonisin B1 [91]. CSF red blood cell counts were mildly increased compared to normal controls (12 RBC/μl vs 0.0), but this difference did not achieve statistical significance [91]. CSF nucleated cell counts appear to be variable, and may be normal or increased, presumably associated with the severity of the CNS necrosis [80, 91, 92].

Postmortem examination finds widespread softening and liquifactive necrosis of cerebral white matter. Lesions vary in size from very small to large cavitations, and are not typically symmetric or bilateral. Lesions may also be seen in the thalamus, brain stem, and medulla. Histologic analysis finds loss of cerebral architecture, primarily white matter necrosis, and perivascular cuffing and proliferation of macrophages [85]. Lesions of the liver may be seen, with hepatomegally and a brownish discolored liver with irregular foci throughout [85]. Histopathologic changes include hepatocyte vacuolation, periacinar necrosis, portal fibrosis, and bile duct proliferation [85].

No specific treatment exists, and supportive care is the only option. Treatment with oral laxatives and/or activated charcoal is not of value due to the long duration of intake necessary for toxicity. The prognosis is grave for severely affected horses, although mildly affected horses have been known to recover. Prevention involves the avoidance of poorly stored grains (humidity > 15%), or those with any questionable appearance. The US Department of Agriculture recommends that feeds contain no more than 5 ppm of fumonisin.

Paspalum staggers

The ergot *Claviceps paspali* infects the seed head of dallis grass (*Paspalum dilatatum*) or bahia grass (*Bahia oppositifolia*). Dallis grass is primarily a warm season grass cultivated in the humid regions of southeastern United States. Toxins produced by the sclerotium of *C. paspali* include a group of compounds that are derivatives of lysergic acid and are collectively referred to as paspalitrems [85, 93]. This group is composed of paspalinine, paspalitrem A, and paspalitrem B [93]. The toxin apparently interferes with the release of the inhibitory neurotransmitter GABA [93]. Loss of inhibitory neurotransmission results in prolonged depolarization facilitating motor end plate activity, which is the ultimate cause of the observed clinical signs [85].

Clinical signs associated with ingestion of the paspalitrems are fine muscle tremors of the head and neck. Stiffness, ataxia, hypermetria, and gross muscle tremors; opisthotonus and seizures may develop. Signs are particularly noticeable when the horse becomes agitated or excited, and may subside if the horse is not handled or stressed.

Diagnosis is based on observation and elimination of other possible causes, associated with the presence of the ergot sclerotium on seed heads. Clinicopathologic examination is unremarkable, showing only nonspecific changes associated with recumbency. No gross or histologic changes are reported in horses. There is no specific antidote, and signs usually resolve within 1–3 weeks

after removal from the infected pasture. Control measures include mowing of pastures to remove the infected seedheads.

Ryegrass staggers

CNS abnormalities associated with the grazing of ryegrass pastures has been recognized in North America, particularly the pacific northwest, Australia, New Zealand, and Europe. Intoxication is the result of infection of the grass with the endophytic fungus *Neotyphodium lolii*, which produces a group of neurotoxic tremorgens known as lolitrem A, B, C, and D [85]. Hot, dry weather with drought stress and overgrazing are the characteristic situation in which this condition is seen. Toxicosis is reported to occur most commonly after a heavy dew or light rain interrupts the dry conditions [85]. Concentrations of the toxin are greatest in the seed; however, the toxin also concentrates in the lower 2 cm of the stem, making ingestion during periods of overgrazing or draught likely [85, 94]. A dose of 2 µg/g of dry matter is considered to cause toxic signs [85].

Earlier reports suggested that the lolitrems cause toxicity by interfering with the release of the inhibitory neurotransmitter GABA [85]. More recent molecular studies have demonstrated that lolitrem B specifically blocks the function of large conductance calcium activated potassium channels [95]. The clinical signs include fine muscle tremors of the head and neck progressing to stiffness, ataxia, hypermetria, gross muscle tremors, opisthotonus, and seizures in severe cases [85, 93, 96]. In a controlled feeding trial with horses carefully observed and fed a standardized amount of lolitrem B, there was noticeable variability in the severity of the clinical signs [97, 98]. All horses demonstrated tremor, and the thoracic musculature seems to be predominately affected, and it was worsened with exercise; blindfolding substantially worsened the ataxia, suggesting cerebellar involvement. Cranial nerve signs were limited to eyeball "tremor." A few horses developed swelling of the distal limbs with heel cracks and nasal discharge, all of which resolved spontaneously after cessation of feeding the lolitrem [97, 98]. Morbidity in affected herds is typically greater than 50% with a low mortality (<10%). Most animals recover within 1 week after removal from the affected premise. Diagnosis is by observation of infected grasses, presence of appropriate clinical signs and elimination of other possible causes. No specific clinicopathological changes are observed, and there are no characteristic postmortem findings. Analysis of affected forage for the presence of the endophyte can be performed.

Locoweed (locoism)

A large variety of plants of the Astragalus and Oxytropis genera have been incriminated in a CNS disorder of the horse known as locoism. There are over 300 species of

Astragalus alone, and not all cause CNS disease, although many have been incriminated [20, 63]. In addition to CNS disease, plants of this genera can cause selenosis and methemaglobinemia, although primarily in cattle. Locoweed is widely distributed in North America from Western Canada as far south as Northern Mexico, and predominately within the Western states [20].

Clinical signs can be seen as quickly as 2 weeks after ingestion of the plant begins, but may take as long as 2 months to be expressed. Although the plant is considered to be unpalatable, once horses do begin to consume it they seek it out and eat it preferentially.

Ingestion of locoweeds by horses leads to clinical signs of a slow staggering gait, depression, weight loss, ataxia and anxiety/nervousness. Changes in behavior are noted, in that the horse may separate itself from the herd and become difficult to handle and unpredictable. Gait abnormalities may become exacerbated with excitement. Difficulty in eating and drinking can be seen, as well as blindness in some cases. Abortion can be seen in pregnant mares, as well as the birth of foals with a variety of limb deformities.

The toxic principle, swainsonine, inhibits alpha-mannosidase—a lysosomal enzyme required for the metabolism of oligosacharides [63]. This metabolic disruption leads to the formation of intracytoplasmic vacuoles which will result in permanent cell damage if persistent. Consumption for as few as 8 days will result in the presence of vacuoles of neurons within the CNS. Vacuoles will regress if feeding is discontinued early, but if consumption continues, vacuolation leads to cell death. Neurologic signs are a direct result of the disruption of cellular function induced by the presence of the vacuoles in Purkinje cells of the cerebellum and cerebral cortex. Associated weight loss is due to vacuolation of numerous other organs, while blindness is likely due to vacuolation of cells of the retina.

Diagnosis is based on observation of consistent clinical signs, and confirmation of access to and consumption of the plant. No specific antemortem test has been described, although biopsy of assessable tissues and histologic examination may reveal the characteristic vacuolation. Clinicopathologic testing is nonspecific and may reflect various organ system dysfunction. Vacuolation may be seen in leukocytes, but the value of this observation as a diagnostic is unknown.

Treatment is dependent on eliminating access of the horse to the plant. This may be difficult in some cases in which the horse seeks out the plant, and requires more than simply providing better quality forage. Early recognition and removal from the plant are key, as mild cases may recover in 1–2 weeks after ingestion ceases. More chronic cases have little chance for full recovery, and may have persistent gait or behavioral deficits making them unsafe for use. Death can result from emaciation and progressively severe neurologic disease may necessitate humane destruction.

Sorghum cystitis

Horses grazing various sorghum species can demonstrate a fairly well-described neurologic syndrome of cystitis and caudal ataxia [99]. Clinical signs are most commonly seen in horses that consume hybrid crosses of sorghum (*Sorghum vulgare*) and sudan grass (*Sorghum vulgare var sudanense*). Other species such as Johnson grass (*Sorghum halepense*) have also been incriminated, but less frequently [100, 101]. Cases have been described in the western and southwestern states of the United States, as well as in northern and western Australia [100, 102, 103]. Sudan or Johnson grass hay that has been well cured does not appear to be toxic [100, 101].

Clinical presentation is a symmetric ataxia and weakness of the rear limbs; flaccid paralysis of the legs or tail may develop abruptly. Urinary incontinence (dribbling of urine) soon follows in about one-half of horses with ataxia [100]. A "bunny-hopping"-type gait is occasionally seen. Backing exacerbates the clinical signs in the pelvic limbs. Clinical examination is unremarkable with the exception of urine scalding, ataxia, and perhaps a flaccid tail. Examination of the bladder may reveal a sabbulous cystitis which may be severe. Clinicopathologic testing is usually unremarkable. CSF results have not been reported.

Diagnosis is supported by the observation of symmetrical ataxia, signs of cauda equina syndrome, and exposure to appropriate feedstuffs. Differential considerations include sacral fractures, equine protozoal myeloencephalitis, osteomyelitis, and bacterial infections. The work-up and differential considerations for cauda equina syndrome are more fully discussed in Chapter 12.

Treatment is supportive, and prompt removal from the toxin source is necessary. Not all horses in an exposed group will be affected; a morbidity of 25% was seen in one study, with a mortality of less than 2% [100, 102]. Drainage of the bladder associated with irrigation to remove sediment is beneficial to prevent distention induced trauma to the detrusor muscle, and aid in the horses comfort.

The toxic principle associated with sorghum intoxication is unknown; however, it has suspected to be associated with the development of cyanide in the plant during periods of rapid lush growth. Most reported cases were associated with a young, green stage of growth and during seasons of medium to high rainfall [100]. In one report, the grazing period prior to development of clinical signs varied among affected cases from 1 week to 6 months [100].

In addition to neurologic disease, fetal abnormalities have been observed in the foals of mares which grazed sorghum. Abortions that may or may not be associated with fetal ankylosis have been observed as well [100, 104].

Postmortem examination usually finds evidence of severe cystitis. Gross changes in the nervous system are not observed; however, histologic examination finds axonal degeneration and demyelination in the ventral funiculus of the cervical, thoracic, lumbar, and sacral segments of the CNS [100].

Miscellanous plant intoxications

Ingestion of various legumes has resulted in neurologic disorders of horses. Ingestion of laburnum (*Laburnum anagyroides*) seeds (0.6 g/kg BW) resulted in signs of excitement, incoordination, convulsions, and death [55]. Consumption of the legume *Lathyrus hissolia* (grass vetchling) was associated with severe ataxia, which resolved following removal of the source [55]. Consumption of Lathyrus has also resulted in laryngeal paralysis and stringhalt.

The black locust tree (*Robinia pseudoacacia*) has been reported to be toxic to horses when they ate bark or trimmed branches. The toxic principle is the plant lectin robin. Clinical signs include depression, anorexia, weakness, mydriasis, irregular tachycardia, diaphragmatic flutter, and posterior paralysis. Treatment is symptomatic.

The poison hemlock (*Conium maculatum*) is found growing in ditches and along roadways in the cooler climates of the United States. The toxic principle is a group of alkaloids including coniine, and *N*-methyl-conine. The pharmacologic action is similar to nicotine, stimulating then paralyzing autonomic ganglia and neuromuscular junctions [63]. Corneal reflexes are spared, but horses are demented and lose awareness, become recumbent and die of respiratory failure. The early growth is most palatable, and as few as five fresh leaves can intoxicate a horse [55]. The toxin is not toxic when dried in hay [63].

Water hemlock (*Cicuta maculate*) is considered one of the most toxic of all plants. It grows only in wet and swampy areas throughout North America. The toxic principle is cicutoxin, which is concentrated in the rootstock, which is the most toxic part of the plant. The toxin is a direct CNS stimulant, leading to apprehension, mydriasis, and convulsions. Death can occur within 30 min of ingestion, but horses that survive 5–6 h usually recover [63].

The western whorled milkweed (*Asclepias subverticillata*) contains neurotoxic cardenolides which can result in CNS stimulation, convulsions and rapid death. The plant remains toxic when dried, and a lethal dose is considered to be 0.05% of BW dry matter in hay [63].

A syndrome of hind-limb ataxia, and limb weakness was noted in horses after long-term grazing of branched onion weed (*Trachyandra divaricata*) [105]. This plant is widely distributed in the southwestern regions of South Africa and the southwestern region of Australia. In South Africa, grazing of a related plant, *Trachyandra laxa*, may cause similar signs [106]. In addition to gait deficits, a crouching posture with diffuse muscle fasciculations was noted. Diffuse muscle weakness becomes prominent, and diffuse muscle wasting had been noted in a flock of sheep which had been similarly intoxicated. Gross postmortem does not reveal any abnormalities, but histopathologic examination finds widespread lipofuscin storage in neurons, brain, and spinal cord [105]. In addition, lipofuscin was noted within the neurons of the autonomic ganglia of the gut, possibly explaining the signs of colic in some animals.

There appears to be no specific treatment, and recovery from the condition has not been observed once clinical signs are noted. The toxic principle has not been identified, but it appears that continuous ingestion over several weeks is required for intoxication. Supplementary feeding of good quality forage for animals housed in pastures with the plant is likely to be protective.

Transient ataxia has been noted following contact with stinging nettles (*Urtica dioica*). Caudal ataxia, associated with mild agitation and an urticarial rash were observed. The signs resolved with empirical treatment within a few hours [107].

A syndrome of ataxia and mental dullness is observed in horses in the Queensland area of Australia, known locally and historically as "coastal staggers" [108]. The illness is due to consumption of the plant *Gomphrena celosioides*. It is reported to be common along the coastal strip of Queensland, extending inland up to 300 miles. It grows on embankments along roads and railways, and on stressed or fallow land. The plant appears to be palatable and readily eaten by horses; however, considerable quantity is required (5–6 lbs/day for 30 days) before clinical signs of ataxia, mental dullness, and eventual recumbency develop. No specific treatment is known, and there are no reported CNS lesions present.

Ingestion of plants of the Indigofera genus has been reported to result in nervous system abnormalities of horses; it has been referred to as Birdsville disease in Australia [109–111]. The primary clinical signs are anorexia, depression, unsteady gait, and ataxia; ocular discharge and blindness have also been observed. A feeding trial using *Indigofera lespedezioides* has produced similar clinical signs in one horse. Postmortem examination found lipofuscin infiltration in the cerebrum, brain stem, spinal cord, and cerebellum [111]. Ultrastructural examination found neuronal and axonal degeneration. Clinical signs may resolve after removal from exposure; however, this is apparently not universal. The toxic principle is not confirmed, but the toxic amino acid indospicine is considered to be the likely cause [111].

Table 34.1 Summary of clinical signs associated with selected equine neurotoxins.

Toxin/syndrome	CNS		Spinal cord signs	Peripheral neuropathy	Muscle fasciculations	Misc
	Stimulation	Depression				
Bracken fern			+++		+	Bradycardia, seizures
Carbamates	+		+		+	Colic, bradycardia
Fluphenazine	+++				+	
Haloxon				+		Roaring
Hypochorius			+++	+		Roaring
Ionophore		+++	+			Sweating
Ivermectin		+	+			Blindness
Lead			+	+++		Dysphagia, roaring
Levamisol	+++				+	
Locoism	+++		+++		+	Weight loss, blindness
Mercury			+++	+++		Dermatitis, weight loss
Metaldehyde	+++				+	Seizures
Moldy corn	+ (seizures)	+++	+++			Blindness
Moxidectin		+++	+		+	Seizures
Nicotine	+++ (early)	+++ (late)	++		+	Tachycardia
Nigropallidal encephalomalacia	+	+				Dysphagia
Organophosphates	+		+		+	Colic, bradycardia
Paspalum staggers	+ (seizures)		+++		+++	
Ryegrass staggers	+ (seizures)		+++		+++	
Sorghum/sudan grass			+++			Cauda equina syndrome
Urea	+++	+++				Dementia

+++ indicates this is a predominant sign or very commonly seen, while + indicates a less commonly seen clinical sign.

References

[1] Brewer, B., Hines, M., Stewart, J.T. *et al.* (1990) Fluphenazine induced Parkinson-like syndrome in a horse. *Equine Vet J*, 22, 136–137.

[2] Kauffman, V.G., Soma, L., Divers, T.J. *et al.* (1989) Extrapyramidal side effects caused by fluphenazine decanoate in a horse. *J Am Vet Med Assoc*, 195, 1128–1130.

[3] Baird, J.D., Arroyo, L.G., Vengust, M. *et al.* (2006) Adverse extrapyramidal effects in four horse given fluphenazine decanoate. *J Am Vet Med Assoc*, 229, 104–110.

[4] McCrindle, C.M., Ebedes, H. and Swan, G.E. (1989) The use of long-acting neuroleptics, perphenazine enanthate and pipothiazine palmitate in two horses. *J S Afr Vet Assoc*, 60, 208–209.

[5] Hautekeete, L.A., Khan, S.A. and Hales, W.S. (1998) Ivermectin toxicosis in a zebra. *Vet Hum Toxicol*, 40, 29–31.

[6] Leaning, W.D. (1983) The efficacy and safety evaluation of ivermectin as a paranteral and oral antiparasitic agent in horses. *Proc Annu Meet Am Assoc Equine Pract*, 29, 319–328.

[7] Swor, T.M., Whittenburg, J.L. and Chaffin, M.K. (2009) Ivermectin toxicosis in three adult horses. *J Am Vet Med Assoc*, 235, 558–562.

[8] Norman, T.E., Chaffin, M.K., Norton, P.L. *et al.* (2012) Concurrent ivermectin and *Solanum* spp. toxicosis in a herd of horses. *J Vet Intern Med*, 26, 1439–1442.

[9] Campbell, W.C. and Benz, G.W. (1984) Ivermectin: a review of efficacy and safety. *J Vet Pharmacol Ther*, 7, 1–16.

[10] Hsu, W.H., Wellborn, S.G. and Schaffer, C.G. (1989) The safety of ivermectin. *Compend Contin Educ Pract Vet*, 11, 584–588.

[11] Roder, J.D. and Stair, E.L. (1998) An overview of ivermectin toxicosis. *Vet Hum Toxicol*, 40, 369–370.

[12] Mealey, K.L., Bentjen, S.A., Gay, J.M. *et al.* (2001) Ivermectin sensitivity in Collies is associated with a deletion mutation of the mdr1 gene. *Pharmacogenetics*, 11, 727–733.

[13] Johnson, P.J., Mrad, D.R., Schwartz, A.J. *et al.* (1999) Presumed moxidectin toxicosis in three foals. *J Am Vet Med Assoc*, 214, 678–680.

[14] Khan, S.A., Kuster, D.A. and Hansen, S.R. (2002) A review of moxidectin overdose cases in equines from 1998 through 2000. *Vet Hum Toxicol*, 44, 232–235.

[15] Cruther, L.R. (1994) Foal Safety Study 0876-E-US-4-94, in *Freedom of Information Summary*, United States Food and Drug Administration Center for Veterinary Medicine, Washington, DC.

[16] Button, C., Barton, R., Honey, P. *et al.* (1988) Avermectin toxicity in calves and an evaluation of picrotoxin as an antidote. *Aust Vet J*, 65, 157–1588.

[17] Bruenisholz, H., Kupper, J., Muentener, C.R. *et al.* (2012) Treatment of ivermectin overdose in a miniature Shetland Pony using intravenous administration of a lipid emulsion. *J Vet Intern Med*, 26, 407–411.

[18] Muller, J.-V.M., Feige, K., Kastner, A.B.R. *et al.* (2005) The use of sarmezil in the treatment of moxidectin intoxication in a foal. *J Vet Intern Med*, 19, 348–349.

[19] Rose, R.J., Hartley, W.J. and Baker, W. (1981) Laryngeal paralysis in Arabian foals associated with oral haloxon administration. *Equine Vet J*, 13, 171–176.

[20] Schmitz, D.G. (1998) Toxicologic Problems, in *Equine Internal Medicine*, 1st edn (eds S. Reed and W. Bayly), W.B. Saunders, Philadelphia, pp. 981–1042.

[21] Drudge, J.H., Lyons, E.T. and Swerczek, T.W. (1974) Critical tests and safety studies on a levamisole-piperazine mixture as an anthelmintic in the horse. *Am J Vet Res*, 35, 67–71.

[22] McClanahan, S., Hunter, J., Murphy, M. *et al.* (1998) Propylene glycol toxicosis in a mare. *Vet Hum Toxicol*, 40, 294–296.

[23] Myers, V.S. and Usenik, E.A. (1969) Propylene glycol intoxication of horses. *J Am Vet Med Assoc*, 155, 1841–1843.

[24] Dorman, D.C. and Hasheck, W.M. (1991) Fatal propylene glycol toxicosis in a horse. *J Am Vet Med Assoc*, 198, 1643–1644.

[25] Amend, J.F., Mallon, F.M., Wren, W.B. *et al.* (1980) Equine monensin toxicosis: some experimental clinicopathologic observations. *Compend Contin Educ Pract Vet*, 2, S173–S182.

[26] Rollinson, J., Taylor, F.G. and Chesney, J. (1987) Salinomycin poisoning in horses. *Vet Rec*, 121, 126–128.

[27] Blomme, E.A.G., La Perle, K.M., Wilkins, P.A. *et al.* (1999) Ionophore toxicity in horses. *Equine Vet Educ*, 11, 153–158.

[28] Shlafer, M., Somani, P., Pressman, B.C. *et al.* (1978) Effects of the carboxylic ionophore monensin on atrial contractility and Ca^{2+} regulation by isolated cardiac microsomes. *J Mol Cell Cardiol*, 10, 333–346.

[29] Shier, W.T. and Dubourdieu, D.J. (1992) Sodium- and calcium-dependant steps in the mechanism of neonatal rat cardiac myocyte killing by ionophores: the sodium-carrying ionophore, monensin. *Toxicol Appl Pharmacol*, 116, 47–56.

[30] Matsuoka, T. (1976) Evaluation of monensin toxicity in the horse. *J Am Vet Med Assoc*, 169, 1098–1100.

[31] Hanson, L.J., Eisenbeis, H.G. and Givens, S.V. (1981) Toxic effects of lasalocid in horses. *Am J Vet Res*, 42, 456–461.

[32] Knight, H.D. and Costner, G.C. (1977) Bromide intoxication of horses, goats, and cattle. *J Am Vet Med Assoc*, 171, 446–448.

[33] Mayhew, I.G. (ed.) (1989) Disorders of Behavior and Personality, in *Large Animal Neurology*, Lea and Febinger, Philadelphia, pp. 73–112.

[34] Gardner, C.A. and Benetts, H.W. (1952) Poison plants of Western Australia. I. Pituri (*Duboisia hopwoodii* [F. Muell]). *J Dep Agric West Aust*3rd ser, 1, 53–56.

[35] Taylor, P. (1980) Ganglionic Stimulating and Blocking Agents, in *The Pharmacological Basis of Therapeutics* (eds A.G. Gilman, L.S. Goodman and A. Gilman), Macmillan, New York, pp. 211–234.

[36] Seawright, A.A., Roberts, M.C. and Costigan, P. (1978) Chronic methylmercurialism in a horse. *Vet Hum Toxicol*, 20, 6–9.

[37] Roberts, M.C., Seawright, A.A. and Ng, J.C. (1979) Chronic phenylmercuric acetate toxicity in a horse. *Vet Hum Toxicol*, 21, 321–327.

[38] Roberts, M.C. and Seawright, A.A. (1978) The effects of prolonged daily low level mercuric chloride dosing in a horse. *Vet Hum Toxicol*, 20, 410–415.

[39] Shuh, J.L., Ross, C. and Meschter, C. (1988) Concurrent mercuric blister and dimethyl sulphoxide (DMSO) application as a cause of mercury toxicity in two horses. *Equine Vet J*, 20, 68–71.

[40] Guglick, M.A., MacAllister, C.G., Chandra, A.M. *et al.* (1995) Mercury toxicosis caused by ingestion of a blistering compound in a horse. *J Am Vet Med Assoc*, 206, 210–214.

[41] Sojka, J.E., Hope, W. and Pearson, D. (1996) Lead toxicosis in 2 horses: similarity to equine degenerative lower motor neuron disease. *J Vet Intern Med*, 10, 420–423.

[42] Burrows, G.E. (1982) Lead poisoning in the horse. *Equine Pract*, 4, 30–36.

[43] Aronson, A.L. (1972) Lead poisoning in cattle and horses following long-term exposure to lead. *Am J Vet Res*, 33, 627–629.

[44] Dollahite, J.W., Rowe, L.D. and Reagor, J.C. (1975) Experimental lead poisoning in horses and Spanish goats. *Southwest Vet*, 28, 40–45.

[45] Goyeri, R.A. (1991) Heavy Metal Toxicities, in *Toxicology* (eds M.D. Amdurr, J. Doull and C.D. Klassen), Pergamon, New York, pp. 623–680.

[46] McSherry, B.J., Willoughby, R.A. and Thompson, R.G. (1971) Urinary delta amino-levulinic acid (ALA) in the cow, dog, and cat. *Can J Comp Med*, 35, 136–140.

[47] Lilly, C.W. (1985) Strychnine poisoning in the horse. *Equine Pract*, 7, 7–10.

[48] Harris, W.F. (1975) Metaldehyde poisoning in three horses. *Mod Vet Pract*, 56, 336–337.

[49] Sutherland, C. (1983) Metaldehyde poisoning in horses. *Vet Rec*, 112, 64.

[50] Edwards, H.G. (1986) Methiocarb poisoning in a horse. *Vet Rec*, 119, 556–557.

[51] Alexander, K.A. (1987) Methiocarb poisoning in a horse. *Vet Rec*, 120, 47–48.

[52] Ray, A.C., Dwyer, J.N. and Fambro, G.W. (1978) Clinical signs and chemical confirmation of 4-aminopyridine poisoning in horses. *Am J Vet Res*, 39, 318–324.

[53] Auer, D.E., Seawright, A.A., Pollitt, C.C. *et al.* (1984) Illness in horses following spraying with amitraz. *Aust Vet J*, 61, 257–259.

[54] Olson, C.T., Keller, W.C., Gerken, D.F. *et al.* (1984) Suspected tremetol poisoning in horses. *J Am Vet Med Assoc*, 185, 1001–1003.

[55] Hahn, C.N., Mayhew, I.G. and MacKay, R. (1999) Nervous System, in *Equine Medicine and Surgery* (eds P.T. Colahan, I.G. Mayhew, A.M. Merritt *et al.*), Mosby, St. Louis, pp. 863–996.

[56] Larson, K.A. and Young, S. (1970) Nigropallidal encephalomalacia in horses in Colorado. *J Am Vet Med Assoc*, 156, 626–628.

[57] Fowler, M.E. (1965) Nigropallidal encephalomalacia in the horse. *J Am Vet Med Assoc*, 147, 607–616.

[58] Young, S., Brown, W.W. and Klinger, B. (1970) Nigropallidal encephalomalacia in horses fed Russian Knapweed (*Centaurea repens* L.). *Am J Vet Res*, 31, 1393–1404.

[59] Farrell, R.K., Sande, R.D. and Lincoln, S.D. (1971) Nigropallidal encephalomalacia in a horse. *J Am Vet Med Assoc*, 158, 1201–1204.

[60] Talcott, P. (2003) Nigropallidal Encephalomalacia, in *Current Therapy in Equine Practice* (ed. N.E. Robinson), Elsevier, Philadelphia, pp. 780–781.

[61] Young, S., Brown, W.W. and Klinger, B. (1970) Nigropallidal encephalomalacia in horses caused by ingestion of weeds of the genus *Centaurea. J Am Vet Med Assoc*, 157, 1602–1606.

[62] Gard, G.P. and de Sarem, W.G. (1973) Nigropallidal encephalomalacia in horses in New South Wales. *Aust Vet J*, 49, 107–108.

[63] Barr, A.C. and Reagor, J.C. (2001) Toxic Plants, in *The Veterinary Clinics of North America: Equine Practice* (ed. A.S. Turner), W.B. Saunders, Philadelphia, pp. 529–546.

[64] Sanders, S.G., Tucker, R.L., Bagley, R.S. *et al.* (2001) Magnetic resonance imaging features of equine nigropallidal encephalomalacia. *Vet Radiol Ultrasound*, 42, 291–296.

[65] Evans, E.T.R., Evans, W.C. and Roberts, H.E. (1951) Studies on bracken poisoning in the horse. *Br Vet J*, 107, 364–371.

[66] Evans, E.T.R., Evans, W.C. and Roberts, H.E. (1951) Studies on bracken poisoning in the horse. II. *Br Vet J*, 107, 399–411.

[67] Cymbaluk, N.F., Fretz, P.B. and Loew, F.M. (1978) Amprolium-induced thiamine deficiency in horses: clinical features. *Am J Vet Res*, 39, 255–261.

[68] Henderson, J.A. (1952) The antithiamine action of Equisetum. *J Am Vet Med Assoc*, 120, 375–378.

[69] Fintl, C. (2003) Idiopathic and Rare Neurologic Diseases, in *Current Therapy in Equine Medicine* (ed. N.E. Robinson), Saunders, Philadelphia, pp. 760–763.

[70] Gay, C.C., Fransen, S., Richards, J. *et al.* (1993) Hypochoeris-associated stringhalt in North America. *Equine Vet J*, 25, 456–457.

[71] Huntington, P.J., Jeffcoat, L.B., Friend, S.C. *et al.* (1989) Australian stringhalt- epidemiological, clinical and neurological investigations. *Equine Vet J*, 21, 266–273.

[72] Gardner, S.Y., Cook, A.G., Jortner, B.S. *et al.* (2005) Stringhalt associated with a pasture infested with *Hypochoeris radicata. Equine Vet Educ*, 7, 154–158.

[73] Galey, F.D. (1991) Outbreaks of stringhalt in Northern California. *Vet Hum Toxicol*, 33, 176–177.

[74] Takahashi, T., Kitamura, M. and Endo, Y. (2002) An outbreak of stringhalt resembling Australian stringhalt in Japan. *J Equine Sci*, 13, 93–100.

[75] Whitton, R.C., Hodgson, D.R. and Rose, R.J. (2000) Musculoskeletal System, in *Manual of Equine Practice* (eds R.J. Rose and D.R. Hodgson), W.B. Saunders, Philadelphia, pp. 95–185.

[76] Cahill, J.I., Goulden, B.E. and Pearce, H.G. (1985) A review and some observations on stringhalt. *N Z Vet J*, 33, 101–104.

[77] Butler, T. (1902) Notes on a feeding experiment to produce leucoencephalitis in a horse with positive results. *Am Vet Rev*, 26, 748–751.

[78] Graham, R. (1936) Cornstalk disease investigations – toxic encephalitis or non-virus encephalomyelitis of horses. *Vet Med*, 31, 46–50.

[79] Wilson, T.M., Ross, F., Rice, L.G. *et al.* (1990) Fumonisin B1 levels associated with an epizootic of equine leukoencephalomalacia. *J Vet Diagn Invest*, 2, 213–216.

[80] Wilkins, P.A., Vaala, W.E., Vivotofsky, D. *et al.* (1994) A herd outbreak of equine leukoencephalomalacia. *Cornell Vet*, 84, 53–59.

[81] Wilson, T.M., Nelson, P.E., Marasis, W.F. *et al.* (1990) A mycological evaluation and in vivo toxicity evaluation of feed from 41 farms with equine leukoencephalomalacia. *J Vet Diagn Invest*, 2, 352–354.

[82] Shier, W.T. (2000) The fumonisin paradox: a review of research on oral bioavailability of fumonisin B1, a mycotoxin produced by *Fusarium moniliforme. J Toxicol Toxin Rev*, 19, 161–187.

[83] Salles-Gomez, T.L., Almeida, P.E., Moreira, M. *et al.* (2003) Equine leucoencephalomalacia caused by commercial horses ration with fumonisin concentration lower than 10 ppm. *ARS Vet*, 19, 267–271.

[84] Marasas, W.F., Kellerman, T.S., Gelderblom, W.C.A. *et al.* (1988) Leukoencephalomalacia in a horses induced by fumonisin B1 isolated from *Fusarium moniliforme*. *Onderstepoort J Vet Res*, 55, 197–203.

[85] Osweiler, G.D. (2001) Mycotoxins, in *Veterinary Clinics of North America: Equine Practice* (ed. A.S. Turner), W.B. Saunders, Philadelphia, pp. 547–566.

[86] Riley, R.T., Showker, J.L., Owens, D.L. *et al.* (1997) Disruption of sphingolipid metabolism and induction of equine leukoencephalomalacia by *Fusarium proliferatum* culture material containing fumonisin B2 or B3. *Environ Toxicol Pharmacol*, 3, 221–228.

[87] Ross, P.F., Nelson, P.E., Owens, D.L. *et al.* (1994) Fumonisin B2 in cultured *Fusarium proliferatum*, M-6104, causes equine leukoencephalomalacia. *J Vet Diagn Invest*, 6, 263–265.

[88] Binkerd, K.A., Scott, D.H., Everson, R.J. *et al.* (1993) Fumonisin contamination of the 1991 Indiana corn crop and its effects on horses. *J Vet Diagn Invest*, 5, 653–655.

[89] Ramasamy, S., Wang, E., Hennig, B. *et al.* (1995) Fumonisin B1 alters sphingolipid metabolism and disrupts the barrier function of endothelial cells in culture. *Toxicol Appl Pharmacol*, 133, 343–348.

[90] Wilson, T.M., Ross, P.F., Owens, D.L. *et al.* (1992) Experimental reproduction of ELEM. *Mycopathologia*, 117, 115–120.

[91] Foreman, J.H., Constable, P.D., Waggoner, A.L. *et al.* (2004) Neurologic abnormalities and cerebrospinal fluid changes in horses administered fumonisin B1 intravenously. *J Vet Intern Med*, 18, 223–230.

[92] McCue, P. (1989) Equine Leukoencephalomalacia. *Compend Contin Educ Pract Vet*, 11, 646–651.

[93] Plumlee, K.H. and Galey, F.D. (1994) Neurotoxic mycotoxins: a review of fungal toxins that cause neurological disease in large animals. *J Vet Intern Med*, 8, 49–54.

[94] Galey, F.D., Tracy, M., Craigmill, A.L. *et al.* (1991) Staggers induced by consumption of perennial ryegrass in cattle and sheep from northern California. *J Am Vet Med Assoc*, 199, 466–470.

[95] Dalziel, J., Finch, S. and Dunlop, J. (2005) The fungal neurotoxin lolitrem B inhibits the function of human large conductance calcium-activated potassium channels. *Toxicol Lett*, 155, 421–426.

[96] Hunt, L.D., Blythe, L. and Holtan, D.W. (1983) Ryegrass staggers in ponies fed processed ryegrass straw. *J Am Vet Med Assoc*, 182, 285–286.

[97] Johnstone, L.K., Mayhew, I.G. and Fletcher, L.R. (2012) Clinical expression of lolitrem B (perinneal ryegrass) intoxication in horses. *Equine Vet J*, 44, 304–309.

[98] Munday, B.L., Monkhouse, I.M. and Gallagher, R.T. (1985) Intoxication of horses by lolitrem-B in ryegrass seed cleanings. *Aust Vet J*, 62, 207.

[99] Roman, W.M., Adams, L.G., Bullard, T.L. *et al.* (1966) Cystitis syndrome of the equine. *Southwest Vet*, 19, 95–99.

[100] Adams, L.G., Dollahite, J.W., Romane, W.M. *et al.* (1969) Cystitis and ataxia associated with sorghum ingestion by horses. *J Am Vet Med Assoc*, 155, 518–524.

[101] Hahn, C.N., Mayhew, I.G. and MacKay, R.J. (1999) Diseases of the Cauda Equina, in *Equine Medicine and Surgery* (eds P.T. Colahan, A.M. Merritt, J.N. Moore *et al.*), Mosby, St. Louis, pp. 972–975.

[102] vanKampen, K.R. (1970) Sudan grass and sorghum poisoning of horses: a possible lathyrogenic disease. *J Am Vet Med Assoc*, 156, 629–630.

[103] Knight, P.R. (1968) Equine cystitis and ataxia associated with grazing of pastures dominated by sorghum species. *Aust Vet J*, 44, 257.

[104] Prichard, J.T. and Voss, J.L. (1967) Fetal ankylosis in horses associated with hybrid Sudan pasture. *J Am Vet Med Assoc*, 150, 871–873.

[105] Huxtable, C.R., Chapman, H.M., Main, D.C. *et al.* (1987) Neurological disease and lipofuscinosis in horses and sheep grazing *Trachyandra divaricata* (branched onion weed) in south Western Australia. *Aust Vet J*, 64, 105–108.

[106] Grant, R.C., Basson, P.A. and Kid, A.B. (1985) Paralysis and lipofuscin-like pigmentation of farm stock caused by the plant, *Trachyandra laxa var. laxa*. *Onderstepoort J Vet Res*, 52, 255.

[107] Bathe, A.P. (1994) An unusual manifestation of nettle rash in three horses. *Vet Rec*, 134, 11–12.

[108] Newton, L.G. (1952) *Gomphrena celosioides*—A plant causing ataxia in horses. *Aust Vet J*, 28, 151–154.

[109] Morton, J.F. (1989) Creeping indigo (*Indigofera spicata* Forsk): a hazard to herbivores in Florida. *Econ Bot*, 43, 314–327.

[110] Lima, E.F., Riet-Correa, F., Gardner, R. *et al.* (2012) Poisoning by *Indigofera lespedezioides* in horses. *Toxicon*, 60, 324–328.

[111] Carroll, A.G. and Swain, B.J. (1983) Birdsville disease in the central high-land area of Queensland. *Aust Vet J*, 60, 316–317.

35 Neonatal Encephalopathy and Related Conditions

Martin Furr

Marion duPont Scott Equine Medical Center, Virginia-Maryland Regional College of Veterinary Medicine, Leesburg, USA

Incidence/occurrence

Noninfectious encephalopathy of neonatal foals has been referred to by various terms that either describe the clinical signs or the putative pathophysiology. Hence, the terms "hypoxic/ischemic encephalopathy" (HIE), "neonatal maladjustment syndrome" (NMS), "barkers", "dummies", "wanderers", and "convulsives" have all been used. Based on similar syndromes in human infants, hypoxic and ischemic (H/I) damage to the central nervous system (CNS) associated with perinatal asphyxia has been considered to be the most likely cause in most cases. Some veterinarians, however, point out that extrapolation from humans is not necessarily appropriate, and no research has demonstrated this particular mechanism of action in foals, and hence prefer to simply refer to this syndrome as "neonatal encephalopathy" (NE). A syndrome of NE that is not associated with asphyxia is recognized in humans, in which the mother has a febrile peripartum illness—certainly a similar clinical situation occurs in horses. It is important, therefore, to recognize that NE in foals not associated with asphyxia can occur. Other potential causes of equine NE include developmental abnormalities, hydrocephalus, metabolic abnormalities, and kernicterus—all of which have been recognized and can result in clinical signs which are, at least at the present, indistinguishable from HIE [1, 2]. Given the similarity of clinical signs, epidemiological evidence, and association of the illness with documented perinatal asphyxia in clinical cases, it is most likely, however, that the combined effects of hypoxia and ischemia (perinatal asphyxia) are involved in many, if not most cases, and this chapter will focus on this aspect of the syndrome.

Perinatal asphyxia is commonly recognized in human neonatal intensive care units, and is becoming more recognizable in equine neonatal units. It is difficult to determine the actual incidence of perinatal asphyxia or HIE, because many foalings are unattended, and perinatal asphyxia is often complicated by other conditions which make recognition difficult. However, one study reported that 52% of foal deaths associated with "respiratory disease" were directly caused by asphyxia [3]. Another study has reported that complications of birth, including dystocia and neonatal asphyxia, were responsible for 19% of 3514 foal deaths at less than 24 h of age [4]. Clearly, perinatal asphyxia is a significant cause of equine neonatal morbidity and mortality. HIE is reported as "a common problem" in horse-breeding areas [5], and was identified as the cause of death in 14% of foals less than 7 days of age in one study [6]. Another study has estimated an incidence of occurrence of HIE/NMS of about 1% of neonates [7].

Etiology and pathophysiology

A number of different pathophysiologic mechanisms have been suggested over the years as the cause of HIE in foals. A strong association with perinatal asphyxia is recognized. Asphyxia is defined as a reduction of tissue oxygenation, which can result from hypoxemia (decreased oxygen content of blood) or ischemia (decreased blood flow and tissue perfusion). Perinatal asphyxia is found in a wide variety of clinical settings that result in decreased umbilical blood flow, uteroplacental perfusion, or tissue oxygenation. Fetal factors, dystocia, placental abnormalities, and maternal illness may all be involved. Additionally, more than one of the above may be involved in an individual case.

Premature clamping or separation of the umbilical cord, with subsequent "blood deprivation" to the foal has been suggested and discussed for many years [8]. While the authors reported that up to 1500 ml of blood could be lost from a prematurely severed umbilical cord, subsequent work has not confirmed this and in fact

Equine Neurology, Second Edition. Martin Furr and Stephen Reed.
© 2015 John Wiley & Sons, Inc. Published 2015 by John Wiley & Sons, Inc.
Companion website: www.wiley.com/go/furr/neurology

demonstrated no progressive blood flow in the umbilical cord, nor any change in the hematology of foals with early cord separation [9]. Hence, the effects of premature clamping or severance of the cord on the development of HIE are probably of very minor importance. Other suggestions have been that dynamic changes in vascular pressures and flow in the head of the foal may be associated [10]. These observations have not been pursued, but initial efforts did not appear to support the concept. Further, the observation of intracranial hemorrhage in foals delivered by caesarian section would appear to invalidate this concept [11]. Some authors have stated that HIE is most often associated with rapid, uncomplicated delivery [12], yet this observation alone does not preclude asphyxial events that are unrecognized. Furthermore, encephalopathy from causes other than H/I must be acknowledged, as noted earlier. HIE is clearly observed in many clinical setting which can result in hypoxia of the fetus, such as dystocia, intrauterine umbilical cord compression, decreased placental blood flow, and premature placental separation. These observations, as well as extrapolation from human medicine provide strong evidence that the pathophysiology must frequently involve asphyxia, while not excluding the possibility that other factors may also contribute.

Energy failure

However it is induced, asphyxia initiates a series of events in the CNS, which result in brain damage and dysfunction. Key elements include energy failure, altered neurotransmitter metabolism, altered calcium metabolism, and alteration in cerebral blood flow, all culminating in neuronal cell death. The primary event is an oxygen deficit, arising from both hypoxia and ischemia. Numerous studies have examined the effects of oxygen deficit upon energy metabolism. Early changes are a decrease in brain glycogen concentration and an increase in lactate (after 2 min of anoxia). Lactate accumulates when glucose is metabolized in the absence of oxygen. High energy phosphate compounds (i.e., ATP) begin to decrease after 2 min of anoxia, and are reduced by 30% after 6 min [13]. While both hypoxia and ischemia will lead to similar effects, the effects of each are magnified when both are present (Figure 35.1).

These effects are "universal"; however, age seems to have a large effect upon the response. Neonates are clearly more resistant to the effects of hypoxia [13]. The reasons for this are numerous, and include the following:
- lower rate of energy utilization
- lower rate of accumulation of toxic products
- increased utilization of lactate
- preservation of cardiovascular function in neonates

While decreased carbohydrate concentrations in the brain exist, the effects of glucose concentration upon brain injury are conflicting [14]. Hyperglycemia results

in greater severity of brain injury in the adult, while hyperglycemia in the neonatal rat is protective [15]. Other investigators have concluded that hyperglycemia is not protective, however, even in neonates [16]. Differences in reported results probably reflect subtle differences in methodology, species or strain, and methods of determining damage. No such work has been reported in the horse (Figure 35.2).

It is important to recognize that a central and fundamental component of brain injury following H/I is energy failure. This energy failure has a number of consequences that lead to neuronal cell dysfunction and death. The energy failure needed to induce these events, however, appears inadequate to be the sole cause of neuronal death. It is further important to recognize that correction of the inciting event (hypoxia, hypoperfusion, or hypoglycemia) does not result in immediate recovery of tissue concentrations of high-energy phosphates—this appears to take up to 72 h (See Figure 35.3).

Role of neurotransmitter metabolism

Alteration in neurotransmitters (particularly glutamate) and its receptors have particular importance in the pathophysiology of brain damage resulting from H/I. In normalcy, glutamate is released from the axon terminus, and it interacts with one of two types of glutamate receptors: ionotropic (NMDA, AMPA, and kainate) and metabotropic (phosphoinositide hydrolysis, protein C activation). Excessive glutamate in the synapse and surrounding tissues is absorbed by the nearby astrocytes, which metabolize the glutamate back to glutamine. AMPA receptors mediate the flux of sodium and potassium, while NMDA receptors mediate the flux of sodium, potassium, and calcium. In addition, calcium will induce the release of glutamate at the presynaptic membrane. In conditions of hypoxia and ischemia, and hypoglycemia, glutamate release is increased, with the end result being accumulation of glutamate. This arises due to (i) increased release from persistent depolarization, (ii) loss of GABAergic inhibitory neurons, (iii) blockade of inhibitory neurons (in neonates, at least), and (iv) reduced re-uptake and recycling of glutamate.

These effects are important, because glutamate is particularly toxic to neurons in vitro at concentrations (500 μmol/l) that can be achieved and demonstrated in vivo [13]. The observation that inhibition of glutamate receptors is protective to hypoxia-induced brain damage lends support to this purported role. There are two forms of cell death associated with excessive tissue concentrations of glutamate. One is a rapid cell death, due to massive sodium influx which is followed by water with subsequent cell swelling and death. Delayed cell death occurs due to the effects of increased intracellular calcium. Most cell death occurs in the period after which the inciting insult has been corrected.

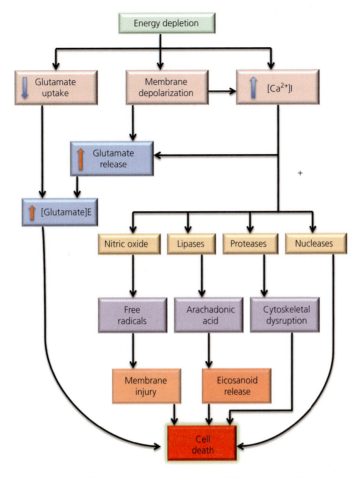

Figure 35.1 Pathophysiologic changes leading to neuronal cellular death following asphyxia.

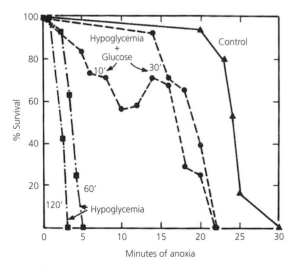

Figure 35.2 Deleterious effect of hypoglycemia on anoxia induced in newborn rats. Hypoglycemia was induced by injection of insulin 1–2 h prior to exposure to hypoxia. One group of rats was pretreated with glucose either 10 or 30 min prior to anoxia. (From Ref. [17], © Wiley.)

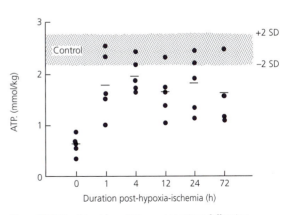

Figure 35.3 Persistent low ATP concentrations following induced hypoxic-ischemic encephalopathy in immature rat pups. Hypoxia/ischemia was induced by unilateral carotid ligation followed by 8% oxygen breathing for 3 h. Note the delay in recovery of high-energy phosphates in brain tissue. (Reproduced with permission from Ref. [18], © Nature.)

Role of calcium

Normal cellular metabolism of calcium is of crucial importance to cell health and viability. In normalcy, the cytosolic calcium concentration is kept very low (10^{-7} M); cellular calcium metabolism is controlled by several mechanisms. There are plasma membrane voltage-dependent calcium channels (VDCC), two agonist-dependent channels (NMDA and metabotropic receptors), ATP-dependent uniporters, the endoplasmic reticulum, and the mitochondrion. These mechanisms are summarized in Figure 35.4.

Energy failure leads to failure of ATP-dependent uniporters resulting in increased cytosolic calcium. In addition, energy failure leads to release of calcium from mitochondrion and the endoplasmic reticulum. Depolarization of the cell membrane results in calcium influx via VDCCs, while stimulation of the NMDA receptor (via glutamate) leads directly to calcium influx. Additionally, stimulation of the glutamate metabotropic receptor stimulates the release of inositol-3-phosphate (IP3), which directly stimulates the release of calcium

from the endoplasmic reticulum. The end result of these processes is an increased cytosolic (but not necessarily blood) calcium concentration. Increased cytosolic calcium has a number of deleterious effects that ultimately lead to the death of the cell (Table 35.1).

Increased intracellular calcium also directly stimulates production of reactive oxygen species (ROS) and nitrogen species (RNS) [19, 20]. Calcium also stimulates nitric oxide (NO) production via neuronal NO synthase (nNOS); NO can, under appropriate conditions, form the toxic RNS peroxynitrite [19]. In one study of sick foals, there was no evidence of oxidative stress, although this was not foals with NE or HIE [21].

Altered blood flow

Asphyxia results in major circulatory alterations. The initial response is a redistribution of cardiac output with subsequent increase in cerebral blood flow (CBF), followed by a rapid loss of cerebral autoregulation (i.e., the ability to maintain normal blood flow over a range of perfusion pressures). Later effects include decreased

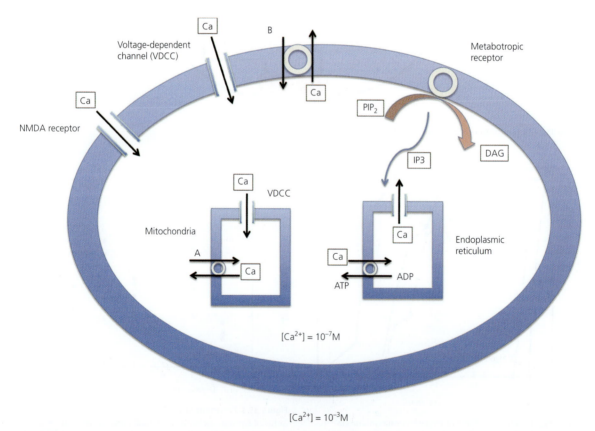

Figure 35.4 Diagrammatic representation of cellular calcium homeostasis. Process labeled as "A" is a sodium/hydrogen coupled exchange pump, while the process at "B" represents an ATPase-dependent pump as well as a sodium/calcium exchange pump.

cardiac output and hypotension with a decreased CBF. Seizure activity is known to increase CBF and induce hypertension and is felt to contribute to CNS parenchymal bleeding. Cerebral blood flow is also important in the postasphyxial period. In experimental models of asphyxia in newborn lambs, cerebrovascular autoregulation is lost when the PaO_2 changed from 70 to 30 mm Hg. This loss of autoregulation occurred after only 20 min of partial asphyxia, and did not return until 7 h after restoring normoxemia [13]. Systemic acidosis also caused a loss in cerebrovascular autoregulation [13]. While similar data have not been generated for neonatal foals, it is reasonable to assume that the responses are similar and have important consequences for treatment of the neonatal foal with HIE.

Table 35.1 Effects of calcium on cellular metabolism.

Calcium effect	Deleterious effects
Activates phospholipases	Cell membrane hydrolysis
Stimulates arachadonic acids and free radicals	Cell membrane hydrolysis
Activates proteases	Cytoskeletal disruption
Activates nucleases	Nuclear injury
Activates Ca ATPase	Increased ATP consumption
Uncouples oxidative phosphorylation	Decrease ATP production
Increases neurotransmitter release	Activates glutamate receptor
Activate nitric oxide (NO) synthase	Increased [NO]

Neuronal cell death

From the foregoing discussion, one can summarize the events that lead to neuronal cell death. Free radicals produced during H/I cause peroxidation of membrane phospholipid, leading to breakdown of the cell membrane and cellular death. Energy depletion increases membrane depolarization and cytosolic calcium. These changes will subsequently increase glutamate release, which also promotes further depolarization and intracellular calcium and cellular swelling [22]. Both glutamate and calcium are cytotoxic (Figure 35.5).

Altered neurosteroid metabolism

Increased concentrations of progesterone, pregnenolone androstenedione, dehydroepiandrosterone, and epitestosterone have been detected in the plasma of foals with NMS, as compared with healthy, age-matched foals [23]. The authors suggested that this occurred due to a delayed or interrupted transition to extra-uterine life and that these compounds may have a role in inducing some of the signs of NMS in foals, as observed from empirical studies [24]. Concentrations were not related to severity of NMS or outcome, and similar changes were also detected in sick, non-NMS affected foals. Hence, it is unclear if these compounds represent a primary cause or if this is simply an epiphenomenon; further studies are warranted to investigate these interesting findings. This may represent a unique pathophysiology for some cases of neonatal encephalopathy that is distinct from perinatal asphyxia.

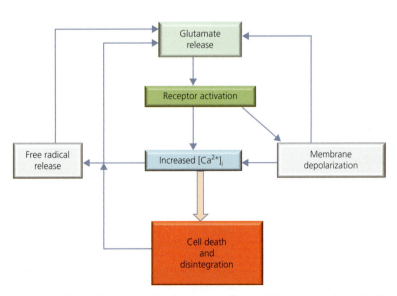

Figure 35.5 Diagrammatic mechanism of glutamate-induced neuronal cell death. Note the central role for alteration in intracellular calcium concentration.

Clinical signs

The clinical signs of HIE in the foal are varied and reflect diffuse cerebrocortical disease. The clinical signs are usually observed in the first 24 h of life, but may be seen anytime during the first week of life. The time of onset has been used to categorize the condition as either category 1 or 2. Category 1 foals are normal at birth with an onset of clinical signs 6–24 h later, while category 2 foals are clinically abnormal from birth. In category 1 foals, the onset of clinical abnormalities is usually abrupt, and typically begins with altered consciousness expressed as loss of affinity for the dam, wandering, and loss of suckling ability. These signs may or may not progress to circling, blindness, abnormal phonations (hence the term

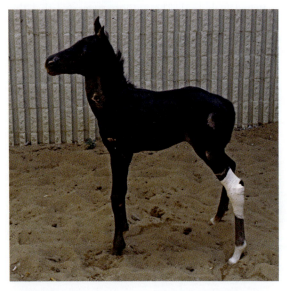

Figure 35.6 A foal demonstrating "star-gazing" behavior associated with cortical blindness secondary to severe HIE. The blindness in this foal was persistent, and it was euthanized at 6 weeks of age.

"barker") and seizures which may be either generalized are partial. Partial seizures include "chewing gum" fits, lip smacking, or nystagmus. Affected foals often become recumbent and semicomatose. Other signs that can be seen include abnormal respiratory patterns, mydriatic pupils, or dysphagia. Dysphagia appears to be fairly common, and probably reflects the complex neurologic control of this reflex. A specific syndrome of pharyngeal dysfunction with paralysis and edema has been described in neonatal foals; about 50% of the affected foals had a concurrent diagnosis of HIE [25]. These foals developed an appropriate swallowing reflex typically within 2 weeks of age, although longer periods were observed in some foals. Overall long-term survival was 81% [25]. Spinal cord signs, such as weakness or loss of specific limb reflexes can also rarely be seen, but are often overshadowed by the CNS abnormalities (Figure 35.6 and Table 35.2) [27].

Diagnosis of NE is made based on the presence of clinical signs and history that are consistent with the syndrome, as well as exclusion of other illnesses with which it may be complicated, such as neonatal sepsis, meningitis, white muscle disease, prematurity, or Tyzzers disease.

The "lavender foal syndrome" must be differentiated from HIE. The lavender foal syndrome, also known as coat color dilution lethal (CCDL), is a tetanic syndrome of Arabian foals of Egyptian breeding. Foals with this syndrome have a characteristic diluted coat color that varies from a striking silver to a pale lavender, pink, or pewter [28]. The syndrome is poorly described in the literature, but it has been recognized among Arabian horse breeders. Tetanic paddling with opisthotonus is present immediately after birth, interspersed with periods of relative normalcy. Routine clinicopathologic evaluation is normal, but may be complicated by failure of passive transfer. Post mortem of the few reported cases does not reveal any changes of the CNS. Treatment success has not been reported in the literature, and affected foals have all been euthanized. The etiology of the syndrome is unknown. Diagnosis is by observation, breeding history and rule-out of other similar conditions.

Table 35.2 Equine Apgar score.[a]

Score	0	1	2
Heart rate	Absent	<60 BPM or irregular	>60 BPM and regular
Respiratory rate	Absent	Irregular	Regular
Muscle tone and postural response	Lateral recumbency, no tone	Some flexion of limbs and muscle tone	Sternal recumbency and attempts to stand
Response to stimuli	No response	Weak ear movement when stimulated, facial grimace	Head shake, sneeze, or cough

[a] 7–8, normal; 4–6, requires some intervention; and 0–3, life-threatening abnormalities [26].

Due to the association with perinatal asphyxia, clinical signs of other body systems may be present and complicate the diagnosis. Severe illness from other diseases may lead to signs of weakness and mental depression that are difficult to distinguish from HIE. Therefore, a careful physical and clinicopathologic examination is necessary to identify all potential abnormalities.

Clinicopathologic findings

As NE is by definition a noninfectious illness, the hemogram and blood chemistry panels are usually normal, or reflect nonspecific stress or dehydration. Hypoxia and acidosis may be present due to concurrent respiratory disease or secondary to seizure activity. Cerebrospinal fluid analysis is often normal, but may show xanthochromia in excess of that seen in normal foals [29]. Mild xanthochromia is normal in foals up to 10 days of age, and its presence neither supports nor refutes the diagnosis of HIE. Cerebrospinal fluid total protein and creatine kinase activity are normal [30]. Recently, the use of two neuronal injury biomarkers has been investigated as a diagnostic aid for HIE in the foal. Results demonstrated that plasma concentrations of ubiquitin C-terminal hydrolase-1 (UCHL1) in affected foals were higher than that of normal age-matched foals (median 6.57 ng/ml vs. 2.52 ng/ml) [31]. The sensitivity and specificity of the test (using a cut-off value of >4.0 ng/ml) was 70 and 94%, respectively. Concentrations of phosphorylated neurofilament H (pNF-H) were not different in affected compared to normal foals [31]. Magnetic resonance imaging or CT scanning of the brain is not readily available, but has been attempted in some cases and may prove to be a useful adjunctive modality in the future.

Electroencephalography (EEG) is commonly used in human neonates with perinatal asphyxia and appears to be a sensitive predictor of outcome [32]. Reports of EEG findings in foals with HIE are rare in the literature; however, the author has noted that such foals frequently have substantial changes in the EEG including focal seizure focus, depressed voltage, and increased slow wave activity. EEG seizures appear to be frequently clinically silent. (Furr M, unpublished observations). Monitoring of the EEG has been of value in the author's practice to help determine the need for continued anticonvulsant therapy, for example. No correlation with outcome has been detected; however; this has not been critically evaluated.

Pathologic examination may find concurrent signs of hypoxia, recumbency or sepsis, and complete and extensive neuropathologic investigations of affected foals are rare. The widely held belief that there are no pathologic changes in the brain of affected foals appears to be erroneous, as one study has reported local hemorrhage and cerebrocortical necrosis in 9 of 18 foals with HIE [33, 34]. In a more recent report of three affected foals, there was gray matter necrosis in the cerebral cortex, caudate nuclei, thalamus, hippocampus, cerebellar cortex, and medulla oblongata; these changes were considered to be consistent with asphyxial brain injury [31]. Evidence of increased intracranial pressure, cerebral edema at the gray–white matter interface, endothelial hypertrophy, congestion, presence of gitter cells, and astrocytosis were seen in another foal with HIE [35]. Pathologic changes associated with perinatal asphyxia have been described in the urinary, respiratory, endocrine, and gastrointestinal system and are variably observed [36, 37]. The failure to find pathologic changes in the brains of some foals with clinical signs of HIE suggests that there may be more than one pathophysiological event leading to similar clinical events.

Treatment and prognosis

Treatment of foals with HIE must address the multisystemic nature of this disease. High-quality nursing care and treatment directed toward correcting hypoxia, hypotension, and hypoglycemia is imperative and must include monitoring of blood gases, cardiac function, renal function, and nutritional status.

Correction of hypoxia (if present) is usually achieved by administration of oxygen by nasal insufflation (10 l/min humidified). Maintaining the foal in sternal recumbency is important to optimize the effects of supplemental oxygen therapy. If atelectasis, sepsis, or meconium aspiration is present, the response to oxygen will be incomplete. If respiratory depression due to CNS lesions is present, treatment may include theophylline, 5–6 mg/kg, intravenously, followed by 1–2 mg/kg q12 h [38]. The therapeutic range for theophylline is narrow, and caution should be exercised not to overdose. Toxicity results in seizures, tachyarrhythmia, and hypotension. Blood concentrations of theophylline should be monitored and the dosage adjusted to maintain therapeutic plasma levels of 5–20 mg/l [38]. Caffeine (7.5–12 mg/kg loading and 2.5–5.0 mg/kg SID, PO) and doxapram (0.02–0.05 mg/kg/h IV) have both been advocated; however in a group of foals with HIE and hypercapnia, there was little effect using caffeine, but rapid correction using doxapram as a continuous rate infusion (CRI) was achieved [39]. If hypercarbia ($PaCO_2$ 60 mm Hg) and hypoxemia ($paO_2 < 50$ mm Hg) persist, mechanical ventilation is necessary.

Appropriate fluid therapy is also important in foals with HIE and perinatal asphyxia. Polyionic isotonic replacement fluids should be given to correct dehydration and expand fluid volume. Overhydration should be avoided due to the failure of cerebral autoregulation and potential to exacerbate cerebral hemorrhage/edema. Metabolic acidosis should be treated with supplemental sodium bicarbonate, based on the results of blood gas analysis. Alternatively, 1–2 mEq of sodium bicarbonate is probably a safe empiric dose if blood gas data are not available. The clinician should be cautious, however, in the use of bicarbonate in a foal with severe respiratory compromise or respiratory depression. In these foals, supplemental sodium bicarbonate can result in worsening of the acidosis, due to CO_2 retention. Specific electrolyte abnormalities should be corrected, as needed, and care should be taken to avoid administration of hyperosmolar fluids. Bolus dosing with hypertonic saline should probably be avoided in foals with HIE due to the risk of exacerbating neurologic damage due to abrupt osmolar shifts.

Seizures are an emergency situation and must be addressed immediately, as the seizure potentiates CNS damage due to excessive depolarization and neurotransmitter release. Furthermore, seizures have profound effects upon blood pressure and CBF, further potentiating neuronal cell death. Diazepam (0.11–0.44 mg/kg IV) is the drug of choice. An effective alternative to diazepam is midazolam, a similar and potent benzodiazepine class pharmaceutical which is also rapidly acting, but short-lived. Midazolam can be administered intravenously, intramuscularly or as a CRI [40, 41]. For immediate seizure control, it has been recommended the drug can be administered IV at a dose of 2–5 mg for a 50 kg foal [40]. For persistent seizures, midazolam can be administered as a CRI at a dose of 1–3 mg/h for a 50 kg foal [40]. Another study has found that midazolam alone at a dose of 0.44 mg/kg IV in healthy pony foals leads to an increase in heart rate and blood pressure, variable effects upon respiratory rate, muscular weakness, lethargy, hyperreactivity to touch, and nystagmus [41]. The importance of these effects in foals with NE is unknown, and appropriate pharmacokinetic studies in foals have not been completed. As a general rule, if more than three doses of diazepam or midazolam are required to control seizure activity, then a longer acting drug such as phenobarbital (2–10 mg/kg slow IV q12 h), or midazolam as a CRI, should be given. Phenobarbital should be maintained for 3–5 days, after which the dose should be incrementally decreased over at least 2 days. Abrupt withdrawal of phenobarbital can lead to recurrence of seizures. The use of other drugs for the control of seizures is further discussed in Chapter 7.

Dimethylsulfoxide (DMSO) (0.5 g/kg IV as a 10% solution) has been advocated to treat cerebral edema, which was identified in 50% of foals in one report [34]. Increased CSF pressure has been recognized only rarely in the author's experience; however, it does occur and

caudal herniation of the brain has been reported in foals [42]. DMSO also has anti-inflammatory properties, which may be beneficial in convulsing neonates. Mannitol has also been used to treat cerebral edema; however, its use in the foal has been limited due to concerns about its potential to exacerbate intracranial hemorrhage. This is probably overly cautious, and mannitol can be used in foals with HIE that do not show gross evidence of hemorrhage on CSF analysis. Antioxidant drugs such as ascorbic acid and Vitamin E have been advocated; however, their penetration of the CNS is questionable, and they may have little value when given after the insult. The effectiveness of antioxidant therapy has not been critically evaluated in foals with HIE or NE.

Intravenous magnesium has been advocated for the treatment of NE in foals [43]. Magnesium blocks calcium entry into the cell, while diminishing glutamate release [44, 45]. Conflicting results have been published, however regarding the efficacy of magnesium in hypoxic injury. As with other agents, the age of the subject and the timing of treatment appear to provide vastly different results. In a model of hypoxia in newborn rats, magnesium treatment was associated with recovery [46]. In another study, however, postasphyxial treatment worsened brain damage in 7-day-old rats [47]. Only limited studies have been reported in humans, and a clear benefit of the use of magnesium for NE has not been established. Notwithstanding the conflicting results observed, doses of magnesium sulfate of 50 mg/kg/h for 1 h, then decreased to 25 mg/kg/h have been advocated for foals with HIE/NMS/NE with anecdotal success [43].

Additional ancillary treatments include nutritional support, treatment of infection if necessary, gastric ulceration prophylaxis, and correction of failure of passive transfer (if present). Good nursing care, with careful attention paid to keeping the foal clean and dry, minimizing decubitus formation, and maintaining intravenous and urinary catheters are critical to successful treatment.

Additional treatment methods in humans are being investigated, including hypothermia, the free radical scavenger desferrioxamine, erythropoietin, melatonin, and xenon gas [48]. Of these, the only modality with well-tested and documented efficacy is hypothermia, which is associated with a significant reduction of mortality, risk of cerebral palsy, visual deficit, or cognitive delay [49]. Application of this treatment modality in foals is challenging and has not been attempted in a controlled fashion. Septic foals are frequently hypothermic, which is known to be a significant risk factor for death [50], so at our present state of knowledge, it seems ill-advised to employ "permissive" hypothermia in such patients in an effort to help the NE.

In the authors' experience, most foals have a minimum of 3 days during which the worst of the clinical signs are present; they will often get worse during the first 48 h in spite of treatment. This is usually followed by gradual return to normalcy over the subsequent 5–7 days. Recovery from NE occurs in somewhat the reverse order of its progression, with return of consciousness, ability to stand, vision, and return of suckling ability usually the last to return. The occasional foal will have prolonged recovery, and lack of nursing ability has been occasionally observed up to 30 days after the illness. Recurrence is rare, but can occur.

Most foals (85%) with uncomplicated NE will survive, assuming appropriate treatment. Foals in category 1 are considered to have a better prognosis than foals in category 2 [51]. In the authors' experience, most foals that survive HIE usually have normal growth patterns and appear to perform equally to their cohorts as they are put into work. Foals with complications such as sepsis, infected joints, or severe respiratory disease have a much lower survival rate and poorer long-term outcome that is dictated in large part by the nature of the complicating condition. Foals that demonstrate signs of cerebral necrosis (e.g., high protein, increased cellularity and RBCs) on CSF examination, or which have refractory convulsions, have a poor prognosis.

References

[1] Johnson, A.L., Gilsenan, W.F. and Palmer, J. (2012) Metabolic encephalopathies in foals—pay attention to the serum biochemistry panel!. *Equine Vet Educ*, 24, 233–235.

[2] Loynachan, A.T., Williams, N.M. and Freestone, J.F. (2007) Kernicterus in a neonatal foal. *J Vet Diagn Invest*, 19, 209–212.

[3] Drummond, W. and Koterba, A. (1990) Neonatal Asphyxia, in *Equine Clinical Neonatology*, 1st edn (eds A. Koterba, W. Drummond and E. Kosch), Lea and Febinger, Philadelphia, PA, pp. 124–135.

[4] Giles, R.C., Donahue, J.M., Hong, C.B. *et al.* (1994) Causes of abortion, stillbirth and perinatal death in horses: 3,527 cases (1986–1991). *J Am Vet Med Assoc*, 203, 1170–1175.

[5] Mayhew, I.G. (ed.) (1989) Disorders of Behavior and Personality, in *Large Animal Neurology*, 1st edn, Lea and Febinger, Philadelphia, PA, pp. 73–112.

[6] Cohen, N.D. (1994) Causes of and farm management factors associated with disease and death in foals. *J Am Vet Med Assoc*, 204, 1644–1651.

[7] Bernard, W., Reimer, J. and Cudd, T. (1995) Historical features, clinicopathologic findings, clinical features, and outcome of equine neonates presenting with or developing signs of central nervous system disease. *Proc Am Assoc Equine Pract*, 41, 222–224.

[8] Rossdale, P.D. and Mahaffey, L.W. (1958) Parturition in the thoroughbred mare with particular reference to blood deprivation in the newborn. *Vet Rec*, 70, 142–152.

[9] Doarn, R.T., Threlfall, W.R. and Kline, R. (1987) Umbilical blood flow and the effects of premature severance in the neonatal foal. *Theriogenology*, 28, 789–800.

[10] Johnson, P. and Rossdale, P.D. (1975) Preliminary observations on cranial cardiovascular changes during asphyxia in the newborn foal. *J Reprod Fertil Suppl*, 23, 695–699.

[11] Palmer, A.C., Leadon, D.P., Rossdale, P.D. *et al.* (1984) Intracranial haemorrhage in pre-viable, premature and full term foals. *Equine Vet J*, 6, 383–389.

[12] Valla, W.E. (1986) Diagnosis and treatment of prematurity and neonatal maladjustment syndrome in newborn foals. *Compend Contin Educ Pract Vet*, 8, S211–S223.

[13] Volpe, J. (ed.) (1995) Hypoxic-Ischemic Encephalopathy: Biochemical and Physiological Aspects, in *Neurology of the Newborn*, 3rd edn, W.B. Saunders, Philadelphia, PA, pp. 211–259.

[14] LeBlanc, M.H., Huang, M. and Vig, V. (1993) Glucose affects the severity of hypoxic-ischemic brain injury in newborn pigs. *Stroke*, 24, 1055–1062.

[15] Hattori, H. and Wasterlain, C.G. (1990) Posthypoxic glucose supplementation reduces hypoxic-ischemic brain damage in the neonatal rat. *Ann Neurol*, 28, 122–128.

[16] Sheldon, R.A., Partridge, J.C. and Ferriero, D.M. (1992) Postischemic hyperglycemia is not protective to the neonatal rat brain. *Pediatr Res*, 32, 489–493.

[17] Vannucci, R.C. and Vannucci, S.J. (1978) Cerebral carbohydrate metabolism during hypoglycemia and anoxia in newborn rats. *Ann Neurol*, 4, 73.

[18] Palmer, C., Brucklacher, R.M., Cristensen, M.A. *et al.* (1990) Carbohydrate and energy metabolism during the evolution of hypoxic-ischemic brain damage in the immature rat. *J Cereb Blood Flow Metab*, 10, 227–235.

[19] Verklan, M.T. (2009) The chilling details: hypoxic-ischemic encephalopathy. *J Perinat Neonatal Nurs*, 23, 59–68.

[20] Mishra, O.P., Enelli, S., Ohnishi, S.T. *et al.* (2000) Hypoxia-induced generation of nitric oxide free radicals in cerebral cortex of newborn guinea pigs. *Neurochem Res*, 25, 1559–1565.

[21] Furr, M., Frellstedt, L. and Geor, R. (2011) Sick foals do not demonstrate evidence of oxidative stress. *J Equine Vet Sci*, 1, 1–3.

[22] Westbrock, G.L. (1993) Glutamate Receptors and Excitotoxicity, in *Molecular and Cellular Approaches to the Treatment of Neurological Disease* (ed. S.G. Waxman), Raven Press, New York.

[23] Aleman, M., Pickles, K.J., Conley, A.J. *et al.* (2013) Abnormal plasma neuroactive progestagen derivatives in ill, neonatal foals presented to the neonatal intensive care unit. *Equine Vet J*, 45, 661–665.

[24] Madigan, J.E., Haggett, E.F., Pickles, K.J. *et al.* (2012) Allopregnanolone infusion induced neurobehavioural alterations in a neonatal foal: is this a clue to the pathogenesis of

neonatal maladjustment syndrome? *Equine Vet J Suppl*, 41, 109–112.

[25] Holcombe, S.J., Hurcombe, S.D., Barr, B.S. *et al.* (2012) Dysphagia associated with presumed pharyngeal dysfunction in 16 neonatal foals. *Equine Vet J Suppl*, 41, 105–108.

[26] Vaala, W.E. (1994) Peripartum asphyxia. *Vet Clin North Am Equine Pract*, 10, 187–210.

[27] Mayhew, I.G. (1982) Observations on vascular accidents in the central nervous system of neonatal foals. *J Reprod Fertil Suppl*, 32, 569–575.

[28] Fanelli, H.H. (2005) Coat colour dilution lethal ("lavender foal syndrome"): a tetany syndrome of Arabian foals. *Equine Vet Educ*, 17, 260–263.

[29] Furr, M. and Bender, H. (1994) Cerebrospinal fluid variables in clinically normal foals from birth to 42 days of age. *Am J Vet Res*, 55, 781–784.

[30] Rossdale, P.D., Falk, M., Jeffcoat, L.B. *et al.* (1979) A preliminary investigation of cerebrospinal fluid in the newborn as an aid to the study of cerebral damage. *J Reprod Fertil Suppl*, 27, 593–599.

[31] Ringger, N.C., Giguere, S., Morresey, P.R. *et al.* (2011) Biomarkers of brain injury in foals with hypoxic-ischemic encephalopathy. *J Vet Intern Med*, 25, 132–137.

[32] Hellstrom-Westas, L. and Rosen, I. (2006) Continuous brain-function monitoring: state of the art in clinical practice. *Semin Fetal Neonatal Med*, 11, 503–511.

[33] Palmer, A. and Rossdale, P.D. (1976) Neuropathological changes associated with the neonatal maladjustment syndrome in the thoroughbred foal. *Res Vet Sci*, 20, 267–275.

[34] Palmer, A.C. and Rossdale, P.D. (1975) Neuropathology of the convulsive foal syndrome. *J Reprod Fertil Suppl*, 23, 691–694.

[35] Wilcox, A.L., Calise, D.V., Chapman, S.E. *et al.* (2009) Hypoxic/ischemic encephalopathy associated with placental insufficiency in a cloned foal. *Vet Pathol*, 46, 75–79.

[36] Furr, M. (1996) Perinatal asphyxia in foals. *Compend Contin Educ Pract Vet*, 18, 1342–1351.

[37] Vaala, W.E. (1999) Peripartum asphyxia syndrome in foals. *Proc Am Assoc Equine Pract*, 45, 247–253.

[38] Koterba, A. (1990) Appendix A, in *Equine Clinical Neonatalogy*, 1st edn (eds A. Koterba, W. Drummond and P. Kosch), Lea and Febinger, Philadelphia, PA, pp. 781–789.

[39] Giguere, S., Slade, J.K. and Sanchez, L.C. (2008) Retrospective comparison of caffeine and doxapram for the treatment of hypercapnia in foals with hypoxic-ischemic encephalopathy. *J Vet Intern Med*, 22, 401–405.

[40] Wilkins, P.A. (2005) How to use midazolam to control equine neonatal seizures. *Proc Am Assoc Equine Pract*, 51, 279–280.

[41] Cornick-Seahorn, J.L. and Seahorn, T.L. (1998) Cardiopulmonary and behavioral effects of midazolam HCL and reversal with flumazenil in pony foals. *Vet Surg*, 27, 169.

[42] Kortz, G.D., Madigan, J.E., Lakritz, J. *et al.* (1992) Cerebral edema and cerebellar herniation in four equine neonates. *Equine Vet J*, 24, 63–66.

[43] Wilkins, P. (2001) Magnesium infusion in hypoxic ischemic encephalopathy. *Proc Annu Meet Am Coll Vet Intern Med*, 242–243.

[44] Berger, R., Garnier, Y. and Jensen, A. (2002) Perinatal brain damage: underlying mechanisms and neuroprotective strategies. *J Soc Gynecol Investig*, 9, 319–328.

[45] Leonard, S.E. and Kirby, R. (2002) The role of glutamate, calcium and magnesium in secondary brain injury. *J Vet Emerg Crit Care*, 12, 17–32.

[46] Seimkowicz, E. (1997) Magnesium sulfate dramatically improves immediate recovery of rats from hypoxia. *Resuscitation*, 35, 53–59.

[47] Sameshima, H., Ota, A. and Ikenoue, T. (1999) Pretreatment with magnesium sulfate protects against hypoxic-ischemic brain injury but post-asphyxial treatment worsens brain injury in 7 day old rats. *Am J Obstet Gynecol*, 180, 725–730.

[48] Dickey, E.J., Long, S.N. and Hunt, R.W. (2011) Hypoxic ischemic encephalopathy—what can we learn from humans? *J Vet Intern Med*, 25, 1231–1240.

[49] Shah, P.S. (2010) Hypothermia: a systematic review and meta-analysis of clinical trials. *Semin Fetal Neonatal Med*, 15, 238–246.

[50] Furr, M., Tinker, M.K. and Edens, L. (1997) Prognosis for neonatal foals in an intensive care unit. *J Vet Intern Med*, 11, 183–188.

[51] Hess-Dudan, F. and Rossdale, P.D. (1996) Neonatal maladjustment syndrome and other neurological signs in the newborn foal. *Equine Vet Educ*, 8, 24–32.

36 Miscellaneous Movement Disorders

Caroline Hahn

Royal (Dick) School of Veterinary Studies, The University of Edinburgh, Midlothian, UK

Medical neurologists define movement disorders "as neurological conditions that affect the speed, fluency, quality, and ease of movement." In this context, abnormal fluency or speed of movement (dyskinesia) may involve excessive or involuntary movement (hyperkinesia) or slowed or absent voluntary movement (hypokinesia). In humans, lesions in areas of the extra-pyramidal upper motor neuronal (UMN) system, particularly in the basal nuclei, commonly cause intermittent disorders of movement, but this has only rarely been recognized in animals. In horses, these are classified as conditions that result in altered muscle tone and movement, which of course includes ataxia, that is, deficits in general or special proprioception (most often due to spinal cord, cerebellar, or vestibular deficits) and generalized changes in muscle tone such as caused by tetanus, tremorgenic mycotoxins, and hyperkalemic periodic paralysis. This section will focus on the most common examples of an enigmatic group of idiopathic disorders causing changes in gait and which do not, for the most part, relate to a focal central nervous system (CNS) lesion and thus do not include paresis and ataxia. These syndromes result from changes in the amount of resting muscle tone and the onset and force of muscle contraction due to a morphologic, or more probably, functional lesion. For the most part, no morbid or biochemical lesions are known or, if lesions have been identified, it is unclear how they result in the resulting movement disorders.

On occasion, horses may present for intermittent muscle spasms of a single limb. Some of these clinical signs then disappear and others remain constant. Partial damage to peripheral nerves or muscles or mild localized spinal cord disease is usually considered as causes, but is mostly not proven. It is also worth remembering that horses with signs of spinal cord disease can have prominent hypermetria in one or both hind limbs with hyperflexion, thus mimicking stringhalt, and a complete neurological examination should be performed on all cases of movement disorders that do not appear to have a classic orthopedic explanation.

In the final analysis, these disorders are due to the imbalance between muscle contraction and muscle relaxation which is regulated via the neuromuscular spindle, Golgi tendon organ, and myotatic reflex arc (Figure 36.1). Muscle stretch is regulated locally by muscle spindles (innervated by gamma motorneurons) whose afferent axons (1a fibers) synapse with lower motor neurons (α-motor neurons) and interneurons (classically 1a inhibitory interneurons). The reflex is important for the automatic maintenance of posture and muscle tone. Alpha and gamma motor neurons are regulated by higher control of through UMNs and a carefully controlled neurotransmitter balance. In addition to this classic view of functional neuroanatomy, it is now known that an autonomous network of interneurons capable of generating a locomotor pattern exists independently of supraspinal inputs. This central pattern generator (CPG) is capable of activating motorneurons in an appropriate sequence as well as setting the excitability of other types of interneurons involved in transmitting information from descending pathways and sensory afferents, so that corrections through these pathways are commensurate with the various phases of the locomotor cycle [1]. It is now evident that a segmental organization of the locomotor generating mechanisms exists whereby rostral and caudal segments may play different roles. In humans, there is some evidence to suggest the involvement of CNS pacemaker neurons and the inappropriate release of CPG motor program may be the basis for several clinical disorders of movement.

Equine Neurology, Second Edition. Martin Furr and Stephen Reed.
© 2015 John Wiley & Sons, Inc. Published 2015 by John Wiley & Sons, Inc.
Companion website: www.wiley.com/go/furr/neurology

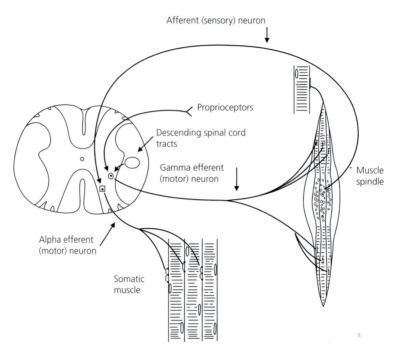

Figure 36.1 Schematic of the mechanism for the maintenance of muscle tone. When a muscle is stretched, a volley of action potentials is triggered in muscle spindle 1a and II afferent axons. These axons activate excitatory synapses on alpha motor neurons in the ventral horn resulting in contraction of the muscle that was stretched. In addition, alpha motor neurons to antagonistic muscles are inhibited via interneurons. The sensitivity of this myotatic reflex is set by gamma motor neurons in the ventral horn that innervate the intrafusal fibers in the muscle spindle. Gamma motor neuron excitability in turn is controlled by descending upper motor neuron tracts from the brainstem. Damage to the descending spinal cord tracts leads to "disinhibition" of the gamma efferent neuron and an increased muscle tonus, expressed clinically as spasticity.

Equine reflex hypertonia (plant associated stringhalt and sporadic stringhalt)

> They have all new legs, and lame ones;
> one would take it,
> That never saw 'em pace before the spavin
> Or springhalt regn'd among 'em.
> Shakespeare Henry VIII Act 1, Scene 3

Stringhalt ("springhalt") is characterized by a sudden, apparently involuntary, exaggerated flexion of one or both hind limbs during attempted movement. Varying degrees of hyperflexion with delayed protraction can occur, ranging from mild, spasmodic lifting, and grounding of the foot when the horse is backed or stopped suddenly, to extreme cases during which the foot can contact the abdomen, thorax, and occasionally the elbow leading to a peculiar bunny-hopping gait (Figure 36.2). Abnormal peripherally or centrally mediated reflex hypertonia and hyperreflexia particularly affects the

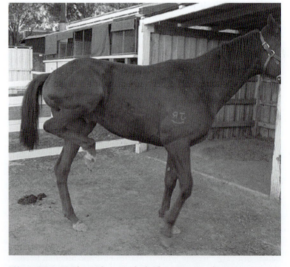

Figure 36.2 Horse with stringhalt showing involuntary hyperflexion of a pelvic limb.

lateral digital extensor muscle, but due to the action of the reciprocal apparatus the whole pelvic limb is involved. Variations in the clinical signs with a lack of forced toe extension and abduction or caudal thrust of the limb at the onset of protraction may well indicate involvement of other muscles in the disease process. Bilateral pelvic limb or additional thoracic limb involvement—usually presenting as extensor hypertonus—is likely to indicate generalized neural involvement such as due to a neurotoxin. In horses with the classical signs of stringhalt two distinct syndromes are recognized, *plant associated* and *sporadic stringhalt*.

Plant-associated stringhalt

Plant-associated, or "Australian" stringhalt is a syndrome most often recognized in Australia [2, 3] but has also been reported in New Zealand [4], North America [5, 6], Chile [7], and Japan [8], and is likely to occur infrequently in other countries. Usually, a number of cases are seen in the one herd, and outbreaks have been associated with the ingestion of the related plants dandelion (*Taraxacum officinal*), flat weed (*Hypochoeris radicata*), and cheese weed (*Malva parviflora*). The active agent, however, has not been isolated and the plants are common the world over. In Australia, cases tend to appear in late summer and are often associated with drier that normal summer; older, taller horses are predisposed [9], and cases are often more severe than seen in classical stringhalt and can progress to debilitating bilateral pelvic limb hyperflexion with delayed protraction during movement. Thoracic limbs can be involved and present as intermittent thoracic limb hypertonia with stumbling. Depending on the chronicity of the disease, there is marked atrophy of the distal limb musculature. Thoracolaryngeal responses are reduced early in disease progression. The majority of animals recover in a few days to up to 18 months (average 6–12 months) when removed from the affected pasture. Mephenesin [2], baclofen [10], and particularly phenytoin (15–25 mg/kg PO, q24h) [11] have been reported to decrease the severity of clinical signs.

Changes on postmortem examination are consistent with those of a distal axonopathy preferentially affecting large axons with a decreased density of myelinated fibers, increases in endoneurial collagen and Büngner's bands (markers of repeated myelination and demyelination). Lesions are likely to be found in the majority of somatic nerves and are most severe in the longest nerve, the recurrent laryngeal. Muscles innervated by affected nerves show degrees of myopathic changes with large group atrophy, small angular fibers, internal nuclei, fatty replacement, dissecting fibrosis, and hypertrophy of intact fibers; convincing central changes have not been reported. The reason for the extraordinary finding that peripheral nerve lesions in these cases result in hyperflexion, rather than the expected paresis with hypometria, has not been explained but is likely to involve specific changes in the fibers innervating the muscle spindles of particularly the lateral digital extensor muscles.

Sporadic stringhalt

The sporadic form occurs worldwide and usually only affects one pelvic limb. The onset can be preceded by trauma to the dorsal tarsal region or the dorsoproximal metatarsus some weeks previously [12]. Etiologies are speculated to include tendon adhesions enhancing tarsocrural joint flexion or abnormalities in the myotatic reflex caused by tendon injury perhaps involving the Golgi tendon organ.

Surgical removal of a section of the myotendinous region, containing the Golgi tendon organs, of the lateral digital extensor muscle relieves the syndrome quite spectacularly in many cases [12, 13]. Interestingly, the gait of some horses does not improve for several days after the surgery, suggesting that the change in gait is not just due to a mechanical effect. Before embarking on surgery, clinicians are urged to carefully examine the affected limb using ultrasonography, radiographs, and scintigraphy as appropriate, in order to rule out and treat any underlying orthopedic lesions. Asymmetric changes have been detected in the digital extensor muscles in some cases. In addition, it is worth remembering that in a retrospective study of 10 horses with sporadic stringhalt there appeared to be no real difference in the follow-up outcomes between four conservatively treated cases and six treated by extensive myotenectomy [12].

There has been no systematic survey of postmortem lesions in sporadic stringhalt cases, but some severely affected animals have had extensive examinations with no evidence of histologic lesions in the CNS or motor unit (A. de Lahunta, pers. commun.). Interestingly, electromyography has demonstrated abnormal activity while standing [14] and even spontaneous activity under anesthesia (personal observation), the absence of neurogenic changes in an affected lateral digital extensor muscle having been confirmed in the latter.

Scandinavian knuckling horses

A neurological disorder referred to as "Scandinavian knuckling horse syndrome" with pathological lesions strikingly similar to plant-associated stringhalt has been documented in Scandinavia for the past decade [15, 16]. At the time of publication, hundreds of horses are known to have been affected in Norway, Sweden, and Finland, but very little has been formally reported. Cases occur during late winter or early spring when

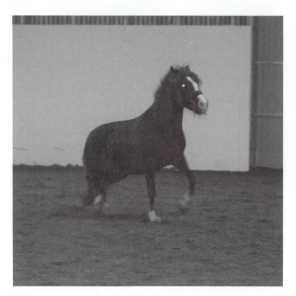

Figure 36.3 Horse with Scandinavian knuckling syndrome showing paresis in the distribution of the peroneal nerve.

horses have been fed with silage preserved in plastic, although not all horses fed the same feed are affected on a premise. More than 50% of horses on individual properties can show clinical signs. Horses have shown varying degrees of usually symmetric knuckling of the metatarsophalangeal joints with stumbling and ataxia (Figure 36.3). In some animals, the clinical signs have worsened within days until horses are unable to rise even when assisted, and mortality rates of between 50 and 100% have been recorded. Cases with milder clinical signs have slowly recovered after convalescence period of 5–6 months. A similar syndrome showing nerve and muscle lesions may be present in Japan [17, 18].

In one well-documented outbreak on a property in Finland, 11 of 17 horses showed clinical signs, which was progressive in seven horses and resulted in euthanasia. The only common feed was fresh ryegrass hay cut from a recently resown field. Horses developed clinical signs of fetlock knuckling due to poor digital extension of the metatarsophalangeal joints and paresis of the pelvic limbs ("dropping of the pelvis"). In the worst cases, clinical signs progressed within 3–4 weeks to severe paresis of the pelvic limbs, with animals "dog-sitting" and being unable to rise. The thoracic limbs appeared to be unaffected. On re-examination 3 months after the onset of clinical signs, the horses showed paresis in the distribution of the peroneal nerve, accentuated by exercise. Careful neurological examinations did not reveal any proprioceptive deficits, overt hypometria, anesthesia of the

peroneal nerve autonomous zone, or muscle atrophy in most of these animals, but one subsequently euthanized case showed prominent ataxia with conscious proprioceptive deficits in both the pelvic and thoracic limbs. Lesion on postmortem examination was limited to the peripheral nerves and muscle. Changes in the muscle were compatible with neurogenic atrophy. Detailed examination of the peroneal and radial nerves showed an evenly distributed, chronic-active, predominantly demyelinating inflammatory polyneuropathy with intracisternal Schwann cell inclusions. Electron microscopy showed spectacular filamentous rough endoplasmic reticulum Schwann cell inclusions pointing toward abnormal posttranslational protein processing [19].

The putative toxin in this disease remains elusive; and despite the fact that the profound axonopathy somehow presents as hyperflexion rather than paresis, it is interesting to speculate whether a similar pathogenesis might be involved in the "knuckling" horses, but principally targeting the peroneal nerve rather than the tibial nerve as in stringhalt. The ataxia observed in some of these cases indicates that proprioceptive axons are also affected. Systematic work detailing the distribution of lesions and a thorough epidemiological investigation is now needed to try and identify the cause of this enigmatic disease.

Shivering (shivers)

A further manifestation of a reflex hypertonia but affecting particularly the flexor muscles of the pelvic limbs is a syndrome referred to as shivering (shivers). The etiology is unknown but again is likely to involve an alteration in the feedback loop between 1a-afferent and gamma-efferent fibers. Other diseases that include shivering as their clinical signs include equine polysaccharide storage myopathy (EPSSM) and "stiff-horse syndrome." Compared to stringhalt cases, the pelvic limbs of shivering horses are flexed, abducted, and held in a spastic state for some time instead of being immediately returned to the ground as in stringhalt.

Classical shivering particularly affects draft breeds [20] and is characterized by involuntary flexion of the pelvic limbs and testicles as well as extension of the tail. Clinical signs are usually noticed when an attempt is made to back or turn the affected horse and may be accentuated by stress or excitement. The pelvic limbs are held off the ground in a flexed and abducted manner while muscles of the upper limb and tail may quiver. After a short time the quivering ceases and the affected limb and tail return to a normal position. The horse then appears to be normal, but clinical signs reappear if attempts are made to turn or back the affected horse. In the early stages, owners often notice that the horse snatches up the hind limbs when they are being picked up to clean the feet or to be shod. Classically, the condition is slowly progressive but there is no way of predicting if or when they will deteriorate.

Even in well-developed shivering cases, signs may not be seen when the horse is standing still. In advanced disease, the affected animal may be unable to move backward more than a few paces, and sometimes this cannot be performed at all. In some horses, there is evidence of involvement of the muscles of the thoracic limbs, neck, or even trunk and face, but it is unclear whether these represent severe cases of classical shivering or represent other myotonic syndromes (i.e., "stiff horse syndrome"). The difficulties backing into traces made this a disease of significant morbidity when draft horses were historically used. A hereditary predisposition is suspected.

Reflex hypertonia could potentially be caused by lesions in the sensory or motor pathways anywhere from the brain stem to the affected muscles and associated joint and tendon sensory receptors. Only rarely, however, have specific lesions, such as focal spinal cord lesions, been identified [21]. Some cases do have histologic evidence consistent with EPSSM [22], and it was hypothesized that horses with shivers might have less stored glycogen and thus deplete their stores more rapidly, leading to localized muscle cramping. Other work, however, was unable to determine a significant association between EPSSM and shivering [23]. In addition to shivering, EPSSM cases should show other clinical signs including generalized weakness, mild to moderately increased serum creatine kinase and abnormal polysaccharide accumulations, particularly in type II muscle fibers [23, 24]. Many of these cases are now known to be caused by a singular gain of function mutation in the equine glycogen synthase 1 gene (*GYS1*) [25, 26]. In the author's experience in the United Kingdom, many shivering draft horses do not have increased muscle fiber polysaccharides but can have prominent myopathic changes (increased fiber size variation with centrally located, euchromatic nuclei), which suggests that some unknown myopathic process is occurring. It is possible that neurotransmitter defects occur to account for some of these baffling syndromes.

There is currently no effective treatment for this syndrome and even though signs may improve after long periods of rest, the condition returns when work is resumed. It has been suggested that dietary treatment of affected draft horses with a high-fat, low carbohydrate feed and a gradually increasing daily exercise program may be beneficial if instituted early in the course of the disease [27]. However, it seems unlikely that a dietary change would benefit cases of classic shivering without EPSSM.

Stiff-horse syndrome

Stiff-man syndrome (recently renamed as the more politically correct "stiff-person syndrome") is a rare neurological disorder in humans characterized by continuous contraction of agonist and antagonist muscles sometimes accompanied by involuntary sudden muscle spasms caused by involuntary motor-unit firing at rest. Variants of the syndrome may involve one limb only ("stiff-leg syndrome"). The disease is thought to be caused by immunological changes leading to a gamma amino butyric acid (GABA) transmission disturbance with antibodies produced against the enzyme glutamic acid decarboxylase (GAD), which is responsible for converting GABA into its active form. The precise pathogenesis, however, is not clear and autoantibodies against GAD are not found in all human patients [28]. Gamma amino butyric acid is an important inhibitory central neurotransmitter, and a reduction in GABA activity can lead to continuous contraction of both agonist and antagonist muscle groups resulting in spasms.

A similar syndrome has been seen in horses in Belgium [29] and was called "stiff-horse syndrome." Clinical signs appear to wax and wane and range from mild muscle stiffness to sudden and often prominent muscle contractions. Mild-to-moderate muscle stiffness may be the only initial clinical sign and can be blamed on exertional rhabdomyolysis. Muscle enzymes, however, stay within normal limits, and there is no apparent weakness or muscle atrophy. Signs appear to be progressive and typically are initiated if the animal is startled, although they may occur spontaneously during voluntary movement. The lumbar and pelvic limb muscles are typically involved with horses appearing to get "stuck" from a few seconds to many minutes during severe episodes. Between episodes the horse may appear normal or generalized myotonia may be evident.

Cases are currently diagnosed by exclusion of other diseases including tetanus, equine motor neuron disease, hyperkalemic periodic paralysis, unusual spinal cord disease, thoracolumbar discospondylosis, and longissimus myopathies. Physical examination is generally unremarkable and a neurological examination will likely fail to detect any abnormalities apart from the intermittent hypertonia. Results of routine blood screening tend to be unremarkable, but it is important to eliminate rhabdomyolysis and electrolyte abnormalities from the differential diagnosis. A muscle biopsy of the semimembranosus or gluteal muscles should be performed in order to rule out exertional rhabdomyolysis and EPSSM.

The confirmatory diagnostic test is detection of antibodies against GAD in serum and cerebrospinal fluid; however, several strongly suspected cases have been negative on this test. Administration of benzodiazepines at an initial dose of 0.05–0.1 mg/kg diazepam, administered by slow intravenous injection, should in theory reduce or alleviate the severity of the muscle spasms and can be used as a crude diagnostic test: pronounced paradoxical excitement on administration has been observed, however.

In humans, drugs that enhance GABA neurotransmission, such as diazepam, vigabatrin, and baclofen, provide mild to modest relief of clinical symptoms. Due to the scarcity of cases and difficulty in making a definitive diagnoses, no studies addressing treatment options in affected horses have been published. Steroid administration (prednisolone PO at 2 mg/kg/day) may be a potential medium to long-term treatment option in the horse. Complications such as laminitis at this dose are a realistic risk but lower doses appear to have little effect (J. Mayhew, pers. commun.).

Stiff man syndrome in humans is a painful condition and it is likely to be the same in horses. Nonsteroidal anti-inflammatory drugs appear to have little effect in alleviating this apparent discomfort and the-long term welfare of affected horses should be considered.

Fibrotic myopathy

Fibrotic myopathy is most commonly caused by either scarring or an induced reflex hypertonia of the semitendinosus and sometimes the gracilis muscle. The pelvic limb hoof is slapped to the ground at the end of the swing phase causing a shortening of cranial phase of the stride [30]. Classically, this is a nonpainful, chronic, progressive, idiopathic, and degenerative disorder caused by mechanical scarring of these muscles, but some cases may be due to an induced reflex hypertonia in the semitendinosus muscle. Three cases of fibrotic myopathy due to a peripheral neuropathy have been described; [31] a very similar syndrome is recognized in dogs. Affected muscles are characterized by contracture and fibrosis and normal tissues are replaced by dense collagenous connective tissue. Most cases are associated with lesions such as muscle tears and injection reactions in the region of the caudal thigh muscles [32] and diagnostic ultrasound is useful to define the nature and extent of the inciting lesion. Surgical release of affected tissues via tenotomy [33–35] produces inconsistent results. Prognosis is guarded due to recurrence.

References

[1] Rossignol S, Bouyer L, Barthelemy D, et al. Recovery of locomotion in the cat following spinal cord lesions. *Brain Res Rev* 2002;40:257–266.

[2] Dixon RT, Stewart GA. Clinical and pharmacological observations in a case of equine stringhalt. *Aust Vet J* 1969;45:127–130.

[3] Huntington PJ, Jeffcott LB, Friend SC, et al. Australian stringhalt—epidemiological, clinical and neurological investigations. *Equine Vet J* 1989;21:266–273.

[4] Cahill JI, Goulden BE, Pearce HG. A review and some observations on stringhalt. *N Z Vet J* 1985;33:101–104.

[5] Galey FD, Hullinger PJ, McCaskill J. Outbreaks of stringhalt in northern California. *Vet Hum Toxicol* 1991;33:176–177.

[6] Gay CC, Fransen S, Richards J, et al. Hypochoeris-associated stringhalt in North America. *Equine Vet J* 1993;25:456–457.

[7] Araya O, Krause A, Solis de Ovando M. Outbreaks of stringhalt in Southern Chile. *Vet Rec* 1998;142:462–463.

[8] Takahashi T, Kitamura M, Endo Y, et al. An outbreak of stringhalt resembling Australian stringhalt in Japan. *J Equine Sci* 2002;13:93–100.

[9] Slocombe RF, Huntington PJ, Friend SC, et al. Pathological aspects of Australian stringhalt. *Equine Vet J* 1992;24: 174–183.

[10] Cahill JI, Goulden BE. Stringhalt—current thoughts on aetiology and pathogenesis. *Equine Vet J* 1992;24:161–162.

[11] Huntington PJ, Seneque S, Slocombe RF, et al. Use of phenytoin to treat horses with Australian stringhalt. *Aust Vet J* 1991;68:221–224.

[12] Crabill MR, Honnas CM, Taylor DS, et al. Stringhalt secondary to trauma to the dorsoproximal region of the metatarsus in horses: 10 cases (1986–1991). *J Am Vet Med Assoc* 1994;205:867–869.

[13] Torre F. Clinical diagnosis and results of surgical treatment of 13 cases of acquired bilateral stringhalt (1991–2003). *Equine Vet J* 2005;37:181–183.

[14] Wijnberg ID, Back W, van der Kolk JH. The use of electromyographic examination as a diagnostic tool and phenytoin sodium as treatment in a case of classic springhalt in a Dutch warmblood horse. *Tijdschr Diergeneeskd* 2000; 125:743–747.

[15] Gustafsson K, Roneus M. Utbrott av neurologisk störning med okänd etiologi hos hästar. (Outbreak of neurological disease with unknown etiology in horses). *Svensk Veterinärtidning (Swedish vet J)* 2000;52:253–259.

[16] Ihler CF, Hanche-Olsen S, Teige J. Extensor weakness due to peripheral neuropathy in horses with possible feed related aetiology. *Proc Br Equine Vet Assoc* 2002;30: 7–8.

[17] Furuoka H, Okamoto R, Kitayama S, et al. Idiopathic peripheral neuropathy in the horse with knuckling: muscle and nerve lesions in additional cases. *Acta Neuropathol (Berl)* 1998;96:431–437.

[18] Furuoka H, Mizushima M, Miyazawa K, et al. Idiopathic peripheral neuropathy in a horse with knuckling. *Acta Neuropathol (Berl)* 1994;88:389–393.

[19] Hahn CN, Matiasek K, Syrja P, et al. Polyneuropathy of Finnish horses characterized by inflammatory demyelination and intracisternal Schwann cell inclusions. *Equine Vet J* 2008;40:231–236.

[20] Mitchell WM. Some further observations on pathological changes found in horses affected with "Shivering" and their significance. *Vet Rec* 1930;10:535–537.

[21] Davies PC. Shivering in a thoroughbred mare. *Can Vet J* 2000;41:128–129.

[22] Valentine BA, Lahunta AD, Divers TJ, et al. Clinical and pathologic findings in two draft horses with progressive muscle atrophy, neuromuscular weakness, and abnormal gait characteristic of shivers syndrome. *J Am Vet Med Assoc* 1999;215:1661–1665.

[23] Firshman AM, Baird JD, Valberg SJ. Prevalences and clinical signs of polysaccharide storage myopathy and shivers in Belgian draft horses. *J Am Vet Med Assoc* 2005;227:1958–1964.

[24] Valentine BA. Equine polysaccharide storage myopathy. *Equine Vet Educ* 2003;15:254–262.

[25] McCue ME, Valberg SJ, Miller MB, et al. Glycogen synthase (GYS1) mutation causes a novel skeletal muscle glycogenosis. *Genomics* 2008;91:458–466.

[26] Stanley RL, McCue ME, Valberg SJ, et al. A glycogen synthase 1 mutation associated with equine polysaccharide storage myopathy and exertional rhabdomyolysis occurs in a variety of UK breeds. *Equine Vet J* 2009;41:597–601.

[27] Valentine BA, Van Saun RJ, Thompson KN, et al. Role of dietary carbohydrate and fat in horses with equine polysaccharide storage myopathy. *J Am Vet Med Assoc* 2001;219:1537–1544.

[28] Levy LM, Dalakas MC, Floeter MK. The stiff-person syndrome: an autoimmune disorder affecting neurotransmission of gamma-aminobutyric acid. *Ann Intern Med* 1999;131:522–530.

[29] Nollet H, Vanderstraeten G, Sustronck B, et al. Suspected case of stiff-horse syndrome. *Vet Rec* 2000;146:282–284.

[30] Adams OR. Fibrotic myopathy and ossifying myopathy in the hindlegs of horses. *J Am Vet Med Assoc* 1961; 139:1089–1092.

[31] Valentine BA, Rousselle SD, Sams AE, et al. Denervation atrophy in three horses with fibrotic myopathy. *J Am Vet Med Assoc* 1994;205:332–336.

[32] Turner AS, Trotter GW. Fibrotic myopathy in the horse. *J Am Vet Med Assoc* 1984;184:335–338.

[33] Bramlage LR, Reed SM, Embertson RM. Semitendinosus tenotomy for treatment of fibrotic myopathy in the horse. *J Am Vet Med Assoc* 1985;186:565–567.

[34] Gomez-Villamandos R, Santisteban J, Ruiz I, et al. Tenotomy of the tibial insertion of the semitendinosus muscle of two horses with fibrotic myopathy. *Vet Rec* 1995;136:67–68.

[35] Adams SB, Fessler JF. *Atlas of Equine Surgery*. Philadelphia: Saunders;2000.

37 Stereotypic and Behavior Disorders

Carissa L. Wickens[1] and Katherine A. Houpt[2]

[1] Department of Animal Sciences, University of Florida, Gainesville, USA
[2] College of Veterinary Medicine, Cornell University, Ithaca, USA

Stereotypies are defined as repetitive, relatively invariant patterns of behavior with no apparent goal or function [1]. Development and continued performance of stereotypic behavior have been linked to suboptimal environments [2, 3]. Specifically, stereotypic behavior can develop within the following contexts: when an animal is unable to execute a behavior pattern that it is highly motivated to perform, such as feeding or foraging behavior, when it cannot escape or avoid a stressful or fearful situation, or when it is kept in confinement or social isolation [1]. Stereotypies have been observed in several species kept in captivity [1, 4]. The performance of stereotypic behavior has been used as an indicator of poor welfare although it is often difficult to determine whether the behavior is the result of poor welfare in the past or due to current adverse conditions [5, 6]. Ethnologist's and welfare scientists have employed a multidisciplinary approach in order to address questions related to stereotypic behavior including the use of behavioral and physiological measures, as well as application of epidemiological research methods.

Studies conducted in Canada [7] and the United Kingdom [8] have reported that greater than 13% of domesticated horses exhibit stereotypies. The primary classifications assigned to stereotypic behavior patterns observed in domestic horses [9, 10] and captive wild horses [11] are *oral* and *locomotor*. Oral stereotypies involve movements of horse's mouth. Locomotor stereotypies involve movements of the horse's head and/or body. Crib-biting and weaving behavior are two of the most widely recognized equine stereotypies [12]. Crib-biting is an example of an oral stereotypic behavior in which the horse anchors its top incisor teeth on a fixed object (e.g., fence, stall, or building structures), pulls backward, contracting the neck muscles, and draws air into the cranial esophagus emitting an audible grunt [13]. Weaving is a locomotor stereotypic behavior pattern characterized by a lateral swaying movement in which the head, neck, forequarters, and sometimes hindquarters are engaged [14]. The average prevalences of crib-biting and weaving behavior in Europe and Canada are 4.1 and 3.3%, respectively [15]. In the United States, the reported prevalence of crib-biting behavior is 4.4% [16]. The exact etiology of equine stereotypic behaviors remains to be elucidated. However, results of recent research suggest that performance of stereotypies may have neurologic, endocrine, and/or gastrointestinal underpinnings. There is substantial evidence to suggest that these behaviors are not simply the result of boredom. Rather, stereotypic and other problem behaviors may develop as a result of neurologic dysfunction or in response to a physiologic condition. Crib-biting, weaving, and other stereotypic behaviors are recognized as both a management and a welfare concern, and many owners attempt to physically prevent horses from engaging in these behaviors [17, 18]. The primary problem with physical prevention, for example, attempting to stop crib-biting using a cribbing collar or by removing crib-biting surfaces, is that this approach fails to address the underlying causes of the behavior and may further reduce equine welfare [19]. Furthermore, these methods of thwarting the behavior do not provide long-term results. Once a cribbing collar is removed, for example, the horse simply returns to performing the behavior. It is important to consider changes in management strategies as a means of mitigating stereotypic behavior prior to, or at least in conjunction with, pharmacological treatment. This chapter will provide the reader with information related to the diagnosis, risk factors, etiology, signs, treatment, and prognosis of equine stereotypical disorders. Additional behavior problems including wood-chewing and abnormal aggression will be addressed.

Equine Neurology, Second Edition. Martin Furr and Stephen Reed.
© 2015 John Wiley & Sons, Inc. Published 2015 by John Wiley & Sons, Inc.
Companion website: www.wiley.com/go/furr/neurology

Weaving

Diagnosis

Observation of the behavior of a horse shifting its weight from one side to other.

Risk factors

The biggest risk factor is box stall confinement, especially in the typical British box with no windows and a Dutch door; another risk factor is breed. In the only large-scale survey of equine stereotypies, Luescher et al. found that 2.5% of horses in Ontario exhibited weaving, but 4% of Thoroughbreds exhibited the behavior, indicating a breed predilection [20]. When owners of pleasure horses on Prince Edward Island were surveyed [21], 4.8% of horses were reported as weavers. Exercise was a risk factor; the more work the horse did, the more likely it was to weave. Redbo et al. also found that, among race horses, Thoroughbreds were more likely to weave than trotters [22]. The prevalence of weaving is almost 10% in British dressage and eventing horses, but only 4% in endurance horses [14]. Age is also a risk factor as is being a stallion. A horse can spend 2 h of a 12-h overnight period weaving, so it would not be surprising if the animal developed musculoskeletal problems, but that has not been investigated [9].

Etiology

One hallmark of weaving behavior is that it occurs at the front of the stall that leads to the hypothesis that it is an intention movement. The intention may be to escape the stall, hence, the location at the only possible exit. Weaving is most likely to occur just prior to feeding. It is the anticipation of feeding rather than hunger level that stimulates weaving because increasing the frequency of feeding increases the frequency and duration of weaving [23]. Horses tethered in tie stalls may also weave. Whether stall walking horses (see below) also weave has not been ascertained.

Signs

The signs are behavioral. The horse shifts its weight from one side to the other, moving its forelimbs and often its hind limbs in a walking pattern, but without forward movement.

Treatment

The classical treatment of weaving, like that of most equine misbehaviors, is to prevent the action physically by blocking access to the space above the stall door with "weaving bars" or stall guards (fabric straps). Preventing the action does not change the horse's motivation, so its frustration may increase or the horse may simply weave farther back in its stall.

There is a treatment that addresses the horse's motivation to be with other horses. Provision of more windows, mirrors, or even a life-size photograph of a horse reduces weaving [23]. Because seeing another horse or its image reduces weaving, the motivation is probably to join the herd, not simply to escape the confines of the stall. Allowing the horse to spend more time outside the stable, for example, by increasing turn out time on pasture, may reduce, or even eliminate the behavior, but this option will depend on the owner's or facility's management regimens, availability of pasture or paddock space, and other considerations including the health, condition, and the use of the horse.

It is best to change the environment, but if that is not possible, antianxiety medications, specifically tricyclic antidepressants such as amitriptyline can be used. There is a single case report of a weaving mare who was improved (>50%) by paroxetine 0.5 mg/kg/day [24].

Prognosis

If the horse must remain in its environment with no modification, the prognosis is poor; but if the horse can be maintained in a run out or other nonconfined situation with other horses, the prognosis is good.

Stall walking

Diagnosis

The diagnosis of stereotypic stall walking is based on the observation of the animal moving around the stall for a period exceeding 5 min or of a track worn in the bedding indicating that the horse circled the stall repeatedly while not observed. Pain as a cause must be ruled out, especially if the onset is acute. The use of closed circuit television can help the owner determine the extent and time patterns of the behavior.

Risk factors

Arabians are the breed most at risk for stall walking. A total of 7% of Arabians and 3% of Thoroughbreds stall walked [20]. The risk of stall walking increases with age [14]. Stall walking is more common in endurance horses than in dressage or eventing horses. Stall walking has a higher prevalence in Thoroughbreds than in trotters [22].

Etiology

The etiology is unknown, but there appears to be one of three motivations for stall walking: stereotypy, claustrophobia, or separation anxiety. Some horses are very active and vocal when by themselves and will settle if a companion is added. Other horses react badly to confinement with or without a companion. Some plod repeatedly around their stall and do not seem agitated. These horses are probably exhibiting stereotypic behavior.

Signs

Walking around the stall, apparently purposelessly, with or without vocalization, defecation, and other signs of agitation.

Treatment

Increasing stall size does not appear to decrease the frequency of stall walking. Placing piles of hay along the horse's path can encourage him to graze rather than walk, and this may help reduce the behavior. Maintaining the horse on pasture or in a run out situation can help. All kinds of stall companions from another horse to a chicken have been reported to help, especially those horses that have separation anxiety. Sometimes, simply changing stalls, preferably to one where the horse lived without stall walking, can help. Mirrors have helped with stall walking as they have with weaving. It is best to change the environment, but if that is not possible, antianxiety medications such as serotonin reuptake inhibitors (e.g., amitriptyline or fluoxetine) can be used. There have been no studies of either the efficacy or side effects of serotonin reuptake inhibitors on horses, but doses of 0.25–0.5 mg/kg orally per day have been suggested for fluoxetine starting with 80 mg and gradually increasing. Gastrointestinal side effects have been seen in small animals so the horse should be carefully monitored for complications [25].

Prognosis

If the horse must remain in its environment with no modification, the prognosis is poor; but if the horse can be maintained in a run out or other nonconfined situation, the prognosis is good.

Stall kicking

Diagnosis

Observation of the horse repeatedly kicking the stall wall.

Risk factors

Arabians (5%) have the greatest prevalence followed by Standardbreds (3%) and Thoroughbreds (1%) [20].

Etiology

Stall kicking can have three etiologies. The first two are causes of nonstereotypic kicking in that there is a function. Horses may stall kick as acts of aggression toward horses in other stalls, or they may have been rewarded for stall kicking by delivery of a meal. Finally, there are horses that stall kick as a true stereotypic-repetitive and functionless behavior. This type of kicking is usually slower and less forceful than aggressive stall kicking. There is the possibility that the sound of the kicking is rewarding and the reward is auditory stimulation, although this is of course speculative.

Signs

The clinical sign is repeatedly striking the walls of the stall with the rear hooves. A few horses may strike with their fore limbs rather than their hind limbs.

Treatment

Treatment for stall kicking varies with the etiology. Separating horses that are aggressive should reduce stall kicking. Horses that have been conditioned to kick in anticipation of food can be counter conditioned with time and patience that nonkicking is rewarded with food. Nourishing the horse with forage rather than highly palatable grain should help. Padding the stall will protect the limb from repetitive injury and eliminate the reward of sound.

Pawing

Diagnosis

Pawing is a normal behavior if the horse is attempting to reach grass covered by snow or water covered by mud, for example. Horses often paw before rolling and when suffering from colic or about to foal. Pawing can be diagnosed as a stereotypic behavior, however, if it has no function and is repetitive.

Risk factors

Pawing is considered a problem primarily of Standardbred race horses. Frustration or anticipation seems to be the greatest risk factor because many horses paw before or while eating and when restrained from moving (e.g., when tied or in crossties).

Etiology

Pawing can be either a displacement behavior when a horse is restrained or an operantly conditioned response when a horse anticipates food. Standardbred horses may stand in the holes they have made by pawing and, in that case, the function may be to take weight off a sore limb.

Signs

There is repetitive pawing on the ground or floor. There can be damage to a dirt floor or damage to the hoof and limb if the floor is concrete.

Treatment

The treatment is to remove sources of frustration or teach the horse that nonpawing will be rewarded. The horse must be taught to stand without pawing for longer and longer periods.

Prognosis

The prognosis is fair. If the horse has free choice hay, no grain to anticipate and as many frustrations are removed as possible the prognosis is fair to good.

Headshaking

Diagnosis

The diagnosis of headshaking is based on observation of repetitive, and sometimes violent bouts of head tossing often accompanied by snorting and nose rubbing. This behavior may be observed in the field and/or during work (e.g., when the horse is ridden under saddle). Bilateral local analgesia of the posterior ethmoidal nerve (PET block) has also been used to diagnose headshaking in horses [26]. Further discussion of headshaking can be found in Chapter 11.

Risk factors

Based on the findings of an owner survey to investigate headshaking in horses, it was found that geldings and Thoroughbreds are overrepresented [27]. This does not necessarily indicate higher prevalence among this sex and breed of horse, but information concerning risk factors for headshaking in horses is limited. Age may also be a factor as the mean age of onset was found to be 9 years [28].

Etiology

The exact pathophysiology of headshaking in horses remains to be determined, but there appear to be two etiologies. Headshaking may be seasonal, with occurrences limited to the spring and early summer and becoming less frequent or even resolving during the fall and winter months. Headshaking may also be caused by trigeminal irritation.

Signs

Clinical signs of headshaking include vertical shaking of the head, snorting or sneezing, acting as if an insect has flown into the nostrils, agitated expression, and rubbing of the nose on the foreleg or nearby objects.

Treatment

Mills and Taylor found that applying a nose net, particularly a half nose net that covers the horse's nostrils, is effective in reducing headshaking behavior [29]. It has been reported by one author that cyproheptadine resulted in improvement of headshaking syndrome in the majority of cases (up to 76%) [27, 28]; however, others have found that cyproheptadine alone was ineffective, but the addition of carbamazepine resulted in 80–100% improvement in 80% of cases. Carbamazepine alone was effective in 88% of cases, but results were unpredictable at predefined dose rates [30].

Prognosis

When the underlying cause of head shaking can be determined and addressed, prognosis is fair to good. Prognosis may depend on the severity and frequency of the condition. Success rate of available treatments is variable and recurrence is possible.

Self-mutilation

Diagnosis

Stereotypic self-mutilation is a diagnosis of exclusion to be made only when all medical causes of the behavior have been eliminated. The lesions produced by biting are usually found on the flank (Figure 37.1), but also can be on the chest or stifle.

Risk factors

Stallions are the sex primarily at risk, although geldings may exhibit the behavior and, very rarely, mares.

Etiology

Pain or discomfort, especially from the pelvic viscera, is a very common cause, but many other illnesses including internal or external parasites, myopathies, and thrombosis can be associated with self-mutilation. Social frustration such as that caused by isolating a stallion from mares, exposing the stallion to other stallions, or housing a gelding with his dam can lead to the behavior. Recently, odor of another stallion or even the stallion's own odors have been hypothesized as triggers of the behavior [31].

Signs

Lesions in the flank, chest, or limbs or observation of the spinning, biting at self, and then kicking usually accompanied by vocalization are the signs of self-mutilation.

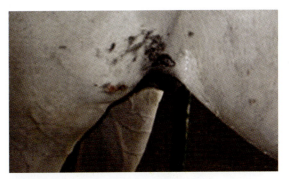

Figure 37.1 Lesions located on the flank of a stallion as the result of self-mutilation behavior.

Treatment

If any cause of pain can be eliminated, then housing the stallion with a mare, reducing or eliminating grain from the affected horse's diet, and eliminating frustration may reduce or eliminate the behavior. Castration of stallions is only effective in a third of cases [32]. Affected geldings should be isolated from mares. The use of serotonin-enhancing medications, including the precursor tryptophan, clomipramine, or fluoxetine has been suggested, but there are no published reports of the efficacy.

Prognosis

The prognosis is usually guarded, especially if the social situation cannot be modified.

Crib-biting and wind sucking

Diagnosis

Horses exhibiting crib-biting behavior anchor their top incisor teeth on a fixed object (Figure 37.2), pull backward, contract the neck muscles, and draw air into the cranial esophagus emitting an audible grunt [8, 13, 33]. The behavior is not known to occur in feral, free-ranging horses, but is observed in domestic [9] and captive wild horses [11]. Performance of crib-biting behavior has been reported to occupy from 15% [34] up to 65% [35] of the daily time budget. Horses exhibiting wind sucking behavior open their mouths, bend their neck and contract the ventral neck muscles, and draw air into the esophagus, but without anchoring their incisor teeth on a solid object. The confusion lies in the fact that sometimes the terms crib-biting and wind sucking are used interchangeably to describe the same behavioral sequence, but they clearly differ slightly in form.

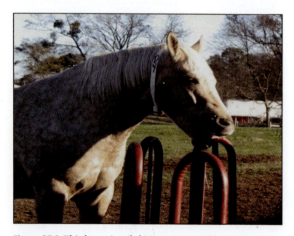

Figure 37.2 This horse is crib-biting on a metal hay ring.

Risk factors

The prevalence of crib-biting behavior reported in horses in Europe and Canada is 2.4–8.3% [14, 20, 36]. Albright et al. reported an overall prevalence of 4.4% in US horses [16]. The prevalence of wind sucking in nonracing horses in North America has been reported to be 3.8% [21]. Survey studies in the United Kingdom and Canada have demonstrated an association between various management practices and stereotypic behavior. For example, a prospective study conducted by Waters et al. found that young Thoroughbred and part-Thoroughbred horses-fed concentrate post-weaning were four times more likely to develop crib-biting behavior than foals not receiving concentrate [37]. Weaning method has also been associated with the performance of crib-biting. In a recent survey of management practices implemented on breeding farms in Europe, North America, and Australia, natural weaning (mare allowed to wean foal) was associated with a decrease in the chance of foals developing abnormal behavior [38]. Post-weaning housing was also associated with the performance of abnormal behavior with decreased risk of abnormal behavior in foals kept exclusively on grass [38]. In eventing and dressage horses in the United Kingdom, increased amounts of time spent outside the stable were associated with a decreased risk of stereotypic behavior [14]. Survey studies conducted to investigate stereotypic behavior in race horses in Sweden [22], and in Swiss horses of multiple breed types and uses [39] found that regular feeding of concentrates increased the risk of performing stereotypic behavior. Specifically, Redbo et al. demonstrated a positive relationship between the amount of concentrate and stereotypic behavior, including crib-biting, and a decreased risk of stereotypy with increased amount of roughage [22].

An experimental study intended to investigate the effect of two different housing conditions on the welfare of young horses exposed to stabling for the first time lends empirical support to the associations between housing, social isolation, and the performance of stereotypic behavior identified using survey methodology [40]. A total of 36 Dutch Warmblood horses, 2 years of age and naïve to stall housing, were enrolled in the study. Upon completion of the 12-week study, 22% of the horses housed individually in 3 × 3.5 m boxes were seen exhibiting crib-biting behavior, whereas horses pair-housed in boxes did not begin performing stereotypic behavior. Although the data were not shown, the authors indicated that after 12 weeks of stabling, performance of stereotypic behavior was still reversible in the majority of the horses [40]. This finding stresses the importance of identifying behavioral problems early so that appropriate management changes can be made before crib-biting and other stereotypic behaviors become established.

Certain breeds of horses may be more likely to exhibit crib-biting behavior than others. This was demonstrated in a survey of stereotypic behavior in Swiss horses in which Warmbloods and Thoroughbreds were at 1.8 and 3.1 times greater risk of performing stereotypic behavior, respectively, compared to other breeds [39]. Albright found that among horses in the United States, Thoroughbreds were three times more likely to exhibit crib-biting behavior than Quarter Horses and five times more likely than Arabians [16]. A genetic component in the performance of stereotypic behavior has been suggested, as evidenced by the finding that one or more relatives in eight families of Thoroughbreds exhibited crib-biting behavior [36]. Luescher et al. found a higher prevalence of crib-biting in geldings and stallions compared to mares, and a greater risk of crib-biting among Thoroughbred horses [20]. Interconnections between genetic and environmental factors, specifically interactions between gender and management, or breed and management, almost certainly play a role in the development of crib-biting behavior.

Crib-biting behavior has been linked to unthriftiness (weight loss and poor condition) in horses. This is thought to be a result of increased energy expenditure and/or a decrease in the amount of time spent eating and grazing during performance of the behavior [9, 19]. The behavior has also been associated with excessive tooth wear [11, 41], which in severe cases may impair the horse's ability to graze or result in dental disease (Figure 37.3) [11, 41]. Two studies have demonstrated an association between epiploic foramen entrapment

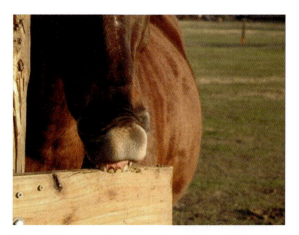

Figure 37.3 Wear of the incisor teeth in a horse with history of crib-biting behavior.

and crib-biting behavior [42]. Despite the latter findings, however, evidence for direct negative consequences of crib-biting behavior on horse health remains largely anecdotal, requiring further empirical investigation and careful documentation.

Etiology

Crib-biting behavior has been a major focus of stereotypic behavior research in horses. However, at present the precise etiology of crib-biting behavior has yet to be elucidated; the causes are likely multifactorial. Several studies have been conducted to investigate the potential biological mechanisms underlying crib-biting behavior. For example, crib-biting has been associated with altered neuroendocrine physiology [43–45] and brain function [46, 47]. There is also some evidence to support a role of gastrointestinal irritation in performance of the behavior [34, 48].

Serotonin reuptake inhibitors have been reported to reduce stereotypic behavior in horses [49]. However, Lebelt et al. expressed uncertainty regarding whether these drugs selectively affect stereotypic behavior or result in changes in behavior by way of a general sedative effect [44]. A trend for lower basal serotonin levels in crib-biting compared to non-stereotypic horses, suggesting that the serotonergic system of crib-biters may differ from that of non crib-biting horses has been observed [44]. The precise role of serotonin in the development or maintenance of the behavior remains unclear, however, and the results obtained by Lebelt et al. have yet to be confirmed or refuted through additional experimental studies of the serotonergic system in crib-biting horses.

Endogenous opioids have been suggested to facilitate and reinforce stereotypic behavior [43, 50, 51]. In one study infusion of opioid antagonists reduced crib-biting behavior, lending support to this hypothesis [50]. In another study, naloxone was demonstrated to result in a reduction in crib-biting behavior, but the authors suggested that a general sedative effect of the opiate antagonist might have influenced performance of the behavior [19]. Measurement of plasma β-endorphin in crib-biting horses has produced conflicting results. Significantly lower baseline concentrations of β-endorphin in crib-biting horses compared to non-crib-biting controls has been described [43], whereas other investigators have found three times higher basal β-endorphin concentrations in crib-biting horses [44]. Other investigators found no significant difference in plasma β-endorphin concentrations between crib-biting and normal horses [52]. It has been proposed that a failure to detect differences in plasma β-endorphin concentrations between crib-biting and normal horses may indicate greater sensitivity of opioid receptors in stereotypic horses. Crib-biting behavior has also been proposed as a means to alleviate a horse's stress; heart rate and nociceptive threshold were lowered in horses during periods of crib-biting [44]. McBride and Cuddeford reported a significant reduction in plasma cortisol concentration following bouts of crib-biting, providing evidence that the act of crib-biting may reduce stress [19]. Higher mean baseline concentrations of cortisol in crib-biting compared to normal horses was seen, but prevention of the behavior via removal of the crib-biting surface did not result in a rise in cortisol concentration, as hypothesized [53]. Subsequent studies have found no significant differences in plasma [52, 54] or salivary [52] cortisol between crib-biting and control horses, suggesting that levels of arousal in stereotypic and normal horses are similar. Horses appear to be as highly motivated to crib as to eat indicating the importance to them of the opportunity to crib [55]. There is some evidence suggesting crib-biting horses react more strongly to acute stressors compared to their non-crib-biting counterparts [35, 56]. Minero and others found that heart rate and general activity of crib-biting horses returned more quickly to basal levels following application of the stressor, providing additional support that the behavior may serve as an adaptive response to stress [56]. Interpretation of the findings obtained from these studies is difficult and remains controversial. Results may be confounded by individual differences in temperament, reactivity, and life experiences of the crib-biting and non-crib-biting horses enrolled in such studies. An inherent limitation in many of these studies is that measurements of cortisol have been obtained in mature horses with an established history of performing the behavior versus horses just beginning to crib.

Research aimed at addressing the role of neuroendocrine physiology and brain function in the development and continued performance of stereotypic behavior is further complicated by the interrelationships between the hypothalamic–pituitary–adrenal (HPA) axis and reward systems within the brain. In mice, stress induces significant changes in dopamine (DA) receptor densities within the mesoaccumbens and nigrostriatal systems [57]. In inbred strains of mice, these stress-induced changes in DA neurophysiology have been associated with the development of stereotypic behavior [58]. Significantly lower DA D1-like receptor subtypes in the caudate nucleus (dorsomedial striatum or DMS) and significantly higher DA D1-like and D2-like receptor subtypes in the nucleus accumbens (ventral striatum) of crib-biting horses as been documented [45]. Due to the involvement of basal ganglia and DA pathways in instrumental task learning, specifically goal-directed learning and response–outcome processes, it was proposed that basal ganglia dysfunction and alterations in DA physiology in crib-biters would be expressed as aberrant or impaired learning task performance [46, 47].

Horses exhibiting crib-biting behavior required significantly more unreinforced trials to reach extinction criterion (i.e., stereotypic horses continued to perform button presses without receipt of the food reward), and it was suggested that this perseverative responding might be indicative of basal ganglia dysfunction [46]. In one study, learning performance within a free-operant instrumental choice paradigm was compared between crib-biting horses and nonstereotypic horses. Crib-biting horses failed to choose a more immediate reinforcer demonstrating difficulty of the crib-biters to effectively learn the response–outcome contingency [47].

Free-ranging horses spend a large proportion of their time grazing and foraging. By contrast, domesticated horses, particularly elite performance horses, are often fed high concentrate, relatively low forage diets in order to meet the increased energy demands associated with their competitive lifestyles. Concentrate and forage rations are often delivered only two times per day, thus subjecting horses to longer periods of feed deprivation. Feed deprivation can result in gastric ulceration due to increased exposure of the squamous mucosal lining to gastric acidity [59]. Gastrin is a potent stimulator of gastric acid secretion [60] and in horses there is a greater and more prolonged gastrin response to the feeding of pelleted and sweet feed diets compared to *ad libitum* hay feeding [61]. Several studies have demonstrated associations between concentrate feeding and crib-biting behavior [22, 37, 43, 62].

It has been suggested that crib-biting behavior may be an adaptive response to gastric acidity and that the act of crib-biting may reduce gastric acidity as a result of increased flow of alkaline saliva [63]. It was demonstrated that salivation is stimulated with crib-biting, which lends support to this theory [64]; however, cribbing does not stimulate salivary flow from the main salivary gland, the parotid [65]. Crib-biting behavior has recently been associated with gastric ulceration in foals, with gastric ulceration and inflammation present in 60% of crib-biting foals compared to 20% of non-crib-biting foals [34]. In addition, crib-biting foals had greater severity of ulceration and inflammation upon initial endoscopic examination [34]. In the same study, the stomach condition of foals consuming a diet containing an antacid improved and there was a trend toward reduced duration of crib-biting in supplemented foals. In mature horses, long-term treatment with antacids has been shown to reduce the frequency of crib-biting, particularly in the period post-feeding [48]. In a study conducted to examine the integrity and function of gastric mucosa in mature horses with a history of crib-biting behavior, there were no differences in the number or severity of squamous mucosal lesions between crib-biting and normal horses maintained on pasture [66]. However, serum gastrin response to concentrate feeding was found to be higher in crib-biting horses compared to controls, providing some additional evidence that gastrointestinal physiology may be altered in horses exhibiting crib-biting behavior [66]. Horses with gastric mucosal injury exhibit bruxism and behavioral signs of colic, thus suggesting that horses are able to detect the pain associated with gastric acidity and mucosal lesions [67]. Pain is known to bring about changes in dopaminergic activity [68] and it was postulated that visceral discomfort in horses may play an important role in the establishment of oral stereotypy through alteration of basal ganglia programming [46]. In a recent publication, it was reported that mean plasma ghrelin concentrations were significantly higher in crib-biting compared to control horses [69]. Ghrelin is a peptide found in the gastric mucosa that is involved with regulation of food intake. Ghrelin also activates systems associated with motivated behavior and reward via the cholinergic–dopaminergic reward system. This was the first study to demonstrate an association between crib-biting behavior and ghrelin concentration. It seems probable that a complex interrelationship between gastrointestinal and brain physiology is involved in the etiology of crib-biting behavior.

Signs

A horse that exhibits crib-biting behavior will be observed anchoring their incisor teeth on a fixed object, pulling back, and contracting the neck muscles. The behavioral sequence is normally accompanied by an audible grunting sound heard when the horse draws air into the cranial esophagus. Some crib-biting horses, particularly older animals with history of performing the behavior, will have hypertrophy of the neck muscles and may have evidence of uneven or excessive incisor tooth wear.

Treatment

Treatments for cribbing include physical prevention of the behavior through removal of crib-biting surfaces (e.g., by applying distasteful paints to fence boards, posts, or stall doors or by electrifying fences) or by applying a cribbing collar that prevents the horse from expanding the larynx. Aversion therapy [70] and the surgical removal of the paired omohyoideus and sternothyrohyoideus muscles (modified Forssell's technique) [71] have also been used to prevent horses from crib-biting, but with varying success. Even with surgery, some recurrence of the behavior is observed. These approaches are expensive and require extra care and time from the owner or farm manager. They also do not take away the motivation to perform the behavior or address the underlying cause of the behavior. Pharmacological agents that target the neurotransmitters DA and serotonin, and the reward systems in the brain, have been used to treat crib-biting behavior with some success [49, 50, 72]. However, pharmacological treatment requires constant infusion/administration, which would increase farm costs and labor. Moreover, the side effects and toxicity levels of such compounds have not been adequately researched in horses. Feeding antacid products may help reduce crib-biting behavior, but there is no evidence to suggest it will completely stop crib-biting in mature horses with established stereotypic behavior. Provision of a stall toy that increased oral activity has been shown to lower the rate of crib-biting at least slightly [73]. Making changes to the horse's diet, feeding, and housing management may produce the best results. Preventing development of crib-biting behavior in young horses is important, and this may be accomplished by minimizing stress at weaning and managing horses under as natural conditions as possible relative to feeding and housing practices.

Prognosis

Unfortunately, the prognosis for horses with established crib-biting behavior (i.e., a long history of crib-biting) is poor. It is extremely difficult to completely stop crib-biting behavior in horses. Even 24-h turn out on pasture with ad libitum access to forage and the company of herd mates may not eliminate the behavior. However, management changes that maximize foraging opportunities, limit grain intake, and allow social interaction, may reduce the frequency or duration of the behavior.

Wood-chewing

Diagnosis

A diagnosis of wood-chewing is made when a horse is observed chewing on wooden materials. The horse bites a wooden surface or object and tears away some of the wood (i.e., the wood disappears). The horse may then proceed to ingest small amounts of the wood. Debate among behavioral scientists and practitioners continues concerning whether or not wood-chewing is a stereotypic behavior or redirected foraging behavior; Nicol has classified it as the latter [15].

Risk factors

High concentrate diets, limited forage, and confinement have been associated with wood-chewing in horses [37, 74]. Wood-chewing may be of concern on facilities that utilize treated wood for fencing. Wood-chewing causes damage to facilities and in some cases, small, sharp pieces of wood may become lodged in the horse's mouth, oral cavity, or esophagus.

Etiology

Fermentation of concentrate feeds in the cecum and large intestine is known to reduce hindgut pH in horses [75]. In one study, increasing the amount of concentrate fed to horses resulted in the appearance of aberrant oral behaviors such as wood-chewing and reductions in fecal pH [74].

Signs

The horse is observed chewing on materials made of wood. This may include tree branches, bark, fence posts or rails, and stall doors or walls. Wood-chewing is sometimes confused with crib-biting; however when a horse wood chews, the horse actually bites off and ingests small pieces of wood. Signs of wood-chewing also include visible damage to farm facilities such as pieces of wood missing from fence rails, posts, trees, stall walls or doors, or from the sides of the shelter.

Treatment

Accumulation of lactic acid in the hindgut of horses has been reduced by the addition of virginiamycin to the diet [75], and supplementation of the diet with virginia-mycin was shown to increase fecal pH and reduce the performance of abnormal oral behavior in horses receiving concentrate [74]. Increasing, the time spent eating and increasing the amount of forage horses receive can reduce incidence of wood-chewing. Applying distasteful paints or electrifying top rails of fences may also discourage wood-chewing and help reduce facility damage. However, a thorough evaluation of the horse's diet and management should be conducted if wood-chewing behavior is observed.

Prognosis

Wood-chewing can be difficult to stop, but the prognosis for reducing wood-chewing is good when horses are provided with adequate foraging opportunities.

Aggressive behavior

Diagnosis

Unexplained aggressive behavior may be described as a sudden change in a horse's behavior, such that a normally amiable horse experiences a marked shift in attitude, displaying agonistic (threat display behavior) or even overt aggression toward herd mates and/or humans. Aggressive behavior may also be described as abnormal in form or frequency, such that a horse exhibits elevated levels of aggression or an increase in the occurrence of aggressive interactions.

Risk factors

Stallions pose the most significant threat with respect to exhibiting aggressive behavior toward humans, but aggressive behavior is also observed in geldings and mares. Horses that have not received appropriate handling or training also may display aggressive behavior.

Etiology

Aggressive behavior in horses can be categorized into several types including fear-induced aggression, pain-induced aggression, intermale aggression, dominance aggression, irritable aggression (as a result of the animal being in chronic pain), redirected aggression, and granulose cell tumors in mares. Horses that have been mistreated by human handlers and horses that have been placed in fearful or pain-inducing situations or environments without a means of escape will act out aggressively. The aggressive behavior may be the result of the horse's inability to withdraw from the inducing stimulus or situation. The horse's memory of the bad experience is retained, leading to subsequent performance of the aggressive behavior. Stallion-like behavior in mares, including heightened levels of aggression has been associated with high levels of androgens with the two most common sources being exogenous steroid hormones and ovarian tumors. Although castration eliminates stallion-like behavior in most geldings, a subset of geldings may retain one or more stallion behaviors, including aggression toward other males and herding of mares [76]. The most abnormal types of aggression are foal-directed aggression by mares [77] and infanticide by stallions, usually not the sire [78].

Signs

Typical signs of offensive aggression in horses include pinning of the ears against the head, clamping or wringing of the tail, crinkling of the lips and nostrils, bearing the teeth, striking, or kicking out. It is important to differentiate offensive aggression from fear-based aggression, in which the horse tucks the tail and holds the ears sideways. These actions may be accompanied by squealing, snorting, or grunting, and may be followed by attempts to bite or lunge at another horse or human. Aggression may be displayed in the field, in the stall, or during specific horse–human interactions (e.g., grooming, tacking-up, during work).

Treatment

Therapeutic intervention requires proper identification of the specific type of aggression and its underlying cause. In the case of fear-induced aggression, gradual exposure of the horse to fearful stimuli using calm and consistent handling while reinforcing desirable behavior with praise or reward will help reduce the inciting fear.

Dominance-aggression and fighting between horses can be minimized by implementing changes in management. For example, make sure all horses in a group at pasture have adequate access to resources such as food, water, and shelter and enough space to withdraw from conflicts with a more dominant herd mate. The process by which new horses are introduced to the group can also reduce aggressive interactions. It is usually recommended to allow the new horse fence-line contact before placing it in a pasture with other horses. There may be some benefit to partnering the new horse with a resident herd member for a period of time. This pair can then be turned out together into the larger group. Progestin treatment and castration have been used as methods to treat intermale aggression with some success, but these therapies may not necessarily resolve fighting behavior. It may be necessary to keep the aggressor separated from other horses. However, it should be kept in mind that social isolation may lead to the development of other problem behaviors including stereotypic behaviors discussed earlier in this chapter. Separation of the offending horse from others should be accomplished without completely eliminating visual and auditory contact with conspecifics. In mares that have been exhibiting aggressive behavior due to granulose cell tumor, removal of the tumor will reduce the behavior, usually within a few weeks, although it may take several weeks for the mare's behavior to return to normal.

Aggression can be treated with drugs using either progesterone 0.4 mg/kg/day IM [55] or fluoxetine, 0.25–0.5 mg/kg orally per day [25]. Foal rejection can be treated with acepromazine 0.04–0.09 mg/kg IM or IV to stimulate prolactin release, or a combination of altrenogest (0.04 mg/kg orally q12 h), domperidone (1.1 mg/kg orally) and estradiol benzoate (10 mg IM q24 h) [79].

Prognosis
When physical pain can be identified as the root cause of the aggressive behavior, treatment of the condition and elimination of the source of pain will most likely eliminate the behavior. Other types of aggression, such as fear-induced aggression, require careful handling and behavior modification. Depending on the experience level of the handler, the guidance of a certified equine behaviorist may be recommended.

References

[1] Mason, G.J. (1991) Stereotypies: a critical review. Anim Behav, 41, 1015–1037.
[2] Ödberg, F. (1987) The influence of cage size and environmental enrichment on the development of stereotypies in bank voles. Behav Proc, 14, 155–173.
[3] Cooper, J.J. and Albentosa, M.J. (2005) Behavioral adaptation in the domestic horse: potential role of apparently abnormal responses including stereotypic behavior. Livest Prod Sci, 92, 177–182.
[4] Mason, G. and Rushen, J. (eds) (2006) A decade-or-more's progress in understanding stereotypic behavior, in Stereotypic Animal Behavior: Fundamentals and Applications to Welfare, CAB International, Wallingford, pp. 5–6.
[5] Broom, D.M. (1983) Stereotypies as animal welfare indicators, in Indicators Relevant to Farm Animal Welfare (ed. D. Schmidt), Martinus Nijhoff, The Hague, pp. 81–87.
[6] Mason, G.J. and Latham, N.R. (2004) Can't stop, won't stop: is stereotypy a reliable animal welfare indicator? Anim Welf, 13, S57–S69.
[7] Luescher, U.A., McKeown, D.B. and Halip, J. (1991) Reviewing the causes of obsessive-compulsive disorders in horses. Vet Med, 86, 527–530.
[8] McGreevy, P., Nicol, C.J., Cripps, P. et al. (1995) Management factors associated with stereotypic and redirected behavior in the thoroughbred horse. Equine Vet J, 27, 86–91.
[9] Houpt, K.A. and McDonnell, S.M. (1993) Equine stereotypies. Compend Contin Educ Equine Pract, 15, 1265–1271.
[10] Mills, D.S. Recent advances in the treatment of equine stereotypic behavior. [Serial online] Animal Behavior Cognition and Welfare Group. Lincoln: University of Lincoln;2002.
[11] Boyd, L. (1986) Behavior problems of equids in zoos. Vet Clin North Am Equine Pract, 2, 653–664.
[12] Kiley-Worthington, M. (1983) Stereotypes in horses. Equine Pract, 5, 34–40.
[13] McGreevy, P., Richardson, J.D., Nicol, C.J. and Lane, J.G. (1995) Radiographic and endoscopic study of horses performing an oral based stereotypy. Equine Vet J, 27, 92–95.
[14] McGreevy, P.D., French, N.P. and Nicol, C.J. (1995) The prevalence of abnormal behaviours in dressage, eventing and endurance horses in relation to stabling. Vet Rec, 137, 36–37.
[15] Nicol, C.J. Stereotypies and their relation to management. Proceedings of the BEVA Specialist Days on Behaviour and Nutrition, London; 1999, pp. 11–14.
[16] Albright, J.D., Mohammed, H.O., Heleski, C.R. et al. (2009) Crib-biting in US horses: breed predispositions and owner perceptions of aetiology. Equine Vet J, 41, 455–458.
[17] McGreevy, P.D. and Nicol, C.J. (1998) Prevention of crib-biting: a review. Equine Vet J, (Suppl 27), 35–38.
[18] McBride, S.D. and Long, L. (2001) Management of horses showing stereotypic behavior, owner perception and the implications for welfare. Vet Rec, 148, 799–802.
[19] McBride, S.D. and Cuddeford, D. (2001) The putative welfare-reducing effects of preventing equine stereotypic behavior. Anim Welf, 10, 173–189.
[20] Luescher, U.A., McKeown, D.B. and Dean, H. (1998) A cross-sectional study on compulsive behavior (stable vices) in horses. Equine Vet J, (Suppl 27), 14–18.

[21] Christie, J.L., Hewson, C.J., Riley, C.B. *et al.* (2006) Management factors affecting stereotypies and body condition score in nonracing horses in Prince Edward Island. *Can Vet J*, 47, 136–143.

[22] Redbo, I., Redbo-Torstensson, P., Ödberg, F.O. *et al.* (1998) Factors affecting behavioral disturbances in race horses. *Anim Sci*, 66, 475–481.

[23] Cooper, J.J., McCall, N., Johnson, S. and Davidson, H.P.B. (2005) The short-term effects of increasing meal frequency on stereotypic behavior of stabled horses. *Appl Behav Sci*, 90, 351–364.

[24] Nurnberg, H.G., Keith, S.J. and Paxton, D.M. (1997) Consideration of the relevance of ethological animal models for human repetitive behavioral spectrum disorders. *Biol Psychiatr*, 41, 226–229.

[25] Crowell-Davis, S.L. (2009) Aggression in horses, in *Current Therapy in Equine Medicine* (eds N. Robinson and K. Sprayberry), Saunders, St. Louis, pp. 112–115.

[26] Roberts, V.L., Perkins, J.D., Skärlina, E. *et al.* (2013) Caudal anaesthesia of the infraorbital nerve for diagnosis of idiopathic headshaking and caudal compression of the infraorbital nerve for its treatment, in 58 horses. *Equine Vet J*, 45, 107–110.

[27] Madigan, J.E. and Bell, S.A. (2001) Owner survey of headshaking in horses. *J Am Vet Med Assoc*, 219, 334–337.

[28] Madigan, J.E. and Bell, S.A. (1998) Characterisation of headshaking syndrome—31 cases. *Equine Vet J*, (Suppl 27), 28–29.

[29] Mills, D.S. and Taylor, K. (2003) Field study of the efficacy of three types of nose net for the treatment of headshaking in horses. *Vet Rec*, 152, 41–44.

[30] Newton, S.A., Knottenbelt, D.C. and Eldridge, P.R. (2000) Headshaking in horses: possible aetiopathogenesis suggested by the results of diagnostic tests and several treatment options used in 20 cases. *Equine Vet J*, 32, 208–216.

[31] McDonnell, S.M. (2008) Practical review of self-mutilation in horses. *Anim Reprod Sci*, 107, 219–228.

[32] Dodman, N.H., Normile, J.A., Shuster, L. and Rand, W. (1994) Equine self-mutilation syndrome (57 cases). *J Am Vet Med Assoc*, 204, 1219–1223.

[33] Dodman, N.H., Normile, J.A., Cottam, N. *et al.* (2005) Prevalence of compulsive behaviors in formerly feral horses. *Intern J Appl Res Vet Med*, 3, 20–24.

[34] Nicol, C.J., Davidson, H.P.D., Harris, P.A. *et al.* (2002) Study of crib-biting and gastric inflammation and ulceration in young horses. *Vet Rec*, 151, 658–662.

[35] Bachmann, I., Bernasconi, P., Herrmann, R. *et al.* (2003) Behavioral and physiological responses to an acute stressor in crib-biting and control horses. *Appl Anim Behav Sci*, 82, 297–311.

[36] Vecchiotti, G.G. and Galanti, R. (1986) Evidence of heredity of cribbing, weaving and stall-walking in Thoroughbred horses. *Livest Prod Sci*, 14, 91–95.

[37] Waters, A.J., Nicol, C.J. and French, N.P. (2002) Factors influencing the development of stereotypic and redirected behaviors in young horses: findings of a four year prospective epidemiological study. *Equine Vet J*, 34, 572–579.

[38] Parker, M., Goodwin, D. and Redhead, E.S. (2008) Survey of breeders' management of horses in Europe, North America and Australia: comparison of factors associated with the development of abnormal behavior. *Appl Anim Behav Sci*, 114, 206–215.

[39] Bachmann, I., Audigé, L. and Stauffacher, M. (2003) Risk factors associated with behavioral disorders of crib-biting, weaving and box-walking in Swiss horses. *Equine Vet J*, 35, 158–163.

[40] Visser, E.K., Ellis, A.D. and Van Reenen, C.G. (2008) The effect of two different housing conditions on the welfare of young horses stabled for the first time. *Appl Anim Behav Sci*, 114, 521–533.

[41] Owen, R.R. (1982) Crib-biting and windsucking—that equine enigma, in *The Veterinary Annual* (eds C.S.G. Hill and F.W.G. Grunsell), Wright Scientific Publications, Bristol, pp. 159–168.

[42] Archer, D.C., Pinchbeck, G.K., French, N.P. and Proudman, C.J. (2008) Risk factors for epiploic entrapment colic: an international study. *Equine Vet J*, 40, 224–230.

[43] Gillham, S.B., Dodman, N.H., Shuster, L. *et al.* (1994) The effect of diet on cribbing behavior and plasma β-endorphin in horses. *Appl Anim Behav Sci*, 41, 147–153.

[44] Lebelt, D., Zanella, A.J. and Unshelm, J. (1998) Physiological correlates associated with cribbing behavior in horses: changes in thermal threshold, heart rate, plasma β-endorphin and serotonin. *Equine Vet J*, (Suppl 27), 21–27.

[45] McBride, S.D. and Hemmings, A. (2005) Altered mesoaccumbens and nigro-striatal dopamine physiology is associated with stereotypy development in a non-rodent species. *Behav Brain Res*, 159, 113–118.

[46] Hemmings, A., McBride, S.D. and Hale, C.E. (2007) Perseverative responding and the aetiology of equine oral stereotypy. *Appl Anim Behav Sci*, 104, 143–150.

[47] Parker, M., Redhead, E.S., Goodwin, D. and McBride, S.D. (2008) Impaired instrumental choice in crib-biting horses (*Equus caballus*). *Behav Brain Res*, 191, 137–140.

[48] Mills, D.S. and Macleod, C.A. (2002) The response of crib-biting and windsucking in horses to dietary supplementation with an antacid mixture. *Ippologia*, 13, 33–41.

[49] McDonnell, S. (1998) Pharmacological aids to behavior modification in horses. *Equine Vet J*, (Suppl 27), 50.

[50] Dodman, N.H., Shuster, L., Court, M.H. and Dixon, R. (1987) Investigation into the use of narcotic antagonists in the treatment of a stereotypic behavior pattern (crib-biting) in the horse. *Am J Vet Res*, 48, 311–319.

[51] Zanella, A.J., Broom, D.M., Hunter, J.C. and Mendl, M.T. (1996) Brain opioid receptors in relation to stereotypies, inactivity, and housing in sows. *Physiol Behav*, 59, 769–775.

[52] Pell, S.M. and McGreevy, P.D. (1999) A study of cortisol and beta-endorphin levels in stereotypic and normal thoroughbreds. *Appl Anim Behav Sci*, 64, 81–90.

[53] McGreevy, P.D. and Nicol, C.J. (1998) Physiological and behavioral consequences associated with short-term prevention of crib-biting in horses. *Phys Behav*, 65, 15–23.

[54] Clegg, H.A., Buckley, P., Friend, M.A. and McGreevy, P.D. (2008) The ethological and physiological characteristics of cribbing and weaving horses. *Appl Anim Behav Sci*, 109, 68–76.

[55] Houpt, K.A. (2011) Behavioral problems, in *Equine Clinical Medicine Surgery and Reproduction* (eds G.A. Munroe and J.S. Weese), Manson, London, pp. 996–1001.

[56] Minero, M., Canali, E., Ferrante, V. *et al.* (1999) Heart rate and behavioral responses of crib-biting horses to two acute stressors. *Vet Rec*, 145, 430–433.

[57] Cabib, S., Giardino, L., Calzá, L. *et al.* (1998) Stress promotes major changes in dopamine receptor densities within the mesoaccumbens and nigrostriatal systems. *Neuroscience*, 84, 193–200.

[58] Cabib, S. and Bonaventura, N. (1997) Parallel strain-dependent susceptibility to environmentally-induced stereotypies and stress-induced behavioral sensitization in mice. *Physiol Behav*, 61, 499–506.

[59] Murray, M.J. and Eichorn, E.S. (1996) Effects of intermittent feed deprivation, intermittent feed deprivation with ranitidine administration, and stall confinement with *ad libitum* access to hay on gastric ulceration in horses. *Am J Vet Res*, 11, 1599–1603.

[60] Katz, J. (1991) Acid secretion and suppression. *Med Clin North Am*, 75, 877–887.

[61] Smyth, G.B., Young, D.W. and Hammond, L.S. (1989) Effects of diet and feeding on postprandial serum gastrin and insulin concentrations in adult horses. *Equine Vet J*, (Suppl 7), 56–59.

[62] Kusunose, R. (1992) Diurnal pattern of crib-biting in stabled horses. *Jpn J Equine Sci*, 3, 173–176.

[63] Nicol, C.J. (1999) Understanding equine stereotypies. *Equine Vet J*, (Suppl 28), 20–25.

[64] Moeller, B.A., McCall, C.A., Silverman, S.J. and McElhenney, W.H. (2008) Estimation of saliva production in crib-biting and normal horses. *J Equine Vet Sci*, 28, 85–90.

[65] Houpt, K.A. (2012) A preliminary answer to the question of whether cribbing causes salivary secretion. *J Vet Behav*, 7, 322–324.

[66] Wickens, C.L., McCall, C.A., Bursian, S. *et al.* (2013) Assessment of gastric ulceration and gastrin response in horses with history of crib-biting. *J Equine Vet Sci*, 33, 739–745.

[67] Murray, M.J. (1998) Gastroduodenal ulceration, in *Equine Internal Medicine* (eds S.M. Reed and W.M. Bayly), W. B. Saunders, Pennsylvania, pp. 615–623.

[68] Wood, P.B. (2004) Stress and dopamine: implications for the pathophysiology of chronic widespread pain. *Med Hypotheses*, 62, 420–424.

[69] Hermann, K., Raekallio, M., Kanerva, K. *et al.* (2012) Circadian variation in ghrelin and certain stress hormones in crib-biting horses. *Vet J*, 193, 97–102.

[70] Baker, G.J. and Kear-Colwell, J. (1974) Aerophagia (windsucking) and aversion therapy in the horse. *Proc Am Assoc Equine Pract*, 20, 127–130.

[71] Delcalle, J., Burba, D.J., Tetens, J. and Moore, R.M. (2002) Nd:YAG laser-assisted modified Forssell's procedure for treatment of cribbing (crib-biting) in horses. *Vet Surg*, 31, 111–116.

[72] Rendon, R.A., Shuster, L. and Dodman, N.H. (2001) The effect of the NMDA receptor blocker, dextromethorphan, on cribbing in horses. *Pharm Biochem Behav*, 68, 49–51.

[73] Whisher, L., Raum, M., Pina, L. *et al.* (2011) Effects of environmental factors on cribbing activity by horses. *Appl Anim Behav Sci*, 135, 63–69.

[74] Johnson, K.G., Tyrrell, J., Rowe, B. and Pethick, D.W. (1998) Behavioral changes in stabled horses given nontherapeutic levels of virginiamycin. *Equine Vet J*, 30, 139–143.

[75] Rowe, J.B., Pethick, D.W. and Lee, M.J. (1994) Prevention of acidosis and laminitis associated with grain feeding in horses. *J Nutr*, 124, 2742–2744.

[76] Linklater, W.L., Cameron, E.Z., Minot, E.O. and Stafford, K.J. (1999) Stallion harassment and the mating system of horses. *Anim Behav*, 58, 295–306.

[77] Juarbe-Diaz, S.V., Houpt, K.A. and Kusunose, R. (1998) Prevalence and characteristics of foal rejection in Arabian mares. *Equine Vet J*, 30, 424–428.

[78] Duncan, P. (1982) Foal killing by stallions. *Appl Anim Ethol*, 8, 567–570.

[79] Vaala, W. (2011) Foal rejection, in *Equine Reproduction* (eds A.O. McKinnon, E.L. Squires, W.E. Vaala and D.D. Varner), Wiley Blackwell, Chichester, pp. 117–120.

38   Miscellaneous Conditions

Martin Furr

Marion duPont Scott Equine Medical Center, Virginia-Maryland Regional College of Veterinary Medicine, Leesburg, USA

Cholesterol granuloma

Cholesterol granulomas are circumscribed, smooth, firm masses found within the choroid plexus of up to 20% of older horses [1]. In one study, cholesterol granulomas represented 1.3% of 21 neoplasms among 1322 horses necropsied [2]. They are also referred to as cholesteatomas or cholesterinic granulomas. Histologically, most masses are composed of cholesterol crystals in a bed of granulation tissue without epithelial elements [3]. The masses appear to be more frequent in the fourth ventricle than in the lateral ventricles; however, it has been stated that the granulomas in the lateral ventricle seem more likely to cause clinical disease. In one report of four horses with clinical abnormalities due to cholesterol granulomas, the mass was present in the lateral ventricles of all four; none was found in the fourth ventricle [4]. The etiology and mechanism of formation for cholesterol granulomas remains unclear, but they are likely to be the result of a granulomatous reaction to cholesterol crystals in the choroid plexus (Figure 38.1).

While most of these benign masses remain clinically silent, they can grow to such a size that they result in clinical illness. This occurs either by obstruction of cerebrospinal fluid (CSF) with secondary hydrocephalus or by direct compression of adjacent nervous tissue. Most reported cases have been seen in middle-aged horses (10–15 years old), and a variety of clinical signs referable to cerebral disease have been reported. Specific signs include depression, reluctance to move forward, stiff gait, seizures, blindness, circling, trembling, odd head movements, somnolence, ataxia, anisocoria, facial nerve paralysis, and syncope [3–6]. Clinical signs are often intermittent with horses being completely normal in between episodes or less frequently persistent once observed.

Serum chemistry and complete blood cell count in reported cases are usually normal and do not demonstrate any consistent pattern of abnormality. CSF evaluation usually reveals fluid that is mildly xanthochromic and with normal or mildly increased total protein concentrations [3, 5]. A mild pleocytosis (i.e., 25–30 nucleated cells/µl CSF) has been reported in some cases. In one case, the monocytes were vacuolated and contained phagocytized basophilic granular material, which were later considered to be phagocytized fragments of the granuloma [3].

Antemortem diagnosis is challenging and the mass is not visualized on routine radiography unless there is extensive mineralization, which does sometimes occur. A mass in one horse was visualized by scintigraphy [5]; however, the ideal imaging modality is CT or MRI. The CT appearance of cholesterol granulomas in horses has been reported [4]. No specific treatment exists; however, treatment with steroids, nonsteroidal anti-inflammatory and anti-edema drugs often provides transient improvement. Diagnosis is made usually on postmortem, at which time the characteristic large, smooth, pearly, and granular mass is noted within the fourth or lateral ventricles (Figure 38.2).

Intracarotid injection

Inadvertent intracarotid injection occurs occasionally in the horse during attempted intravenous injections. The clinical event that follows is variable in its severity and depends upon the nature of the compound injected and the volume. One author report 24 cases of intracarotid injection, in which there were five fatalities [7]. It was also reported that individual animals had varying responses to intracarotid injection of the same drug [7]. While this suggests some component of individual animal sensitivity, the variable response might also have arisen from incomplete delivery of the dose, due to the method of injection. In most cases, the signs occur within seconds of the intracarotid injection but may be

Equine Neurology, Second Edition. Martin Furr and Stephen Reed.
© 2015 John Wiley & Sons, Inc. Published 2015 by John Wiley & Sons, Inc.
Companion website: www.wiley.com/go/furr/neurology

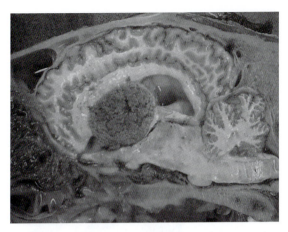

Figure 38.1 Sagittal view of a cholesterol granuloma. Note the internal hydrocephalus present as a result of blockage of flow of cerebrospinal fluid.

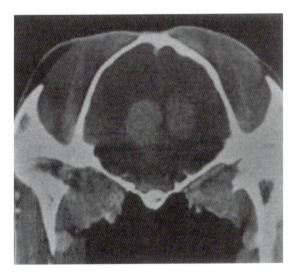

Figure 38.2 Transverse contrast image at the hypophyseal region. There is homogenous contrast enhancement of masses within both lateral ventricles. (Reprinted from Ref. [4], © Wiley.)

delayed for a few minutes. Signs can occur abruptly and violently or be preceded by a few moments of progressive anxiety and trembling prior to collapse and convulsions. Systemic signs such as arrhythmias, changes in blood pressure, and "blowing" respiration can be seen. With water soluble compounds such as xylazine, acepromazine, and butorphanol, horses usually regain consciousness within an hour, although full recovery may take up to 1 week. During this time, clinical abnormalities such as facial hypalgesia, blindness, and mild hemiparesis may be seen. If the injection occurs with viscous or irritant drugs, drug suspensions, or oil-based compounds, then the reaction is more acute, and the outcome is worse. Seizures, coma, and prolonged recumbency can occur, with euthanasia as a common outcome. In an experimental setting, three of five horses given 3.3 ml/800 lb body weight of promazine were euthanized after 20 h of recumbency [7]. Another animal given 50 ml of 20% calcium gluconate solution by intracarotid injection collapsed, convulsed, and then died 6 min after completion of the injection [7].

Treatment is primarily symptomatic; anticonvulsant medication is appropriate, as is intravenous dimethyl sulfoxide or mannitol, and dexamethasone. Postmortem examination finds signs of cerebral edema and vascular endothelial damage, with necrosis and vacuolation in subcortical white matter [7].

Prevention is achieved by careful placement of syringes for intravenous injection. Ideally, an 18 gauge needle should be used and directed down the vessel (toward the heart). If the carotid artery is entered with an 18 gauge needle, the blood usually spurts only a few inches; with a 20 gauge needle, the blood only drips even if it is within the carotid artery. Color of the blood is suggestive but can be misleading. If infusions are needed, placement of an intravenous catheter is advised.

Air embolism

The widespread use of intravenous catheters has led to several cases of air embolism, which typically occur when the catheter becomes disconnected and air is aspirated by the catheter. The volume of air required to lead to clinical abnormalities in the horse is unknown, as prospective trials have not been reported. In dogs, a dose of 0.75 ml/kg of air injected into the carotid artery resulted in some deaths and cerebral lesions were found [8]. In horses, 4 l of air by intravenous injection can result in death [9]. It is often impossible clinically to determine how long the catheter has been disconnected, or how much air might have been aspirated.

Clinical signs reflect diffuse cerebral irritation, and horses typically are anxious, tremble, and pace the stall; mild ataxia may be seen. In severe cases, horses can become manic, crashing into the stall and falling; this may progress to death or horses may be found dead in the stall with a disconnected catheter. Seizures and blindness can be seen. In addition to the neurologic signs, most horses have an elevated heart rate and abnormal respiration.

Treatment is nonspecific and in mild cases no specific treatment is required. In more severe cases, the use of corticosteroids, nonsteroidal anti-inflammatory drugs and dimethyl sulfoxide (DMSO) is potentially beneficial. Of those horses that survive the initial onset, most appear to recover within 1–2 h; however, in severe cases blindness has persisted for several days.

Spinal hematoma

A syndrome of spinal compression associated with hemorrhage and hematoma development has been observed and described [10]. Although a very limited number of cases have been formally reported, in general, an abrupt onset of caudal ataxia of variable severity has been observed [10]. Signs of cervical pain are often present. In reported cases (as well as one seen by the author), moderate to severe caudal ataxia was seen [10]; the author has observed an additional case in which the presenting sign was acute recumbency associated with a large and rapidly progressive hematoma. All cases reported in the literature as well as those observed by the author have been found in the caudal cervical spine; however, lesions at other spinal levels can likely occur.

The pathophysiology of these lesions is not known. The degree of mobility of the cervical spine associated with the site of the reported lesions may lead to spontaneous rupture of the vessels; trauma could also play a role, although obvious or observed trauma was not reported in the published cases. In humans, trauma, vascular malformations, and inherited or acquired bleeding disorders have been associated in some, but not in all cases. Vascular malformations have been reported in the horses causing weakness and ataxia and may have a role in some cases (Figure 38.3) [11].

In affected horses, routine clinicopathologic evaluation is normal, and in published cases, the CSF is usually also normal, reflecting the epidural nature of the hematoma [10]. In one severe case seen by the author, the CSF was grossly bloody and dissection found the hemorrhage to arise from a ruptured artery as it penetrated the dura. Hence, bloody CSF may be seen but is apparently uncommon. Routine radiography is unremarkable unless there is associated trauma and fractures; myelography may demonstrate a soft tissue compressive mass that is focal or spans several vertebrae. Magnetic resonance imaging or CT is preferred; however, these modalities are unavailable currently except for perhaps small ponies.

Treatment in humans often involves emergency decompressive surgery; however, this is not a very realistic option for most horses, and furthermore the duration of compression prior to diagnosis may be associated with a poor outcome for neurologic recovery. Conservative medical management including stall rest, anti-inflammatory drugs, and perhaps corticosteroids can be attempted; however, the long-term prognosis for soundness is guarded.

Pathologic examination finds a focal or diffuse, coalescing area of hemorrhage sometimes with associated fibrin or granulation tissue within the epidural space [10]. Microscopic examination of the spinal cord demonstrates signs consistent with focal compressive myelopathy. One postmortem report describes marginal

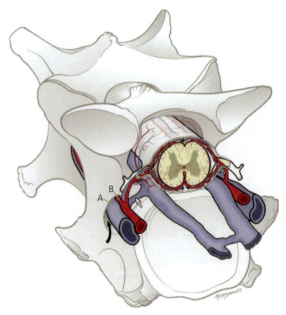

Figure 38.3 Drawing depicting the vascular supply at the cervical intervertebral space in the horse. A and B are the vertebral vein and artery coursing through the transverse foramen (solid arrow). Spinal branches of the vertebral artery and the intervertebral vein are shown entering and exiting (vein) the intervertebral space. The internal venous plexus is shown at both 5 and 7 o'clock on the floor of the vertebral canal with communicating branches. The venous plexus elevates off the floor at each intervertebral space toward the intervertebral vein where it communicates (open arrow). (Reprinted from Ref. [10], © Wiley.)

siderosis associated with chronic hemorrhage from a mass [12].

Uremic encephalopathy

Diffuse encephalopathy arising secondary to renal failure has been described in a variety of species but has only rarely been documented in horses [13, 14]. In one retrospective study of 332 horses with renal failure, only five had conclusive signs of neurologic abnormalities that could not be attributed to other causes such as sever colic, hepatic disease, endotoxemia, or electrolyte abnormalities. A total of 40 of the 332 horses had some type of neurologic abnormality identified, however [14]. Progressive anorexia associated with altered mentation, head pressing, seizures, and lethargy have been reported [13, 14]. Findings of CSF examination are reported for only one horse, which was normal.

The pathophysiologic mechanisms that result in encephalopathy in animals with renal failure are unknown; however, imbalances in amino acid concentrations and their metabolites are observed in laboratory animals. Damage to the blood–brain barrier and associated endothelial cell transport mechanisms may also contribute [15–17].

In one horse with uremic encephalopathy, histopathologic examination of the CNS found a marked and diffuse reactive astrocytosis with marked cellular swelling. In this case, the horse was markedly azotemic (BUN 166 mg/dl and creatinine 8.2 mg/dl) and was also hypochloridemic and hypokalemic [13]. It is unclear if the associated electrolyte abnormalities had any impact upon the development of neurologic signs in this case, or at what magnitude of azotemia, encephalopathy becomes a risk.

Horses with severe azotemia associated with a variety of serious illnesses commonly demonstrates signs of depression and abnormal mentation; these signs are usually attributed to general malaise from illness, fever, or pain. However, there may be a component of uremic encephalopathy associated with these signs. In most cases, these signs resolve associated with treatment of the primary illness. Furthermore, among horses that do not survive, it is not very common to closely examine the brain unless gross neurologic abnormalities are present; hence, the incidence of uremic encephalopathy in horses remains completely undetermined.

Specific treatments for horses with uremic encephalopathy are not recognized but empirical treatment such as correction of hydration and electrolyte abnormalities, treatment for cerebral edema, and anti-inflammatory drugs is likely to be beneficial.

References

[1] Maxie MG. The nervous System. In: Maxie MG, ed. *Jubb, Kennedy, and Palmers Pathology of Domestic Animals*, 5th ed. Philadelphia, PA:Elsevier Saunders;2007:281–457.

[2] Sundberf LJP, Burstein T, Page E, et al. Neoplams of equidae. *J Am Vet Med Assoc* 1977;170:150–152.

[3] Johnson PJ, Lin TL, Jennings DP. Diffuse cerebral encephalopathy associated with hydrocephalus and cholesterinic granulomas in a horse. *J Am Vet Med Assoc* 1993; 203:694–697.

[4] Vink-Nooteboom M, Junker K, van den Ingh, T, Dik KJ. Computed tomography of cholesterinic granulomas in the choroids plexus of horses. *Vet Radiol Ultrasound* 1998;39:512–516.

[5] Jackson CA, deLahunta A, Dykes NL, Divers TJ Neurological manifestation of cholesterinic granulomas in three horses. *Vet Rec* 1994;135:228–230.

[6] Duff S. Cholesterinic granulomas in horses. *Vet Rec* 1994;135:288.

[7] Gabel AA, Koestner A. The effects of intracarotid artery injection of drugs in domestic animals. *J Am Vet Med Assoc* 1963;142:1397–1403.

[8] Worman LW, Siedel B. Treatment of cerebral air embolism in the dog. *Am J Surg* 1966;111:820.

[9] Gabel A. Air embolism. *J Am Vet Med Assoc* 1970;156:283.

[10] Gold JR, Divers TJ, Miller AJ, et al. Cervical vertebral spinal hematomas in 4 horses. *J Vet Intern Med* 2008;22:481–485.

[11] Miller LM, Reed SM, Gallina AM, Palmer GH. Ataxia and weakness associated with fourth ventricle vascular anomalies in two horses. *J Am Vet Med Assoc* 1985;186:601–603.

[12] Huxtable CR, de LaHunta A, Summers BA, Divers T. Marginal siderosis and degenerative myelopathy: a manifestation of chronic subarachnoid hemorrhage in a horse with a myxopapillary ependymoma. *Vet Pathol* 2000; 37:483–485.

[13] Bouchard PR, Weldon AD, Lewis RM, Summers BA. Uremic encephalopathy in a horse. *Vet Pathol* 1994; 31:111–115.

[14] Frye MA, Johnson JS, Traub-Dagartz J, et al. Putative uremic encephalopathy in horses: five cases (1978–1998). *J Am Vet Med Assoc* 2001;218:560–566.

[15] Biasioli S, D'Andrea G, Feriani M, et al. Uremic encephalopathy: an updating. *Clin Nephrol* 1986;25:57–63.

[16] Jeppsson B, Freund HR, Gimmon Z, et al. Blood-brain barrier derangement in uremic encephalopathy. *Surgery* 1982;92:30–35.

[17] Seifter JL, Samuels MA. Uremic encephalopathy and other brain disorders associated with renal failure. *Semin Nephrol* 2011;31:139–143.

Index

Acanthomoeba spp., 316
acepromazine, 52
  in anesthesia, 185
acetazolamide (in HYPP), 376
acyclovir, 48
air embolism, 485
akathisia, 437
albumin quotient, 38
allopurinol, 88
Alzheimer's type 2 cells, 211, 345
amebic encephalitis-pathology, 208
aminoglycosides, 48
ammonia, 343
AMPA receptor, 456
amphotericin B, 315
androstenedione, 459
Angiostrongylus cantonensis, 308
anisocoria, 112
antibody index, 41, 43
anticonvulsants for CNS trauma, 421
Antoni A areas, 209
Antoni B areas, 201
aquaporins, 370
arboviruses, 233
Asclepius subverticulata, 450
ascorbic acid (in NE), 462
astrocytes, 37
Aujesky's disease, 267
  pathology, 206
autonomic nervous system, 18
axonotmesis, 429
azithromycin, 57

baclofen (for stringhalt), 467
bacterial meningitis
  agents of, 273
  treatment, 280
Balamuthia mandrillaris, 316
basal ganglia (in cribbing), 478
benztropine (in fluphenazine toxicity), 437
bethanechol (for urinary incontinence), 143
Blastomycosis, 315
blindness, 113
blood–brain barrier, 21, 36, 38, 46
  in neonatal encephalopathy, 343
Borna disease virus encephalitis, 265
Borrelia burgdorferi, 154

botulism, 149, 150
  grass sickness, 336
brachial intumescence, 77
Bracken fern, 445
brainstem auditory evoked response, 104, 157, 168
branched chain amino acids (in HE), 347
bromide-anticonvulsant, 51, 86
Büngner's bands (in stringhalt), 467
  in EMND, 334
Bunyaviridae, 248
buspirone, 53
butorphanol (in anesthesia), 185

Cache Valley virus encephalitis, 248
caffeine (in NE), 461
carbamazepine-anticonvulsant, 52
  for headshaking, 135
  in hyponatremia, 369
cauda equina neuritis, 434
cauda equina syndrome, 144
central pattern generator, 465
cephalosporin, 47
cerebellar abiotrophy, 338
  pathology, 201
cerebellar degeneration, 337
cerebellar hypoplasia, 404
cerebellar peduncles, 9, 10
cerebral blood flow, 409
  in anesthesia, 184
cerebral necrosis-post anesthetic, 187
cerebral perfusion pressure-in trauma, 417
  in anesthesia, 184
  in hyponatremia, 369
cerebrospinal fluid
  B cells, 38
  cauda equina neuritis, 94, 116, 141, 145, 434
  collection, 31
  composition, 24
  electrophoresis, 28
  formation, 22
  hypoglycorrhacia, 29
  lymphocytes, 38
  T cells, 38
  total protein, 26
  in verminous encephalitis, 309, 310
Chiari malformation, 200
chloramphenicol, 47

Equine Neurology, Second Edition. Martin Furr and Stephen Reed.
© 2015 John Wiley & Sons, Inc. Published 2015 by John Wiley & Sons, Inc.
Companion website: www.wiley.com/go/furr/neurology